INTERVENTIONAL NEURORADIOLOGY

INTERVENTIONAL NEURORADIOLOGY

■ STRATEGIES AND PRACTICAL TECHNIQUES

J. J. Connors III, M.D.

Associate Professor of Clinical Radiology
Director, Interventional Neuroradiology
Louisiana State University Medical Center
New Orleans, Louisiana

Joan C. Wojak, M.D.

Department of Radiology
Our Lady of Lourdes Regional Medical Center
Lafayette, Louisiana
Clinical Assistant Professor
Department of Radiology
Louisiana State University Medical Center
New Orleans, Louisiana

W.B. SAUNDERS COMPANY
A Division of Harcourt Brace & Company
Philadelphia   London   Toronto   Montreal   Sydney   Tokyo

W.B. SAUNDERS COMPANY
A Division of Harcourt Brace & Company

The Curtis Center
Independence Square West
Philadelphia, Pennsylvania 19106

Library of Congress Cataloging-in-Publication Data

Interventional neuroradiology: strategies and practical techniques / J.J. Connors III,
Joan C. Wojak.

p.   cm.

ISBN 0-7216-7147-0

1. Brain—Interventional radiology   2. Nervous system—Interventional radiology.
I. Wojak, Joan C.   II. Title. [DNLM: 1. Cerebrovascular Disorders—
radiography.   2. Cerebrovascular Disorders—therapy.   3. Radiography,
Interventional—methods.   4. Embolization, Therapeutic—methods.
WL 355 C752i 1998]

RD594.15.C66 1999   617.4′8—DC21

DNLM/DLC   97–28810

INTERVENTIONAL NEURORADIOLOGY   ISBN 0–7216–7147–0

Printed in the United States of America.

Last digit is the print number: 9   8   7   6   5   4   3   2   1

To everyone who encouraged us, supported us, listened to us complain,
and remained our friends during the past three years

Contributors

V. A. ALETICH, M.D.
Assistant Professor, Department of Neurosurgery
and Radiology, University of Illinois at Chicago,
Chicago, Illinois
*Intracranial Arteriovenous Malformations: The
Approach and Technique of Cyanoacrylate
Embolization*

A. AYMARD, M.D.
Department of Neuroradiology and Therapeutic
Angiography, Hôpital Lariboisière, Paris, France
*Endovascular Therapy for Vertebral Artery
Arteriovenous Fistulae; Embolization of Spinal
Vascular Malformations; Current Management of
Cervicofacial Superficial Vascular Malformations
and Hemangiomas; Percutaneous Direct
Embolization of Head and Neck Vascular Tumors;
Endovascular Test and Permanent Occlusion of
Extracranial and Intracranial Cerebral Vessels:
Indications, Techniques, and Management*

P. T. BA HUY, M.D.
Professor of Otorhinolaryngology, University of
Paris VII, School of Medicine; Professor of Otorhino-
laryngology, Chief of Otorhinolaryngology Depart-
ment, Hôpital Lariboisière, Paris, France
*Percutaneous Direct Embolization of Head and Neck
Vascular Tumors*

C. BELLEC, M.D.
Department of Anesthesiology, Hôpital Lariboisière,
Paris, France
*Medical Management of Vasospasm and
Hemodynamic Alterations in the Neurosurgical ICU*

B. L. BERGER, M.D.
Director, Interventional Neuroradiology Stroke
Service, Centennial Medical Center, Nashville,
Tennessee
*Treatment and Prevention of Acute Ischemic Stroke
by Endovascular Techniques: A Network-Based
Community Model*

A. S. CALLAHAN III, M.D.
Clinical Assistant Professor of Medicine, Meharry
Medical College; Medical Director, Stroke Service,
Centennial Medical Center, Nashville, Tennessee
*Treatment and Prevention of Acute Ischemic Stroke
by Endovascular Techniques: A Network-Based
Community Model*

A. E. CASASCO, M.D.
Associate Professor, University of Paris VII; Chief,
Department of Neuroradiology and Therapeutic
Angiography, Hôpital de la Pitie Salpetrière, Paris,
France
*Endovascular Therapy for Vertebral Artery
Arteriovenous Fistulae; Embolization of Spinal
Vascular Malformations; Endovascular Therapy and
Long-Term Results for Intracranial Dural
Arteriovenous Fistulae; Current Management of
Cervicofacial Superficial Vascular Malformations
and Hemangiomas; Percutaneous Direct
Embolization of Head and Neck Vascular Tumors;
Endovascular Test and Permanent Occlusion of
Extracranial and Intracranial Cerebral Vessels:
Indications, Techniques, and Management*

R. CHAPOT, M.D.
Department of Neuroradiology and Therapeutic
Angiography, Hôpital Lariboisière, Paris, France
*Endovascular Therapy for Vertebral Artery
Arteriovenous Fistulae; Endovascular Therapy and
Long-Term Results for Intracranial Dural
Arteriovenous Fistulae; Current Management of
Cervicofacial Superficial Vascular Malformations
and Hemangiomas*

JACQUES CHIRAS, M.D.
Chief of Neuroradiology, Hôpital de la Pitie
Salpetrière, Paris, France
*Intra-Arterial Chemotherapy for Central Nervous
System Tumors*

C. COGNARD, M.D.
Interventional Neuroradiology Department,
Foundation Ophtalmologique Rothschild, Paris,
France
*Endovascular Therapy and Long-Term Results for
Intracranial Dural Arteriovenous Fistulae*

J. J. CONNORS III, M.D.
Associate Professor of Clinical Radiology, and
Director, Interventional Neuroradiology, Louisiana
State University Medical Center, New Orleans,
Louisiana
*Tools of the Trade; Future Devices and Procedures;
Tricks of the Trade; General Principles of*

Embolization; Meningiomas; Juvenile Nasopharyngeal Angiofibromas; Paragangliomas; Tumors of the Vertebral Bodies and Other Bones; Epistaxis; Soft Tissue Tumoral Hemorrhage in the Head and Neck; Arteriovenous Fistulae and Traumatic Vascular Lesions; Treatment of Carotid-Cavernous Sinus Fistulae; Intracranial Arteriovenous Malformations: General Considerations; Intracranial Aneurysms: General Considerations; Interventional Neuroradiologic Procedure for Wada Testing; Temporary Test Occlusion of the Internal Carotid Artery; Permanent Occlusion of the Internal Carotid Artery; Inferior Petrosal Sinus Sampling; Nerve Blocks and Discectomy; General Concepts of Brachiocephalic Angioplasty for Atherosclerosis; General Technique of Extracranial Angioplasty and Stenting; General Considerations for Endovascular Therapy of the Extracranial Internal Carotid Artery at the Bifurcation; Other Extracranial Locations Amenable to Angioplasty and Stenting; Intracranial Angioplasty; Endovascular Therapy of Postsubarachnoid Hemorrhage Vasospasm; General Considerations in Emergency Stroke Therapy; Current Directions in Emergency Stroke Therapy; Radiology of Emergency Stroke Therapy; Strategic Considerations Concerning Emergency Stroke Treatment; Specific Stroke Situations, Territories, and Guidelines for Therapy; Specific Technical Procedure of Emergency Intracranial Fibrinolysis; Problems, Complications, and Solutions in Embolization; Rupture of a Vessel, Aneurysm, or Arteriovenous Malformation; Other Problems, Complications, and Solutions

J. COPHIGNON, M.D.
Professor of Neurosurgery, University of Paris VII; Consulting Professor; Department of Neurosurgery, Hôpital Lariboisière, Paris, France
Medical Management of Vasospasm and Hemodynamic Alterations in the Neurosurgical ICU

M. E. CRONQVIST, M.D.
Assistant Professor, University of Lund; Section of Neuroradiology, Department of Radiology, University Hospital of Lund, Lund, Sweden
Detachable Coil Embolization of Intracranial Aneurysms

F. CULICCHIA, M.D.
Clinical Associate Professor, Department of Neurological Surgery, Tulane Medical School, New Orleans, Louisiana
Surgical Alternatives to Interventional Neuroradiology

G. M. DEBRUN, M.D.
Chief, Interventional Neuroradiology, Department of Neurosurgery and Radiology, University of Illinois at Chicago, Chicago, Illinois
Intracranial Arteriovenous Malformations: The

Approach and Technique of Cyanoacrylate Embolization

C. DEMATONS, M.D.
Department of Anesthesiology, Hôpital Lariboisière, Paris, France
Medical Management of Vasospasm and Hemodynamic Alterations in the Neurosurgical ICU

C. DEPRIESTER, M.D.
Radiology Department A, Hôpital Nord, Amiens, France
Percutaneous Vertebroplasty: Indications, Technique, and Complications

H. DERAMOND, M.D.
Professor of Radiology, Chief, Department of Radiology, University Hospital, Amiens, France
Percutaneous Vertebroplasty: Indications, Technique, and Complications

L. DO, M.D.
Department of Neurosurgery, Hôpital Lariboisière, Paris, France
Medical Management of Vasospasm and Hemodynamic Alterations in the Neurosurgical ICU

BRUCE FISCH, M.D.
Director, Clinical Neurophysiology Laboratories and Fellowship Program, Professor of Neurology, Louisiana State University, School of Medicine, New Orleans, Louisiana
The Intracarotid Amobarbital (Wada) Test: Neurology Perspective

J. C. FLICKINGER, M.D.
Professor of Radiation Oncology, University of Pittsburgh Medical Center, Pittsburgh, Pennsylvania
The Role of Embolization in Combination with Stereotactic Radiosurgery in the Management of Pial and Dural Arteriovenous Malformations

P. GALIBERT, M.D.
Professor of Neurosurgery, University Hospital; Chief, Department of Neurosurgery, Hôpital Nord, Amiens, France
Percutaneous Vertebroplasty: Indications, Technique, and Complications

A. GAUDRIC, M.D.
Professor of Ophthalmology; Chairman, University of Paris VII, School of Medicine; Chief, Department of Ophthalmology, Hôpital Lariboisière, Paris, France
Technique of Superselective Intraophthalmic Artery Fibrinolytic Therapy Using Urokinase for Central Retinal Vein Occlusion

B. GEORGE, M.D.
Professor of Neurosurgery, University of Paris VII, School of Medicine; Professor of Neurosurgery, Chief, Department of Neurosurgery, Hôpital Lariboisière, Paris, France
Percutaneous Direct Embolization of Head and Neck Vascular Tumors; Medical Management of Vasospasm and Hemodynamic Alterations in the Neurosurgical ICU

J.-P. GUICHARD, M.D.
University of Paris VII, School of Medicine; Department of Neuroradiology and Therapeutic Angiography, Hôpital Lariboisière, Paris, France
Embolization of Spinal Vascular Malformations

D. HERBRETEAU, M.D.
Department of Neuroradiology, Hôpital Bretonneau, Tours, France
Embolization of Spinal Vascular Malformations; Current Management of Cervicofacial Superficial Vascular Malformations and Hemangiomas; Percutaneous Direct Embolization of Head and Neck Vascular Tumors

RANDALL T. HIGASHIDA, M.D.
Director, Division of Interventional Neuroradiology, Clinical Professor of Radiology and Neurological Surgery, University of California, San Francisco, Medical Center, San Francisco, California
Treatment of Carotid-Cavernous Sinus Fistulae

E. HOUDART, M.D.
Associate Professor, University of Paris VII, School of Medicine; Associate Professor, Department of Interventional Neuroradiology, Hôpital Lariboisière, Paris, France
Endovascular Therapy for Vertebral Artery Arteriovenous Fistulae; Embolization of Spinal Vascular Malformations; Endovascular Therapy and Long-Term Results for Intracranial Dural Arteriovenous Fistulae; Current Management of Cervicofacial Superficial Vascular Malformations and Hemangiomas; Percutaneous Direct Embolization of Head and Neck Vascular Tumors; Endovascular Test and Permanent Occlusion of Extracranial and Intracranial Cerebral Vessels: Indications, Techniques, and Management

S. IYER, M.D.
Associate Director of Endovascular Therapy, Lenox Hill Hospital; New York Cardiac and Vascular Institute, New York, New York
Cervical Carotid Angioplasty and Stent Placement for Atherosclerosis

S. P. JAIN, M.D.
Cardiology Fellow, Ochsner Clinic, New Orleans, Louisiana
Clinical Applications of Intravascular Ultrasound

H. S. JHAVERI, M.D.
Department of Neuroradiology and Therapeutic Angiography, Hôpital Lariboisière, Paris, France
Endovascular Therapy for Vertebral Artery Arteriovenous Fistulae; Embolization of Spinal Vascular Malformations; Endovascular Therapy and Long-Term Results for Intracranial Dural Arteriovenous Fistulae; Current Management of Cervicofacial Superficial Vascular Malformations and Hemangiomas; Percutaneous Direct Embolization of Head and Neck Vascular Tumors; Percutaneous Vertebroplasty: Indications, Technique, and Complications; Endovascular Test and Permanent Occlusion of Extracranial and Intracranial Cerebral Vessels: Indications, Techniques, and Management; Technique of Superselective Intraophthalmic Artery Fibrinolytic Therapy Using Urokinase for Central Retinal Vein Occlusion

R. KACHEL, M.D.
Professor of Radiology/Neuroradiology, Teaching Hospital of the University Jena; Head of MRI and Neuroradiology, Department of Diagnostic Radiology, University Hospital Erfurt, Erfurt, Germany
Current Status and Future Possibilities of Balloon Angioplasty in the Carotid Artery

C. W. KERBER, M.D.
Professor of Radiology and Neurosurgery, University of California, San Diego, San Diego, California
A Treatment for Head and Neck Cancer by Direct Arterial Infusion

D. KONDZIOLKA, M.D., M.Sc., F.R.C.S.(C.)
Associate Professor, Department of Neurological Surgery, University of Pittsburgh Medical Center, Pittsburgh, Pennsylvania
The Role of Embolization in Combination with Stereotactic Radiosurgery in the Management of Pial and Dural Arteriovenous Malformations

DONALD LARSEN, M.D.
Associate Professor of Radiology and Neurological Surgery, University of Miami, School of Medicine; Interventional Neuroradiologist, Jackson Memorial Hospital, Miami, Florida
Treatment of Carotid-Cavernous Sinus Fistulae

G. LOT, M.D.
University of Paris VII; Department of Neurosurgery, Hôpital Lariboisière, Paris, France
Medical Management of Vasospasm and Hemodynamic Alterations in the Neurosurgical ICU

L. D. LUNSFORD, M.D., F.A.C.S.
Professor and Chairman, Department of Neurological Surgery; Professor of Radiation Oncology and Radiology, University of Pittsburgh Medical Center, Pittsburgh, Pennsylvania
The Role of Embolization in Combination with

Stereotactic Radiosurgery in the Management of Pial and Dural Arteriovenous Malformations

J.-J. MERLAND, M.D., Ph.D.
University of Paris VII, School of Medicine;
Professor of Radiology, Chief, Department of
Neuroradiology and Therapeutic Angiography,
Hôpital Lariboisière, Paris, France
*Endovascular Therapy for Vertebral Artery
Arteriovenous Fistulae; Embolization of Spinal
Vascular Malformations; Endovascular Therapy and
Long-Term Results for Intracranial Dural
Arteriovenous Fistulae; Current Management of
Cervicofacial Superficial Vascular Malformations
and Hemangiomas; Percutaneous Direct
Embolization of Head and Neck Vascular Tumors;
Endovascular Test and Permanent Occlusion of
Extracranial and Intracranial Cerebral Vessels:
Indications, Techniques, and Management; Medical
Management of Vasospasm and Hemodynamic
Alterations in the Neurosurgical ICU; Technique of
Superselective Intraophthalmic Artery Fibrinolytic
Therapy Using Urokinase for Central Retinal Vein
Occlusion*

P. MOHANAKRISHNAN, Ph.D.
Assistant Professor, Louisiana State University
Medical Center, New Orleans, Louisiana
Radiology of Emergency Stroke Therapy

J. MORET, M.D.
Professor, Faculty of Medicine, Xavier-Bichat; Chief,
Department of Interventional Neuroradiology, La
Fondation Rothschild, Paris, France
*Detachable Coil Embolization of Intracranial
Aneurysms*

K. L. MOURIER, M.D.
Professor of Neurosurgery, Universite de Bourgogne,
School of Medicine; Professor of Neurosurgery,
Department of Neurosurgery, Centre Hospitalier de
Dijon, Dijon, France
Embolization of Spinal Vascular Malformations

PIOTR OLEJNICZAK, M.D.
Assistant Professor of Neurology, Staff Physician,
Clinical Neurophysiology Laboratories and
Fellowship Program, Louisiana State University
School of Medicine, New Orleans, Louisiana
*The Intracarotid Amoborbital (Wada) Test:
Neurology Perspective*

C. PAOLETTI, M.D.
Department of Anesthesiology and Critical Care,
Hôpital Lariboisière, Paris, France
*Medical Management of Vasospasm and
Hemodynamic Alterations in the Neurosurgical ICU*

P. PAQUES, M.D.
Fellow, Department of Ophthalmology, Assistant,
University of Paris VII, School of Medicine; Hôpital
Lariboisière, Paris, France

*Technique of Superselective Intraophthalmic Artery
Fibrinolytic Therapy Using Urokinase for Central
Retinal Vein Occlusion*

J. C. PARODI, M.D.
Department of Vascular Surgery, Instituto
Cardiovascular de Buenos Aires, Buenos Aires,
Argentina
*Endovascular Treatment of Traumatic Lesions in
Supra-Aortic Vessels with Stent-Grafts*

M. PARKS, M.D.
Director of Interventional Laboratories, St.
Vincent's Hospital, Birmingham, Alabama
*Cervical Carotid Angioplasty and Stent Placement
for Atherosclerosis*

D. PAYEN DE LA GARANDERIE, M.D.
Professor of Anesthesiology and Critical Care
Medicine; Chairman, Department of Anesthesiology
and Critical Care, Hôpital Lariboisière, Paris,
France
*Medical Management of Vasospasm and
Hemodynamic Alterations in the Neurosurgical ICU*

B. E. POLLOCK, M.D.
Assistant Professor, Department of Neurological
Surgery, Mayo Clinic, Rochester, Minnesota
*The Role of Embolization in Combination with
Stereotactic Radiosurgery in the Management of Pial
and Dural Arteriovenous Malformations*

Z. QIAN, M.D.
Assistant Professor, Department of Radiology,
Louisiana State University, Medical Center, New
Orleans, Louisiana
Tools of the Trade

J. L. RAGGUENEAU, M.D.
Department of Anesthesiology, Hôpital Lariboisière,
Paris, France
*Medical Management of Vasospasm and
Hemodynamic Alterations in the Neurosurgical ICU*

S. R. RAMEE, M.D.
Director, Cardiac Catheterization Laboratory,
Ochsner Clinic, New Orleans, Louisiana
Clinical Applications of Intravascular Ultrasound

D. REIZINE, M.D.
University of Paris VII, School of Medicine;
Department of Neuroradiology and Therapeutic
Angiography, Hôpital Lariboisière, Paris, France
*Endovascular Therapy for Vertebral Artery
Arteriovenous Fistulae; Embolization of Spinal
Vascular Malformations*

K. T. ROBBINS, M.D.
Professor of Otolaryngology, University of
Tennessee, Memphis, Tennessee
*A Treatment for Head and Neck Cancer by Direct
Arterial Infusion*

D. V. RODRIGUEZ, M.D.
Assistant Professor of Neurology, Director, Stroke
Program, Louisiana State University, School of
Medicine, Department of Neurology, New Orleans,
Louisiana
*Neurological Correlates of Cerebrovascular
Occlusions*

G. ROUBIN, M.D.
Director of Endovascular Therapy, Lenox Hill
Hospital, New York, New York
*Cervical Carotid Angioplasty and Stent Placement
for Atherosclerosis*

C. J. SCHÖNHOLZ, M.D.
Department of Interventional Neuroradiology,
Clinica la Sagrada Familia, Buenos Aires,
Argentina
*Endovascular Treatment of Traumatic Lesions in
Supra-Aortic Vessels with Stent-Grafts*

P. Y. SANTIAGO, M.D.
Fellow, Department of Ophthalmology, Assistant,
University of Paris VII, School of Medicine; Hôpital
Lariboisière, Paris, France
*Technique of Superselective Intraophthalmic Artery
Fibrinolytic Therapy Using Urokinase for Central
Retinal Vein Occlusion*

S. SLABA, M.D.
Fellow, Department of Neuroradiology and
Therapeutic Angiography, Hôpital Lariboisière,
Paris, France
*Current Management of Cervicofacial Superficial
Vascular Malformations and Hemangiomas*

J. G. THERON, M.D.
Professor, Department of Radiology, Caen Medical
School; Chief of Service, Centre Hospitalier
Regional et Universitaire, Cote De Nacre, Caen,
France
*Percutaneous Treatment of Cervical and Lumbar
Disc Herniations; Protected Angioplasty and
Stenting of Atherosclerotic Stenosis at the Carotid
Artery Bifurcation*

J. R. TOMPKINS, M.D.
Resident, Department of Neurological Surgery,
Tulane Medical School, New Orleans, Louisiana
*Surgical Alternatives to Interventional
Neuroradiology*

P. TOUSSAINT, M.D.
Department of Neurosurgery, Hôpital Nord, Amiens,
France
*Percutaneous Vertebroplasty: Indications, Technique,
and Complications*

M. TOVI, M.D.
Fellow, Department of Neuroradiology and
Therapeutic Angiography, Hôpital Lariboisière,
Paris, France

*Technique of Superselective Intraophthalmic Artery
Fibrinolytic Therapy Using Urokinase for Central
Retinal Vein Occlusion*

J. N. VALLEE, M.D.
Assistant Fellow, Clinical Interventional
Neuroradiology, University of Paris VII, School of
Medicine; Hôpital Lariboisière, Paris, France
*Endovascular Test and Permanent Occlusion of
Extracranial and Intracranial Cerebral Vessels:
Indications, Techniques, and Management;
Technique of Superselective Intraophthalmic Artery
Fibrinolytic Therapy Using Urokinase for Central
Retinal Vein Occlusion*

J. VITEK, M.D.
Lenox Hill Hospital, New York, New York
*Cervical Carotid Angioplasty and Stent Placement
for Atherosclerosis*

V. WADLINGTON, M.D.
Assistant Professor of Radiology, University of
Alabama at Birmingham, Birmingham, Alabama
*Cervical Carotid Angioplasty and Stent Placement
for Atherosclerosis*

M. WASSEF, M.D.
Associate Professor, University Paris VII, School of
Medicine; Consultant Pathologist, Department of
Pathology, Hôpital Lariboisière, Paris, France
*Percutaneous Direct Embolization of Head and Neck
Vascular Tumors*

L. A. WEISBERG, M.D.
Director of Neurology, Vice-Chairman, Department
of Neurology and Psychiatry, Tulane Medical School,
New Orleans, Louisiana
Medical Aspects of Cerebral Ischemia

J. C. WOJAK, M.D.
Department of Radiology, Our Lady of Lourdes
Regional Medical Center, Lafayette; Clinical
Assistant Professor, Department of Radiology,
Louisiana State University Medical Center, New
Orleans, Louisiana
*Tools of the Trade; Future Devices and Procedures;
Tricks of the Trade; Pharmacology in Interventional
Neuroradiology; Fundamental Neurovascular
Anatomy; General Preprocedure and Postprocedure
Orders; General Principles of Embolization;
Meningiomas; Juvenile Nasopharyngeal
Angiofibromas; Paragangliomas; Tumors of the
Vertebral Bodies and Other Bones; Epistaxis; Soft
Tissue Tumoral Hemorrhage in the Head and Neck;
Arteriovenous Fistulae and Traumatic Vascular
Lesions; Intracranial Arteriovenous Malformations:
General Considerations; Intracranial Aneurysms:
General Considerations; Interventional
Neuroradiologic Procedure for Wada Testing;
Inferior Petrosal Sinus Sampling; Nerve Blocks and
Discectomy; Endovascular Therapy of
Postsubarachnoid Hemorrhage Vasospasm; General*

*Considerations in Emergency Stroke Therapy;
Cerebral Protection; Current Directions in
Emergency Stroke Therapy; Radiology of Emergency
Stroke Therapy; Strategic Considerations
Concerning Emergency Stroke Treatment; Specific
Stroke Situations, Territories, and Guidelines for
Therapy; Specific Technical Procedure of Emergency
Intracranial Fibrinolysis; Management of
Intracranial Hemorrhage During Thrombolysis;
Problems, Complications, and Solutions in
Embolization; Rupture of a Vessel, Aneurysm, or
Arteriovenous Malformation; Other Problems,
Complications, and Solutions*

W. H. M. WONG, D.O.
Associate Professor of Radiology, University of
California, San Diego; Staff Radiologist, San Diego
V.A. Medical Center, San Diego, California

*A Treatment for Head and Neck Cancer by Direct
Arterial Infusion*

J. YADAV, M.D.
Associate Professor of Cardiology & Neurology,
Cleveland Clinic, Cleveland, Ohio
*Cervical Carotid Angioplasty and Stent Placement
for Atherosclerosis*

W. F. J. YAKES, M.D.
Director, Vascular Malformation Center, Radiology
Imaging Associates, P.C., Colorado Neurological
Institute, Englewood, Colorado
*Ethanol Endovascular Management of Brain
Arteriovenous Malformation: Initial Experience;
Management of Extracranial Head and Neck and
Paraspinal Vascular Malformations*

Preface

Improvements in diagnostic and therapeutic capability have allowed the interventional neuroradiologist to offer a steadily increasing variety of services to clinicians and patients. This progress has been driven by three factors: the need for effective treatment of certain therapeutically challenging diseases, the continuing advancement of technical capabilities, and the corresponding growth in knowledge and skills of those practicing in this field.

Originally, interventional neuroradiologic procedures were primarily for treatment (occlusion) of arteriovenous fistulae and intracranial arteriovenous malformations. The role of endovascular therapy in the treatment of intracranial vascular lesions has been expanded by the emerging field of therapy for intracranial aneurysms. Advancements in the therapy for a wide variety of head and neck pathologies are being made as well.

An area of great potential is that of brachiocephalic revascularization, encompassing both extracranial and intracranial angioplasty and stenting and the emergent endovascular therapy of stroke. Because of the lack of organized information currently available, we have placed special emphasis on these topics. In-depth discussion of the evolution of these therapies is provided along with the rationales, specific techniques, controversies, and potential complications of these procedures.

As with any therapy, optimal outcome is most likely to occur when interventional neurologic procedures are performed in the proper environment by physicians with the knowledge, skills, and experience to accomplish these tasks. To best accomplish this goal, adequate preparation is necessary. We believe that this mandates knowledge of the potential difficulties and complications that can be encountered in these procedures and have stressed this aspect of treatment. Although the acquisition of skill and experience is by necessity a gradual process, it is our goal to make procurement of the necessary knowledge less arduous than it has been in the past.

J. J. CONNORS III, M.D.
JOAN C. WOJAK, M.D.

Acknowledgments

We wish to thank Wilfrido R. Castañeda-Zuniga, M.D., for furnishing the initial motivation to take on this project; our colleagues, John N. Joslyn, M.D., Albert E. Alexander, Jr., M.D., Hugh J.F. Robertson, M.D., and Jessica Borne, M.D., for providing continuing encouragement, support, and understanding; my (JJC) nurse and chief executive officer, Karen Walker, for her invaluable help with every step of this project and without whom it would not have been finished; Lori Nicholson and Hobbes for providing stress relief, sympathetic ears, and a reminder that high goals can be reached; and Harish S. Jhaveri, M.D., for acting as international liaison.

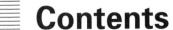

Contents

FUNDAMENTALS

Tools of the Trade

J.J. Connors III / J.C. Wojak / Z. Qian

The successful completion of interventional neuroradiology cases requires a wide array of specialty products and technology. The availability of specific catheters, guidewires, and other tools can determine whether a case is completed successfully or even at all. In the past, it was a major challenge to accomplish even the most basic procedures, but the widespread availability of high-quality equipment has made the job much easier. Even so, the proper equipment greatly aids in the performance of the more difficult cases attempted today and decreases the complication rate. Evolving technology makes specific recommendations transient at best; therefore, rationales for specific tools are discussed as well as particular products. Table 1–1 lists several of the manufacturers of products described here and elsewhere in this text.

ROUTINE SUPPLIES FOR INTERVENTIONAL NEURORADIOLOGY CASES

The following is the routine set-up of supplies for interventional neuroradiology cases at our institution:

Angiography tray (prepackaged):
  (1) Patient drape with transparent fluid catchment sides (to see table and digital subtraction angiography [DSA] controls)
Syringes—*separate size syringes are used for each specific purpose; intermingling is never permitted*
  (3) 20-cc syringes (all saline for regular catheters and guide catheters)
  (3) 10-cc syringes (all contrast for regular catheters and guide catheters)
  (3) 5-cc syringes (all saline for microcatheters)
  (3) 3-cc syringes (all contrast for microcatheters)
—Additional 3-cc syringes are taped and labeled when used for particulate (PVA) injection
  (1) 12-cc syringe for local anesthetic (or *any* drug)
—Additional 12-cc syringes as needed. All drugs (nitroglycerin, papaverine, urokinase, and so on) are placed in 12-cc syringes, never in any other size. This prevents inadvertent injection of drug. Each

separate 12-cc syringe for each pharmaceutical is separately taped and labeled
Bowls
  (1) Large bowl for guidewires
  (3) Small bowls (one to hold wet 4 × 4's; two to hold syringes during the case)
Accessories
  (1) Sharps holder
  (2) Sterile gowns
  (40) 4 × 4 sterile sponges
  (1) Scalpel
  (1) 25-gauge needle (1″) for local anesthesia
  (1) 20-gauge needle (2″) for local anesthesia
  (1) Large, clear fluoroscopy shield cover
  (3) Towel clips
  (4) Medium sterile covers (for x-ray tubes, image intensifiers, and table controls)
Additional material not in prepackaged angiogram tray:
  (1) Micropuncture set (Cook, Inc.) to prevent large back wall or errant vascular puncture; to be used when abciximab, long-term heparin, or urokinase use is anticipated
Fluid systems materials
  (2) Pall Set Saver air filters with microbore extension tubing (placed in line just before Y connectors to eliminate any possible bubbles)
  (1) Mini-volume extension set tubing (for use during inflation of any angioplasty catheter)
  (1) Closed tubing system for flush and contrast
  (2) Nonvented fluid delivery systems (for use with pressure bags)
  (3) 1000 ml normal saline with 5000 U heparin added—one for flush and two for pressurized flush
  (2) 1000-ml IV pressure bags
  (1) Flow switch
  (2) Three-way stopcocks
Vascular sheath
A 45-cm braided vascular sheath (Arrow International) used with the FasGUIDE catheter (Target Therapeutics). This length of sheath facilitates introduction of diagnostic catheters and guide catheters. (When using any larger guide catheter, no sheath is used; all sizes of Cook, Inc., Lumax Neuroguide catheters come with matching dilators.)

T A B L E   1 - 1   Manufacturers of Products Used in Interventional Neuroradiologic Procedures

Abbott Laboratories
Abbott Park, IL 60064
1-800-851-0108

Boston Scientific Corp.
One Boston Scientific Place
Natick, MA 01760-1537
1-800-221-1542

Cook, Inc.
P.O. Box 489
Bloomington, IN 47402
1-800-457-4500

Cordis Corporation (division of Johnson & Johnson
Interventional Systems)
P.O. Box 025700
Miami, FL 33102-7714
1-800-327-7714

DVI (division of Guidant, Inc.)
3200 Lakeside Drive
Santa Clara, CA 95054
1-800-288-7525

Johnson & Johnson Interventional Systems
40 Technology Drive
P.O. Box 4917
Warren, NJ 07059-0917
1-800-228-5547

Mallinckrodt Medical
511 E. John Carpenter Freeway
Suite 190
Irving, TX 75062
1-800-696-3636

Medi-Tech, Inc. (division of Boston Scientific Corp.)
One Boston Scientific Place
Natick, MA 01760-1537
1-800-225-3238

Medtronic, Inc.
7000 Central Avenue NE
Minneapolis, MN 55432
1-800-328-2518

MicroTherapeutics, Inc. (MTI)
1062-F Calle Negocio
San Clemente, CA 92673
1-800-684-6733

MicroInterventional Systems (MIS)
(division of Medtronic, Inc.)
680 West Maude Avenue
Suite 2
Sunnyvale, CA 94086
1-800-647-6116

Microvena
3600 LaBore Road
Suite I
Vadnais Height, MN 55110
612-773-7605

Navarre Biomedical Ltd.
2545 Fernbrook Lane North
Plymouth, MN 55447

Neurovena (division of Microvena)
1875 Buerkle Road
White Bear Lake, MN 55110
1-800-716-6700

Nycomed, Inc.
101 Carnegie Center
Princeton, NJ 08540
1-800-292-8514

Schneider (USA), Inc.
Pfizer Hospital Product Group
5905 Nathan Lane
Minneapolis, MN 55442
1-800-822-6822

SciMed (division of Boston Scientific Corp.)
One SciMed Place
Maple Grove, MN 55311-1566
1-800-344-0979

Target Therapeutics (division of Boston Scientific Corp.)
47201 Lakeview Boulevard
P.O. Box 5120
Fremont, CA 94537
1-800-895-8969

PUNCTURE SYSTEMS

Standard Seldinger technique puncture using an 18- or 19-gauge arterial needle is employed in most cases. For specific circumstances, however, a micropuncture set is helpful. Cook, Inc. makes two triaxial puncture sets, both of which have a 21-gauge needle and an 0.018″ Chiba-type stainless steel guidewire with a coil tip (Fig. 1–1). After the artery is punctured, the guidewire is advanced and the needle withdrawn. A dilator loaded within either a 4-Fr. or 5-Fr. outer sheath is then advanced; this can then take either an 0.035″ or 0.038″ wire when the inner dilator is removed.

This system is excellent for use in children or in patients with axillary or brachial punctures and is also useful to obtain access to the vascular tree when a large hole in the back wall of the artery is not desirable (e.g., when fibrinolysis is planned). It is also useful when the vessel is stenotic or fibrotic.

HEMOSTATIC DEVICES

Devices are being developed that effectively occlude the arterial puncture site, allowing early removal of the sheath or catheter and mobilization of the patient, even if the patient remains on anticoagulants or antiplatelet agents. Of these, the most effective appears to be the Angio-Seal (Sherwood Davis & Geck). This ingenious device consists of a biodegradable anchor that sits against the inner surface of the vessel wall, connected by a suture to a collagen wad that sits against the outer wall of the vessel. The existing sheath or catheter is exchanged over a supplied wire for the enclosed 8-Fr. sheath and inner dilator. The delivery unit is then advanced through the sheath and positioned. The Angio-Seal device is deployed. The deployment procedure allows the anchor and collagen wad to be drawn firmly together and the suture snugged down. Tension is kept on the suture for 20 minutes by a supplied tension spring; the suture is then cut at the skin surface and allowed to retract. The kit even comes with its own timer. The Food and Drug Administration (FDA) has approved mobilization of the patient in 3 hours with use of this device and is considering lowering this limit to 1 hour. Hemostasis is obtained regardless of the patient's coagulation status.

Other devices on the market rely on collagen in-

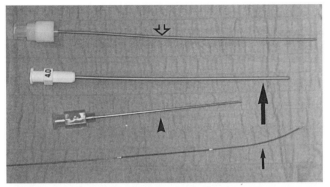

Figure 1-1 The micropuncture set manufactured by Cook, Inc. The components include a 21-gauge, single wall puncture needle *(arrowhead)*, an 0.018″ Chiba-type wire (stainless steel or nitinol) with a coil tip *(small arrow)*, an inner dilator *(open arrow)*, and a 4- or 5-Fr. sheath *(large arrow)*. After arterial puncture is made with the needle, the wire is advanced, and the needle is exchanged for the dilator and sheath, which lock together and are advanced as a unit. The inner dilator and wire are then removed. The outer sheath is now capable of accepting an 0.035″ or 0.038″ standard guidewire.

serted into the tract without a tensioning anchor or are more complicated to use, requiring actual placement of sutures.

GUIDEWIRES

0.035″ Specialty Wires

General Selecting Wires

For standard practice, there are multitudes of wires on the market that are suitable for use. The angle-tip Terumo Glidewire (Medi-Tech, Inc.) and the Roadrunner (Cook, Inc.) are two hydrophilic-coated wires available in a variety of shaft stiffnesses and floppy distal segment lengths. These are the wires that we use most frequently for diagnostic work and routine vessel selection.

Under certain circumstances, other wires may be useful. The Tapered Torque (Medi-Tech, Inc.) has an 0.035″ shaft that tapers to an 0.018″ distal tip. The tip is not precurved but is shapable. This can allow selection of tortuous vessel origins; the wire tends to track safely downstream and the stiffer proximal shaft supports advancement of the catheter. The Storq (Cordis Corp.) is a hydrophilic-coated wire with a shapable tip that is extremely easy to steer and that has nearly one-to-one torque transmission. This guidewire can help tremendously in navigation of extremely tortuous great vessels.

Exchange Wires

One of the most necessary specialty wires is a good, safe exchange wire. This is used for placement of either a guide catheter or a temporary occlusion catheter. No available wire is ideal for head and neck work. For this reason, many different wires are used by different interventional neuroradiologists. Cook, Inc. is developing an exchange version of the hydrophilic-coated Roadrunner wire with a soft J tip, the "Connors neuro-exchange wire." This wire does not have hydrophilic coating on the proximal portion, making it easier to grip and control.

The standard angle-tip hydrophilic-coated exchange wire is unsuitable for several reasons and is probably the most dangerous exchange wire on the market. It is difficult to hold during catheter advancement or withdrawal because of its hydrophilic coating. The catheter and wire combination develops occasional bends in the aorta or elsewhere during catheter advancement because of lack of sufficient stiffness, causing the tip to drift forward and backward too easily, potentially damaging the vessel or (more likely) causing an intimal tear. The third reason is that the angled tip is guaranteed to be up against the wall of the vessel and is too stiff to be allowed to poke uncontrollably during exchange for a guide catheter or other tool.

A straight Bentson-type wire also can easily cause an intimal tear or perforation when the tip reaches an abrupt curve in the vessel; its coiled design and lack of bend allow it to act like a stack of quarters when it comes to an abrupt curve. The TAD wire (Mallinkrodt Medical, Inc.) is suitable for certain circumstances.

A Rosen-type exchange-length wire is a suitable general-purpose alternative. Although the tip is not ideal (the J tip is slightly too large and hard and can cause vasospasm), once it "forms up" in the vessel, it is safe. The shaft gives adequate support for almost all exchanges, and the tight curl at the end renders true vascular damage almost impossible.

A wire with a true "noodle" tip tapering to a stiff shaft would be ideal, but is unavailable commercially. The wire under design and construction by Cook, Inc. should be ideal for exchanges because it has an extremely soft, atraumatic tip and a shaft stiff enough for easy exchange of any guide catheter or other tool.

Downstream Wires

A guidewire that can go downstream safely and stay in the main lumen without selecting vulnerable side branches is sometimes necessary. This is particularly useful for catheterizing the vertebral artery with its typically tortuous origin, or even for getting downstream around corners to intrahepatic branches when doing peripheral work. This wire has a soft, tight C curve, a soft, distal 3- to 5-cm shaft that tapers to a stiffer normal shaft, and a hydrophilic coating. This construction makes it capable of following curves easily and staying in the main vessel without selecting diverting or vulnerable side branches.

For catheterization of difficult vessels, however, technique is more important than technology. "Safe Catheterization of Difficult and/or Tortuous Vessels" in Chapter 3 addresses this issue.

Microwires

General Selecting Wires

Guidewire technology is undergoing rapid evolution, and what was good last year may not be next year. The platinum coil tip types are the safest, particularly if they do not have a stiff weld on the end, but even they can cause endovascular damage in certain circumstances. The original Seeker Standard guidewire

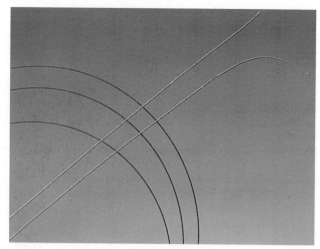

Figure 1-2 The Preceder guidewire (Medi-Tech, Inc.) has a platinum coil tip, is shapable, and is now hydrophilic coated.

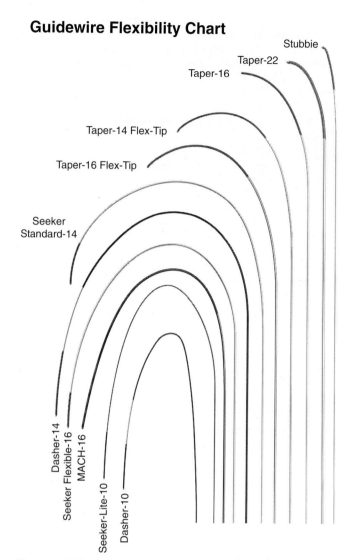

Guidewire Flexibility Chart

Figure 1-4 Example of the wide variety of guidewires available from Target Therapeutics. Other manufacturers have their own particular wires, but none has this spectrum of choices. Note the position of the Seeker Standard guidewire in the middle of the range; this wire is one of the most widely used in the world. Also note the Stubbie wire, the stiffest of the selection; this would be suitable for stiff support and comparable with the Platinum Plus microwire from Medi-Tech, Inc.

(Target Therapeutics) is still an excellent general-purpose wire and practically an industry benchmark.

The new hydrophilic-coated wires, such as the gold-tipped Terumo Micro Glidewire, perform best but may be the most dangerous. The tip needs to be custom shapable to a small radius; a straight metal bead found on the tip of some types of hydrophilic wires renders them incapable of making tight distal turns. These types are generally preshaped and are not considered as useful as the custom-shapable type. In addition, the frictionless ease of advancement renders tactile feedback minimal; when the tip comes to an abrupt curve, it can easily go straight. For difficult distal subselection, however, this type of wire is best, as long as caution and good technique are employed.

The state-of-the-art microguidewire for distal tortuous access is the Transcend (Medi-Tech, Inc.) and its new cousin the Transcend-EX; Medi-Tech, Inc. produces the Preceder wire, which has a shapable tip and a hydrophilic coat (Fig. 1–2). New models have been released by Target Therapeutics (Mach) (Figs. 1–3 and 1–4) and are being designed by Cordis Corp. and Medtronic, Inc./MicroInterventional Systems (MIS).

Exchange Microwires

The Platinum Plus guidewire (Medi-Tech, Inc.) is a useful wire for exchange purposes but is not a primary access neurovascular guidewire. For angioplasty with catheters requiring an 0.018″ system, however, the Platinum Plus is valuable. In addition, it is useful in the safe catheterization of tortuous vessels, as described in Chapter 3. The Transcend-EX is an interesting new design intended for exchange when the catheter is in a distal location. It

Figure 1-3 Close-up of the tip of the MACH 16 (0.016″) microguidewire from Target Therapeutics. This is one of the few nitinol core guidewires on the market with a coil tip.

uses a magnet to hold the wire in place while the catheter is exchanged.

Coil Pusher Microwires

Two wires have been designed for pushing microcoils through microcatheters: the Coil Pusher (Target Therapeutics) and the Trupush coil pusher (Cordis Corp.). The original Coil Pusher from Target Therapeutics rapidly fatigues with use, however, and often several are necessary for one case. It is imperative to have multiple Coil Pushers on hand for any case in which multiple coils are to be used. These wires can develop an amazing amount of friction during use and often develop buckles in the distal section while pushing coils, destroying the vectors of force necessary for pushing. If this happens, the operator should switch to another Coil Pusher immediately.

An interesting alternative for this purpose is the gold-tipped Terumo Micro Glidewire mentioned previously. This wire has a bead on the end that is ideal for pushing a coil, and the hydrophilic coating facilitates this process. The construction of this wire renders it far less likely to buckle than the Coil Pusher.

The new Trupush coil pusher from Cordis Corp. is designed specifically for this purpose. The nitinol core and lubricious coating are welcome additions. This coil pusher comes in a version with two distal markers, for use with the microcatheters with two tip markers designed for Guglielmi detachable coils. The distal tip marker of a microcatheter or coil pusher is sometimes difficult to see when it is embedded in a mass of coils. The proximal marker, however, is almost always visible. Alignment of the proximal marker on the coil pusher with that on the catheter ensures that the coil has been completely deployed, regardless of whether the distal tip and the coil are visible.

NEURO-SHEATHS

When a sheath is necessary for interventional neuroradiologic work, the use of one that is relatively stiff and extends to the level of the diaphragm (about 45 cm) is not only sensible but also frequently advantageous. A neuro-sheath gives added support to the shaft of the guide catheter so that it does not tend to snake in the aorta but rather maintains a relatively straight course. The positioning of the end hole of the sheath in the descending *thoracic* aorta allows easy exchange of another catheter through it. This type of sheath probably should be used for all diagnostic neuroangiography cases in which a sheath is necessary. The neuro-sheath allows easy manipulation of the diagnostic catheter even in tortuous iliac vessels.

Neuro-sheaths are available from Cook, Inc. (custom and stock products), Cordis Corp. (custom product), Arrow International, and probably other manufacturers.

GUIDE CATHETERS

For years, there was no suitable guide catheter for interventional neuroradiologic use. As with exchange wires, each operator had his or her favorite catheter. New guide catheters have been appearing, however, that represent vast improvements over the original design. The task-specific role of the guide for a microcatheter is to provide a stable platform for the deployment of the microcatheter and to be atraumatic to the surrounding vessel by whatever means possible. This can be achieved by anchoring the catheter in the vessel by a preset shape, by matching the vessel perfectly (patently impossible, particularly in a moving environment), or by having a forgiving tip (extremely soft and noodle-like) that allows the cath-

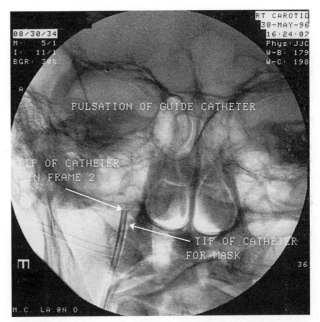

Figure 1-5 During a static run, it is possible to see the extensive movement of the guide catheter, solely due to cardiac pulsation. It is for this reason that it is absolutely mandatory to place the guide catheter in a comfortable position and to use a guide catheter that not only has a soft tip but also has a distal shaft capable of adapting to the vessel shape easily. A guide catheter with a distal curve used for selecting a vessel is incapable of adapting to a vessel shape on its own. The demonstration of the motion caused by cardiac pulsation, not to mention respiration, indicates that it is not possible to place a curved catheter in a matching curve of a vessel and have it maintain this position indefinitely.

eter to sit for prolonged periods atraumatically in this moving environment (i.e., through respiration and cardiac pulsation). The guide catheter *does* move during the case (Fig. 1–5).

There is no need for the guide catheter to have an independent role other than to get the microcatheter to the desired location. A variable-stiffness catheter with smooth transitions from the stiffness of a superstiff guidewire to a noodle end would be ideal. The location can be reached by means of a task-specific, vessel-selecting diagnostic catheter. This is then exchanged for the task-specific guide catheter. In the past, this exchange involved risk to the patient because of inadequate exchange wires and guide catheters, along with poor technique, but is safer now with the use of a good exchange wire and good technique.

The Vinuela catheter (Cook, Inc.) formerly was one of the most popular guide catheters; however, technology has advanced considerably. At present, the Envoy (Cordis Corp.), Omniguide and Omniguide-Flx (Medtronic/MIS) (Fig. 1–6), Guidezilla (Schneider, Inc., Minneapolis, MN), Lumax and Lumax Neuroguide (and other guide catheters from Cook, Inc.; Figs. 1–7 and 1–8), FasGUIDE (Target Therapeutics; Fig. 1–9), and Platform (Medi-Tech, Inc., Fig. 1–10) are good guide catheters, although none is perfect. The FasGUIDE is hydrophilic coated inside and out,

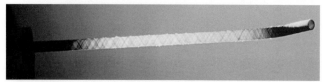

Figure 1-6 The Omniguide-Flex (Medtronic/MIS) is one of the largest-lumen and smallest outer-diameter guide catheters available. It is steamable and shapable, and the 4-Fr. model can carry a microcatheter, which is ideal for use in children.

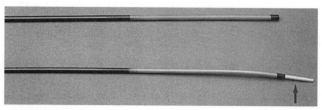

Figure 1-7 The Lumax guide catheter (Cook, Inc.) comes in either a 7-Fr. (0.073″ inner diameter [ID]) or an 8-Fr. size (0.086″ ID); a matched dilator is available *(arrow).*

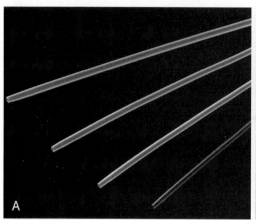

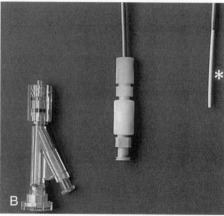

Figure 1-8 *A* and *B,* Cook, Inc. manufactures an array of guide catheters, including 4.8-Fr. (0.043″ ID), 5.8-Fr. (0.053″ ID), 6.8-Fr. (0.061″ ID), and 7.8-Fr. (0.070″ ID). They are all soft with a tapered tip; a good dilator (white core, *asterisk*) is supplied with the set. The body is not as stiff as that of other guide catheters.

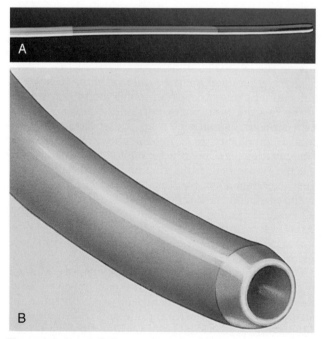

Figure 1-9 *A* and *B,* The FasGUIDE guide catheter from Target Therapeutics offers a variable stiffness design (as do all good guide catheters intended for head and neck work) as well as a very blunt end *(B)* designed to dwell atraumatically in a vessel for considerable periods.

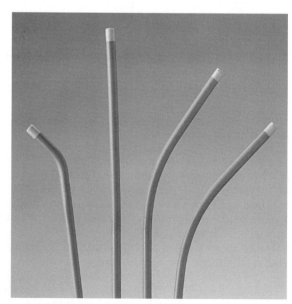

Figure 1-10 The Platform neuro-guide catheter (Medi-Tech, Inc.) has several available shapes and a relatively stiff shaft.

has reasonable tip softness (although not soft enough!), and has a good tip bevel. The Envoy and Omniguide have large lumens and good variable stiffness. None is stiff enough in its proximal shaft or soft enough distally, but all are functional and represent vast improvements over prior choices. The new Lumax Neuroguide has an excellent stiff shaft. The distal shaft has an acceptably soft tip (although not perfect!) and is a welcome addition. Cook, Inc. also has a prototype guide catheter that is based on the Lumax Neuroguide but that has a softer, floppier distal 5 to 6 cm and hydrophilic coating on the distal 50 cm of the catheter. It is being tested in a 9-Fr. size. This catheter has a matched dilator for direct percutaneous introduction over a guidewire.

Any tip that is stiff enough to be used for selection of a vessel is too stiff to be placed in a fragile distal location (such as the internal carotid artery or distal vertebral artery). The operator should beware of placement of a guide catheter in a curve in a vessel where there appears to be a perfect fit; it will not be perfect for long. Respiratory motion moves the tip up and down (or back and forth), whether the procedure does so or not. The vessels in which these guide catheters sit commonly are fragile (old and atherosclerotic), and dissections can occur. Although these guide catheters represent vast improvements over past choices, continuing improvements are being made. Caution is advised with their use.

Matched dilators are available for other guide catheters, allowing direct percutaneous introduction without the use of a sheath (see Chapter 3).

FLOW CONTROL CATHETERS

Flow control catheters are a general group of double-lumen catheters with a latex or silicone occlusion balloon at the tip. They range in size from 3-Fr. to 9.4-Fr. Their purposes are varied, but they can be very useful. The Zeppelin guide catheter (Medtronic/MIS) is one such catheter (Fig. 1–11). The larger sizes can be used for delivery of detachable balloons, and they are *highly* recommended for this purpose.

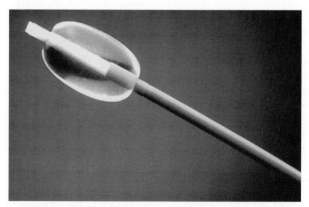

Figure 1-11 The Zeppelin flow control and guide catheter (Medtronic/MIS) has a soft silicone balloon with a relatively atraumatic tip. Newer models can be made with the balloon closer to the tip.

During the balloon detachment process, the flow in the target vessel can be halted to prevent inadvertent detachment or distal embolization. In addition, after the first detachable balloon has been placed, flow arrest can allow time for placement of additional detachable balloons to ensure stability of the occlusion balloons.

When used as guide catheters, these catheters can help to control flow in high-flow diagnostic situations or to slow flow during embolic procedures. In addition, the balloon can allow stabilization of the catheter tip or can be partially inflated to keep the tip off the vessel wall for protection purposes.

For carotid bifurcation angioplasty or stent placement, a flow control guide catheter placed in the common carotid artery can give cerebral protection (see Chapter 43). While the balloon is inflated in the common carotid artery, there is flow reversal in the internal carotid artery, with antegrade flow out of the external carotid artery. This is caused by the higher pressure of the intracranial circulation compared with the external carotid distribution in this circumstance; the bed of the external carotid artery is a sump. This does not apply if the distribution of the internal carotid artery is isolated or if the patient cannot withstand a temporary test occlusion, a relatively rare occurrence that is easily tested. The angioplasty catheter is placed through the occluding guide catheter (e.g., the Zeppelin) and into the intended angioplasty site. This procedure is described in detail in "Ideal Cerebral Protection Technique for Internal Carotid Angioplasty" in Chapter 43.

For intracranial work, new temporary occlusive microcatheters can give aid in high-flow situations or proximal protection during distal embolization. One such catheter, the Grapevine (Medtronic/MIS), has double-lumen design with a distal silicone balloon.

TEMPORARY TEST OCCLUSION BALLOON CATHETERS

Although temporary test occlusion appears to be one of the most straightforward procedures done by an interventional radiologist or neuroradiologist, it has been observed to be one of the more dangerous procedures performed. This is due in part to the technologic limitations of the previously available systems and to the preexisting diseased vessels in many of these patients. The newer temporary occlusion balloons are much improved. Medi-Tech, Inc. makes three models (all require a 7-Fr. sheath) of varying shaft and taper characteristics. The balloon is latex and thus distensible, and it needs considerable room to get into and out of the vessel or sheath (thus requiring the 7-Fr. sheath). The tip of the catheter protrudes too far past the balloon and can impale the vessel wall during occlusion, but the manufacturer is releasing an improved version (with a shorter tip) and an even better model to follow in the near future.

The Zeppelin (Medtronic/MIS) is capable of going straight through the skin over a wire (or over a dilator and a wire), has a beautiful transition at its silicone balloon, and has a safer, less traumatic tip. It primarily was designed as a flow control guide catheter rather than as a test occlusion balloon, but the manufacturer is working on a task-specific model for temporary carotid occlusion. An added bonus is that the silicone balloon on the Zeppelin is capable of being purged by simply instilling fluid and waiting for 5 to 10 minutes for the residual air bubble to diffuse through the silicone balloon! See Chapter 3 for further discussion on purging latex balloons and detachable balloons.

Interventional Therapeutics Corporation (ITC) has been acquired by Target Therapeutics. Target Therapeutics makes a soft (silicone) temporary occlusion balloon mounted on a TRACKER catheter but with the balloon on the very tip (nondetachable silicon balloon, or NDSB, now called the Endeavor). This is a non–end-hole microcatheter and thus requires a guide catheter. With this type of non–end-hole catheter, it is not possible to infuse past the balloon while it is inflated nor is it possible to use a guidewire for steering. Use of a soft microcatheter for balloon transport is ideal for distal occlusion testing. This is the same type of balloon and catheter used for vasospasm angioplasty, but with a slightly different balloon shape. The one used for vasospasm angioplasty is 4 × 10 mm inflated, whereas the other occlusion balloons are larger, measuring 7 × 13 mm, 8 × 21 mm, or 10 × 23 mm; the balloon chosen depends on the target vessel.

The Grapevine balloon catheter described previously can be used for temporary occlusion, over-the-wire applications, and intracranial temporary test occlusions.

ANGIOPLASTY BALLOON CATHETERS

Many available angioplasty catheters are suitable for use in the extracranial brachiocephalic vessels. Some of the more commonly used angioplasty balloon catheters include the Blue Max, Ultrathin, Sub-4, and Symmetry (Medi-Tech, Inc.); Opta-5 (Cordis Corp.); Total Cross (Schneider, Inc.); and Bandit (SciMed, now part of Boston Scientific). The Opta-5 works especially well as a delivery balloon for the Palmaz stent (Johnson & Johnson Interventional Systems).

MICROCATHETERS
Over-the-Wire Microcatheters

The advent of the TRACKER-18 heralded a new era in microvascular work. The new generation of variable-stiffness, hydrophilic-coated microcatheters has permitted even greater ease of access to distal sites (Fig. 1–12). Target Therapeutics has produced numerous variants of their basic microcatheter (Fig. 1–13) in different sizes with variable tip lengths and flow characteristics, along with a model (the Fas-TRACKER-18 MX) designed to undergo less crimping or "ovalling" (i.e., assuming an oval shape when making tight turns) at the end, and therefore more resistant to jamming during embolization. High-perfor-

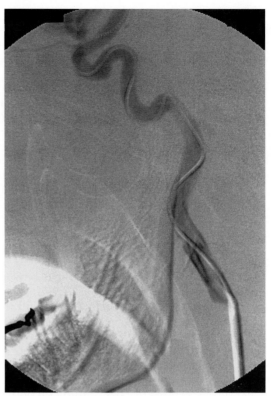

Figure 1-12 A good example of the loss of vectors of force due to the tortuous path a catheter has to take to get to its ultimate location. Note how the microcatheter follows the outside of every curve. A significant amount of friction builds at the outside of each curve. Any force applied from below simply increases the curve of the catheter, and the lateral vectors of force increase, rather than those along the direction of catheter travel. The increasing tortuosity further diverts the vectors of force away from the downstream direction and further increases the friction. The development of hydrophilic coatings greatly influenced the ability to access distal locations by reducing friction.

mance products are also available from Medtronic/MIS, ranging from 2-Fr. (0.010″ lumen), to 3-Fr., 4-Fr., and 5-Fr. variable-stiffness catheters. Medi-Tech, Inc. (Venture) (Fig. 1–14), Microvena (Wanderer), and Cook, Inc. (Microferret and Rufenacht-Merland; Figs. 1–15 and 1–16) also have microcatheters. In addition, Target Therapeutics (TurboTRACKER-18 MX), Cordis Corp. (Transit, Rapid Transit), Medtronic/MIS (Jetstream; Fig. 1–17), and Navarre Biomedical, Ltd. (N-fuser) make microcatheters that contain a braid in the wall to help prevent luminal collapse around tight curves, thus delivering coils and particles with less jamming. Cordis Corp. has introduced a new microcatheter, the Prowler, in two different sizes: 0.010″ and 0.014″. These have a proximal braid and a distal coil for reinforcement and kink prevention.

Multisidehole infusion catheters are available from Target Therapeutics (Softstream, 3.5 Fr., and Micro-Softstream, based on the TRACKER), Cordis Corp., and MicroTherapeutics, Inc. (Fig. 1–18). These are useful in certain situations, such as when infusing thrombolytic agents into a large quantity of thrombus in the internal carotid artery.

Contrast Solution Flow Rates

Catheter Model	Shaft Length	Dead Space Volume	Approximate Flow Rate at 100 PSI (690 kPa)		
			Water	60% Ionic Contrast	76% Ionic Contrast
FasTRACKER-10	155 cm	0.30 cc	0.30 cc/sec.	0.10 cc/sec.	0.04 cc/sec.
Tracker-10	155 cm	0.30 cc	0.30 cc/sec.	0.10 cc/sec.	0.04 cc/sec.
FasTRACKER-18	150 cm	0.49 cc	0.90 cc/sec.	0.20 cc/sec.	0.10 cc/sec.
Tracker-18	100 cm	0.34 cc	1.10 cc/sec.	0.30 cc/sec.	0.20 cc/sec.
Tracker-18 Unibody	135 cm	0.43 cc	0.90 cc/sec.	0.20 cc/sec.	0.10 cc/sec.
Tracker-18 Hi-Flow	135 cm	0.53 cc	1.30 cc/sec.	0.40 cc/sec.	0.20 cc/sec.
	150 cm	0.60 cc	1.30 cc/sec.	0.40 cc/sec.	0.20 cc/sec.
Tracker-25	70 cm	0.45 cc	2.50 cc/sec.	1.10 cc/sec.	0.40 cc/sec.
	135 cm	0.83 cc	2.30 cc/sec.	0.90 cc/sec.	0.30 cc/sec.
	150 cm	0.90 cc	2.10 cc/sec.	0.80 cc/sec.	0.30 cc/sec.
Tracker-38	105 cm	1.20 cc	7.50 cc/sec.	4.40 cc/sec.	2.40 cc/sec.
	120 cm	1.40 cc	6.60 cc/sec.	4.00 cc/sec.	2.10 cc/sec.
Tracker-38 NYL	120 cm	0.96 cc	4.00 cc/sec.	2.10 cc/sec.	2.00 cc/sec.
Zephyr	165 cm	0.37 cc	0.40 cc/sec.	0.14 cc/sec.	0.07 cc/sec.

			Approximate Flow Rate at 300 PSI (2,070 kPa)		
			Water	60% Ionic Contrast	76% Ionic Contrast
FasTRACKER-325	105 cm	0.42 cc	2.6 cc/sec.	1.3 cc/sec.	0.7 cc/sec.

BALT Magic	155 cm	0.3 mL	Approximate Saline Flow Rate at 100 PSI: 0.5 mL/sec.

			Approximate Flow Rate at 300 PSI *	
			Water	Non-Ionic Contrast / 300 mgI/ml
FasGUIDE 6F	90 cm	0.6 cc	7.6 cc./sec.	Not Available
FasGUIDE 6F	100 cm	0.7 cc	6.9 cc./sec.	1.87 cc./sec.

*Flow rate around an intraluminal FasTRACKER-18

Figure 1-13 Sample chart of flow rates for Target Therapeutics catheters. This information is provided by the vendor but is not similarly available for other vendors; the data would perhaps be similar. Note that the flow rate for the guide catheter injection is measured while injecting around a typical microcatheter. The pressures exerted by a "hand injection" with a 3-cc syringe easily can exceed 20 atmospheres (i.e., greater than the 100 psi at which the catheters are rated). Therefore, the maximal flow rates may be slightly higher than those given for typical hand injections, but the catheters are not rated for the extreme pressures exerted during these injections. Because of the potentially extremely high pressures capable of being exerted during a hand injection, occluded catheters have been known to burst.

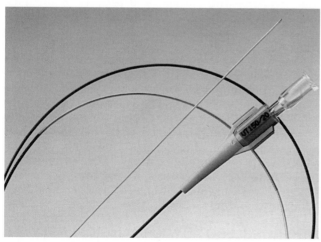

Figure 1-14 The Venture microcatheter was originally marketed by SciMed but is now distributed by Medi-Tech, Inc. It has a multisegmented construction with more firm proximal support than any other microcatheter on the market.

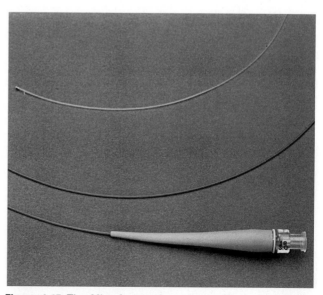

Figure 1-15 The Microferret microcatheter (Cook, Inc.) has an excellent strain relief at the hub.

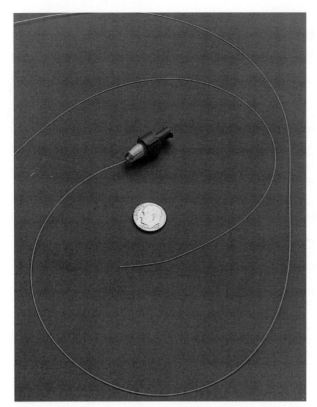

Figure 1-16 The Rufenacht-Merland Teflon microcatheter (Cook, Inc.) is one of the smallest catheters in the world (1.0-Fr., or one third of a millimeter!).

Target Therapeutics produces specific catheters for delivery of their detachable coils (see "Electrolytically Detachable Platinum Microcoils" below) as well as catheters with markers at varying distances from the tip for other specialty applications, such as for the delivery of detachable balloons. Cordis Corp. produces a version of the Transit and Rapid Transit with two tip markers, for use with detachable coils.

Flow-Directed Microcatheters

Flow-directed microcatheters are more flexible and smaller (1.5- to 1.8-Fr.) than over-the-wire catheters. They are designed to be carried distally by flowing blood, especially in high-flow situations such as in the feeding vessels of an arteriovenous malformation. They are thus capable of travelling more distally

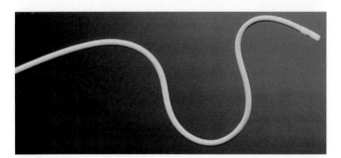

Figure 1-17 The Jetstream microcatheter (Medtronic/MIS) is steamable and braided.

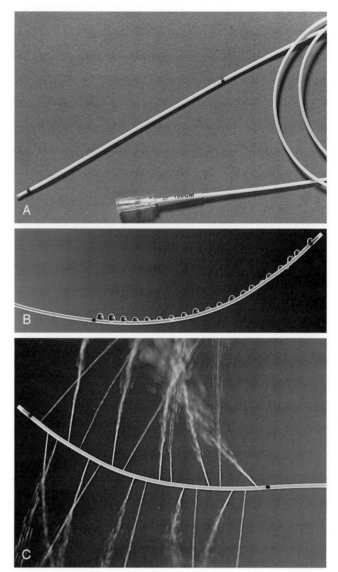

Figure 1-18 *A* to *C,* Multisidehole infusion catheter made by MicroTherapeutics, Inc.

than over-the-wire catheters, especially in tortuous anatomy. They are most frequently used for embolization with liquid agents such as cyanoacrylates, when delivery must be as close to the nidus as possible (even to the point of impacting the catheter in the vessel). The Magic (Balt Extrusion, Montmorency, France; distributed by Target Therapeutics), Zephyr and Spinmaker (Target Therapeutics), Ultralight (Medtronic/MIS), Regatta (Cordis Corp.), and Eddy (Medi-Tech, Inc.) are all good examples; the Zephyr, Spinmaker, Ultralight, Regatta, and Eddy were designed with hydrophilic coatings to be easier to retrieve from tortuous vessels in the presence or absence of vasospasm; hydrophilic coating has been added to the Magic as well.

ATHEROSCLEROTIC MICROANGIOPLASTY CATHETERS

Several microangioplasty catheters are available, mostly for cardiac applications. Only two are capable

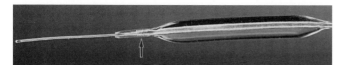

Figure 1-19 Magnification view of the tip of the FasSTEALTH single-lumen balloon dilation system from Target Therapeutics. The kit includes the hydrophilic-coated catheter, the 0.014″ valve wire, a torque device for the wire, and two rotating hemostatic valves. Note the occlusive point of the valve wire *(arrow)*.

of true intracranial work: the STEALTH (Target Therapeutics) and the Stratus (Medtronic/MIS), both single-lumen designs with hydrophilic coating.

The original STEALTH design was capable of accessing the circle of Willis region, and now that it is hydrophilic coated (FasSTEALTH), its use has become even easier (Fig. 1–19). The FasSTEALTH is a single-lumen catheter that uses a dedicated occluding guidewire to allow infusion of fluid through a Tuohy-Borst–type rotating hemostatic valve around the wire for inflation of the balloon. The wire has a bead near its tip that occludes the distal end of the catheter at the catheter tip just past the balloon. The occlusion guidewire can be backloaded (placed rear-end first through the catheter tip before the angioplasty catheter is introduced) or used as a normal guidewire; alternatively, a normal guidewire can be used and exchanged for the occlusion wire when the catheter has been positioned. Once the guidewire nears its distal location, however, some subtle catheter feel is lost. A curve needs to be placed on the guidewire tip before introduction to prevent impaction of the wire at a sharp curve of the vessel and therefore to allow easy bending of the wire through the turn.

The Stratus (Medtronic/MIS) is similar in design to the STEALTH, other than the fact that it uses a guidewire that does not require a bead near the end to occlude the catheter tip (Fig. 1–20). Instead, it has

a slip fit at the proximal end of the balloon that is watertight and a small side channel opening into the balloon proximal to the slip fit. This allows balloon inflation around the wire in a fashion similar to the STEALTH. The ability to inflate the balloon with the wire at any position is convenient; it is not necessary to advance the locked balloon catheter and guidewire apparatus, which has poor control and feel.

VASOSPASM MICROANGIOPLASTY CATHETERS

The original vasospasm balloon was the STEALTH; a hard (noncompliant) angioplasty balloon that is now used primarily for atherosclerotic dilation but that can be used for "resistant" (more long-standing or tougher than usual) vasospasm. Several years ago, ITC/Target Therapeutics introduced the previously described NDSB (or Endeavor) in various sizes. One size, when inflated, becomes about 4 × 10 mm. This size is useful for vasospasm angioplasty, and the soft silicone of the balloon is the preferred type for this pathology. The treatment of vasospasm is discussed in Chapter 51.

In addition, Medtronic/MIS has developed two silicone balloon microcatheters capable of distal work; one has a double-lumen design (the Grapevine) and the other a single-lumen design (the Solstice; Fig. 1–21). The latter is capable of more distal work because of its single-lumen design. Its occlusion method is similar to that used for the Stratus, that is, a dedicated guidewire (the Quicksilver) goes through a slip ring proximal to the balloon but distal to a side channel leading to the balloon to occlude it so that the balloon can be inflated by injecting around the guidewire. This catheter has a silicone balloon as well.

VENTING CATHETERS

Interventional Therapeutics Corporation/Target Therapeutics makes a small microtube for use with their nondetachable silicone balloon. It is designed to be placed coaxially into a microcatheter and to

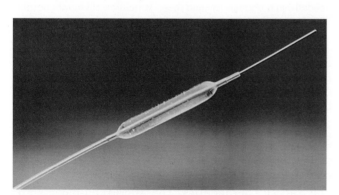

Figure 1-20 The Stratus microangioplasty balloon (Medtronic/MIS) is a hard (noncompliant) balloon that uses single-lumen design and an occlusive wire and was designed for atherosclerotic angioplasty in distal, difficult, or tortuous locations or for treatment of resistant vasospasm. This wire does not have an actual occlusion point, as does the FasSTEALTH occlusion wire, but rather has a tight fit down the entire wire tip, allowing occlusion with the wire extruded to variable lengths. The wire occludes the balloon at its proximal end rather than at the tip of the catheter.

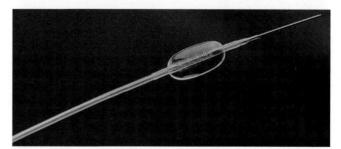

Figure 1-21 The Solstice microangioplasty balloon (Medtronic/MIS) is a soft (silicone) angioplasty balloon (silicone) that uses a single-lumen design, hydrophilic coating, and an occlusive wire; it is thus steerable. It is primarily intended for treatment of vasospasm. The occlusion mechanism is similar in design to the Stratus, thus allowing a variable length of wire to be external to the catheter tip.

infuse contrast into the balloon and allow air to reflux out of the microcatheter around the venting tube. This simplifies preparation of the balloon and permits minimal inflation (inflation will permanently enlarge a latex balloon and thus make it harder to introduce into the guide catheter). It is intended to allow preparation of a small-volume balloon that is too small to allow enough air–fluid exchange to remove all the intrinsic air, such as might occur with the 4 × 10 mm vasospasm balloon (Endeavor).

TEMPORARY STENTING CATHETERS

Temporary stenting catheters are specialty products needed in only particular situations. There are two different types: standard size and microcatheters. The standard size should be available for any angioplasty involving the great vessels of the head and neck. These are catheters with multiple proximal sideholes and distal holes designed to bridge a gap. They are intended for use in failed angioplasty cases to maintain distal perfusion until open surgery can be performed (Figs. 1–22 and 1–23). Cook, Inc. manufactures a custom catheter for this purpose, but one can be made on the spot in an emergency by taking a nonbraided guide catheter (such as that made by ITC/Target Therapeutics or the Ferguson introducer by Cook, Inc.), punching multiple large holes over a 10- to 15-cm distance, and using this to bridge the gap. In this way, distal perfusion can be maintained until either surgery is performed or a permanent metallic stent is placed.

A catheter useful for microstenting is intended for an entirely different purpose. This is a sidehole microcatheter typically used for infusion of fibrinolytic agents, but it can be used for bridging a gap as well. There is one instance in which bridging a gap may be necessary: an embolus to the distal internal carotid artery with occlusion of the middle cerebral

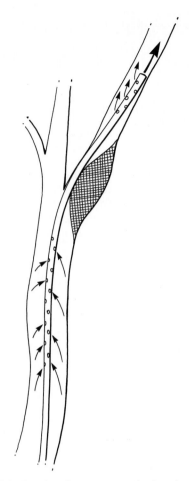

Figure 1-23 This drawing demonstrates the function of a stenting catheter. This is a large-lumen catheter with multiple proximal and distal sideholes as well as the end hole. It is used in an emergency situation (such as failed angioplasty with resultant cerebral vascular insufficiency) to allow time to prepare definitive rescue measures (e.g., stenting, surgery). The catheter is advanced over the guidewire that has been left in place across the stenosis during the angioplasty. Blood flows in the proximal sideholes and out the distal sideholes and end hole, perfusing the downstream structures. A large volume flow is not needed—just enough to keep these structures alive until normal flow can be restored.

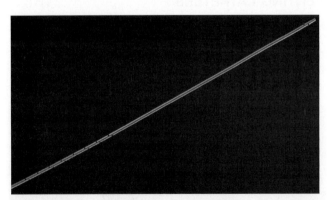

Figure 1-22 Note the sideholes on this "stenting" catheter, which is available for emergency use during a failed angioplasty. The distal end and sideholes are placed through the occluded segment (over a wire). The multiple proximal sideholes allow inflow of blood into the large lumen and out of the distal holes to the downstream structures. This distal perfusion allows time for preparation for any anticipated rescue effort, either surgery or stenting. The presence of this device is recommended in any laboratory practicing head and neck angioplasty. This is a custom product supplied by Cook, Inc., based on their Ferguson guide catheter.

artery by a large volume of thrombus. While the internal carotid artery is being cleared, a stenting catheter such as this can carry a small amount of blood downstream to the most ischemic territory.

SNARES

For emergency retrieval of catheters, coils, or other foreign bodies, snares are available from Microvena and Target Therapeutics. The Microvena models are available in micro as well as macro sizes and have the ability to turn at right angles to the vessel lumen when deployed. They are supplied in either a 2-mm or 4-mm circular snare size for use through a microcatheter (Fig. 1–24). The snare is relatively invisible within the microcatheter (Fig. 1–25). When the snare is deployed, it assumes a right angle to the axis of the catheter (Fig. 1–26).

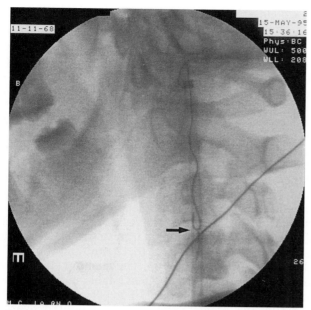

Figure 1-24 An errant platinum coil is retrieved by means of a Microvena snare. The large guide catheter is the Zeppelin by Medtronic/MIS. This particular catheter has a 7-Fr. lumen with a flow control silicone balloon at the end (see text). The snare was deployed distal to the coil and dragged back past the coil, catching the end of the coil in the loop. Once snagged, the snare has a good grip, which is tightened by withdrawing the snare wire slightly. The coil wire should not be withdrawn too forcefully, because it can break.

The Target Therapeutics model (the Retriever; Fig. 1–27) is somewhat softer and is capable of more distal access but is slightly more difficult to use. See "How to Use a Snare" in Chapter 3 for discussion of particulars concerning snare use.

EMBOLECTOMY DEVICES

The snares described in the previous section can be used to retrieve an embolus from a vessel, particularly if it is an old, hard (white) thrombus. In addition, Medtronic/MIS is developing a dedicated re-

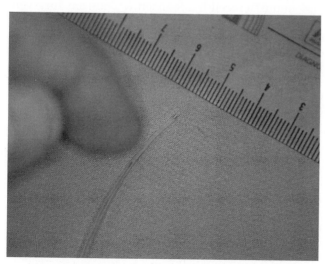

Figure 1-25 Microvena snare within a microcatheter.

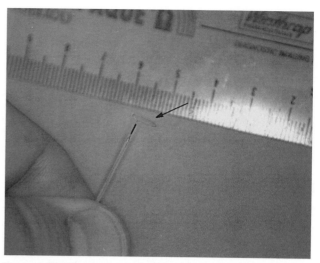

Figure 1-26 Microvena snare deployed. Note that the loop assumes a right angle to the axis of the catheter *(arrow)*.

trieval device for use with microcatheters. This is a nitinol wire with a spiral mounted on it that tapers from 5 to 2 mm distally. Beyond this is a short, straight segment. The catheter and wire are advanced with only the distal short segment exposed, so that the spiral portion of the wire is past the thrombus. The catheter is then slowly withdrawn, releasing the spiral. The catheter can be withdrawn to expose the appropriate amount of the spiral for the size of the vessel and thrombus. The wire and microcatheter are then withdrawn together into the guide catheter, bringing the thrombus with them.

COMMERCIAL AND INVESTIGATIVE METALLIC STENTS

This section reviews many of the stents in use or being developed worldwide. Of these, the Palmaz-

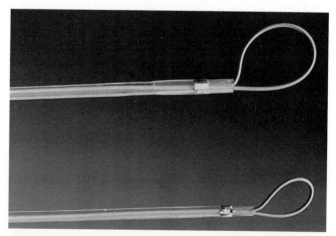

Figure 1-27 The Retriever (Target Therapeutics) is a single-piece snare incorporated into the body of the FasTRACKER-18 and the FasTRACKER-10. Through the lumen of the catheter is a single wire that is doubled back on itself only over the last 2 cm, at which point it becomes part of the distal marker for the catheter. Opening and closing of the snare is performed by advancing and withdrawing the wire. The FasTRACKER body allows the catheter to advance distally with ease, and the size of the loop allows a flexible approach to retrieval.

Schatz, Wiktor, Radius, MultiLink, Gianturco-Rou-bin Flex, and Gianturco-Roubin II are approved for coronary use in the United States. The Palmaz stent is approved for peripheral vascular and biliary use; the Wallstent has limited approval for these applications as well as for tracheal and esophageal use. The Wallstent and Integra stent are in clinical trials in the United States for use in the carotid artery. Table 1–2 provides a summary of the characteristics of various stents.

Palmaz Balloon-Expandable Stent

The Palmaz balloon-expandable stent (Johnson & Johnson Interventional Systems) was developed in 1985.[1] The stent is one of the few devices approved by the FDA for arterial placement. The device was intended to allow for dilation and simultaneous placement of an intraluminal stent to support the wall, preventing elastic arterial recoil. The initial design of the stent was a continuous, woven, stainless steel, 150-micron diameter wire. The cross-points of the wire mesh were soldered to give the stent high resistance to radial collapse.[1] Lossef et al.[2] found that the 4- to 9-mm Palmaz stent had 30% more resistance to deformation than the 8- to 12-mm stent.

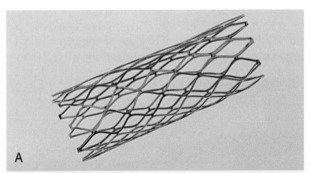

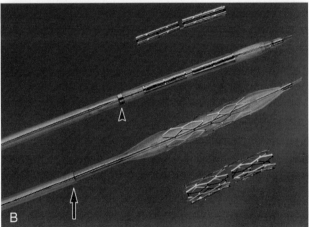

Figure 1-28 *A* and *B,* This expanded Palmaz stent *(A)* demonstrates the diamond-shaped openings. The illustration *(B)* shows the nonexpanded Palmaz-Schatz stent mounted on the balloon with the protective sheath in place (note the marker band on the sheath, just proximal to the proximal balloon marker, *arrowhead*), the sheath withdrawn *(arrow)* with the stent expanded on the balloon, and the expanded stent.

The stent design was changed by replacing the woven mesh with a lath design produced by electro-mechanical etching of thin-walled, stainless steel tubing.[3] The etching produces a stent with parallel rows of staggered rectangular slots, allowing for a smaller diameter and thinner walls (Fig. 1–28A). In expanded form, the rectangular slots open up to form diamond-shaped spaces. This design offers the advantage of a larger open area (90%), which theoretically decreases thrombogenicity and promotes rapid endothelialization. The unique diamond-shaped structure provides not only more precise sizing of stent to vessel but also the possibility of further expansion of diameter after deployment. The Palmaz stent comes in two size ranges: large and medium. The 0.005″, thinner-walled, large stents are available in an expansion range of 8 to 12 mm and are available in lengths up to 30 mm. The medium stent, with an 0.0055″ wall thickness, is available in ranges of 4 to 9 mm in diameter and 10 to 39 mm in length. Initially, the stents needed to be mounted over a "wrapped" balloon using a combination of finger crimping and crimping with the special tool. Because of the tendency of the stent to slip back on the balloon, the stent and balloon assembly needs to be protected during introduction through the hemostatic valve by a stainless steel introducer. A newer version of the stent is available premounted on a 5-Fr. balloon catheter in a choice of 4, 5, 6, and 7 mm sizes, eliminating the need for mounting. These premounted stents can be introduced through a 7-Fr. sheath, so they maintain a low profile during delivery. The Palmaz stent, however, is still often mounted manually by the operator as needed.

Stenting with the Palmaz stent has been proved safe and effective in the iliac arteries; disadvantages, such as its lack of longitudinal flexibility, may limit its application in the tortuous supra-aortic vessels.

Palmaz-Schatz Stent

The Palmaz-Schatz stent is a variant of the Palmaz stent specifically designed for coronary use and is also manufactured by Johnson & Johnson Interventional Systems. This stent is one of the few designed to be balloon expandable but delivered within a covered sheath. It is sold as a complete unit, with a premounted stent, angioplasty balloon, and covering sheath. The entire unit is 5-Fr. The sheath allows the unit to be placed through curves that could dislocate the stent but also increases the stiffness of the unit.

The Palmaz-Schatz stent is articulated; in other words, instead of being one large piece of metal, there are sections (in this case, two) which are connected only at a certain point (see Fig. 1–28B). Articulation improves the rigidity of these stents. The stent has minimal immediate thrombosis and a good record for minimal restenosis. It is not as flexible as some of the newer coronary stents, and it is extremely difficult to see once deployed (the marker bands are on the balloon catheter, not the stent).

T A B L E 1 - 2 Comparison of Characteristics of Various Stents

Stent Name	Manufacturer	Basic Design	Material and Characteristics	Sizes Available	Current Use	Delivery Characteristics	Approval
AngioStent	AngioDynamics	Balloon-expandable; sinusoidal wire; helically wrapped with longitudinal member	Platinum; high radiopacity; nonferromagnetic; 9.4%–12.5% metallic surface area; 0.005" strut thickness; excellent flexibility; 7% shortening; good radial strength; 7% recoil; high biocompatibility; low thrombogenicity	3, 3.5, 4 mm diameter; 15, 25, 35 mm length	Coronary	Nonexpanded profile 1.60 mm (RE), 1.78 mm (OTW); minimum guide catheter 6-Fr. (RE), 8-Fr. (OTW); premounted; protective sheath (OTW); marker center (RE), proximal/distal (OTW); semicompliant balloon, 12–15 atmospheres (initial), up to 16 atmospheres (second); further balloon expansion optional; good recrossability	Not approved in U.S.
Cragg stent	MinTech/Boston Scientific Corp.	Self-expanding; round wire; zigzag pattern of loops tied together	Nitinol; moderate radiopacity; nonferromagnetic; 0.27-mm strut thickness; excellent flexibility; 9% shortening; moderate radial strength	6 mm diameter; 40 mm length	Iliac, femoral	Nonexpanded profile 8-Fr.; premounted; protective sheath; proximal/distal markers; further balloon expansion not recommended; good recrossability	Not approved in U.S.
Crown stent	Cordis Corp.	Balloon-expandable; slotted tube; scalloped strut pattern	Stainless steel (316L); medium radiopacity; nonferromagnetic; 0.069-mm strut thickness; good flexibility; good radial strength 3%–15% shortening; good radial strength	3, 3.5, 4 mm diameter; 15, 22, 30 mm length	Coronary	Nonexpanded profile 4-Fr.; minimum guide catheter 6-Fr.; premounted; no protective sheath; no markers; non-compliant balloon; further balloon expansion not recommended; good recrossability	Not approved in U.S.
Gianturco-Rösch Z stent	Cook, Inc.	Self-expanding; round wire; zigzag pattern; segments linked by strut or suture	Stainless steel (304); medium radiopacity; ferromagnetic; 10% metallic surface area; 0.01"–0.018" strut thickness; medium flexibility; high radial strength; 0% shortening; 0% recoil	6, 8, 10, 12 mm diameter; 1.5, 3, 4.5, 6, 7.5, 9 cm length (biliary); 15, 20, 25, 30, 35, 40 mm diameter; 50 mm length (tracheo-bronchial)	Biliary, esophageal; tracheo-bronchial	Nonexpanded profile 8.5–18-Fr.; not premounted; protective sheath; marker on tip of sheath; further balloon expansion optional; good recrossability	Approved in U.S. for tracheo-bronchial and biliary use
Gianturco-Roubin Flex stent	Cook, Inc.	Balloon-expandable; wire; interdigitating zigzag pattern	Stainless steel; low radiopacity; slightly ferromagnetic; 10% metallic surface area; excellent flexibility; no shortening; good radial strength	2.0, 2.5, 3.0, 3.5, 4.0 mm diameter; 12, 20 mm length	Coronary	Minimum guide catheter 7-Fr.; premounted; no protective sheath; proximal/distal markers; low compliance balloon; good recrossability	Approved in U.S. for coronary use

Table continued on following page

T A B L E 1 - 2 Comparison of Characteristics of Various Stents *Continued*

Stent Name	Manufacturer	Basic Design	Material and Characteristics	Sizes Available	Current Use	Delivery Characteristics	Approval
Gianturco-Roubin II stent	Cook, Inc.	Balloon-expandable; flat wire; interdigitating zigzag pattern with longitudinal spine	Stainless steel; excellent radiopacity (gold end markers); nonferromagnetic; 15%–20% metallic surface area; excellent flexibility; no shortening; good radial strength	2.5, 3.0, 3.5, 4.0 mm diameter; 20, 40 mm length	Coronary	Minimum guide catheter 6–7-Fr.; premounted; no protective sheath; proximal/distal markers on stent; minimally compliant balloon; good recrossability	Approved in U.S. for coronary use
Global stent	Global Therapeutics, Inc.	Balloon-expandable; round wire; trapezoidal spiral pattern	Stainless steel (316L); moderate radiopacity; nonferromagnetic; 0.024″ strut thickness; excellent flexibility; 1% shortening; moderate radial strength	6 mm diameter; 40 mm length	Peripheral vascular	Nonexpanded profile 9-Fr.; not premounted; no protective sheath; balloon expansion not recommended	Not approved in U.S.
Memotherm stent	Global Technology Center/Bard, Inc.	Self-expanding; diamond pattern	Nitinol; moderate radiopacity; nonferromagnetic; 0.16–0.18 mm strut thickness; moderate flexibility	4, 5, 6, 7, 8 mm diameter; 20–120 mm length (10 mm increments)	Iliac, femoral arteries	Nonexpanded profile 7-Fr.; minimum guide catheter 7-Fr.; premounted, protective sheath; marker at proximal end of stent; further balloon expansion not recommended; good recrossability	Limited approval in U.S.
Nitinol Hexagonal stent	Boston Scientific Corp.	Self-expanding; wire; welded hexagonal cells	Nitinol; moderate radiopacity; metallic surface area 19%; 0.008″–0.009″ strut thickness; moderate flexibility; good radial strength	4–14 mm diameter; 2, 4, 6 mm length	Peripheral vascular	Nonexpanded profile 7-Fr.; premounted; protective sheath; markers proximal/distal; further balloon expansion optional; good recrossability	Not approved in U.S.; in trial in Europe
Palmaz stent	Johnson & Johnson Interventional Systems	Balloon-expandable; slotted tube; diamond-shaped openings	Stainless steel (316L); moderate radiopacity; negligibly ferromagnetic; metallic surface area 10%; 0.005″–0.0055″ strut thickness; low flexibility; 10%–20% shortening; high radial strength; minimal recoil	4–8 mm diameter; 10–39 mm length (premounted); 4–12 mm diameter; 12–39 mm length (unmounted)	Coronary, femoral, iliac, renal, biliary, TIPS	Nonexpanded profile 2.1–3.1 mm; minimum guide catheter 6–7-Fr.; premounted or unmounted; protective sheath (Palmaz-Schatz); markers proximal/distal; noncompliant delivery balloon; 8 atmospheres; further balloon expansion optional; good recrossability	Approved in U.S.; Palmaz-Schatz approved for coronary use in U.S.

Stent	Manufacturer	Design	Material/Properties	Dimensions	Application	Delivery Features	Approval Status
Radius/Integra stent	SciMed/Boston Scientific Corp.	Self-expanding; zigzag loops with cross-links	Nitinol; moderate radiopacity; negligibly ferromagnetic; excellent flexibility; moderate radial strength	3.0–4.0 mm diameter; 14–21 mm length (Radius); 6.0–7.0 mm diameter; 20–31 mm length (Integra)	Coronary (Radius); carotid (Integra)	Nonexpanded profile 4.6-Fr. (Radius), 0.089" (Integra); minimum guide catheter 7-Fr. (Radius), 9-Fr. (Integra); premounted; protective sheath; markers proximal/distal; further balloon expansion optional; good recrossability	Radius approved in U.S. for coronary use; Integra in clinical trial for carotid use
Strecker stent	Medi-Tech, Inc./ Boston Scientific Corp.	Balloon-expandable; knitted wire mesh	Tantalum; excellent radiopacity; nonferromagnetic; 0.1 mm strut thickness; excellent flexibility; negligible shortening; low radial strength; 0.5–1.0 mm recoil	4–12 mm diameter; 20–80 mm length	Peripheral vascular	Nonexpanded profile 8–9-Fr.; premounted; protective sheath; markers proximal/distal; noncompliant delivery balloon; further balloon expansion optional	Not approved in U.S.; in trial in Europe
Strecker Nitinol stent	Medi-Tech, Inc./ Boston Scientific Corp.	Self-expanding; wire; woven; distal stabilization anchors	Nitinol; moderate radiopacity; negligibly ferromagnetic; 0.13 mm strut thickness; excellent flexibility; 35% shortening; moderate radial strength	8, 10 mm diameter; 40, 60 mm length	Biliary, colorectal, esophageal	Nonexpanded profile 10-Fr.; premounted; protective sheath; markers proximal distal and middle (showing proximal end after expansion); moderate recrossability	Not approved in U.S.; in trial in Europe
VascuCoil stent	InStent, Inc.	Self-expanding; round wire; spring-shaped coil	Nitinol; moderate radiopacity; nonferromagnetic; 0.01"–0.013" strut thickness; moderate flexibility; 30% shortening; high radial strength	4–9 mm diameter; 40 mm length	Coronary, peripheral vascular	Nonexpanded profile 7-Fr.; premounted; no protective sheath; markers proximal/distal; further balloon expansion not recommended; good recrossability	Not approved in U.S.
Wallstent	Schneider, Inc.	Self-expanding; wire; braided mesh	Stainless steel; moderate radiopacity; nonferromagnetic; 0.005" strut thickness; excellent flexibility; 25%–40% shortening; moderate radial strength; no recoil	5–25 mm diameter; 20, 40, 60, 80 mm length	TIPS, biliary; peripheral vascular; esophageal; tracheo-bronchial	Nonexpanded profile 7-Fr.; minimum guide catheter 8-Fr.; premounted; protective sheath; markers proximal/distal; good recrossability	Limited approval in U.S.; ongoing trial in carotid use in U.S.
Wiktor stent	Medtronic, Inc.	Balloon-expandable; sinusoidal-shaped wire in a helical pattern	Tantalum; good radiopacity; nonferromagnetic; 0.005" wire thickness; excellent flexibility; minimal shortening; high radial strength; ~8% recoil	3.0, 3.5, 4.0, 4.5 mm diameter; 16 mm length	Coronary, peripheral vascular	Minimum guide catheter 8-Fr.; premounted; no protective sheath; marker center; compliant delivery balloon; good recrossability	Approved for coronary use in U.S.

OTW, over-the-wire; RE, rapid-exchange; TIPS, transjugular intrahepatic portacaval shunt.

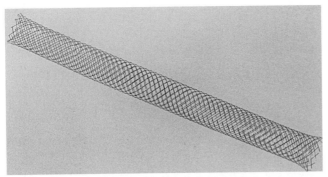

Figure 1-29 The self-expanding Wallstent is shown, demonstrating the woven crisscross pattern of wire filaments.

Wallstent

The self-expanding Wallstent (Schneider, Inc.) is composed of 20 filaments (surgical-grade, stainless steel alloy), each 100 microns in diameter, woven in a crisscross pattern to form a tubular braid configuration (Fig. 1–29). The 77% macroporosity of the device permits rapid endothelialization and good patency of collateral vessels bridged by the stent. The filament crossing points are not fixed but are free to slide or pivot over each other. Its unique design renders the stent self-expanding, pliable, and highly longitudinally flexible. Therefore, the stent can be moderately stretched to a smaller diameter and spontaneously recovers its original diameter when released into the vascular lumen, owing to the spring characteristics of the individual filaments. This also makes the stent resistant to collapse when subjected to extrinsic compression because the cylindrical braid springs back. The constant expansile force against the vessel wall, however, has been thought to result in the increased neointimal reaction within the stented segment.[4, 5] This theory has been challenged by the results of Vorwerk and colleagues' animal study,[6] which indicated that the self-expanding Wallstent does not induce additional neointimal growth in the dog model and that less radial force does not necessarily reduce the thickness of neointimal build-up.

When mounted on the 7-Fr. delivery catheter, the stent is constrained by a double-over rolling membrane that is progressively retracted by the operator. The Wallstent originally was deployed by a delivery system that required lubrication in the space between catheter and membrane by hand injection of diluted contrast medium before deployment. The manufacturer has changed its design to the Unistep system, which eliminates lubrication. While the membrane is being unrolled, the stent expands radially, molding itself to the vessel wall; its longitudinal flexibility allows perfect adaptation to vessel curvature. As long as the stent is partially within the membrane, the membrane can be readvanced, and the stent then repositioned as needed. The stent is loaded at the distal end of the delivery catheter. The caliber of the delivery catheter varies according to

the stent diameter (5- to 9-Fr.). The introducer catheter can be used over guidewires of 0.014″ to 0.035″ diameter. The delivery catheter is highly flexible, permitting advancement through tortuous vessels. The catheter tip is flexible despite the presence of the mounted stent. One of two major disadvantages of the Wallstent is the poor fluoroscopic visibility, especially in obese patients.[7, 8] For convenience and precise deployment, three metal markers on the stent delivery catheter indicate the distal and the proximal ends of the stent and proposed position of the distal end after shortening during deployment. The release of the constrained stent leads to a spontaneous return to the initial shape, the diameter and length of which are predetermined. Stent shortening is the other main drawback. When the membrane is 50% retracted, the stent achieves 90% of its eventual shortening. This allows more accurate positioning; the membrane can be readvanced and the stent repositioned if needed.

Among the commercially available large vascular stents, the Wallstent possesses the greatest degree of shortening, with 30% to 40% shortening during deployment, compared with 17% shortening with the Palmaz stent and 19% with the Strecker stent.[7] (The Gianturco-Roubin stents do not shorten.) Choosing a proper size of stent is crucial to successful stent placement.

Wallstents are sold for use with transjugular intrahepatic portacaval shunt (TIPS) procedures, esophageal dilation, iliac stenting, enteral endoprosthesis, and tracheobronchial stenting. The tracheobronchial stents have been used "off-label" for stenting in carotid angioplasty procedures.

The Wallstent is undergoing a clinical trial for carotid use in the United States.

Strecker Balloon-Expandable Stent

The tantalum balloon-expandable stent (Strecker stent, Medi-Tech, Inc.) was first described by Strecker in 1988. Most of the reported clinical experience with the Strecker stent was obtained from Germany because the stent is not yet available for sale in the United States.[9, 10]

The Strecker stent consists of a knitted, tubular, flexible metal wire mesh structure, which is made of a single tantalum filament 0.1 mm in diameter. Because of its loose structure of connected wire loops, the stent offers a high degree of longitudinal and radial flexibility (Fig. 1–30). It has been reported that the Strecker stent has greater flexibility than the Wallstent because knitting forms a looser fabric than weaving. The unique knitted design permits the stent to adapt to tight vascular curves to ease negotiation of tortuous anatomy and facilitates a contralateral approach over the aortic bifurcation, if it becomes necessary. The slightly softened edges at the stent ends allow a natural transition to the native vessel wall. The dimensions are determined by the number and size of loops (1.5 to 2.5 mm), and the inside diameter depends on the diameter of the core.

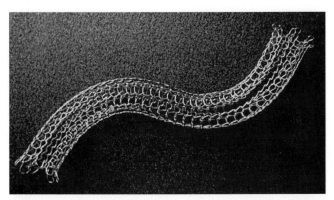

Figure 1-30 The Strecker balloon-expandable stent. The expanded stent is shown, demonstrating its excellent flexibility.

Like the Palmaz stent, the Strecker stent has no spring action of its own; it needs to be expanded passively over a balloon, up to six times its collapsed introducing dimensions to a predetermined diameter, and it has no tendency to increase its diameter after placement, in contrast to the self-expanding stent. To prevent displacement of the stent over the balloon caused by friction with the introducer sheath or with the inner arterial wall, both ends of the stent are attached to the balloon by silicone sleeves. When the balloon is inflated, the silicone sleeves slide back and thus release the stent. A 0.5- to 1.0-mm recoil was observed after stent expansion during laboratory tests.[11] Shortening of the stent on expansion is negligible.[12]

The loops of the Strecker stent are made of tantalum, which is regarded as a highly biocompatible, inert metal. The advantages of tantalum over stainless steel and other alloys include (1) high radiopacity, which allows good visualization under fluoroscopy; (2) corrosion resistance, which was confirmed by the long-term studies of orthopedic implants and surgical clips; and (3) its nonferromagnetic properties, which permit magnetic resonance imaging (MRI) or magnetic resonance angiography with minimal artifact. To further decrease thrombogenicity, the wire is chemically electroplated. By this process, the oxide film on the metal surface is fully removed, and microscopic irregularities are eliminated. These measures ensure that the metal oxidation that will occur in the bloodstream will lead to a "uniform" oxide film surface. The thin layer of inert tantalum pentoxide, which creates an electrically negative surface charge, prevents the adhesion of platelets, which are negatively charged as well.

The Strecker stent is available in 7 sizes, from 4 to 12 mm in diameter in expanded form and 4 cm in length. The stent is mounted on a 5-Fr. (for stents 6 to 8 mm in diameter) or 5.8-Fr. (for stents 9 to 12 mm in diameter) balloon catheter with a usable length of 95 cm (Ultra-Thin ST, Medi-Tech, Inc.). The stent and balloon catheter assembly easily can be introduced through an 8-Fr. (for stents 6 to 8 mm in diameter), 9-Fr. (for stents 9 to 11 mm in diameter), or 10-Fr. (for stents 12 mm in diameter) introducer sheath.

A disadvantage of the Strecker stent appears to be lack of hoop strength. Among the commercially available stents, including the Palmaz stent, the Wallstent, and the Gianturco stent, the Strecker stent has the least stress–strain resistance. Kuhn and colleagues[13] claimed that the Strecker stent would be completely collapsed when the external force applied to the stent exceeded 0.2 to 0.3 atmospheres of pressure.

Strecker Nitinol Self-Expanding Stent

The modified Strecker stent (Elastally, Boston Scientific Corp.) was first reported in 1994 for biliary application.[14] It has been widely used in the gastrointestinal and urinary systems in Europe. The basic structure of the stent is similar to that of the tantalum version. The nickel and titanium alloy gives the stent remarkable flexibility, elasticity, and radial hoop strength. Initially, the stent was made of a nitinol wire with thickness of 0.10 mm; this was changed to 0.15 mm and finally to 0.13 mm to reach a good balance among hoop strength, radiopacity, and low profile. The dimensions of the stent are 10 mm in diameter and 6 cm in length in full expansion. The stent can be deployed through a 10-Fr. delivery system that can be advanced over an 0.038″ guidewire. The stent is released by withdrawing the outer sheath (Fig. 1–31). The major drawbacks of this device are low radiopacity and significant shortening (35%). Highly radiopaque markers have been used to indicate the proximal and distal ends of the constrained stent as well as the proximal end of the stent at expanded form (Fig. 1–32). This stent is not commercially available.

Gianturco-Rösch Z Stent

The Gianturco-Rösch Z stent (Cook, Inc.) is made of 0.010″ stainless steel wire, which is bent in a zigzag pattern to form a cylinder (Fig. 1–33A), thereby possessing self-expanding characteristics. These stents are commercially available in several sizes, including 15-, 20-, 25-, 30-, and 35-mm expanded diameters, and are 5 cm in length. If longer lesions are treated, multiple stents joined either by stainless steel wire struts (Gianturco type) or by a nylon monofilament

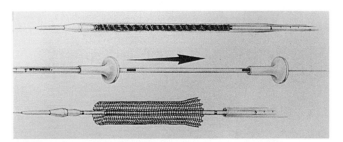

Figure 1-31 The self-expanding Strecker nitinol (Elastally) stent comes premounted on a delivery catheter. When the stent is properly positioned, the protective sheath is withdrawn (arrow), and the stent expands.

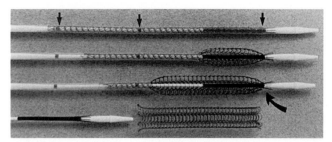

Figure 1-32 Radiopaque markers on the delivery catheter indicate the proximal and distal ends of the self-expanding Strecker nitinol stent as well as the proximal end of the fully expanded stent *(arrows)*. The curved arrow indicates how the distal end of the stent remains attached to the delivery catheter until fully deployed.

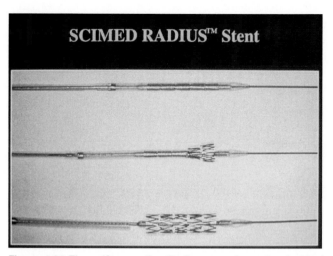

Figure 1-34 The self-expanding Radius stent is made of nitinol loops in a zigzag pattern. It is designed for coronary use. The Integra stent, in clinical trial for carotid use, is based on this design.

suture (Gianturco-Rösch type) can be used in tandem. The tandem configuration reduces stent slippage and enables exertion of a greater expansile force. The expansile force exerted by the stent increases in proportion to the number of legs in the stent, the leg bends, and the diameter of wire used. The expansile force decreases with the length of each stent. In most cases, the diameter of stents used in the venous system is 15% to 25% over the estimated normal diameter of the vessel. In concentric stenoses, oversizing by 25% to 50% may produce an expansile force. The stents are compressed and introduced through an 8- to 12-Fr. Teflon catheter, depending on the caliber of the wire and the diameter of the stent.

Several modifications of the original design have been made. The bends of the wire legs may be soldered to form circles that are then connected with surgical suture, to ensure a fixed final expanded diameter after deployment. A wire skirt was added to one or both ends of the stent by Rösch. This reduces the tendency of the stent to migrate forward during deployment. When a single skirt is used, this is located at the forward end of the stent. Small hooks oriented in the direction of stent introduction help to stabilize stent position. Irie and associates[15] modified the Gianturco stent, allowing it to be repositioned and retrieved.

Radius Stent

The Radius stent (SciMed/Boston Scientific Corp.) is a self-expanding stent made of nitinol and designed

for coronary applications. It is multisegmented and constructed of a series of rings bent in a zigzag pattern with cross-links (Fig. 1–34). The stent is available in 3.0-, 3.5-, and 4.0-mm diameters and in 14- and 20-mm lengths. The stent comes premounted on a delivery catheter and sheath system and requires a guide catheter with an inner diameter of at least 0.072″. The Radius stent has been approved by the FDA for coronary use in the United States.

Integra Stent

A variant of the Radius stent, the Integra (Boston Scientific Corp.) has been designed for carotid use and is in clinical trial in the United States. This stent is similarly designed with a zigzag pattern and is available in 6.0- and 7.0-mm diameters and in 20- and 31-mm lengths. The stent comes mounted on a delivery system like that used for the Radius stent; however, a larger guide catheter is needed (9-Fr.). The Integra is self-expanding and appears to offer a reasonable alternative to the dilemma of choosing the proper stent for carotid angioplasty.

Memotherm Stent

The Memotherm stent (Angiomed, Karlsruhe, Germany; sold by Bard, Inc. in the United States) is self-

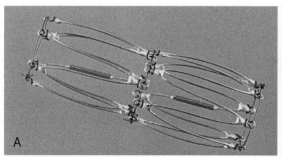

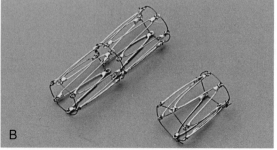

Figure 1-33 *A,* The fully expanded Gianturco-Rösch stent, demonstrating the joining of segments with monofilament suture. *B,* Single-segment and multisegment stents are shown.

expanding and made of nitinol alloy, which has a temperature-dependent shape memory. The material varies its form in reaction to the surrounding environmental temperature. The stent remains in collapsed form at 0°C and is fully expanded, with diamond-shaped openings, at 35°C (Fig. 1–35). The Memotherm stent is negatively charged, which hinders early thrombus formation. Its one-wall design eliminates filament crossing, and the minimal width of the lattice minimizes the profile and surface area. The stent is deployed through a 7-Fr. delivery system connecting to a gunlike controller, so placement of the stent easily can be accomplished by manipulating the controller with one hand. The dimensions of the stents range from 4 to 10 mm in diameter and from 20 to 120 mm in length. A clinical trial has been conducted by Starck et al.[16, 17] in iliac and femoral arterial applications, which demonstrated 100% primary angiographic success and 96.8% clinical success after stent placement. Lifetable analysis indicated 96% clinical patency in the iliac artery and 56% in the femoral artery 14 months after placement.

Cragg Nitinol Stent

The Cragg stent (MinTech, Bahamas) was developed in 1993. It is made of 0.27-mm nitinol wire that is longitudinally bent on a metal mandrel in a zigzag configuration (Fig. 1–36). The distance between bends is about 4 mm. The apices of each abutting loop are tied with 7-0 polypropylene sutures to form a tube. The stent length can be changed by winding more wire, and the diameter can be set by using different diameters of the mandrel. The stent can be deformed to be preloaded in a Teflon capsule in ice water, in which the nitinol becomes soft, without loss of the memorized shape. As soon as deployed into the vessel, the stent resumes its pre-programmed shape at body temperature. The stent is deployed through an 8-Fr. delivery system consisting of a 30-cm-long introducer sheath, a blunt positioning catheter, and a Teflon cartridge in which the stent is loaded. The purported advantages of the Cragg stent include high radiopacity, minimal shortening (7%), good longitudi-

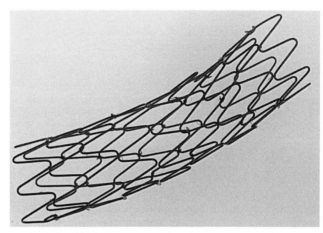

Figure 1-36 The Cragg stent is constructed of multiple loops of nitinol wire, each bent in a zigzag pattern. The adjacent loops are connected by polypropylene suture.

nal flexibility, and greater expansion ratio because of thermal memory. Results of hoop strength analysis conducted by Cragg et al.[18] showed that the external forces required to reduce the stent diameter by 33%, 44%, 55%, and 66% were 49, 110, 166, and 690 mm Hg, respectively, for the Cragg stent, compared with 132, 242, 320, and 754 mm Hg, respectively, for the Wallstent.

Nitinol Hexagonal Stent

The self-expanding nitinol Hexagonal stent (Boston Scientific) is made of a single strand (0.009″ in diameter) of nitinol wire with a pattern of hexagonal cells axially arranged in six columns in each direction. The vertical sides of the hexagonal cells are welded together to form an integral cylindrical structure. The properties of nitinol confer the stent softness and pliability at low temperature (such as ice water), so that the stent can be compressed into a low profile (7-Fr.) delivery system. After introduction to the vascular system and release from the constraining sheath, the stent promptly recovers its memory shape, which matches the size of the target vessel. The stents range from 8 to 10 mm in diameter and are 4 cm in length. The stent metal area is 16.5% for 10-mm stents and 18.4% for 8-mm stents. A company publication claims that the radial hoop strength of the nitinol Hexagonal stent compares favorably to that of the Wallstent. Experimental observations in a swine model revealed ease of deployment through a 7-Fr. sheath, no migration when sized to at least 10% oversizing, and mild intimal proliferation 30 and 60 days after deployment. No clinical data are available on this stent.[19]

Wiktor Stent

A sinusoidal-shaped wire wound into an open helical pattern is used to make the Wiktor stent (Medtronic, Inc.) highly longitudinally flexible and adaptable to vascular segments of differing diameters and

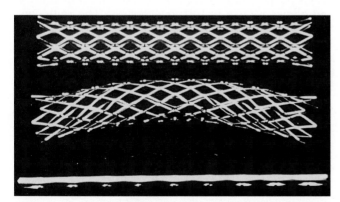

Figure 1-35 The self-expanding Memotherm stent is made of nitinol and has a single-wall structure, without crossing filaments. It assumes its expanded shape when released at body temperature.

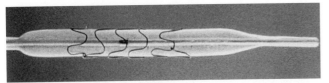

Figure 1-37 The Wiktor stent is composed of a sinusoidal-shaped stainless steel wire that is wound into an open helical pattern. It is balloon expandable. Its design renders it susceptible to both shortening and lengthening during delivery.

lengths. Because of the low radiopacity of the original Wiktor stent, the 0.279-mm stainless steel wire was replaced by tantalum, without an apparent effect on thrombogenicity. The new Wiktor stent is composed of a single strand of tantalum wire (0.005″ in diameter), which greatly increases its radiologic visibility and allows precise placement of the stent at the desired location (Fig. 1–37).

The stent is mounted and manually crimped onto a nonprofile Prime balloon. For precise placement, the balloon and stent assembly is advanced through an 8-Fr. guide catheter into the target artery. Because of its sinusoidal configuration, the stent can be expanded to a slightly larger diameter than that of the vessel. Although a slightly overexpanded (10% to 15% larger than the diameter of the artery) stent is used, the Wiktor stent does not induce an excessive proliferative response of smooth muscle cells and fibrous tissue. Histologic results revealed that early intimal thickening peaks 4 weeks after placement and subsequently decreases to a minimal thickness 32 weeks after placement. The stent was found to be completely re-endothelialized at 32 weeks.[20]

It has been hypothesized that the Wiktor stent may possess less scaffolding properties than the other stents because the Wiktor stent is made of a single loose interdigitating tantalum wire and the other commercially available stents generally have a stronger mesh structure. A clinical review of 77 patients undergoing Wiktor stent placement in coronary arteries, however, indicated that acute recoil after placement averaged 8.2%, compared with 3.5% to 17.7% with the Palmaz stent and 20% with the Gianturco stent.[21]

In coronary applications, procedure-related complications with the Wiktor stent have been noted by Vogt et al.[22] One complication is stent shortening (50% of its original length), which occurred when the stent was immobilized and continual force advanced the delivery balloon partially from the stent. The other was stent elongation, attributable to impaction of a balloon catheter within the stent. This stent has been approved by the FDA for coronary use in the United States.

Cook Prototype Stent

The Cook balloon-expandable stent (Cook, Inc.) was first reported on by Fontaine in 1995[23] and was intended for vascular and biliary applications. The prototype stent is constructed of tantalum with a honey-comb pattern. When fully expanded, each honeycomb cell of the stent assumes a boxlike configuration, with two vertical and two nearly horizontal struts. The horizontal struts efficiently resist extrinsic force. This design purportedly offers high hoop strength at full expansion. Flexibility is achieved by means of changes in cellular configuration. The expansion ratio and shortening of the stent are 6:1 and about 35%, respectively.

The Cook stent is available in several sizes, 4 to 12 mm in diameter and 1.5 to 6 cm in length. The stent is preloaded on a 3.5-Fr. balloon catheter, which is concurrently being developed. The stent and balloon catheter assembly can be introduced over an 0.018″ stiff nitinol guidewire through a 7-Fr. sheath.

The Cook stent has not yet been used in humans. The results of animal studies, reported by Fontaine et al.,[24] showed no evidence of occlusion and that the stents were completely covered by smooth neointima, with mean thickness of 354 ± 175 microns, during an 8- to 24-week period. Stented bile ducts demonstrated varying degrees of nonobstructive epithelial hyperplasia that extended to the bile duct lumen adjacent to stent struts.[25]

Cook, Inc. has also developed a self-expanding version, primarily for carotid arterial stenting. It is made of 0.005″ to 0.0065″ nitinol wire with a Z pattern (Fig. 1–38). The metallic surface area is about 9% to 13% in expanded form. No significant shortening was observed after expansion. The stent is preloaded in a 6- or 7-Fr. delivery catheter. Available stent sizes include 4- to 12-mm diameters in 2-mm increments and 10- to 60-mm lengths. This stent is in an investigative stage and not available for sale. Clinical or experimental results with this stent are not available.

Global Balloon-Expandable Stent

The Global balloon-expandable stent (Global Therapeutics, Inc.) is constructed with a single continuous strand of stainless wire (0.0024″ in diameter). The wire is folded back and forth to form a tubular structure with a trapezoid spiral pattern (Fig. 1–39), which purportedly offers high longitudinal flexibility and allows its use in tortuous vessels. The radiopacity of the stent is similar to that of the Palmaz stent and higher than that of the Wallstent and the Strecker balloon-expandable stent. The shortening of the stent on expansion is about 1%. The external forces required to reduce the stent diameter by 20%

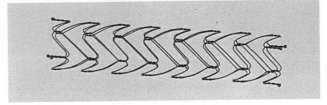

Figure 1-38 The self-expanding prototype stent from Cook, Inc. is made of nitinol wire bent in a Z pattern.

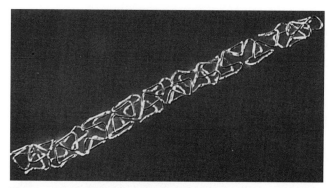

Figure 1-39 The balloon-expandable Global stent is made of a single strand of stainless steel wire, folded in a complex spiral pattern. It has excellent flexibility.

and 50% are 225 and 340 mm Hg, respectively, for the Global stent, compared with 750 and 1320 mm Hg, respectively, for the Palmaz stent and 135 and 170 mm Hg, respectively, for the Wallstent.[26]

The stent is mounted on a 5-Fr. balloon catheter. The stent and balloon assembly can be introduced through a 9-Fr. sheath. Mid-term observations in an animal model revealed a high patency rate in the iliac arteries without evidence of neointimal hyperplasia.[26] The stent is not commercially available.

VascuCoil Self-Expanding Nitinol Stent

The VascuCoil nitinol stent (InStent, Inc./Medtronic, Inc.) is a simple, spring-shaped coil with balls at the two ends of the coil (Fig. 1–40). It is constructed of an 0.01″ or 0.013″ nitinol wire. The coil density can be adjusted to reach a desirable radial hoop strength. The stent metal surface area when expanded is 7% to 15%, depending on the wire size and coil density. It is premounted on a specially designed delivery catheter and is restrained at the two terminal balls of the stent with string ties, which are released by a single wire connecting to the handle at the proximal

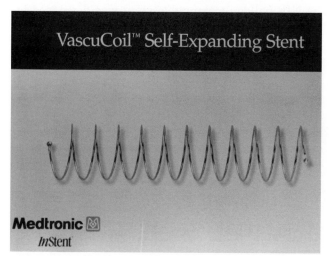

Figure 1-40 The VascuCoil stent is a simple, spring-shaped coil. Note the balls at the ends of the coil; these help restrain the coil on its delivery catheter.

end of the delivery catheter. The whole system can be introduced over an 0.035″ guidewire through a 7- to 9-Fr. sheath, depending on the size of the stent. The delivery system is available in two types: fixed tip delivery and fixed center delivery. With the fixed tip type, the proximal end of the stent initially is released by pulling the first handle on the system. Release of the distal end subsequently is achieved by slowly dragging the second handle. This gradual deployment process facilitates precise positioning, especially for tandem stenting. With the fixed center type, the two ends of the stent are released simultaneously by pulling the first handle. The central portion is then released by dragging the second handle. This allows precise centering of the stent to cover a lesion. The latter type of delivery system is available only for nonvascular applications at present. Beyar et al.[27] reported that the stent could be retrieved through a catheter after deployment by dragging the stent wire. The dimensions of the VascuCoil stents are 4 to 9 mm in expanded diameter and 40 mm in length. The average shortening rate on expansion is 30%.

A study on coronary stent placement in 23 dogs revealed that the VascuCoil stent can be deployed safely and reliably and that histologic responses to this stent are similar to those observed with the Palmaz stent.[27] Limited clinical experience with the stent in vascular applications has been reported.[27] The stent is not commercially available in the United States.

AngioStent

The AngioStent balloon-expandable stent (AngioDynamics, Inc.) is composed of a single platinum wire (0.005″ in diameter), which is folded six times in sinusoidal fashion and connected end to end by a longitudinal member (Fig. 1–41). This single-wire design provides great longitudinal flexibility with about a 7% shortening rate on expansion. The stent is available in several dimensions: 3.0 mm, 3.5 mm, and 4.0 mm in diameter; and 15 mm, 25 mm, and 35 mm in length. The stent is preloaded on a catheter with a high-pressure (up to 15 atmospheres) balloon, which can be advanced through a 6- or 8-Fr. guide

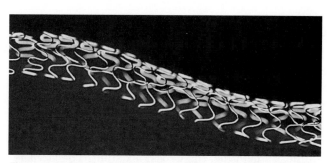

Figure 1-41 The AngioStent is a balloon-expandable stent composed of a single sinusoidal platinum wire bent in a spiral pattern with a connecting longitudinal element, which offers stability combined with flexibility. The expanded stent is shown here.

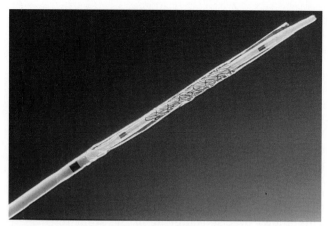

Figure 1-42 The AngioStent is supplied premounted. There are two delivery systems: over the wire and rapid exchange. The over-the-wire system is shown here, with the protective sheath in place. This is retracted before balloon expansion.

catheter or sheath, depending on the model of the delivery system being used. The delivery systems available are a rapid-exchange model and an over-the-wire model. With the rapid-exchange system, the stent is mounted on a Cruiser II coronary dilation balloon, which can be passed through a 6-Fr. guide catheter. With the over-the-wire model, the stent is protected by a thin sheath (0.001″), which should be retracted through the proximal hub of the catheter before the stent is deployed. The over-the-wire model can be introduced through an 8-Fr. guide catheter (Fig. 1–42). Metal material surface areas are 12.5% for the 3-mm, 10.7% for 3.5-mm, and 9.4% for 4-mm stent.

Experimental observations on coronary, renal, and carotid stenting in an atherogenic swine model demonstrated that the AngioStent was easily placed, had superior visibility under fluoroscopy, and provided excellent short-term patency without anticoagulation; whereas 29% (2 of 7) stented coronary arteries showed intrastent luminal stenoses larger than 20% 20 and 52 weeks after stent placement.[28] Histopathology revealed an average neointimal thickness ranging from 325 to 650 microns at the stent sites. At present, the stent is predominantly used in coronary application but is not yet available for sale in the United States.

Cordis Balloon-Expandable Stent

The Cordis balloon-expandable stent (Cordis Corp.) consists of a single-strand wire that is folded into a sinusoidal pattern and is helically wrapped. Two types of the Cordis stent are available: one is made of 0.005″ tantalum wire and the other of 0.006″ stainless steel wire. The Cordis tantalum stent is being phased out of the market and replaced with the stainless steel type, the CrossFlex stent. The stent is mounted on a Duralyn balloon catheter (Cordis Corp.), which accommodates an 0.014″ guidewire. Recoil and shortening on expansion are minimal, with

15% metal surface area. The Cordis tantalum stent has been used in coronary applications.[29] Although tantalum offers great radiopacity to facilitate the precise positioning of the stent in the target segment, strongly radiopaque stent struts may negatively affect the quantitative evaluation of intrastent restenosis by angiography. The Cordis stent has not been approved for clinical use in the United States.

AVE Microstent

The AVE Microstent is being considered for development as a *dedicated intracranial stent*. It is a promising design for this purpose.

The AVE stent (Arterial Vascular Engineering, Inc.) is a balloon-expandable device made of 0.008″ stainless steel wire that is bent in a sinusoidal fashion to form a 3-mm segment (Fig. 1–43). The stent consists of several elements that are laser fused at selected end points. This design purportedly offers great flexibility; the metal surface area in the expanded form is about 14.5% for a stent with 3.5-mm diameter.

Clinical uses of the AVE stent were reported in Europe and Japan.[30, 31] The results of early experience in coronary stenting in 20 patients showed a 96% technical success rate and an 85% event-free rate 30 days after stent placement.[30] The study found about 16% stent recoil on initial stent deployment; however, this could be managed by stent re-expansion with a high-pressure balloon (14.6 ± 3.5 atmospheres). Initial clinical results in 17 patients with hypertension resulting from renal arterial stenosis revealed 100% immediate technical success without procedural complication.[31] Short-term clinical outcome after AVE stent placement is comparable to that after Palmaz stent placement. Long-term clinical results with this stent are not available. The AVE stent has not been used in the United States.

NIR Stent

The NIR balloon-expandable stent was developed by Medinol/Boston Scientific for coronary application. It

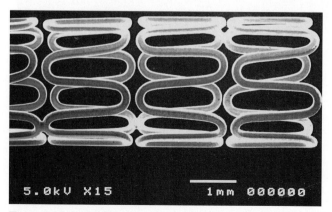

Figure 1-43 The AVE stent, shown expanded, is constructed of stainless steel wire hoops bent into a zigzag pattern. Adjacent segments are welded together. It is balloon expandable.

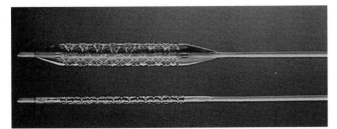

Figure 1-44 Unexpanded and expanded views of the NIR stent, demonstrating its multicellular design.

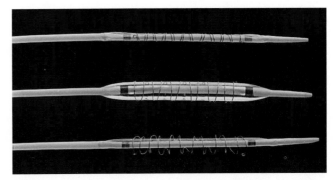

Figure 1-46 Unexpanded and expanded views of the Gianturco-Roubin Flex stent.

is made of stainless steel with a unique multicellular rectangular design, which offers superior flexibility, high radial hoop strength, and increased conformability (Fig. 1–44). In the expanded form, its metal surface area is 11% to 18%. The stent's design purportedly eliminates any possibility of kinks, transverse ridges, or internal flare points that could cause vessel damage during tracking or recrossing. There is no shortening on expansion. The stent can be premounted on a VIVA! Primo delivery balloon catheter (SciMed/Boston Scientific), which accommodates an 0.014″ guidewire. The NIR stent comes in several dimensions, 3.0 to 5.0 mm in diameter and 9, 16, and 32 mm in length. The stent is not available in the United States.

MultiLink Stent

The MultiLink balloon-expandable stent (Advanced Cardiovascular Systems) was designed for coronary use. It is made of 0.0022″ stainless steel struts with a multiple-ring design. Twelve corrugated rings linked by 33 articulations offer high longitudinal flexibility (Fig. 1–45). This design overcomes some of the disadvantages of the first-generation rigid stent. The delivery balloon is covered by an elastic membrane, and the stent and balloon assembly is protected by a 5-Fr. sleeve that can be retracted immediately before stent deployment. The metallic surface

area in expanded form is less than 15%. The other potential advantages of the stent include minimal interstrut gaps and symmetric expansion because of the elastic membrane on the stent. Available dimensions of the stent are 3.0, 3.5, and 4.0 mm in diameter and 15 mm in length. Early clinical results with the MultiLink stent in 40 patients with a total of 44 lesions showed a high technical success rate (100%) and minimal complications.[32]

Gianturco-Roubin Flex and Gianturco-Roubin II Stent

The Gianturco-Roubin Flex stent is a balloon-expandable stent made of interdigitating stainless steel loops (Fig. 1–46). The Gianturco-Roubin II stent is the second generation of this stent. Because the interdigitating loops are made of flat wire, its radial hoop strength is augmented. An axial spine has been added to limit stent distortion (Fig. 1–47). The Gianturco-Roubin II stent can be readily identified under fluoroscopy because of two gold radiopaque markers at the ends of the stent. The metallic surface coverage of the Flex stent is 10%; that of the Gianturco-Roubin II stent is between 15% and 20%, with no shortening on expansion of either stent. Both stents have been approved for coronary use in the United States and come in diameters ranging from 2.5 to 4.0 mm and in 20- and 40-mm lengths (Gianturco-Roubin II) or 12- and 20-mm lengths (Flex stent).

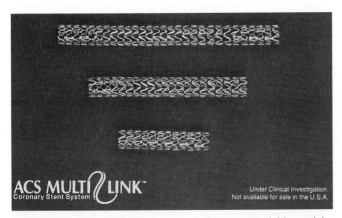

ACS MULTI LINK™
Coronary Stent System

Under Clinical Investigation.
Not available for sale in the U.S.A.

Figure 1-45 The MultiLink stent is balloon expandable and is composed of multiple corrugated rings linked by a series of articulations. It is less rigid than many earlier balloon-expandable stents. The collapsed and expanded stents are shown here; note that there is relatively little shortening.

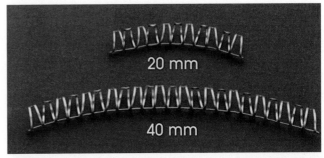

20 mm

40 mm

Figure 1-47 The Gianturco-Roubin II stent is made of flat wire and offers excellent radial strength. The spine limits distortion. Gold radiopaque marker beads are located at either end of the stent.

Other Investigative Stents

Crown Stent

The Crown stent (Cordis Corp.) is a modified version of the Palmaz-Schatz stent for coronary application. It purportedly maintains the same radial strength, accuracy of placement, and geometric openness as the Palmaz-Schatz stent, except with greater longitudinal flexibility. The stent is premounted on the PowerGrip delivery system (Cordis Corp.), which takes an 0.014″ guidewire. The crimped stent profile measures about 4-Fr.

BeStent

The BeStent (Medtronic, Inc.) is a balloon-expandable coronary stent. Its serpentine design features rotating, stress-free junctions with an orthogonal self-locking mechanism. The unique design renders this device highly flexible without shortening on expansion. The stent comes in sizes ranging from 15 to 35 mm in length in increments of 10 mm.

Paragon Stent

The Paragon stent (Progressive Angioplasty Systems, Inc.) is constructed of a martensitic nitinol metal with a honeycomb design (Fig. 1–48). The stent is deployed using a balloon catheter at as low as 4 atmospheres of pressure. Surface area coverage is more than 23% with 4-mm diameter and 36% with 3-mm diameter. Available stent sizes include 3.0, 3.5, and 4.0 mm in diameter and 15 to 16 mm in length.

Freedom Stent

The Freedom stent (Global Therapeutics, Inc.) is a balloon-expandable stent designed for coronary use. The stent is constructed with an 0.18-mm 316 LVM stainless wire that is folded in concentric loops. The strut thickness is 0.008″ and the metallic surface area approximates 11%, with no shortening on stent expansion. The stent recoils about 7% on delivery. It is available in sizes including 2.5 to 4.5 mm in diameter and 12 to 40 mm in length. The stent can be deployed through a 6-Fr. guide catheter.

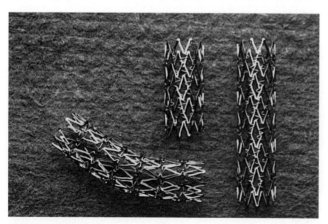

Figure 1-48 The Paragon stent is a nitinol, balloon-expandable stent.

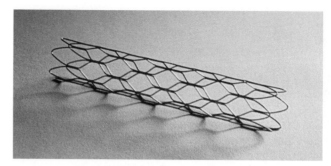

Figure 1-49 The Symphony nitinol stent.

Symphony Stent

The Symphony nitinol stent is a version of the nitinol Hexagonal stent designed for transhepatic biliary use. The stent is stiff and uses the inherent qualities of nitinol to expand to its unrestrained diameter (Fig. 1–49). It is delivered in standard nitinol fashion with a covered sheath using an 0.035″ guidewire. The delivery catheter has five marker bands; two narrow bands at the ends of the stent and three wide markers that identify the movement of the outer sheath.

Bard XT Stent

The XT stent (Angiomed, Karlsruhe, Germany; sold by Bard, Inc., in the United States) is another of the multisegment concentric circle designs, and uses a single continuous backbone to link the segments. Each segment is a wavy line with four peaks in the complete circle. It is made from 316 LVM stainless steel, with each strut and the spine 0.006″ in diameter. Each modular ring is 2.15 mm in length. For a 3-mm diameter stent, the metal surface area is 19%.

Iris II Stent

The Iris II stent (Uni-Cath, Inc.) has nonbending struts; all flexion occurs at C-shaped joints. This produces increased rigidity in the expanded stent. The profile of the crimped and compressed stent is 1.0 mm, allowing introduction through very small guide catheters.

Pura-Vario-A Stent

The Pura-Vario-A stent (Devon Medical, Hamburg, Germany) has a complex shape, in some respects similar to the Paragon stent. The varying direction of the segments allows some degree of flexibility.

V-Flex Coronary Stent

The V-Flex coronary stent is another stent manufactured by Global Therapeutics, Inc. This is another stent constructed of a series of concentric rings linked by longitudinal arms. This allows for essentially no shortening on deployment. It is manufactured from 316 L stainless steel and is nonferromagnetic. Strut thickness is 0.0025″. The recoil is less than 1%, and shortening is negligible.

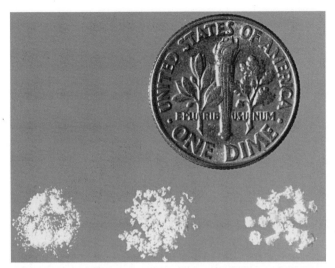

Figure 1-50 Sizing of PVA particles made by ITC/Target Therapeutics (Contour Emboli). Note the irregularity of the particles themselves.

PARTICULATE EMBOLIC AGENTS

Polyvinyl Alcohol Particles

Polyvinyl alcohol (PVA) particles are available in varying sizes (50 to 150, 150 to 250, 250 to 350, 350 to 500, 500 to 750, and 750 to 1000 micron diameters and larger; Fig. 1–50). They are available from ITC/Target Therapeutics (Contour Emboli), Cook, Inc., and Ivalon, Inc. PVA particles produce an initial inflammatory reaction followed by a giant cell foreign-body reaction.[33, 34] They are considered permanent, but recanalization can and does occur. In other words, the particles may be permanent, but the occlusion may not be.

Gelfoam

Gelfoam (gelatin) sponge (Upjohn) is supplied in sheets, cut into appropriately sized pieces, and used for occlusion of small to medium-sized vessels as well as for protection of normal vascular territory by proximal occlusion before particulate or liquid use.[35, 36] This is not considered to be a permanent agent, with recanalization occurring in 7 to 30 days. Due to its bulk, it has minimal use in the microcirculation and therefore is of only ancillary use in interventional neuroradiology. Its use has been largely supplanted by Avitene (see below). Other sections of this text discuss its use in appropriate situations.

Gelfoam Powder

Gelfoam powder (Upjohn) is useful for small vessel embolization because of its small (40 to 60 microns) particle size. It is a temporary agent but can produce severe ischemia (or necrosis) of the embolized tissue because of its ability to penetrate to the capillary level.[37] Larger, presized particles can be useful for temporary occlusion of a large vascular trunk for protection purposes.

Avitene

Avitene (Alcon Laboratories) is composed of microfibrillar collagen of bovine origin. It achieves a particle size of 75 to 150 microns (and clumps of even larger size) in suspension and is used for small vessel occlusion.[38] Its activity is complex; it produces significant ischemia as a result of distal penetration but also promotes platelet agglutination and granulomatous arteritis. Avitene is considered a temporary agent. It can be combined with PVA particles in a slurry for a more effective thrombogenic agent, but the duration is questionable (see Chapter 3). It also can be combined with ethanol for a more permanent occlusion.[39] Avitene appears to be more thrombogenic than most agents and can cause the occlusion of large vascular channels, although of questionable duration.

Angiostat

Angiostat (Collagen Corp.) consists of glutaraldehyde cross-linked microfibrillar collagen of bovine origin. Particle size averages 75 microns. This agent works by mechanical obstruction alone and is used for small vessels.[40]

Surgical Sutures

Silk or polypropylene surgical sutures, usually 6-0, can be cut to appropriate lengths (generally 3 to 10 mm) and used to embolize small fistulae or in conjunction with other embolic agents.[41] Silk has long been known to incite an intense inflammatory response. It is not visible in and of itself, and its eventual location frequently is not known.

Autologous Clot

Autologous clot is useful for temporary occlusion of vessels.[42] The duration of occlusion is highly variable. The clot can be stabilized for longer life by treating with ε-aminocaproic acid (Amicar, Lederle Laboratories) or oxidized cellulose. This agent is perhaps underused in the field of interventional neuroradiology, particularly for protective embolization of vital vessels (see below). It is a perfect temporary agent, easily lasting for the duration (about an hour) of proximal embolization when the main trunk is to be protected. The tendency (or at least the possibility), however, of the injected clot material to reach very small vessels (capillaries) and thus cause true tissue ischemia is unknown. For proximal occlusion for protective purposes, the capillary bed of the area to be preserved should remain intact. With the injection of clot material, this could be a problem.

Pulsar Particles

Pulsar particles have been developed by Medtronic/MIS for embolization. They are made from a proprietary hydrogel material and contain tantalum for radiopacity (Fig. 1–51). They are delivered in desic-

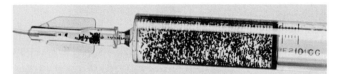

Figure 1-51 Pulsar embolization particles (Medtronic/MIS), which are optically and radiographically visible.

cated form and, after hydration, swell by about 40%. Their desiccated size, however, is what is used to judge embolization size because they are compressible when used. Pulsar particles yield a benign tissue reaction but are not biodegradable; once in place, they are permanent. In addition, early results indicate that they may fill the lumen better than PVA particles and thus may be more resistant to vascular recanalization. Their size range is similar to that of PVA particles: 150 to 1400 microns.

Cellulose Porous Beads

Cellulose porous beads are solid embolic agents undergoing clinical trial.[43, 44] They are exceptionally uniform in size, flow readily through microcatheters without jamming, and have a specific gravity similar to blood. They appear to suspend evenly, partly owing to their uniform size and specific gravity and partly to their net positive charge. They are thus capable of penetrating far into the vascular tree, with a relatively homogeneous distribution and tight packing. The positive charge attracts negatively charged blood components, facilitating thrombus formation. Cellulose porous beads do not, however, induce an inflammatory reaction. The tight packing and thrombus formation fill the vessel, lessening the chance of recanalization.

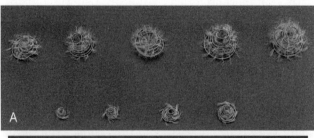
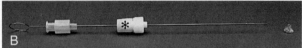

Figure 1-52 *A* and *B*, Tornado coils (Cook, Inc.) are complex and offer excellent deliverability and occlusion qualities. The sizes all taper in their spiral down to 2 mm and tend to fill the lumen of a vessel well. The larger the outer loop, the longer is the coil length, with a corresponding increase in the difficulty in pushing the coil down the lumen of a microcatheter, as is typical of all longer coils. Note the middle hub on the delivery device *(asterisk)*; this is for locking the introducer to the hub of the microcatheter during delivery.

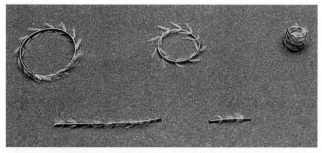

Figure 1-53 Hilal microcoils (Cook, Inc.) come in a variety of sizes, either straight or with simple cylindrical coil shapes.

MECHANICAL EMBOLIC AGENTS

Platinum Microcoils

Platinum microcoils are available from Cook, Inc. (Tornado and Hilal; Figs. 1–52 to 1–54) and Target Therapeutics (complex helical coils, Vortx coils, and Braided Occlusion Device coils; Fig. 1–55) and have been introduced by ITC/Target Therapeutics (Bungi; Fig. 1–56) and Cordis Corp. (Trufill Pushable Coils). They are available in a wide variety of sizes and shapes, allowing proper sizing for a wide range of vessels (Fig. 1–57). Most coils contain Dacron fibers to enhance thrombogenicity.[45, 46] These coils are MRI compatible and highly visible fluoroscopically. The coils from Target Therapeutics have the widest range of sizes, with some truly complex shapes. In addition, a new spherical coil shape (Sphericoils, Target Therapeutics) is being tested. The Tornado coils from Cook, Inc. pack particularly well.

Stainless Steel Coils

The Gianturco stainless steel coils are macro sized, have attached Dacron fibers, and are more thrombogenic than platinum coils. Presoaking the coils in thrombin further enhances their thrombogenicity.[47] Because of their large size, they require a larger delivery catheter (0.038″). They are used for large vessel occlusion (e.g., vein of Galen malformations, dural sinuses, and other large vessels).[48, 49] Like plati-

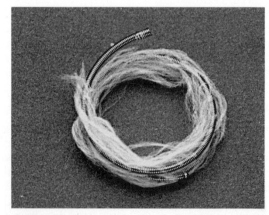

Figure 1-54 Large-size platinum microcoil (Cook, Inc.) used for vein of Galen occlusion.

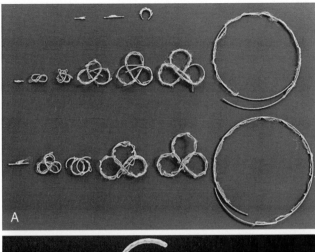

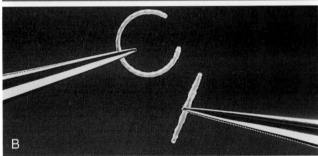

Figure 1-55 *A* and *B*, Sampling of platinum embolic coils available from Target Therapeutics. Note the predominant complex shapes for these coils *(A)*. These are good for filling large spaces, but packing into a typical vessel can be difficult because of their overall large size. The simple spiral (4 × 30 mm), the third from the left in the bottom row, is a good, standard-use coil. The fibers embedded in these coils make them thrombogenic, much more so than the unfibered Guglielmi detachable coil (GDC). Note the huge loop coils intended for vein of Galen use. The three coils at the top are ultrathin coils intended for use with the TRACKER-10 system (i.e., they are less than 0.010″). The others on the page are all for use with typical 0.018″ microcatheters. *B*, The braided occlusion device (BOD) coils.

num coils, they have been manufactured in a wide variety of shapes and sizes. They are not generally considered to be MRI compatible; they produce susceptibility artifacts and may shift position as a result of effects of the magnetic field.[50]

Electrolytically Detachable Platinum Microcoils

Guglielmi Detachable Coils (GDC; Target Therapeutics) are platinum microcoils soldered to the end of an insulated stainless steel guidewire (Fig. 1–58); a short segment at the solder joint is exposed. After the coil is positioned, detachment is effected by passing a direct current through the wire, which evokes an

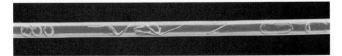

Figure 1-57 An example of proper sizing of a coil *(left)* as opposed to incorrect sizing of a coil *(right)* in a vessel.

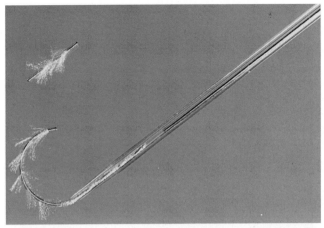

Figure 1-56 A Bungi coil is shown being extruded from the introducer supplied by ITC/Target Therapeutics. Note the clear plastic construction, allowing visualization of the coil before and during delivery.

electrolytic process at the exposed distal solder tip of the wire[51] (Fig. 1–59). This system permits withdrawal of the coil before final placement, a major advantage over any other mass embolic agent. Target Therapeutics is manufacturing these coils in an increasing array of shapes and sizes.

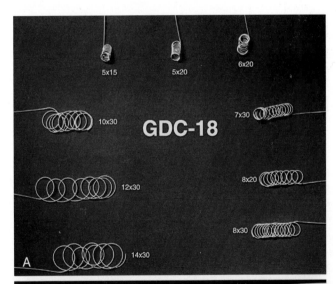

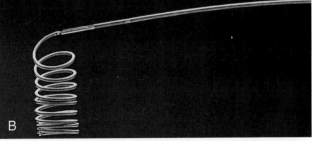

Figure 1-58 *A* and *B,* These detachable platinum coils (GDC) from Target Therapeutics are made in two diameters for use with the two primary microcatheter sizes and are available in numerous coil diameters to custom fit into individual aneurysms. They are easily extruded from the catheter and can be withdrawn back into the catheter just as easily.

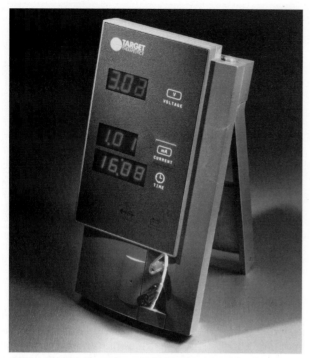

Figure 1-59 The coil can be detached by means of an electrolytic current passed through the wire. The current generator for the detachment process is shown.

Mechanically Detachable Coils

Retrievable coils are in use that detach electrolytically. These will be more widely available in the future. Also available are coils that can be detached mechanically rather than electrolytically. These may be easier to use. The method of detachment can be an interlocking mechanism or an electrically controlled gripping device.

The available models have been developed by Target Therapeutics and Cook, Inc. (Fig. 1–60) and have a simple interlocking mechanism released by placement and turning. The device formerly was easier to

use than the GDC-type release, but now that the GDC is more advanced, the electrolytic process appears to be an elegant method and is working well.

Coils of different materials will become available, some with different thrombogenic characteristics, retrieval characteristics, or thermal characteristics.

Liquid Coils

Liquid coils are made from extremely fine platinum wire and thus are very supple; they are intended to be flow directed. They are made by Target Therapeutics and are in limited release. Their primary application is in the treatment of arteriovenous malformations in conjunction with cyanoacrylates; they are used to reduce the flow rate through the arteriovenous malformation before embolization with glue.

Amplatz Vascular Obstructing Devices (Spiders)

Amplatz spiders are interesting structures, designed to spring open in a short space and impale themselves into the wall of the vessel for secure anchorage, similar to the anchors of vena cava filters (Fig. 1–61). Once the device is in location, coils can pile behind it without the risk of migrating. These vascular obstructing devices are made by Cook, Inc. and are available in sizes for vessels up to 9, 13, 15, or 20 mm in diameter. They are supplied as a kit with a sheath, guidewire, delivery catheter (8-Fr.), and positioning guidewire.

Detachable Balloons

Detachable balloons are made of latex or silicone. They either have self-sealing valves or are attached to the catheter and sealed with a latex string (latex balloons only). ITC/Target Therapeutics manufactures a well-designed silicone balloon (detachable silicone balloon) with a good, self-sealing valve (Fig. 1–62). Ingenor of Paris manufactures latex balloons

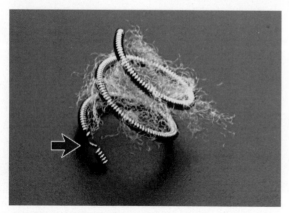

Figure 1-60 A mechanically detachable coil produced by Cook, Inc. These are made for use with catheters capable of accepting an 0.038″ guidewire. Note the notch at one end of the coil *(arrow)*. This is the site of engagement with the steering and release mechanism.

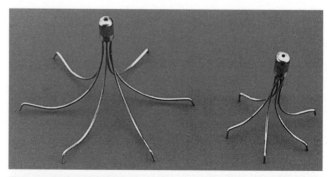

Figure 1-61 Amplatz vascular obstructing devices (spiders) (Cook, Inc.) are designed to deploy similarly to a Greenfield filter, with their legs anchoring to the walls of the blood vessel. They form a stable base for coil occlusion of the vessel, retaining the coils in position and preventing them from embolizing distally. They come in various sizes and are supplied as a kit that includes a sheath, guidewire, delivery catheter, and positioning guidewire.

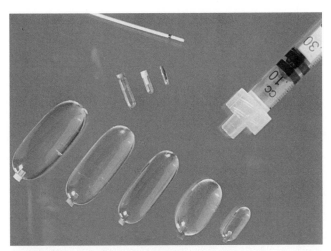

Figure 1-62 The detachable balloons manufactured by ITC/Target Therapeutics come in a variety of sizes and shapes and can be delivered with the pictured catheter or one supplied by Target Therapeutics. Their release strength also varies.

(Gold Valve balloons); none of these has been approved by the FDA. Silicone balloons are semipermeable; therefore, they must be inflated with iso-osmolar contrast medium (see below).[52] Latex balloons are impermeable.[53] Silicone balloons are softer and tend to deflate more slowly. Both are manufactured in a variety of sizes and shapes. Generally, guide catheters must be at least 7 to 9-Fr. for these balloons.

LIQUID EMBOLIC AGENTS

Cyanoacrylates

Cyanoacrylates (glues) are not widely available in the United States but are undergoing clinical evaluation. N-butyl-2-cyanoacrylate (Histoacryl, B. Braun Melsungen A.G.) is being used elsewhere around the world.[54] It is capable of reaching distal small vessels and therefore requires skillful and careful handling. Exposure of this glue to ionic solutions results in polymerization. The rate of polymerization can be slowed by the addition of iophendylate (Pantopaque, Lafayette Pharmacal) or glacial acetic acid,[55, 56] although the exact guidelines for use of these agents have not been established. Additional opacification can be achieved by the addition of tantalum or bismuth powder. Cordis Corp. has developed a preparation of N-butyl-2-cyanoacrylate that is opacified with tantalum powder. The speed of polymerization is controlled by the addition of ethiodol, according to a supplied table. This agent is undergoing clinical testing in the United States.

The behavior of cyanoacrylates is unpredictable. The risks associated with the use of these agents include stroke or cranial nerve dysfunction due to occlusion of branches other than the desired branches, obstruction of venous outflow, and cementing of the catheter in the vessel. Polymerization is accompanied by heat production, which may lead to a degree of angionecrosis. Cyanoacrylates are con-

sidered permanent agents, but when large amounts of oily contrast (e.g., Pantopaque) are added, their permanency is questionable.

A new cyanoacrylate, 2-hexyl cyanoacrylate (Neuracryl; Prohold Technologies, Inc.) has been developed and is undergoing clinical trials in the United States. This glue is supplied in two vials. The first contains purified liquid 2-hexyl cyanoacrylate monomer; the second contains a thick, yellowish-brown mixture of 2-hexyl cyanoacrylate polymer, finely powdered (5 microns) pure gold, and a biologically metabolizable esterified fatty acid. After a microcatheter is positioned in the vessel to be embolized, the monomer is introduced into the glass vial containing the mixture and shaken for 1 minute. The mixture is then drawn up into the syringe used to transfer the monomer and injected through the catheter. Neuracryl is a single viscosity agent. It has less adhesiveness but more viscosity than N-butyl-2-cyanoacrylate and hardens more predictably in arterial structures, before penetrating to the veins. In addition, it has decreased cohesiveness, permitting catheter withdrawal even after it has partially hardened. Neuracryl is also discussed in Chapter 2.

Methylmethacrylate

Methylmethacrylate is used mainly by orthopedic surgeons, specifically for placement of joint prostheses. It can be used as an intraosseous injection to bolster vertebral bodies that are undergoing progressive compression secondary to degenerative changes with associated pain, or even pathologic compression fractures caused by tumors. Percutaneous access is made with a large-bore bone biopsy needle, and the toothpaste-like consistency material is infused. This polymerizes into a mass that is extremely hard. Fears concerning the heat generated during curing appear to be unfounded; the human body has the capacity to remove large amount of excess heat with no apparent difficulty.

2-Hydroxyethylmethacrylate

In 1980, Taki et al.[57] presented information concerning a new polymerizing agent called HEMA. This is a liquid polymerizing agent used inside of a detachable balloon for permanent occlusion. It can react adversely with latex, however, with fissuring or rupture of the balloon.[58]

The characteristics of this substance are interesting. It is of low enough viscosity to inject through a microcatheter. It will "cure" in 15 to 60 minutes (operator variable). It can mix with blood (or water) and still become 100% solid (up to about 30% water). It does not expand when polymerizing like hydrogels do. The components need to be mixed (i.e., it is like an epoxy); the monomer (HEMA) is mixed with polyethelene glycol dimethacrylate (PEGDM) and hydrogen peroxide, which has to be exposed to its polymerizing agent (ferrous ammonium sulfate). This material was supplied in a kit but has been unavailable for a number of years.

Dehydrated Ethanol

Absolute or dehydrated ethyl alcohol (ethanol, 96%) (Abbott Laboratories) is an extremely dangerous agent and must be used with caution. It produces both a cytotoxic reaction in the target organ and sclerosis of the arterial walls with resultant thrombosis.[59-61] Ethanol is capable of causing extensive necrosis. It can be used intra-arterially or through direct puncture of the lesion.[62] Ethanol may be diluted with liquid contrast or used undiluted; in the latter case, opacification with powdered contrast material is possible (see Chapter 3). Ethanol can be very painful.

Sodium Tetradecyl Sulfate (Sotradecol)

Sodium tetradecyl sulfate (Sotradecol, Elkins-Sinn) is a sclerosing agent that can be used either transarterially or by direct puncture.[63] Unlike alcohol, it is a painless agent; therefore, less sedation is required for its use. It can be opacified by diluting it 1:1 with nonionic contrast material.

Ethibloc

Ethibloc (Ethicon) is a mixture of corn protein (zein), sodium amidotrizoate, oleum papaveris, and propylene glycol in a 60% alcohol solution[64]; it is not available in the United States. Zein is not water soluble; as the alcohol dissolves into the blood, the zein precipitates and forms a gummy mass. The rate of precipitation can be controlled by preinjection of 40% glucose. This mixture is capable of distal penetration and produces a marked local inflammatory reaction. Like ethanol, it is painful. The mixture is viscous and difficult to use with microcatheters.

Hydrogels

Hydrogel polymers are undergoing investigation. They are not available for use in the United States. Hydrogels are available in either liquid (1% to 10% solution in DMSO) or 100- to 1000-micron particles (see "Pulsar Particles" above). They form a soft, shapeless mass when exposed to water and do not elicit an inflammatory response. Hydrogels are similar to EVAL. They are considered permanent agents but do not attach themselves to the wall of the vessel. A cast of the vessel therefore must be made for the material to stay in place, which is a potential liability (Fig. 1–63). The material is intriguing to use, can be delivered easily through microcatheters, and may find a use in the future in the field of aneurysm therapy. The author (JJC) has experimented with the use of hydrogel as an embolic agent for a number of years (Hypan, Panaphase, Kingston Technologies), both in vascular occlusions and to fill aneurysms. For embolization of arteriovenous malformations, some

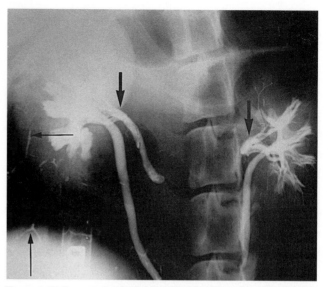

Figure 1-63 Demonstration of liquid hydrogel used as an embolic agent in a dog. Note the cast of the renal arteries *(thick arrows)*. Powdered barium was added for opacification, which in limited quantities worked much better than powdered iodine contrast agents. Note the streaks of material in the abdomen *(thin arrows)*; this is the result of further embolization in the mesenteric vessels. Notice how it did not maintain its integrity, but instead broke up; some of the material migrated distally, whereas some remained proximal. Hydrogel does not stick to the vessel walls as glue does and is soft enough to ooze downstream.

degree of inflammatory response is advisable; retention of a healthy vascular malformation simply filled with a gelatinous mass is not ideal conceptually.

Variations in the formulation permit different properties to manifest themselves. In general, all of these materials are mostly water with a matrix of material within. Therefore, there is a large coefficient of expansion (water absorption) when they are used, making certain applications unpredictable.

These materials probably will be used in the future not only as embolic agents but also as basic construction materials for certain devices, including catheters. They are lubricious, soft, strong, and extremely flexible.

Copolymers

MicroTherapeutics, Inc. has developed a copolymer similar to the cyanoacrylates but without adhesive properties. It is delivered as a liquid but polymerizes to form a rubbery substance. It is basically a dissolved plastic but does not precipitate nearly as fast as hydrogels, nor does it harden nearly as fast as cyanoacrylates. It is in the early stages of clinical testing, but its clinical use would be different from either of the two mentioned above because of its slow coagulation.

EVAL

EVAL is a mixture of ethylene vinyl alcohol copolymer and metrizamide powder (Amipaque, Nycomed,

Inc.) dissolved in DMSO.[65] It is similar to the abovementioned hydrogels. It is not available in the United States. On entering the bloodstream, the DMSO diffuses *extremely* rapidly, leaving the EVAL–metrizamide mixture, which forms a spongy mass. This mass acts as a pure mechanical obstruction and produces no inflammatory reaction. It is of low viscosity, is permanent, and poses no risk of gluing the catheter into place.

Fibrin Glue

Fibrin glue (or fibrin adhesive) is a mixture of autologous cryoprecipitate and thrombin, which forms a solid fibrin clot. This has seen limited use; its use in the embolization of facial arteriovenous malformations has been described.[66] Ongoing research may lead to more widespread applications.

Boiling Contrast

The use of boiling contrast as an embolic agent has been investigated. In experimental studies, contrast was heated to boiling and injected through a temporary occlusion balloon catheter. One minute after injection, the catheter was flushed and the balloon deflated. This technique produced complete occlusion of the perfused territory with coagulation necrosis, hemorrhagic infarction, and arterial thrombosis. The advantages of this technique are that it can penetrate to small vessels, is rapidly rendered nontoxic by cooling, and requires no further opacification. Disadvantages include the technical difficulty of injecting the contrast while it is still heated and that infarction of the affected territory appears to be gradual and progressive.[67] It may take days or weeks for the results to manifest, rendering intraprocedural judgment difficult. Because increased distance from the catheter tip, flow rate, and other factors can render the material ineffective, however, it may offer an alternative to the treatment of lesions thought unapproachable by other means.

The availability of delivery catheters capable of flow control may increase the usefulness of this technique. Previously, boiling contrast or any other substance (saline) has been useful only in a controlled infusion situation because of the rapid dissipation of the heat contained within the fluid. In such a small volume of tissue as exemplified by an intracranial arteriovenous malformation, however, the strategic concept of an embolic material that is capable of delivering a focal destructive blow with downstream harmlessness may prove not only efficacious but also safer and easier to employ than the available "permanent" agents such as cyanoacrylates and ethanol.

Plastics

As strange as this may sound, plastics are being developed as liquid embolization materials. The exact nature of these are not public knowledge at present, but they would be delivered in a liquid form that would harden after delivery. The potential for these materials is enormous; almost any physical characteristics necessary can be designed into the materials. Their potential use could range from arteriovenous malformation embolization to aneurysm therapy.

AIR FILTERS

It is nearly impossible to remove all air from the tubing of arterial flush systems. An air filter placed immediately proximal to the rotating hemostatic valve ensures an air-free fluid delivery system. Several air-eliminating filters are available, such as the micropore air filters available from Baxter Healthcare Corp. and Pall Biomedical Products Corp.

MICROTUBING

When working with certain connections, it is advantageous to have small, flexible, soft tubing that is too small to allow trapped air bubbles to remain. The microtubing lumen diameter flushes bubbles as it is filled because of the normal surface tension of water. This pediatric microtubing, made by numerous manufacturers, is used in many situations by our team. Specifically, it is used to connect angioplasty balloon ports to inflating devices to allow more convenient maneuvering of the angioplasty catheter and visualization of a bubble-free column of fluid that is intended to enter the balloon (Fig. 1–64). It also can be used as a convenient extension tube that is easier to maneuver than typical intravenous tubing.

LARGE-BORE Y CONNECTORS

In some cases, there is no substitute for a rotating hemostatic valve–type Y connector with a truly large

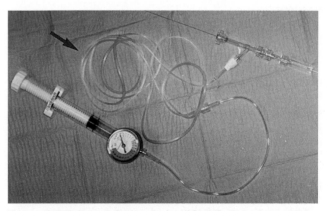

Figure 1-64 Balloon inflation device (Medi-Tech, Inc.) attached to the sideport of a rotating hemostatic valve. This is the set-up used to inflate a single-lumen microangioplasty balloon. Note the occlusion wire protruding from the O ring of the valve. The long segment of interposed microtubing *(arrow)* allows easier manipulation of the catheter and inflation device and helps prevent introduction of an air bubble into the system (these are nearly impossible to eliminate from the device and its gauge).

bore. This product is available from several manufacturers because of its demand (primarily for stent work). For detachable balloons or nondetachable vasospasm angioplasty balloons, these are essential.

STEAMERS

In the practice of neuroradiology, many specialized items are needed, and one of these is a good source of steam. The typical hot plate with a kettle on top is no match for a dedicated, self-contained boiling kettle such as is made by Presto Industries, Inc. This unit boils water faster than a microwave and shuts itself off automatically when it runs out of water.

ISOTONIC ISO-OSMOLAR NONIONIC CONTRAST

The use of a totally benign contrast agent occasionally is required. When an isotonic, iso-osmolar nonionic contrast agent is needed (to fill a latex balloon or to inject into vulnerable territory), the usual choice by most interventionalists is half contrast, half saline.

This does not work. Saline itself is isotonic. If any dilution is to be made, it must be with sterile water, and even then one does not know what tonicity one has achieved. If a dilution is to be made, at least 20 ml of water and 20 ml of contrast should be used just to get the mixture to a reasonable degree of accuracy.

Fortunately, a solution to this problem is available with the introduction of the first truly isotonic, iso-osmolar nonionic contrast agent, the dimer iodixanol (Visipaque, Nycomed). Iodixanol has been shown to be safe and to provide acceptable opacification in trials involving coronary, aortofemoral, and cerebral angiography, with generally fewer adverse effects than are reported with standard nonionic contrast.[68–70] Although the use of this agent is not necessary or indicated in all procedures, having it available for uses such as those indicated above is prudent.

Most particularly, it is prudent to use this agent in cases of acute cerebral ischemia in which there may be endothelial (or cerebral) damage. There is a proven tendency for deposition of contrast material in an extravascular location in these cases, and a material that is not hyperosmolar may prove to be of significant advantage. Serious concerns have been raised by principal investigators in the local intra-arterial fibrinolysis stroke trials about the overuse of contrast during these procedures, specifically because of its hyperosmolar nature and the fear of potential negative influence on cerebral edema and postfibrinolysis hemorrhage.

This contrast agent has idiosyncrasies concerning its use. It is more viscous than the typical agents used. It requires heating to body temperature for reasons beyond patient comfort, such as decreasing viscosity. Iodixanol is one of the most, if not the most, well-tolerated agents by patients in terms of pain or discomfort; the heating is primarily for ease of

injection during use. It gives excellent opacification, possibly because it is somewhat syrupy and does not dilute as rapidly as other agents.

TEMPORARY PACEMAKERS

Symptomatic bradycardia is a potential complication of manipulation of the carotid bulb, especially during angioplasty and stenting in this location. Although this often can be managed medically, it is prudent to have some form of temporary pacemaker available in the angiography suite *at the beginning of the procedure*. Options include transvenous, transcutaneous, and transesophageal systems. Each has advantages and disadvantages.

Temporary transvenous pacing is the most comfortable and well-tolerated form of pacing in an awake patient. Central venous access, however, is required for electrode placing; this can cause problems in an emergent situation. In addition, positioning the electrode properly within the right ventricle to achieve capture can be difficult. Some interventionalists recommend establishing central venous access at the beginning of angioplasty and stenting procedures involving the carotid bulb if this form of temporary pacing will be employed (should the need arise).

Transcutaneous pacing electrodes are easy to apply rapidly and do not require precise placement. This form of temporary pacing is uncomfortable for the patient, however, and may produce an unacceptable amount of patient movement if it is employed in an awake patient. Transesophageal temporary pacing requires insertion of an electrode into the esophagus. This requires slightly more precise positioning than transcutaneous electrodes and is uncomfortable for an awake patient.

VERTEBRAL BODY BIOPSY NEEDLES

The Geremia biopsy kit (Cook, Inc.) is excellent for deep biopsy of vertebral body masses (Fig. 1–65). This kit comes with a long micropuncture needle (22-

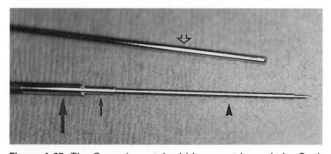

Figure 1-65. The Geremia vertebral biopsy set is made by Cook, Inc. The lesion is localized with the Chiba needle, which has a removable hub and is shown with its stylet in place *(arrowhead)*. The biopsy needle *(large arrow)* and its dilator *(small arrow)* are then loaded coaxially over the Chiba needle after an extended stiffening mandrel has been inserted and the hub removed. Note the serrated distal tip of the biopsy needle. The Chiba needle, mandrel, and dilator are withdrawn and the biopsy performed. The needle is withdrawn, and the blunt-tipped stylet provided *(open arrow)* is used as a plunger to expel the specimen.

gauge) to access the deep site safely. The stylet is then removed and replaced with a long, stiff introducer guide that helps load the coaxial biopsy needle. The hub of the microneedle is removable, and the coaxial biopsy set is placed over the microneedle shaft and guide. This results in *four* tubes loaded in a coaxial fashion (the microstylet, the microneedle, the stylet for the biopsy needle [19-gauge], and the 16-gauge cutting biopsy needle). Once in position, the microstylet, microneedle, and stylet for the biopsy needle are removed. The cutting needle is then rotated (forcefully, if necessary!) to enter the vertebral body, and is removed in the standard fashion. The kit contains a "rammer" to push any material out of the biopsy needle that may have been obtained.

This kit is also useful for interventional techniques (as opposed to biopsy techniques) involving vertebral bodies (see Chapter 12).

REFERENCES

1. Palmaz JC, Sibbitt RR, Reuter SR, et al. Expandable intraluminal graft: a preliminary study. *Radiology* 1985;156:73–77.
2. Lossef SV, Lutz RJ, Mundorf J, Barth KH. Comparison of mechanical deformation properties of metallic stents with use of stress-strain analysis. *J Vasc Interv Radiol* 1994;5:341–349.
3. Palmaz JC, Sibbitt RR, Tio FO, et al. Expandable intraluminal vascular graft: feasibility study. *Surgery* 1986;99:199–205.
4. Schatz R. A view of vascular stents. *Circulation* 1989,79:445–457.
5. Rousseau H, Puel J, Joffre F, et al. Self expanding endovascular prosthesis: an experimental study. *Radiology* 1987; 164:709–714.
6. Vorwerk D, Redha F, Neuerburg J, et al. Neointima formation following arterial placement of self-expanding stents of different radial force: experimental results. *Cardiovasc Intervent Radiol* 1994;17:27–32.
7. Hausegger KA, Lammer B, Hagen F, et al. Iliac artery stenting: clinical experience with the Palmaz stent, Wallstent, and Strecker stent. *Acta Radiol* 1992;33:292–296.
8. Dyet JF, Shaw JW, Cook AM, Nicholson AA. The use of the Wallstent in aortic-iliac vascular disease. *Clin Radiol* 1993;48:227–231.
9. Liermann DD, Strecker EP, Peters J. The Strecker stent: indications and results in iliac and femoropopliteal arteries. *Cardiovasc Intervent Radiol* 1992;15:295–305.
10. Strecker EP, Hagen B, Liermann D, et al. Iliac and femoropopliteal vascular occlusive disease treated with flexible tantalum stents. *Cardiovasc Intervent Radiol* 1993;16:158–164.
11. Barth KH, Virmani R, Strecker EP, et al. Flexible tantalum stents implanted in aortas and iliac arteries: effects in normal canines. *Radiology* 1990;175:91–96.
12. Echenagusia A, Camunez F, Simo G, et al. Variceal hemorrhage: efficacy of transjugular intrahepatic portosystemic shunts created with Strecker stents. *Radiology* 1994;192:235–240.
13. Kuhn FP, Kutkuhn B, Torsello G, Modder U. Renal artery stenosis: preliminary results of treatment with the Strecker stent. *Radiology* 1991;180:369–372.
14. Bezzi M, Orsi F, Salvatori F, Maccioni F. Self-expandable nitinol stent for the management of biliary obstruction: long-term clinical results. *J Vasc Interv Radiol* 1994;5:287–293.
15. Irie T, Furui S, Yamauchi T, et al. Relocatable Gianturco expandable metallic stents. *Radiology* 1991;178:575–578.
16. Starck E. First clinical experience with the Memotherm vascular stent. In: Liermann DD (ed). Stents: State of the Art and Future Development. Morin Heights: Polyscience Publications, 1995, pp. 59–62.
17. Starck E, Knaupp D, Dukiet C, et al. Memotherm and tantalum stents in femoropopliteal arteries. Paper presented at the Fifth International Interdisciplinary Symposium on Endoluminal Stents and Grafts, Washington, DC, 1996.
18. Cragg AH, De Jong SC, Barnhart WH, et al. Nitinol intravascular stent: results of preclinical evaluation. *Radiology* 1993;189:775–778.
19. Venbrux AA, Brown PR, Prescoot CA, et al. A new self-expanding nitinol stent: experimental observations. Paper presented at the Fifth International and Interdisciplinary Symposium on Endoluminal Stents and Grafts, Washington, DC, 1996.
20. White CJ, Ramee SR, Banks A, et al. A new balloon-expandable tantalum coil stent: angiographic patency and histologic findings in an atherogenic swine model. *J Am Coll Cardiol* 1992;19:870–876.
21. de Jaegere P, Serruys P, van Es G-A, et al. Recoil following Wiktor stent implantation for restenotic lesion of coronary arteries. *Cathet Cardiovasc Diagn* 1994;32:147–156.
22. Vogt P, Eeckhout E, Stauffer J-C, et al. Stent shortening and elongation: pitfalls with the Wiktor coronary endoprosthesis. *Cathet Cardiovasc Diagn* 1994;31:233–235.
23. Fontaine AB, Dos Passos SB. Design analysis of stent prototype: in vitro comparison with current devices and in vivo models of peripheral vascular applications. *Radiology* 1995;197(P):382.
24. Fontaine AB, Dos Passos SB. Prototype stent: in vivo evaluation. Paper presented at the SCVIR 21st Annual Scientific Meeting. Seattle, WA, 1996.
25. Fontaine AB, Dos Passos S. Vascular stent prototype: results of preclinical evaluation. *J Vasc Interv Radiol* 1996;7:29–34.
26. Qian Z, Xu HB, Wholey M, et al. A new balloon expandable stent: experimental observations. Paper presented at the Fifth International and Interdisciplinary Symposium on Endoluminal Stents and Grafts, Washington, DC, 1996.
27. Beyar R, Shofti R, Grenedier E, et al. Self-expandable nitinol stent for cardiovascular applications: canine and human experience. *Cathet Cardiovasc Diagn* 1994;32:162–170.
28. Hijazi ZM, Homoud M, Aronovitz MJ, et al. A new platinum balloon-expandable stent (Angiostent) mounted on a high pressure balloon: acute and late results in an atherogenic swine model. *J Invas Cardiol* 1995;7:127–134.
29. Ozaki Y, Keane D, Nobuyoshi M, et al. Coronary lumen at six-month follow-up of a new radiopaque Cordis tantalum stent using quantitative angiography and intracoronary ultrasound. *Am J Cardiol* 1995;76:1135–1143.
30. Ozaki Y, Keane D, Ruygrok P, et al. Acute clinical and angiographic results with the new AVE micro coronary stent in bailout management. *Am J Cardiol* 1995;76:112–116.
31. Henry M, Amor M, Porte JM, et al. First clinical experience with the AVE stent in renal arteries. Paper presented at the Fifth International and Interdisciplinary symposium on Endoluminal Stents and Grafts, Washington, DC, 1996.
32. Wong P, Wong C-M, Cheng C-H, et al. Early clinical experience with multi-link coronary stent. *Cathet Cardiovasc Diagn* 1996;39:413–419.
33. Lanman TH, Martin NA, Vinters HV. Pathology of cerebral arteriovenous malformations treated by prior embolotherapy. *Neuroradiology* 1988;30:1–10.
34. Quisling RG, Mickle JP, Ballinger WB, et al. Histopathologic analysis of intra-arterial polyvinyl alcohol microemboli in rat cerebral cortex. *AJNR* 1984;5:101–104.
35. Matsumoto AH, Suhocki PV, Barth KH. Technical note: superselective Gelfoam embolotherapy using a highly visible small caliber catheter. *Cardiovasc Intervent Radiol* 1988;11:303–304.
36. Berenstein A, Russell E. Gelatin sponge in therapeutic neuroradiology: a subject review. *Radiology* 1981;141:105–112.
37. Kunstlinger F, Brunelle F, Chaumont P, Doyon D. Vascular occlusive agents. *AJR* 1981;136:151–156.
38. Kumar A, Kaufman SI, Patt J, et al. Preoperative embolization of hypervascular head and neck neoplasms using microfibrillar collagen. *AJNR* 1982;3:163–168.
39. Lee DH, Wreidt CH, Kaufmann JCE, et al. Evaluation of three embolic agents in pig rete. *AJNR* 1989;10:773–776.
40. Strother CM, Laravuso R, Rappe A, et al. Glutaraldehyde cross-linked collagen (GAX): new material for therapeutic embolization. *AJNR* 1987;8:509–516.

41. Eskridge JM, Hartling RP. Preoperative embolization of brain AVMs using surgical silk and polyvinyl alcohol [Abstract]. *AJNR* 1989;10:882.

42. Barth KH, Strandberg JD, White RI. Long-term follow-up of transcatheter embolization with autologous clot, Oxycel, and Gelfoam in domestic swine. *Invest Radiol* 1977;12:273–280.

43. Hamada J-I, Ushio Y, Kazekawa K, et al. Embolization with cellulose porous beads. I. An experimental study. *AJNR* 1996;17:1895–1899.

44. Hamada J-I, Kai Y, Nagahiro S, et al. Embolization with cellulose porous beads. II. Clinical trial. *AJNR* 1996;17:1901–1906.

45. Yang PJ, Halbach VV, Higashida RT, Hieshima GB. Platinum wire: a new transvascular embolic agent. *AJNR* 1988;9:547–550.

46. Hilal SK, Khandji AG, Chi TL, et al. Synthetic fiber-coated platinum coils successfully used for endovascular treatment of arteriovenous malformations, aneurysm and direct arteriovenous fistulae of CNS [Abstract]. *AJNR* 1988;9:1030.

47. McLean GK, Stein EJ, Burke DR, Mearnze SG. Steel occlusion coils: pretreatment with thrombin. *Radiology* 1986,158:549–550.

48. Braun IS, Hoffman JC Jr., Casarella WJ, Davis PC. Use of coils for transcatheter carotid occlusion. *AJNR* 1985;6:953–956.

49. Hanner JS, Quisling RG. Transtorcular embolization of vein of Galen aneurysm: technical aspects. *Radiographics* 1988;8:935–946.

50. Spickler E, Dion JE, Lufkin R, et al. The MR appearance of endovascular embolic agents *in vitro* with clinical correlation. *Comput Med Imag Graphics* 1990;14:415–423.

51. Guglielmi G, Vinuela F, Spetka I, Macellari V. Electrothrombosis of saccular aneurysms via endovascular approach. I. Electrochemical basis, technique, and experimental results. *J Neurosurg* 1991;75:1–7.

52. Higashida RT, Halbach VV, Dormandy B, et al. Endovascular treatment of intracranial aneurysms with a new silicone microballoon device: technical considerations and indications for therapy. *Radiology* 1990;174:687–691.

53. Hawkins TD, Szaz KF. The permeability of detachable latex rubber balloons: an in-vitro study. *Invest Radiol* 1987;22:969–972.

54. Brothers MF, Kaufmann JCE, Fox AJ, Devekis JP. N-butyl-2-cyanoacrylate: substitute for IBCA in interventional neuroradiology—histopathologic and polymerization time studies. *AJNR* 1989;10:777–786.

55. Cromwell LD, Kerber CW. Modification of cyanoacrylate for therapeutic embolization: preliminary experience. *AJR* 1979;132:799–801.

56. Spiegel SM, Vinuela F, Goldwasser MJ, et al. Adjusting polymerization time of isobutyl-2-cyanoacrylate. *AJNR* 1986;7:109–112.

57. Taki W, Handa H, Yamagata S, et al. Radio-opaque solidifying liquids for releasable balloon technique: a technical note. *Surg Neurol* 1980;13:140–142.

58. Monsein LH, Debrun GM, Chazaly JR. Hydroxyethyl methacrylate and latex balloons. *AJNR* 1990;11:663–664.

59. Yakes WF, Haas DK, Parker SH, et al. Symptomatic vascular malformations: ethanol embolotherapy. *Radiology* 1989;170:1059–1066.

60. Pevsner PH, Klara P, Doppman J, et al. Ethyl alcohol: experimental agent for interventional therapy of neurovascular lesions. *AJNR* 1983;4:388–390.

61. Choi IS, Berenstein A, Scott J. Use of ethyl alcohol in the treatment of malignant brain tumors. *AJNR* 1985;6:462.

62. Berenstein A, Choi IS. Treatment of venous angiomas by direct alcohol injection [Abstract]. *AJNR* 1983,4:1144.

63. Chow KJ, Williams DM, Brady TM, et al. Transcatheter embolization with sodium tetradecyl sulfate: experimental and clinical results. *Radiology* 1984;153:95–99.

64. Dubois JM, Sebag GH, DeProst Y, et al. Soft tissue venous malformations in children: percutaneous sclerotherapy with Ethibloc. *Radiology* 1991;180:195–198.

65. Taki W, Yonekawa Y, Iwata H, et al. A new liquid material for embolization of arteriovenous malformations. *AJNR* 1990;11:163–168.

66. Luedke MD, Pile-Spellman JM, Ecker MH. Percutaneous treatment of facial arteriovenous malformations with cryoprecipitate: adjunct to surgery. *AJNR* 1989;10:882.

67. Cragg AH, Rosel P, Rysavy JA, et al. Renal ablation using hot contrast medium: an experimental study. *Radiology* 1983;148:683–686.

68. Kløw NE, Levorstad K, Berg KJ, et al. Iodixanol in cardioangiography in patients with coronary artery disease: tolerability, cardiac and renal effects. *Acta Radiol* 1993;34:72–77.

69. Albrechtsson U, Lárusdótter H, Norgren L, Lundby B. Iodixanol—a new nonionic dimer—in aortofemoral angiography. *Acta Radiol* 1992;33:611–613.

70. Palmers Y, DeGreef D, Grynne BH, et al. A double-blind study comparing safety, tolerability and efficacy of iodixanol 320 mg I/ml and ioxaglate 320 mg I/ml in cerebral arteriography. *Eur J Radiol* 1993;17:203–209.

ADDITIONAL READINGS

Alcohol

Buchta K, Sands J, Rosenkrantz H, Roche WD. Early mechanism of action of arterially infused alcohol U.S.P. in renal devitalization. *Radiology* 1982;145:45–48.

Ellman BA, Parkhill BJ, Curry TS III, et al. Ablation of renal tumors with absolute ethanol: a new technique. *Radiology* 1981;141:619–626.

Ellman BA, Parkhill BJ, Marcus PB, et al. Renal ablation with absolute ethanol: mechanism of action. *Invest Radiol* 1984;19:416–423.

Lee MJ, Mueller PR, Dawson SL, et al. Percutaneous ethanol injection for the treatment of hepatic tumors: indications, mechanism of action, technique, and efficacy. *AJR* 1995;164:215–220.

Yakes WF, Parker SH, Gibson MD, et al. Alcohol embolotherapy of vascular malformations. *Semin Intervent Radiol* 1989;6:146–161.

Balloons

Goto K, Halbach VV, Hardin CW, et al. Permanent inflation of detachable balloons with a low-viscosity hydrophilic polymerizing system. *Radiology* 1988;169:787–790.

Miyachi S, Negoro M, Handa T, et al. Histopathological study of balloon embolization: silicone versus latex. *Neurosurgery* 1992;30:483–489.

Contrast

Latchaw R. The cost of low-osmolality contrast media: can we minimize the economic impact? *AJNR* 1990;11:850–851.

Rasuli P, McLeish WA, Hammond DI. Anticoagulant effects of contrast materials: in vitro study of iohexol, ioxaglate, and diatrizoate. *AJR* 1989;152:309–311.

Stormorken H, Skalpe IO, Testart MC. Effect of various contrast media on coagulation, fibrinolysis, and platelet function in an in vitro and in vivo study. *Invest Radiol* 1986;21:348–354.

Ethibloc

Wright KC, Bowers T, Chuang VP, Tsai C-C. Experimental evaluation of Ethibloc for nonsurgical nephrectomy. *Radiology* 1982;145:339–342.

Glue

Berenstein A, Hieshima G. Clinical versus experimental use of isobutyl-2-cyanoacrylate [Letter]. *J Neurosurg* 1987;67:318–319.

Nagino M, Hayakawa N, Kitagawa S, et al. Interventional embolization with fibrin glue for a large inferior mesenteric-caval shunt. *Surgery* 1992;111:580–584.

Vinters HV, Galil KA, Lundie MJ, Kaufmann JCE. The histotoxicity of cyanoacrylates. *Neuroradiology* 1985;27:279–291.

Widlus DM, Lammert GK, Brant A, et al. In vivo evaluation of iophendylate-cyanoacrylate mixtures. *Radiology* 1992;185:269–273.

Woodward SC, Herrmann JB, Cameron JL, et al. Histotoxicity of cyanoacrylate tissue adhesive in the rat. *Ann Surg* 1965;113–122.

Polyvinyl Alcohol Particles

Castaneda-Zuniga WR, Sanchez R, Amplatz K. Experimental observations on short and long-term effects of arterial occlusion with Ivalon. *Radiology* 1978;126:783–785.

Chuang VP, Tsai C-C, Soo C-S, et al. Experimental canine hepatic artery embolization with polyvinyl alcohol foam particles. *Radiology* 1982;145:21–25.

Horton JA, Marano GD, Kerber CW, et al. Polyvinyl alcohol foam-Gelfoam for therapeutic embolization: a synergistic mixture. *AJNR* 1983;4:143–147.

Jack CR, Forbes G, Dewanjee MK, et al. Polyvinyl alcohol sponge for embolotherapy: particle size and morphology. *AJNR* 1985;6:595–597.

Kerber CW, Bank WO, Horton JA. Polyvinyl alcohol foam: prepackaged emboli for therapeutic embolization. *AJR* 1978;130:1193–1194.

Szwarc IA, Carrasco H, Wallace S, Richli W. Radiopaque suspension of polyvinyl alcohol foam for embolization. *AJR* 1986;146:591–592.

Wright KC, Anderson JH, Gianturco C, et al. Partial splenic embolization using polyvinyl alcohol foam, dextran, polystyrene, or silicone. *Radiology* 1982;142:351–354.

Snares

Graves VB, Rappe AH, Smith TP, et al. An endovascular retrieving device for use in small vessels. *AJNR* 1993;14:804–808.

Smith TP, Graves VB, Halbach VV, et al. Microcatheter retrieval device for intravascular foreign body removal. *AJNR* 1993;14:809–811.

Sodium Tetradecyl Sulfate (Sotradecol)

Cho KJ, Williams DM, Brady TM, et al. Transcatheter embolization with sodium tetradecyl sulfate. *Radiology* 1984;153:95–99.

Stents

Bailey S, Kiesz R. Intravascular stents: current applications. *Curr Probl Cardiol* 1995;9:618–678.

Becker GJ, Benenati JF, Zemel G, et al. Percutaneous placement of a balloon-expandable intraluminal graft for life-threatening subclavian arterial hemorrhage. *J Vasc Interv Radiol* 1991;2:225–229.

Becker GJ, Palmaz JC, Rees CR, et al. Angioplasty-induced dissections in human iliac arteries: management with Palmaz balloon-expandable intraluminal stents. *Radiology* 1990;176:31–38.

Buchwald AB, Unterberg C, Nebendahl K, et al. Low-molecular-weight heparin reduces neointimal proliferation after coronary stent implantation in hypercholesterolemic minipigs. *Circulation* 1992;86:531–537.

Eeckhout E, Stauffer J-C, Vogt P, et al. Unplanned use of intracoronary stents for the treatment of a suboptimal angiographic result after conventional balloon angioplasty. *Am Heart J* 1995;130:1164–1167.

George B, Voorhees W, Roubin G, et al. Multicenter investigation of coronary stenting to treat acute or threatened closure after percutaneous transluminal coronary angioplasty: clinical and angiographic outcomes. *J Am Coll Cardiol* 1993;22:135–143.

Lau KW, Gunnes P, Williams M, et al. Angiographic restenosis after successful Wallstent stent implantation: an analysis of risk predictors. *Am Heart J* 1992;124:1473–1477.

Long AL, Page PE, Raynaud AC, et al. Percutaneous iliac artery stent: angiographic long-term follow-up. *Radiology* 1991;180:771–778.

Marin ML, Veith FJ, Panetta TF, et al. Percutaneous transfemoral insertion of a stented graft to repair a traumatic femoral arteriovenous fistula. *J Vasc Surg* 1993;18:299–302.

Moss JG, Laborde JC, Clem MC, et al. Vascular occlusion with a balloon-expandable stent occluder. *Radiology* 1994;191:483–486.

O'Brien CJ, Rankin RN. Percutaneous management of large-neck pseudoaneurysms with arterial stent placement and coil embolization. *J Vasc Interv Radiol* 1994;5:443–448.

Piana RN, Moscucci M, Cohen DJ, et al. Palmaz-Schatz stenting for treatment of focal vein graft stenosis: immediate results and long-term outcome. *J Am Coll Cardiol* 1994;23:1296–1304.

Painter J, Mintz G, Wong S, et al. Serial intravascular ultrasound studies fail to show evidence of chronic Palmaz-Schatz stent recoil. *Am J Cardiol* 1995;75:398–400.

Palmaz J, Laborde J, Rivera F, et al. Stenting of the iliac arteries with the Palmaz stent: experience from a multicenter trial. *Cardiovasc Intervent Radiol* 1992;15:291–297.

Rosenblum JD, Leef JA, Kostelic JK, Boyle CM. Angioplasty and intravascular stents in peripheral vascular disease. *Surg Clin* 1995;75:621–631.

Sapoval MC, Long AL, Pagney J-Y, et al. Outcome of percutaneous intervention in iliac artery stents. *Radiology* 1996;198:481–486.

Vorwerk D, Gunther RW. Stent placement in iliac arterial lesions: three years of clinical experience with the Wallstent. *Cardiovasc Intervent Radiol* 1992;15:285–290.

Zollikofer C, Antonucci F, Pfyffer M, et al. Arterial stent placement with use of the Wallstent: midterm results of clinical experience. *Radiology* 1991;179:449–456.

Future Devices and Procedures

J.J. Connors III / J.C. Wojak

PAVING

Early work is now being done on lining the inside of vessels with biocompatible materials, some fibrillar in nature and others being membranes. These are not a true substitute for stents but rather an alternative to be used in certain situations. Specifically, when significant vascular motion is required, a new lining can potentially work better than a hard stent and be more permanent. In addition, a soft flexible liner can be easier to deliver (more flexible). An internal liner such as this may be an endovascular treatment for intracranial aneurysms.

STENTS

Continuing work is being done with numerous types of stents made of various materials (see Chapter 1). Stents are being made smaller and more flexible, as well as potentially retrievable. None is currently truly capable of intracranial work, but there has been placement of a metallic stent as far as the distal vertebral artery and internal carotid artery proximal to its bifurcation. Eventual uses for intracranial stents could be for angioplasty or endovascular treatment of aneurysms. In addition, a covered stent may eventually be the tool of choice for the treatment of a vascular perforation or pseudoaneurysm, particularly in the neck.

Currently, stents are being placed by some physicians in a primary fashion for therapy for carotid bifurcation disease (see Chapter 43), but this is still considered controversial by the neurovascular community. Initial results for this particular use may be acceptable, but long-term results are still unknown. The incidence of intimal hyperplasia would seem to be high in a moving vessel of this nature. The key to this statement is the realization that the long-term results are not actually known.

Intracranial stents are under development but are currently too stiff to routinely advance to a distal location. These will have to be shorter than any used in the periphery to aid in the navigation of sharp turns. Another reason for the short length is the necessity of accurate placement without occlusion of any vital branches. Also, various new mechanisms for detachment and retrieval have to be developed, some of which are already known but are proprietary at this time.

SPHERICAL COILS AND THREE-DIMENSIONAL COILS

New coil shapes are being investigated by several companies, as well as new materials. The need for the coils to assume a spherical shape renders them stiffer than usual coils, the Guglielmi detachable coils (GDC) in particular. However, the goal of covering the outer walls of an aneurysm could make these variations most valuable. Deployment could render the aneurysm a sealed chamber, allowing further packing without the worry of coil protrusion or extravasation into the lumen of the parent vessel.

Three-dimensional coils are a variant of the spherical coils but are not truly spherical. They are formed by having segments that are mostly straight with periodic abrupt 90-degree curves. This design forces the coils to assume a more random, boxlike configuration upon deployment, thus filling the aneurysm more thoroughly.

ADVANCED EMBOLIC AGENTS

DMSO-Dissolved Embolic Agents

Various embolic agents formed by dissolving materials in the potent solvent DMSO have been formulated, including hydrogels, plastics (Embolyx, Microtherapeutics Inc.), ethylene vinyl alcohol copolymer (EVOH), cellulose acetate polymer (CAP), and urethane copolymer (UCO). These have been evaluated for purposes ranging from vascular occlusion to aneurysm occlusion.

The lack of adhesiveness and slow "hardening" of these agents are detriments to vascular occlusion, and these products have not been used for this purpose. However, their ability to fill a void may make them useful for aneurysm occlusion. The characteristics of these materials differ somewhat. EVOH is the least viscous, followed by UCO, and then CAP. This means that flow control is more necessary when using EVOH than with the others. EVOH also forms a more deformable mass. UCO is less cohesive than the others, resulting in possible fragmentation. However, the cohesiveness also causes the catheter to adhere to the mass, producing stretching and "tailing" as the catheter is withdrawn.

Hydroxyapatite

Hydroxyapatite is an insoluble crystalline material and is the mineral component of bone. This material can be ground, purified, and separated into particles suitable for use as an embolic agent. It has low inflammatory potential and good biocompatibility.

Neuracryl

Since the advent of NBCA (*n*-butyl-2-cyanoacrylate), there has been very little advancement in the science of "superglue" embolization of vascular structures, primarily arteriovenous malformations (AVMs). Certain properties of superglue are advantageous for embolization, such as cohesiveness (sticking to itself) and adhesion (sticking to other things, such as vessel walls). However, these properties can be detrimental when present to an excessive degree. Rapid polymerization allows the material to set in flowing blood without passing through small channels into venous structures.

A new cyanoacrylate with slightly different properties, 2-hexyl-cyanoacrylate, has been developed. It has less cohesiveness but more viscosity and hardens more predictably in arterial structures, before penetrating to the veins. In addition, it has decreased adhesiveness, permitting catheter withdrawal even after it has partially hardened. It is not commercially available.

"Multipurpose Ointment"

An entirely new concept of embolization material has been developed by Ji and Guglielmi at UCLA Medical Center. The concept is simple: sclerotherapy is an effective means of vascular occlusion if the contact time between the vessel wall and the agent is sufficient. They have developed a sclerosing agent that incorporates all the assets necessary for effective embolization: visibility, immediate vascular occlusion, permanency, and the ability to be delivered through a microcatheter.

The agent, a "multipurpose ointment," is a semi-solid-semiliquid composed of a mixture of 30 mg albumin, 50 mg tetracycline, 0.2 ml Omnipaque, and 0.8 ml Ethiodol. Tetracycline is the active sclerosing agent. The viscosity of the mixture causes it to be stopped by small vessels. The mixture has several advantageous properties: (1) easy delivery through a microcatheter, (2) friction with the vascular wall to facilitate stasis, and (3) prolonged contact of the tetracycline with the vessel wall. In addition, all components of the mixture are biodegradable.

A trial involving embolization of pig rete was performed to evaluate the effectiveness of this mixture. Mixtures with and without tetracycline were prepared. In all cases, the vessels embolized without tetracycline recanalized while those embolized with tetracycline were permanently occluded.

MONITORING GUIDEWIRES

Truly micro devices are on the horizon that may allow future potentials undreamed of now. In use at this time, however, are ultrasound guidewires capable of modest intracranial use. Fiberoptic guidewires probably will not be useful for routine intracranial intravascular work any time in the near future. Boston Scientific Corp. produces a pressure-monitoring 0.018″ guidewire capable of distal delivery and intended for evaluation of angioplasty results.

MICROMINIATURIZED TOOLS

With the demise of the military-industrial complex, new products of incredible miniaturized complexity are beginning to surface. Grasping forceps controllable by microcurrents have been made on the order of microns and are capable of being attached to the end of microwires. None of this technology is currently of practical significance, but with these capabilities the implications are astounding. The amount of force these microtools can apply on a micro-scale is awesome, easily capable of holding, releasing, or retrieving various objects. It is up to the interventional neuroradiologic community to help guide these scientists in their pursuits.

PERCUTANEOUS DILATION OF AQUEDUCTAL STENOSIS

The concept of dilation of stenosis of the aqueduct of Sylvius has for years appeared to be an obvious treatment for a common and troublesome problem, congenital aqueductal stenosis. This procedure has undergone early animal trials and clinical trials in Japan. This form of treatment can change the approach to therapy for typical aqueductal stenosis. Access to the point of stenosis (the cerebral aqueduct of Sylvius) can be by either a retrograde approach via the foramina of Luschka or an antegrade approach by means of an indwelling ventriculostomy shunt catheter. Currently, most work has been by means of a fiberoptic system through a ventriculostomy, but theoretically a fluoroscopic system could allow a smaller access hole.[1] Currently available microwires and microangioplasty catheters are ideal for this purpose; the technique, however, has yet to be perfected.

ALTERNATIVE INFLATION METHODS FOR ANGIOPLASTY BALLOONS

A new angioplasty balloon designed for use in the coronary circulation (Rebel, SciMed/Boston Scientific Corp.), utilizes a novel method of inflation. Instead of using an inflating device with fluid delivered from the region of the hub of the angioplasty balloon catheter, inflation of the balloon is achieved by advancing a guidewire ("contrast displacement wire") downstream into the inner lumen of the catheter. This wire displaces the distal column of contrast into the balloon, thus inflating it. The effective moving fluid column is thus greatly shortened, allowing much more rapid inflation and deflation. Indeed, the balloon will essentially deflate and inflate as fast as the wire can be moved back and forth, which is almost instantly.

Perhaps of more practical significance, however, is the resultant decrease in "stored" energy. What this means is that when an angioplasty balloon is pressurized to the point at which the vessel begins to stretch, the entire lumen of the catheter actually expands microscopically and elastically, storing some of the infused liquid and subsequent energy. When the balloon starts to expand and the vessel begins to stretch, the catheter deflates slightly, keeping the pressure in the balloon relatively constant. In contrast, the small amount of fluid utilized by the new system produces much less stored energy. As the balloon begins to expand, the pressure within the balloon actually drops. This allows much more precise control of the angioplasty, avoiding excessive trauma to the vessel wall.

This is particularly important in view of the growing volume of data indicating that restenosis is directly related to the amount of vascular damage caused during angioplasty, particularly high-pressure inflation.

BETA RADIATION DELIVERY CATHETER SYSTEM

Catheters and stents that contain radioactive material are being used in an effort to reduce restenosis after angioplasty. The interest in the ability of radiation to prevent restenosis is based on the effect of radiation on cells. While other methods aimed at killing replicating cells have been used (e.g., lasers), radiation has a different effect on these cells. In previous studies, cells responded to radiation by apoptosis (programmed cell death) rather than by necrosis. Rather than simply dying, these cells lost the ability to reproduce because of damage to their DNA.

Two types of radiation, gamma and beta, are currently under consideration for use in this regard. Gamma radiation is the type generally used for radiography and has great penetrating power. Beta radiation is the result of an energized electron and is absorbed within a few millimeters from its source. The intrinsic difference between these two radiation types mandates completely different delivery strategies. A substantial dose of beta radiation can be delivered in a short time with essentially no exposure to the operator, whereas gamma radiation requires a longer delivery time and the operator has to leave the room (and the patient).

The Beta-cath (Novoste), which contains a sealed beta source (^{90}Sr), is a device specifically designed to deliver radiation. After angioplasty, the delivery catheter is advanced into the angioplasty site. This catheter is sealed at the end so that no blood comes into contact with the inner lumen. A small "radiation source train," with the beta source at the end, is then placed through this delivery catheter into the lesion and left for up to 5 minutes to irradiate the angioplasty site.

This method of deactivating the replicating endothelium has shown promise, decreasing restenosis rates by 50% or more.

RADIOACTIVE STENTS

An alternative method of delivering radiation to an angioplasty site is by means of a radioactive stent.

Numerous methods have been used to achieve this goal, most often by treating commercially available stents to produce alpha-, beta-, or gamma-emitting stents.[2] Impregnation of stents with a pure beta-particle–emitting isotope such as ^{32}P results in minimal penetration and rapid decay. In one study, Palmaz-Schatz stents (Johnson & Johnson Interventional Systems) treated with ^{32}P were implanted in a rabbit model. Stents with an initial activity of 13 μCi inhibited neointima formation, while those with an initial activity of 4 μCi did not, indicating a dose-response curve or at least a threshold dose needed to achieve this result.[3]

CUTTING BALLOONS

Small vertical razors have been placed on the surface of an angioplasty balloon. These small cutters are placed longitudinally in three locations around the balloon. When the balloon is inflated, they slice a very shallow groove, perforating to a depth of only a few microns and not even penetrating the media. Once the angioplasty has been performed, the resultant micro-injury results in delayed remodeling of the vessel wall, with gradual stretching of the incised points yielding an overall increase in lumen diameter.

INFILTRATING ANGIOPLASTY BALLOONS

Small, nearly microscopic needles have been placed onto the surface of an angioplasty balloon. When the balloon is inflated, the needles puncture the surface of the vessel wall and allow direct injection of a pharmaceutical agent. This strategy is mostly applicable to the prevention of restenosis by injection of some yet-to-be-determined drug.

This method of drug delivery is reportedly far more efficient at delivery of the agent than simple infusion of the drug into the vessel. These needles yield an effective delivery of over 90% of the drug compared with less than 10% with other methods (e.g., using a semipermeable balloon to instill the material into the vessel wall).

MULTIBALLOON ANGIOPLASTY SYSTEMS

A new angioplasty balloon system has been developed with multiple angioplasty balloons on the same catheter tip (Intella Interventional Systems, Inc.). The most distal balloon is a small-diameter predilation balloon, which prepares the vessel for a stent. The stent is mounted on the larger second balloon, which is about 5 mm proximal to the distal balloon.

After the stent is delivered, a third angioplasty balloon, located within the more proximal balloon, allows for further inflation and imbedding of the stent in the vessel wall. This complex design allows all steps of stenting to be performed by one device.

EXCIMER LASER ABLATION VASCULAR RECANALIZATION

Lasers have been used in the past for vascular recanalization, without beneficial results. Two different approaches have previously been used, direct and indirect. The direct method (utilizing neodymium:yttrium-aluminum-garnet lasers) allows laser energy to directly impact on the vascular tissues, while the indirect method allows the laser energy to heat the tip of a blunt probe, essentially burning a hole through the obstruction. Unfortunately, the thermal damage results in very poor healing and a high restenosis rate, and these methods of recanalization have been abandoned.

The excimer laser utilizes ultraviolet light in the 193- to 351-nm wavelength range. For coronary application, only the 308-nm xenon/hydrogen chloride (XeCl) devices are used. The excimer laser utilized by the Vitesse-C and CVX-300 systems (Spectranetics) reportedly achieves recanalization without excessive heating. However, during early use there was apparent generation of excessive thermoacoustic pressure waves, in the range of several hundred atmospheres. This effect has been greatly reduced by infusing saline during lasing.

The technique of laser use involves establishing a channel utilizing the laser and following this with a simple balloon angioplasty. Utilizing the laser as an initial step reduces the recoil of the vessel after the angioplasty.

REFERENCES

1. Oka K, Yamamoto M, Ikeda K, Tomonaga M. Flexible endoneurosurgical therapy for aqueductal stenosis. *Neurosurger* 1993;33:236–243.
2. Carter AJ, Laird JR. Experimental results with endovascular irradiation via a radioactive stent. *Int J Radiat Oncol Biol Phys* 1996; 36:797–803.
3. Hehrlein C, Stintz M, Kinscherf R, et al. Pure beta-particle–emitting stents inhibit neointima formation in rabbits. *Circulation* 1996; 93:641–645.

CHAPTER 3

Tricks of the Trade

J.J. Connors III / J.C. Wojak

DIAMOX CHALLENGE TEST

Acetazolamide (Diamox) can be used in conjunction with ^{133}Xe tomography to evaluate cerebrovascular reserve and the adequacy of collateral circulation.

Acetazolamide is a carbonic anhydrase inhibitor that blocks conversion of carbonic acid to CO_2 and H_2O in the brain, producing carbonic acidosis and lowering pH (see Chapter 4 for further information).[1] This results in vasodilation. Acetazolamide does not lower peripheral blood pressure, which would confuse the test results.

As originally described, this test was, and is, used to assess cerebrovascular reserve in patients with significant carotid artery disease (especially occlusion), and to predict those patients who might benefit from revascularization. A ^{133}Xe scan is obtained to assess the baseline cerebral blood flow (CBF). Acetazolamide (1 gm) is then injected intravenously and the scan is repeated 15 to 20 minutes later. Blood pressure is monitored during the course of the procedure to make sure that any observed changes in CBF are not due to changes in blood pressure.[1, 2] The baseline and postacetazolamide scans are compared with each other and with a baseline computed tomographic (CT) scan. The response to acetazolamide varies from patient to patient. What is important is not the absolute CBF response, but the development of, or change in, asymmetry in regions that do not demonstrate CT abnormality (and are thus presumably not infarcted).[1]

In normal patients, there is a diffuse increase in CBF without evidence of redistribution. In patients with compromised supply to a region (e.g., internal carotid artery occlusion with poor collateral supply), perfusion pressure is decreased and there is a *baseline* degree of focal vasodilation. This compensatory vasodilation may be sufficient to allow the baseline scan to appear normal. However, *these vessels have a limited ability to dilate further in response to acetazolamide.* The postacetazolamide scan will therefore reveal redistribution to the *unaffected regions,* and possibly even steal from the affected region. Patients with adequate collateral supply should have a normal response to acetazolamide, without redistribution.

This test has also been used to evaluate areas of decreased perfusion surrounding vascular malformations that have preserved vasoreactivity. These regions are especially prone to normal perfusion pressure breakthrough (see "Normal Perfusion Pressure Breakthrough" in Chapter 64) after surgical or endovascular treatment of the malformation, and are associated with poor prognosis.[3]

With the advent of intracranial angioplasty, tests such as this may prove to be valuable in predicting which patients may benefit from these procedures.

HOW TO TEST A VESSEL BEFORE EMBOLIZATION (PROVOCATIVE TESTING)

General Considerations

Before occlusion, it may be necessary to determine whether a vessel can be safely sacrificed. This can be determined by one of two ways—temporary occlusion of the vessel or injection with a neuroleptic drug—depending on which outcome is to be simulated. If the entire capillary bed is to be destroyed, simulation by drug injection can duplicate this outcome. If only the main supply vessel is to be occluded, temporary occlusion will give a more accurate reproduction of this outcome than drug injection.

This is because peripheral collateral supply after proximal occlusion is more closely simulated by not infusing the capillary bed with a drug. Drug injection will simulate total destruction of all downstream structures, whereas proximal occlusion (by a detachable balloon or mass of coils) will very likely spare these structures.[4-7]

General Technique

Amobarbital (Amytal) or methohexital (Brevital) can be used to test the functionality of certain vessels before sacrifice. From a cosmic viewpoint, all intracranial structures actually have a function, but some appear to be more important than others. From a diagnostic standpoint, an amobarbital test is most useful when it is positive. This is directly important information. A negative test leaves one with the knowledge that whatever was clinically tested for was not what that structure (or vessel) affected, but it may still have some (undetected) function that might possibly be eradicated with the embolization. However, in all likelihood the structure does have a function.

For intracranial segmental vascular testing, 25 to 75 mg amobarbital or 3 to 10 mg methohexital injected as a bolus should be used[4, 5, 8] (40 mg methohexital is nearly enough in some people to induce general anesthesia). Methohexital is potentially more useful owing to its extremely short half-life. The dose used by anesthesiologists for induction is 1 to 2 mg/kg every 8 to 10 minutes intravenously (older patients need a longer interval owing to metabolic abilities, i.e., 1 to 2 mg/kg every 10 to 20 minutes).

The patient should have appropriate neurologic testing performed before the injection (depending on the particular vascular distribution being tested), and again after the bolus. A dose of 25 mg amobarbital is enough for distal vessels supplying only a small portion of the brain (e.g., a branch supplying less than 25% of the middle cerebral artery [MCA] distribution). The amobarbital should be slightly diluted; 50 mg/ml is usually too strong (potentially toxic), but if the catheter tip is in a high-flow arteriovenous malformation (AVM) feeder, a short rapid bolus with this concentration may be needed to overcome the streaming character of the flow (see Chapter 22). In addition, although mixing amobarbital with contrast can demonstrate where the drug is going, mixing with any strength of contrast greater than or equal to 1:1 dilution with saline can cause *precipitation of the contrast*. When performing this maneuver, one should use weaker contrast (30%). In a small vessel such as the anteroinferior cerebellar artery (AICA), 50 mg amobarbital is too large a dose and can be toxic; one should use 25 mg.

Blood flow rate should be tested by a contrast injection before amobarbital injection, particularly when dealing with an AVM. The amobarbital injection should be forceful enough to fill the vessel and all its branches. Laminar flow streaming can give false-negative results. This method works best in smaller vessels. For any larger vessel, 50 to 75 mg should be used. For repeated tests, it may be necessary to pause during the procedure to allow recovery from the systemic effects of the drug; unfortunately, the half-life of amobarbital combined with repeated injections can mean a pause of 1 to 2 hours.

Caution should be used when working in the posterior fossa. Amobarbital injection can cause respiratory arrest or other hemodynamic effects. In addition, neurologic testing of the subtle but vital functions of certain cerebellar vessels (testing for ataxia, for instance) is difficult to perform, particularly while the patient is on the table. While cranial nerve function can be assessed, other tests will probably not yield accurate results.

When extracranial vessels are tested, amobarbital does not work nearly as well or as thoroughly as lidocaine. Peripheral nerves have different receptors than central neurons, yielding false-negative results. This is also true of the retina.[9] Care should be taken not to trust a potentially false-negative result from a test injection of the retina, peripheral nerves, or skull base with amobarbital. Typically, 1 to 2 ml 1% lidocaine (10 to 20 mg, without epinephrine) is injected into the vessel in question when testing extracranial vessels, although the use of up to 30 to 60 mg 2% lidocaine has been reported.[10] Cardiac lidocaine is the preferred agent, as it contains no potentially adverse preservatives and has a more physiologic pH.

It is important to thoroughly evaluate the arteriogram before injection of lidocaine. If there is an anastomotic connection between the extracranial branch to be tested and the internal carotid artery, a seizure may be induced by lidocaine injection.[10]

Methohexital Versus Amobarbital

The 1993 article by Peters et al stimulated interest in the possible use of sodium methohexital for provocative testing as well as Wada testing.[8] The obvious advantage is that of an extremely short half-life (about half that of thiamylal and thiopental, or less), permitting repeat testing if necessary. In addition, during a Wada test, there may not need to be the standard delay in the middle of the examination to allow the effects of amobarbital to wear off. The clinical effects of amobarbital are not as long-lived as the hypnotic effects, and repeated doses of amobarbital have a cumulative hypnotic effect. When amobarbital is used, the accuracy of the later tests is questionable owing to generalized cerebral dysfunction and thus possibly resulting in poor cooperation. Methohexital is also about twice as potent (on a weight basis) as amobarbital.

Once amobarbital is mixed for use, its shelf life is only 30 minutes. This is probably not widely appreciated; indeed, for most Wada testing, the interval between mixing the amobarbital preparation and the final usage is probably 1 hour. Methohexital has a longer shelf life after reconstitution.

Methohexital has been ignored for many years because of the fear that intra-arterial injection of this agent would cause direct arterial injury. Thiopentone has been shown to cause severe vasospasm and tissue necrosis. Similarly, methohexitone (a similar, but not the same, drug) has been shown to cause tissue necrosis when injected into rabbit ear arteries. These problems, however, arose from use of stronger concentrations than the 1% solution produced by reconstitution of 500 mg in 50 ml sterile water (specifically not bacteriostatic nor containing preservatives). The final solution is alkaline with a pH between 10.6 and 11.6, similar to that of amobarbital (9.6 to 10.4). Reports of epileptogenicity have not been verified.

A verbal report from Peters indicates that methohexital may be acceptable for Wada testing; doses between 3 and 10 mg administered in a bolus in the internal carotid artery in a fashion similar to the administration of amobarbital can be used. The extremely short clinical effect, however, may require repeat dosing, which is a drawback. In addition, the correct dose for Wada testing is not firmly established. For provocative testing, however, the active clinical duration of approximately 3 minutes is adequate, and the dose is 1 to 5 mg of 1% solution, depending on pedicle size.

Neurophysiologic Testing

Neurophysiologic testing can be used in conjunction with clinical assessment to delineate more fully the effect of amobarbital injection. Electroencephalography (EEG) can be used, but there are limitations to its usefulness. EEG records cortical function; it cannot be used to evaluate a vessel supplying deep structures. In addition, it is affected by the use of anesthetic agents. EEG, however, is the only available neurophysiologic method for evaluating the motor cortex.

Somatosensory evoked potentials (SSEPs) can also be used. The advantages to this method of testing are several. Interruption of function anywhere along the sensory pathway will result in a change in the recorded signal; its usefulness is not limited to the evaluation of vessels supplying the cortex. SSEPs are less sensitive to anesthetic agent use and can be used in conjunction with general anesthesia. Fewer electrodes are required than for EEG recording, and the waveforms are easier to interpret; changes in amplitude, latency, and waveform are readily detected as they occur. It is easy to obtain a baseline recording and serial comparisons during the procedure. The major drawback to the use of SSEPs is implied in the name; this method is useful only for evaluation of the effect of amobarbital injection on the somatosensory pathway. Although motor evoked potentials have been explored, a clinically useful system has never been developed.

HOW TO MIX PARTICLES

Whenever particulate matter is used for embolization, an entirely separate set-up of syringes, flush, and contrast is necessary. Each syringe should be clearly labeled as to particle size. This can be done with, for example, a sterile pen or strips of sterile tape. Unless otherwise stated, all syringes for embolization are 3 cc. Contrast diluted by 30% to 50% with heparinized saline for a less viscous injection material (but still mostly contrast) is used to suspend the particles. In other words, two parts contrast and one part saline is used. It is important to be able to accurately watch for any subtle reflux, hence the density of the contrast. It is still hyperosmolar, however, since it is diluted with saline, not water.

Newer packaging permits some particles to be mixed in their container. The most practical of these appears to be the PVA particles introduced by Cordis Corp. in 1997. This permits a safer, less easily contaminated solution that can be kept for however long the procedure lasts.

Different-brand particles tend to mix and float or sink differently. Contour Emboli from ITC/Target Therapeutics appear to mix and stay in solution very well, but other preparations are available that are at least as good (see "Particulate Embolic Agents" in Chapter 1). No thorough scientific comparison of the mixing properties of the various agents has been performed.

The smaller the particles, the denser the mixture can be without jamming in the catheter or hub. Practice makes perfect in this area. Remember, however, in this era of nonionic contrast agents, *it is usually not the amount of contrast injected during embolization* that is the limiting factor for procedures; therefore, dilute mixtures of particles within the contrast are safer and easier to use and produce less catheter jamming even though this may require more syringes of embolic particles.

When the particles are drawn up into the syringe, further dilution can be made with a separate syringe containing two thirds contrast and one third saline with a large-sized plastic Angiocath-type intravenous catheter attached (to stick down into the 3-cc syringe). This will allow accurate specific dilutions for different-sized particles.

During injection, frequent rolling or shaking of the syringe is necessary to prevent settling of the particles in the funnel of the catheter hub. Frequent puffs of particles allow observation of the *washout* of contrast to determine when stasis or slowing has been reached. If any clumping in the catheter hub starts to occur at all, these clumped particles then filter out *all the remaining particles* being injected, and thus none actually get through. If any clumping in the catheter hub starts, the syringe should be immediately detached and the catheter hub rinsed. After each syringe is injected, a forceful squirt of saline into the catheter hub is used to rid the hub of any pile-up of embolic particles.

A good technique for hub rinsing is to use the plastic outer part of an 18-gauge Angiocath-type intravenous needle on a 20-cc syringe filled with saline; this can be introduced into the hub of the catheter to flush it. Otherwise, forceful squirting into the hub with a nonattached saline syringe can wash out most remaining particles between each syringeful of particles used.

If a catheter becomes clogged with particles, it is at one of three places: the hub, any curved portion of the catheter where the lumen may become oval, or a transition point in the catheter construction. See "Catheter Occlusion" in Chapter 64 for further discussion.

Reports have been made concerning the possibility of decreased "jamming" or occlusion of the catheter if a small amount of ethanol is mixed into the solution with the PVA particles. Other information indicates this to be untrue. Newer catheter hub designs have been stated to decrease the incidence of particle jamming, specifically fluting or rifling of the lumen. Experience with the use of this design is limited, unfortunately.

In the past, there were reports of permanent cranial nerve palsies as well as other ischemic effects caused by the use of small particles (150 to 250 microns). This was thought to be due to the presence of much smaller particles within these mixtures (i.e., down to the 2- to 10-micron range). Tests indicate that the presence of ultrasmall particles (less than 30 microns) mixed into the larger particles is no longer a problem, even with the 50- to 150-micron particles, so the risk of permanent nerve damage associated with the use of small particles is lessened. Indeed, manufacturers now supply particles in the 50-micron range consistently, and much more uniform products are available. Particles in the 50-micron range, however, are certainly more capable of severe devascularization and should be used only in an appropriate territory.

HOW TO MIX AND USE AVITENE

Avitene (microfibrillar collagen) is available as a large clump of material in a container or compressed into a sheet. A small amount should be picked up with a needletip or forceps and mixed by vigorous swirling in half-strength contrast. After thorough mixing, the solution should be repeatedly aspirated and injected (back and forth) into a syringe without a needle on the end. The final mixture to be injected should be aspirated through a 16- to 20-gauge needle to filter any clumps before injection. The Seldinger needle works adequately, but a 20-gauge needle is preferred so that a more uniform small particle size is obtained.

This Avitene mixture can be combined with PVA particles to make a truly effective slurry. Absolute alcohol can also be added to produce a very effective, if nasty, mixture.[11] There is no clear recommendation for exact proportions of this mixture.

Avitene is extremely thrombogenic and, if given the opportunity, will cause sludging and occlusion of rather large vessels. The duration of this occlusion, however, can be short. The addition of ethanol can render this occlusion permanent but also increases the risk of a permanent complication.

HOW TO LOAD SILK FOR EMBOLIZATION

Silk is used for embolization for two reasons: (1) it stimulates an aggressive tissue reaction, thus potentially rendering a more permanent occlusion, and (2) it is very thrombogenic and can precipitate occlusion when it would otherwise be difficult to achieve stasis. Delivery of the silk is a challenge, however.

The simplest way to achieve this is by delivering the silk in the form of "torpedoes." These are individually loaded little bombs about 4 to 8 mm long. In the past, these were cut up by a scalpel on a table top and placed by means of a needle into the barrel of a syringe.

An easier method is to run a length of 3-0 silk through an Angiocath-type intravenous catheter (with the needle of the Angiocath removed). The length of silk is pulled out the tip of the plastic sheath, leaving about 5 mm of silk still within the tube. This is then trimmed with very sharp scissors, leaving this 5-mm length of silk within the plastic Angiocath. The Angiocath is then placed tip to tip against the barrel of the 1- or 3-cc syringe (previously filled with dilute contrast), and the previously removed needle of the Angiocath is then used to push the silk into the tip of the syringe. It is now ready for delivery.

HOW TO USE ALCOHOL

Ethanol is the most dangerous embolic agent currently in use. No one should attempt the use of this material without training or practice in its use; complications are unfortunately not infrequent. The use of ethanol for intracranial AVM embolization and the treatment of craniofacial vascular malformations (e.g., hemangiomas) is covered in Chapters 22 and 27.

Absolute alcohol can be injected either with or without opacification, either percutaneously into soft tissue or bone marrow, or intravascularly. It is far more effective undiluted and far more dangerous. When injected intravascularly, actual contact with the wall of the vessel must be made; dribbling of alcohol through the catheter does no good. A full column of injected alcohol is necessary for permanent vascular obliteration, but reflux must be avoided. Meticulous control of the rate of injection is therefore necessary.

If the intrinsic flow in the target vessel is too rapid and streaming is thus occurring, it may be possible to slow the flow for more accurate infusion control by several means. Perhaps the easiest is proximal flow control with either a flow control guide catheter (such as Zeppelin, described in Chapter 1) or a flow control microcatheter (the Grapevine by Medtronic/MIS). In addition, partial embolization with coils or particles can slow the flow enough to allow better control of infusion.

Opacification of the alcohol is possible with contrast agents such as powdered metrizamide (Amipaque) or powdered iohexol (Omnipaque). Each of these renders the mixture far more viscous, and a truly massive amount of powder is necessary to see the mixture fluoroscopically. Stirring the powder into the alcohol can be done with any instrument and it takes robust stirring to dissolve it all. A "glob" will invariably form on the end of this stirrer. This is fine. Aspiration of the final solution through a small-gauge needle (23 to 25 g) will filter out any remaining particles. The final density of the mixture is confirmed fluoroscopically *in the syringe* before use (hold this syringe under the image intensifier externally). After a satisfactory amount of powdered contrast has been added (a massive amount, remember), the mixture will have about the same viscosity as normal contrast, unfortunately. The incredible bulk of powdered contrast necessary for visualization is what dilutes the actual effectiveness of the opacified ethanol mixture.

Alcohol not only destroys vascular endothelium but also red cells and other structures. In addition, it can be terribly painful. If the vessel is one with sensory supply, general anesthesia may be necessary to control patient discomfort. Conversely, if the vessel is in an appropriate location, preinjection with lidocaine may help greatly, but often not enough. Conscious sedation and analgesia also may be increased temporarily during the periods of alcohol injection.

The alcohol injection itself can cause severe vasospasm, making assessment of the efficacy of the occlusion difficult. It may appear that the embolization procedure is working satisfactorily when in fact all that is being observed is spasm. After injection of alcohol, effects can manifest themselves up to *days* later. Patience is needed. After approximately 15 minutes, a repeat contrast injection can be performed; this will usually show a gradual change in the appearance and flow characteristics of the structure being insulted, to the point of total occlusion. We have observed that even when use of alcohol is ceased with some channels still open, complete obliteration is demonstrated on follow-up angiography months later.

There are also certain idiosyncratic results observed with the use of ethanol. Occasionally, acute pulmonary hypertension ensues, apparently caused by pulmonary arteriolar spasm (although this mech-anism is unproved at this time). For this reason, Yakes, a pioneer in this field and one of the most experienced users of ethanol in the world, uniformly uses a Swan-Ganz catheter to monitor pulmonary artery pressure during these procedures. If any rise in pulmonary artery pressure is detected, an immediate infusion of massive amounts of nitroglycerin is started directly into the main pulmonary artery through the Swan-Ganz catheter (200 µg/ml, infused at a "wide open" rate). The infusion is titrated according to the pulmonary artery pressure response as well as the peripheral blood pressure response. See Chapter 64 for a thorough discussion of the acute cardiopulmonary response and its treatment.

The use of alcohol anywhere in the body is fraught with danger. Nerve and/or vascular damage frequently results even in locations thought to be totally safe. The operator is advised to beware.

EMBOLIZING WITH COILS

Coils can be deposited by a coil pusher or by forceful injection of saline. However, a coil should never be injected if the catheter is even close to being wedged (i.e., jammed into a vessel the same size as the catheter). Even though the coil goes downstream, when it reaches its end point most of the saline has to suddenly come back beside the catheter, and if the catheter is wedged, this can rupture the vessel.

Injecting coils by a bolus of saline is a good technique for rapid placement of a pile of coils downstream where there is plenty of room and no vital structures to be protected. Even though *exact positioning is not possible* with this technique, it does get the coils downstream well and allows quick placement of a large number.

Target Therapeutics recommends using a continuous flush when deploying platinum microcoils. Red cells can be large enough to actually jam the coil in the lumen of the microcatheter, particularly if the catheter tip is highly curved near the end and thus potentially oval in shape. If meticulous technique is used, however, continuous flush is usually not necessary. It is actually the flattening or ovaling of the distal tip of the catheter in its last few curves that hinders the coils. This problem is far less with the use of braided microcatheters.

Embolizing without a continuous flush of saline is possible. The catheter should be filled with saline and the coil immediately introduced. It should then be advanced approximately 20 to 40 cm using the *back end* of the pusher wire; this is stiffer and far easier to use to get the coil started, and provides room in the catheter to advance the floppy part of the pusher wire before it hits the coil. As the back end of the wire is being removed, the hub should be continuously filled with saline, and then the syringe should be hooked up and about 0.5 ml of saline *very* slowly injected into the catheter (around and past the coil) to refill the catheter with saline and flush any blood out of the end of the catheter. While this is being done, the coil pusher wire is reversed. The front end of the pusher is then introduced into the catheter and used to advance the coil to the intended location.

The tips of coil pushers made by Target Therapeutics are notorious for "accordioning" (crinkling) with any forceful push at all. If any trouble in advancing the coil is encountered, switching without hesitation to a fresh coil pusher is strongly recommended. "Accordioning" greatly affects the vectors of force and only tends to get worse as more force is applied. In addition, the vectors of force become directed more laterally, and it is not unheard of for the pusher wire to rupture the side wall of the microcatheter.

Use of a gold-tipped Micro Glidewire (Terumo) for the pusher wire can potentially solve the problem of crinkling of the tip. This wire is hydrophilic and made of nitinol, and thus does not kink. The gold bead on the end acts as a good ramrod. Additionally, this wire does not fatigue the inside of the catheter (scratch it), like the plastic coil pusher can.

Cordis Corporation has developed a hydrophilic-coated nitinol coil pusher (Trupush) that does not "accordion" and that does not tend to scratch the inside of the catheter. In addition, this pusher is available with two markers at the tip, for microcatheters designed for use with Guglielmi detachable coils (GDC). These catheters also have two distal markers to assist in positioning the coil properly for detachment. The markers on the pusher and the catheter align when the tip of the pusher reaches the tip of the catheter, indicating deployment of the coil. This is especially helpful when the marker at the tip of the catheter cannot be seen because it is in the midst of a tangle of coils; alignment of the proximal markers on the pusher and catheter can be used to determine when the coil has exited from the catheter. The wire tapers to a very flexible end with a ramming bead on the tip, an effective design.

The topic of coil jamming is discussed further in "Catheter Occlusion" in Chapter 64. If a coil becomes jammed, it is probably due to the lumen of the catheter becoming oval at a sharp bend, thus decreasing the cross-sectional diameter. If the coil is partially deployed and the microcatheter is slowly withdrawn, there is no guarantee that the coil will not free itself when the lumen again becomes round. Aspiration during withdrawal is theoretically a good idea but probably does not really help.

Coil jamming secondary to the catheter becoming oval can be alleviated to some degree by presteaming the catheter at the point where the bend will occur. This may preserve a round lumen at this point and thus prevent the coil from becoming wedged. This is particularly important with the use of GDC. Newer catheters with braiding or coils within their walls are very effective at preventing this problem. These include all but the original TRACKER catheters (Target Therapeutics).

Infusion of saline while using a new coil pusher may free a jammed coil. In addition, a forceful injection may dislodge the coil (possibly by microscopically ballooning the microcatheter at the tight spot).

However, rupture of the side wall of the catheter (proximal to the jammed coil) is not unheard of, either by forceful pushing of the coil pusher or by a vigorous injection of saline. Again, braided microcatheters have practically eliminated this problem.

If the entire catheter tip breaks off with the coil within it, this may be no problem, depending on the location. After all, this was where the coil was intended to go. However, if the catheter ruptures but is still attached, removal can be tricky (see Chapter 64).

If the broken piece of catheter needs to be removed, see "How to Use a Snare" below. Frequently, however, a piece of remaining catheter will cause no real harm, just as a single errant coil may not. If flow can be maintained for a week or so (by means of aggressive anticoagulation and antiplatelet therapy combined with hemodilution), in most cases the coil (or catheter) will become endothelialized (or not) and blend into the surroundings.

HOW TO MOUNT A DETACHABLE BALLOON

As stated in the chapters discussing specific procedures, the use of a guide catheter with flow control capability is highly recommended for any case involving detachable balloon use; one such catheter is the previously described Zeppelin (Chapter 1). If there is no antegrade flow owing to the temporary flow arrest, the detachable balloon does not tend to flap around as it would otherwise and any misplaced detachment can be dealt with. In addition, the placement of the first balloon is stable until a second can be placed. It is most disturbing to have the first balloon in perfect position only to see it slowly pushed downstream by pulse pressure before a second balloon can be placed. A flow control guide catheter also greatly lowers the pulse rate of the interventional neuroradiologist.

Detachable balloons are not approved by the Food and Drug Administration (FDA) for manufacture in the United States. Three kinds are currently available worldwide (see Chapter 1 for further details). The self-sealing valve varieties are preferable. ITC/Target Therapeutics (silicone) and Ingenor (latex) are continuing to manufacture high-quality detachable balloons overseas.

Trying to seat the tiny balloon on the tip of the microcatheter can be a challenge. This is made far easier if the stiff end of a 0.018″ guidewire is allowed to protrude from the tip of the microcatheter by 2 to 4 mm (Fig. 3–1A). After the balloon has been slipped onto the wire (Fig. 3–1B), it can then be forced over the end of the catheter to its final position (Fig. 3–1C). An 0.018″ guidewire is recommended because if an 0.014″ wire is used, the catheter tip can accordion back onto the wire.

Use of a catheter with the marker band right at the tip (as is usual) renders detachment more difficult; the marker band itself is larger than the catheter tip (which, before the advent of the flow control guide catheter, was probably helpful!). A TRACKER catheter with a marker band 5 mm from the tip is

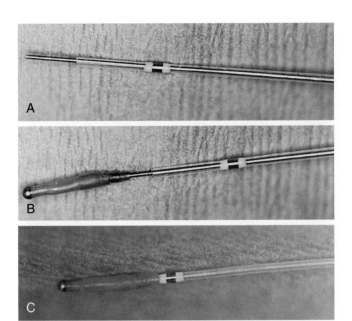

Figure 3-1 A TRACKER-18 Unibody microcatheter (Target Therapeutics) with a 0.5-cm extended tip is utilized for deployment of detachable balloons. This is not a hydrophilic-coated catheter. A 0.018″ straight guidewire is advanced until the distal 3 to 4 mm protrudes from the catheter *(A)*. The latex Gold Valve balloon (Ingenor) is then mounted on the guidewire *(B)*. The wire is slowly withdrawn and the balloon is forced onto the tip of the catheter *(C)*.

available from Target Therapeutics, as well as one with the marker 2 cm from the tip. Hydrophilic-coated catheters are not recommended for use with detachable balloons, as this makes detachment unpredictable.

Latex balloons that are hand-tied onto the catheter can give a certain feeling of security to the practiced user; a tight knot is always possible (a latex string is wrapped multiple times around the balloon neck, which has been placed over the catheter tip to hold it in place and act as a seal after detachment). Detachment usually requires the use of an outer sleeve over the microcatheter to push the balloon off the tip when it has been positioned. Although the sleeve renders the device stiffer and more difficult to use, it certainly adds a margin of safety not present otherwise owing to the firm resistance of the balloon to premature detachment. This feeling of security can also be achieved with a regular valved balloon when a flow control guide catheter is used.

PREPPING A BALLOON

Test filling and preparing a balloon is recommended for all detachable balloons as well as temporary occlusion balloons for test occlusion. Unfortunately, this stretches latex balloons beyond their original deflated size, thus increasing the necessary size of the guide catheter up to a truly large diameter.

A venting tube microcatheter is available from ITC/Target Therapeutics (see Chapter 1) which greatly aids in removing air from the balloon on the tip of a catheter. The tiny (microscopic) tube is simply inserted into the catheter until the tip is in the balloon, and contrast mixed with saline is injected until it fills the balloon. The air will reflux around the tube and out of the catheter, although very slowly.

This venting tube is not nearly so effective for purging the air from temporary test occlusion balloons, which have their balloon ports on the side of the catheter. Some air can be removed this way, but a small amount must be worked out of the catheter in the standard manner. The balloon is filled and all air is collected in one bubble. The vent hole of the balloon is then located, and the air is forced out by putting pressure against the balloon over the hole and pushing the air out before any of the contrast exits, thus leaving enough contrast in the balloon and catheter lumen to carry the offending bubble out of the catheter.

Silicone balloons are far easier to prepare for use: they eventually purge themselves of air if one just fills them up and waits. This pertains to the Zeppelin catheter and the ITC/Target Therapeutics detachable silicone balloon in particular. Figure 3–2 demonstrates an example of a bubble in a silicone balloon and one in a latex balloon allowed to sit for a period of about 10 minutes.

After all the contained air has been removed from the balloon and catheter system, the balloon is left inflated with contrast mixed with saline while the final syringe is mounted on the catheter hub. This allows ideal (airless) connection because of ongoing reflux from the catheter and balloon during syringe hook-up (just as when connecting a catheter to a power injector during an aortogram).

STEERING A DETACHABLE BALLOON

Sometimes it is necessary to steer the balloon during a procedure, and placement of a curved guidewire tip within the balloon is possible. The use of a rotating hemostatic valve is then necessary (to seal around the wire and allow inflation of the balloon), and the same meticulous care is required to remove all air bubbles from the valve set-up. A guidewire should *never* be introduced into a catheter with a balloon mounted on the tip while the catheter is in the patient. The wire tip must be seen accurately when it exits the catheter into the balloon. This is not possible fluoroscopically. Therefore, the guidewire must be placed while the apparatus is still external. When the guidewire tip is in an ideal location, bending the shaft of the wire where it exits the rotating hemostatic valve will prevent inadvertent advancement of the guidewire during manipulation, and thus possible premature detachment of the balloon.

Before mounting the balloon, steam curving the tip of the delivery catheter is possible (see "How to Steam a Catheter" below). A *very* tight curl has to be steamed for this maneuver to work. In certain cases this maneuver can snatch victory from the jaws of defeat. While this sounds like a great idea, the catheter-balloon system is actually very poorly torqueable,

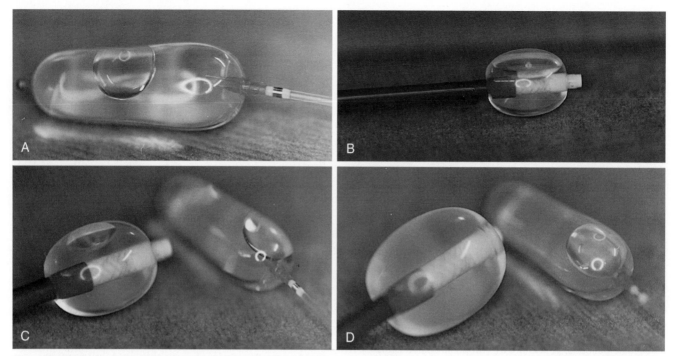

Figure 3-2 Demonstration of the difference between latex and silicone balloons. *A* shows a latex Gold Valve balloon mounted on the end of a TRACKER-18 extended-tip catheter, as described in Figure 3-1. Note the air bubble. This balloon must be purged before use. The venting tube microcatheter made by ITC/Target Therapeutics can be used for this purpose. In *(B)*, the silicone balloon of a Zeppelin catheter (Medtronic/MIS) has been inflated. Again, note the bubble. In *(C)*, note that the bubbles in the two balloons are approximately the same size initially. After a wait of 10 minutes, note that the air has disappeared from the semipermeable silicone balloon of the Zeppelin, while the bubble in the latex balloon is still the same size *(D)*. The Zeppelin does not require the rigorous preparation that is needed when latex balloons are utilized; time performs the trick of purging the balloon.

and still may not go where the operator wants it to. The indwelling guidewire, however, can be torqued, and this is what allows actual steering, albeit limited. The balloon itself is fairly stiff and straight (and *long*, believe it or not), and, depending on the particular model, will yield a straight segment of 5 to 8 mm on the tip of the catheter. This straight segment can be a real problem if a tight curve has to be negotiated.

The simplest way to steer a detachable balloon is to let the balloon lead the way in a flowing stream. This requires having the latex (or silicone) balloon barely mounted on the catheter so that it can follow its own course. In addition, some slight filling of the balloon can allow it to "catch the breeze."

HOW TO USE A SNARE

There are several types of snares on the market. However, for microvascular work, the simple loop snares by Target Therapeutics and Microvena are the two most commonly available. Target Therapeutics manufactures only "micro" snares; Microvena makes micro and macro snares.

The Microvena snare has a shape that may aid in encircling the object. It automatically assumes a round shape at right angles to the vessel lumen when extruded from its catheter, and therefore helps encircle the lost object. It is, however, stiffer than the Target snare, and thus more dangerous.

The Microvena snare can be used through any typical microcatheter. It is actually just a wire with a loop on the end. The Target Therapeutics snare is an entire system, i.e., the catheter is integrated. The Microvena snare can be advanced through a microcatheter that has been preplaced, utilizing standard catheter and guidewire technique. Once the microcatheter is in place, the guidewire can be exchanged for the Microvena snare and into the intended location, thus greatly facilitating its use.

Both snares require a large lumen for retrieval of the object, but not necessarily for distal placement of the snare. If a large guide catheter is in place through a sheath (i.e., the sheath has at least a 6-Fr. lumen), it may be possible to withdraw the retrieved object back into the sheath without actually getting it into the guide catheter. If not, one should plan ahead by placing a larger retrieval sheath system (see "Preparing a Large-Lumen Intravascular Withdrawal System for a Foreign Body" below).

Snares can be advanced past the object to be retrieved before deployment. This works well if the object is not straight against a side wall and the Microvena snare can open up perpendicularly. Alternatively, the large loop of the Target snare can be greatly extended and the huge loop then dragged across the entire object from distal to proximal. Wherever the object (such as a coil) is best positioned away from the vessel wall is the best place to attack. However, even when the coil radiographically appears to be away from the vessel wall, it probably is actually adjacent to the vessel wall on a tangential view. Patience and luck are as much help as technical skill.

Retrieval of an errant coil is demonstrated in Figure 3–3. A Microvena snare was utilized to grasp a coil hanging into the subclavian artery. An additional case demonstrating retrieval of a coil is shown in Chapter 1.

The operator should be aware that these are rela-

tively traumatic instruments that may do more harm than good. Also, it is sometimes not necessary to retrieve a malpositioned coil at all (see Chapter 64).

PREPARING A LARGE-LUMEN INTRAVASCULAR WITHDRAWAL SYSTEM FOR A FOREIGN BODY

An appropriately sized system must be chosen. If exchange over a guidewire is possible, simply placing

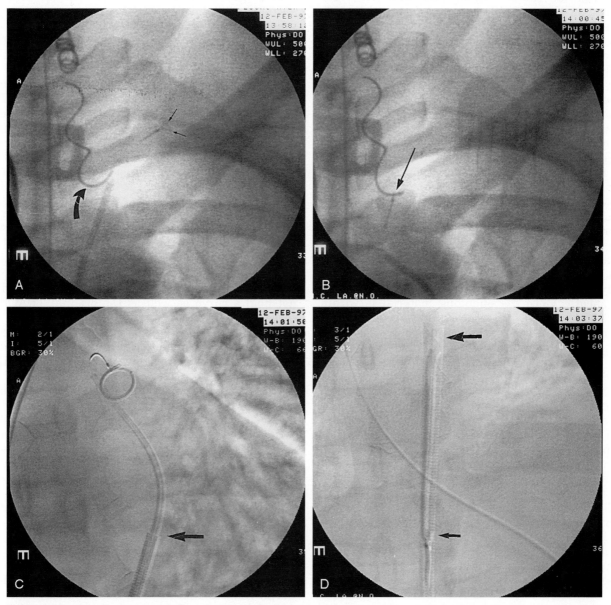

Figure 3-3 *A,* A young man who was shot through the neck had a damaged vertebral artery with episodic neurologic symptoms (visual). Occlusion of the vertebral artery was performed utilizing large coils (with proximal flow arrest during coil embolization, of course). The last coil was too large and inadvertently pushed the catheter (and coil tip) out into the subclavian artery *(curved arrow* at the vertebral artery origin). While the slight amount of coil hanging into the vessel would in all likelihood be no problem, it is aesthetically unappealing (it might also cause blue finger syndrome). The two small arrows point at the snare deployed distal to the dangling coil in an effort to retrieve this last coil.

B, The coil has been snared by the loop *(arrow).*

C, The free coil is now in the descending thoracic aorta, held by the snare and the tip of the microcatheter, coming out of the 5-Fr. catheter. Note the 45-cm-long neuro-sheath *(arrow)* in the midthoracic aorta, which is used on all interventional neuroradiological cases. This allows a good channel from which the coil can exit.

D, The pulsations of the aorta are well demonstrated in the shaking of the sheath with the snared coil within it *(arrows).*

a huge sheath is possible. However, if the guide catheter cannot be moved, for example, because of a coil in its tip, the maneuver becomes more difficult.

If the guide catheter in place is 6-Fr., for instance, a set is prepared using the outer portion (the sheath) of a long (25- to 45-cm) 6-Fr. sheath set and the outer sheath of a short 8-Fr. sheath set. The 8-Fr. sheath is inserted *over* the 6-Fr. outer sheath, so that the 6-Fr. sheath is like a giant dilator for the 8-Fr. sheath. This will yield a fairly snug-fitting unit that can be advanced over the indwelling 6-Fr. guide catheter (with the hub cut off) through the skin. The hubs are cut off the indwelling microcatheter and guide catheter system, and the new sheath system is slid over it into the femoral artery. The 6-Fr. sheath (which was hugging the catheter and allowed smooth entry into the vessel) is then withdrawn, leaving the 8-Fr. sheath in place with the cut-off 6-Fr. guide catheter within it.

An even larger lumen for withdrawal can be made by using the outer sheath of a 10-Fr. set as the external final "sheath" and making a triaxial system. The long (45-cm) 6-Fr. piece is kept as is, a long (25-cm) 8-Fr. sheath (just the outer sheath) is placed over this, and the outer sheath part of the short 10-Fr. set is placed *over this*. Once in position, the two inner liners are withdrawn, leaving only the largest outer sheath in place. This yields a huge 10-Fr. lumen through which to withdraw any foreign body, but also a 12-Fr. hole in the vessel.

At this point, the entire microcatheter/guide catheter system is slowly withdrawn into the 8-Fr. (or 10-Fr.) sheath. Once the offending material is within the 10-Fr. sheath, the entire unit is pulled. This maneuver almost invariably retrieves all the offending materials.

In addition, it is possible to load a microsnare over the 6-Fr. guide catheter, advance it through the 10-Fr. sheath (a large stent introducer may be required to get it through the valve), and follow the guide catheter and then the microcatheter until the snare is in place. Once the snare has grabbed the object (such as a broken catheter or a coil protruding from the microcatheter), the guide catheter/snare/object assembly can be pulled into the 10-Fr. sheath.

If the entire tip of a microcatheter is broken off, retrieval by snare or open surgical means is possible. Alternatively, depending on the location, it may be left in place. Numerous microcatheters have been glued in place in the past with no long-term effects (although admittedly some have yielded adverse effects) (see Chapter 66).

HOW TO STEAM A CATHETER

An electric tea kettle, such as that made by Presto Industries, Inc., has many advantages over the hot plate/tea pot combination used by most people (see Chapter 1). It can boil water extremely rapidly (less than 1 minute for modest amounts of water) and has an automatic shutoff when it runs out of water.

Both standard catheters and microcatheters can be steamed. The Vinuela catheter (Cook, Inc.) is specifically designed for steaming and comes preloaded with a malleable mandrel. It requires 5 to 15 seconds over steam to take its shape and takes heat well, but it does shrink slightly during steaming. It also loses some of its curve after removal of the mandrel and some more after being in the body for a few minutes; hence, the need to *overcurve* the steamed shape. It is very useful for any procedure requiring adaptation or needing a somewhat different curve from typical stock items for selection of a particular vessel.

Most microcatheters are also capable of being steam shaped, but they are far more sensitive. With steam-curved microcatheters, the guidewire is still the tool used for selecting vessels; the catheter curve is intended primarily to allow it to follow the guidewire more easily. Note that even though these are soft catheters, the steamed curve at the tip can be amazingly stiff and hard. Unfortunately, a TRACKER-18 catheter can shrink in length as well as diameter. This can become critical when GDC coils are used; the marker bead of a GDC delivery catheter (Target Therapeutics) can measurably change distance from the tip after steaming. Only a brief blast of steam is usually necessary (about 1 second for the TRACKER catheter).

The microcatheters from Medtronic/MIS and Cordis Corp., as well as the new TurboTRACKER (Target Therapeutics), have a braid within the wall (as discussed in Chapter 1) and do not shrink as much as the original TRACKER-18. These catheters require more aggressive steaming to hold a curve and do not hold a curve as well as the original TRACKER catheter. For steaming any of these catheters, the steaming mandrel supplied by the company is recommended. Before the mandrel is removed, the catheter should be cooled externally with saline, and then flushed.

Most catheters lose some of their steamed curve after removal of the mandrel, so exaggeration of the desired curve is necessary when steaming. For microcatheters, simple, very small arcs are usually sufficient (they are not truly torqueable, no matter what the manufacturers claim). In steaming microcatheters, it should be remembered that the vessels to be worked in are very small and the turns are frequently very tight. This is even true with large catheters; the vessels are amazingly small.

HOW TO USE THE INTIME CATHETER

The design of the Intime catheter (Boston Scientific Corp.) renders this catheter somewhat awkward to use, although its placement is fast and simple. It is designed as a one-piece unit with a fixed internal guidewire. The designers intended this to be placed directly through a diagnostic catheter, which is indeed possible. Although not needing to use a true guide catheter allows rapid placement of the Intime, it prevents adequate injection of contrast around the microcatheter to evaluate the results of treatment. The Intime catheter itself has a very small lumen owing to the presence of the fixed indwelling guide-wire and cannot be used for contrast injections. Therefore, we recommend placing a true guide catheter prior to use of the Intime.

It is impossible to inject adequate contrast through the lumen of the Intime, so do not try. In addition, it is not possible to flush the catheter adequately due to the inability to aspirate blood. For this reason, the Intime microcatheter should be hooked up to a pressurized flush setup using pediatric microtubing while the catheter is still outside the patient; the saline can be switched to urokinase when the catheter is in position. Placement of the Intime can then be performed by using roadmapping or contrast injections through the guide catheter.

STEERING A FLOW-DIRECTED CATHETER INTO THE ANTERIOR RATHER THAN THE MIDDLE CEREBRAL ARTERY

Occasionally, while treating an arteriovenous malformation (AVM) in the midline supratentorially, it is difficult to get the catheter to choose the anterior cerebral artery (A1) rather than the middle cerebral artery (M1) when advancing it from the internal carotid artery. This difficulty can be overcome by compressing the contralateral common carotid artery, inducing a steal from the ipsilateral anterior cerebral territory, and thus increasing flow from the internal carotid artery into the A1. This makes the catheter tend to enter the A1 segment.

HOW TO INTRODUCE A GUIDE CATHETER DIRECTLY THROUGH THE SKIN

In the past, all guide catheters needed to be inserted through sheaths. The need to use large guide catheters (up to 9-Fr.) for certain procedures (e.g., angioplasty, stent placement) meant that large sheaths had to be used, creating huge (11-Fr.) holes in vessels.

Some companies have begun to manufacture matched dilators for their guide catheters, allowing direct percutaneous introduction without a sheath. Medtronic/MIS currently has dilators available for certain sizes of their Omniguide and Zeppelin catheters (Fig. 3–4). Cook, Inc. is now marketing a dilator for their Lumax and Lumax Neuroguide catheters (Fig. 3–5). In addition, the dilators supplied by Devices for Vascular Intervention, Inc. (DVI) for their

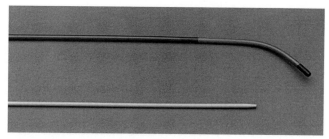

Figure 3-5 A Lumax Neuroguide catheter (Cook, Inc.) with its matched dilator.

atherectomy catheters can be used for percutaneous introduction of appropriately sized guide catheters from other manufacturers.

The 9-Fr. Brite-Tip catheter (Cordis Corp.) is a useful platform for angioplasty and stent procedures. At the present time, no dilator is available for this catheter. However, a 7-Fr., 110-cm Berenstein catheter (USCI Cardiology & Radiology Division, CR Bard) fits snugly within this catheter, providing a smooth transition from guidewire to diagnostic catheter to guide catheter (Fig. 3–6). The hubs of the catheters are held together manually and the catheters are advanced as a unit.

In most cases, when it is possible to introduce a 9-Fr. guide catheter percutaneously, this is far preferable to placing an 8-Fr. guide through a sheath, which results in a 10-Fr. hole in the femoral artery but only an 8-Fr. guide catheter to work through. We therefore use a 9-Fr. guide catheter for almost all cases requiring anything larger than a 6-Fr. guide catheter. The hole in the vessel produced by the 6-Fr. guide is 8-Fr. (a 6-Fr. sheath is used), whereas the hole produced by Lumax Neuroguide catheters is the same as the guide catheter size.

DEALING WITH UNWANTED HYDROPHILIC COATING

Although hydrophilic coating has made many procedures easier (or even possible), there are circumstances under which it is a decided disadvantage. This is not uncommonly encountered when one is trying to manipulate a hydrophilic-coated guidewire in order to selectively catheterize a difficult vessel—during attempts to rotate the wire, the resistance

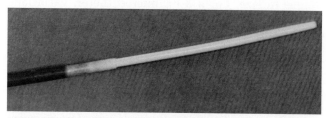

Figure 3-4 A Zeppelin (Medtronic/MIS) flow-control catheter with its matched dilator. Note the snug fit and smooth transition between the dilator and catheter.

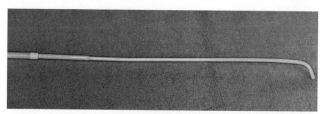

Figure 3-6 A 9-Fr. Brite-Tip catheter (Cordis Corp.) with a 7-Fr. Berenstein catheter (USCI) through it. The catheters are advanced together over a guidewire; the snug transition between the Berenstein and Brite-Tip catheter allows the Brite-Tip to be introduced percutaneously without the use of a sheath.

can be so great that the proximal portion of the wire spins in the operator's fingers rather than transmitting the torque down the wire.

Improved traction can be achieved by several means. Sterilized microfine emery cloth squares have been used to roughen the hydrophilic coating on the proximal portion of the wire. The wire must be carefully wiped down after this to remove any fine particles. Alternatively, the offending portion of the wire can be scrubbed with a sterile alcohol wipe; this also degrades the hydrophilic coating. Some coatings are amazingly resistant to this approach. The alcohol must be fully rinsed from the wire and/or allowed to evaporate. Perhaps an equally effective method is wiping with a dry cloth.

Amazingly, some manufacturers either will not or cannot remove this unwanted coating from the proximal portion of their guidewires, although this would greatly improve their product! Cook, Inc. now manufactures their Roadrunner guidewire without a hydrophilic coating on the proximal shaft.

Another instance when the ability to remove unwanted coating is helpful is in working with detachable balloons. As noted below, these must be mounted on noncoated catheters. However, there are circumstances when hydrophilic coating will aid greatly in the delivery of the balloon to its final location (or when the only catheters available are coated). The distal tip of the catheter can be scrubbed with a sterile alcohol wipe to strip the coating, giving a secure surface for mounting the balloon. If the last centimeter of any microcatheter could be left uncoated to mount a detachable balloon on, this would be ideal.

The most common reason to remove hydrophilic coating is when one is mounting a stent onto an angioplasty balloon that has a hydrophilic coating. The balloon can be rubbed with an alcohol wipe and then with a wet sponge. This allows the stent to be mounted without fear of its movement before deployment.

ACCURATE MEASUREMENT OF A VESSEL, STENOSIS, ANEURYSM, OR OTHER STRUCTURE

For microvascular work, truly accurate measurement is necessary. Catheter marker bands (placed typically at every centimeter) can be erroneous if the catheter is not truly in the plane of measurement. An accurate method of measurement is by means of an external circular marker, such as a coin. A quarter is 24 mm in diameter; a dime is 17 mm (Fig. 3–7).

The greatest dimension of the coin shadow on the screen can *never* be less than the actual coin size if the coin is placed *over the lesion on one view and measured on the orthogonal view* (and thus has the same object-intensifier distance).

Interestingly, many practitioners, primarily cardiologists, use a metal ball similar to that found in a pinball machine. This is totally unnecessary; the geometry of the situation requires only a coin.

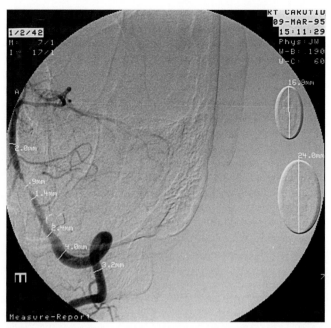

Figure 3-7 Demonstration of external markers (a dime and a quarter) for measurement purposes. A quarter measures 24 mm and a dime 17 mm (±0.1 mm). When the coin is placed tangentially (orthogonally) directly over a lesion (i.e., when one is looking from a plane 90 degrees from the intended measuring view), the greatest dimension can never be less than correct. The measurement can either yield true units of measure (e.g., millimeters) or the number of pixels from which a calculation can be made (depending on the software supplied with the angiography equipment). It is not necessary to place a ball bearing on the head, as some angiographers do.

Although the marker bands on catheters may not be accurate, the diameter of the tip of the catheter can be used as a reference standard (if the catheter is nontapered and if the final French size of the taper is known). If the tip of the catheter is adjacent to the structure to be measured, it should be in the same plane (i.e., have the same object-intensifier distance). By definition, 3-Fr. = 1 mm; this calibration factor can be used to measure the object. Note, however, that this method is extremely inaccurate!

Unfortunately, many of the measurements necessary for interventional neuroradiology require a degree of accuracy that is probably beyond the limits of resolution for most equipment used today. Even the high-resolution 1024 × 1024 matrix leaves a significant degree of uncertainty in dealing with measurements of a fraction of a millimeter. Simply measuring the catheter and then the vessel can yield wild ranges in size. For a 3-Fr. microcatheter, variations in measured size can be by only one pixel but still cause a discrepancy of as much as 20%. For example, in one case a microcatheter was used to measure a vessel for angioplasty. The catheter was measured for calibration, then the vessel measured, and finally an external quarter was measured. In three attempts, the size of the quarter was shown to be 28 mm, 17 mm, and 40 mm; a huge degree of inaccuracy! For this reason, measuring a larger object such as a quarter is far more accurate.

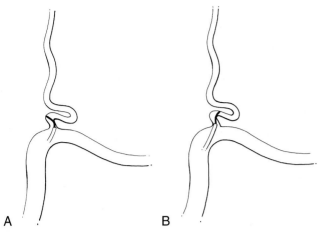

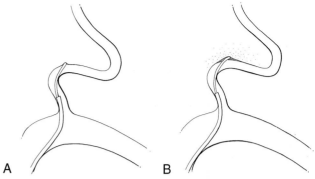

Figure 3-9 Safe catheterization of a tortuous vessel (continued). Close-up images demonstrate the result when attempts are made to forcibly advance the wire downstream. The wire impacts into the wall of the vessel along the outside of the curve (A); if forward pressure is continued, dissection or frank perforation can occur (B).

A

B

Figure 3-8 A and B, Safe catheterization of a tortuous vessel. These figures illustrate what happens when an attempt is made to select a tortuous vessel using the standard Terumo-type "glide" wire. The wire is aimed in the direction necessary to select the vessel (A); however, this results in the tip impacting into the outside of the first acute curve. No matter how the wire is rotated, the short segment protruding from the catheter (which is aimed into the orifice of the vessel) cannot negotiate the series of curves.

PUNCTURE THROUGH A GRAFT

Owing to the toughness of an artificial graft, it may be difficult to obtain access. If use of heparin or urokinase is a possibility, a clean puncture without a hole in the back wall is desirable. This is best achieved by using a micropuncture set (Cook, Inc.). The 21-gauge needle makes a clean puncture through the graft, and it does not matter if there is transgression of the back wall.

Once the small needle is in the vessel lumen, the monofilament wire usually leads the triaxial dilator system into position. However, if this is not possible because the toughness of the wall of the graft resists advancement of the plastic dilators, success can be achieved by using a 19-gauge Angiocath intravenous-type catheter as a dilating system. The steel needle of the Angiocath follows the wire and carries its plastic catheter into the vascular lumen. The plastic Angiocath is then used to introduce a 0.035″ stiff wire (Amplatz-type), over which a standard dilator and sheath or catheter can be advanced.

SAFE CATHETERIZATION OF DIFFICULT AND/OR TORTUOUS VESSELS

This technique is useful only for those experienced enough to recognize danger when they see it. Disastrous dissections during catheterization of the origin of the vertebral artery or a really tortuous distal internal carotid will truly make one appreciate safe technique and equipment.

While the advent of the newer hydrophilic-coated guidewires makes certain catheterizations more feasible, the angled tips of the commonly available types are not suitable for going around tight curves and can easily cause a dissection, particularly in a patient

with hard or brittle vessels (Figs. 3–8 and 3–9). A *very* soft and floppy tipped guidewire with a small tight C curve and a hydrophilic coating is ideal and will be commercially available from Cook, Inc. The standard-sized (3-mm) J curve guidewire without a hydrophilic coating can safely go downstream but is too large (actually larger than 3 mm) and too stiff for certain locations (e.g., the vertebral artery origin). In addition, most J curves are straight for their initial 3 to 4 mm before the curve actually starts, thereby complicating their safe and easy deployment from the catheter lumen into the vessel lumen. (They tend to jut sideways into the wall of the vessel before curling adequately.)

A truly safe way to access a distal territory is via a multistage approach (Figs. 3–10 to 3–14). The standard diagnostic catheter is placed near the origin of the vessel to be catheterized. First, a Seeker Standard (Target Therapeutics) type microguidewire with

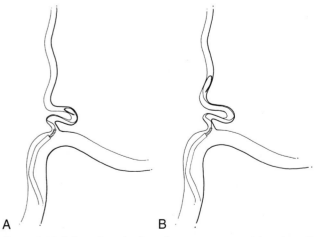

Figure 3-10 Safe catheterization of a tortuous vessel (continued). This vessel can be safely catheterized, however. The diagnostic catheter is left in a comfortable position in the parent vessel and a microcatheter and microwire are advanced through it. The vessel is selected with the microwire (with an appropriately shaped tip) (A). This wire will tend to stay within the lumen and advance downstream (B).

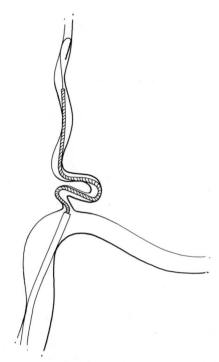

Figure 3-11 Safe catheterization of a tortuous vessel (continued). Once the wire is advanced safely downstream, the microcatheter is advanced over the wire until it is past the tortuous section and is sitting comfortably in the vessel.

a tight C curve or P curve is advanced downstream (not a hydrophilic-coated monofilament type— e.g., a gold-tipped Glidewire—unless it has a very tight C curve). Once this wire is safely into a straight segment of the target artery downstream (e.g., the vertebral artery at about the C3 or C4 level), a hydrophilic-coated microcatheter is advanced over it until the two are safely together (near the C3 level in the case of vertebral artery catheterization). The original

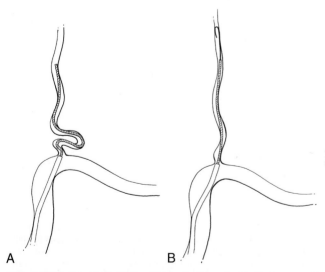

A   B

Figure 3-12 *A* and *B*, Safe catheterization of a tortuous vessel (continued). The microwire is then withdrawn and replaced with a stiff microwire, which straightens out the curves of the vessel. Again, this wire should have an atraumatic tip.

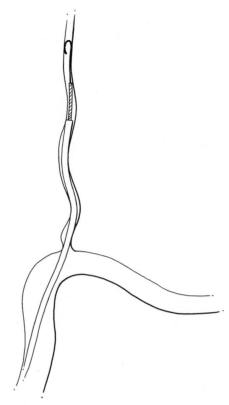

Figure 3-13 Safe catheterization of a tortuous vessel (continued). The diagnostic catheter can next be advanced over the stiff microwire and microcatheter into the distal vessel. One of the newer hydrophilic-coated catheters should be used.

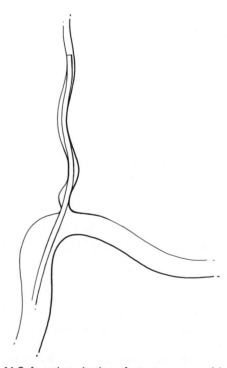

Figure 3-14 Safe catheterization of a tortuous vessel (continued). Once the diagnostic catheter is in position, the microwire and microcatheter are withdrawn, leaving the diagnostic catheter in location. This can then be exchanged for a true guide catheter, using a true neuroexchange wire, if desired.

microguidewire is then exchanged for a Platinum Plus–type microguidewire (Medi-Tech, Inc.). This has a very stiff 0.018″ shaft with a soft platinum coil tip. Once this wire is in place, the (soft) full-sized catheter that the microcatheter system has been placed through (such as the Vinuela or any other soft, diagnostic type of catheter) can follow over the microcatheter/Platinum Plus system until it is safely downstream. Once the standard-sized catheter is safely downstream, the microcatheter and microguidewire can be pulled. The standard-sized catheter can then be used for injection, or a full-sized (0.035″) *safe* exchange wire can be placed and a true guide catheter positioned for any further work.

PROTECTIVE EMBOLIZATION OF VITAL VESSELS

If accurate and safe direct catheterization of a specific side branch to be embolized is not possible, it may still be feasible to effectively embolize this side branch even when superselective catheterization cannot be achieved. This situation usually occurs when there is a small feeding branch originating at an acute angle from a normal parent vessel in a fashion not allowing the microcatheter to enter it directly, or when the branch is physically too small for the catheter to enter.

If this is the case, the microcatheter can be advanced past the target branch, and this distal normal parent vessel can then be occluded with coils. This will prevent any emboli from coursing distally into the normal distribution during the procedure. In the external circulation, this is almost uniformly tolerated. Knowledge of collateral supply to vital territories is necessary, however.

Once occlusion of the main vessel distal to the target side branch has been achieved, embolization with microparticles is then possible while the microcatheter remains within the parent vessel just proximal to the target branch. There is now no danger of perfusion of the vital distal capillary bed with embolic particles. After particulate embolization has been performed, coil embolization of the parent vessel just over the origin of the target branch is carried out. This completes the occlusion of the target vessel and adds no further hemodynamic alteration to the parent vessel than has already been achieved.

Attempts have been made to use a temporary agent to occlude the parent vessel. This has proved difficult, however, and it has been shown that permanent agents are entirely acceptable.

PREVENTION OF CATHETER-INDUCED SPASM

This is another of the examples of when the best therapy is to avoid the problem. The manner in which to address this problem can be either prospective or retrospective. A certain group of interventional neuroradiologists use sublingual nifedipine before a procedure, while others use a strip of nitroglycerin paste on the upper anterior chest wall to give a constant infusion of the drug.[10] The amount of this paste varies from 1″ to 5″. Reports have indicated that there are at least a few failures with only 1″ of nitroglycerin paste, but there is an almost guaranteed headache after the use of 5″ (albeit with apparent success as far as spasm is concerned!). Perhaps a happy medium of 2″ to 3″ of nitroglycerin paste will allow most procedures to be performed without difficulty. This is our preference.

For treatment of catheter-induced vasospasm after it occurs, there are several approaches. The use of inhaled amyl nitrite is described in Chapter 66. This is easy to administer but causes generalized systemic effects, possibly affecting normal vessels more than abnormal ones. Direct infusion of papaverine is described in Chapter 66 as well as in chapters discussing specific procedures; for acute local episodes of vasospasm, about 30 to 60 mg infused over about 3 to 10 minutes will suffice to relieve the problem.

Alternatively, nitroglycerin can be infused directly intra-arterially, usually with excellent results. A typical solution is 50 μg/ml of saline to be infused over approximately 20 to 90 seconds, but other doses can be used. We mix 2.5 ml of the standard 5 mg/ml solution into 250 ml of normal saline to produce this dilution. A commercially available preparation of 200 μg/ml is available but only in a large bottle. This can be diluted, however, to a slightly more reasonable concentration.

SPINAL ANGIOGRAPHY

Proper performance of spinal angiography requires both an organized approach with attention to detail and a thorough understanding of the vascular anatomy of the spinal cord. The vascular anatomy of the spinal cord is reviewed in Chapter 5.

As can be seen from Chapter 5, it is necessary to evaluate the vertebral arteries, ascending and deep (posterior) cervical arteries, iliolumbar arteries, middle sacral artery and/or lateral sacral arteries, and intercostal and lumbar arteries, depending on the part of the cord to be studied and the reason for performing the examination. Attention to detail with meticulous thoroughness is required. The method is detailed below.

The patient should be positioned on the table with a yardstick containing radiopaque markers, such as the type used for evaluating leg length, under the length of the spine, but 5 to 8 cm off center. This can be adjusted to lie on either side of the spine as needed to avoid interfering with the study. The position along the yardstick of each vertebral level (vertebral body) is recorded by an assistant and documented with spot films before any angiograms are performed. This permits assessment and confirmation when the angiograms are reviewed later.

Access is then gained to the arterial system (usually via the common femoral artery) and a short sheath is inserted. The short sheath will allow for extensive manipulation of the catheter without interfering with selection of lower lumbar or iliac branches.

Although many different catheters have been utilized for spinal angiography, we prefer to shape our own from a 5.5-Fr. Vinuela catheter (see "How to Steam a Catheter" above). The desired final curve produces a tip at a right angle to the vessel wall, with the horizontal tip slightly longer (about 1 cm) than the diameter of the aorta at the level(s) to be studied, so that it will fall into any orifice. This allows the catheter to brace against the opposite wall of the aorta, and permits selection of branches while both advancing and withdrawing the catheter.

Remember that the aorta tapers as it descends; the catheter will have to be reshaped during the procedure if many levels are being studied. This is another reason for placing a sheath—ease of catheter exchange. As the steamed curve relaxes slightly when the mandrel is removed and on introduction into the body, it is necessary to exaggerate the curve slightly into a gentle arc (beyond 90 degrees) when steaming the catheter.

Since the catheter relaxes somewhat during the procedure, it may be desirable to start at the larger part of the aorta while most of the curve is still present. By the time the lower aorta is reached, the catheter may have lost most of its curve but still be working correctly. Once the appropriate curve is obtained, the orifices of the left and right intercostal (and/or lumbar) arteries at each level of interest are selected, using the predetermined position of each vertebral segment along the ruler as a guide. Remember that the intercostal and lumbar arteries arise from the posterolateral walls of the aorta; the lumbar arteries in particular may arise either very closely together or even as one trunk. In addition, as a person ages, the aorta can rotate, resulting in both vessels arising from one side or the other.

A careful test injection is performed to confirm the position of the catheter, properly position the patient, and make sure that the vessel is not occluded by the catheter, if possible. Contrast is then gently injected by hand while digital subtraction images are obtained. These are small vessels! Only 0.5 to 2 ml of contrast is needed. Images should be obtained in the posteroanterior plane at a minimum, along with any necessary oblique views. If a biplane unit is being used, one plane can be set at the posteroanterior position and the other at a 60-degree oblique position, or lateral where possible. An assistant should keep track (with note of the corresponding ruler level) of which arteries have been studied as the examination progresses, so that none are inadvertently omitted.

CAROTID COMPRESSION PROCEDURE FOR CAROTID-CAVERNOUS FISTULAE

This is actually a combined carotid-jugular compression technique. This procedure is discussed in Chapter 19. It is primarily used for the treatment of minimally symptomatic or asymptomatic carotid-cavernous fistulae, or ones that have been incompletely treated.

The goal of this therapy is to give the body the chance to heal itself. The idea behind this is that if the flow through the fistula can be stopped for a time, the venous side (or small holes) may thrombose, thus stopping the leak. This is obviously possible only if the arteriovenous shunting is very slow.

The patient is instructed to compress the carotid artery on the side of the pathology by using the opposite hand. The opposite hand is used in case intracranial ischemia develops (the arm will become weak, thus releasing the artery). This procedure should be done with the patient sitting comfortably, and should last 30 to 300 seconds. There is no controlled study indicating that a particular duration or frequency of compression works better than any other. However, patience can be rewarded, and this procedure can be performed relatively safely for weeks, with eventual success.

The act of compressing the carotid artery also compresses the jugular vein, thus hopefully rendering stasis of flow within the cavernous sinus and the fistula on both an arterial and a venous basis. This can thus allow thrombus formation in the cavernous sinus and potentially cure the fistula. This maneuver has resulted in at least one reported inadvertent death, but this was considered an aberration, and the technique has been employed successfully for years.[12]

Any drugs interfering with clotting are to be avoided during this time (typically antiplatelet agents such as aspirin and nonsteroidal anti-inflammatory drugs). This procedure is also contraindicated in any patient with cortical venous drainage (the increased venous pressure may induce a cortical venous infarct) or with a hypercoagulable state (the carotid stasis may allow thrombi to form). Also, patients with atheromata in the carotid bifurcation should not risk disruption of this with subsequent intracranial embolization. Success may be noted by the patient if there is a change in any audible bruit that may be present (the noise may either stop or change in pitch).

When thrombosis of the cavernous sinus occurs, there may be a transient worsening of any cavernous sinus syndrome symptoms owing to the mass effect of the thrombus; this generally improves after a matter of days.

This same maneuver can be performed by compressing the superior ophthalmic vein as it exits the orbit above the eye.

DIRECT PUNCTURE OF THE CAROTID ARTERY

On occasion, it is necessary to obtain access to the carotid system directly through the neck. This vessel is incredibly tough and thick walled. Direct puncture of the carotid artery for angiography was formerly routine, and, amazingly, is relatively safe. For simple angiography, the old technique of simply puncturing the vessel and injecting directly through the needle is perhaps still the most efficient means (although perhaps not the safest) to accomplish this task, particularly if care is taken to place the needletip safely under fluoroscopic guidance and secure the needle carefully to the skin. A single-wall puncture is far preferable to a double-wall puncture for hemostatic purposes; the back wall is not compressed at all by external pressure without totally occluding the vessel, and it may bleed throughout the procedure. This has apparently been of minimal consequence in the past, however.

For interventional purposes, access to the carotid artery should be achieved with as little trauma to the vessel as possible. The puncture site is likely to be used for several hours; any endothelial damage may be worsened by the indwelling catheter and hemostasis will either not be easily possible or be inadvertently overlooked.

The micropuncture set from Cook, Inc. should be utilized (see Chapter 1). A single-wall stick is possible; the small 21-gauge needle punctures the artery with more finesse than larger 18- to 19-gauge needles. A low puncture site should be chosen; a Trendelenburg position, either at the time of the procedure or beforehand, will help localize the jugular vein if there is doubt regarding its location. The jugular vein lies in a variable position posterior and lateral to the carotid artery. The anterior jugular veins are superficial to the carotid sheath and may or may not be present; they may be large, or invisibly in the line of puncture. The internal jugular vein itself may be huge and nearly unmissable. The sternocleidomastoid muscle is anterolateral to the vascular bundle, giving support to the puncture site. The point of maximal impulse is usually at or near the carotid bifurcation; thus, a puncture site well below this point is indicated. Approximately 1″ to 2″ above the clavicle is a reasonable location. In the "old days," ultrasound was not available to help evaluate the normal architecture, but is useful whenever this procedure is to be performed.

If the head is maximally extended, the external carotid artery can be directly punctured if an entry point slightly cephalad is used. Usually the indication for direct puncture, however, is entry into the internal carotid artery or access to the region of the bifurcation; therefore, a low puncture into the common carotid artery is necessary, as described above.

The angle of puncture should be about 20 degrees lateral to a vertical (anteroposterior) line as viewed on an axial slice and about 30 degrees from the horizontal (with the needle aimed cephalad, obviously). This somewhat anterior approach will help avoid the jugular vein, if it can be avoided at all, because it will tend to be lateral to the carotid artery.

A low approach, i.e., comfortably over the clavicle, helps ensure that the entry site is below the carotid bifurcation; entry directly into the internal carotid artery is to be avoided owing to the incidence of preexisting atheromatous disease in the proximal internal carotid artery. Obviously, if direct entry is made into one of the two vessels (the internal or external carotid arteries), it will invariably be the other vessel that is the intended target.

The wire that comes with the micropuncture set allows safe advancement until the stiff monofilament shaft is reached, thus allowing easier entry of the dilator set. The wire should be fluoroscopically observed before removal of the needle and replacement with the dilator set, which should also be observed as it is advanced. Caution should be used when advancing the sheath set; it may be longer than the cervical internal carotid artery. After it has reached a comfortable location, the inner sleeve can be removed and contrast injection can be utilized to ascertain its position. A curved guidewire can then be used to select the particular branch needed, either the internal carotid artery or any external carotid branch.

Dilators should always be used before upsizing a catheter; the carotid artery is very tough, and possible intimal damage from the forceful insertion of a blunt catheter tip must be avoided. A working sheath can be placed, but the smaller the puncture site the better. The use of a guide catheter without a sheath is recommended (i.e., one that has its own dilator [see "How to Introduce a Guide Catheter" above]). This yields only a 6-Fr. hole (or 4-Fr. if the 4-Fr. Omniguide [Medtronic/MIS] is used).

Pediatric sizes of guide catheters and microcatheters are available. One must make sure the lengths used are compatible. Short (pediatric) TRACKER catheters are available; care should be taken not to use a guide catheter longer than the microcatheter.

USEFUL MEASUREMENTS AND CONVERSIONS

The information in Tables 3–1 and 3–2 is useful for trying to figure out what size catheters and wires will work with each other and what size guide catheter is needed for a certain balloon or stent, and for estimating the relative size of structures and objects seen fluoroscopically. Now that certain companies are providing a coherent set of catheters, guidewires, dila-

T A B L E 3 - 1 Equivalence of Inches, Millimeters, and French Sizes

French*	Millimeters (OD)	Inches (OD)
1	0.33	0.013
2	0.67	0.026
3	1.0	0.039
4	1.33	0.053
5	1.67	0.066
6	2.0	0.079
7	2.33	0.092
8	2.67	0.105
9	3.0	0.118
10	3.33	0.131
12	4.0	0.158
14	4.67	0.184
15	5.0	0.197
16	5.33	0.210
18	6.0	0.236

*By definition, 3-Fr. = 1 mm ~ 0.0394″.
OD, outer diameter.

T A B L E 3 - 2   Catheter and Needle Sizing

French*	OD (inches)	Gauge (inches)	Needle ID (inches)	Guide Catheter ID (inches)	Sheath OD (inches)
1	0.013	29	0.008		
2	0.026	~23	0.014		
3	0.039	~19.5	0.026		
4	0.053	~17.7	0.043		
5	0.066	~16	0.052	~0.039–0.042	~0.088
6	0.079	~14.4	0.067	~0.062–0.066	~0.101
7	0.092	~13.3	0.074	~0.052–0.066	~0.114
8	0.105	~12.3	0.087	~0.063–0.079	~0.125
9	0.118	~11.2	0.098	~0.084–0.092	~0.152
10	0.131	~10.2	0.111		
12	0.158	~ 8.4	0.136		
14	0.184	~ 6.8			

*By definition, 3-Fr. = 1 mm ~ 0.0394".
OD, outer diameter; ID, inner diameter.

tors, stents, and so forth, this information may not be as useful as it once was. Nevertheless, the reader may want to copy it and put it on a wall.

As mentioned previously, coins can be used to measure structures accurately:

$$\text{Diameter of a quarter} = 24 \text{ mm}$$

$$\text{Diameter of a dime} = 17 \text{ mm}$$

Other useful measurements and conversions:

$$1 \text{ pound} = 454 \text{ gm} \qquad 1 \text{ kg} = 2.2 \text{ lb}$$

$$1 \text{ ml} = 0.034 \text{ oz} \qquad 1 \text{ oz} = 29.6 \text{ ml}$$

$$1 \text{ qt} = 947 \text{ ml} \qquad 1 \text{ L} = 1.1 \text{ qt}$$

REFERENCES

1. Vorstrup S, Brun B, Lassen NA. Evaluation of the cerebral vasodilatory capacity by the acetazolamide test before EC-IC bypass surgery in patients with occlusion of the internal carotid artery. *Stroke* 1986;17:1291–1298.
2. Rogg J, Rutigliano M, Yonas H, et al. The acetazolamide challenge: imaging techniques designed to evaluate cerebral blood flow reserve. *AJR* 1989;153:605–612.
3. Batjer HH, Devous MD. The use of acetazolamide-enhanced regional cerebral blood flow measurement to predict risk for arteriovenous malformation patients. *Neurosurgery* 1992; 31:213–217.
4. Cross DT. Interventional neuroradiology. *Curr Opin Neurol* 1993;6:891–899.
5. Berenstein A, Lasjaunias P. Surgical Neuroangiography, Vol 4: Endovascular Treatment of Cerebral Lesions. New York: Springer-Verlag, 1992, pp 195–196.
6. Rauch R, Vinuela F, Dion J, et al. Preembolization functional evaluation in brain arteriovenous malformations: the superselective Amytal test. *AJNR* 1992;13:303–308.
7. Rauch R, Vinuela F, Dion J, et al. Preembolization functional evaluation in brain arteriovenous malformations: the ability of superselective Amytal test to predict neurological dysfunction before embolization. *AJNR* 1992;13:309–314.
8. Peters KR, Quisling RG, Gilmore R, et al. Intraarterial use of sodium methohexital for provocative testing during brain embolotherapy. *AJNR* 1993;14:171–174.
9. Horton JA, Dawson RC III. Retinal Wada test. *AJNR* 1988;9:1167–1168.
10. Kurata A, Miyasaka Y, Tanaka C, et al. Prevention of compli- cations during endovascular surgery on the external carotid arteries, with special reference to use of nitropaste and the lidocaine test. *Intervent Neuroradiol* 1996;2:193–200.
11. Lee DH, Wreidt CH, Kaufmann JCE, et al. Evaluation of three embolic agents in pig rete. *AJNR* 1989;10:773–776.
12. Halbach VV, Higashida RT, Hieshima GB, et al. Dural fistulas involving the cavernous sinus: results in treatment of 30 patients. *Radiology* 1987;163:437–442.

ADDITIONAL READINGS

Arteriogram

Alhalabi M, Moore PM. Serial angiography in isolated angiitis of the central nervous system. Neurology 1994;44:1221–1226.
Slavotinek J, Kendall SW, Flower CDR, et al. Radiological evaluation of the ascending aorta following repair of type A dissection. *Cardiovasc Intervent Radiol* 1993;16:293–296.
Tsai FY, Wadley D, Angle JF, et al. Superselective ophthalmic angiography for diagnostic and therapeutic use. *AJNR* 1990;11:1203–1204.

Diamox Challenge Test

Mandai K, Sueyoshi K, Fukunaga R, et al. Acetazolamide challenge for three-dimensional time-of-flight MR angiography of the brain. *AJNR* 1994;15:659–665.
Muller M, Voges M, Piepgras U, Schimrigk K. Assessment of cerebral vasomotor reactivity by transcranial Doppler ultrasound and breath-holding: a comparison with acetazolamide as vasodilatory stimulus. *Stroke* 1995;26:96–100.
Piepgras A, Schmiedek P, Leinsinger G, et al. A simple test to assess cerebrovascular reserve capacity using transcranial Doppler sonography and acetazolamide. *Stroke* 1990;21:1306–1311.
Ringelstein EB, Van Eyck S, Mertens I. Evaluation of cerebral vasomotor reactivity by various vasodilating stimuli: comparison of CO_2 to acetazolamide. *J Cereb Blood Flow Metab* 1992;12:162–168.
Sorteberg W, Lindegaard K-F, Rootwelt K, et al. Effect of acetazolamide on cerebral artery blood velocity and regional cerebral blood flow in normal subjects. *Acta Neurochir* 1989;97:139–145.
Yonas H, Smith H, Durham S, et al. Increased stroke risk predicted by compromised cerebral blood flow reactivity. *J Neurosurg* 1993;79:483–489.

How to Test a Vessel

Katsuta R, Morioka T, Hasuo K, et al. Discrepancy between provocative test and clinical results following endovascular obliteration of spinal arteriovenous malformation. *Surg Neurol* 1993;40:142–145.

Pharmacology in Interventional Neuroradiology

J.C. Wojak

Many types of medications are routinely employed before, during, and after interventional neuroradiologic procedures. These include drugs administered as part of a procedure (e.g., thrombolysis, treatment of vasospasm, functional testing), those given as part of the patient's periprocedural management (e.g., sedation, analgesia), and those administered as part of the patient's long-term management (e.g., anticoagulants, antiplatelet drugs). Interventional neuroradiologists should be thoroughly familiar with the drugs they use during the course of procedures and during the periprocedural period, and should have a working knowledge of those drugs that may be employed as part of the ongoing management of patients.

The following is not meant to be an exhaustive review of commonly used drugs; the reader is referred to a pharmacology text for this information. What is presented here is a brief overview of the types of medications routinely employed and what they are used for, along with a chart outlining pertinent information concerning the most utilized drugs in each group, such as doses, duration of action, primary effects, adverse reactions, and reversal (Tables 4–1A and B).

EMBOLIC AGENTS

Ethyl alcohol and sodium tetradecyl sulfate are sclerosing agents used in the embolization of vascular malformations. The use of ethyl alcohol is described in Chapter 3 and in specific chapters dealing with the embolization of brain arteriovenous malformations and vascular malformations of the head and neck. Its use is accompanied by hazards such as tissue necrosis and cardiopulmonary collapse; these are discussed in Chapter 64.

As described in Chapter 1, sodium tetradecyl sulfate (Sotradecol) is a sclerosing agent that can be used either transarterially or via direct puncture. Unlike alcohol, it is a painless agent; therefore, less sedation is required for its use. It can be opacified by diluting 1:1 with nonionic contrast material.

LOCAL ANESTHETICS

Local anesthetic agents are used to provide analgesia at the site of percutaneous needle or catheter entry during a procedure. They are also utilized in the performance of nerve blocks for diagnostic and therapeutic purposes. The most commonly used local anesthetic agents are lidocaine (Xylocaine) and bupivacaine (Marcaine, Sensorcaine). Lidocaine has a more rapid onset of action; bupivacaine has a longer duration of activity.

SEDATION

Although many different classes of drugs are used for sedation, benzodiazepines are among the most frequently utilized. Midazolam (Versed) is a very-short-acting benzodiazepine and is often used for intravenous (IV) sedation during procedures. It is easily titrated and often given in conjunction with a short-acting opioid such as fentanyl citrate (Sublimaze). Lorazepam (Ativan) has a longer duration of action and can be given IV or intramuscularly (IM); unfortunately, it tends to cause paradoxical agitation in elderly patients and in individuals who are agitated because of alterations in neurologic function (e.g., patients with subarachnoid hemorrhage). The authors therefore tend to avoid lorazepam. Diazepam (Valium) is a long-acting benzodiazepine. It is unreliable if given IM owing to variable absorption. When given IV, diazepam can be difficult to titrate, leading to repeated administration of small doses without apparent effect until the total dose administered becomes substantial and the patient suddenly becomes profoundly sedated. The drug is slowly cleared from the body and can accumulate in body fat, leading to prolonged and fluctuating drug effect, which may be problematic when neurologic status must be followed closely.

Other agents used for sedation include diphenhydramine hydrochloride (Benadryl) and hydroxyzine hydrochloride (Vistaril). Hydroxyzine is usually given IM in conjunction with meperidine hydrochloride (Demerol) as a premedication for short procedures in which the need for prolonged sedation and titration of sedation is not anticipated. It is also useful as an antiemetic, as noted below.

When reversal of action of benzodiazepines is required (because of overdosage or a need to assess the patient's neurologic status), flumazenil (Romazicon) can be administered IV. When long-acting benzodiazepines (e.g., diazepam) have been given, a repeat dose of flumazenil may be needed in 1 to 2 hours.

ANALGESIA

For relatively short procedures in which repeated doses are not expected to be needed and in which

T A B L E 4 – 1A   Commonly Used Drugs Listed by Type

Analgesics

Ketorolac tromethamine (Toradol)
Meperidine (Demerol)

Antibiotics

Cefazolin sodium (Ancef)
Ceftriaxone sodium (Rocephin)
Cephalexin monohydrate (Keflex)
Vancomycin (Vancocin)

Anticoagulants

Dalteparin sodium (Fragmin)
Enoxaparin (Lovenox)
Heparin sodium
Warfarin sodium (Coumadin)

Anticonvulsants

Fosphenytoin (Cerebyx)
Phenobarbital
Phenytoin sodium (Dilantin)

Antiemetics

Droperidol (Inapsine)
Hydroxyzine HCl (Vistaril)
Ondansetron HCl (Zofran)
Promethazine HCl (Phenergan) (also a sedative)

Antihypertensives

Labetalol HCl (Normodyne, Trandate)
Sodium nitroprusside (Nipride)

Antiplatelet Agents

Abciximab (ReoPro)
Acetylsalicylic acid (aspirin)
Dipyridamole (Persantine)
Ticlopidine HCl (Ticlid)

Antiulcer Agents

Ranitidine HCl (Zantac)
Sucralfate (Carafate)

Cardiovascular Agents

Dobutamine HCl (Dobutrex)
Dopamine HCl (Dopastat, Inotropin)
Levarterenol (norepinephrine) bitartrate (Levophed)
Metaraminol bitartrate (Aramine)
Phentolamine mesylate (Regitine)

Drugs for Neurologic Testing

Acetazolamide (Diamox)
Amobarbital (Amytal)
Methohexital (Brevital)

Embolic Agents

Ethanol
Sodium tetradecyl sulfate (Sotradecol)

Local Anesthetics

Bupivicaine (Marcaine, Sensorcaine)
Lidocaine HCl (Xylocaine)
Procaine HCl (Novocain)

Miscellaneous Agents

Low-molecular-weight dextran (Rheomacrodex)
Mannitol
Probucol

Neuroprotectants

Dexamethasone sodium phosphate (Decadron Phosphate)
Methylprednisolone (Medrol)
Methylprednisolone sodium succinate (Solu-Medrol)
Nimodipine (Nimotop) (also a vasodilator)

Prothrombotic Agents/Reversal of Anticoagulation

ϵ-Aminocaproic (Amicar)
Protamine sulfate
Vitamin K_1 (phytonadione) (AquaMEPHYTON)

Sedative Reversal

Flumazenil (Romazicon)
Naloxone (Narcan)

Sedatives

Diazepam (Valium)
Diphenhydramine HCl (Benadryl)
Fentanyl (Sublimaze)
Midazolam (Versed)
Morphine sulfate

Thrombolytic Agents

Streptokinase (Streptase)
Tissue-type plasminogen activator (alteplase) (Activase)
Urokinase (Abbokinase)

Vasodilators

Amyl nitrite
Nifedipine (Procardia) (also an antihypertensive)
Nitroglycerin (Nitro-Bid) (also an antihypertensive,
   cardiovascular agent)
Papaverine hydrochloride
Prostacyclin (epoprostenol) (Flolan)
Prostaglandin E_1 (alprostadil)

---

reversal of sedation or analgesia is not anticipated (for functional testing or temporary test occlusion), meperidine can be utilized, usually in conjunction with hydroxyzine hydrochloride. It has a slightly shorter duration of action than morphine sulfate and a more rapid onset of action.

When titration of analgesia and sedation is required (e.g., prolonged procedures, need for reversal during the procedure, need for transient increase in analgesia during embolization with alcohol), fentanyl citrate is a good choice. It is rapid in onset of activity, short acting, and readily titrated. It is often used in conjunction with midazolam, as noted above. This is the combination of drugs preferred by most anesthesiology personnel for conscious sedation and analgesia.

For postprocedure analgesia, we prefer ketorolac tromethamine (Toradol), a nonsteroidal anti-inflammatory drug available in both oral and injectable forms. It is a potent analgesic but has no effect on central nervous system function, allowing for accurate evaluation of neurologic function. Because of its anti-inflammatory and antipyretic effects, it is an excellent agent for the treatment of the postemboli-

Text continued on page 73

T A B L E 4 – 1B Commonly Used Drugs

Drug	Class	Half-Life	Dosage/Route of Administration/ How Supplied	Primary Effects	Side Effects*	Contraindications	Treatment of Toxicity
Abciximab (ReoPro)	Fab antibody fragment	30 min	IV: 0.25 mg/kg bolus prior to PTCA, then 10 μg/min for 12 hr (no other doses established). 2 mg/ml (5-ml vials)	Binds to receptor sites on platelets, blocking fibrinogen-associated aggregation	Bleeding, thrombocytopenia, arrhythmia, dizziness, disorientation	Active or recent GI or GU bleed, bleeding disorder, recent stroke, hypertension, thrombocytopenia, recent surgery, intracranial vascular abnormality, sensitivity	Supportive
Acetazolamide (Diamox)	Carbonic anhydrase inhibitor	?	IV: 1 gm for challenge test. 500-mg vials (reconstituted with 5 ml sterile water)	CNS carbonic acidosis resulting in vasodilation via autoregulation	Hypokalemia, hyperglycemia, drowsiness, anxiety, nausea/vomiting, rash/ urticaria	Sensitivity to sulfonamides, electrolyte imbalance, severe renal/hepatic disease	Correct electrolytes and hydration
ε-Aminocaproic acid (Amicar)	Antifibrinolytic	2 hr	IV: 4–5 gm over first hour, then 1 gm/hr for total of 8 hr or until bleeding is controlled. PO: 5 gm in first hour, then 1–1.25 gm/hr for 8 hr or until controlled. 250 mg/ ml (20-ml vials)	Inhibits plasminogen activation, antiplasmin activity	Nausea, hypotension, dizziness, tinnitus, headache, rash, myopathy	Active intravascular clotting (DIC), sensitivity	Supportive
Amobarbital (Amytal)	Barbiturate	?	Intra-arterial: ≈60–115 mg for Wada, 25–75 mg for functional testing of a vessel. 500-mg vials (for reconstitution)	Depresses CNS activity	CNS depression, nausea/ vomiting, rash/urticaria, hypotension, bradycardia, respiratory depression	Sensitivity to barbiturates, respiratory depression, liver impairment	Supportive
Amyl nitrite	Nitrate	5–10 min	Inhalation: 0.15 or 0.3 ml as needed, may repeat in 3–5 min. 0.15- and 0.3-ml ampules	Vascular smooth muscle relaxation	Tachycardia, headache, dizziness, nausea/ vomiting, flushing, hypotension	Sensitivity to nitrates, increased intracranial pressure, hypertension	Supportive
ASA (Aspirin)	Prostaglandin inhibitor	15–20 min	PO: One tablet (325 mg) daily for therapy of thromboembolic diseases. 325-mg (5-grain) tablets	Inhibits prostaglandin-mediated platelet aggregation	Thrombocytopenia, neutropenia, nausea/ vomiting, GI bleeding, rash/urticaria, tinnitus/ hearing loss, wheezing, hypoglycemia, hyponatremia	Sensitivity to salicylates, GI bleeding, bleeding disorders, vitamin K deficiency, peptic ulcer, children under 3 yr of age or with flulike symptoms	Supportive

Table continued on following page

61

T A B L E 4 – 1B Commonly Used Drugs *Continued*

Drug	Class	Half-Life	Dosage/Route of Administration/ How Supplied	Primary Effects	Side Effects*	Contraindications	Treatment of Toxicity
Atropine sulfate	Anticholinergic	?	IV: 0.5–1.0 mg, may repeat every 5 min up to 2 mg; IM: 0.4–0.6 mg 45–60 min prior to procedure as prophylaxis. 0.5–1.2 mg/ml (1 ml vials)	Inhibits acetylcholine at parasympathetic junctions, blocks vagal effect on SA node	Headache, restlessness, coma, insomnia, dizziness, tachycardia, palpitations, angina, blurry vision, mydriasis, dry mouth, constipation	Glaucoma, obstructive uropathy, GI obstruction, myasthenia gravis, ileus, toxic megacolon	Physostigmine, supportive
Bupivacaine (Marcaine, Sensorcaine)	Amide-type local anesthetic	2.7–3.5 hr	Injectable: Total dose depends on route and site. 0.25%, 0.5%, 0.75% with and without epinephrine and preservative (5- and 30-ml ampules; 10-, 30-, and 50-ml vials)	Competes with calcium for nerve membrane sites, blocks action potential	Anxiety, restlessness, drowsiness, myocardial depression, arrhythmia, hypotension, nausea/ vomiting, rash/urticaria, blurry vision, tinnitus, asthma	Sensitivity to amide-type local anesthetics, severe liver disease	Supportive
Cefazolin sodium (Ancef)	Semisynthetic cephalosporin	1.8–2 hr	IV/IM: 500 mg–1 gm every 6–8 hr. 500-mg and 1-gm vials (reconstitute with 2 ml sterile water)	Inhibits cell wall synthesis	Thrush, pseudomembranous enterocolitis, nausea, vomiting, rash/urticaria, Stevens-Johnson syndrome, leukopenia, thrombocytopenia	Sensitivity to cephalosporins (caution in patients with sensitivity to penicillin)	Supportive, oral vancomycin for pseudomembranous enterocolitis
Ceftriaxone sodium (Rocephin)	Semisynthetic cephalosporin	5.8–8.7 hr	IV/IM: 1 gm single dose (preop) or 1–2 gm every 12 hr. 250 mg/ml (250-, 500-, and 1-gm vials)	Inhibits cell wall synthesis	Thrush, pseudomembranous enterocolitis, nausea, vomiting, rash/urticaria, Stevens-Johnson syndrome, leukopenia, thrombocytopenia/cytosis, eosinophilia, elevated liver enzymes	Sensitivity to cephalosporins (caution in patients with sensitivity to penicillin)	Supportive, oral vancomycin for pseudomembranous enterocolitis
Cephalexin (Keflex)	Semisynthetic cephalosporin	≈4 hr	PO: 250–500 mg every 6 hr. 250- and 500-mg capsules, 25, 50, and 100 mg/ml oral suspension (100- and 200-ml bottles)	Inhibits cell wall synthesis	Thrush, pseudomembranous enterocolitis, nausea, vomiting, rash/urticaria, Stevens-Johnson syndrome, leukopenia, thrombcytopenia	Sensitivity to cephalosporins (caution in patients with sensitivity to penicillin)	Supportive, oral vancomycin for pseudomembranous enterocolitis
Dalteparin sodium (Fragmin)	Anticoagulant (low-molecular-weight heparinoid)	3.5 hr	Subcutaneous: 2500–5000 U daily. 2500- and 5000-U syringes	Enhances inhibition of factor X_a by antithrombin	Local hematoma, thrombocytopenia, bleeding	Sensitivity to heparins or pork, major bleeding, heparin-induced thrombocytopenia, bleeding disorder, hemorrhagic stroke, intracranial surgery	Protamine, supportive

Drug	Classification	Half-life	Dosage	Action	Side effects	Contraindications	Treatment
Dexamethasone sodium phosphate (Decadron Phosphate)	Synthetic adrenocorticoid	?	IV: 0.75–50 mg every 6 hr; PO: 0.75–16 mg every 6 hr. 4 mg/ml (1-, 5-, 25-ml vials)	Free radical scavenger, inhibits lipid peroxidation, stabilizes cell membranes, reduces cerebral edema	Fluid/electrolyte disturbances, muscle weakness, peptic ulcer, bowel perforation, pancreatitis, impaired healing, rash/urticaria, vertigo, headache, psychosis, seizure, hyperglycemia, increased intraocular pressure, myocardial rupture with recent infarction	Sensitivity, fungal sepsis	Supportive
Diazepam (Valium)	Benzodiazepine	20–70 hr	IV: ≈5–20 mg as needed for adequate sedation; generally in 5 to 10-mg doses. 5 mg/ml (2- and 10-ml vials)	Potentiates action of GABA in CNS	CNS depression, paradoxical stimulation, nausea/vomiting, rash, hypotension, blurry vision, tinnitus, respiratory depression	Sensitivity to benzodiazepines, narrow-angle glaucoma, psychosis, <18 yr of age	Flumazenil, supportive
Diphenhydramine HCl (Benadryl)	Histamine (H_1) blocker	6–8 hr	IV/IM: 25–50 mg, repeat as needed (up to 400 mg over 2 hr). 50 mg/ml (1 ml syringes and ampules, 10-ml vials)	Antihistamine, anticholinergic	Drowsiness, dizziness, discoordination, urinary retention, urticaria/rash, chills, thickened secretions	Sensitivity, MAO inhibitor therapy, asthma	Supportive
Dipyridamole (Persantine)	Non-nitrate vasodilator	10–12 hr	PO: 50–100 mg 3–4 times daily for treatment of TIAs and/or platelet inhibition. 25-, 50-, and 75-mg tablets	Coronary vasodilation; inhibits platelet adhesion	Hypotension, headache, dizziness, nausea/vomiting, rash	Hypersensitivity, hypotension	Phenylephrine, supportive
Dobutamine HCl (Dobutrex)	β-Adrenergic agonist	2 min	IV: 2.5–10 μg/min as needed to optimize cardiac output. 12.5 mg/ml (20-ml vials)	Decreases preload and afterload	Headache, tachycardia, hypertension, angina, arrhythmias, nausea/vomiting, dyspnea	Sensitivity, idiopathic hypertrophic subaortic stenosis	Supportive
Dopamine HCl (Dopastat, Inotropin)	Dopaminergic, α- and β-adrenergic agonist	?	IV: 2–5 μg/kg/min, titrate at 10–30 min intervals. 40–160 mg/ml (1-ml vials); 0.8–3.2 mg/ml in D_5W (250-ml bags)	Stimulates sympathetic receptors	Headache, arrhythmia, hypotension, nausea/vomiting	Tachyarrhythmia, pheochromocytoma, ventricular fibrillation	Supportive
Droperidol (Inapsine)	Neuroleptic/antiemetic	2.2 hr	IV/IM: 0.625 mg as needed (as antiemetic). 2.5 mg/ml (1-, 2-, and 5-ml vials)	Centrally acting antiemetic	Hypotension, tachycardia, dysphoria, drowsiness, paradoxical agitation, dystonia, hallucination, dizziness, chills, wheezing, malignant hyperthermia	Sensitivity	Anticholinergic for dystonia, dantrolene for hyperthermia, supportive

Table continued on following page

T A B L E 4 – 1B Commonly Used Drugs *Continued*

Drug	Class	Half-Life	Dosage/Route of Administration/ How Supplied	Primary Effects	Side Effects*	Contraindications	Treatment of Toxicity
Enoxaparin sodium (Lovenox)	Anticoagulant (low-molecular-weight heparinoid)	4.5 hr	SC: 30 mg every 12 hr. 30-mg syringes	Enhances inhibition of factor X_a by antithrombin	Local hematoma, thrombocytopenia, bleeding	Sensitivity to heparins or pork, major bleeding, heparin-induced thrombocytopenia, bleeding disorder, hemorrhagic stroke, intracranial surgery	Protamine, supportive
Ethyl alcohol (dehydrated)	Sclerosing/ neurolytic agent	?	Ganglion block: 0.5–1.5 ml; Intra-arterial: up to 1.0 ml/kg (preferably 0.5 ml/kg or less). 1, 2, 5-ml ampules	Dehydration of cells and precipitation of protoplasm	Cardiopulmonary collapse, thrombosis, tissue edema and necrosis, neural damage, post-injection neuritis	Pregnancy	Nitroglycerin for cardiopulmonary collapse, supportive
Fentanyl citrate (Sublimaze)	Synthetic opiate	3.6 hr	IV: 0.05–0.1 mg as needed for analgesia/ sedation. 1 mg/ml (2-ml ampules, 10-ml vials)	Inhibits CNS pain pathways	Dizziness, delirium, nausea/ vomiting, blurry vision, bradycardia, hypotension, respiratory depression	Sensitivity to opiates, myasthenia gravis	Naloxone, supportive
Flumazenil (Romazicon)	Benzodiazepine receptor antagonist	41–79 min	IV: 0.2 mg over 15 sec every 60 sec as needed (up to 1 mg) for reversal; 0.2 mg over 30 sec, followed by 0.3 mg at least 30 sec later (over 30 sec), followed by 0.5 mg over 30 sec every 1 min (up to 3 mg) for overdose. 0.1 mg/ml (5-ml vial)	Inhibits activity of benzodiazepine recognition site on GABA/ benzodiazepine receptor complex	Blurry vision, tinnitus, hypertension, palpitations, arrhythmia, chest pain, nausea/vomiting, dizziness, agitation, seizure, headache, rigors	Sensitivity to flumazenil or benzodiazepines, patients receiving benzodiazepines for epilepsy or other conditions	Supportive
Fosphenytoin (Cerebyx)	Anticonvulsant	12–29 hr	IV: 15–20 mg phenytoin equivalents (PE)/ kg (22.5–30 mg/kg) given no faster than 150 mg equivalents/min, followed by 4–6 mg PE/kg/day; IM: 10–20 mg PE followed by 4–6 mg PE/kg/day. 75 mg (50 mg PE)/ml (2- and 10-ml vials)	Modulates sodium channels in neurons	Cardiovascular collapse, hypertension, nystagmus, dizziness, pruritus, paresthesias, headache, somnolence, ataxia, fever, constipation, thrombocytopenia, pancytopenia, hyperreflexia, dysarthria, rash, taste disturbance, hepatotoxicity	Sensitivity, cardiac arrhythmias, pregnancy	Supportive

Drug	Classification	Half-life	Dose	Mechanism	Side effects	Contraindications	Treatment
Heparin sodium	Anticoagulant	1 hr	IV: Bolus up to 10,000 U as needed during procedure; infusion ≈1000 U/hr (titrated) to maintain anticoagulation. 1000, 2500, 5000, and 10,000 U/ml (0.5- and 1-ml syringes; 1-, 4-, 10-, and 30-ml vials)	Enhances inhibitory effects of antithrombin III	Nausea/vomiting, diarrhea, hematuria, rash, urticaria, fever/chills, bleeding, thrombocytopenia	Sensitivity, bleeding disorders, peptic ulcer, severe hepatic or renal disease, severe hypertension, endocarditis, acute nephritis	Protamine sulfate
Hydroxyzine HCl (Vistaril)	Antiemetic/anxiolytic	3 hr	IM: 25–100 mg every 6 hr as needed as antiemetic, 25–100 mg for premedication (usually with meperidine HCl). 25 mg/ml (1-ml vials) and 50 mg/ml (1- and 2-ml vials)	Central antiemetic, subcortical effect on CNS	Drowsiness, dry mouth, tremor	Sensitivity	Supportive
Ketorolac tromethamine (Toradol)	Nonsteroidal anti-inflammatory	3.5–9.2 hr	IV/IM: 30–60 mg initially, then 30 mg every 6 hr (up to 5 days); PO: 10 mg every 6 hr; 10-mg tablets, 15 mg/ml (1-ml syringes), 30 mg/ml (1- and 2-ml syringes)	Inhibits prostaglandin synthesis	GI bleeding, peptic ulcer, hypertension, renal dysfunction, edema, rash/urticaria, nausea/vomiting, wheezing, headache, drowsiness	Sensitivity to NSAIDs, peptic ulcer, renal or hepatic disease, bleeding disorder, active bleeding, congestive heart failure, hypertension	Supportive
Labetalol HCl (Normodyne, Trandate)	α_1-, and β-blocker	5.5 hr	IV: 20 mg over 2 min, then repeat doses 40–80 mg at 10-min intervals (up to 300 mg). 5 mg/ml (20- and 40-ml vials)	α_1- and β-adrenergic blockade	Hypotension, sweating, flushing, dizziness, nausea/vomiting, arrhythmia, somnolence, wheezing	Sensitivity, asthma, congestive heart failure, heart block, bradycardia	Supportive, pressors, atropine, epinephrine, inotropes
Levarterenol (norepinephrine) bitartrate (Levophed)	α- and β_1-adrenergic agonist	?	IV: 8–12 μg/min initially, titrate as needed to maintain blood pressure. 1 mg/ml	Stimulates sympathetic receptors	Headache, anxiety, weakness, tremor, bradycardia, hypertension, arrhythmias, decreased cardiac output, oliguria, respiratory distress, fever, hyperglycemia	Hypoxia, hypercapnia, hypovolemia, mesenteric or peripheral arterial thrombosis	Supportive, atropine for bradycardia, phentolamine for hypertension, propranolol for arrhythmias

Table continued on following page

65

T A B L E 4 – 1B Commonly Used Drugs *Continued*

Drug	Class	Half-Life	Dosage/Route of Administration/How Supplied	Primary Effects	Side Effects*	Contraindications	Treatment of Toxicity
Lidocaine HCl (Xylocaine)	Amide-type local anesthetic	≈1.5 hr	Intra-arterial: 10–20 mg of "cardiac" formulation for functional vessel testing; injectable: total dose depends on route and site. 10 and 20 mg/ml ("cardiac," 5-ml ampules and syringes); 0.5%, 1%, 1.5%, and 2% with and without epinephrine and preservative (2-, 5-, 10-, 20-, and 30-ml ampules and vials, 50-ml vials)	Competes with calcium for nerve membrane sites, blocks action potential	Headache, dizziness, confusion, seizure, tremor, tinnitus, blurry vision, nausea/vomiting, hypotension, bradycardia, heart block, dyspnea, rash/urticaria, fever	Sensitivity to amide-type local anesthetics, heart block, SVT, Wolff-Parkinson-White or Adams-Stokes syndrome	Supportive, dopamine for hypotension, diazepam for seizure
Low-molecular-weight dextran (Rheomacrodex)	Plasma volume expander	3 hr	IV: As needed to maintain blood pressure/filling pressures; up to 20 mg/kg/day first 24 hr, 10 mg/kg/day subsequently (up to 5 days total). 10% in normal saline or 5% dextrose (500-ml bags)	Draws fluid from interstitial to intravascular space	Coagulopathy, rash/urticaria, wheezing, hypotension, renal failure, hyponatremia, nausea/vomiting, elevated liver enzymes	Sensitivity, renal failure, congestive heart failure, dehydration	Supportive
Mannitol	Osmotic diuretic	100 min	IV: 25–50 gm for protection against renal failure related to administration of contrast. 25% (50-ml vials and syringes)	Increases osmolarity of glomerular filtrate	Diuresis, dizziness, headache, seizure, confusion, nausea/vomiting, diarrhea, hypotension, tachycardia, fever, chills, fluid/electrolyte imbalance, dehydration, blurry vision, hearing loss	Sensitivity, anuria, severe pulmonary congestion, dehydration	Correct electrolytes and hydration, supportive
Meperidine HCl (Demerol)	Synthetic opiate	4 hr	IV/IM: 25–100 mg every 3–4 hr as needed 10, 25, 50, 75, and 100 mg/ml (1-ml ampules and syringes)	Inhibits CNS pain pathways	Tachycardia, respiratory depression, seizure, dizziness, drowsiness, nausea/vomiting, hypotension, rash/urticaria	Sensitivity to opiates, MAO inhibitor therapy, respiratory depression	Naloxone, supportive

Drug	Class	Half-life/duration	Action	Dose	Adverse effects	Contraindications	Treatment
Metaraminol (Aramine)	Sympathomimetic amine	?	Positive inotropic agent, peripheral vasoconstriction	IV: 15–100 mg in 500 ml D₅W or normal saline, 0.5–5.0 mg bolus followed by continuous infusion titrated to maintain desired pressure. 10 mg/ml (1-ml ampules)	Arrhythmias, exacerbation of malaria, hypertension	Sensitivity, halothane or cyclopropane anesthesia	Phentolamine, antiarrhythmics
Methohexital (Brevital)	Barbiturate	1.5–5 hr	Depresses CNS activity	Intra-arterial: 3–6 mg for either Wada test or functional testing of a vessel. 1% solution	Respiratory depression, amnesia/somnolence, tachycardia, hypotension, arrhythmia, chills, shivering, coughing, bronchospasm	Sensitivity, severe asthma, porphyria	Supportive
Methylprednisolone (Medrol), Methylprednisolone sodium succinate (Solu-Medrol)	Synthetic adrenocorticoid	80–90 min	Free radical scavenger, inhibits lipid peroxidation, stabilizes cell membranes, reduces cerebral edema	IV/IM: 4–250 mg every 4–6 hr; PO: 4–64 mg every 6 hr. (Both PO and IV/IM up to 72 hr to avoid adrenal suppression). 2-, 4-, 8-, 16-, 24-, and 32-mg tablets; 40-mg, 125-mg, 500-mg, 1-gm, and 2-gm vials)	Fluid/electrolyte disturbances, muscle weakness, peptic ulcer, bowel perforation, pancreatitis, impaired healing, rash/urticaria, vertigo, headache, psychosis, seizure, hyperglycemia, increased intraocular pressure, myocardial rupture with recent infarction	Sensitivity, fungal sepsis	Supportive
Midazolam (Versed)	Benzodiazepine	≈2.5 hr	Potentiates action of GABA in CNS	IV: 0.5–1.0 mg, titrated as needed to achieve and maintain sedation. 1 mg/ml (1-, 2-, and 5-ml vials)	CNS depression, paradoxical stimulation, headache, coughing, bronchospasm, hypotension, arrhythmia, tachycardia, blurry vision, nystagmus, nausea/vomiting, rash/urticaria	Sensitivity to benzodiazepines, narrow-angle glaucoma	Flumazenil, physostigmine, supportive

Table continued on following page

T A B L E 4 – 1B Commonly Used Drugs *Continued*

Drug	Class	Half-Life	Dosage/Route of Administration/ How Supplied	Primary Effects	Side Effects*	Contraindications	Treatment of Toxicity
Morphine sulfate	Opiate	1.5–2.0 hr	IV: 2–3 mg slowly, titrate up to 0.2 mg/kg; IM: 1 mg/10 kg as premedication. 0.5 and 1 mg/ml (2-ml ampules, 10-ml ampules and vials); 1 and 2 mg/ml (60-ml vials), 1, 2, 4, 5, 8, 10, and 15 mg/ ml (1-ml ampules, syringes, and vials)	Blocks CNS pain pathways	Respiratory depression, seizure, nausea/vomiting, hypotension, bronchospasm, urinary retention, elevated bile duct pressure	Sensitivity to opiates, acute asthma, biliary obstruction, hepatic disease	Naloxone, supportive
Naloxone HCl (Narcan)	Narcotic antagonist	60–100 min	IV/IM: 0.4 mg, repeat every 2–3 min as needed, up to 2 mg. 0.4 mg/ml (1-ml vials)	Competes with narcotics at receptor sites	Drowsiness, nervousness, nausea/vomiting, tachycardia, hypertension	Sensitivity	Supportive
Nifedipine (Procardia)	Calcium channel blocker	2 hr	PO/sublingual: 10–20 mg at start of procedure to prevent vasospasm; 10–20 mg as needed to control blood pressure. 10-mg capsules	Vascular smooth muscle relaxation	Arrhythmia, edema, hypotension, tachycardia, MI, pulmonary edema, nausea/vomiting, polyuria, rash/urticaria, flushing, cough, fever/chills, headache, dizziness, drowsiness, tinnitus, blurry vision	Sensitivity	Atropine, supportive
Nimodipine (Nimotop)	Calcium channel blocker	1–2 hr	PO: 30–60 mg PO at start of procedure; 60 mg every 4 hr for 21 days for vasospasm prophylaxis. 30-mg capsules	Vascular smooth muscle relaxation	Arrhythmia, edema, heart block, nausea/vomiting, diarrhea, elevated liver enzymes, rash/pruritus, headache, depression	Sensitivity, hypotension	Atropine, supportive
Nitroglycerin (Nitro-Bid)	Nitrate	1–4 min	IV: 5–640 µg/min for control of blood pressure or pulmonary vasodilatation; intra-arterial: ≈50 µg for treatment of vasospasm; transdermal: 1″–5″ paste for spasm prophylaxis. 5 mg/ ml (1-, 5-, and 10-ml vials); 2% (≈15 mg/inch) ointment (1-gm pouches; 3-, 30-, and 60-gm tubes)	Vascular smooth muscle relaxation; pre- and afterload reduction	Hypotension, tachycardia, syncope, dizziness, headache, nausea/ vomiting, rash, flushing, sweating	Sensitivity, anemia	Supportive

Drug	Classification	Half-life	Dosage	Action	Adverse effects	Contraindications	Overdose treatment
Omeprazole (Prilosec)	Gastric acid secretion inhibition	0.5–1 hr	PO: 20 mg daily. 10-mg and 20-mg delayed-release capsules	Blockade of gastric acid (proton) pump	Headache, dizziness, abdominal pain, nausea/vomiting, diarrhea, constipation, rash, cough	Sensitivity	Supportive
Ondansetron HCl (Zofran)	Serotonin blocker (HT_3)	3.5–5.5 hr	IV: 0.15 mg/kg every 4 hr. 2 mg/ml (2-ml vials)	Antiemetic	Headache, diarrhea	Sensitivity	Supportive
Papaverine HCl	Alkaloid	0.5–2.0 hr	Intra-arterial: 30–50 mg over several minutes for catheter-induced spasm; 300–600 mg/hr for SAH-related vasospasm. 30 mg/ml (10-ml vials)	Smooth muscle relaxation	Tachycardia, hypertension, hyperpnea, headache, dizziness, drowsiness, nausea, flushing, sweating, rash	Sensitivity, complete heart block	Supportive
Phenobarbital	Anticonvulsant	79 hr	IV or PO: Initial dose of 120 mg followed by 60–240 mg daily in 2–3 divided doses. 30, 60, 130 mg/ml (1-ml vials and syringes); 15-, 30-, 60-, 100-mg tablets; 0.4 gm/100 ml elixir	CNS depression	CNS depression, irritability, respiratory depression, circulatory collapse, facial swelling, Stevens-Johnson syndrome, nausea/vomiting, headache, constipation, hepatotoxicity	Sensitivity, porphyria, liver dysfunction, respiratory disorders	Supportive
Phentolamine mesylate (Regitine)	α-Adrenergic blocker	19 min	IV/IM: 2–5 mg for hypertensive crisis, followed by 1 mg as needed. 5 mg/ml (1-ml vials)	Complete block of catecholamine effects	Dizziness, weakness, flushing, shock, hypotension, arrhythmias, tachycardia, angina, nasal stuffiness, diarrhea, nausea/vomiting, hypoglycemia	Angina, coronary artery disease	Supportive, norepinephrine for hypotension
Phenytoin sodium (Dilantin)	Anticonvulsant	7–42 hr	PO: 400 mg followed by two 300-mg doses at 2-hr intervals, then 300–600 mg/day in 1–3 doses. 100-mg capsules	Modulates sodium channels in neurons	Nystagmus, ataxia, slurred speech, confusion, nausea/vomiting, constipation, hepatotoxicity, rash, Stevens-Johnson syndrome, lymphadenopathy, thrombocytopenia, pancytopenia, gingival hyperplasia	Sensitivity	Supportive

Table continued on following page

T A B L E   4 – 1B   Commonly Used Drugs *Continued*

Drug	Class	Half-Life	Dosage/Route of Administration/ How Supplied	Primary Effects	Side Effects*	Contraindications	Treatment of Toxicity
Probucol (Lorelco)	Antioxidant	?	PO: 500 mg twice daily. 250- and 500-mg tablets	Suppresses neointimal formation and vascular remodeling	Diarrhea, abdominal pain, ventricular arrhythmias, headache, dizziness, paresthesias, tinnitus, eosinophilia, anemia, thrombocytopenia, pruritus, ecchymosis, impotence	Sensitivity, recurrent or progressive myocardial damage, cardiac syncope, serious ventricular arrhythmias	Supportive
Procaine HCl (Novocain)	Local anesthetic	1.5–2.0 hr	Injectable: Total dose depends on route and site. 1% (2- and 6-ml ampules, 30-ml vials); 2% (30-ml vials)	Prevents transmission of nerve impulses	CNS excitation, drowsiness, seizure, blurry vision, dizziness, hypotension, bradycardia, rash/urticaria	Sensitivity	Supportive, diazepam for seizure
Promethazine HCl (Phenergan)	Phenothiazine derivative, anticholinergic, and histamine (H₁) blocker	?	IV/IM: 12.5–25 mg every 4 hr. 25 and 50 mg/ml (1-ml vials)	Centrally acting antihistamine/ anticholinergic	Drowsiness, extrapyramidal reactions, dizziness, tachy/ bradycardia, hypotension, nausea/vomiting, urticaria, wheezing, leukopenia	Sensitivity, coma, CNS depression	Supportive, levarterenol or phenylephrine for hypotension, diphenhydramine for extrapyramidal effects
Prostacyclin (epoprostenol) (Flolan)	Hormone	3–6 min	IV: Start at 2 ng/kg/ min, titrate until dose-limiting effects (bradycardia, hypotension) occur. 0.5- and 1.5-mg vials (for reconstitution)	Vascular smooth muscle relaxation, platelet aggregation inhibition	Headache, nausea/vomiting, hypotension, anxiety, chest pain, dizziness, bradycardia, abdominal pain, musculoskeletal pain, dyspnea, tachycardia	Sensitivity, severe left ventricular systolic dysfunction	Supportive, decrease dose or stop briefly
Prostaglandin E₁ (alprostadil)	Hormone	5–10 min	IV: Titrate up to 0.4 μg/kg/min to maintain ductus patency; use in vasospasm not yet specified. 0.5 mg/ ml (1-ml ampules)	Vascular smooth muscle relaxation	Sepsis, hypo/hyperkalemia, hypoglycemia, apnea, wheezing, DIC, thrombocytopenia, fever, seizure, lethargy, diarrhea, anuria, brady/tachycardia, hypotension, shock, flushing, edema	Sensitivity, respiratory distress syndrome	Supportive
Protamine sulfate	Low-molecular-weight protein	0.5–6.0 hr	IV: 1 mg for every 100 U heparin/ heparinoid given (if >30 min since heparin, 0.5 mg/ 100 U), slowly (up to 5 mg/min). 10 mg/ml (5-ml ampules, 25-ml vials)	Binds to heparin, making it ineffective	Hypotension, tachycardia, nausea/vomiting, rash/ urticaria	Sensitivity	Supportive

Drug	Classification	Half-life	Dosage	Action	Side effects	Contraindications	Treatment
Ranitidine HCl (Zantac)	Histamine (H₂) blocker	2–2.5 hr	IV: 50 mg every 8 hr; PO: 150 mg every 12 hr. 75- and 150-mg tablets; 50 mg/ml (1-ml vials)	Inhibits acid secretion	Malaise, dizziness, confusion, agitation, arrhythmia, constipation, diarrhea, rash/urticaria, nausea/vomiting, leukopenia, elevated liver enzymes	Sensitivity, porphyria	Supportive
Sodium nitroprusside (Nipride)	Nitrate	2 min	IV: 0.5–8 µg/kg/min for control of blood pressure. 50-mg vials	Vascular smooth muscle relaxation; preload reduction	Nausea/vomiting, dizziness, headache, agitation, tinnitus, blurry vision, sweating	Sensitivity	Amyl nitrite, IV sodium nitrate, sodium thiosulfate
Sodium tetradecyl sulfate (Sotradecol)	Sclerosing agent	?	Intra-arterial/IV: No more than 10 ml of 1% solution (generally diluted 1:1 with nonionic contrast). 1% and 3% solution (2-ml vials)	Causes intimal inflammation and thrombus formation with subsequent formation of fibrous tissue	Urticaria, pain, tissue necrosis, headache, nausea/vomiting, bronchospasm, anaphylaxis	Sensitivity, use of anovulatory agents, systemic diseases such as diabetes, tuberculosis, asthma, sepsis, hyperthyroidism, or bleeding disorders	Supportive
Streptokinase (Streptase)	Enzyme	20–25 min	Intra-arterial: ≈500,000 U/hr for local intracranial thrombolysis. 250,000-, 750,000-, and 1,500,000-U vials (reconstitute with 5 ml sterile normal saline or 5% dextrose in water)	Activates conversion of plasminogen to plasmin	Bleeding, rash/urticaria, flushing, fever, headache, nausea, bronchospasm, hypertension, arrhythmia	Sensitivity, active bleeding, recent surgery, hypertension, intracranial lesions (tumor/vascular), colitis, severe renal or hepatic disease, bleeding disorder, COPD, endocarditis	Supportive
Sucralfate (Carafate)	Antiulcer agent	?	PO: 1 gm every 6 hr on empty stomach. 1-gm tablets	Coats and protects ulcers and erosions	Constipation, diarrhea, nausea, vomiting, rash/urticaria, dizziness, insomnia	None	Supportive
Ticlopidine HCl (Ticlid)	Platelet aggregation inhibitor	8–12 hr	PO: 250 mg twice daily. 250-mg tablets	Inhibits ADP-induced effects on platelet aggregation	Rash, nausea/vomiting, hepatitis, cholestatic jaundice, bleeding, thrombocytopenia, neutropenia	Sensitivity, acute liver disease, bleeding disorder	Supportive
Tissue-type plasminogen activator (alteplase) (Activase)	Enzyme	<5 min	IV: 0.9 mg/kg (10% as bolus, remainder over 1 hr (recent NINDS trial for acute stroke therapy). 1 mg/ml (20-, 50-, and 100-ml vials)	Fibrin-enhanced conversion of plasminogen to plasmin	GI bleeding, hematuria, rash/urticaria, nausea/vomiting, hypertension, hypotension, fever	Sensitivity, bleeding disorder, recent surgery, pericarditis, endocarditis, hepatic disease	Supportive

Table continued on following page

71

T A B L E 4 – 1B Commonly Used Drugs *Continued*

Drug	Class	Half-Life	Dosage/Route of Administration/ How Supplied	Primary Effects	Side Effects*	Contraindications	Treatment of Toxicity
Urokinase (Abbokinase)	Enzyme	20 min	Intra-arterial: 250,000–750,000 U/hr for local intracranial thrombolysis. 50,000 U/ml (5-ml vials)	Enhances conversion of plasminogen to plasmin	Bleeding, rash/urticaria, flushing, headache, fever/ chills, nausea, bronchospasm, back pain, hypertension, arrhythmia	Sensitivity, acute bleeding, recent surgery, hypertension, intracranial lesions (tumor/vascular), colitis, severe renal or hepatic disease, bleeding disorder, COPD, endocarditis	Supportive
Vancomycin HCl (Vancocin)	Glycopeptide antibiotic	4–6 hr	IV: 500 mg every 6 hr. 50 mg/ml (10- and 20-ml vials)	Inhibits cell wall synthesis	Anaphylactoid reaction, renal failure, ototoxicity, neutropenia, phlebitis, Stevens-Johnson syndrome	Sensitivity	Supportive
Vitamin K₁ (phytonadione) (AquaMEPHYTON)	Fat-soluble vitamin	?	IM: 2.5–10 mg 4 hr before procedure to reverse warfarin; may repeat in 6–8 hr if needed. 10 mg/ml (1-ml vials)	Restores ability to synthesize factors II, VII, IX, X	Headache, nausea, hemolytic anemia, rash/urticaria, hemoglobinuria	Sensitivity, severe hepatic disease	Supportive
Warfarin sodium (Coumadin)	Anticoagulant	1.5–2.5 days	PO: 10–15 mg daily × 3, then titrate to therapeutic level. 1-, 2-, 2.5-, 4-, 5-, 7.5-, and 10-mg tablets	Inhibits synthesis of factors II VII, IX, X in liver	Diarrhea, nausea/vomiting, stomatitis, hepatitis, hematuria, rash/urticaria, fever, bleeding, neutropenia	Sensitivity, peptic ulcer disease, leukemia, severe hepatic disease, bleeding disorder, endocarditis, hypertension, nephritis	Vitamin K, supportive

*Note that hypersensitivity reaction has been reported with nearly every drug listed in this table; this is not listed separately under the side effects of each drug.

ADP, adenosine diphosphate; CNS, central nervous system; COPD, chronic obstructive pulmonary disease; DIC, disseminated intravascular coagulation; GABA, gamma-aminobutyric acid; GI, gastrointestinal; GU, genitourinary; IV, intravenous; IM, intramuscular; MAO, monoamine oxidase; MI, myocardial infarction; NINDS, National Institute of Neurological Diseases and Stroke; NSAIDs, nonsteroidal anti-inflammatory drugs; PO, oral; PTCA, percutaneous transluminal coronary angioplasty; SA, sinoatrial; SAH, subarachnoid hemorrhage; SC, subcutaneous; SVT, supraventricular tachycardia; TIAs, transient ischemic attacks.

zation syndrome of fever and local pain (see Chapter 64). For maximal benefit, this drug must be given as a loading dose followed by maintenance doses every 6 hours, rather than prn.

When narcotic analgesia is required, morphine sulfate or meperidine hydrochloride can be used. Which drug is chosen depends on the duration of action and potency desired, as well as the preference of the interventionalist.

For patients who may require further (short-term) analgesics after discharge from the hospital, we prefer the oral form of ketorolac tromethamine to narcotics.

When reversal of narcotic analgesia is required, naloxone hydrochloride (Narcan) can be administered IV. Repeat doses may be needed every 1 to 2 hours, depending on the narcotic agent and dosage being reversed.

ANTICONVULSANTS

Seizures are a known complication of aneurysms, arteriovenous malformations, and other intracranial pathology (e.g., strokes, central nervous system tumors). Many patients are maintained on anticonvulsants. For certain procedures, such as intra-arterial chemotherapy of brain tumors and stereotactic radiosurgery of arteriovenous malformations, prophylactic anticonvulsants are recommended. The most commonly used agents are phenytoin sodium (Dilantin) and phenobarbital. For IV use, Dilantin has been replaced by fosphenytoin (Cerebyx), whose active metabolite is phenytoin.

ANTIEMETICS

Commonly used antiemetic agents include hydroxyzine hydrochloride (Vistaril), promethazine hydrochloride (Phenergan), and droperidol (Inapsine). All can be administered IM; droperidol and promethazine hydrochloride can be given IV. These drugs act on the central nervous system and produce sedation. A fourth antiemetic that is becoming more widely used is ondansetron hydrochloride (Zofran). This is a serotonin (HT_3) blocker and is administered IV. It does not produce sedation but can cause headache or extrapyramidal reactions.

ANTIBIOTICS

Antibiotics are generally used for prophylaxis against infection, usually with skin organisms. We usually administer an antibiotic during procedures in which there is increased risk of contamination (e.g., with an agitated, uncooperative patient) or when there is prolonged catheterization (especially when embolization is being performed). Antibiotics are administered to any patient with a sheath left in place until the sheath is removed. The most commonly used antibiotic for prophylaxis is cefazolin sodium (Ancef). This drug has good broad-spectrum coverage against common skin microbes. If a broader

spectrum agent is needed, ceftriaxone sodium (Rocephin) can be utilized. In patients who are sensitive to cephalosporins, vancomycin hydrochloride (Vancocin) can be used. If a patient does develop a local infection at the puncture site, this can usually be treated with a 10-day course of cephalexin (Keflex).

ANTIHYPERTENSIVES

For control of blood pressure in patients receiving thrombolytic therapy and other patients in whom adequate control of blood pressure is necessary, the guidelines provided by the American Heart Association for patients receiving tissue-type plasminogen activator (t-PA) are useful (see Chapter 7).[1] Sublingual nifedipine can also be used for control of blood pressure, especially during relatively short procedures such as diagnostic angiography.

ANTIULCER AGENTS

Any patient receiving a nonsteroidal anti-inflammatory agent or glucocorticoid should be placed on ulcer prophylaxis. Generally, a histamine (H_2) blocker is administered. We prefer ranitidine (Zantac) to cimetidine (Tagamet) owing to the lower incidence of confusion and agitation associated with its use. Another useful agent is sucralfate (Carafate), which works by creating a protective coating over erosions and ulcers.

NEUROPROTECTANTS

Neuroprotectant agents are those drugs that help protect the brain from the effects of ischemia and reduce cerebral edema (these agents are discussed more fully in Chapter 54). At this time, only a limited number of these agents are available for use, other than as part of investigational protocols. As discussed below (see "Vasodilators"), nimodipine (Nimotop) is routinely administered to patients suffering from subarachnoid hemorrhage to help reduce vasospasm and help the brain withstand the ischemia associated with vasospasm.

The other widely available neuroprotectant agents are glucocorticoids. These act as free radical scavengers, inhibiting lipid peroxidation and thereby stabilizing cell membranes to interrupt the ischemic cascade of injury. They are also effective in reducing cerebral edema. The glucocorticoids most commonly used for these purposes include dexamethasone sodium phosphate (Decadron Phosphate), methylprednisolone (Medrol), and methylprednisolone sodium succinate (Solu-Medrol). The major side effects associated with short-term use of glucocorticoids are hyperglycemia, peptic ulcers, and gastrointestinal perforation.

CARDIOVASCULAR AGENTS

Manipulation of paragangliomas can lead to a hypertensive crisis. This is managed by administration of the α-adrenergic blocker phentolamine.

In the majority of cases, the goal of blood pressure management is to keep the pressure from becoming too elevated. However, there are circumstances when pressure support is indicated. Agents such as dopamine, levarterenol, and metaraminol can be employed. If an increase in cardiac output is desired, dobutamine can be administered. Dopamine is used to raise systemic pressure in the medical management of vasospasm (see Chapter 52).

Patients undergoing carotid angioplasty and stenting in the region of the carotid bulb require careful monitoring and management of their cardiovascular status. Pretreatment with atropine can help prevent bradycardia. If symptomatic bradycardia does occur, medical management with volume expansion and metaraminol may be attempted. However, these patients may require temporary pacing, and it is prudent to have some form of temporary pacemaker (transvenous, percutaneous, transesophageal) available.

DRUGS FOR FUNCTIONAL NEUROLOGIC TESTING

The most commonly utilized agent for functional neurologic testing (Wada test) is amobarbital (Amytal), as discussed in Chapter 3. Methohexital (Brevital) is also used for this purpose.

For testing of a vessel before occlusion, the agent chosen depends on the location of the vessel. For evaluation of vessels supplying the brain, either amobarbital or methohexital can be used. When the vessel to be tested may supply cranial nerves, injectable lidocaine hydrochloride ("cardiac" lidocaine) is utilized.

ANTICOAGULANTS AND ANTIPLATELET DRUGS

Heparin sodium is commonly used as an anticoagulant. It works by combining with antithrombin III to inactivate thrombin. Heparin does not lyse existing clot. It is mixed in flush solutions and administered IV during certain procedures (temporary test occlusion of the internal carotid artery, inferior petrosal sinus sampling, or any procedure in which prolonged catheterization of a vessel is expected and anticoagulation is not contraindicated). Under certain circumstances, patients may be maintained on a constant heparin infusion after a procedure (e.g., coil or balloon malposition; vessel dissection during a procedure; indwelling catheter, such as for treatment of venous sinus thrombosis). The nomogram for heparinization is given in Chapter 7. In addition, if a sheath is left in place after a procedure, heparinized flush is maintained through the sheath.

When reversal of heparinization is needed, protamine sulfate can be administered IV (slowly); when this is given at the end of a procedure during which the patient has received heparin, it is better to wait approximately 10 minutes after administration before removing the catheter/sheath.

Low-molecular-weight heparinoids (enoxaparin sodium [Lovenox], dalteparin sodium [Fragmin]) are a more recent development. The half-life of these agents is approximately twice as long as that of heparin. One drawback of these drugs is that their anticoagulant effect cannot be monitored by activated partial thromboplastin time (aPTT) and produces barely any effect on activated clotting time (ACT). An antifactor X_a assay is needed to measure effect. Fortunately, the anticoagulant activity of these agents is more predictable than that of heparin, and it has been shown that patients being maintained on low-molecular-weight heparinoids do not require the frequent monitoring of prothrombin time (PT)/aPTT required in conjunction with heparin or warfarin use. In addition, there is a superior benefit:risk ratio associated with these drugs; fewer hemorrhagic complications are associated with their use than with heparin. The use of these agents in the management of stroke is the subject of much current interest.

Warfarin sodium (Coumadin) is used when long-term anticoagulation is required. This drug inhibits synthesis of clotting factors II, VII, IX, and X. Like heparin, warfarin prevents the formation of new clot but does not lyse existing clot. Because of its mechanism of action, the onset of effective anticoagulation is 2 to 7 days after the loading dose, and several days are required for coagulation function to normalize when the drug is stopped. If the patient must be maintained on anticoagulation during this time, an IV heparin drip can be utilized. If rapid reversal of the effect of warfarin is needed, vitamin K_1 can be administered IM approximately 4 hours before the procedure. This will interfere with re-establishment of adequate anticoagulation with warfarin for up to 3 weeks after administration.

Antiplatelet drugs are usually employed in patients with ongoing atherosclerotic disease. They can also be used when needed to prevent platelet plugs from forming and embolizing downstream (such as in the case of malposition of a coil with a portion dangling into the parent vessel). Aspirin is the prototypical antiplatelet agent. It acts by inhibiting prostaglandin-mediated effects on platelet aggregation. The onset of its antiplatelet activity is within minutes of administration if the chewable form is given. One tablet per day (325 mg) is used for prophylaxis for coronary artery disease and cerebrovascular disease.

Dipyridamole (Persantine) is a coronary vasodilator and platelet inhibitor used for treatment of transient ischemic attacks and in coronary artery disease. Ticlopidine hydrochloride (Ticlid) is a newer agent that inhibits adenosine diphosphate (ADP)-mediated effects on platelet aggregation. It has a longer duration of action than either aspirin or dipyridamole.

An exciting antiplatelet agent is abciximab (ReoPro). This is the Fab fragment of an antibody that binds to platelets at a major receptor site involved in platelet aggregation. This prevents platelet aggregation by preventing binding of fibrinogen and other factors involved in aggregation. This agent is currently being used as an adjunct to percutaneous transluminal coronary angioplasty (PTCA) to prevent acute cardiac ischemia in patients at high risk for abrupt closure of the treated vessel, and it is used in conjunction with heparin and aspirin. It is administered IV as a bolus 10 to 60 minutes before PTCA followed by a continuous infusion for 12 hours. Reo-Pro has been shown to add to the activity of heparin, increasing the ACT by 30 to 40 seconds. The bolus dose gives activity for at least 2 hours, and residual activity after administration of the entire protocol dose can last up to 96 hours. An increased incidence of hemorrhagic complications is associated with its use (as compared with the same procedure without its use). In addition, there is a risk of development of thrombocytopenia, which appears to be greater in thin patients. Although no clinical trials have been completed to evaluate this agent as an adjunct to brachiocephalic (or peripheral) angioplasty, it may prove to be of great use in controlling the tendency to develop local thrombosis after angioplasty, which is so bedeviling to interventional neuroradiologists.

All antiplatelet agents and anticoagulants are associated with increased incidence of gastrointestinal bleeding, hematuria, and other hematologic complications. Patients taking these medications should be monitored closely, especially if both an anticoagulant and an antiplatelet agent are being given.

VASODILATORS

Vasodilators are used by interventional neuroradiologists primarily for the prevention or treatment of catheter-induced vasospasm or for the treatment of vasospasm secondary to subarachnoid hemorrhage. They can also be used to lower systemic blood pressure in conjunction with temporary test occlusion of the internal carotid artery. Elective vasodilation can also be helpful during certain procedures. This might be used to allow more distal passage of a catheter for embolization, to allow particles to penetrate more distally, or to provoke hyperemia to aid in the identification of a bleeding source (e.g., when treating epistaxis).

As described in Chapter 3, many interventional neuroradiologists apply 1″ to 5″ of nitroglycerin paste to the chest wall at the beginning of any procedure in which catheter-induced vasospasm might be anticipated; some prefer to administer oral nifedipine (Procardia), a calcium channel blocker, instead. Once vasospasm has occurred, nitroglycerin or papaverine (an alkaloid with peripheral vasodilatory activity) can be administered through the catheter to relieve this spasm. Alternatively, inhaled amyl nitrite can be used for this purpose.

We have used intracatheter papaverine, intracatheter nitroglycerin, and inhaled amyl nitrite for elective vasodilation. Different patients respond better to one or another of these drugs both in the setting of catheter-induced vasospasm and in the setting of elective vasodilation. Do not be afraid to try another agent if the first one does not produce the desired effect.

Vasospasm associated with subarachnoid hemorrhage continues to be a major source of morbidity and mortality. The treatment of this condition is covered in great detail in Chapter 51. Currently, it is accepted practice in the neurosurgical community to place patients with aneurysmal subarachnoid hemorrhage on the calcium channel blocker nimodipine to help decrease the incidence and sequelae of vasospasm. Once vasospasm has occurred and intra-arterial therapy is instituted, papaverine is the drug of choice. The doses recommended for the treatment of vasospasm have been steadily increasing in recent years; some practitioners state that there is no hard-and-fast limit. Some early work has been done with the use of prostaglandin E_1 (alprostadil) for the treatment of vasospasm. This drug is utilized in neonates to maintain patency of the ductus arteriosus by vascular smooth muscle relaxation.

Sodium nitroprusside (Nipride) can be used to lower systemic blood pressure in conjunction with temporary test occlusion of the internal carotid artery. Alternatively, labetalol (Normodyne), a β-blocker, can be administered. Nipride is utilized as titrated drips and probably should be administered by anesthesia personnel.

Infusion of nitroglycerin directly into the pulmonary arterial tree (via a Swan-Ganz catheter) has been used to treat acutely symptomatic pulmonary embolization associated with the use of particulate embolization agents, as well as in the treatment of cardiopulmonary collapse associated with alcohol embolization. In either event, the patient's cardiovascular and pulmonary status is obviously fragile, and anesthesia personnel should be actively involved in the management of these conditions.

Prostacyclin (epoprostenol, Flolan) is an agent that produces direct vasodilatation of the pulmonary and systemic vascular beds and inhibits platelet aggregation. This agent can also be utilized in the setting of acutely symptomatic pulmonary embolization associated with the use of particulate embolization agents, as well as in the treatment of cardiopulmonary collapse associated with alcohol embolization. Again, owing to the implicitly unstable condition of the patient, anesthesia personnel should be directly involved in the management of the situation. The inhibition of platelet aggregation makes this agent especially appealing in the setting of acute pulmonary embolism, in which further thrombosis could worsen an already serious situation. In addition, this agent can be used for a prolonged period of time, thus allowing the patient's system more time to adapt to the insult.

THROMBOLYTIC AGENTS

The treatment of acute stroke by means of thrombolysis (fibrinolysis) is an area of ongoing research. The fibrinolytic agents currently available work by converting plasminogen to plasmin, an enzyme that causes degradation of fibrinogen and fibrin. Most of the clinical stroke trials have focused on the use of IV t-PA or local intra-arterial urokinase. Some early trials employed streptokinase, but this agent has fallen out of favor owing to a high rate of allergic reactions.

t-PA causes fibrin-enhanced conversion of plasminogen to plasmin. IV administration for the treatment of stroke has been approved by the Food and Drug Administration. Urokinase is an enzyme that converts plasminogen to plasmin; it is approved for intra-arterial use and is also undergoing continued clinical evaluation. Studies employing both drugs have shown promising results; the ideal drug, route of delivery, timing, and dosage are by no means certain at this time. Newer forms of urokinase, such as prourokinase, are also being developed and evaluated. Prourokinase is a single-chain form of urokinase that is more clot specific—it preferentially causes degradation of thrombus-associated fibrin. It is currently undergoing clinical trials.

All thrombolytic agents are associated with bleeding complications, both intracranially and systemically. Systemic complications are less common in trials utilizing local intra-arterial infusion, unless the dose administered is large enough to result in a significant systemic concentration of the drug. Careful screening of patients (including history, PT/aPTT, fibrinogen level) and careful evaluation of the computed tomographic scan before treatment (to exclude those patients with recent infarction or intracranial bleed) are needed to minimize the risks of subsequent catastrophic intracerebral hemorrhage or systemic hemorrhagic complication.

MISCELLANEOUS PHARMACEUTICALS

Acetazolamide

Acetazolamide is a carbonic anhydrase inhibitor. Its primary clinical use is in the treatment of increased intraocular pressure (due to glaucoma). In the field of interventional neuroradiology, it is used in conjunction with cerebral blood flow imaging studies to evaluate cerebrovascular reserve and to aid in predicting those patients at risk for normal perfusion pressure breakthrough (see Chapters 3 and 64).

ε-Aminocaproic Acid

ε-Aminocaproic acid (Amicar) is an antifibrinolytic agent that inhibits plasminogen activators and has antiplasmin activity. It is used to enhance hemostasis in any condition in which there is abnormally increased fibrinolysis. It has been employed in patients with aneurysmal subarachnoid hemorrhage who are unable to undergo immediate surgery, in an attempt to avoid potentially fatal rebleeding. It has also been used in conjunction with carotid compression to produce thrombosis of carotid-cavernous fistulae.

Low-Molecular-Weight Dextran

Low-molecular-weight dextran (Rheomacrodex) is a plasma volume expander that draws fluid from interstitial spaces into the intravascular space. It is utilized in the medical management of vasospasm secondary to subarachnoid hemorrhage. Caution is advised, as prolonged use can lead to diminished platelet function and increased bleeding.

Mannitol

Mannitol is a potent osmotic diuretic used to prevent or treat oliguria, to induce diuresis in patients suffering from drug intoxication, and to treat elevated intraocular and/or intracranial pressure. Administration of mannitol is recommended in patients with compromised renal function to help clear contrast and decrease the risk of contrast-associated renal failure. We routinely administer mannitol during any procedure in which the contrast volume administered exceeds 500 ml.

Probucol

Probucol (Lorelco) is an antioxidant that was originally marketed as a cholesterol-lowering agent. It was superseded by more effective medications, and production was stopped in 1996. However, a trial published in 1997 demonstrated its effectiveness in reducing the rate of restenosis following coronary angioplasty.[2] The company is considering restarting production at this time. Further work needs to be done, but this drug may be useful in lowering the restenosis rate following intracranial angioplasty as well.

REFERENCES

1. Adams HP Jr, Brott TG, Furlan AJ, et al. Guidelines for thrombolytic therapy for acute stroke: a supplement to the guidelines for the management of patients with acute ischemic stroke. A statement for healthcare professionals from a special writing group of the Stroke Council, American Heart Association. *Stroke* 1996;27:1711–1718.
2. Tardif JC, Cote G, Lesperance J, et al: Probucol and multivitamins in the prevention of restenosis after coronary angioplasty. Multivitamins and Probucol Study Group. *N Engl J Med* 1997;337:365–372.

ADDITIONAL READING

Faulds D, Sorkin EM. Abciximab (c7E3 Fab): a review of its pharmacology and therapeutic potential in ischemic heart disease. *Drugs* 1994;48:583–598.

CHAPTER 5

Fundamental Neurovascular Anatomy

J.C. Wojak

It is essential that the interventional neuroradiologist be thoroughly familiar with vascular neuroanatomy and have an in-depth understanding of the territory and anastomoses of the branches of the internal and external carotid arteries and the vertebral arteries. Certain structures (such as cervical roots and cranial nerves) receive supply directly from external carotid artery branches, rendering these vessels potentially dangerous to embolize. In addition, certain congenital variants in anatomy result in dangerous anastomoses between internal and external carotid artery branches. These dangerous anastomoses, particular vessels, and variants are described below,[1-3] along with the vascular supply to the spinal cord.[4] In addition, the functional aspects of vascular neuroanatomy are reviewed.

DANGEROUS EXTRACRANIAL-INTRACRANIAL ANASTOMOSES

The potential anastomoses described below are summarized in Figure 5–1.

Ascending Pharyngeal Artery

The meningeal branch of the ascending pharyngeal artery enters the cranium via the foramen lacerum; supplies the dura of the clivus and cerebellopontine angle; and anastomoses with the meningohypophyseal trunk and petrous branches of the internal carotid artery, the middle meningeal artery, and the meningeal and segmental branches of the vertebral artery.

Occipital Artery

The occipital artery can form anastomoses with the superficial temporal artery, posterior auricular artery, muscular branches of the vertebral artery, costocervical and thyrocervical trunks, and transverse cervical artery. The latter two can be important in cases of subclavian steal.

Facial Artery

The terminal (angular) branch of the facial artery anastomoses with the ophthalmic artery (dorsal nasal branch). This can provide a major collateral pathway to bypass an occlusion of the internal carotid artery proximal to the origin of the ophthalmic artery.

Superficial Temporal Artery

The anterior branch of the superficial temporal artery may form anastomotic connections with terminal branches of the ophthalmic artery (dorsal nasal, supratrochlear, supraorbital) over the frontal scalp.

Internal Maxillary Artery

This is the largest terminal branch of the external carotid artery. It originates near the condylar process of the mandible and passes medial to it before coursing upward to the posterior portion of the pterygopalatine fossa.

Branches of the Internal Maxillary Artery

The numerous branches of the internal maxillary artery are divided into three groups based on the portion from which they arise: the mandibular, the pterygoid, or the pterygopalatine portion. The mandibular group includes the anterior tympanic, deep auricular, middle meningeal, accessory meningeal, and inferior alveolar arteries. The pterygoid group includes the deep temporal (posterior, middle, anterior), pterygoid, masseteric, and buccal arteries. The pterygopalatine group includes the posterior superior alveolar, infraorbital, greater (descending) palatine, pharyngeal, and sphenopalatine arteries, as well as the artery to the foramen rotundum and the artery of the pterygoid canal.

Dangerous Anastomoses

The internal maxillary artery forms several potentially dangerous anastomoses. Tiny branches of the middle meningeal artery, which supply the tensor tympani, anastomose with the stylomastoid branch of the internal carotid artery in the facial canal. Both the middle meningeal and the accessory meningeal arteries form anastomoses with dural branches of the cavernous internal carotid artery and vertebral artery, along with the meningeal branch of the posterior cerebral artery (artery of Davidoff and Schechter) when present. Pial collaterals between meningeal branches and the underlying brain can be found in a variety of clinical settings.

The lacrimal and/or muscular anastomotic branches of the anterior deep temporal artery connect with the lacrimal branch of the ophthalmic artery and potentially the globe or intracranial internal carotid artery. These branches enter the orbit either via the inferior orbital fissure or by perforating the malar bone directly.

The infraorbital artery gives off lacrimal, muscular, and palpebral branches, all of which anastomose with corresponding ophthalmic artery branches. The sphenopalatine artery branches form connections with the anterior and posterior ethmoidal branches

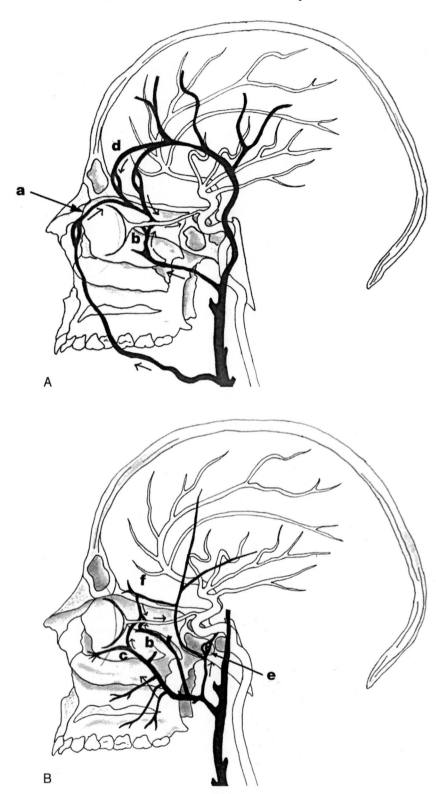

Figure 5-1 *A* to *C*, Potential anastomoses between the external carotid artery, the vertebral artery, and the internal carotid artery, including the angular branch of the facial artery to the dorsal nasal branch of the ophthalmic artery (a); the anterior deep temporal branch of the internal maxillary artery (IMAX) to lacrimal and muscular branches of the ophthalmic artery (b); the infraorbital branch of IMAX to lacrimal and muscular branches of the ophthalmic artery (c); the superficial temporal artery to terminal branches of the ophthalmic artery (d); branches of the middle meningeal artery supplying the tensor tympani to the stylomastoid artery (arising from the petrous portion of the internal carotid artery) (e); branches of the middle meningeal supplying the dura over the orbit to terminal branches of the ophthalmic artery (f); the ascending pharyngeal artery to the meningohypophyseal trunk, petrous internal carotid artery, and middle meningeal artery (g); the posterior auricular artery to the cervical vertebral artery and occipital artery (h); the occipital artery to the posterior auricular artery, vertebral artery, and ascending and/or posterior (deep) cervical artery (i); and the ascending and/or posterior (deep) cervical artery to the vertebral artery and occipital artery (j).

of the ophthalmic artery, and thus also potentially with the intracranial internal carotid artery and globe. In addition, meningeal branches of the ethmoidal branches form anastomoses with dural branches of the internal carotid artery and with branches of the middle meningeal artery. The artery of the pterygoid canal is a continuation of the vidian artery and thus is a potential anastomosis with the petrous portion of the internal carotid artery. The pharyngeal branch anastomoses with cavernous branches of the internal carotid artery. The artery of the foramen rotundum may connect to branches of the inferolateral trunk of the cavernous segment of the internal carotid artery.

Figure 5-1 *Continued*

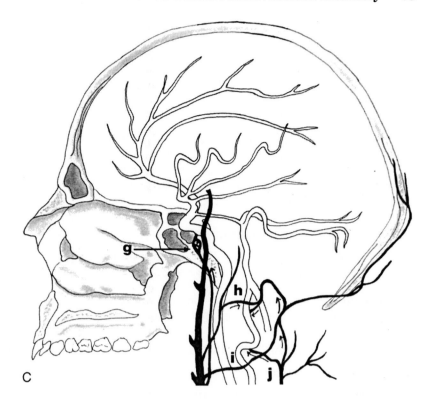

C

Posterior Auricular Artery

This vessel can give rise to meningeal supply to the posterior fossa, anastomosing with branches of the vertebral and occipital arteries. It can also anastomose with the internal carotid artery via the stylomastoid artery.

Ascending Cervical Artery

The ascending cervical artery arises from the thyrocervical trunk and provides the C3 and C4 nerve root anastomotic branches that connect with branches of the vertebral artery, external carotid artery, ascending pharyngeal artery, and posterior (deep) cervical artery.

Posterior (Deep) Cervical Artery

The posterior cervical artery arises from the costocervical trunk and provides C2, C3, and C4 nerve root anastomotic branches that connect with branches of the vertebral artery, external carotid artery, ascending pharyngeal artery, and anterior cervical artery.

PERSISTENT PRIMITIVE ANASTOMOSES FROM THE ANTERIOR CIRCULATION TO THE POSTERIOR CIRCULATION

The possible persistent fetal anterior to posterior circulation anastomoses presented below are illustrated in Figure 5–2.

Primitive Trigeminal Artery

This is the most common persistent anastomotic artery (Fig. 5–2a). It arises from the internal carotid artery proximal to the meningohypophyseal trunk and travels posteriorly to join the basilar artery between the anterior inferior cerebellar arteries (AICAs) and the superior cerebellar arteries. The ipsilateral posterior communicating artery may be hypoplastic.

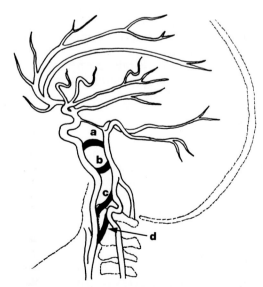

Figure 5-2 Potential persistent fetal (primitive) connections between the internal carotid artery and the vertebrobasilar system include the trigeminal artery (a), the acoustic (otic) artery (b), the hypoglossal artery (c), and the proatlantal segmental artery (d).

Primitive Acoustic (Otic) Artery

This is a rare vessel connecting the petrous portion of the internal carotid artery with the basilar artery at the level of the AICAs or to the AICA itself (Fig. 5–2b).

Primitive Hypoglossal Artery

This is also a rare finding. The artery originates from the internal carotid artery at C1 or C2 and joins the lower basilar artery (Fig. 5–2c). The ipsilateral vertebral artery may be hypoplastic. This artery may supply the brainstem.

Persistent Proatlantal Segmental Artery

This is an extremely rare vessel that arises from the internal carotid artery (or, even more rarely, the external carotid artery) and runs upward and backward through the foramen magnum to join the vertebral artery (Fig. 5–2d). It may also supply the brainstem.

INTRINSICALLY DANGEROUS VESSELS

External Carotid Artery

The external carotid artery gives rise to a collateral branch directly supplying the C4 nerve root.

Ascending Pharyngeal Artery

The ascending pharyngeal artery has many branches that supply vital structures. The superior pharyngeal (or carotid) branch supplies the gasserian ganglion and the parasympathetic (pericarotid) plexus. The jugular artery (or lateral clival branch) supplies cranial nerves VI, IX, X, and XI. The hypoglossal branch supplies cranial nerve XII; the C3 nerve root; and variably cranial nerves IX, X, and XI. The musculospinal branch supplies the C3 and C4 nerve roots and cranial nerve XI; the lateral spinal artery supplies the C1 and C2 nerve roots, the medulla, and the upper spinal cord. The inferior tympanic artery supplies Jacobson's nerve.

The posterior inferior cerebellar artery may rarely arise directly from the ascending pharyngeal artery as the pharyngocerebellar artery.

Occipital Artery

The occipital artery supplies the C1 and C2 nerve roots via anastomotic branches. The stylomastoid branch, arising from either the occipital or the posterior auricular artery, supplies cranial nerve VII and can anastomose with the vertebral system.

Internal Maxillary Artery

The internal maxillary artery and its branches supply many important structures. The middle meningeal artery supplies the first division of cranial nerve V via the meningo-ophthalmic branch, and the gasserian ganglion and the second division via the cav-

ernous ramus. The middle meningeal artery can also give rise to the ophthalmic artery.

The accessory meningeal artery supplies the second and third divisions and the motor part of cranial nerve V via its cavernous ramus. The ophthalmic artery may rarely arise from the accessory meningeal artery, as may the anterior cerebral artery. If there is accessory meningeal dominance to the cavernous sinus, cranial nerves III to VII will be supplied by this artery rather than the inferolateral trunk of the cavernous internal carotid artery.

The artery of the foramen rotundum supplies the second division of cranial nerve V and anastomoses with the artery of the inferior cavernous sinus (inferolateral trunk or lateral mainstem). The artery of the pterygoid canal (vidian artery) supplies the vidian nerve. The anterior tympanic artery supplies the chorda tympani.

Ascending Cervical Artery

The ascending cervical artery supplies the C3 and C4 nerve roots via anastomotic branches.

Posterior (Deep) Cervical Artery

The posterior cervical artery supplies the C2, C3, and C4 nerve roots via anastomotic branches.

VASCULAR SUPPLY TO THE SPINAL CORD

The following is an overview of spinal arterial anatomy. An in-depth discussion of this topic, beyond the scope of this text, is presented by Lasjaunias and Berenstein.[4]

The spinal cord is supplied by one anterior and two posterior spinal arteries (Fig. 5–3). The anterior spinal artery extends the length of the cord in the midline and supplies the anterior two thirds of the cord. The posterior spinal arteries extend along the posterolateral aspects of the cord and supply the remaining posterior third of the cord. They can be discontinuous.

The anterior spinal artery is formed at its most superior (cephalad) aspect by the junction of the anterior spinal branches of the vertebral arteries, which arise between the origins of the posterior inferior cerebellar arteries and the vertebrobasilar junction. The anterior spinal artery then receives contributions from radicular arteries. In the cervical region, these arise from the vertebral, ascending cervical, and deep (posterior) cervical arteries. At the thoracic and lumbar levels, they arise from the posterior intercostal arteries and lumbar arteries (which in turn arise from the aorta). Not all radicular arteries supply the cord; most merely supply the nerve roots in the neural foramina. The larger ones (radiculomedullary arteries) give off meningeal branches and anterior branches that ascend and descend to supply the anterior spinal artery. Usually, six to ten radicular arteries supply the anterior spinal artery. An average of three cervical radicular arteries give supply, but only one upper-midthoracic radicular artery (~ T4 or

Arteries of Spinal Cord

Anterior view

Posterior view

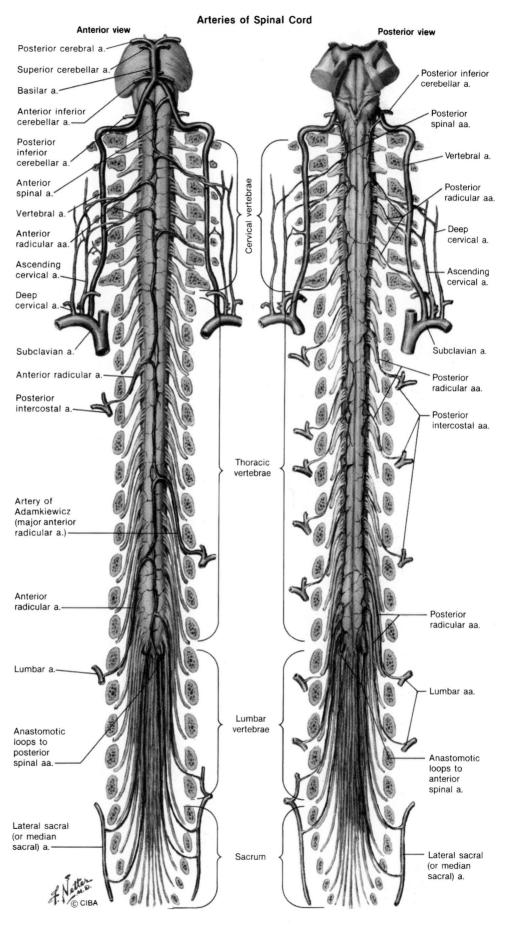

Posterior cerebral a.

Superior cerebellar a.

Basilar a.

Anterior inferior cerebellar a.

Posterior inferior cerebellar a.

Anterior spinal a.

Vertebral a.

Anterior radicular aa.

Ascending cervical a.

Deep cervical a.

Subclavian a.

Anterior radicular a.

Posterior intercostal a.

Artery of Adamkiewicz (major anterior radicular a.)

Anterior radicular a.

Lumbar a.

Anastomotic loops to posterior spinal aa.

Lateral sacral (or median sacral) a.

Posterior inferior cerebellar a.

Posterior spinal aa.

Vertebral a.

Posterior radicular aa.

Deep cervical a.

Ascending cervical a.

Subclavian a.

Posterior radicular aa.

Posterior intercostal aa.

Posterior radicular aa.

Lumbar aa.

Anastomotic loops to anterior spinal a.

Lateral sacral (or median sacral) a.

Cervical vertebrae

Thoracic vertebrae

Lumbar vertebrae

Sacrum

Figure 5-3 Illustration of the arterial supply to the spinal cord. (Drawings by Frank Netter. © Copyright 1996. CIBA-GEIGY Corporation. Reprinted with permission from the Ciba Collection of Medical Illustrations illustrated by John Craig or Frank Netter, M.D. All rights reserved.)

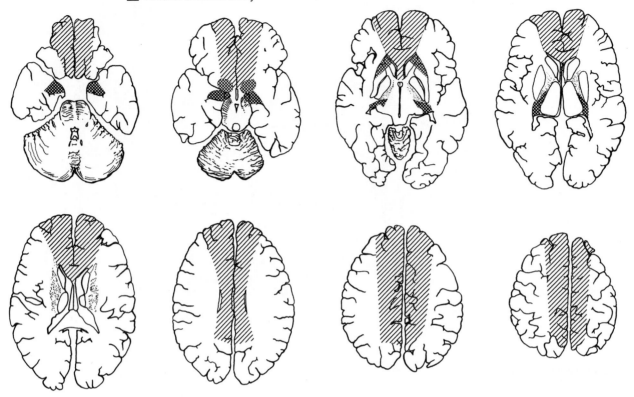

Territory of anterior cerebral artery
Perforators of anterior cerebral artery (medial lenticulostriates; recurrent artery of Heubner)
Anterior choroidal artery

Figure 5-4 Territory of the anterior cerebral artery and its perforators.

Territory of middle cerebral artery
Perforators of middle cerebral artery (lateral lenticulostriate arteries)

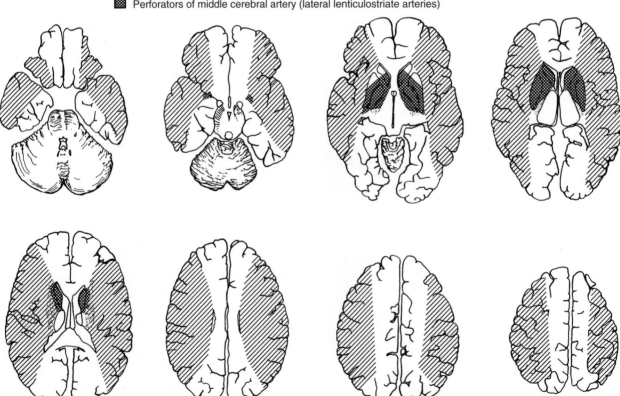

Figure 5-5 Territory of the middle cerebral artery and its perforators.

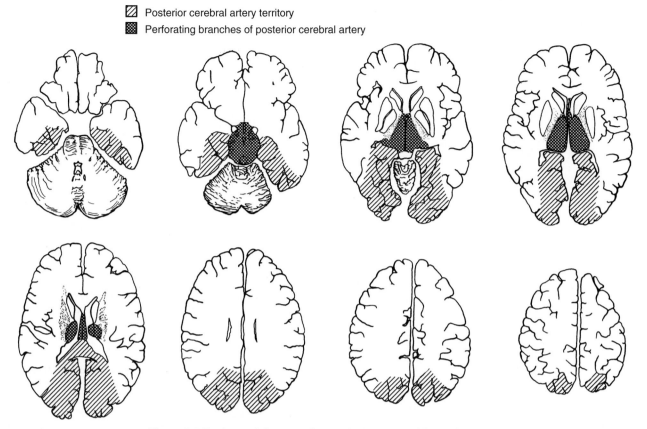

◩ Posterior cerebral artery territory
▨ Perforating branches of posterior cerebral artery

Figure 5-6 Territory of the posterior cerebral artery and its perforators.

T5). Below T8, the major supply is via the artery of Adamkiewicz, which arises most often from a left-sided intercostal artery (80%) between T9 and L2 (85%). This is a large radicular artery with a prominent anterior and smaller posterior branch. The anterior branch reaches the anterior aspect of the cord, then ascends a short distance, makes a hairpin turn, and descends as the terminus of the anterior spinal artery. At the conus, it forms anastomotic loops with the posterior spinal arteries. The cauda equina receives supply from lumbar, iliolumbar, lateral sacral, and/or middle sacral arteries.

The posterior spinal arteries are formed superiorly by posterior spinal branches of the vertebral arteries, arising just proximal to the origins of the posterior inferior cerebellar arteries. They are supplied by posterior branches of multiple radicular arteries. In the cervical and upper thoracic region, there is supply from one or both radicular arteries at nearly every level. Below T4 or T5, there is supply from one radicular artery an average of every other level, including the posterior branch of the artery of Adamkiewicz.

INTRACRANIAL VASCULAR TERRITORIES

Knowledge of the vascular territories as seen on a computed tomographic scan is helpful in the diagnosis and treatment of any vascular pathology but perhaps most important in the newly developing fields relative to the emergency treatment of stroke. Not only can the vessel involved be determined, but the pattern of involvement of its territory may yield information as to the status of collateral supply as well as the location of the occlusion within the vessel (see Chapter 59). Figures 5–4 to 5–6 illustrate the territories of the anterior, middle, and posterior cerebral arteries, along with their perforators.

REFERENCES

1. Lasjaunias P, Berenstein A. Surgical Neuroangiography, Vol 1: Functional Anatomy of Craniofacial Arteries. New York: Springer-Verlag, 1987, pp 239–244.
2. Osborn AG. Introduction to Cerebral Angiography. Philadelphia: Harper & Row, 1980.
3. Huber P. Cerebral Angiography, 2nd ed. New York: Thieme, 1982.
4. Lasjaunias P, Berenstein A. Surgical Neuroangiography, Vol 3: Functional Vascular Anatomy of Brain, Spinal Cord and Spine. New York: Springer-Verlag, 1990, pp 15–87.

ADDITIONAL READINGS

Ahn HS, Kerber CW, Deeb ZL. Extra- to intracranial arterial anastomoses in therapeutic embolization: recognition and role. *AJNR* 1980;1:71–75.
McLennan JE, Rosenbaum AE, Haughton VM. Internal carotid origins of the middle meningeal artery, the ophthalmic-middle meningeal and stapedial-middle meningeal arteries. *Neuroradiology* 1974;7:265–275.
Quisling RG, Seeger JF. Orbital anastomoses of the anterior deep temporal artery. *Neuroradiology* 1975;8:259–262.
Russell EJ. Functional angiography of the head and neck. *AJNR* 1986;7:927–936.

Neurologic Correlates of Cerebrovascular Occlusions

D.V. Rodriguez

The focus for the neurologist when seeing a patient is to localize the lesion by way of a thorough and directed history and neurologic examination. If a vascular cause is presumed, the vessel involved is inferred from the site of the lesion. On the other hand, the interventional neuroradiologist usually has one or more studies to peruse, and the cerebral vessel involved is often visualized rather than inferred. The purpose of this chapter is to give the interventional neuroradiologist a practical knowledge of the signs and symptoms resulting from an occlusion of a particular cerebral vessel: for example, what a patient lying on the angiography table with a proximal middle cerebral artery (MCA) occlusion will look like. Several important points need to be addressed. First, the descriptions found herein are those most likely to be seen; variations can and do occur. Second, the signs and symptoms described are those most easily observed and tested. Further, the etiologic mechanism of occlusion is not discussed, as a decrease in or loss of blood flow yields a pattern of deficits regardless of whether the occlusion is due to an in situ thrombus or embolus. Finally, this discussion is not intended to focus on the anatomic basis for neurologic deficits. A lesion in a circumscribed region of the brain usually gives a typical deficit, but occasionally a variation of the deficit or no deficit is seen. In addition, similar deficits can be seen with lesions in different areas of the brain. Again, the aim here is to associate the findings on an angiogram with the most common presentation in a patient.

A framework for considering the signs and symptoms of cerebrovascular occlusion is in terms of large vessels, small vessels, or both. In general, the cortex is supplied by larger or "cortical" branches and the deeper, subcortical regions are supplied by small vessels. Typically, occlusions in large vessels yield deficits that tend to be distinct from deficits due to small vessel occlusions. Thus, the term *cortical deficits* refers to those disturbances of higher level functioning resulting from occlusions of large vessels. While this is a distinctly useful concept, it is important to keep in mind that there can be deficits of "higher cortical functioning" as a result of small vessel occlusions because a "higher cortical" deficit can be due to damage to the cortex or due to an interruption of the cortical pathways.

SPECIFIC VESSELS AND ASSOCIATED FINDINGS

Anterior Circulation

Figure 6–1 provides a general overview of the anatomic regions affected by various anterior circulation vascular occlusions.

Internal Carotid Artery

Internal carotid artery occlusion often may not be associated with any symptoms or signs, depending on the rate at which the occlusion occurred and the degree of collateral flow to the territory in question. If symptoms do occur secondary to occlusion, they generally mimic an M1 (MCA stem) occlusion.

Posterior Communicating Artery

This is the largest of the terminal branches of the internal carotid artery. It usually decreases in size to some degree during life. It generally has two to ten small perforating branches, even if the vessel itself appears to be hypoplastic. The vessel can usually be clipped with impunity, but if the branches (usually called the anterior thalamoperforating arteries) are affected, the neurologic results can be devastating. They supply the inferior optic chiasm, optic tract, tuber cinereum, subthalamus, posterior hypothalamus, anterior ventral portion of the thalamus, and mamillary bodies.

Infarction related to this vessel is present only if there is involvement of the anterior thalamoperforating arteries. Symptoms include mild to moderate hemiparesis and hemisensory loss. More striking are the findings related to neuropsychological factors, apathy, memory disturbance, transcortical aphasia, and learning difficulty. The short-term memory problem can be very disabling.

Anterior Choroidal Artery

This is the last major branch of the internal carotid artery, arising just distal to the posterior communicating artery (PCoA). It is smaller than the PCoA averaging about 1.0 mm, while the PCoA is about 1.4 mm on average. While originating just distal to the PCoA, it can have more than one trunk or even have another vessel arise between it and the PCoA.

The anterior choroidal artery is divided into two

Occlusion of Middle and Anterior Cerebral Arteries

Lesion	Artery occluded	Infarct, surface	Infarct, coronal section	Clinical manifestations
Middle cerebral artery — Entire territory	Anterior cerebral; Superior division; Lenticulostriate Medial Lateral; Internal carotid; Middle cerebral; Inferior division			Contralateral gaze palsy, hemiplegia, hemisensory loss, spatial neglect, hemianopsia Global aphasia (if on left side) May lead to coma secondary to edema
Deep				Contralateral hemiplegia, hemisensory loss Transcortical motor and/or sensory aphasia (if on left side)
Parasylvian				Contralateral weakness and sensory loss of face and hand Conduction aphasia, apraxia and Gerstmann's syndrome (if on left side) Constructional dyspraxia (if on right side)
Superior division				Contralateral hemiplegia, hemisensory loss, gaze palsy, spatial neglect Broca's aphasia (if on left side)
Inferior division				Contralateral hemianopsia or upper quadrant anopsia Wernicke's aphasia (if on left side) Constructional dyspraxia (if on right side)
Anterior cerebral artery — Entire territory				Incontinence Contralateral hemiplegia Abulia Transcortical motor aphasia or motor and sensory aphasia Left limb dyspraxia
Distal				Contralateral weakness of leg, hip, foot and shoulder Sensory loss in foot Transcortical motor aphasia or motor and sensory aphasia Left limb dyspraxia

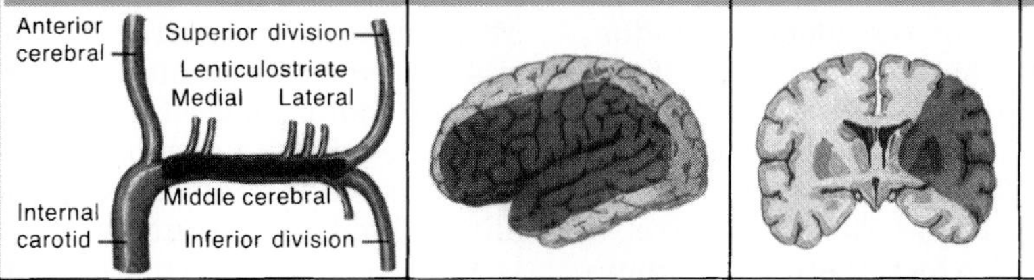

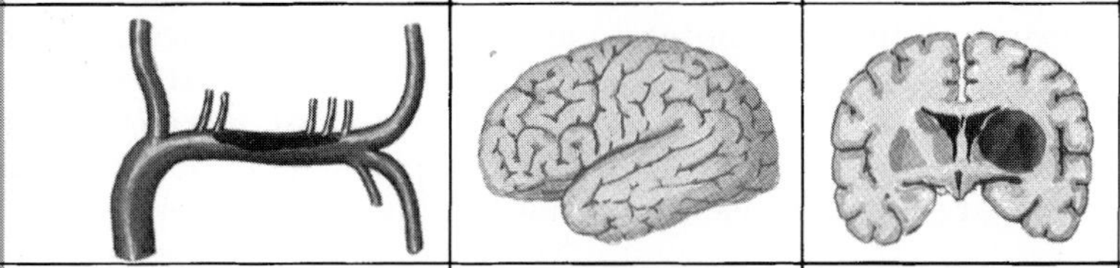

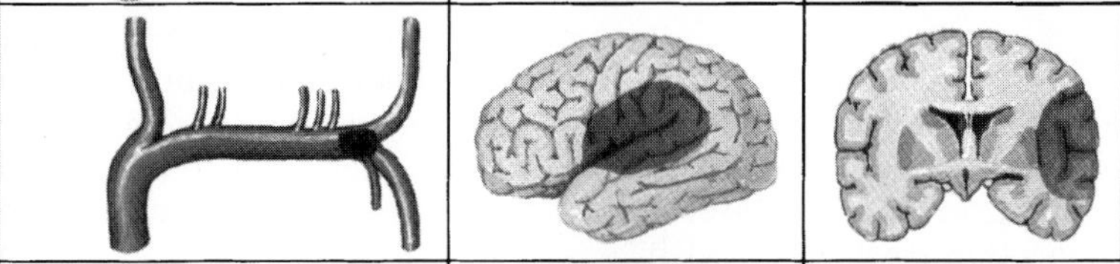

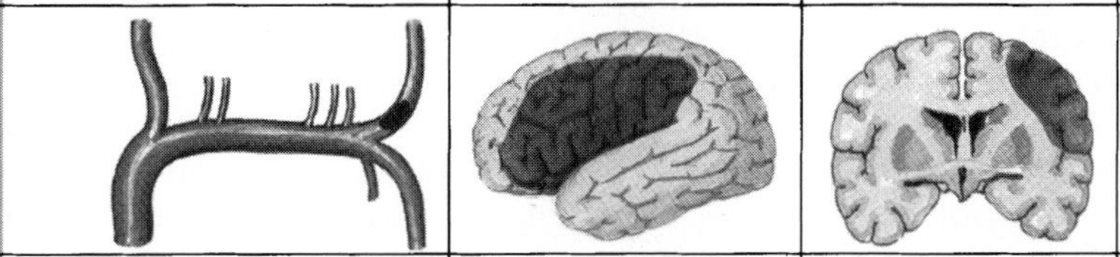

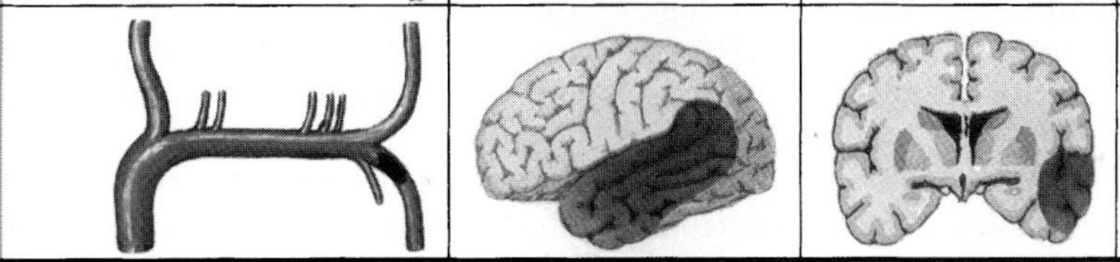

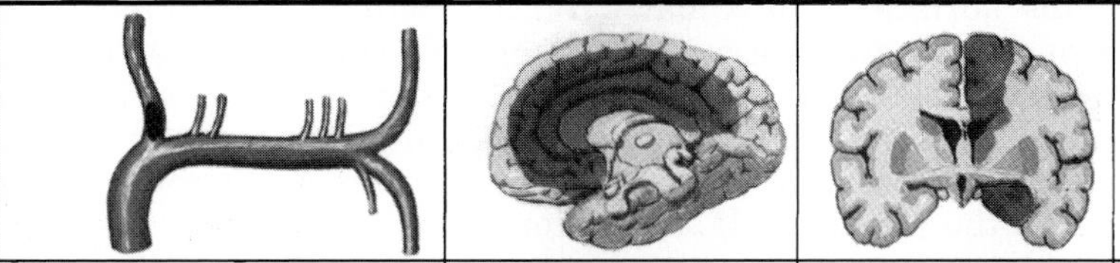

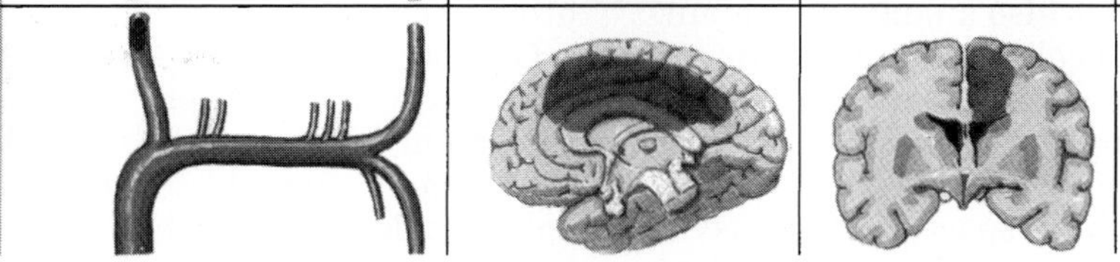

Figure 6-1 Table outlining the anatomic location of infarctions produced by various anterior circulation arterial occlusions and the resultant neurologic deficits. (Drawings by Frank Netter. © Copyright 1996. CIBA-GEIGY Corporation. Reprinted with permission from the Ciba Collection of Medical Illustrations illustrated by John Craig or Frank Netter, M.D. All rights reserved.)

segments, the cisternal and the plexal. The cisternal segment extends from the origin of the vessel from the internal carotid artery to the choroidal fissure; the plexal segment is the terminal portion of the vessel past this point.

The cisternal segment is the primary functional portion of the anterior choroidal artery, supplying between eight and 13 branches to the optic tract, cerebral peduncle, lateral geniculate body, uncus, and anterior perforated substance. The plexal segment sends branches to the choroid plexus and collateralizes with the posterior choroidal artery to supply this structure as well as a small amount of supply to the thalamus, lateral geniculate body, cerebral peduncle, and optic tract.

In addition to the anastomoses with the posterior choroidal artery, there are anastomoses *through* or on the lateral geniculate body, thalamus, or temporal lobe. *In general, the structures supplied by the choroidal segment of the anterior choroidal artery are protected from ischemia from proximal occlusion of the anterior choroidal artery by these distal anastomoses, but not usually the proximal branches.*

Deficits resulting from occlusion of the anterior

choroidal artery have not been studied in great detail. The territory includes the posterior aspects of the posterior limb of the internal capsule and the optic tract, medial portions of the globus pallidus, the lateral choroid plexus, the uncus, the tail of the caudate, and superficial aspects of the thalamus.[1] Occlusion most often results in a hemiparesis with a hemisensory disturbance and some degree of visual field loss (usually incomplete).[2] Although rare, a "quadruple-sectoranopia" in which there is a homonymous hemianopia with sparing of the horizontal sector is very suggestive of an anterior choroidal artery occlusion.[3]

In addition, disturbances of consciousness, long-term memory loss, and aphasia are possible results of an insult to this territory.

Middle Cerebral Artery

The largest portion of the anterior circulation consists of the MCA. This vessel supplies most of the supratentorial territory, including most of the lateral frontal, parietal, and superior temporal lobes with their corresponding deep white matter; most of the basal ganglia and the internal capsule; and the lateral aspects of the thalamus.

The MCA is divided into four segments. The M1 segment courses just over, posterior, and parallel to the sphenoid ridge and is called the sphenoidal segment. The bifurcation (or trifurcation) of the MCA is generally at the region of the insula where the insular segment begins (M2). M3 (the opercular segment) courses over the frontoparietal and temporal operculum. The M4 portion comprises all the cortical branches that spread over the surface. A proximal occlusion of the MCA involving the lenticulostriates and the distal cortical branches leads to weakness and sensory deficit of the face, arm, and leg along with a same-sided visual hemi-field defect and a gaze preference or deviation opposite the weakness. If the left MCA is involved, there is also a language impairment; that is, the patient may be awake, look around, and track objects but does not speak (or speak intelligently) or respond appropriately to speech. Occlusion of the right MCA leads predominantly to a disturbance of orientation to self and space, particularly of the left side of the body. The patient may even deny the presence of deficits or not have appropriate insight into the severity of deficits. If there is adequate leptomeningeal collateral flow and/or a timely partial lysis of the occlusion leading to sparing of the distal territory, the patient may present with weakness and sensory deficits with minimal higher cortical deficits, or there may be cortical deficits that improve rapidly in relation to the motor and sensory findings.[4]

Occlusion of the superior division of the MCA leads to a brachiofacial predominant hemiparesis (face = arm > leg) as well as varying degrees of conjugate gaze abnormality.[5] There may be mild sensory decrements, but visual fields are intact. With left superior MCA occlusion, there is defective production of speech (decreased output, word substitution, paucity of articles, word searching) but a relative sparing of comprehension. There may be varying degrees of orobuccal apraxia—inability to protrude tongue, form a whistle, or puff out cheeks. With right superior MCA disease, there are often no other obvious deficits. There may be mild left-sided neglect or inattention or motor neglect (underutilizing the left arm and/or leg despite adequate strength).

Disease in the inferior division of the MCA is usually without significant weakness. Primary sensation is relatively preserved as opposed to a disturbance of higher sensory function such as the inability to distinguish objects, letters, and numbers by feel, and loss of two-point discrimination. Also present is a hemianopia or superior quadrantanopia. With inferior left MCA occlusion, the patient will often appear "confused." In fact, the patient has significant language comprehension difficulties and some mild deficit of speech output. In some cases it may be almost impossible to elicit other deficits. Visual non-language cues tend to be spared, so that the patient may not respond to the command "Shake my hand" but will readily reach out to shake if the examiner smiles and extends his or her hand. If there is a milder degree of comprehension deficit, one might be able to demonstrate various combinations of right/left confusion, problems with calculations, difficulties with writing, and defective ability to identify the names of fingers (finger agnosia); this is the Gerstmann triad. Right inferior MCA occlusions lead to a left-sided neglect or inattention as well as difficulty with copying figures.[6]

Descriptions of syndromes resulting from occlusion of the distal branches of the MCA are mostly based on the anatomic region involved; thus, variations are likely.[7] The most likely syndromes are described here.

Occlusion of the prefrontal branch can result in apathy, abulia, a transcortical motor aphasia in dominant hemisphere lesions, and motor neglect in nondominant hemisphere lesions. Hemiparesis is not prominent.

Occlusion of the precentral branch may yield a contralateral weakness with upper extremity involvement (proximal > distal). Dominant hemisphere involvement may also result in a transcortical motor aphasia. Central branch occlusion leads to the typical face = arm > leg contralateral weakness.

Parietal branch occlusions are predominated by contralateral sensory deficits; the anterior branch by pansensory deficits and the posterior by discriminative, graphesthesia, and stereognosis deficits. Angular branch occlusion is typically related to loss of contralateral optokinetic response and an occasional contralateral hemi- or inferior quadrantanopia. In the dominant hemisphere there may be part or all of the Gerstmann triad, and in the nondominant hemisphere predominantly neglect or inattention and constructional deficits.

Occlusion of the temporal branches to the most posterior territory (temporo-occipital and posterior temporal branches) generally yields a contralateral superior quadrantanopia or hemianopia with minimal motor or sensory deficits. In the dominant hemisphere a Wernicke-type aphasia is typically present, while in the nondominant hemisphere a contralateral neglect and possibly a confusional state result.

Anterior Cerebral Artery

Acute occlusion of the anterior cerebral artery (ACA) is less common. The cortical branches of the ACA supply the medial surfaces of the frontal and parietal lobes and the adjacent deep white matter as well as most of the corpus callosum. There are also small branches of the ACA that supply parts of the caudate, internal capsule, globus pallidus, and anterior diencephalon. The presentation of an ACA occlusion can be described in terms of motor, psychomotor, and language deficits.[8] The characteristic weakness is crural (leg > arm = face). A spectrum of psychomotor deficits occur, ranging from an akinetic mutism (basically a state of unresponsiveness in a seemingly alert patient) to a more common abulic state (decreased spontaneous motor and verbal output, increased latency of responses, and mild impersistence). Some patients exhibit a grasp reflex. In terms of language, a muteness that rapidly improves is common, and there may be a transcortical aphasia with normal comprehension and repetition but abnormal spontaneous speech.[9]

One important variation of the pattern of weakness is a face = arm = leg or even face = arm > leg pattern. This occurs most likely as a consequence of occlusion of either the small penetrators off the proximal segment of the ACA supplying portions of the genu and adjacent posterior limb of the internal capsule and the rostral thalamus or the recurrent artery of Heubner that supplies the anterior aspects of the head of the striatopallidum and the anterior hypothalamus.[10, 11]

Recurrent Artery of Heubner

This is the largest branch of the first portion of the anterior cerebral artery, but interestingly enough, it actually originates from the A2 segment about three fourths of the time and from A1 or the anterior communicating artery in the remainder. It is approximately 1 mm in size and is unique in that it doubles back along the length of its parent artery to supply its region. This would appear to be because it originally supplies its region but gets stretched as the anterior cerebral trunk becomes displaced farther and farther anteriorly during development.

This artery supplies the anterior internal capsule, the anterior third of the putamen, the adjacent region of the globus pallidus, and the anterior caudate nucleus. Some researchers suggest that owing to its limited supply area, this vessel is not the one responsible for hemiparesis after sugery in this region, but this is probably not the case: some people may have a modest amount of additional coverage, with consequently more severe effects from occlusion of this vessel.

Posterior Circulation

Occlusions of the major vessels in the posterior circulation are generally characterized by crossed findings (weakness and/or sensory change in the face *opposite* the body), conjugate horizontal or vertical gaze palsies, and upper and lower motor neuron cranial nerve abnormalities. Patients often complain of some combination of nausea, vomiting, diplopia, vertigo, incoordination, ataxic gait, dysphagia, and dysarthria. These constellations of signs and symptoms localize to the posterior circulation.

Vertebral Artery

Vertebral artery occlusion results most commonly in ataxia, Horner's syndrome, and contralateral loss of pinprick sensation. In addition, there are combinations of hoarseness, dysphagia, hiccuping, nystagmus, a lower motor–type facial nerve palsy, and loss of pinprick over the face (ipsilateral to the Horner's). This is the lateral medullary, or Wallenberg's, syndrome.[12–16]

Basilar Artery

Occlusion of the basilar artery (BA) in its proximal course leads to hemiparesis or quadriparesis, facial weakness, dysarthria, eye movement abnormalities such as nystagmus and gaze pareses (horizontal), often decreased level of consciousness, and lack of clear cerebellar and sensory findings.[17]

Occlusion of the distal basilar gives a "top of the basilar" syndrome that can be considered as deficits of four types: motor function, consciousness, cognition, and oculomotor nerve function.[18] Most commonly seen are vertical gaze pareses, retraction nystagmus, convergence spasms, large non- or minimally reactive pupil, ptosis, marked drowsiness, and amnesia.

Posterior Cerebral Artery

The occipital, inferior and medial temporal, and posterior inferior parietal lobes, as well as some of the midbrain and thalamus, are supplied by the posterior circulation via the posterior cerebral arteries (PCAs). The supratentorial portions are supplied by larger branches, and the potions of the midbrain and thalamus by small penetrators. Proximal occlusion of the PCA before the posterior communicating artery (PCoA) is characterized most notably by weakness. In addition, there are often vertical gaze abnormalities, cranial nerve III palsy, and a depressed level of consciousness.[19] If there is inadequate collateral flow through the PCoA, the more distal territory is compromised and there are dysesthesias, hemianopia (often macular sparing), and attentional (right hemisphere) or language (left hemisphere) abnormalities. Occlusions just distal to the PCoA are primarily without weakness; otherwise, there are dysesthesias, hemianopia, decreased level of consciousness, and possibly attentional or language deficits.[20, 21] More distal occlusions lead to visual deficits, the most obvious and consistent being a field cut in which the macular vision is spared. Occlusions of the named branches of the PCAs lead to various visual deficits. One interesting finding is the ability to write normally but inability to read secondary to occlusion of the distal PCA branches of the dominant hemisphere involving the left occipital lobe and splenium of the corpus callosum.

Posterior Choroidal Artery

The deficits arising from posterior choroidal artery (PChA) occlusion, like those associated with the AChA, have not been extensively characterized. PChA territory includes the choroid plexus of the lateral ventricle; the pulvinar; the lateral geniculate body; the hippocampus and the mesial temporal lobe; portions of the medial and dorsolateral thalamic nuclei; and small, varying portions of the upper midbrain. Most likely to be seen is a visual field defect (either sectoranopia, quadrantanopia, or incomplete hemianopia) and a hemisensory defect.[22] Neuropsychiatric abnormalities, such as a transcortical aphasia or visual or verbal memory disturbances, are uncommon but do occur. Notably, hemiparesis is uncommon and usually mild and transient.

Superior Cerebellar Artery

The superior cerebellar artery (SCA) is not commonly involved in isolation, but rather as part of occlusion of the distal BA. However, in cases reported, the syndrome is notable for a lack of significant weakness, a contralateral hemisensory impairment usually not involving the face, truncal and appendicular ataxia, and dysarthria.[23–25]

Anterior Inferior Cerebellar Artery

The anterior inferior cerebellar artery (AICA) is most often involved as part of a BA occlusion. In patients with isolated occlusion, an ipsilateral hearing decrement, an ipsilateral sensory decrement of the face, cerebellar findings, and a contralateral pin/temperature sensory loss over the body can be demonstrated. Patients most frequently complain of vertigo, nausea, and tinnitus.[25, 26]

Posterior Inferior Cerebellar Artery

Isolated posterior inferior cerebellar artery (PICA) occlusion is uncommon but may present as Wallenberg's syndrome (see above) or with vertigo and headache, and signs of truncal and appendicular ataxia as well as nystagmus.[12, 25] Typically, PICA occlusion is caused by distal vertebral artery occlusion and can result in severe symptoms.

REFERENCES

1. Mohr JP, Steinke W, Timsit SG, et al. The anterior choroidal artery does not supply the corona radiata and the lateral ventricular wall. *Stroke* 1991;22:1502–1507.
2. Helgason C, Caplan LR, Goodwin J, Hedges T. Anterior choroidal artery–territory infarction. Report of cases and review. *Arch Neurol* 1988;43:681–686.
3. Frisen L. Quadruple sectoranopia and sectorial optic atrophy: a syndrome of the distal anterior choroidal artery. *J Neurol Neurosurg Psychiatry* 1979;42:590–594.
4. Saito I, Segawa H, Shiokawa Y, et al. Middle cerebral artery occlusion: correlation of computed tomography and angiography with clinical outcome. *Stroke* 1987;18:863–868.
5. Althemus RL, Roberson GH, Fisher CM, Pessin M. Embolic occlusion of the superior and inferior divisions of the middle cerebral artery with angiographic-clinical correlation. *AJR* 1976;126:576.
6. Caplan LR, Kelly M, Kase CS, et al. Infarcts of the inferior division of the right middle cerebral artery. *Neurology* 1986;36:1015–1020.
7. Waddington MM, Ring BA. Syndromes of occlusion of the middle cerebral artery branches: angiographic and clinical correlation. *Brain* 1968;91:685–696.
8. Bogousslavsky J, Regli F. Anterior cerebral artery territory infarction in the Lausanne Stroke Registry: clinical and etiologic patterns. *Arch Neurol* 1990;47:144–150.
9. Ross ED. Left medial parietal lobe and receptive language functions: mixed transcortical aphasia after left anterior cerebral artery infarction. *Neurology* 1980;30:144–151.
10. Dunker PO, Harris AB. Surgical anatomy of the proximal anterior cerebral artery. *J Neurosurg* 1975;43:359–367.
11. Perlmutter D, Rhoton AL Jr. Microsurgical anatomy of the anterior cerebral–anterior communicating–recurrent artery complex. *Surg Form* 1976;27(62):464–465.
12. Fisher CM, Karnes WE, Kubik CS. Lateral medullary infarction—the pattern of vascular occlusion. *J Neuropathol Exp Neurol* 1961;20:323–379.
13. Currier RD, Giles CL, Dejong RN. Some comments on Wallenberg's lateral medullary syndrome. *Neurology* 1961; 11:778–790.
14. Norrving B, Cronqvist S. Lateral medullary infarction: prognosis in an unselected series. *Neurology* 1991;41:244–248.
15. Peterman AF, Siekert RG. The lateral medullary (Wallenberg) syndrome: clinical features and prognosis. *Med Clin North Am* 1960;44:887–895.
16. Sacco RL, Freddo L, Bello J, et al. Wallenberg's lateral medullary syndrome. Clinical–magnetic resonance imaging correlations. *Arch Neurol* 1993;50:609–614.
17. Kubik CS, Adams RD. Occlusion of the basilar artery—a clinical and pathologic study. *Brain* 1946;69:73–121.
18. Caplan LR. "Top of the basilar" syndrome. *Neurology* 1980;30:72–79.
19. Castaigne, P, Lhermitte F, Buge A. Paramedian thalamic and midbrain infarcts: clinical and neuropathological study. *Ann Neurol* 1981;10:127–148.
20. Fisher CM. The posterior cerebral artery syndrome. *Can J Neurol Sci* 1986;13:232–239.
21. Goto K, Tagawa K, Yemura K, et al. Posterior cerebral artery occlusion: clinical, computed tomographic, and angiographic correlation. *Radiology* 1989;132:357–368.
22. Neau J-P, Bogousslavsky J. The syndrome of posterior choroidal artery territory infarction. *Ann Neurol* 1996;39:779–788.
23. Amarenco P, Hauw J-J. Cerebellar infarction in the territory of the superior cerebellar artery: a clinicopathologic study of 33 cases. *Neurology* 1990;40:1383–1390.
24. Struck CK, Biller J, Bruno A, et al. Superior cerebellar artery territory infarction. *Cerebrovasc Dis* 1991;1:71–75.
25. Kase CS, Norrving B, Levine SR, et al. Cerebellar infarction. Clinico-anatomic correlations. *Stroke* 1993;24:76–83.
26. Amarenco P, Rosengart A, Dewitt LD, et al. Anterior inferior cerebellar artery territory infarcts: mechanisms and clinical features. *Arch Neurol* 1993;50:154–161.

CHAPTER 7

General Preprocedure and Postprocedure Orders

J.C. Wojak

PREPROCEDURE ORDERS

1) NPO after midnight before the procedure (may have oral medications with sips of water)
2) IV: 0.45 normal (half normal) saline with 20 mEq KCl/L @ 75 ml/hr
3) Foley catheter inserted in early AM or just before call to Radiology
4) Complete blood count with platelets, serum electrolytes, BUN/creatinine, PT/aPTT
5) Electrocardiogram and chest radiograph for all adult patients if participation by Anesthesiology is expected
6) Elbow and heel protectors placed on the patient on call to Radiology

POSTPROCEDURE ORDERS

1) Activity: Bedrest, flat (may logroll prn) for 6 hours, then increase head of bed to 30 degrees, and out of bed in AM with assistance. (If sheath is left in place, head of bed may be raised to 30 degrees when patient returns to nursing unit; keep legs straight.)
2) Vital signs: Pulse, blood pressure, respiratory rate, neurologic check, peripheral pulse assessment, puncture site assessment every 15 minutes (×4), then every 30 minutes (×4). Hourly after this while in Recovery or ICU or hourly (×4) and then every 4 hours if patient returned to ward
3) Pulse oximeter continuously while in Recovery or ICU
4) Nursing: Foley to gravity drainage
   Intake and output monitored and recorded every shift
   Antiembolism stockings and/or sequential compression devices on both lower legs (to mid-thigh level) while patient in bed
   (If sheath is in place, maintain transparent occlusive dressing)
5) Respiratory: Nasal cannula/mask as needed to keep oxygen saturation above 98%
   (If on ventilator, initial settings per anesthesia, adjust according to goals—hyperventilation, weaning, etc.)
6) Diet: Advance as tolerated to preprocedure diet
7) IV: 0.45 normal saline with 20 mEq KCl/L @ 75 ml/hr; adjust on basis of intake and output
   (If multiple lines, a total of at least ~75 ml/hr should be maintained)
   (If long femoral sheath is in place, normal saline

with 1000 U heparin/L @ 50 ml/hr should be administered through sheath—this will require an infusion pump with the high-pressure alarm set above systolic pressure)
   (If a standard arterial line (e.g., radial or femoral) is in place, normal saline with 1000 U heparin/L is administered via a standard flush/monitor apparatus at ~3 ml/hr)
Medications: Resume previous medications unless contraindicated
   Antipyretic/analgesic: Acetaminophen, 1000 mg PO or rectally every 6 hours as needed for pain or temperature >38.5°C
   Analgesic: If acetaminophen is ineffective, ketorolac (Toradol), 60 mg IM initially, then 30 mg IM or 10 mg PO every 6 hours (up to 48 hours), unless patient is anticoagulated
   (If this is ineffective, morphine sulfate, 2 to 10 mg IV every 2 hours as needed [give with antiemetic])
   Antiemetic: Droperidol (Inapsine), 0.625 mg IV prn
   (Or promethazine HCl [Phenergan], 12.5 to 25 mg IV/IM every 4 hours prn)
   (Or ondansetron [Zofran], 4 mg IV every 4 hours prn)
   Antibiotic: If sheath is left in place, if the procedure was prolonged and involved extensive embolization, or if contamination is feared, cefazolin (Ancef), 1 gm IV every 8 hours for 24 hours or until sheath is removed
   (If patient is allergic to cephalosporins, vancomycin [Vancocin], 500 mg IV every 6 hours for 24 hours or until sheath is removed)
   Miscellaneous: Temazepam (Restoril), 15 mg PO at bedtime as needed; may repeat once after 1 hour
Laboratory tests: Complete blood count with platelets, serum electrolytes, BUN/creatinine, and PT/aPTT in Recovery and the following AM
   (If patient is on heparin drip, PT/aPTT per nomogram: see below)
   Electrocardiogram and chest radiograph in Recovery if indicated
Notify MD for: Temperature >38.5°C, pulse >120 or <55 beats/min, systolic blood pressure >170 or <105 mm Hg, diastolic blood pressure >95 mm Hg, respiratory rate <8 or >20 breaths/min, respiratory distress, oxygen saturation <95%, change in neurologic examination, change in pulses, bleeding/hematoma at puncture site, urine output <30

ml/hr for 2 consecutive hours, pain not controlled by medication, abnormal laboratory results

ADDITIONAL MEDICATIONS (AS NEEDED FOR SPECIFIC CASES)

Maintenance of Vessel Patency

When vessel patency is a concern:

> Heparin (see nomogram below)
> Abciximab (ReoPro): if bolus was given during procedure, continuous infusion at 10 μg/min is maintained for 12 hours—7.2 mg mixed in 250 ml normal saline at a rate of 21 ml/hr. If postprocedure bolus is indicated, 0.25 mg/kg IV is given, followed by continuous infusion
> (Or aspirin, 325 mg PO daily)
> (Or ticlopidine [Ticlid], 250 mg PO bid)

Heparin Nomogram

Heparin (25,000 U in 500-ml normal saline; 50 U/ml) titrated as follows to keep aPTT 2.5 to 3 times control:

1) Bolus 5000 U heparin IV (adjust depending on amount received during case)
2) Start drip at 24 ml/hr (1200 U/hr).
3) Obtain aPTT in 6 hours and adjust drip as follows:
   - If <40, bolus 3000 U heparin IV and increase drip by 4 ml/hr (200 U/hr), repeat aPTT in 4 hours
   - If 40 to 60, increase drip by 2 ml/hr (100 U/hr), repeat aPTT in 4 hours
   - If 60 to 90, repeat aPTT in 8 hours
   - If 90 to 100, decrease drip by 2 ml/hr (100 U/hr), repeat aPTT in 4 hours
   - If 100 to 120, stop heparin for 30 minutes, then decrease drip by 2 ml/hr (100 U/hr) when restarting, repeat aPTT in 4 hours
   - If >120, stop heparin for 1 hour, then decrease drip by 4 ml/hr (200 U/hr) when restarting, repeat aPTT in 4 hours
4) Repeat step 3 after every subsequent aPTT is obtained.

Reversal of Abciximab

The platelet count should be monitored during abciximab administration. If it falls below 60,000, the heparin and aspirin are stopped. If the platelet count drops below 50,000 or uncontrollable bleeding occurs, the following steps are taken:

1) Obtain bleeding time.
2) Administer platelets until bleeding is controlled or platelet count is acceptable.

Management of Blood Pressure

Control of Intraprocedural Hypertension

For control of blood pressure in patients receiving thrombolytic therapy and other patients in whom adequate control of blood pressure is necessary, the guidelines provided by the American Heart Association for patients receiving t-PA are useful:[1]

1) Monitor arterial blood pressure during the first 24 hours after starting treatment:
   - Every 15 minutes for 2 hours after starting the infusion, then
   - Every 30 minutes for 6 hours, then
   - Every 60 minutes until 24 hours after starting treatment.
2) If systolic blood pressure is 180 to 230 mm Hg or if diastolic blood pressure is 105 to 120 mm Hg for two or more readings 5 to 10 minutes apart:
   - Give IV labetalol, 10 mg over 1 to 2 minutes. The dose may be repeated or doubled every 10 to 20 minutes up to a total dose of 150 mg.
   - Monitor blood pressure every 15 minutes during labetalol treatment and observe for development of hypotension.
3) If systolic blood pressure is >230 mm Hg or if diastolic blood pressure is in the range of 121 to 140 mm Hg for two or more readings 5 to 10 minutes apart:
   - Give IV labetalol, 10 mg over 1 to 2 minutes. The dose may be repeated or doubled every 10 minutes up to a total dose of 150 mg.
   - Monitor blood pressure every 15 minutes during labetalol treatment and observe for development of hypotension.
   - If no satisfactory response, infuse sodium nitroprusside (0.5 to 10 μg/kg/min).
   - Continue monitoring blood pressure.
4) If diastolic blood pressure is >140 mm Hg for two or more readings 5 to 10 minutes apart:
   - Infuse sodium nitroprusside (0.5 to 10 μg/kg/min).
   - Monitor blood pressure every 15 minutes during infusion of sodium nitroprusside and observe for development of hypotension.

Continuous arterial monitoring is advised if sodium nitroprusside is used. The risk of bleeding secondary to an arterial puncture should be weighed against the possibility of missing dramatic changes in pressure infusion.

Periprocedural Hypertension

For periprocedural hypertension, the same protocol is used as for intraprocedural hypertension. The standard orders for sodium nitroprusside infusion are:

1) Sodium nitroprusside (50 mg) in 250 ml 5% dextrose (200 μg/ml).
2) Begin infusion at 0.5 μg/kg/min.
3) Monitor arterial pressure continuously.
4) Titrate infusion to maintain desired systemic pressure.

Hypotension

For systemic hypotension requiring pharmacologic support, or to induce hypertension as part of medical management of vasospasm:

1) Dopamine (400 mg) in 250 ml 5% dextrose (1600 μg/ml).

2) Begin infusion at 5 μg/kg/min.
3) Monitor arterial pressure continuously.
4) Titrate infusion to maintain desired systemic pressure.

Management of Diabetic Patients

General Orders

If a Short Procedure Is Planned Early in the Day

Preprocedure:
1) NPO after midnight except medications with sips of water.
2) Hold insulin or oral hypoglycemic agents.
3) IV 0.45 normal saline at 75 ml/hr.

Postprocedure:
1) Capillary blood glucose and/or serum glucose in Recovery.
   • If needed, give 50% dextrose for hypoglycemia. If hyperglycemic, the patient may need to be placed on sliding-scale insulin (see below) until stabilized.
2) Once patient is able to eat/drink, give AM insulin/oral agent.
   • If patient does not resume oral intake until midday, one half of the usual AM dose should be given.

If a Longer Procedure Is Planned, or in Brittle Diabetics

Preprocedure:
1) NPO after midnight except medications with sips of water.
2) Give one half of normal AM insulin or oral agent.
3) IV 2.5% dextrose in 0.45 normal saline at 75 ml/hr.

Postprocedure:
1) Capillary blood glucose and/or serum glucose in Recovery, then capillary blood glucose every 4 hours until patient is on preprocedure medication with a stable blood glucose.
   • If glucose is <60, give 50% dextrose (one ampule).
   • If glucose >200, begin sliding-scale insulin coverage (see below).

Sliding-Scale Insulin Coverage

1) Capillary blood glucose every 4 hours.
2) If <60, give 50% dextrose (1 ampule) and contact physician.
3) If 60 to 200, nothing needs to be done.
4) If 200 to 250, give 2 U regular insulin subcutaneously.
5) If 250 to 300, give 4 U regular insulin subcutaneously.
6) If 300 to 350, give 6 U regular insulin subcutaneously.
7) If >350, give 8 U regular insulin subcutaneously and contact physician.

These doses may need to be adjusted if the patient is relatively insulin-resistant.

Patients on Glucophage

Preprocedure:
1) Stop glucophage 48 hours before procedure.
   • Substitution of another oral agent or sliding-scale insulin may be needed.

Postprocedure:
1) Obtain serum BUN/creatinine before restarting glucophage.
2) Restart glucophage 48 hours after procedure.

REFERENCE

1. Adams HP Jr, Brott TG, Furlan AJ, et al: Guidelines for thrombolytic therapy for acute stroke: A supplement to the guidelines for the management of patients with acute ischemic stroke. A statement for healthcare professionals from a special writing group of the Stroke Council, American Heart Association. *Stroke* 1996;27:1711–1718.

PART II

EMBOLIZATION

CHAPTER 8

General Principles of Embolization

J.J. Connors III / J.C. Wojak

Owing to the nature of the procedures performed in interventional neuroradiology, there is no true "cookbook" method that can be recommended for each and every treatment. *Knowing* what to do is frequently far more difficult than actually doing it. This is the challenge as well as the reward associated with work in this field. As opposed to performing a hysterectomy, for instance, no two embolizations will be exactly alike; therefore, a thorough understanding of the pathologic process, hemodynamics, goals, and therapeutic options is necessary for every case. For this reason, the focus of this discussion is more on strategy and rationale than on "show and tell" of what can be done with pretty preprocedure and postprocedure pictures.

Some general statistics and "facts" will be stated without documentation from any large series of cases. Portions of this field are too new for some of this information to be totally accurate or to have reached a large enough number of cases to be statistically significant, but some idea of the nature of the work, early trends concerning efficacy and risks, and techniques believed to be useful will be presented.

Vascular pathologies requiring embolization can be grouped into a few categories that can be analyzed. These will be discussed broadly concerning rationale for therapy and then more specifically to cover additional strategic points.

Embolization, broadly speaking, is the "plugging up" of a "tube or tubes," most commonly a vascular channel (but theoretically, a sinus, ureter, or other tract). This can be done either by filling the channel with material of some sort or by actual destruction of the channel or walls thereof. In interventional neuroradiology, embolization almost always refers to occlusion or obliteration of a vascular channel.

Numerous factors determine the technique and material to be used for any embolization procedure. Differences in the location and structure of the target to be embolized require variations in technique and materials. In addition, the goal of embolization (e.g., whether preoperative, palliative, permanent) also affects technique. Factors such as flow dynamics, intrinsic danger related to the location of the disorder, and ease of access also affect the choice of therapeutic strategy.

For these reasons, while angioplasty may be technically difficult, embolization is a far more complex strategic procedure with a greater number and variety of potential failures and/or complications. Only with appropriate training and experience should certain of these procedures be undertaken. Unfortunately, however, without this experience a false sense of confidence may be present. Being able to make an incision and sew a stitch is not sufficient authorization to perform heart transplants. Nor should simply being able to perform an angiogram be deemed all the training necessary to perform embolotherapy (or even angioplasties). Numerous unforeseen technical difficulties and complications can occur, and unfortunately have done so. It has been only from lessons learned the hard way by pioneers in the field and ongoing improvements in technique that knowledge has advanced to its current level.

Just when one thinks one has seen everything, something never dreamed of occurs. It is in the patient's best interest, as well as the interventionist's, not to have to "reinvent the wheel" by rediscovering hazards and complications over and over.

PATHOLOGIES AMENABLE TO ENDOVASCULAR EMBOLOTHERAPY

Five basic types of abnormal vascular structures can be treated by embolization: a simple straight tube (a fistula), a network of channels without an intervening filter (an arteriovenous malformation [AVM]), a vascular bed with a capillary network (a tumor), a "dural" type of arteriovenous (AV) fistula (a large venous sump supplied by innumerable small arteriolar feeders), and a postcapillary venous (cavernous) angioma (or its variant, a lymphangioma). In addition, several other bizarre entities, such as intraosseous hemangiomas, represent additional unique challenges. Treatment of each of these lesions may require vastly different strategies and techniques. The strategic approach to each of these is described below.

Fundamental Limitations of the Science

With any of the procedures about to be described, if it were possible to be absolutely perfect in accuracy and performance, many of the adaptations employed by interventional neuroradiologists would not be necessary and subsequent surgery would not be mandated by limitations. However, intravascular therapy is not perfect and current technique does have limitations. It is for this reason that judgment is required concerning catheter location, embolic agent, particle size, embolization target, and ultimate goal. Unfortunately, it is sometimes not possible to cure the patient completely because it is not possible either to access the target microvessel or to completely and *permanently* obliterate the vessel or structure.

Vascular Protection

A useful technique to know is how to protect nontarget areas. A very common situation is when the target vessel is a small side branch of a parent vessel that needs to be preserved. It may not be possible to select the small side branch to be sacrificed; the vessel may be either too small or at an angle too acute for the catheter to select. If this is the case, occlusion of this main vessel (distal to the target branch) by a protective coil can allow proximal embolization, with the small particles only going out the desired side branch. This is covered in some detail in "Protective Embolization of Vital Vessels" in Chapter 3.

Alternatively, if there is a branch leading to a dangerous location or a vascular territory that needs to be preserved, this branch can be protectively embolized prior to embolization of the target vessel. This can be done if for no other reason than to protect against accidental reflux into the nontarget territory. In the case presented in Figures 8–1, 8–2, and 8–3, injection into the internal maxillary artery revealed flow through the deep temporal artery into the orbital contents and then into the retinal artery. Even though this vessel was not in the area to be embolized, it was felt to be prudent to occlude this vessel prior to the more distal embolization of the internal maxillary artery. This case is discussed at length in the figure legends.

Ideally, it would be nice to be able to only *temporarily* occlude the distal normal territory of a branch, such as with a temporary occlusion balloon. Practically speaking, this is not currently possible. Previous attempts have been made to occlude the normal territory with temporary agents, but at present these techniques are inaccurate or inconvenient, or both. Injection of autologous clot as well as air has been performed, but both are extremely difficult to control and the results are not worth the risk. Even though a platinum coil is permanent, the occlusion is accurate and the long-term results are acceptable. Normal tissue will revascularize downstream around this occlusion to an acceptable degree. The key to an acceptable protective embolization is preservation of the *capillary bed* of the vital territory distal to the occlusion site (not necessarily the feeding arteries), and thus preservation of the tissue and its function

(see "Protective Embolization of Vital Vessels" in Chapter 3).

General Technique of Embolization

Numerous methods are used for embolization along with numerous materials. Most interventional neuroradiologists use "over-the-wire" catheter technique for almost all cases, but about one third use flow-directed catheters at least when using cyanoacrylates to treat AVMs.

Over-the-wire microcatheter technique requires years of practice for proficiency in its use, as does flow-directed catheter technique. It is beyond the scope of this book to describe how to use a microcatheter; hands-on training and extensive practice is required. *Knowing what to do*, as stated previously, is far more difficult than simply being able to do it.

Suffice it to say that good equipment (e.g., guide catheters, microcatheters, microguidewires) can make procedures far easier. Good digital subtraction angiographic equipment is almost mandatory also.

General Preoperative Procedure

The standard preprocedure laboratory tests should be obtained (see Chapter 7). Respiratory and cardiac evaluation should be performed as indicated.

Depending on the target of embolization, additional steps may be necessary. See the specific discussions of each particular pathology for recommendations concerning these needs (e.g., general anesthesia, premedication with steroids, cerebral protectants).

Intraprocedural Vasospasm

The prevention and treatment of intraprocedural vasospasm are covered in detail elsewhere (see "Prevention of Catheter-Induced Spasm" in Chapter 3 and "Intraprocedural Vasospasm" in Chapter 66). Extensive catheter manipulation is required for many of these procedures, and prophylaxis against vasospasm should be routine. There have been reports of severe intraprocedural vasospasm in patients who are prone to migraine headaches; perhaps increased aggressiveness in prophylactic control is necessary in these patients. Microcatheters have actually been held in place by the spastic vessel! This is particularly troublesome when soft, breakable flow-directed catheters are being used. The Magic catheter (Balt, distributed by Target Therapeutics) has a high friction coefficient, while the Zephyr (Target Therapeutics) and the Eddy (Medi-Tech, Inc.) are designed to be more slippery and are easier to retrieve with or without vasospasm.

Extracranial-Intracranial Anastomoses

There are several potentially dangerous extracranial-intracranial anastomoses; these are described in Chapter 5. It is important to be aware of these at all times. In addition, it is important not to allow the

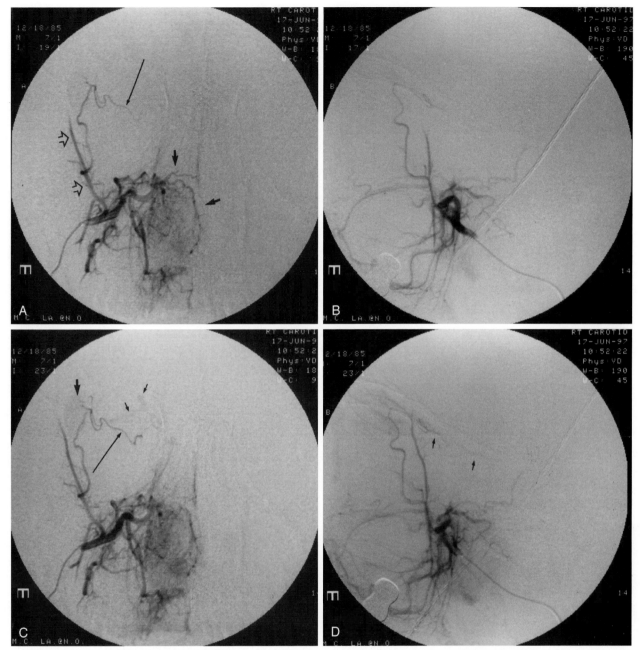

Figure 8-1 Early posteroanterior (PA) and lateral views (*A* and *B*) and late PA and lateral views (*C* and *D*) of a selective injection of the internal maxillary artery demonstrate a mass in the distribution of this vessel *(short arrows, A)* with another vessel coursing superiorly *(open arrows, A)*. This ascending vessel is the anterior deep temporal artery. The artery coursing medially *(long narrow arrow, A and C)* from the anterior deep temporal artery is leading to the intraorbital contents. Note the blush of the lacrimal gland *(short arrow, C)*. Note also in *C* and *D* the very faint shadow of a large vascular structure in the region of the apex of the orbital cone—the superior orbital vein *(small arrows)*—confirming the supply to intraorbital contents.

Even though the globe itself cannot be seen, the implication is that some blood is reaching vessels in the same arterial network that supplies the globe and retina, and lack of visualization of a specific vessel is essentially meaningless under these circumstances. *Case 1 continues*

pCO$_2$ to rise during the case. Hypercapnia directly causes cerebral vasodilation, lowering intracranial arterial pressure. This allows the intracranial vessels to act as a sump and may open dangerous anastomoses.

Vascular Access

The use of the smallest catheter access system possible is recommended. A 6-Fr. sheath system produces the largest hole practically ever necessary. When truly large guide catheters or temporary balloon occlusion guide catheters (e.g., the Zeppelin) are used, a dilator for the *specific catheter* should be utilized to allow direct percutaneous placement, thus avoiding the necessity of a huge sheath. These guide catheters and dilators are now widely available. Vascular damage, postprocedural bleeding, and pseudoaneurysm formation are directly related to puncture hole size,

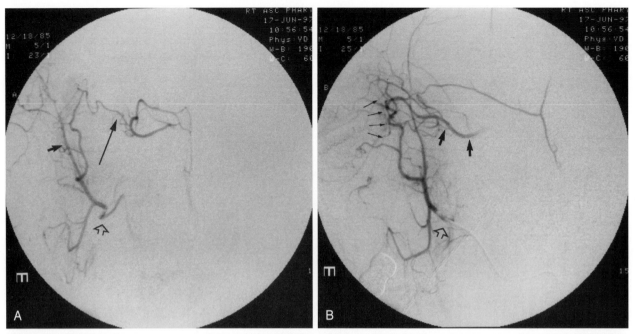

Figure 8-2 *A* and *B,* PA and lateral views of the (almost) selective injection of the anterior deep temporal artery; the catheter is right at its origin *(open arrow),* and some contrast still fills the internal maxillary artery. Note in *A* that the same artery in the roof of the orbit is seen *(long arrow).*
Note in *B* the blush of the retina *(thin arrows).* The ophthalmic artery is now seen also *(thick arrows).*

and anything above 9-Fr. (at the most) should be avoided.

Materials for General Endovascular Occlusion

This topic is discussed in detail in the separate section on embolic agents in Chapter 1.

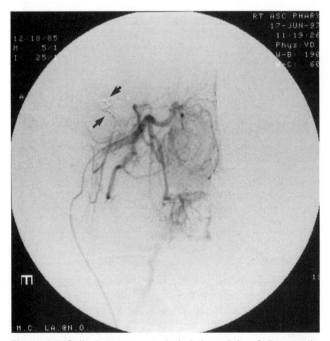

Figure 8-3 Coils have now occluded the origin of the anterior deep temporal artery *(arrows).* Injection of the internal maxillary artery now demonstrates no flow into the region of the orbit. It is now safe to embolize the distal internal maxillary artery without worrying about reflux into any critical territory.

Particulate embolic agents (primarily PVA) have improved considerably over the years. At one time, it was not unusual for patients to suffer cranial nerve palsies with the use of certain particles (in addition to the standard risk of liquid agents). For this reason, recommended particle size was kept over the 300-micron level for most procedures. It is now thought that these problems were due to inadequate quality control related to these preparations with subsequent inclusion of particles in the 2- to 100-micron range (and subsequent penetration to the capillary level and tissue and nerve death). Current preparations have been analyzed and found to be much more uniform, and the use of small particles (150 to 250 microns) has been almost always safe when adequate strategy and technique are used.

Several other particulate agents are now available (see Chapter 1) and have certain advantages and disadvantages. Avitene is extremely thrombogenic and can cause very effective occlusion of relatively large structures, but it is not a permanent agent and the thrombus it stimulates is easily broken down. It also contains particles in the <50-micron range, that is, capable of causing tissue necrosis and cranial nerve damage.

Gelfoam is available as presized microparticles (powder) and sheets. It is also biodegradable. Typically, for intravascular embolization, it is cut into pieces and utilized as separate chunks (torpedoes) injected through a 0.038″ catheter. This is technically not an easy feat with microcatheters.

Cyanoacrylates have their role primarily in the treatment of AVMs, but they have been employed in several other circumstances (e.g., percutaneous tumor embolization). This material is tricky and should be used with caution.

Methylmethacrylate has been used for years for open surgical procedures and in recent years for percutaneous vertebral body infiltration to provide structural support. It has no current role in intravascular embolizations.

Ethanol is an emerging agent useful for certain situations, although it is almost always controversial and/or dangerous. For certain dural arteriovenous fistulae feeders, it works wonders. It can be curative for AVMs, but it must be used extremely precisely. It has been used for percutaneous tumor ablation, percutaneous superficial vascular malformation treatment, and treatment of hemangiomas (see relevant chapters).

Detachable balloons are primarily used for elective arteriovenous fistulae occlusion, carotid-cavernous fistulae, and elective carotid artery occlusion. Their use is primarily restricted to space-occupying tasks and to abrupt occlusion needs. Their propensity to deflate unpredictably, as well as to move from their intended location, makes their use somewhat exciting (see Chapter 35). Silicone balloons can be very slippery and can migrate more readily than latex balloons even when fully inflated; this may produce an unpredictable result and necessitates the use of multiple balloons or balloons stabilized with coils. The increasing use of fibered coils is reducing the need for balloons.

Guglielmi detachable coils (GDC) are intended primarily for intracranial aneurysm therapy. Their cost, cumbersomeness, and poor thrombogenicity render these not the material of choice for simpler pathologies, although more and more uses are being found for them. They are very safe compared with simple pushable coils. The new mechanically detachable coils from Cook, Inc. are straightforward in their use, cheaper than GDC, and suitable for occlusion of a proximal vessel. They are not available for use with a standard microcatheter, however. No coils should ever be used to occlude the vascular supply to central nervous system structures without total flow arrest by means of a flow-control guide catheter (see Chapter 1).

EXTRA-AXIAL TUMORS

General Considerations

This category (tumors) can cover a huge range. If the science of interventional neuroradiology offered wonderful solutions to everything, this category *would* cover a huge range. There are certain situations in which this field has specific benefits, however. Hypervascular masses presenting technical difficulties during excision are one example. Most tumors currently treated by endovascular embolotherapy are outside the cranium (meningiomas being the exception), but the technique of endovascular therapy is the same. General strategies will be discussed first.

Goal of Therapy: Definitive Cure vs. Presurgical Aid

The luxury of having a capillary bed filter renders embolization of tumors perhaps the most technically straightforward of the various forms of embolotherapy. The primary consideration for this procedure should be the *goal* of the embolotherapy, not necessarily what can theoretically be accomplished. This goal is primarily determined by whether or not the treatment is aimed at a definitive cure or is simply presurgical.

The aim of endovascular therapy is to do as little as possible as safely as possible while accomplishing the goal (definitive cure vs. presurgical aid). Therefore, strategic decisions are limited to the choice of embolic agent (e.g., permanent versus nonpermanent, tissue destruction versus simple occlusion), the approach (e.g., percutaneous, transarterial), and the exact sites (vessels) to be occluded.

Most tumor embolization is presurgical. The goal should thus be to simply render surgery safer and easier, but not at the expense of adding another potentially dangerous procedure to the dangers already associated with the surgery. This is achieved by rendering the tumor easier to manually manipulate (e.g., less friable or rupturable) as well as by selectively devascularizing the surgical field and thus allowing more accurate dissection. Too much devascularization, however, can lead to inadvertent destruction of surrounding normal structures and/or poor healing after surgery. This appears to be a less common result than would initially be thought, but in certain circumstances overaggressive embolization can be harmful (and, unfortunately, in many cases the interventional neuroradiologist may be unaware of the postoperative results, or even of when the surgery was done!).

Simply filling the capillary bed of a tumor with embolic material (either particulate or solidified liquid—e.g., glue) may actually be counterproductive. While it may make the final angiogram appear satisfactory, it can make the tumor difficult to manipulate and still preserve the vascular supply to the operative region, thereby retaining the potential for excessive bleeding during surgery. Conversely, simply occluding the main large feeding vessel(s) (e.g., by proximal coil placement) may also yield a nice appearance on a postembolization angiogram, but may result in a persistent near-normal transtumoral blood flow due to recruitment of collateral arterial supply. Even if no significant arterial collaterals develop by the time of surgery, the lack of intratumoral vascular occlusion can result in a bloody tumor during surgery because of preservation of these vessels and extensive retrograde filling from the venous side. Ideal embolization should prevent the tumor from recruiting new vascular supply, as well as block intratumoral vascular communication that might render the dissection excessively bloody. In addition, it should be accurate enough to preserve the normal vascular supply to the surrounding normal tissues, which will be necessary for ideal healing.

This goal is accomplished by thorough filling of the precapillary intratumoral arterioles followed by occlusion of the significant tumoral supply vessels. The tumor can thus remain somewhat soft (owing to the capillary bed *not* being filled with particles or hard glue), and the operative field can be kept dry. The availability of numerous agents for preoperative embolization and of technically sophisticated catheterization materials and radiographic equipment now renders this task much easier than was previously the case.

Cooperation and close association with the surgeons involved in these cases is very helpful, even to the experienced endovascular therapist. Feedback concerning which vessels were adequately treated and which may not have been is valuable information. The true test of the effectiveness of the interventionist's job is not pretty postangiographic images and a self-congratulatory slap on the back, but rather any clinical and/or surgical benefit he or she may have rendered.

Preservation of the Surrounding Tissue

Superselective embolization is necessary for ideal results. Simply flooding the external carotid arterial bed or internal maxillary artery distribution is unacceptable, even if the immediate postembolization results appear satisfactory and are achieved without apparent complications. The inexperienced interventionist would not even know that postoperative healing will be impaired. He or she might blame any deficiency in the postsurgical result on the surgical procedure, not realizing that the preceding endovascular procedure is the real cause of a less than ideal outcome.

Specifically, for extracranial embolizations, preservation of the superficial temporal and deep temporal arteries is of great significance to the surgeon, while being of minor consequence to the endovascular therapist as far as the postprocedure angiographic results and complications are concerned. Embolization of these vessels can be performed routinely without any significant consequence as long as nothing further is done to their territories, such as *surgery*! These vessels supply broad areas of skin and muscle, and while devascularization may be tolerated, the effect of embolization on surgical healing or wound infection may be unacceptable.

The temporalis muscle (as well as other structures) is supplied by the deep temporal artery(ies). This muscle is used for certain reconstructive flaps after extensive paranasal tumor resection. It is placed under the middle and/or anterior cranial fossa after paranasal tumor resection to separate the contaminated paranasal sinus region from the intracranial contents; otherwise, meningitis and/or encephalitis may result. Devascularization of this area can adversely affect any reconstructive procedure. The same holds true for facial artery branches, scalp branches, and meningeal branches.

Strategic Choice of Agents for Endovascular Tumor Embolization

Currently, particulate agents are the safest and easiest to use for preoperative embolization purposes, and the widespread commercial availability of high-quality PVA particles in numerous sizes renders this the ideal choice (see "Particulate Embolic Agents" in Chapter 1).

For most preoperative treatment of head and neck tumors, initial embolization is begun with particles in the 150- to 250-micron range. If, however, distal access to the specific feeder in a position close to the tumor is not possible, a larger (safer) size may be indicated. For dural feeders of a meningioma, PVA particles 50 to 150 microns in size will allow better downstream penetration without any significant risk to vital structures. These particles will flow all the way to the tumor and penetrate well into its vascular bed, causing significant capillary and precapillary occlusion with resultant cell death. These particles will also penetrate into other territories supplied by the feeding meningeal vessel, but with little chance of harm (depending, of course, on the territory supplied by this vessel). Preembolization lidocaine testing (for non–central nervous system territories) can be performed if there is any question, but it must be known what finding (symptom) is to be tested *for.* These extremely small particles can cause true cell death (read "nerve damage"), hence their effectiveness *and* danger. Particles in the 50-micron range should not be used in the region of the skull base.

If access to a spot very close to the tumor is not possible or if there is potential supply to vital structures (e.g., cranial nerves), particles of 150 to 250 microns are still routinely used but are not as absolutely safe; therefore, particles of 250 to 350 or 350 to 500 microns can be used. If diluted sufficiently, they do not clump. They may not penetrate as well all the way to the tumor vascular bed and may simply occlude the feeder in a location somewhat too proximal, but they are safer. They rarely cause true cell death, but they do devascularize a region. This is particularly true if the interventionist is working in vessels near the skull base (see "Intrinsically Dangerous Vessels" in Chapter 5).

Particles in the size range mentioned above (150 to 350 microns) are adequate to produce complete occlusion in most tumors. Depending on the tumor type, however, there may be large arteriovenous shunts, and continued infusion of small particles may simply flood the lungs (see Chapter 64). For this reason, careful evaluation of the changing flow characteristics of the tumor should be made during the procedure, and the size of the particles should be increased if it is judged that the particles of chosen size are simply traversing the tumor. Indeed, for certain tumors (e.g., glomus tumors), the size of these shunts may be extraordinary, rendering particulate embolization difficult and possibly unfeasible. These tumors can have arteriovenous shunts larger than 1 mm.

If shunting is considerable, it is possible to be successful by employing several maneuvers. Making a slurry of PVA and Avitene can allow very large vessels to be rapidly occluded, but the duration of this occlusion is questionable. Avitene is very thrombogenic, causing rapid platelet aggregation, sometimes amazingly so. Injecting small coils or silk suture is also possible, but these may or may not reach the intended site, or may not stay there if they make it. In addition, the ultimate location of the silk sutures is frequently unknowable, and very small pieces are difficult to use. Straight platinum coils measuring 2 or 5 mm or braided occlusion device (BOD, Target Therapeutics) coils can be used and piled on top of one another, but they may not stay where intended while high flow continues or before an effective coil mass is present. They may pile up in a location too proximal or go completely through a really large shunt. Liquid coils (Target Therapeutics) can be individually injected and can be effective.

Cyanoacrylates have been used for occlusion of shunts, but this is difficult because of the high flow and short tube length. In experienced hands, however, this can be an effective technique.

New liquid embolic materials (e.g., liquid hydrogels) may render occlusion of large intratumoral shunts easier in the future but cannot be recommended at this time. This mass has no ability to stick to the walls and is so malleable that it can slither through vessels with relative ease. A slurry of PVA particles, Avitene, and alcohol has also been described,[1] as noted in Chapter 3; this is a very aggressive mixture. Slowing flow with a proximal coil and injecting a slurry through this can produce stasis. The duration of this occlusion is not known, but, as stated above, Avitene and PVA can be effective occlusive agents, and alcohol could make this occlusion permanent. Final proximal occlusion with coils can render the distal occlusion obtained by the Avitene and PVA more stable and long-lasting. Fibered coils are more thrombogenic than nonfibered, and coil packing and time are allies. The addition of a small piece of silk suture can help complete occlusion. In addition, dipping or soaking a coil in thrombin can render it truly effective.

Temporary proximal flow occlusion can also allow thrombus to form at the site of embolization, particularly in high flow situations (see "Embolizing with Coils" in Chapter 3). Proximal flow control is a rarely used tool that can be of vast help in certain high flow situations, but it is technically more complicated than what has formerly been practiced and could lead to unforeseen complications in inexperienced hands (branch vessels may have stagnant flow, thrombus could form, and, most discouraging, there could be reversal of flow in some downstream vessels). However, newer, more technologically advanced guide catheters with flow control capability are now becoming available (such as the Zeppelin described above).

If total cure of a tumor or palliation without surgical resection is desired, an obliterative agent such as ethanol can be used. This is acceptable only for a vascular territory in which necrosis and liquefaction are tolerable, and in which there is known to be no supply to vital structures. This is most typically the case with meningiomas. Further discussion of this technique is beyond the scope of this chapter; remember that the use of ethanol is a dangerous therapy that should be approached with extreme caution.

Occlusion of Vascular Supply After Intratumoral Embolization

After successful occlusion of intratumoral flow, it is necessary to occlude the feeding arteries that may be difficult for the surgeon to reach. This preserves a dry operative field. Surgical technique has improved considerably over the years, and with proper care it is possible for a skilled surgeon to resect almost any mass without excessive bleeding or damage to nearby structures. However, the technical difficulty can be greatly lessened by preoperative occlusion of the vessels that are hard to reach. This implies knowledge of which vessels are the difficult ones for the surgeons to reach and requires either close cooperation with the surgeon, or preferably, an adequate knowledge of what is necessary. Frequently, the easiest vessel to occlude intravascularly is the one that is easiest for the surgeon to access and is thus unnecessary to be dealt with preoperatively.

Depending on the size of the target tumoral parent vessel, the most common means of final preoperative occlusion is the use of platinum microcoils. Sizing of coils is an art in itself and depends on the vessel size and shape, vascular flow rate, and the specific brand of coil. In general, too small a coil size is better than too large for this specific purpose, particularly for the first coil. Usually, the vessel to be occluded is one in which the catheter has traveled some distance and is tapering to the arteriolar feeders that have just been embolized with particulate agents. Coils that may be too small will travel only to a more distal location and impact where they will. This is not a problem. A multitude of these coils will eventually accomplish the task at hand. A coil that is too large will be too long, and thus may force recoil of the catheter tip to an unsuitable proximal location.

True difficulty in coil selection and placement arises only when the parent vessel to be occluded (i.e., the one feeding the tumor) has a very short trunk beyond its origin from another vascular pedicle that needs to be preserved. The classic example is the meningohypophyseal trunk when it supplies a meningioma at the skull base. Plugging the meningohypophyseal trunk may be intended, but the segment available for occlusion is usually extremely short.

A coil that is intrinsically "nonretaining" (i.e., "straight"), which will just sit in a vessel without any built-in curve to retain its position, is hazardous when placed just within the orifice of a branch from a major vessel. In other words, one should not put a 2-mm straight coil in the origin of the meningohypophyseal trunk from the internal carotid artery; any change in head position or gravity, or even a simple cough, could dislodge this coil back into the main vessel (the internal carotid artery), whence it would then travel to the brain.

REFERENCE

1. Lylyk P, Vinuela F, Vinters HV. Use of a new mixture for embolization of intracranial vascular malformations. Preliminary experimental evidence. Neuroradiology 1990;32:304–310.

ADDITIONAL READINGS

Halbach VV, Higashida RT, Hieshima GB, Hardin CW. Embolization of branches arising from the cavernous portion of the internal carotid artery. AJNR 1989;10:143–150.
Kerber CW. Flow-controlled therapeutic embolization: a physiologic and safe technique. AJR 1980;134:557–561.

CHAPTER 9

Meningiomas

J.J. Connors III / J.C. Wojak

EPIDEMIOLOGY

Meningiomas represent 15% of all primary central nervous system neoplasms.[1] They originate from cellular elements that form the meninges, but also may come from pial or dural fibroblasts. They are more common in females and have been shown to contain estrogen and/or progesterone receptors.[2] These lesions can calcify or ossify. They are found as part of neurofibromatosis type 2 along with bilateral acoustic neuromas and schwannomas; this is an autosomal dominant trait. They can be seen up to 25 years after cranial radiation therapy; these particular tumors tend to be more aggressive, recurrent, and multiple.[3] They typically affect adults aged 25 to 65 with a peak age of about 45 years. Multiple meningiomas are present in approximately 1% to 2% of cases, but this is usually associated with the central form of neurofibromatosis.

Meningiomas are typically benign but rarely can be malignant. They are occasionally found incidentally at autopsy. They are well-circumscribed lesions that tend to be round, with or without lobulations. Typically, they eventually compress adjacent structures.

As is typical of most vascular tumors, meningiomas do not tend to necrose and characteristically remain cellular throughout their growth rather than develop cysts or hemorrhage. They are slow growing and do not invade local structures, specifically the brain. They do, however, parasitize nearby structures for their vascular supply. Hyperostosis of the overlying calvarium is not uncommon accompanying meningiomas (Case 1, Figs. 9–1 to 9–10). There may be frank bony or scalp invasion with more aggressive lesions (Case 2, Figs. 9–11 to 9–26).

Common presenting symptoms associated with meningiomas include headaches, visual changes, and seizures. These symptoms are almost exclusively related to mass effect. Depending on where the mass effect is located, this can cause vascular occlusion or hormonal disturbance (pituitary).

Malignant meningiomas can be very invasive, to the point of being considered a sarcoma. They indeed invade nearby structures and characteristically can invade the brain. Distant metastases have been reported, but by far the most common behavior is local recurrence. Hemangiopericytomas can be considered a variant of a malignant meningioma with angiomatous characteristics.

Meningiomatosis refers to a pathology also called meningeal sarcoma. This is a spreading malignancy, usually multifocal at presentation and without a specific nidus. This tumor presents at an early age for meningioma and also behaves far more aggressively.

En plaque meningiomas are another subtype. They are highly osteogenic but do not compress surrounding structures as badly as do the more focal types of meningioma. They can resemble hyperostosis if located in the typical places but do not respect the midline as is typical for frontal hyperostosis. They occur even more frequently in females than do the garden variety of meningiomas.

The most common sites of involvement tend to be related to a dural sinus and are more often in the anterior cranial fossa than in the posterior. Intraventricular meningiomas are rare and tend to arise in the lateral ventricles. Ocular meningiomas are often the en plaque variety, with primary occurrence in the meninges associated with the optic nerve or spreading from an intracranial location. They can cause exophthalmos or slowly deteriorating vision and/or optic atrophy.

Meningiomas may also arise from sites not typically considered as locations in which they would be capable of forming. Specifically, cranial nerves may be a locus of formation, most typically those near the foramen magnum.

RADIOGRAPHIC EVALUATION

The postcontrast computed tomographic (CT) scan is the gold standard for detection of these tumors. Magnetic resonance imaging (MRI) can delineate their margins very well and help classify them as

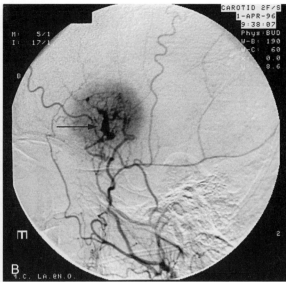

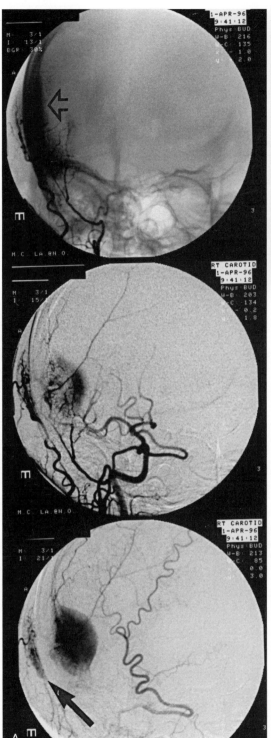

Figure 9-1 Case 1. *A* and *B,* Posteroanterior (PA) (slightly oblique to yield a tangential view of the tumor and overlying skull) and lateral views of a right external carotid injection in a patient with a known intracranial tumor reveal a classic meningioma with hyperostosis *(open arrow)* and transosseous growth *(arrow)*. Note the vascular dysplasia *(thin arrow)* associated with the intense blush.

Case 1 continues

extra-axial tumors, but the first line of defense is the CT scan. Noncontrast MRI can be misleading because these tumors have signal characteristics typical of brain on all sequences. Contrast-enhanced MRI is a very sensitive study for detection of small en plaque lesions, particularly with fat suppression.

On CT examination, meningiomas are typically the same density as brain or slightly higher. About one in 10 are actually lower in density than brain. About the same percentage contain calcification. After contrast administration, they uniformly enhance with distinct margins. Tumor necrosis or cyst formation is rare.

Meningiomas typically have a broad base near a dural surface and "buckle" the gray/white junction beneath them (best seen on MRI). Selective angiogra-

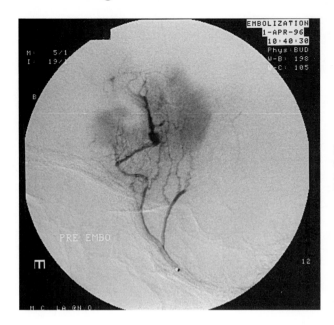

Figure 9-2 Lateral superselective injection of the middle meningeal artery shows the extensive recruitment from the branches of the middle meningeal artery, with a beautiful demonstration of their abnormal corkscrew appearance. Note also the dysplastic arterial varix.

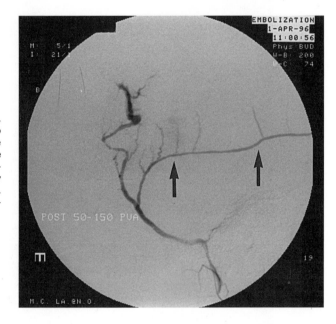

Figure 9-3 After embolization with 50- to 150-micron PVA particles, the tree is pruned but not eliminated. These particles were used to try to penetrate into the tumor and thus eliminate later extensive recruitment from different meningeal or other sources. Note the more distal extension of the posterior branch of the middle meningeal artery *(arrows)*, previously not seen in Figure 9-2, presumably because of the elimination of the sump effect of the tumor bed. Further embolization with 150- to 250-micron particles is now performed to occlude the arteriolar supply.

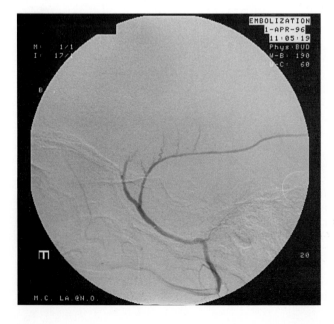

Figure 9-4 Lateral view of the result of additional embolization of the middle meningeal artery with 150- to 250-micron particles. The vessel leading to the tumor is now eliminated, but the posterior branch of the middle meningeal artery is preserved. This is not actually necessary, but it may aid in healing of the operative site.

Case 1 continues

phy used to be performed to evaluate whether these were extra-axial or not, but MRI is uniformly capable of this task, with rare exceptions. In addition, MRI can reveal the presence of vessel voids (flow voids) within the mass, indicative of the degree of hypervascularity.

Angiography reveals the supply typically seen for meningiomas in certain locations (Table 9–1). In general, selective internal and external carotid injections are necessary, frequently bilaterally. In addition, vertebral artery injections reveal auxiliary meningeal supply. While supply is uniformly present from meningeal/dural vessels, the amount of this supply is variable. Skull base lesions frequently have minimal hypervascularity. Pial supply does not necessarily indicate invasion by the tumor of the brain itself. In addition, simple compression of underlying brain can cause a rim of hyperemia seen on digital subtraction angiography (DSA).

One of the primary reasons to perform angiography is not to evaluate the arterial supply, but to study the effect the tumor has had on the venous sinuses and normal cerebral drainage. If a convexity meningioma has obliterated the superior sagittal sinus, it is far easier for the neurosurgeon to remove than if it has simply abutted and compressed this structure. If this is the case, preservation of the sinus is necessary because, while the brain may survive a gradual venous occlusion, an abrupt venous occlusion is usually not well tolerated. For this reason, sensitive DSA is vital for these studies.

T A B L E 9 - 1	**Typical Vascular Supply to Meningiomas by Location**
Location of Tumor	**Supply**
Convexity	Middle meningeal artery
	Artery of anterior falx
	Scalp arteries (e.g., superficial temporal artery)
	Pial branches (anterior and middle cerebral arteries)
Sphenoid wing	Middle meningeal artery
	Meningohypophyseal trunk
Tentorium/cerebellopontine angle	Tentorial artery (artery of Bernasconi and Cassinari)
	Posterior middle meningeal artery
Olfactory groove	Ophthalmic artery branches
Foramen magnum/clivus	Dorsal meningeal artery
	Meningeal branches of vertebral artery
	Occipital artery branches
	Ascending pharyngeal artery

PREOPERATIVE EMBOLIZATION

Preoperative embolization of meningiomas is routinely done in some medical communities; in others, it is almost never performed. Vascular neurosurgical techniques are improving, and preoperative embolization is not necessarily mandatory (Case 3, Figs. 9–27 to 9–30; Case 4, Figs. 9–31 and 9–32; and Case 5, Figs. 9–33 to 9–39). In addition, if a neurosurgeon has not operated on an embolized meningioma, he or

Text continued on page 115

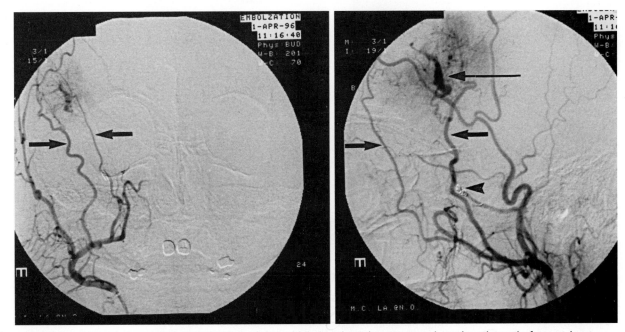

Figure 9-5 PA and lateral views after embolization of the middle meningeal artery reveal continued supply from at least two branches *(small arrows)* both thought to represent deep temporal arteries. Note that the position of the larger of the two is extracranial (see the original PA view, above) and is the primary supply to the extracranial tumor. Note that the intracranial varix is again filling *(long arrow)*. Also note the platinum microcoils in the more proximal occluded middle meningeal artery *(arrowhead)*, placed there to eliminate any deep source of bleeding at the time of surgery.

Case 1 continues

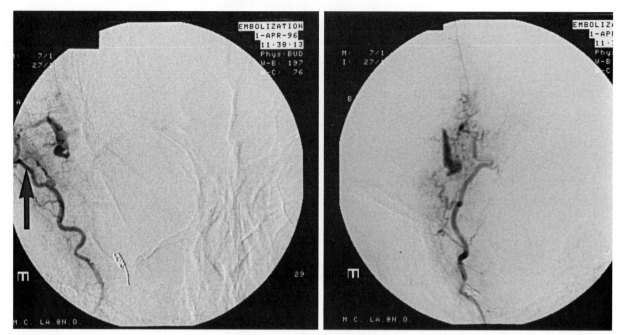

Figure 9-6 PA and lateral views of superselective injection of the large (posterior) deep temporal branch, demonstrating the extracranial tumor blush *(arrow),* as well as the transosseous supply to the large intratumoral dysplastic artery. Note that on the oblique PA view there is no supply to any intraorbital structure. This was embolized with 250- to 350-micron particles followed by platinum coils in order not to devascularize the tissues too extensively.

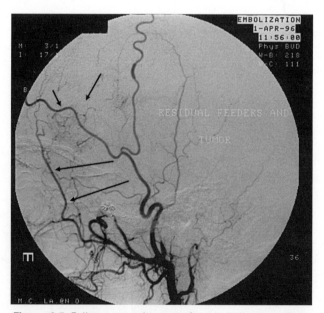

Figure 9-7 Follow-up angiogram after embolization of the larger of the two deep temporal arteries. There is minimal continued supply to the tumor bed *(short arrows)* by way of the remaining anterior deep temporal artery *(long arrows).* The procedure could have been terminated at this point, but this was a particularly compulsive day.

Case 1 continues

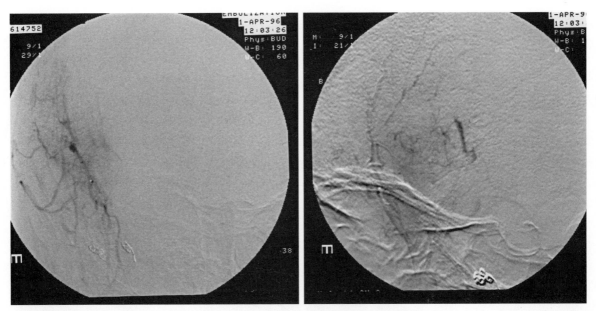

Figure 9-8 The microcatheter has been advanced to a far distal location where this angiogram was obtained. Embolization at this point was then performed with larger 250- to 350-micron particles.

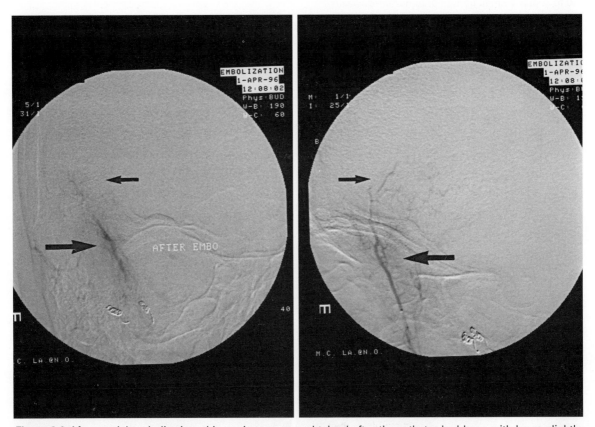

Figure 9-9 After partial embolization, this angiogram was obtained after the catheter had been withdrawn slightly. The goal was not to devascularize the area but to cut down on intraoperative bleeding. Note that there is a continued tissue blush *(large arrows)* proximal to where the catheter tip had been, but no further supply to the tumor bed *(small arrows)*. A small coil will be placed at the location of the catheter tip for final occlusion.

Case 1 continues

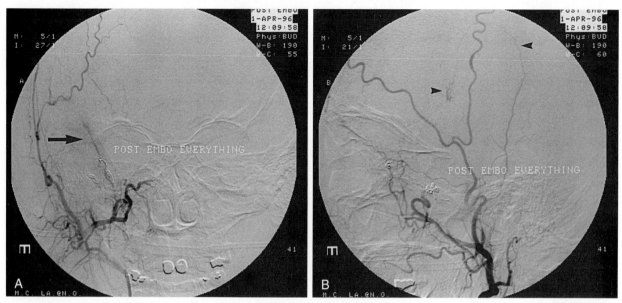

Figure 9-10 *A* and *B,* Final external carotid artery injection, PA and lateral views. The primary supply to the tumor has been eliminated, with excellent preservation of the remaining external carotid branches. Note the preservation of the blush to the deep temporal territory *(arrow),* advantageous for postoperative healing. Also note the recurrent meningeal branch looping around to supply a small portion of tumor *(arrowheads).*

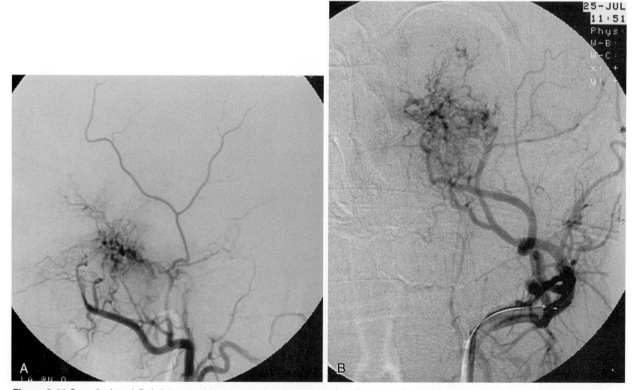

Figure 9-11 Case 2. *A* and *B,* A 54-year-old man, previously operated on for a meningioma, returned with a massive abnormality of the face and eye. A left external carotid artery injection reveals a huge hypervascular mass (supraethmoidal, retroglobal) filling from multiple external sources. The angioarchitecture of the mass is extremely abnormal. Note the gross irregularity of the vessel lumina with the appearance of pooling and beading.

Case 2 continues

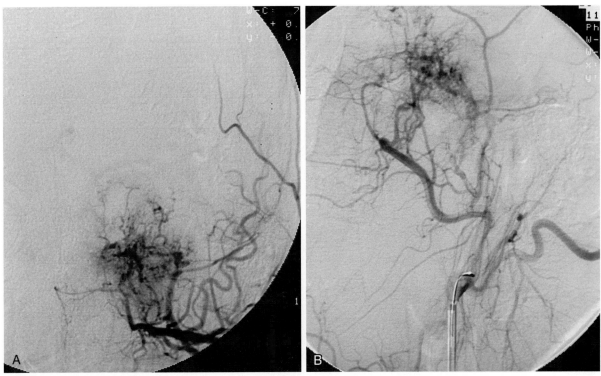

Figure 9-12 *A* and *B,* Magnified view of the extremely abnormal appearance of the feeders from the external carotid artery (mostly from the internal maxillary branches).

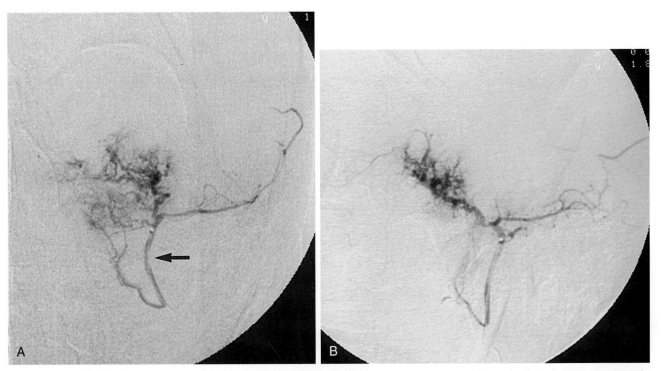

Figure 9-13 *A* and *B,* Selection of the middle meningeal artery *(arrow)* clearly demonstrates the extension of this tumor into the infraconal/superior maxillary region. Indeed, the tumor was much larger than this. Note the characteristic ascending curve and the infratemporal branch; the grossly abnormal swirl in the medial and anterior direction (to the infraorbital area) is not characteristic. Initial embolization of the tumor was from this vessel.

Case 2 continues

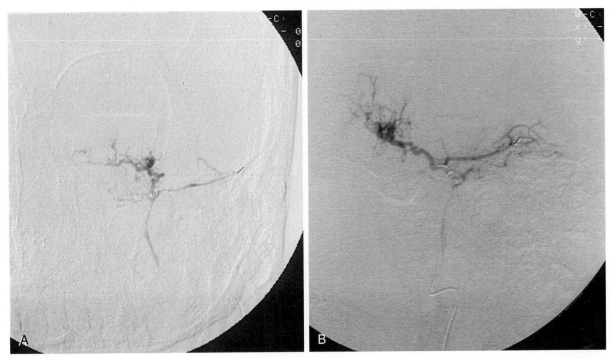

Figure 9-14 *A* and *B,* After partial embolization of the feeders to the tumor, only a minimal amount of tumor blush was left. Further embolization was performed followed by coil occlusion.

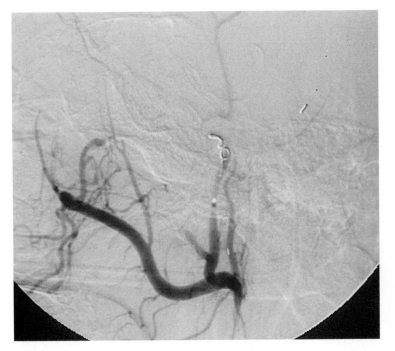

Figure 9-15 After embolization of the feeders from the external carotid artery to the tumor, it appears that this source has been successfully occluded. This is good and bad. If true intranidal/intratumoral penetration by particles has not been achieved, the tumor will still fill by whatever means possible. The postembolization appearance looks good from this view, however.

Case 2 continues

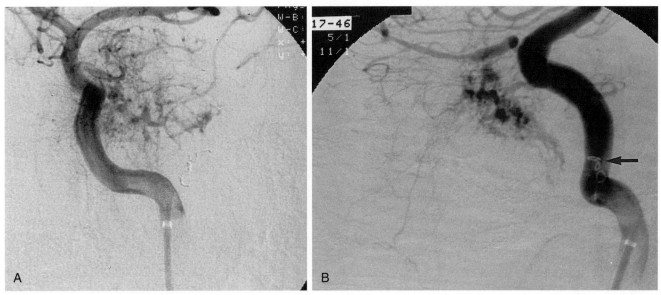

Figure 9-16 *A* and *B,* PA and lateral views of the internal carotid artery injection. This appearance is almost predictable. Elimination of the external supply will render the tumor mass dependent on internal carotid supply, which is achieved with regularity in this location. The internal carotid injection clearly demonstrates a massive tumoral supply with grossly abnormal vessels. On this particular injection, it is difficult to determine whether the supply is coming from the ophthalmic artery, the meningohypophyseal trunk (or other cavernous branch), or both. Note the small coils overlying the internal carotid artery on the lateral view from the previous embolization of the middle meningeal artery *(arrow).*

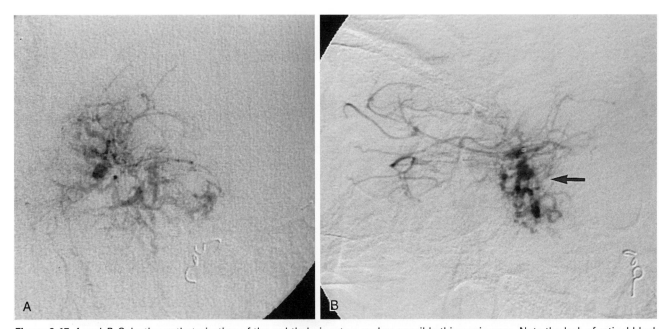

Figure 9-17 *A* and *B,* Selective catheterization of the ophthalmic artery makes possible this angiogram. Note the lack of retinal blush (nonspecific: it could be supplied by the external carotid artery, but the patient had now been totally blind for some time). Again note the extremely abnormal vessels within the tumor *(arrow).* These vessels do not necessarily delineate the extent of the tumor, however.

Case 2 continues

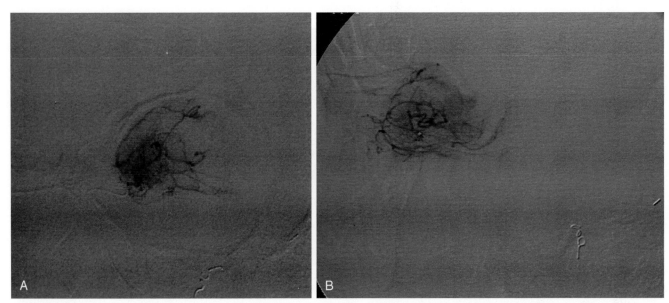

Figure 9-18 *A* and *B,* The catheter is now placed farther out into the ophthalmic artery. A repeat injection no longer reveals the extensively abnormal tumor mass; the catheter tip is beyond the feeders. Even though the patient has been totally blind for a number of months, it is still unwise to feel free to embolize the ophthalmic trunk; the surgeons may want to preserve the patient's external aesthetic appearance, and other branches arising from this vessel nourish surrounding intraconal tissues necessary for healing. Protective occlusion of the distal ophthalmic artery is achieved with straight platinum coils.

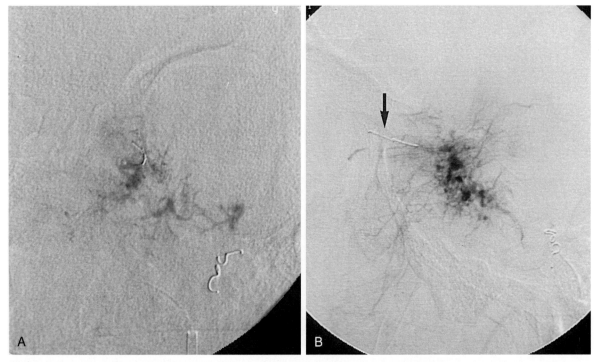

Figure 9-19 *A* and *B,* The occlusive, protective coils are well seen *(arrow)* and now the injection reveals the tumor mass (or at least this portion of its bizarre vasculature) clearly. No flow is seen past the protective coils; therefore, it is now possible to embolize with microparticles from this location (being careful to avoid reflux into the internal carotid artery).

Case 2 continues

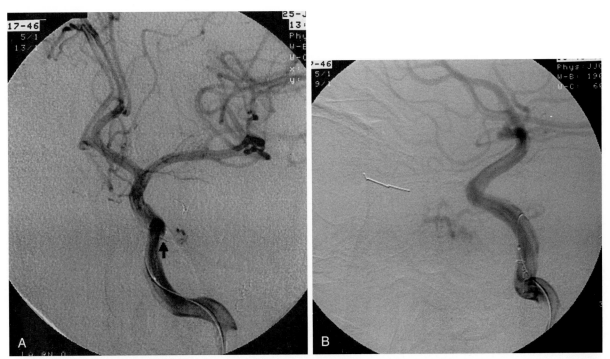

Figure 9-20 *A* and *B,* A repeat injection of the internal carotid artery revealed that significant filling of the tumor did arise from the meningohypophyseal trunk. This film was obtained during the attempt to catheterize this vessel. Note the wire tip at the orifice on the lateral view, while actually external to the carotid trunk on the PA view *(arrow).* The size of the trunk of this vessel reveals what flow it has been sending to this tumor.

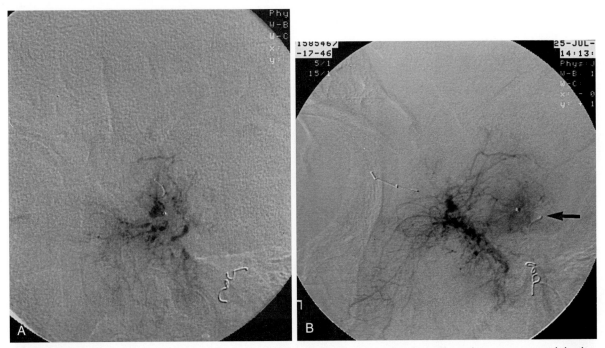

Figure 9-21 *A* and *B,* After successful catheterization of the trunk of the meningohypophyseal artery, contrast injection reveals this picture. Not only is there normal tissue stain, but there are probably cranial nerves supplied by this vessel. A test injection with lidocaine or amobarbital could be performed at this point but could possibly overstate the significance of this supply. Total embolization is not planned for this vessel, and a positive test would scare the operator to death. A secure position has been obtained: note the curve around the corner on the lateral view *(arrow).* Large particles are used (350 to 500 microns) followed by a small coil. This will help control bleeding from this deep supply.

Case 2 continues

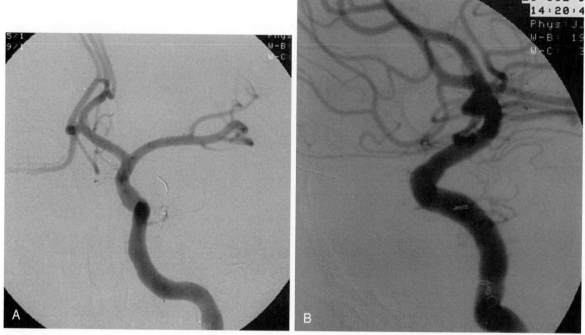

Figure 9-22 *A* and *B,* Follow-up internal carotid angiogram demonstrates the previously placed coils in the ophthalmic artery, as well as the newly placed coil in the meningohypophyseal trunk. As stated elsewhere, caution should be used when placing a small straight coil in the orifice of a minor vessel originating from the internal carotid artery; a simple cough or sneeze may dislodge this. Ideally, a self-retaining curved coil should be used, but since this placement is around the sharp bend in the trunk of this vessel, it was deemed adequately stable. The angiogram now shows nearly complete obliteration of supply from the internal carotid artery.

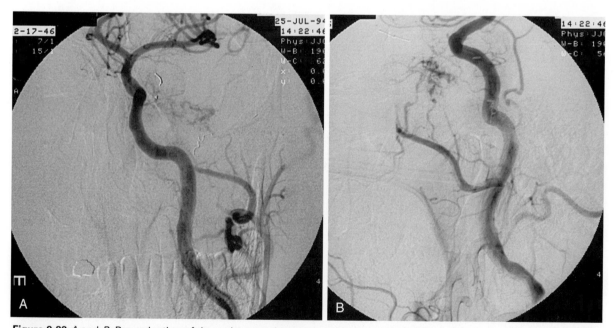

Figure 9-23 *A* and *B,* Re-evaluation of the entire vascular supply to the anterior skull base/face is now made. The catheter is pulled back and a common carotid injection is made. There it is! The external carotid has done it again. There are new feeders already present, arising from the internal maxillary artery in its sphenopalatine portion. The internal carotid does not appear to supply any significant residual (at least not *yet*).

Case 2 continues

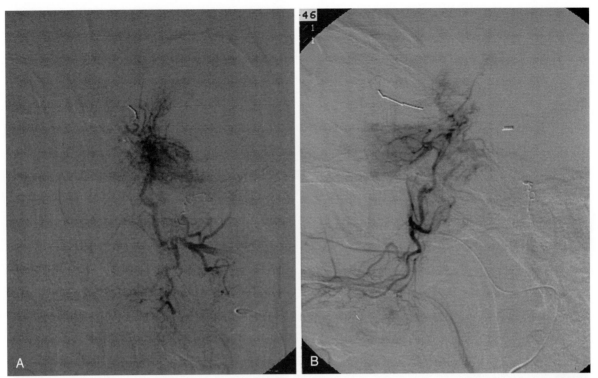

Figure 9-24 *A* and *B,* It would be simple to just flood the trunk of the internal maxillary artery with small particles followed by larger particles, followed by coils. This would yield a truly wondrous angiographic picture of devascularization. However, the surgical site might never heal, or even worse, might break down into a mess. Superselective embolization is again called for. The most distal branch supplying the tumor is selected first. The injection reveals some supply to normal tissue as well as tumor. Sacrifice (or more accurately, devascularization) of a small amount of normal tissue in this location (deep infraorbital in a blind eye) is acceptable to the surgeons since some reconstruction will be necessary anyway. The normal tissue supplied by this vessel is in any case essentially nonfunctional (not the palate, however).

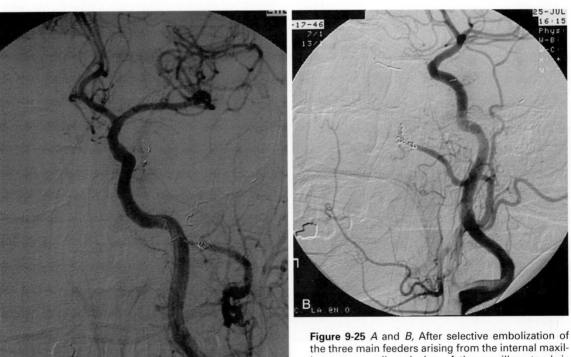

Figure 9-25 *A* and *B,* After selective embolization of the three main feeders arising from the internal maxillary artery, coil occlusion of the maxillary trunk is carried out. Even though this blocks direct flow to the palate, no small embolic material was delivered to this territory. This area will be supplied adequately by collateral vessels (e.g., the opposite external carotid branches, the ipsilateral facial artery, and the ipsilateral ascending pharyngeal artery).

Case 2 continues

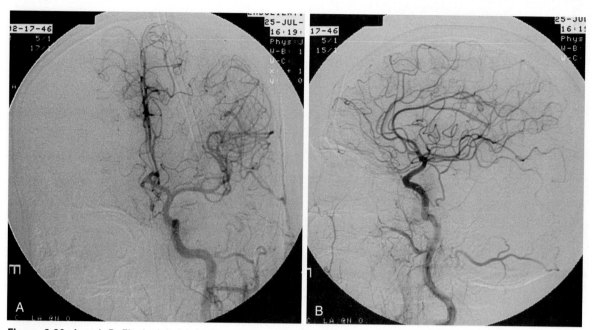

Figure 9-26 *A* and *B,* Final global injection of the entire internal and external carotid systems reveals excellent devascularization of the tumor mass, with (hopefully) preservation of the surrounding tissues necessary for healing. In fact, this patient was taken to surgery 3 days later, and there was still some significant oozing from a deep unknown source.

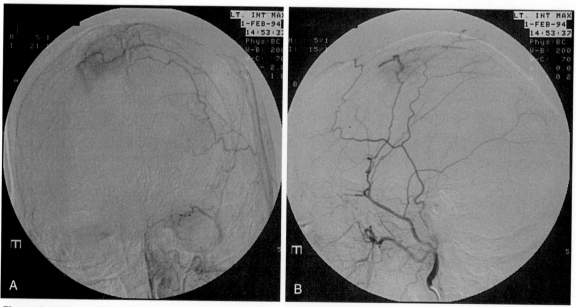

Figure 9-27 Case 3. *A* and *B,* A woman who presented with a large right parasagittal meningioma. Angiographic evaluation was desired with devascularization, if possible. Contralateral internal maxillary artery injection reveals significant supply across the midline via middle meningeal vessels.

Case 3 continues

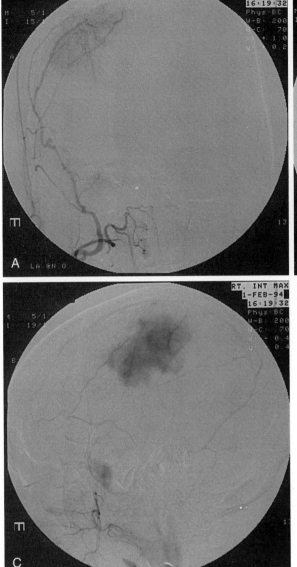

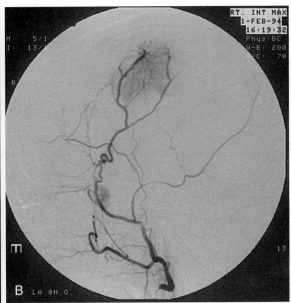

Figure 9-28 *A* to *C,* Ipsilateral external carotid artery injection reveals a dense blush in the tumor, as well as an additional blush in the retro-orbital region (found to be a second tumor). Note the prolonged blush of both masses into the late capillary phase. Note also the irregular margins of the parasagittal blush; this is unusual for a meningioma because of the typically well-circumscribed nature. This implies the possibility that the true sharp margins (which should be present) are being supplied by other vessels (e.g., pial branches).

Case 3 continues

she may be unaware of the benefits of this procedure. The number of preoperative embolizations appears to be decreasing; this is due at least in part to these factors.

Certain intracranial locations are far harder for a neurosurgeon to access and treat than others; this holds true for the endovascular therapist also. In addition, meningiomas that arise in certain locations are typically far more vascular than those that arise in other locations (most convexity meningiomas are hypervascular, while skull base tumors frequently are not); but tumor size, age, and idiosyncrasies can vary this generalization considerably. The vascular supply to the more commonly encountered meningiomas is given in Table 9–1.

Most practitioners premedicate patients who have large meningiomas with steroids before the procedure, but this is not of proved benefit. Anticonvulsants are probably also indicated before embolization of large tumors.

The goal and technique of embolization for most meningiomas is similar to that described above for tumors in general (see Chapter 8). The intratumoral vasculature should be eliminated as much as possible, followed by elimination of the supply to the operative field. PVA particles are typically used[4]; if safe distal access can be obtained, 50- to 150-micron particles can be used, followed by 150 to 250 and then larger. The scalp vessels should be spared to allow optimal healing.

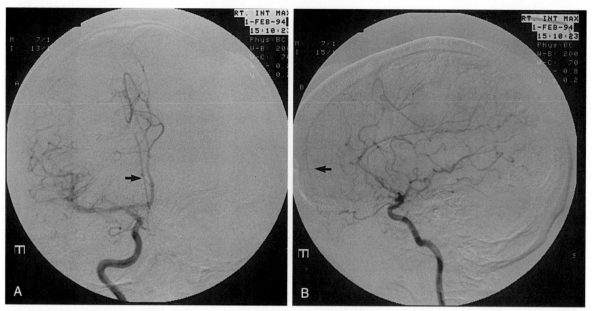

Figure 9-29 *A* and *B,* The right internal carotid artery injection gives a beautiful demonstration of the artery of the anterior falx (*arrows* on both PA and lateral views). In addition, the marginal branches of the anterior cerebral artery are displaced, irregular in size, and draped around the mass. Note the blush from the anterior cerebral artery supply.

Case 3 continues

Intratumoral flow should be stopped as well as supply from the parent vessel(s). This may be difficult or impossible if the supply is from small direct meningeal feeders originating from the internal carotid artery, such as the marginal artery of the tentorium (artery of Bernasconi and Cassinari) or the meningohypophyseal trunk. Attempts have been made to embolize these small perforators arising from major parent vessels that cannot be directly reached, such as branches arising from the cavernous carotid artery. Occlusion distal to the feeders by means of an occlusion balloon with proximal infusion of microparticles has been attempted, but this has resulted in residual particles within the temporarily occluded parent vessel lumen (internal carotid artery) and, after deflation of the occlusion balloon, subsequent distal migration and stroke. Occlusion proximal to the branch (e.g., in the internal carotid artery) with a flow control guide catheter has been proposed, but this distorts normal flow patterns, may produce reversal of flow in the intended vessel, and causes stasis in the main trunk, with the same potential embolic complications.

Of particular concern in dealing with meningeal vessels are branches leading to the petrous temporal bone (the petrous branch of the middle meningeal artery) where they can anastomose with the supply to the facial nerve (cranial nerve VII) and any other branches leading to the orbit. Meticulous evaluation for these anastomoses has to be performed, particularly if liquid embolic agents or the new 50-micron particles are to be used.

In superficial vessels such as the temporal or occipital arteries, as well as in small meningeal branches, an initial small bolus of nitroglycerin (50 µg) can result in far better distal penetration of the PVA particles. Extreme care must be taken with the occipital artery, however, owing to its dangerous anastomoses with the vertebral artery (see "Dangerous Intracranial-Extracranial Anastomoses" in Chapter 5).

Complications of preoperative embolization are usually secondary to poor mechanical technique or inadequate evaluation of potential collaterals from external branches to internal carotid (pial) vascular supply. Additionally, as is true in many areas of this work, the enemy of good is better, and overzealous embolization may lead to trouble.

INOPERABLE TUMORS

For tumors difficult or impossible to surgically remove (e.g., postradiation meningiomas, "malignant" meningiomas, en plaque unresectable tumors), more aggressive therapy may be appropriate. If the vascular supply can be accessed adequately and supplies a nonvital territory, it is possible to cause extensive tissue necrosis and liquefaction by alcohol embolization. This can either render surgery far easier (the tumor can frequently be simply aspirated) or shrink the tumor enough so that surgery may no longer be needed. Again, this therapeutic choice should be made only as a team decision. The surgical, chemotherapeutic, radiation, and benign neglect options should be considered as a whole by the medical team, the patient, and the family.

Skull Base and Cavernous Meningiomas

Tumors in these locations are extremely difficult to deal with even with a coordinated, combined embolization and surgical approach. They can invade and surround all structures in the cavernous sinus (e.g.,

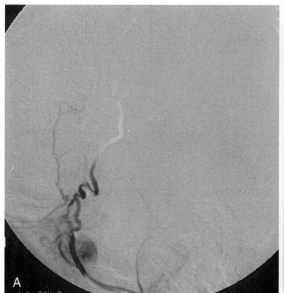

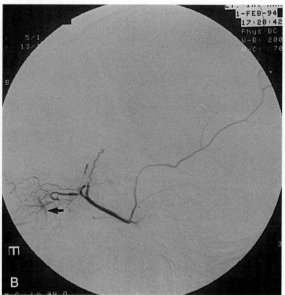

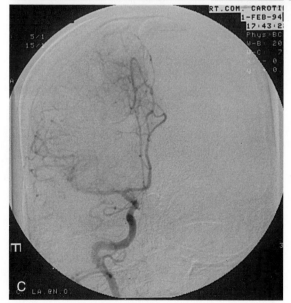

Figure 9-30 *A* to *C,* Magnification view of the embolized distal segment of the middle meningeal artery with a subsequent whole head run. Careful embolization of the middle meningeal artery was necessary; note the postembolization retinal blush *(arrow).* This supply had been identified before the embolization procedure by careful analysis of the films. Pre-embolization lidocaine (not amobarbital, see text) testing would have revealed the same finding. Simple random flooding of the distribution of the middle meningeal artery would have had disastrous consequences. Note the residual tumor blush supplied from the anterior cerebral and anterior falx arteries.

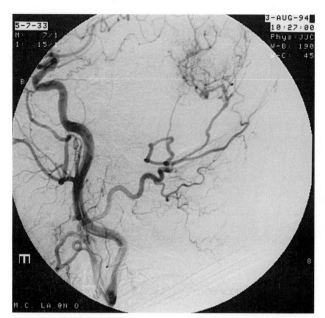

Figure 9-31 Case 4. Typical appearance of meningeal supply to a meningioma, although in an interesting location. This intracranial branch of the occipital artery was embolized with 150- to 250-micron PVA particles.

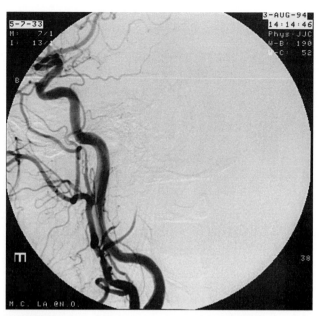

Figure 9-32 Postembolization lateral common carotid angiogram. Note the absence of perfusion of the distal extracranial occipital artery territory in addition to the occlusion of meningeal supply. It was not possible to selectively catheterize the direct feeders from the peripheral occipital artery, and therefore the entire distal distribution of this vessel was embolized (after selective angiography and pharmacologic testing determined that there was no supply to the vertebral artery or its territory).

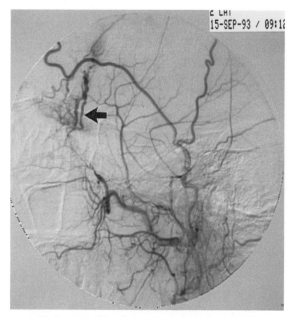

Figure 9-33 Case 5. Classic presentation of a cribriform plate meningioma. This lateral view during injection of the left internal maxillary artery demonstrates extensive filling of the tumor from midline ethmoidal branches. Note the spectacularly abnormal appearance of the intratumoral branches *(arrow)*.

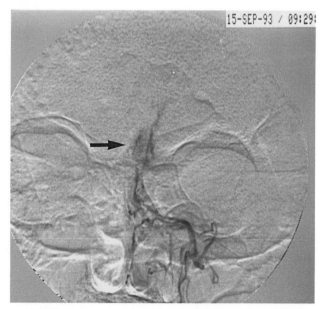

Figure 9-34 PA view of injection of the distal left internal maxillary artery reveals the typical nasal septum blush as well as filling of the intracranial tumor *(arrow)*. It would be possible to embolize from this point, although more distal subselection would be more ideal.

Case 5 continues

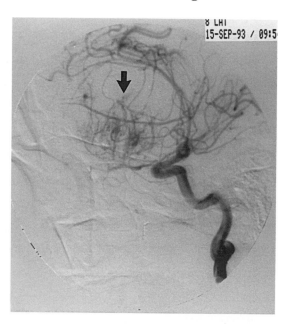

Figure 9-35 Left internal carotid artery injection reveals the typical difficulty in dealing with these tumors; there is extensive meningeal supply to the tumor via the ophthalmic artery. Worse, there is direct evidence of retinal blush from this same vessel; this implies that there is no significant supply to the retina from any vessel distal to the meningeal feeders, or else *that* vessel would supply the retina. In other words, if there were a distal external carotid artery branch feeding the ophthalmic artery, the flow from that vessel should be divided between the retina and the demand from the tumor, thus flowing *toward* the tumor from its entry point into the ophthalmic artery. This would prevent the downstream flow from the origin of the ophthalmic artery from the internal carotid artery from reaching the retina. Therefore, no protective occlusion of the retinal artery with a coil should even be contemplated; this would potentially (probably) devascularize the retina. There is also noted *(arrow)* an abnormal vascular appearance to the superior aspect of the tumor, fed by the anterior cerebral artery. The surgeon wanted to approach this tumor via a subfrontal approach (to access the cribriform plate supply), and to achieve embolization of the feeder from above.

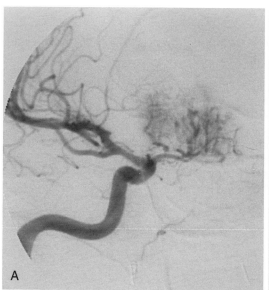

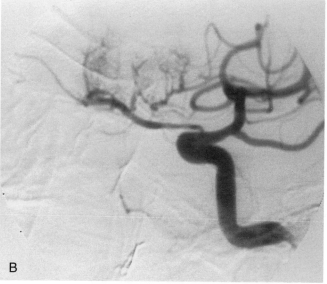

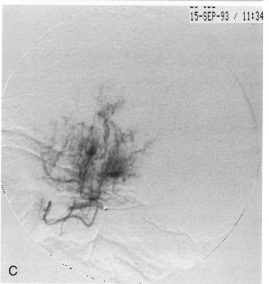

Figure 9-36 *A* to *C,* Right anterior oblique view and lateral view during internal carotid artery injection, and lateral view of selective ophthalmic artery injection, demonstrating similar findings upon injection of the right internal carotid artery as described above. The selective injection demonstrates the extensive supply from the right ophthalmic artery but no direct evidence of filling of the retina. A lidocaine test was performed at this point to evaluate the safety of coil occlusion before embolization of the proximal trunk and the feeders. This proved to be positive. Total embolization of the ophthalmic feeders is not indicated with the current technique and skills. Surgical technique allows satisfactory removal of the tumor mass with low morbidity and mortality. This should be remembered when planning a therapeutic strategy.

Case 5 continues

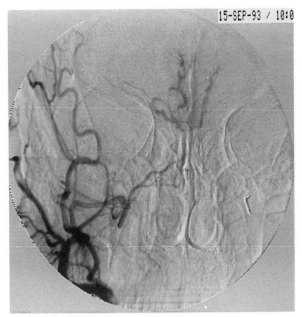

Figure 9-37 Injection of the external carotid artery on this right side also displayed filling of the tumor bed.

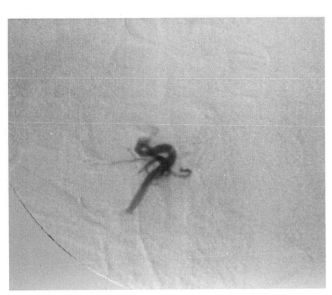

Figure 9-38 After embolization with 250- to 350-micron PVA particles in the ethmoidal branches of the left internal maxillary artery, no further supply to the tumor is noted. This same procedure was then carried out on the other side.

cranial nerves III, IV, VI, internal carotid artery) and compress the optic nerve and other nearby structures. Stripping the tumor from the internal carotid artery can lead to perforation or occlusion of this vessel; therefore preoperative test occlusion is mandatory (see Chapter 34).

Frequently, the best option for tumors in this location is removal en bloc, necessitating sacrifice of the internal carotid artery. Sacrifice of the internal carotid artery can be performed preoperatively with minimal morbidity (see Chapter 35). If the test occlu-

sion is a failure, preocclusion extracranial-intracranial bypass is necessary and can be a standard superficial temporal artery to middle cerebral artery bypass or one of several high-flow bypasses (see Chapter 49 for a discussion of these bypass options).

Although embolization of the middle meningeal artery can be performed for tumors in this location, some of the supply to these tumors arises from direct meningeal feeders arising from the internal carotid artery, such as the inferolateral trunk and the meningohypophyseal trunk. As stated previously, we feel

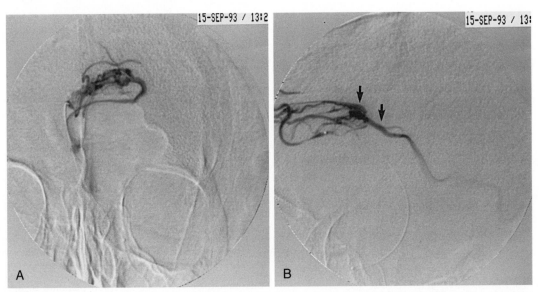

Figure 9-39 *A* and *B*, Access to the anterior cerebral artery supply via the left internal carotid artery was attained. Note the arteriovenous shunt in one portion of the tumor *(arrows)*. Embolization with large particles (250 to 350 microns) was then performed, followed by occlusion of the main branch by a coil. No further embolization was performed, leaving the extensive supply from both ophthalmic arteries. This limited embolization was all that could safely be performed in this case, demonstrating the concept of knowing when to say "when."

routine embolization of these vessels to be too risky to attempt unless they are greatly enlarged. The origins of these vessels are very short and tortuous, resulting in precarious catheter position. Particulate embolization can easily result in reflux, and any coil placed in this location is insecure and can be dislodged by something as simple as a cough.

Percutaneous ethanol ablation or cyanoacrylate infusion is perhaps a more reasonable approach for skull base tumors that are extremely difficult to approach (see Chapter 28). This innovative technique opens possibilities for treatment not previously available.

REFERENCES

1. Russell DS, Rubenstein LJ. Pathology of Tumors of the Nervous System, 4th ed. Baltimore: Williams & Wilkins, 1977.
2. Donnell MW, Meyer GA, Donegan WI. Estrogen-receptor protein in intracranial meningiomas. *J Neurosurg* 1979;50:499–502.
3. Canale DJ, Bebin J. Von Recklinghausen disease of the nervous system. In Vinken PJ, Bruyn GW (eds): Handbook of Clinical Neurology: The Phakomatoses, Vol 14. Amsterdam: North-Holland, 1972, pp 132–162.
4. Wachloo A, Juengling F, Velthoven V, et al. Extended preoperative polyvinyl alcohol microembolization of intracranial meningiomas: assessment of two embolization techniques. *AJNR* 1993;14:571–582.

ADDITIONAL READINGS

Black PM. Meningiomas. *Neurosurgery* 1993;32:643–657.
Dean BL, Flom RA, Wallace RC, et al. Efficacy of endovascular treatment of meningiomas: evaluation with matched samples. *AJNR* 1994;15:1675–1680.
Geoffray A, Lee Y-Y, Jing B-S, et al. Extracranial meningiomas of the head and neck. *AJNR* 1984;5:599–604.
Grand C, Bank WO, Baleriaux D, et al. Gadolinium-enhanced MR in the evaluation of preoperative meningioma embolization. *AJNR* 1993;14:563–569.
Latchaw RE. Preoperative intracranial meningioma embolization: technical considerations affecting the risk-to-benefit ratio. *AJNR* 1993;14:583–586.
Nelson PK, Setton A, Choi IS, et al. Current status of interventional neuroradiology in the management of meningiomas. *Neurosurgery Clinics* 1994;5:235–259.
Rostomily RC, Eskridge JM, Winn HR. Tentorial meningiomas. *Neurosurg Clin* 1994;5:331–348.
Wakhloo AK, Juenging FD, Van Velthoven VV, et al. Extended preoperative polyvinyl alcohol microembolization of intracranial meningiomas: assessment of two embolization techniques. *AJNR* 1993;14:571–582.

CHAPTER 10

Juvenile Nasopharyngeal Angiofibromas

J.J. Connors III / J.C. Wojak

EPIDEMIOLOGY

Juvenile nasopharyngeal angiofibromas (JNAs) are classically seen in young males, with the peak incidence at 14 to 17 years.[1] Although they have been seen in females and in older male patients, other tumors should be considered in these individuals. Chromosomal analysis has been recommended when this tumor is diagnosed in a female. Possible lesions that may be confused with this tumor are angiomatous polyps and (rarely) a true carcinoma. No ethnic or geographical predilection has been reported.

CLINICAL PRESENTATION

Generally, patients present with recurrent epistaxis and nasal obstruction. Sinusitis or otitis may be present if drainage of these structures is impeded. Anosmia, proptosis, facial or temporal swelling, and extraocular movement palsies may be seen, depending on the direction of spread. Upon physical examination, a lobulated, reddish-gray mass can be seen in the nasal cavity.

PATHOLOGY

Location and Behavior

JNAs are benign, fibrovascular tumors that are locally aggressive. Malignant conversion is extremely rare in tumors that have not been irradiated. Spontaneous regression has been described but is also extremely rare.

It is generally agreed that these tumors arise from the lateral margin of the posterior nasal cavity, near the sphenopalatine foramen.[2] They do not generally frankly invade bone, but rather remodel it and erode it. Multifocal tumors have not been reported. However, these tumors can spread extensively, and spread tends to be along natural tissue planes. This may be anteriorly into the nasal cavity, medially toward the opposite nasal cavity (deforming and eroding the septum), or posteriorly and inferiorly into the oropharynx (displacing the soft palate). Superiorly, spread into the sphenoid sinus, sella, cavernous sinus, and/or middle cranial fossa is possible. Lateral spread into the pterygomaxillary fossa and maxillary sinus, sphenopalatine fossa and infratemporal region, orbit, and/or parapharyngeal space may also be seen.[1]

Invasion of the paranasal sinuses is fairly common. Intracranial spread is generally seen in advanced tumors and in older patients. The tumor usually remains extradural. Intraorbital spread tends to remain extraconal.

Staging of Tumors

Several classification or grading schemes have been proposed. Sessions et al defined stages on the basis of the spread of the tumor[3]:

Ia. Limited to the nasal cavity and/or nasopharynx
Ib. Extension into paranasal sinuses
IIa. Involvement of pterygopalatine fossa
IIb. Involvement of pterygomaxillary fossa
IIc. Involvement of infratemporal fossa
III. Intracranial extension

The staging system developed by Chandler et al is similar[4]:

I. Tumor limited to the nasopharynx
II. Extension into the nasal cavity and/or sphenoid sinus
III. Extension into the maxillary or ethmoid sinuses, pterygomaxillary or infratemporal fossae, orbit, or cheek
IV. Intracranial extension

Vascular Supply

These lesions are generally supplied by branches of the internal maxillary (sphenopalatine and descending palatine branches) and ascending pharyngeal arteries. As spread occurs, there is recruitment of other supply, including branches of the facial, ophthalmic (ethmoidal branches), and internal carotid arteries (via the vidian and other arteries arising from the petrous portion, as well as the meningohypophyseal trunk and inferolateral trunk).

Relationship to Sex Hormones

These tumors are known to be hormonally sensitive. Increase in size after testosterone administration and decrease in size after estrogen therapy have been seen. Estrogen therapy produces fibrosis and thrombosis within the tumor, which is a typical response of blood vessels to exogenous estrogens, rather than a response mediated by specific estrogen receptors within the tumor.

Nasal mucosal tissue itself has been shown to be hormonally sensitive. Premenstrual epistaxis is thought to be due to a response to endogenous estrogens. In addition, ectopic rests of tissue within the nasal mucosa that resemble erectile tissue have been shown to exist. It is believed that the response of this tissue to increasing levels of testosterone at puberty causes this tumor to develop, while the fibrous component may be due to an associated hypersensitivity to estrogens, resulting in recurrent hemorrhage and formation of granulation tissue.[1]

EVALUATION

Both computed tomography (CT) and magnetic resonance imaging (MRI) have roles in the assessment of these tumors. Axial and coronal CT images with bone windows best demonstrate the degree of bone remodeling and erosion. Pre- and postcontrast MRI demonstrates the extent of the tumor and its vascularity, and also allows differentiation between sinusitis secondary to obstruction and frank sinus invasion. The presence or absence of intracranial invasion is also best assessed by multiplanar MRI.

Angiography is generally performed in conjunction with preoperative embolization. The tumor classically has a dramatic appearance with fast flow (arteriovenous shunting), very dense capillary blush, and increased visibility of prominent veins (Case 1, Figs. 10–1 to 10–13). The angiomatous polyp resembles the JNA angiographically, but a carcinoma typically is not hypervascular unless it was originally a JNA and had malignant degeneration. A rare nasal carcinoma (squamous cell) in a child (Case 2, Fig. 10–14) can present with mass effect and nosebleed and lead to angiography; in other words, it can be clinically similar to a true JNA. The angiogram, however, is very different. In the case presented, even though the vasculature is somewhat more prominent than usual with some minimal microtortuosity, it is not much different from the range of normal for turbinates. There is some mass effect, however.

The presence or absence of internal carotid artery supply is important to note, as this affects the surgical management, but not necessarily the embolization. If the internal carotid artery provides extensive supply and/or is enveloped in intracranial tumor (rare), sacrifice of the vessel may be proposed (rarely necessary). If encroachment on the internal carotid artery may be necessary during surgery, a temporary test occlusion should be performed (see Chapters 34 and 36).

ENDOVASCULAR THERAPY

Goals of Therapy

The goal of treatment of a JNA is eradication of the tumor. The definitive treatment is surgical resection. This may require a combined carniofacial approach if there is intracranial spread. Surgical resection may be technically difficult owing to the size of the tumor and excessive bleeding. Bleeding may obscure the surgical field, resulting in an incomplete resection and increased risk of complications. In an attempt to reduce intraoperative bleeding to a minimum (thereby reducing the risks involved in the procedure and improving visibility), embolization of these tumors is often undertaken preoperatively (see Figs. 10–1 to 10–13).[5] Radiation therapy can be useful as an adjunct in tumors in which complete resection is

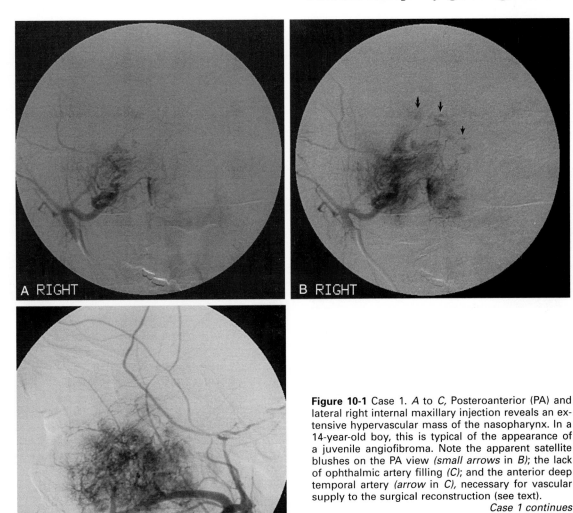

Figure 10-1 Case 1. *A* to *C,* Posteroanterior (PA) and lateral right internal maxillary injection reveals an extensive hypervascular mass of the nasopharynx. In a 14-year-old boy, this is typical of the appearance of a juvenile angiofibroma. Note the apparent satellite blushes on the PA view *(small arrows* in *B);* the lack of ophthalmic artery filling *(C);* and the anterior deep temporal artery *(arrow* in *C),* necessary for vascular supply to the surgical reconstruction (see text).

Case 1 continues

not possible. However, radiation has been associated with induction of malignancy and should be used with caution. Estrogen administration can reduce the size of the tumor, but its use in pubertal males is risky and should be avoided.

Technique of Embolization

Embolization needs to be both thorough and *intratumoral.* Once one feeder is occluded, the tumor will aggressively tend to recruit supply from other sources. These newly recruited collaterals may be more difficult to reach for embolization purposes as well as to control at surgery. Intratumoral embolization prevents this recruitment. Superselective catheterization needs to be performed, infiltrating the tumor mass with particles at least as small as the 150- to 250-micron range, or smaller (50 to 150 microns) if accurate superselection has been achieved.

Thorough preembolization evaluation of the vascular supply from both external carotid arteries is nec-

essary even for a tumor that is purely unilateral. This will reveal the degree of parasitization of the particular tumor as well as any potentially dangerous collaterals from either side. After embolization of the vascular supply on the side of the tumor, abundant recruitment is often seen from vessels originating from the contralateral external or internal carotid artery. These then need to be embolized. Vertebral artery evaluation should also be performed to assess for any aberrant supply to the skull base or connections to external carotid branches.

The endovascular therapist tends to occlude the largest suppliers first; these typically are branches from the internal maxillary artery. This is both good and bad. These vessels are usually safe to embolize and easy to reach; however, once they are embolized, other supply becomes very visible (depressingly so!). Even though more thorough embolization would be possible if the internal maxillary branches were left until the end, it is usually easier to catheterize the other, often bizarre feeders once they enlarge toward

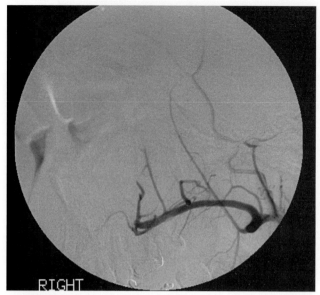

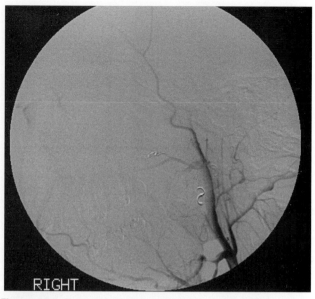

Figure 10-2 After superselective embolization of distal internal maxillary branches with 150- to 250-micron particles, there is good devascularization of this source. The distal trunk of the internal maxillary artery is now occluded with platinum coils to prevent supply to the surgical bed during the operative procedure. The deep temporal artery is untouched (as is confirmed in Fig. 10–7).

Figure 10-4 Postembolization angiogram of the right external carotid artery demonstrates excellent control of the supply to the tumor from this source. Some of this devascularization may be temporary, as shown in Figure 10–7.

Case 1 continues

the end of the embolization. This is a good reason to use very small particles *from very distal (near the tumor) locations* in order to obtain true intratumoral occlusion from the beginning; this prevents gross recruitment from alternative sources.

Care must be taken to be *acutely* aware of dangerous collaterals to the intracranial/intraorbital contents. Simple random flooding of the internal maxillary artery is unacceptable. An illustration of this

concept as pertaining directly to this pathologic process is demonstrated in Figs. 8–1 to 8–3, where a branch of the internal maxillary artery is seen to supply the intraorbital contents and the retina.

Once the external carotid artery supply is occluded, it will be seen that any supply from the internal carotid artery is increased (if it was previously present at all). These vessels are almost uniformly difficult to reach, particularly the vidian artery, which usually arises on the inferior wall of the horizontal (intrapetrous) portion of the internal

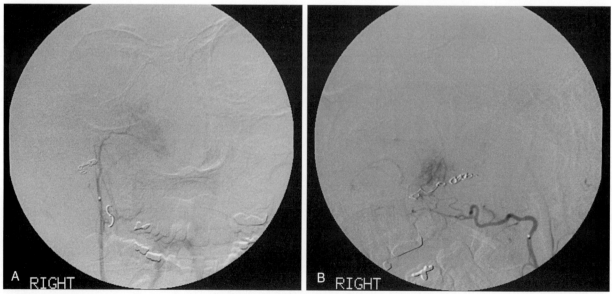

Figure 10-3 *A* and *B,* PA and lateral views of the right ascending pharyngeal artery, which is seen to supply a residual portion of the tumor. This is a typical appearance of the anterior extent of this vessel to the nasopharynx. This vessel is embolized with 150- to 250-micron PVA followed by coils. Note also the size of the vessel (slightly larger than a standard microcatheter), typical for an ascending pharyngeal artery (see Fig. 10–10).

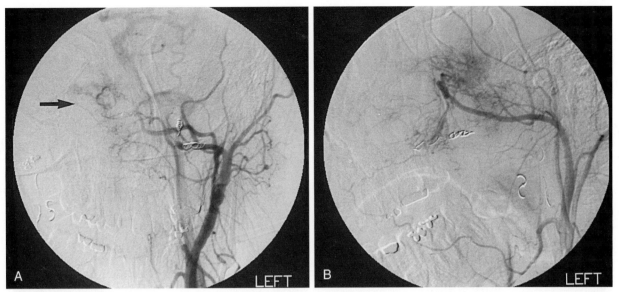

Figure 10-5 *A* and *B,* Left external carotid artery injection demonstrates supply across the midline to the tumor via ethmoidal and sphenopalatine collaterals from the internal maxillary artery *(arrow).* These should be embolized also, since this supply will be deep to the surgical approach.

carotid artery. Catheterization of the vidian artery necessitates a complete 180-degree turn of the microcatheter in a space of only 5 to 7 mm within a 4-mm vessel (see Fig. 10–11). Even when the origin of this vessel can be selected by a guidewire, any advancement of the microcatheter must be exactly opposite to the vectors of force. This maneuver is therefore very difficult. Unfortunately, this deep supply is the last to be reached by the surgeons, and this can result in significant ongoing bleeding during surgery. However, if good intratumoral vascular occlusion has been achieved by the previous embolization efforts,

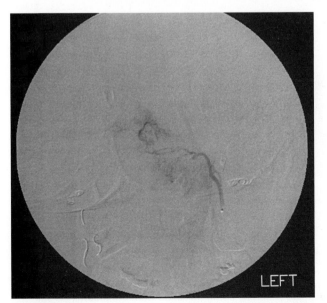

Figure 10-6 PA view of the left (contralateral) ascending pharyngeal artery demonstrates the typical intercommunication between the two ascending pharyngeal arteries, with continuing supply to the tumor.

Case 1 continues

the oozing or hemorrhage from this deep vascular supply during resection will not be of any great amount until the end of the surgical resection, and therefore may be of minimal consequence. It is for this reason that good intratumoral penetration and occlusion during the initial stages of the embolization is necessary, to prevent an even worse situation than before embolization owing to abundant recruitment from these deep direct internal carotid artery feeders. The surgeons should be forewarned before the surgical procedure of any deep vessel(s) that may still be present.

Embolization of any feeders from the internal carotid artery is rarely attempted in these cases. The surgeons, if forewarned, can usually deal with this supply adequately and with greater safety than the interventional neuroradiologist.

An alternative to intra-arterial embolization that has been used by some interventional neuroradiologists is direct percutaneous embolization with cyanoacrylate (see Chapter 28).

Deep Temporal Arteries

Owing to the extensive reconstruction of the posterior nasal cavity after surgical resection, as well as potential involvement of the skull base, it is necessary to spare as much normal surrounding tissue as possible, particularly the superficial temporal, anterior deep temporal, and middle meningeal arteries. Preservation of these vessels will aid the surgeon greatly. Random devascularization is inelegant and leads to inadequate wound healing.

After extensive resection of a large JNA, the surgeon may need to place a viable temporalis muscle flap at the posterior paranasal sinus surgical defect to prevent infection of the meninges or intracranial

Text continued on page 130

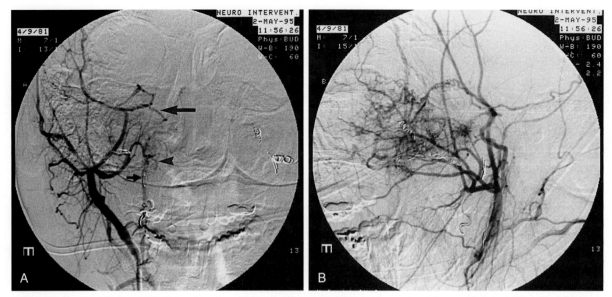

Figure 10-7 *A* and *B,* In view of the duration of the procedure and the contrast load, it was deemed necessary to bring the patient back for completion 2 weeks later. The right external carotid angiogram demonstrates distal occlusion of the internal maxillary feeders previously embolized, with excellent residual filling of the important deep temporal artery. In addition, however, the angiogram now reveals some new arterial recruitment, not previously seen. Note the meningeal feeder *(large arrow)* arising from the middle meningeal artery, coursing along the floor of the middle cranial fossa and supplying the posterior nasopharynx. Note also the internal maxillary collateral now present *(arrowhead).* In addition, flash filling of the previously embolized and coiled ascending pharyngeal artery is present (*small arrow* pointing at coil within ascending pharyngeal artery). Obviously, not enough coils were used!

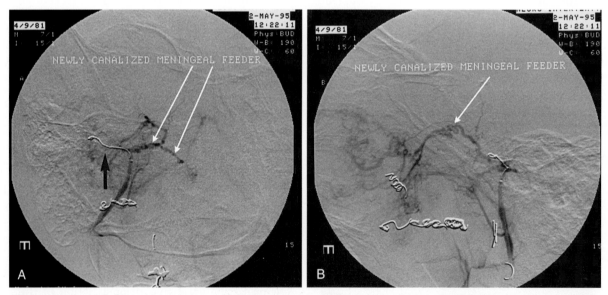

Figure 10-8 *A* and *B,* PA and lateral views of injection into the middle meningeal artery demonstrate protective embolization of the lateral infratemporal trunk (*black arrow* indicates a protective coil). This protective embolization was performed to preserve the vascular supply to the meninges on the lateral surface of the brain in order to optimize postsurgical healing. The vessel heading medially *(white arrows)* can potentially anastomose with the meningohypophyseal trunk and thus the internal carotid artery. Great care should be taken when evaluating this position for embolization. Even if no internal carotid artery is seen, filling of this vessel could still be present and not seen owing to rapidity of flow in the vessel with subsequent dilution and washout of contrast. A slow infusion of methohexital or amobarbital may reveal some intracranial supply, but the amount of flow reaching the brain may be too little to detect by pharmacologic means, albeit clearly evident after particulate embolization (later, unfortunately). Normal hemodynamics would cause the direction of flow to be toward the tumor both from this meningeal branch and from any communication from the internal carotid artery. Therefore, it is crucial not to overcome this dynamic by any forceful embolization.

Very dilute particles of 250 to 350 microns were used to occlude this vessel in order to reduce the risk of microcollateral communications. A very small amount is necessary and *no forceful injection should be made (which could lead to opening of these pathways).* This is followed by coil occlusion of the trunk of the middle meningeal artery.

Case 1 continues

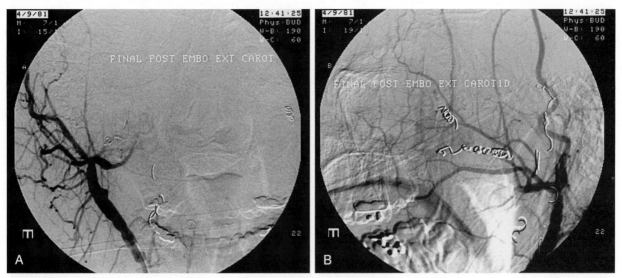

Figure 10-9 *A* and *B,* Final angiogram of the internal maxillary trunk now demonstrates effective occlusion of this supply (again!). Note the preservation of the deep temporal artery (under the "T" of "CAROTID" in *B*).

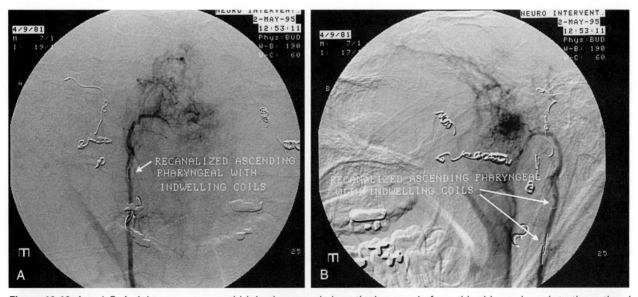

Figure 10-10 *A* and *B,* A right common carotid injection revealed continuing supply from this side, and much to the authors' surprise it is seen to arise from the (previously embolized) ascending pharyngeal artery (see comment in Fig. 10–7 legend concerning the insufficient number of coils). Note the greatly increased size of this vessel compared with previously, with the small coils now "blowing in the breeze" *(arrows).* Note also that curved coils were chosen rather than straight coils owing to their self-retaining nature. The ascending pharyngeal artery is seen to supply a substantial amount of flow to the tumor at this time. It was re-embolized with 150- to 250-micron particles and repacked with coils.

Case 1 continues

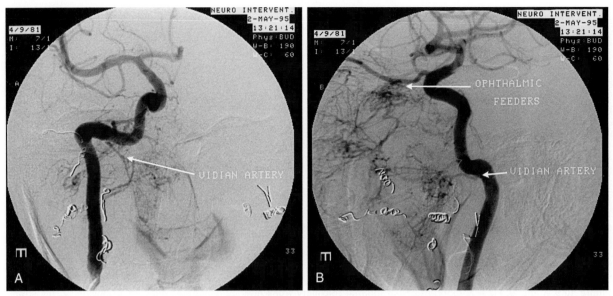

Figure 10-11 *A* and *B,* Final internal carotid artery injection demonstrates a fine example of the vidian artery (a primitive communication between the petrous internal carotid artery and the internal maxillary system). Ophthalmic supply is also seen from the standard collaterals between this vessel and the internal maxillary territory.

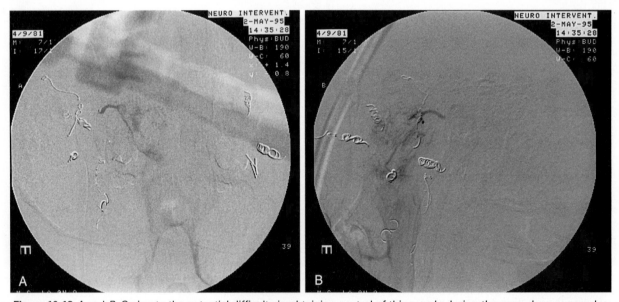

Figure 10-12 *A* and *B,* Owing to the potential difficulty in obtaining control of this supply during the procedure, superselective embolization of the vidian artery was attempted. Steaming a sharp curve into the tip to help make the turn in the petrous carotid artery allowed catheterization of this vessel. Even though the vessel was successfully selected, the 180-degree turn precluded advancement of the catheter into the vessel to a distance considered safe for embolization. Therefore, embolization was not performed! The surgeons were notified of the residual supply.

Case 1 continues

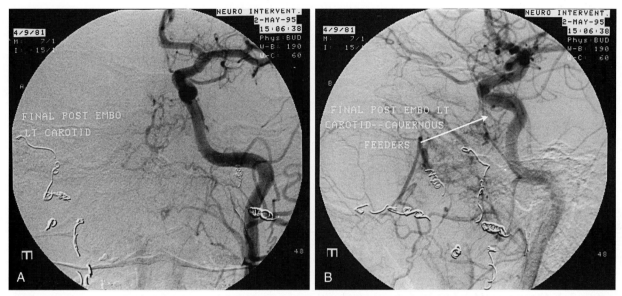

Figure 10-13 *A* and *B,* Final injection of the left common carotid artery displays some residual supply from the cavernous segment of this contralateral internal carotid artery *(arrow).* This supply also cannot be safely embolized; in fact, it will cause only a minor amount of bleeding, and once again the surgeons should be notified of this residual.

Figure 10-14 Case 2. A 10-year-old boy with recurrent epistaxis. A previous biopsy was attempted, but an inadequate specimen was obtained owing to excessive friability. In view of the clinical appearance and history, it was thought reasonably certain that the boy had a juvenile nasopharyngeal angiofibrema, and an embolization was requested before surgical resection. Selective injection of the internal maxillary artery demonstrates a very mildly abnormal pattern with some mass effect *(arrows)* and tortuousity/beading of microvessels. No real arteriovenous shunting is seen. No truly abnormal *hypervascular* mass is seen. At the time of angiography, the referring otolaryngologist was informed that the angiographic picture was not consistent with the diagnosis of angiofibroma and was asked whether the embolization was still desired. Since there was a history of epistaxis with a previous aborted biopsy, embolization was still desired and was performed. (Note the collateral vessel to the orbital contents *(thin arrow)*—later shown to be to the globe. This was the anterior deep temporal artery and was protectively embolized before embolization of this tumor mass.) The tumor was subsequently demonstrated to be a true nasal squamous cell carcinoma.

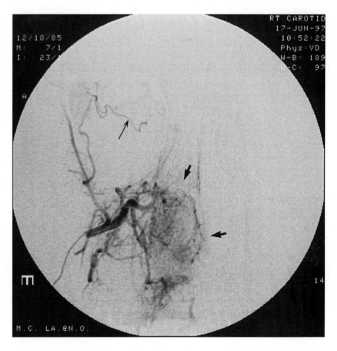

contents from the surgical defect and sinuses. The temporalis muscle flap is supplied by the deep temporal arteries. It is therefore crucial not to devascularize this territory during the preoperative embolization.

RECURRENCE

Recurrence rates as high as 30% have been reported, most being due to incomplete removal of the tumor, resulting in fairly rapid regrowth. This is most commonly seen in patients with intracranial spread, which may not be completely resectable (as in the case of cavernous sinus involvement). If recurrent tumor is surgically accessible, re-embolization may

be undertaken before resection (if the feeders have not previously been proximally occluded).

REFERENCES

1. Lasjaunias P, Berenstein A. Surgical Neuroangiography, Vol 2: Endovascular Treatment of Craniofacial Lesions. New York: Springer-Verlag, 1987.
2. Gullane PJ, Davidson J, O'Dwyer T, Forte V. Juvenile angiofibroma: a review of the literature and a case series report. *Laryngoscope* 1992;102:928–933.
3. Sessions RB, Bryan RN, Naclerio RM, et al. Radiographic staging of juvenile angiofibroma. *Head Neck Surg* 1981;3:279–283.
4. Chandler JR, Goulding R, Moskowitz L, et al. Nasopharyngeal angiofibromas: staging and management. *Ann Otol Rhinol Laryngol* 1984;93:322–329.
5. Deschler DG, Kaplan MJ, Boles R. Treatment of large juvenile nasopharyngeal angiofibroma. *Otolaryngol Head Neck Surg* 1992;106:278–284.

CHAPTER 11

Paragangliomas

J.J. Connors III / J.C. Wojak

Paragangliomas are vascular tumors arising from neural crest tissue belonging to the amine precursor uptake and decarboxylation (APUD) system and can secrete vasoactive substances such as catecholamines and serotonin. They can be found in the locations of normal, preexisting paraganglia or may be ectopic. The most common locations (in decreasing order) are tympanic, jugular, carotid, vagal, laryngeal, orbital, and nasopharyngeal. The mean age of presentation is in the fifth decade, but the range is extensive, especially in carotid tumors. Of the most common types listed above, tympanic, jugular, vagal, and nasopharyngeal tumors are more common in females (2.5:1), while the others are evenly distributed. Paragangliomas have been associated with other tumors of the APUD system, including carcinoid tumors, pheochromocytomas, pituitary adenomas, and thyroid carcinomas.

These tumors can be found as part of a familial syndrome of APUDomas; there is autosomal dominant inheritance and variable expression. Thirty percent of these patients have multicentric disease. Among spontaneously occurring lesions, 2.8% are bilateral and 10% are multifocal. Carotid (15%) and vagal (10%) tumors are most likely to be multicentric. In most cases of multicentric tumors, two tumors are identified (84%); three (13%), four (2%), and five (1%) tumors are much less common.[1] Secretory activity and multicentricity are associated with an increased incidence of malignancy.

It is important to understand the vascular architecture of these lesions. There may be one or more distinct compartments of the tumor, each fed by one or more arteries. These compartments have distinct capillary beds and venous drainage. There are also small, direct arteriovenous connections within the tumor. Owing to the encapsulated nature of these tumors, they do not tend to recruit arterial supply from adjacent territories until they are quite large. Therefore, a large paraganglioma that demonstrates an arterial supply typical of two different lesions most likely represents a confluent, multicentric lesion (i.e., two lesions that have grown together). This is particularly seen with tympanic and jugular paragangliomas. A large tumor supplied by both tympanic branches and the jugular branch of the neuromeningeal division of the ascending pharyngeal artery most likely represents a confluence of these two tumors.[2]

Although these lesions are slow growing and most are "benign" at presentation, there is evidence to show that these tumors all have malignant potential and should be aggressively treated. In one series, the survival of patients with temporal (jugular or tympanic) paragangliomas was analyzed.[3] The average age at presentation was 45 years. At 5 years after diagnosis, 71% of patients were alive and well; the number decreased to 29% at 10 years, 17% at 15 years, and 10% at 20 years. In other words, in a person who had one of these tumors at age 45, his or her chance of being alive at age 55 was less than 1 in 3. These are certainly not "benign" numbers.

TYMPANIC PARAGANGLIOMAS

Tympanic paragangliomas typically present with pulsatile tinnitus, occasionally intermittent but usually

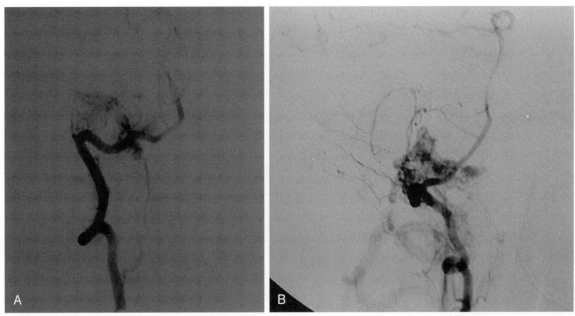

Figure 11-1 Case 1. *A* and *B,* Posteroanterior (PA) and lateral views of a left vertebral artery injection show extensive supply to a hypervascular mass at the skull base. This patient presented with a neck mass and cranial nerve deficits. Note that most of the flow goes to the tumor, not intracranially. While posterior inferior cerebellar artery (PICA) arises distal to the visible part of the mass on these images, the mass clearly extends at least to the junction between the skull base and C1, and is possibly intimately involved with the dura.

Note the arteriovenous shunting with extensive venous filling even during the arterial and capillary phases. The vertebral artery itself appears to be intimately involved with the tumor mass and may have to be sacrificed at the time of surgery. A test occlusion can be performed with a small ITC/Target Therapeutics Endeavor balloon (see Chapter 1) if there is any doubt as to the capability of the opposite vertebral artery to handle the flow necessary. The test occlusion should be done with the balloon *past* the bulk of the tumor mass, or a false result may be obtained owing to steal by the tumor.

Case 1 continues

progressively worsening. Disappearance of the tinnitus heralds cochlear destruction. Conductive hearing loss, vertigo, bleeding into the ear, palsy of cranial nerve VII, and bluish or reddish bulging of the tympanic membrane are also typical. Further growth of the tumor leads to mass in the external canal, parapharyngeal space, and petrous apex. Extension toward the mastoids leads to retroauricular pain. Figures 11–1 to 11–11 illustrate the case of a paraganglioma that involves the territory of both a typical tympanic and jugular tumor.

JUGULAR PARAGANGLIOMAS

Jugular paragangliomas present with paralysis of cranial nerves IX, X, and XI (Vernet's syndrome), resulting in hoarseness, swallowing difficulty, deviation of the soft palate to the unaffected side, weakness of the upper trapezius and sternomastoid muscles, and anesthesia of the posterior pharyngeal wall. At this stage, the tumor is already large. A history of preceding intermittent tinnitus and hypoglossal neuralgia (spasm of the tongue) may be elicited in retrospect. With further growth, impairment of cranial nerves XII (paralysis of the affected side of the tongue) and VII (paralysis of the ipsilateral facial muscles and possibly loss of taste over the anterior two thirds of the tongue) can be seen. The tumor can extend toward the tympanic cavity or intracranially.

Extension toward the tympanic cavity may produce symptoms similar to those associated with tympanic tumors. Occlusion of the internal jugular vein by intraluminal tumor growth is not usually symptomatic.

Differential Diagnosis of Temporal (Jugular and Tympanic) Paragangliomas

The differential diagnosis of temporal (jugular and tympanic) paragangliomas includes many different entities, ranging from anatomic variants to other neoplastic processes. This includes a prominent jugular bulb, intratympanic course of the internal carotid artery, stapedial artery persistence, dural arteriovenous (AV) fistula, aneurysm, tympanic granuloma (cholesteatoma), neurogenic tumor, meningioma of the temporal bone, metastatic lesion at the jugular foramen, chondroid tumor/chordoma, and hemangioma.[1] *The first six entities listed above are capable of producing tinnitus.*

In the case of extension to the petrous apex, the differential diagnosis includes other lesions that occur in this location, such as epidermoid cyst, mesenchymal tumor, eosinophilic granuloma, mucocele, osteomyelitis, meningioma, nasopharyngeal carcinoma (from the clivus), neurogenic tumor, metastatic carcinoma, and internal carotid artery aneurysm.[4]

Text continued on page 137

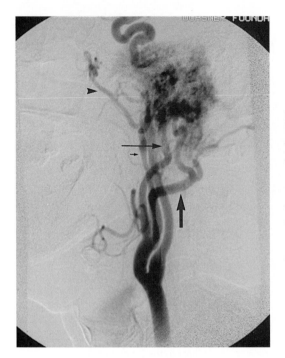

Figure 11-2 Lateral right common carotid injection reveals an enormously hypervascular mass in the sigmoid sinus region. This covers the territory of a jugular foramen and/or a tympanic glomus. Note that the ascending pharyngeal artery *(small arrow)* and the occipital artery *(thick arrow)* are nearly the size of the internal carotid artery. The proximal trunk of the internal maxillary artery *(long arrow)* is also too large; it becomes more normal in size in its horizontal portion *(arrowhead)*.

The black spots amid the vascular pooling are indicators of possible shunts. This appearance has been recognized in tumors that have been difficult to occlude with PVA particles, even the largest size injectable through a standard microcatheter. Glomus tumors are known to contain vascular lakes that may not be true large-caliber shunts, but they are also notorious for these huge shunts.

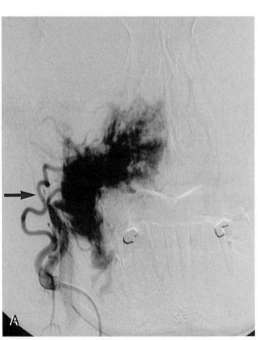

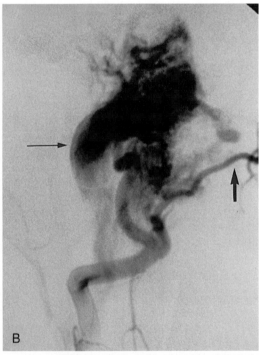

Figure 11-3 *A* and *B*, PA and lateral selective occipital artery injection. The peripheral branches *(thick arrows)* are seen to continue past the huge stylomastoid branch to their normal territory. A massive shunt is seen to opacify an enormous venous drainage structure (the internal jugular vein) *(long arrow)*. The stylomastoid branch appears to end in the tumor blush, as indeed it would. The amount of flow through this vessel is incredible (look at the size of its trunk!). Before embolization, a test injection of lidocaine can give warning of the presence of a potentially vulnerable cranial nerve. However, in cases such as this, there is often preexisting cranial nerve palsy. In addition, full removal of these tumors not infrequently results in cranial nerve palsy.

If the test injection with lidocaine is positive, what does one do? Nothing? The author (JJC) thinks not. Large-size particles are uniformly tolerated, even when directly embolizing a feeding vessel. This should be what is utilized in this case (i.e., 350 microns and greater). This can be accompanied by fibered coils.

Case 1 continues

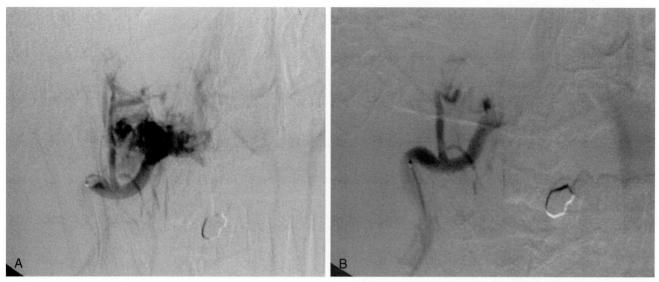

Figure 11-4 *A* and *B,* Partial embolization has been performed by *A* and continued embolization by *B.* Embolization of this vessel was started with PVA particles in the 250- to 350-micron range; anything smaller would almost assuredly wash right through, and the chance of causing ischemic damage to a cranial nerve has to be considered. As the embolization progresses, the particle size should be increased quickly to the 750+-micron range. The feeder trunk can then be occluded with coils to prevent bleeding into the surgical bed during dissection (according to the personal preference of the interventional neuroradiologist as well as the surgeon).

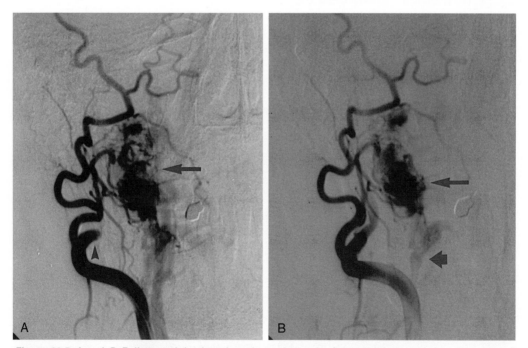

Figure 11-5 *A* and *B,* Follow-up injections into the main trunk of the occipital artery reveal continued supply to the tumor from another branch. Note the early tumoral filling *(arrows),* the early draining vein *(fat arrow),* and the stub of the stylomastoid branch already embolized *(arrowhead).* Additional embolization of this branch should be carried out, with every attempt made to spare the normal posterior occipital branch visualized. At the least, if superselective catheterization of the remaining feeding branch cannot be made, protective embolization of the normal branch can be made (see "Protective Embolization" in Chapter 3). The normal branch should be spared in order to optimize postsurgical healing.

Case 1 continues

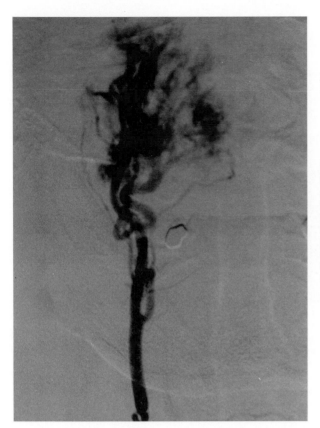

Figure 11-6 PA right ascending pharyngeal injection. Massive supply to the skull base tumor is present. The normally thin branches are very dilated and tortuous. Beading is also seen in some of the vessels. Embolization of this vessel should be performed in the same manner as that described above for the occipital artery, with final occlusion of the trunk performed by means of coils. Selection of each vascular pedicle should be performed, rather than just random infusion of particles into the main trunk. Not only would random infusion of particles be a sledgehammer, inelegant approach to therapy, but it is not possible to see where the flow is carrying the particles.

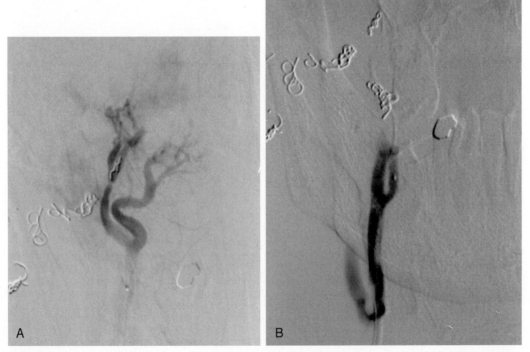

Figure 11-7 *A* and *B,* Follow-up injections after partial embolization and full embolization of the ascending pharyngeal artery. The trunk should be occluded with coils after the tumor bed is filled, to obtain a dry surgical field. Coil packing should be performed at a point proximal to the tumor bed, not within it.

Case 1 continues

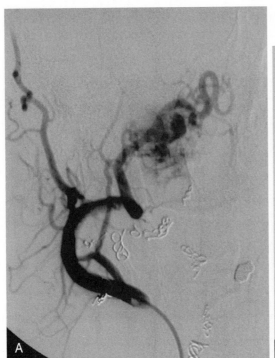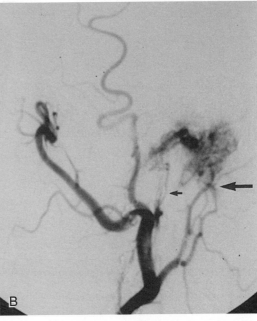

Figure 11-8 *A* and *B,* Injection of the internal maxillary artery demonstrates continued supply to the tumor from the posterior auricular artery *(large arrow)* and the anterior tympanic artery *(small arrow).* This is another example of how intratumoral penetration with embolic material can make the later stages of the procedure easier, as well as the surgery. The collateral supply to the tumor would have been much greater if the previously embolized vessels had been occluded only at their proximal trunks. Free intratumoral supply from this vessel would have allowed continued extensive permeation. Once these vessels are embolized in the above-described manner, the likelihood of any significant hemorrhage during the operative procedure is further decreased.

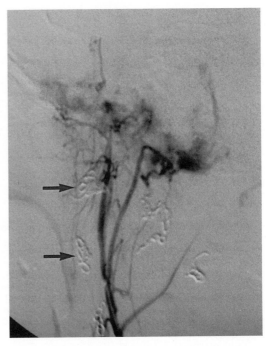

Figure 11-9 Lateral view of a selective injection of the opposite (left) ascending pharyngeal artery reveals supply across the midline to the tumor. Note the coils in the bed of the opposite ascending pharyngeal artery *(arrows).* Note also the apparent filling of the tumor from both the neuromeningeal branch of this vessel and the muscular pharyngeal division. Embolization of this vessel should be undertaken with caution, but it needs to be done. This area will be the last to be controlled by the unwary surgeon and is a potential source of significant intraoperative hemorrhage. Pre-embolization cranial nerve testing can be performed utilizing cardiac lidocaine, not amobarbital (see text). This vessel can supply cranial nerves VI, IX, X, XI, and XII, as well as the PICA, brainstem, and cervical nerve roots.

Owing to the contralateral devascularization, larger PVA particles (>350 microns) should probably be used, not only for neural protection but also to facilitate postoperative healing.

Case 1 continues

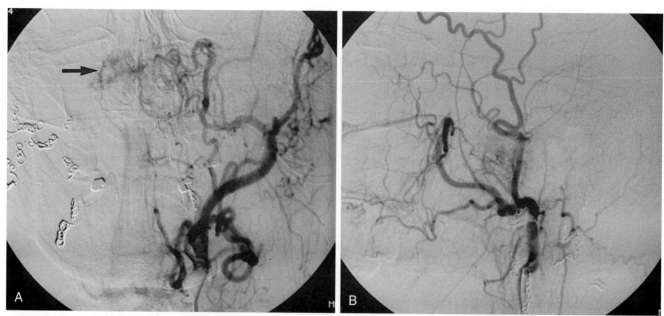

Figure 11-10 *A* and *B,* Note the filling of tumor *(arrow)* across the midline during injection of the contralateral external carotid artery. Again, this could be a real problem for the surgeon to control without preoperative occlusion of these feeders. Even though it looks as if the supply may be coming from the internal maxillary artery on the PA view, reason tells us this is not the case; rather, these are retropharyngeal collaterals, just as were seen above involving the ascending pharyngeal artery.

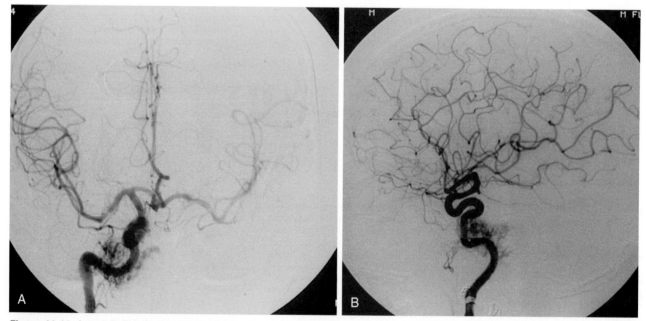

Figure 11-11 *A* and *B,* The final selective internal carotid artery injection displays a significant amount of residual tumor filling from the internal carotid artery. This is probably from intrapetrous branches (vidian artery) as well as cavernous branches (e.g., clival branch of the meningohypophyseal artery). These feeders are too numerous, difficult, and dangerous to be dealt with lightly. Choices in this circumstance include (1) preoperative test balloon occlusion and (2) preemptive balloon occlusion before surgery. If preoperative balloon occlusion is to be performed, the surgeon should be cautioned not to compress this vessel at the time of surgery; otherwise, inadvertent distal migration of balloon/clot mass can occur (and has been reported). In addition, after the first balloon has been placed in the standard distal cavernous location (proximal to the ophthalmic artery), the remainder of the cavernous and intrapetrous internal carotid artery should probably be occluded with coils. This not only occludes the orifices of the feeder vessels but also may make the embolic/clot mass more immobile. Proximal occlusion of the cervical internal carotid artery should also be performed, as usual. We did not occlude this vessel in this case.

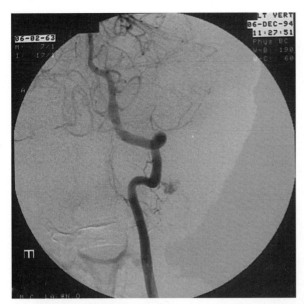

Figure 11-12 Case 2. This 31-year-old man has a known carotid body tumor. Thorough preoperative, preembolization angiographic evaluation reveals a small blush arising from a muscular branch of the vertebral artery. This is coursing toward the tumor mass in the region of the carotid bifurcation, indicating a multi-compartmented tumor as discussed in the text.

CAROTID PARAGANGLIOMAS

Carotid paragangliomas usually present as a pulsatile, expansile mass (Case 2, Figs. 11–12 to 11–22). Involvement of the parapharyngeal space, oral cavity, or larynx is thought to represent multicentricity. Tumor invasion into the internal carotid artery wall may result in occlusion of the artery. In a large series, 19% of patients reported pain, 11% dysphagia, 9%

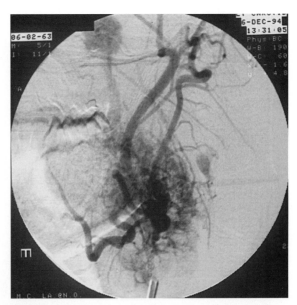

Figure 11-14 Selective injection of the external carotid artery reveals the previously seen massive blush. Arterial anatomy is difficult to unravel in an image such as this. Further subselection will allow better, more accurate analysis.

syncope, 8% hoarseness, 7% Horner's syndrome, and 2% cranial nerve XII deficit, as described above.[1] Cranial nerve involvement (XII and the superior laryngeal nerve, which arises from cranial nerve X and supplies sensation to the larynx) is associated with large, multicentric tumors.

VAGAL PARAGANGLIOMAS

Vagal (cranial nerve X) tumors present with cervical or pharyngeal mass. Cranial nerve involvement is

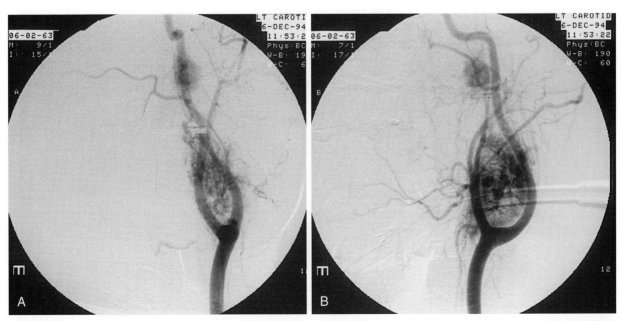

Figure 11-13 *A* and *B,* PA and lateral views of the left common carotid artery display the typical appearance of a carotid body chemodectoma (paraganglioma). Note the characteristic widening of the carotid bifurcation and dense *inhomogeneous* blush. The inhomogeneity is due to the fact that different areas of the tumor mass contain varying sizes of shunts. Note the additional tumor blush at the skull base indicative of multiple tumors (see text).

Case 2 continues

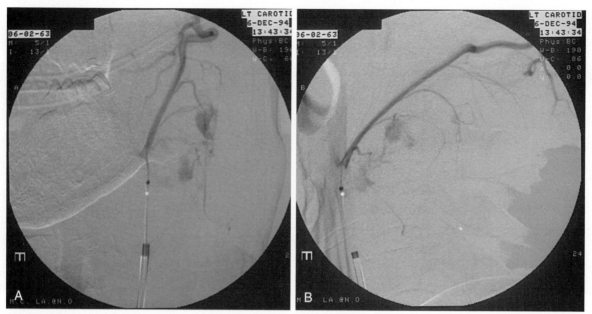

Figure 11-15 *A* and *B*, PA and lateral views of the occipital artery reveal significant supply to the tumor from above. It is not possible to select these small twigs with the microcatheter, but embolization of the tumor masses is possible if the downstream occipital artery is protected.

seen in 30% of patients.[2] The nerves most frequently affected are cranial nerve X (24%), XII (14%), IX (11%), and XI (8%); 11% have Horner's syndrome.[2] Pharyngeal pain is common. The tumor can arise intravagally (at or below the inferior or nodose ganglion of the nerve) or extravagally. Intravagal tumors lead to rapid impairment of vagal nerve function. Extravagal tumors can grow larger before cranial nerve impairment develops. These tumors can extend to the skull base or intracranially.

Differential Diagnosis of Cervical (Carotid and Vagal) Paragangliomas

The differential diagnosis of cervical paragangliomas (carotid and vagal) also includes a wide range of entities, including lymphadenitis, branchial cleft cysts, metastases, neurogenic tumors, and carotid artery aneurysms.

Among the less common paragangliomas, nasopharyngeal lesions are often misdiagnosed as carcino-

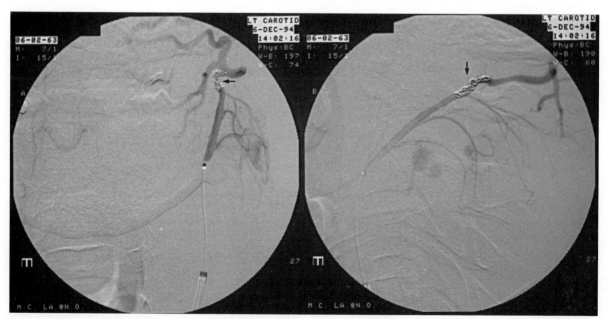

Figure 11-16 Coils have been placed in the midportion of the occipital artery *(arrows),* distal to the branches to the tumor masses. However, the coils have not caused occlusion of the vessel at this time. Catheterization of additional feeders will be performed, and this vessel will be returned to when occlusion of the occipital artery via thrombosis is complete.

Case 2 continues

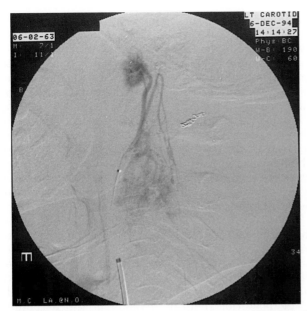

Figure 11-17 Injection of the ascending pharyngeal artery displays the typical "drooping lily" appearance due to the supply to the upper portion of the carotid body tumor mass. The contrast is diluted by the extremely fast wash-in of unopacified blood caused by the rapid arteriovenous shunting.

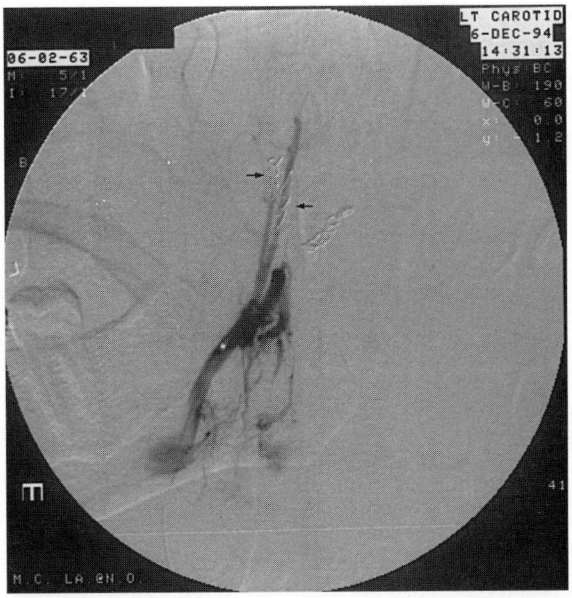

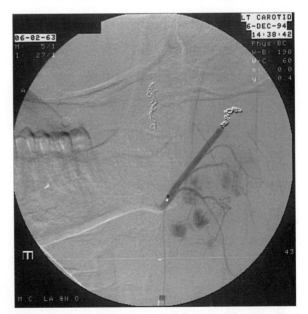

Figure 11-19 After additional embolization of the upper tumor mass, the supply is occluded permanently with coils (arrows) to prevent excessive bleeding in the surgical bed during resection. The intratumoral particles will prevent bleeding from the tumor itself due to arterial collaterals or retrograde venous flow.

mas; there may be delay in instituting proper therapy. Impairment of cranial nerve V (third division), resulting in anesthesia over the affected side of the mandible and possibly masseter and pterygoid paralysis, and diplopia have been described with these lesions. Laryngeal paragangliomas tend to present early as a result of hoarseness (70%), dyspnea (43%), and pain. Orbital paragangliomas are difficult to differentiate from other orbital tumors; they are intraconal and present with proptosis and decreased vision. These tumors tend to be locally invasive, recurrent, and metastatic.

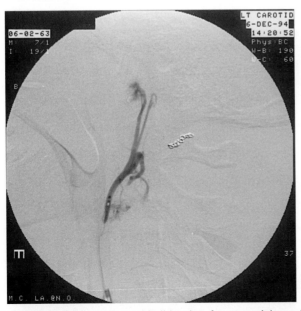

Figure 11-18 After testing with lidocaine for potential cranial nerve damage secondary to embolization, particulate embolization of this vessel was begun with PVA particles in the 150- to 250-micron range. Note the significant increase in contrast density on this injection owing to the slowing of the arteriovenous shunting. Note also the previously placed coils in the occipital artery.

Figure 11-20 Returning to the occipital artery, it can be seen that the coil embolization has effectively occluded the distal territory of this vessel, and the supply to the tumor is clearly demonstrated. Note the lack of any evidence of flow to any intracranial structures. This can be confirmed by a bolus injection of amobarbital or methohexital. Embolization of the branches can now be performed by use of small or medium-sized particles (250 to 500 microns).

Case 2 continues

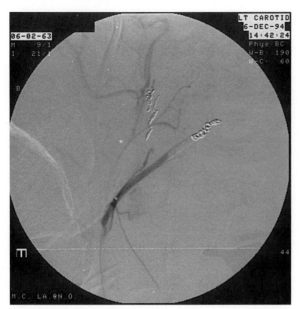

Figure 11-21 Follow-up angiogram of the embolized occipital artery displays occlusion of the branches to the tumor with preservation of the main trunk. Note the reflux into the internal maxillary branches on this injection. This is due to the lack of any downstream runoff in the occipital artery; there is thus nowhere for the contrast to go.

SECRETORY ACTIVITY OF PARAGANGLIOMAS/HYPERTENSIVE CRISIS

Secretory activity of paragangliomas is manifested by headache, hypertension, palpitations, diaphoresis, and anxiety; this is seen in approximately 5% of patients. Owing to the activity of these tumors, manual palpation (massage or during surgery) or angiography may precipitate a hypertensive crisis. The hypertensive crises seen during angiography have been associated with the use of hypertonic ionic contrast material. Therefore, the use of nonionic contrast media is recommended. Blockade of α-receptors with phenoxybenzamine before and/or during manipulation is helpful. Phentolamine mesylate, nitroprusside, and labetalol HCl can be helpful for treating a hypertensive crisis (see "Hypertensive Crisis" in Chapter 64). Hypotensive episodes during tumor manipulation are less common; these usually cease when devascularization is complete. Other associated problems include increased vagal tone (bradycardia, hypotension) after embolization of a carotid body tumor; this responds to atropine.

The difficult surgical dissection is helped considerably by devascularization. As stated under the general discussion of tumoral embolization, however, endovascular treatment of these tumors is sometimes difficult due to the size of the AV shunts. In addition, there are frequently multiple vessels to be accessed.

The posterior (neural) division of the ascending pharyngeal artery (seen to the right in Figure 11–9) is one of the riskier vessels to treat. Typically, embolization can be performed with particles in the 150- to 250-micron range without difficulty, but there have been reported cases of cranial nerve damage after this embolization. Smaller particles or liquids (ethanol or pure glue) should not be used. Caution should also be maintained when working with the occipital artery (as usual); it can send supply to the vertebral artery. Indeed, any vessel going to the region of the skull base should be handled with care.

General Goal of Endovascular Therapy for Paragangliomas

Embolization of glomus tumors is not only a technical challenge but a challenge to patience. Theoretically,

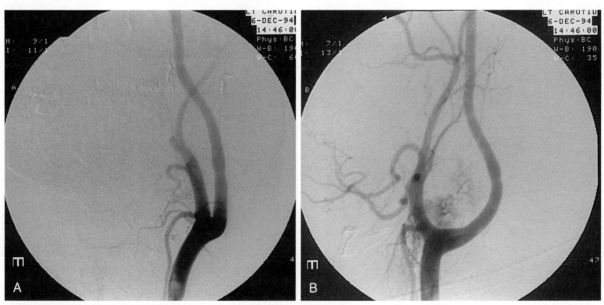

Figure 11-22 A and B, Final appearance of the embolized tumor mass during common carotid artery injection. The residual supply is from microvessels arising from the bifurcation region or proximal external carotid branches. It is not necessary to treat these vessels; the surgeons should be capable of dealing with the minimal amount of residual supply at the time of surgery.

these tumors (any size or location) could be removed without a significant deficit by excellent surgical technique, but drying the operative field for the surgeon is of major benefit. The interventional neuroradiologist's task is to make the operative procedure easier and safer.

These particular tumors can have such an amazing number of vessels supplying them, as well as such a high flow rate, that it is almost incredible that they are resectable *without* embolization! Cases have been observed in which it appeared that at least 10% to 25% of the entire supply to the head and neck was going to the tumor! In addition, some of the AV shunts can be far larger than 1 mm. (The lumen of a typical microcatheter is about 0.5 mm, or 0.018 to 0.022″.) Occlusion of these large AV shunts becomes a real challenge, particularly when they are at the skull base, and the vascular supply should not be occluded randomly. It is at this point that injection of short straight coils or BOD coils (Target Therapeutics) can help control the flow. Once the flow has slowed to a reasonable degree, PVA mixed with Avitene can result in occlusion (for how long is still in question).

This aggressiveness is necessary only for tumors at the skull base. For carotid body tumors, there is usually a vascular supply from "drooping lily"–appearing vessels coming from the ascending pharyngeal artery (Fig. 11–16) (and the occipital artery via the stylomastoid branch) (Fig. 11–17), curving over the top of the tumor, and supplying it from above. Usually, any supply from the ascending pharyngeal artery is from branches originating from this vessel after it has passed the tumor. At this point, other vital branches of the ascending pharyngeal are present, however, and simple random embolization of this vessel is unsafe, unnecessary, and technically inelegant. It will be apparent which small side branches have been cannibalized to supply the tumor, and before any embolization is performed, either these branches should be specifically selected or protective distal vessel occlusion should be performed.

Other vascular supply to a carotid body glomus tumor is variable. There can be supply from the posterior auricular or occipital arteries as well as other branches, and there is usually some residual minimal supply arising from microbranches at the bifurcation of the internal and external carotid arteries, which are technically untreatable by endovascular means and of minimal consequence to the surgeon (Fig. 11–22*B*). Simply pointing these out to the surgeon before the open surgical procedure will suffice.

An alternative to the intra-arterial embolization described here is direct percutaneous embolization. This is described in Chapter 28.

ELECTIVE PRESURGICAL INTERNAL CAROTID ARTERY OCCLUSION

For extensive tumors with known arterial invasion, the surgeon may choose to request elective presurgical internal carotid artery occlusion. This can be performed as described in Chapters 34 and 35. A note of caution should be made, however: the internal carotid artery will be a closed tube, and manipulation by the surgeon after preoperative occlusion could mash thrombus or other material downstream into the brain. A continuous line of silicone balloons would perhaps be the easiest to move. A cavernous balloon followed by tightly packed coils in the petrous carotid artery and another balloon just below the skull base is perhaps the best way to achieve some anchoring of the mass (0.038″ coils are the most thrombogenic and inflammatory and probably offer the greatest degree of stability). Again, occlusion with coils alone in the carotid artery without proximal flow arrest during the occlusion is very dangerous; it may allow thrombus to break off as the coils are being placed and embolize to the brain before occlusion is complete. See the technique described in Chapter 35.

REFERENCES

1. Zak FG, Lawson W. The paraganglionic chemoreceptor system. Physiology, pathology and clinical medicine. New York: Springer-Verlag, 1982.
2. Lasjaunias P, Berenstein A. Surgical neuroangiography, Vol 2: Endovascular treatment of craniofacial lesions. New York: Springer-Verlag, 1987.
3. Harrison K. Glomus jugulare tumors: their clinical behavior and management. *Proc R Soc Med* 1974;67:264–267.
4. Flood LM, Kemink JL. Surgery in lesions of the petrous apex. *Otolaryngol Clin North Am* 1984;17:565–575.

ADDITIONAL READINGS

George B. Jugulare foramen paragangliomas. *Acta Neurochir* 1992;118:20–26.
Herdman RCD, Gillespie JE, Ramsden RT. Facial palsy after glomus tumour embolization. *J Laryngol Otol* 1993;107:963–966.
Lack EE, Cubilla AL, Woodruff JM, Farr HW. Paragangliomas of the head and neck region: A clinical study of 69 patients. *Cancer* 1977;39:397–409.
LaMuraglia GM, Fabian RL, Brewster DC, et al. The current surgical management of carotid body paragangliomas. *J Vasc Surg* 1992;15:1038–1045.
Rock JP, Mahmood A, Cramer HB. Giant cell tumor of the skull base. *Am J Otol* 1994;15:268–272.
Sharma PD, Johnson AP. Whitton AC. Radiotherapy for jugulotympanic paragangliomas. *J Laryngol Otol* 1984;98:621–629.
Wax MK, Briant DR. Carotid body tumors: A review. *J Otolaryngol* 1992;21:277–285.

CHAPTER 12

Tumors of the Vertebral Bodies and Other Bones

J.J. Connors III / J.C. Wojak

Numerous types of intraosseous tumors may benefit from interventional treatment, including hypervascular metastases (e.g., renal cell carcinoma), hemangiomas, and primary bone tumors of a destructive (osteolytic) or hypervascular nature.

Endovascular transarterial embolization of intraosseous tumors is not curative (at least with present techniques) and hardly beneficial except as a preoperative aid in certain situations. Particles do not appear to accomplish much of a permanent nature other than blocking access for later procedures. Ethanol can be used intra-arterially to truly kill tumor tissue, but it is usually not totally curative and is potentially dangerous when used from this approach without great skill and care (in neuroradiology, all osseous structures are intimately associated with neural structures). Cyanoacrylates have been used percutaneously to occlude vascular tumors and even to try to strengthen bone that has been destroyed by tumor. Various types of methylmethacrylates have been used from a percutaneous approach to try to bolster vertebral bodies that have been weakened by tumor, and they appear to be useful in cases of progressive vertebral body collapse due to degenerative osteoporosis as well as tumor. This percutaneous cementing procedure stops the progressive collapse and subsequent chronic pain. Unfortunately, other vertebral bodies may then collapse, necessitating further therapy. Under certain circumstances, however, this may yield a solution not otherwise available.

TRANSARTERIAL VERTEBRAL BODY TUMOR EMBOLIZATION

For preoperative embolization (e.g., before an attempt by a surgeon to remove at least a portion of a hypervascular vertebral body tumor mass for decompressive purposes), the guidelines concerning embolization of tumors described in Chapter 8 are appropriate. The vascular supply to the vertebral body and the spinal cord should be thoroughly evaluated. Frequently, the surgeon may not plan to do a total excision, but rather only a therapeutic subtotal resection for control of nerve root compression or mass effect (Case 1, Figs. 12–1 to 12–6). True intratumoral permeation with embolic material and vascular occlusion should not be necessary for these procedures. However, good control of the vascular supply to the region should be obtained, because hemostasis may

be difficult during surgery, with remaining vascularized tumor present and bone blocking the way to any deep arterial supply so that the surgeon cannot reach it for hemostasis.

PERCUTANEOUS ETHANOL ABLATION OF INTRAOSSEOUS VERTEBRAL BODY HEMANGIOMAS

Of interest is the report of work utilizing ethanol via a direct percutaneous intraosseous approach. This appears to destroy tumor but leave a matrix of bone for osteoblasts to invade into and then regenerate normal bone.[1] This innovative approach appears promising, but there are many unknown factors concerning the specifics of this therapy and possible sequelae (Case 2, Figs. 12–7 to 12–11).

A large percutaneous bone-puncturing or biopsy needle is used for access under computed tomographic (CT) guidance (see "Vertebral Body Biopsy Needles" in Chapter 1). The needle may be extremely easy to advance into the tumor, the cortical shell being greatly softened by the tumor mass. Once the needle has bored into the core of the tumor, there will usually be a plug of material occluding the nee-

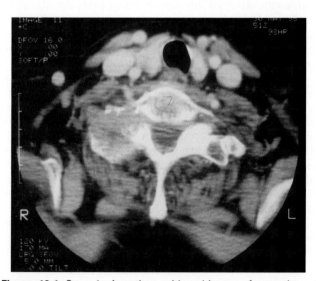

Figure 12-1 Case 1. A patient with a history of resection of a lower extremity hemangiopericytoma now presents with a destructive lesion involving the transverse processes of two lower cervical vertebral bodies, with resultant nerve root compression inducing pain and cervical instability. Surgical resection/decompression is planned, with preoperative embolization.

Case 1 continues

dle lumen. It is necessary to use the "ramrod" supplied with the kit to clear the lumen. This is important. Pulsatile blood return can then be observed, but usually without a high flow rate. It should be possible to aspirate blood, but this is variable, depending on the size and structure of the tumor.

A chosen quantity of dilute contrast (approximately one-half strength) is then infused and a repeat CT scan performed to evaluate the extent of permeation of the tumor. The volume of a sphere is πr^3, and this formula can be used to help with the approximation of the volume to be infused. (The dilution percentage is chosen to yield a material appreciably different from the density of bone so that the area of permeation is highly visible on CT.) The amount of pure ethanol is then adjusted to fill the appropriate amount of tumor space.

The tumor bed can hold varying amounts of material. Typically, a hemangioma will contain large vascular lakes, but filling these lakes can be difficult, either because of resistance encountered during infusion (limited venous drainage generating high intraosseous pressure) or because of the multitude of communicating spaces rendering adequate filling difficult (i.e., the ethanol will become diluted by the volume of stagnant blood encountered). This latter is generally not a significant problem if the tumor is not too tremendous in size (30 ml of ethanol can fill a huge volume of tumor). Remember, however, that

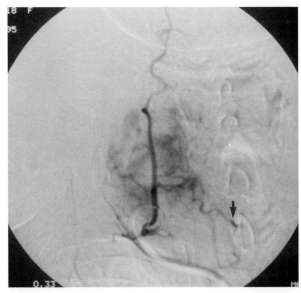

Figure 12-3 Selective catheterization with a microcatheter and injection of the proximal trunk of the posterior cervical artery clearly shows the vascular supply to the tumor and the medially coursing vessel previously seen (*arrow* near spinous process). Oblique projections should be performed to evaluate this vessel's true destination. The somewhat curvilinear inferior course and caudad "hook" after the vessel nears the midline is atypical for a spinal artery, but its territory should nevertheless be absolutely determined (and, if need be, tested by lidocaine injection). The trapezius has muscular insertions on the spinous processes. In addition, the en passant nature of the supply to the tumor will necessitate embolization from within the posterior cervical artery itself rather than selective embolization within each feeder. This will necessitate protective occlusion of the distal territory of the posterior cervical artery.

Case 1 continues

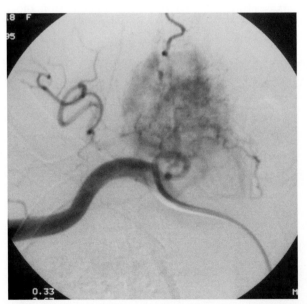

Figure 12-2 Initial injection of the right subclavian artery reveals a hypervascular mass originating from the costocervical trunk. Note the posterior (deep) cervical artery coursing "through" the tumor as viewed on this projection. Note also the diminished contrast within this deep (posterior) cervical artery at the level of the tumor due to the sump effect of the tumor, with increased runoff compared with the distal portion of the vessel. Also note the small vessel extending medially toward the spinal canal (supply to the cord?). Selective injection of the thyrocervical trunk and vertebral arteries was made to exclude any supply from these sources. The location of the mass suggested that supply should be from the "posterior" branch of the subclavian artery (the costocervical trunk), and possibly from musculoskeletal branches arising from the vertebral artery.

the maximal amount of ethanol to be infused at any one time should not exceed 1 ml/kg.

Theoretically, once the volume of hemangiomatous venous lakes has been determined, pure ethanol is infused and allowed to sit. Instead of trying to later aspirate this quantity or plug the hole made by the puncture needle (e.g., with Gelfoam), the ethanol is simply allowed to slowly diffuse and be washed out by normal flow. After 30 minutes, the needle can be simply removed. Alternatively, for increased safety, a relatively large volume of saline (e.g., 20 ml) can be infused very slowly to flush the area and absolutely ensure the absence (or at least the significant dilution) of retained ethanol. The needle can then be removed.

The technique originally described[1] contains no solution for the above-described problems of high-resistance infusion pressure and subsequent potential need for end-of-procedure dilution of the ethanol. If ethanol is injected too forcefully into a closed space or in too large a volume, inadvertent or errant extravasation of ethanol may occur with unknown consequences. In addition, in the case presented, 1 hour after infusion of a large volume of contrast (10 ml) (which had puddled in several pockets), there was no evidence of significant clearing on CT, raising a question concerning the validity of the concept of

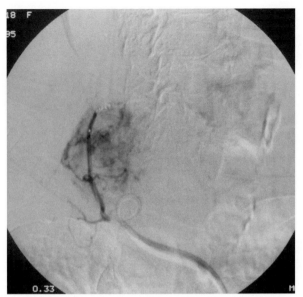

Figure 12-4 After protective embolization of the distal portion of the posterior (deep) cervical artery by three platinum coils, an oblique projection confirms occlusion and reveals the worrisome vessel to project posterior to the spinous process and represent a muscular branch (note the inferior hook of the vessel below and to the left of the tumor mass). Dense tumoral blush is present even though the catheter is still in the distal portion of the occluded vessel. Initial embolization was performed from this location with PVA particles in the 150- to 250-micron range.

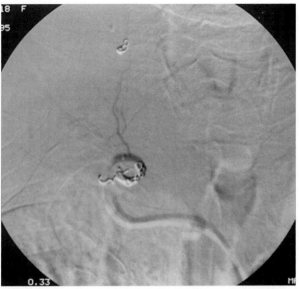

Figure 12-6 After near-cessation of flow in the main trunk, the proximal trunk was occluded with multiple platinum coils. The final selective angiogram confirms no further supply to the tumor, with a small costocervical branch still present. (The last injection, in the subclavian artery, confirmed no further supply.)

PREABLATION TESTING

Early work has shown this direct infusion of ethanol into a vertebral body hemangioma to be apparently confined to the tumor volume (in the small number of cases studied) with resultant destruction of the lesion that produced the expansile and erosive osse-

"washing out" of ethanol over a period as brief as 30 minutes. This is the rationale for the above maneuver of further infusion of saline to ensure the dilution of any remaining ethanol and hopefully prevent its leakage from the needle tract.

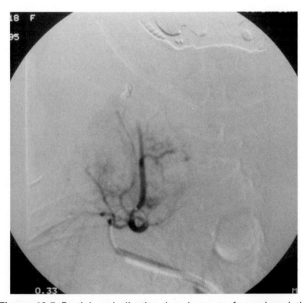

Figure 12-5 Partial embolization has been performed and the microcatheter is withdrawn to a somewhat more proximal location. Note the "leafless" or "bare" tree appearance of the vasculature. Tumoral supply is still present, particularly from more proximal vessels, and continued embolization was performed, first with 150- to 250-micron and then with 250- to 350-micron PVA particles.

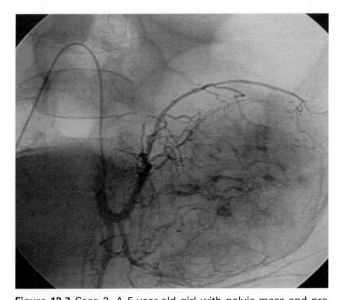

Figure 12-7 Case 2. A 5-year-old girl with pelvic mass and progressive neurologic deficits. Selective internal iliac injection reveals vascular pooling and staining typical of a hemangioma. This lesion had been embolized on multiple previous occasions with minimal, if any, response. Steroids and interferon therapy had been utilized for years. The patient's symptoms had progressed to include bowel and bladder incontinence, three fifths to four fifths strength in the left leg with varying episodes of severe pain (chronically treated with massive doses of codeine), and recently increasing right leg pain and weakness.

Case 2 continues

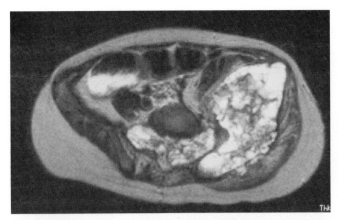

Figure 12-8 Magnetic resonance imaging (MRI) scan reveals the massive nature of this lesion. Note that the original iliac lesion has crossed the sacroiliac joint and now extensively involves the posterior elements of the sacrum. The thecal sac cannot be identified as a separate structure on any imaging sequence and is probably involved (hence the bowel and bladder dysfunction). The massive nature of the iliac involvement was not clearly appreciated on the angiogram.

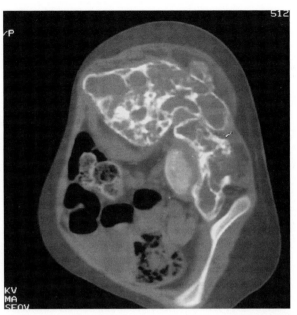

Figure 12-9 Representative image obtained immediately before the start of direct percutaneous intraosseous ethanol ablation therapy. The huge "caverns" are well demonstrated throughout the involved regions.

ous changes.[1] Long-term results and the number of patients are limited, but as stated above, there is some evidence that this technique leads to the ability of the bone to actually reossify. In the case presented, the tumor appeared to be intimately involved with the structures surrounding nerve roots, and there was considerable concern about these roots. A trial with lidocaine was negative, and no neurologic deficit developed after thorough perfusion of the mass.

To try to give a further margin of safety concerning any possible danger to neural structures in the area of coverage of the ethanol, a volume of saline containing 3 mg/kg of "cardiac" lidocaine can be infused

through the needle before embolotherapy with ethanol. The total volume of this fluid should be slightly more than the volume of ethanol to be used, to err on the safe side, as the total area reached by diffusion of fluid containing lidocaine should be greater than the area affected by the volume of ethanol. For example, after appropriate preliminary neurologic testing, 25 to 100 mg of lidocaine (depending on patient weight) can be diluted in 5 to 25 ml of normal saline (depending on the appropriate volume of ethanol to

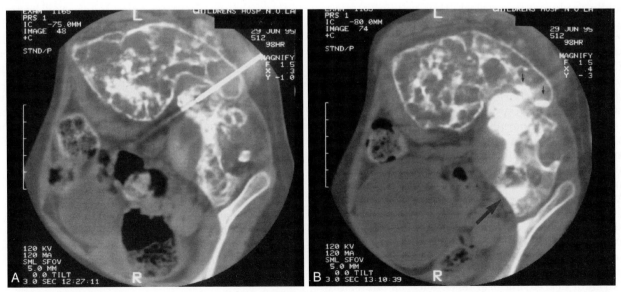

Figure 12-10 *A* and *B*, Direct puncture through the ilium and sacroiliac joint and into the lateral portion of the sacrum has been performed (utilizing a Geremia needle [Cook, Inc.]) *(A)* and dilute contrast injected *(B)*. Note the layering of contrast in the *opposite* side of the sacrum *(large arrow)*, as well as in the ilium *(small arrows)*; it had apparently refluxed back along the needle itself. This reflux around the needle where it had pierced the bone was a dramatic demonstration of the pressure generated during infusion of the contrast. Also note that thus high-density contrast has settled to the bottom of each pool.

Case 2 continues

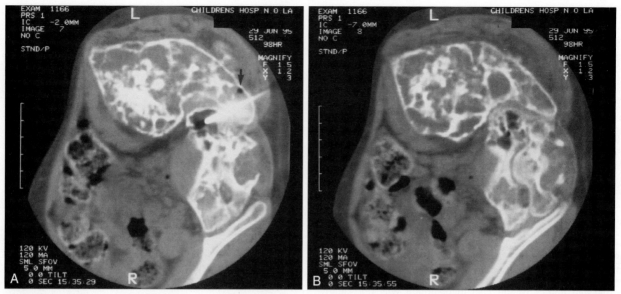

Figure 12-11 *A* and *B,* Dehydrated ethanol has now been infused (see text). The low-density material around the needletip is the alcohol—not air, although there is an air bubble in the ilium *(arrow).* Ethanol is less dense than blood or water and thus has this computed tomographic appearance. It also behaves in exactly the opposite manner from contrast; it floats rather than sinks, thus potentially distributing to different areas than were demonstrated with the contrast material. It is for this reason that the lidocaine infusion test is used (see text).

be used) and this mixture gradually infused into the target area. After a few minutes, a repeat neurologic examination can be performed that may warn of any potential pitfalls to the injection of ethanol (e.g., the lidocaine injection may result in a local nerve block, indicating a possibility of disaster if ethanol is injected). If this test is negative, this will add even greater weight to the advisability and acceptability of infusing a lesser volume of ethanol into the same space. Unfortunately, the amount of lidocaine reaching a specific nerve root may not be enough to actually produce a nerve block, thus yielding a false-negative result. For this reason, an amount of lidocaine equal to the upper limits of the intravenous dose range should be used to perform this test.

The tumor shown in Figure 11–8 is far larger than any in the limited number presented in case reports, and a prolonged therapeutic procedure with very slow evidence of efficacy is expected. In addition, the presence of the abnormal mass exterior to the osseous framework raises concern for the limits of extension of the ethanol infusion (it will not be completely contained within osseous walls and the periosteal limits may be violated).

An additional concern regarding this form of therapy is the probable destruction of the draining veins of the lesion. This can lead to delayed thrombosis of these veins with subsequent edema of normal structures, which may be of considerable significance. Medication with high-dose intravenous steroids followed by a decreasing oral dose (such as one of the standard tapering "dose packs") may be of some benefit.

Whenever ethanol is to be used, note should be made of possible complications (see "Postethanol Embolization Cardiopulmonary Collapse" in Chapter

64). Even if there is no real cardiopulmonary "collapse," there is usually a significant cardiopulmonary response (tachycardia, at least, even under general anesthesia). Caution should always be used when dealing with ethanol.

After the procedure, depending on patient size and volume of ethanol used, the patient may be intoxicated or experience a "hangover" in addition to postanesthesia, postprocedure nausea. Local pain should not be severe unless there was extravasation into surrounding soft tissues.

Even though these vascular lakes may be under significant pressure, there is usually no high flow present in these lesions. However, when the needle was removed in one case, an arterial squirt was observed to erupt from the puncture site, and pressure was held for 15 minutes. Hemostasis should not be difficult, but depending on location, direct pressure may be suboptimal. For this reason, preoperative coagulation studies should be obtained to verify normal clotting function.

PERCUTANEOUS VERTEBROPLASTY

This innovative technique involves injecting a cement (typically methylmethacrylate) into bones to add pure structural strength. This does not kill tumor per se, but it is used mostly for buttressing osteoporotic bones. This technique is covered in detail in Chapter 29.

REFERENCE

1. Doppman JL. Percutaneous treatment of symptomatic vertebral hemangiomas by direct injection of alcohol. Paper presented at the 1995 Course in Interventional Neuroradiology of

the American Society of Interventional and Therapeutic Neuroradiology, Chicago.

ADDITIONAL READINGS

Dick H, Bigliani L, Michelsen J, Johnston A, Stinchfield F. Adjuvant arterial embolization in the treatment of benign primary bone tumors in children. *Clin Orthop* 1979;139:133–141.

Feldman F, Casarella W, Dick H, Hollander B. Selective intraarterial embolization of bone tumors. *Clin Orthop* 1979;123:130–139.

Glasscock ME, Smith PG, Nissen AJ, Schwaber MK. Clinical aspects of osseous hemangiomas of the skull base. *Laryngoscope* 1984;94:869–873.

Murphy W, Strecker W, Schoenecker P. Transcatheter embolization therapy of an ischial aneurysmal bone cyst. *J Bone Joint Surg* 1982;64-B:166–168.

Radanovic B, Simunic S, Stojanovic J, et al. Therapeutic embolization of aneurysmal bone cyst. *Cardiovasc Intervent Radiol* 1990;12:313–316.

Rowe DM, Becker GJ, Rabe FE, et al. Osseous metastases from renal cell carcinoma: Embolization and surgery for restoration of function. *Radiology* 1984;150:673–676.

Suby-Long T, Bos G, Rosch J. Biopsy proven eradication of an aneurysmal bone cyst treated by superselective embolization: A case report. *Cardiovasc Intervent Radiol* 1988;11:292–295.

Wallace S, Granmayeh M, DeSantos L, et al. Arterial occlusion of pelvic bone tumors. *Cancer* 1979;43:322–328.

CHAPTER 13

Epistaxis

J.J. Connors III / J.C. Wojak

Intractable nosebleed is fortunately a rare occurrence but one that occasionally may be difficult for a primary care physician to manage. However, simple epistaxis is not uncommon, with up to 50% to 60% of the population suffering from at least one episode in their lifetime and as many as 6% presenting for medical attention.[1] Conversely, epistaxis is simple to treat from an endovascular approach (Case 1, Figs. 13–1 to 13–3).

Anterior epistaxis is a common occurrence in chil-

dren and rarely of major consequence, whereas posterior epistaxis can be life threatening and occurs not uncommonly in an older age group. Conservative therapy begins with local pressure and nasal spraying of vasoconstrictors. More aggressive therapy constitutes nasal packing (anterior/posterior) as well as possible blood transfusions.

Intractable epistaxis is defined as any nosebleed that does not respond to those conservative measures. The otolaryngologist is then forced to perform

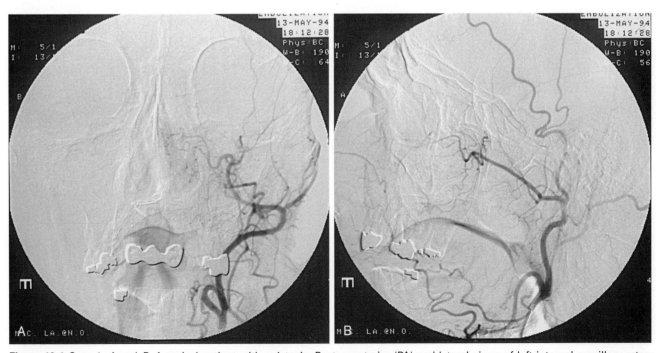

Figure 13-1 Case 1. *A* and *B,* A typical patient with epistaxis. Posteroanterior (PA) and lateral views of left internal maxillary artery injection reveal no abnormal blush, hyperemia, beading, or arteriovenous shunting.

Case 1 continues

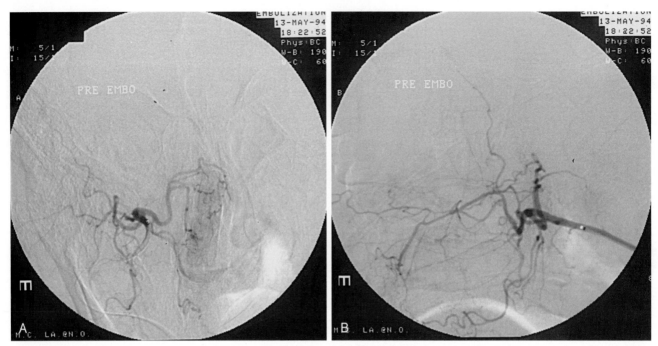

Figure 13-2 *A* and *B,* The right internal maxillary artery does display the changes typical for this condition. Note the "beading" of the arterioles, representing alternating bands of vasodilatation and constriction. Angiographically, this is the side that has been the problem.

more aggressive and invasive forms of therapy, including cautery, percutaneous injection (into the sinus/nasal passages) of hemostatic agents, and vascular ligation.[1-4]

These maneuvers are distasteful, painful, and not without their complications. In addition, they do not succeed in many cases; nasal packing has a failure rate as high as 25% to 50%. Packing can cause alar necrosis as well as sinus infection. Surgical clipping of the maxillary artery can result in infraorbital nerve injury, sinusitis, and other cranial nerve palsies.[1]

Endovascular embolization has been used successfully for the treatment of epistaxis since at least

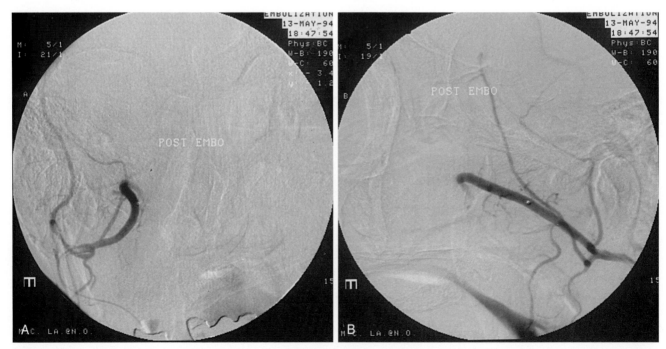

Figure 13-3 *A* and *B,* Treatment of this condition is usually straightforward (however, see the next case of a patient with Osler-Weber-Rendu syndrome). PVA particles of 150 to 250 microns were used to occlude the arterioles, resulting in this postembolization picture. This is generally all that is required.

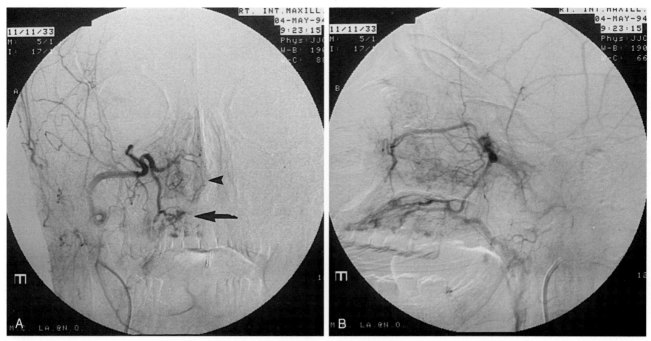

Figure 13-4 Case 2. *A* and *B,* A 60-year-old man with a history of multiple episodes of epistaxis from known Osler-Weber-Rendu syndrome. Initial PA and lateral views of right internal maxillary artery injection reveal extensive vascularity in the nose as well as the palate. Note the abnormal puddles *(arrow)* as well as the hypervascularity in the nasal turbinates *(arrowhead).* Arteriovenous shunting is noted, with an abnormal draining vein on the lateral view.

1974. Merland et al[5] reported on 54 patients with 94% success rate in 1980; catheters and techniques have only improved since that time. Several reports[6-8] give success rates ranging from 96% to 100%, and recommendations now exist to consider embolization as the preferred method of therapy if simple packing does not succeed.

The usual cause of intractable epistaxis is uncontrolled hypertension with or without some focal superficial disease of the nasal passages. Rarely, uncommon pathology such as Osler-Weber-Rendu syndrome can be the cause of repeated episodes of nosebleed (or other internal bleeding) (Case 2, Figs. 13–4 to 13–15).

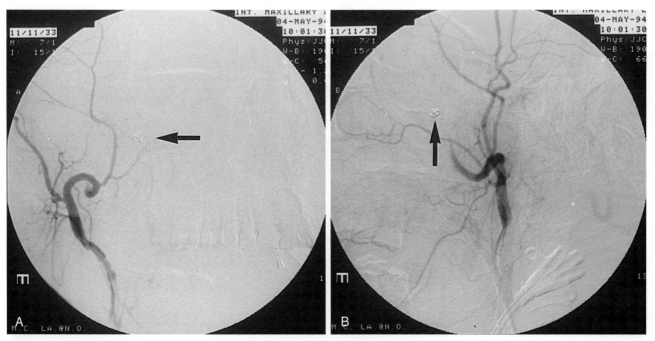

Figure 13-5 *A* and *B,* These images were obtained after embolization with 150- to 250-micron PVA particles followed by placement of a coil in the distal ethmoidal region *(arrows).* Obviously, we had not encountered this particular pathology before, or we would not have used a coil at this time.

Case 2 continues

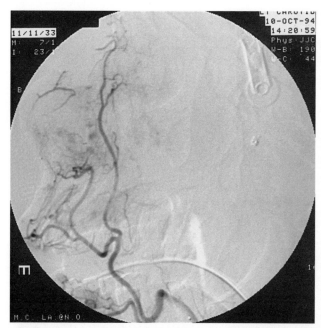

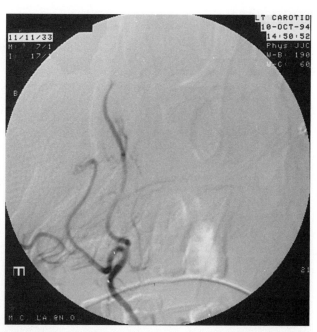

Figure 13-6 *Six months later, the patient returned with recurrent epistaxis. Selective injection of the left facial artery reveals extensive recruitment of the facial artery to supply the paranasal region and palate. The abnormal vascular puddling is again seen, indicative of the fact that this pathologic capillary bed was not occluded.*

Figure 13-7 *After 150- to 250-micron PVA particles were slowly floated downstream, the abnormal vasculature is no longer seen. Embolization was ceased at this point in this vessel because of fear of devascularizing the nasal tip and facial skin.*

RATIONALE FOR THE THERAPEUTIC APPROACH TO EPISTAXIS

The typical nosebleed will heal itself if given the chance, and thus the strategy for treatment is simply to *reduce the arterial pressure head to the region*

without causing any ischemic damage. Usually, the side of bleeding is known, but the angiogram does not demonstrate ongoing extravasation. This is because the patient typically arrives in the angiography suite with nasal packing in place and with some degree of control of the active process. In addition, these nosebleeds are frequently episodic in nature. However, abnormal vessels are frequently seen, ap-

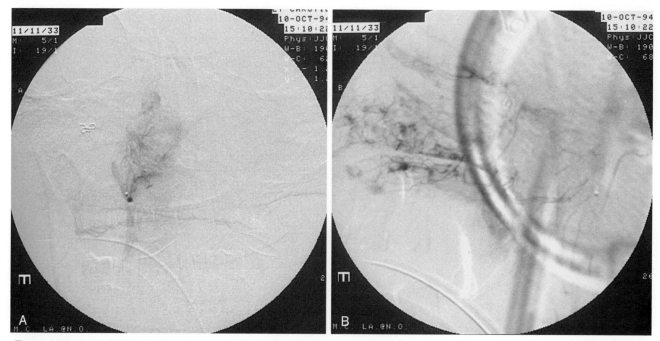

Figure 13-8 *A and B, PA and lateral views of the ascending pharyngeal artery now demonstrate supply to an area of hyperemic nasal mucosa as well as the previously identified abnormal palate. Again, embolization with first 150- to 250-micron and then 250- to 350-micron PVA particles was performed.*

Case 2 continues

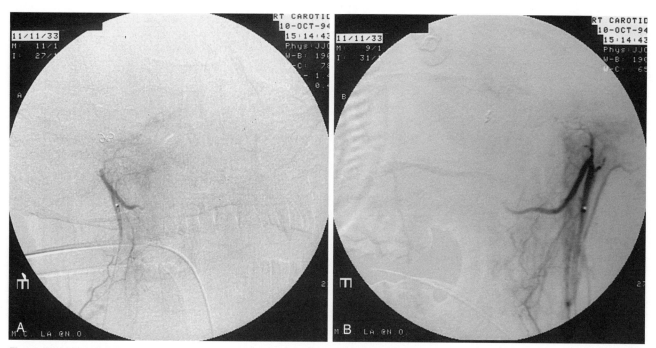

Figure 13-9 *A* and *B*, Postembolization injection of the ascending pharyngeal artery reveals a typical retropharyngeal blush. The abnormal downstream distribution is no longer seen.

pearing dilated, beaded, and tortuous. In the case of a bleeding necrotic tumor, active extravasation may be more often seen.

If the bleeding is caused by the typical hypertensive or microvascular abnormality and not by intrinsic tumor, the goal of therapy is to decrease the pressure head to the region and allow the body to heal itself. This can be done by occlusion of proximal

arterioles without true capillary devascularization. This is accomplished by using particles in the 250- to 350-micron or 350- to 500-micron range. This will effectively decrease perfusion to the area embolized but must be administered *superselectively, not regionally.*

If the underlying problem is a superficial tumor, the goal of therapy is altered: the capillary bed itself

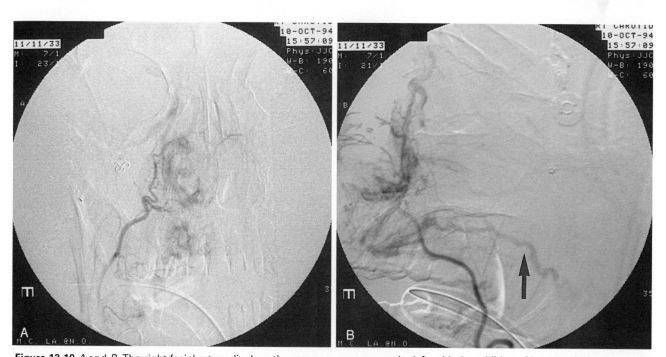

Figure 13-10 *A* and *B*, The right facial artery displays the same appearance as the left, with the addition of hyperemic arteriovenous shunting. Note the large early draining vein, similar to that previously seen *(arrow).*

Case 2 continues

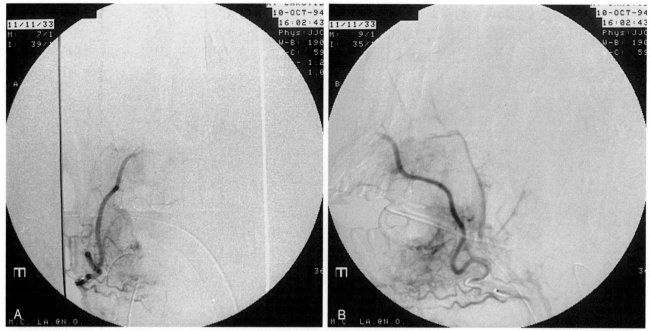

Figure 13-11 *A* and *B,* Again, PVA particles were floated out, this time in the 250- to 350-micron range. No further evidence of hypervascularity is seen, but it is almost guaranteed that the particles did not penetrate to the abnormal arteriolar/capillary level.

must be eliminated. The tumor is not bleeding secondary to hypoperfusion ("tumor necrosis") but because the vessels themselves are intrinsically abnormal. In these cases, true microdevascularization must be performed. This is accomplished by superselective, distal microembolization utilizing dilute particles (to prevent clumping) in the 150- to 250-micron range.

Rarely, the cause of epistaxis is rupture of an internal carotid artery aneurysm into a sinus, typically the sphenoid. This can be a life-threatening emergency. Treatment can be performed by coil emboliza-

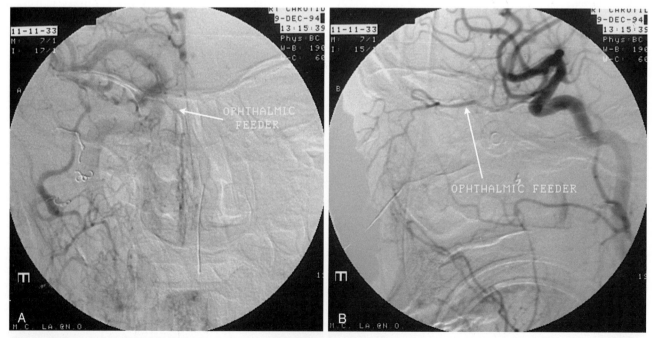

Figure 13-12 *A* and *B,* Two months later, the patient again returned. The right common carotid injection reveals extensive supply to the nasal septum and turbinates from the ophthalmic artery *(arrow)*: a fine example of not quite sufficient penetration to the abnormal arteriolar/capillary bed. However, the blush does not appear to be excessively hyperemic, and there is no evidence of abnormal puddling.

Case 2 continues

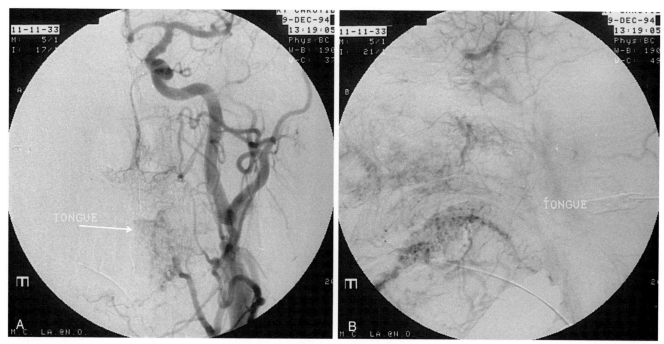

Figure 13-13 *A* and *B,* The left common carotid artery injection reveals findings similar to those shown in Figure 13–12. In addition, note the impressively abnormal tongue.

tion of the aneurysm or sacrifice of the internal carotid artery itself. For a discussion of these maneuvers, see Chapters 24, 25, 34, 35, and 36.

TECHNIQUE OF THERAPY FOR EPISTAXIS

All interventional neuroradiologic cases should be started with a control angiogram of the intracranial vasculature. This is useful if needed later and helps

visualize any aberrant vascularity that may be important (e.g., absent ophthalmic artery, implying possible supply from the external carotid artery to the globe).

Guide Catheter

The common carotid artery is selectively catheterized with a standard diagnostic catheter. Utilizing a safe

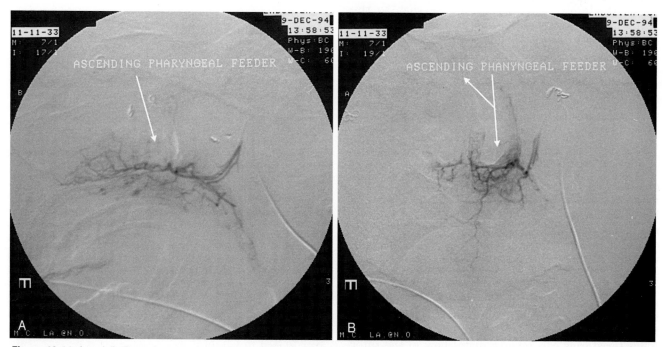

Figure 13-14 *A* and *B,* The left ascending pharyngeal artery was finally determined to be the culprit this time. This is practically the only vessel not previously embolized. PVA particles of 150 to 250 microns were used to occlude these feeders, followed by small coils.

Case 2 continues

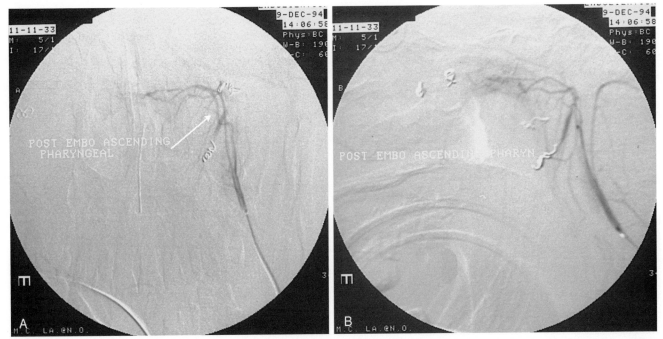

Figure 13-15 *A* and *B,* Final postembolization images demonstrate early recruitment of vessels to the area. The abnormal capillary bed has been very difficult to treat, with continued evidence that at least a portion has remained open after each embolization and recruited further supply. Total obliteration of the capillary bed of normal structures is not desired, however, and treatment of this type of pathology is difficult.

neuro-exchange wire (Cook, Inc.), the diagnostic catheter is exchanged for a "neuro" guide catheter. Since there is no need for major support, and spasm is to be avoided, we use a 90-cm FasGUIDE (Target Therapeutics) with a 5-cm tip because of its very safe atraumatic nature.

The origin of the external carotid or internal maxillary artery is then carefully catheterized with this neurovascular guide catheter. A true guide catheter is not absolutely necessary for a case such as this owing to the clear goal (needing to reach only proximal locations), relatively constant anatomy, and limited adaptation typically necessary. However, "neuro" guide catheters are optimized for their purpose—sitting safely in a brachiocephalic vessel and deploying a microcatheter—and we choose to use one in every interventional neuroradiologic procedure.

Vasospasm

Nitropaste (about 2″) may be placed on the patient's chest before the procedure, but this may be asking for trouble in an already bleeding circumstance. It is better to have a premixed solution of nitroglycerin ready (50 μg per ml normal saline) to be used in the event of vasospasm secondary to catheter or wire manipulation, which is common in these circumstances.

Careful catheterization is necessary to prevent vasospasm of the external carotid artery and its branches. If proximal vasospasm occurs, the natural hemodynamics are shifted; distal anastomoses from other territories can reverse distal flow in the internal maxillary artery (IMAX), and any embolization

will not flow to the intended sites. In addition to failing to reach the intended location, injection may force open anastomoses to the intracranial circulation.

Therefore, any vasospasm should be treated before further manipulation or embolization is performed (see "Prevention of Catheter-Induced Spasm" in Chapter 3 and "Intraprocedural Vasospasm" in Chapter 66).

Angiographic Evaluation

A control angiogram of the catheterized external carotid artery is performed to look for any potentially dangerous collateral supply to the intracranial structures. IMAX branches may anastomose with the ophthalmic artery, cavernous or petrous branches of the internal carotid artery (e.g., vidian artery), meningeal vessels, and other intracranial vessels and thus be a source of emboli to vital cerebral structures (see "Intrinsically Dangerous Vessels" in Chapter 5).

A microcatheter is then advanced into the IMAX and the tip placed distal to the origin of the middle meningeal artery, accessory meningeal artery, and deep temporal artery(ies) (their origins are close together and the vessels extend straight superiorly from the IMAX). The IMAX is a complex vessel with varying supply to the intraorbital (or retro-orbital) region, sphenoid and cavernous sinus areas, maxillary sinus walls, nasal turbinates, sphenoid sinus, hard palate, and nose and other facial areas. It can send collateral supply to the retina also (see Figs. 8–1 to 8–3 in Chapter 8).

The portion of the IMAX of concern to the interventional neuroradiologist in the treatment of epistaxis is usually the pterygopalatine division, which supplies the region typically affected by posterior epistaxis (the sphenopalatine artery, greater palatine artery, posterior superior alveolar artery, and pharyngeal and vidian arteries). These are all seen to be medial to the ramus of the mandible on the postero-anterior view, and they course medially and anteriorly toward the region of the nose. They arise beyond the origins of the superficial temporal and anterior deep temporal arteries and the middle meningeal artery. The middle meningeal artery typically arises about 1 to 3 cm distal to the point where the IMAX suddenly turns from its ascending direction to a horizontal and anterior course; the IMAX continues on a medial and anterior course while the middle meningeal takes an abrupt upward turn. The vidian artery has an anastomosis with the petrous internal carotid artery and should be closely observed.

Once the microcatheter is in position, another control angiogram is performed through the microcatheter. This is again to look for dangerous collaterals to the intracranial circulation or direct supply to the globe and to check for normal hemodynamics. If dangerous communications are present, protective embolization of these branches is possible with small microcoils (see Chapter 3 and Fig. 8–1 to 8–3 in Chapter 8). This will prevent any possible reflux into these vessels and allow more thorough particulate embolization of the target territory.

Embolization

As stated above, in a typical nosebleed case, if the nasal mucosal bleeding is stopped for a brief period (hours to days) and the lesion is allowed to heal, the problem is solved. Occlusion with a nonpermanent agent that occludes small arterial branches and large arterioles would therefore be ideal; the optimal particle size would be about 200 to 700 microns. This would occlude small arterioles and allow low-pressure distal collateral reperfusion of the nasal mucosa.

Unfortunately, no true temporary agent is commercially prepared and readily available in this size range. Gelfoam would be the ideal agent but is not available in pre-sized batches. Gelfoam torpedoes, which work well in full-sized 0.038″ inner-diameter catheters, are not truly (or easily) usable with microcatheters and have to be prepared individually. Other temporary agents, such as Avitene or Gelfoam powder, contain particles that are far smaller than necessary and thus may give unpredictable results (e.g., tissue necrosis, nerve damage) and may possibly pass through small dangerous collaterals.

For this reason, depending on factors such as catheter location, speed of flow, and degree of hemorrhage, PVA particles measuring 250 to 500 microns or 500 to 750 microns are used. Even though this is supposedly a "permanent" agent, the vasculature of the nose and face adapts to these occlusions easily, and the territory embolized is not rendered truly *permanently* ischemic. In addition, there is usually

recanalization of a certain percentage of these embolized vessels.

As the embolization proceeds, serial angiograms are performed as needed to carefully monitor flow. This procedure should not require a large amount of particles: usually one or two syringes are all it takes in these small vessels. Once the territory distal to the anterior deep temporal and meningeal vessels is occluded (has become nearly stagnant), a repeat bilateral evaluation of the external carotid arteries is performed.

Occasionally, additional supply to the nose or posterior nasal turbinates can be seen, typically arising from the ascending pharyngeal artery or facial artery. Rarely, supply may be seen to arise from other collateral vessels. Not infrequently, collateral supply may be seen to arise from across the midline, and this needs to be superselectively embolized. The ascending pharyngeal artery supply will be overlooked if not actively sought, however. It should therefore be specifically selected for evaluation.

If microparticulate embolization is necessary in bilateral IMAX territories, the use of *small* particles on both sides simultaneously should be avoided. It is safe to use 150- to 250-micron particles on one side if only larger particles are used on the other (e.g., 500 to 750 microns). Alternatively, 350- to 500-micron particles can be used in small territories on both sides, since the larger the area devascularized, the greater is the potential problem with ischemia. Superselective catheterization is therefore required.

After embolization, the nasal packing can be removed on the angiography table to confirm the adequacy of embolization. This is not usually done, however, because of space and personnel limitations and because the endovascular therapy, if performed adequately, is reliably effective. Occlusion of the above-described vessels is almost always permanently successful unless bilateral bleeding is present or an underlying mucosal abnormality exists.[9] If there is an underlying mucosal abnormality (primarily neoplastic in origin), therapeutic maneuvers need to be altered somewhat, as described in Chapter 14.

Problems, Complications, and Solutions

Acute Ischemia

If worries about true ischemia are raised after bilateral microparticulate embolization, but before the procedure is concluded, some relief can be obtained by superselective infusion of nitroglycerin at the end of the procedure, at a strength of 50 μg/ml. This will open auxiliary channels in the microcirculation and increase perfusion, just as is performed to treat the "no-reflow" phenomenon in the heart. This is what the body will do anyway, but it speeds up the process.

Postprocedure Ischemia

If there is evidence of ischemia or concern for this after the procedure, certain measures can be undertaken to increase the perfusion of the embolized territory. This is best achieved by local efforts. Heat is the first line of defense; this can be by means of a warm water pack or warm towels placed over the face and nose. This usually suffices. Further vasodilation can be obtained by intranasal application of nitropaste (placed with a cotton swab). Even inhalation of amyl nitrate can succeed.

Postprocedure Pain

Postembolization *aching pain* is a common phenomenon and not necessarily indicative of a true problem. It can be treated with ketorolac tromethamine (10 mg orally qid) with good success. Cimetidine (300 mg orally qid) should also be given to avoid the gastrointestinal side effects of ketorolac. This aching pain is usually self-limiting and resolves in 1 to 3 days.

Cranial Nerve Damage

If a cranial nerve deficit is noted after the procedure, immediate steroid therapy should be instituted (250 mg methylprednisolone [Solu-Medrol] intravenously q6h). If particles of the sizes recommended above were utilized, any cranial nerve deficit should be temporary and due to swelling around this nerve rather than true nerve death. Steroid administration usually relieves this, and the deficit will improve over a period of days to weeks.

Stroke

No one wants to even think about this. Embolization of epistaxis should be routinely safe. However, if the unthinkable occurs, certain measures can be taken. The treatment of stroke on the operating table is discussed in Chapter 59.

Oxygen should be administered immediately. The stroke will probably be due to a *microembolus* to a vital territory (e.g., internal capsule), not a large embolus. For this reason, urokinase will probably not be of any use. However, a very thorough evaluation of the intracranial circulation should be performed (this is why a baseline cerebral angiogram should be taken before any procedure).

Once this is done, if no major branch occlusion can be found, the reason for the deficit is thought to be the embolic material itself, with or without some attendant thrombus. Immediate heparinization is therefore indicated, to prevent further occlusion if for no other reason.

At this point, therapy becomes nonspecific. The mean arterial pressure should be raised (by about 20 to 40 mm). This can usually be accomplished by rapid administration of intravenous normal saline. If available, a hyperbaric chamber can be used to saturate the tissues with oxygen. This last step may be of benefit, but there has been no formal study of its use in these circumstances.

REFERENCES

1. Shaw CB, Wax MK, Wetmore SJ. Epistaxis: a comparison of treatment. *Otolaryngol Head Neck Surg* 1993;109:60–65.
2. Quine SM, Gray RF, Rudd M, et al. Microscope and hot wire cautery management of 100 consecutive patients with acute epistaxis: a superior method to traditional packing. *J Laryngol Otol* 1994;108:845–848.
3. Wurman LH, Sack JG, Flannery JV, et al. Selective endoscopic electrocautery for posterior epistaxis. *Laryngoscope* 1988;98:1348–1349.
4. Gluckman JL, Portugal LG. Modified Young's procedure for refractory epistaxis due to hereditary hemorrhagic telangiectasia. *Laryngoscope* 1994;104:1174–1177.
5. Merland JJ, Melki JP, Chiras J, et al. Place of embolization in the treatment of severe epistaxis. *Laryngoscope* 1980;90:1694–1704.
6. Breda SD, Choi IS, Persky MS, et al. Embolization in the treatment of epistaxis after failure of internal maxillary artery ligation. *Laryngoscope* 1989;99:809–813.
7. Hicks JN, Vitek G. Transarterial embolization to control posterior epistaxis. *Laryngoscope* 1989;79:1027–1029.
8. Elahi MM, Parnes LS, Fox AJ, et al. Therapeutic embolization in the treatment of intractable epistaxis. *Arch Otolaryngol Head Neck Surg* 1995;121:65–69.
9. Elden L, Montanera W, Terbrugge K, et al. Angiographic embolization for the treatment of epistaxis: a review of 108 cases. *Otolaryngol Head Neck Surg* 1994;111:44–50.

CHAPTER 14

Soft Tissue Tumoral Hemorrhage in the Head and Neck

J.J. Connors III / J.C. Wojak

If an underlying mucosal abnormality exists (e.g., a necrotic tumor mass), the strategy of treatment is very different from that for epistaxis, or simple bleeding from a wound. Instead of trying to give normal mucosa a chance to heal, as with epistaxis, a direct attack on the abnormal mucosa/tumor is necessary. The goal of typical epistaxis therapy is simply to decrease the pressure head and let healing occur; unfortunately, this does not typically happen with abnormal neoplastic mucosa. Decreasing the pressure head can be accomplished by means of relatively proximal occlusion with moderate-sized microparticles. True capillary devascularization, however, is necessary to stop tumor oozing.

Abnormal bleeding mucosa occurs for two primary reasons: a necrotic tumor mass or an underlying angiomatous lesion. In both of these circumstances, the target of embolization is therefore *the superficial bleeding surface itself*. In addition, the use of a more permanent agent is warranted, PVA particles being the agent of choice (not Gelfoam) (Case 1, Figs. 14–1 to 14–8).

RATIONALE FOR THERAPY

No large series have been reported comparing different techniques and results for endovascular treatment of oozing necrotic tumors; anecdotal experience must therefore suffice. Superficially, it seems that if a necrotic tumor mass already exists, devascularization would make it worse. However, this does not appear to be the case. The "necrotic" tumor is *not bleeding secondary to "lack of blood"* and therefore ischemic necrosis, but is bleeding because of *basically normal perfusion to intrinsically sick tissue, which then bleeds*. The blood vessels in the tumor mass are themselves not normal and do not have the ability to respond in a normal manner to hemodynamic forces. Decreasing the pressure head coming to this abnormal superficial tissue will not necessarily prevent further oozing unless the surface is truly dried out.

True devascularization at the arteriolar/capillary level is therefore necessary to treat a bleeding necrotic tumor. *Simply blocking a proximal feeder may not stop the actual oozing going on at the mucosal level.* "Drying up" of the mucosa is necessary. Thorough embolization with particles in the 150- to 250-micron range is necessary (or even 50 to 150 microns, depending on the catheter tip location and tissue being embolized). This can be followed with larger particles until the main supply branches to the tumor are occluded. Permanent occlusion with microcoils is

then an option, but since this disease process may necessitate a return for additional treatment at a later date, this is not recommended. Blocking the access for return is a short-sighted action that can return to haunt the unwary operator.

CONTINUED BLEEDING FROM THE TUMOR MASS DUE TO COLLATERAL SUPPLY

For treatment of a superficial angiomatous problem, some difficulty is often encountered. If occlusion has been too proximal, the abnormal mucosal oozing con-

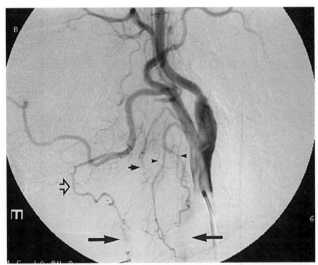

Figure 14-1 Case 1. Lateral view of left common carotid injection in a patient presenting with bleeding from a necrotic squamous cell carcinoma of the throat. A tracheostomy had previously been placed because of chronic respiratory problems secondary to repeated bleeding as well as mass effect constricting the air passage. Embolization was requested for control of the bleeding. Two large branches of the superior thyroidal artery *(arrowheads)* as well as a branch of the lingual artery *(small arrow)* and facial artery *(open arrow)* are seen to course inferiorly toward the mass *(large arrows)*.

Bleeding from a necrotic tumor is caused by an abnormal capillary bed, not an excessive pressure head (as is typical of nosebleeds). For nosebleeds, elimination of the main vascular supply without primary attack of the capillary bed is effective. For bleeding tumor masses, the capillary bed can continue oozing blood unless it is actually dried out by superselective embolization with very small particles (150 to 250 microns) and elimination of nearly all the microvascular supply, including small collaterals. This necessitates very accurate superselective embolization to avoid widespread tissue ischemia. Care must be taken to identify the specific location of embolization in order not to cause any inadvertent cranial nerve damage.

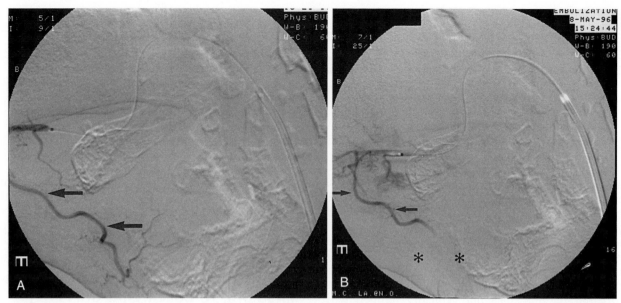

Figure 14-2 *A* and *B,* Initial microcatheterization of the facial artery branch was performed, demonstrating the suspicious descending branch *(large arrows).* No active extravasation was observed, but this vessel provides collateral supply to the tumor. After the catheter was advanced into this branch, it was embolized with 150- to 250-micron PVA particles; the catheter was then withdrawn back to the more proximal position. The repeat angiogram now reveals the more inferior portion of this branch to be occluded *(asterisks)* with preservation of the more proximal portion *(small arrows).*

tinues and supply is simply recruited from elsewhere. In the region of the nose, this supply can arise from collaterals from the ipsilateral facial artery, ascending pharyngeal artery, ophthalmic artery, internal maxillary artery branches, lingual artery, and/or any of these same vessels from the contralateral side.

In the neck, vascular supply can arise not only from external carotid branches but also from thyrocervical, costocervical, or muscular branches from the vertebral artery.

Occlusion (true capillary devascularization) has been necessary in a truly astounding manner for

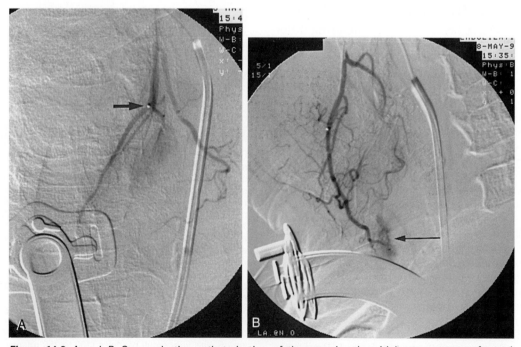

Figure 14-3 *A* and *B,* Superselective catheterization of the superior thyroidal artery was performed. Posteroanterior (PA) and lateral views demonstrate two branches, both of which are to be embolized. Note the abnormal blush in the lower branch on the lateral view, behind the tracheostomy *(thin arrow),* not well seen through the tracheostomy on the PA view. Injection of particles in the catheter location demonstrated *(thick arrow)* is initially relatively safe owing to the ability of any refluxed particles to be siphoned into the more proximal branch.

Case 1 continues

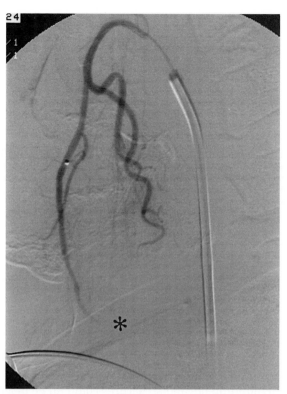

Figure 14-4 After partial embolization, the distal portion of the vessel is gone, eliminating the previously identified blush *(asterisk).*

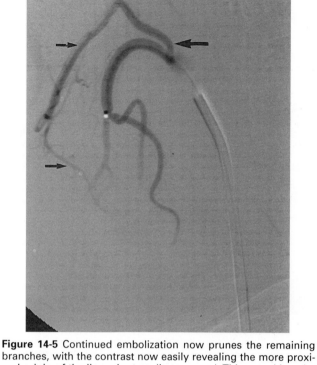

Figure 14-5 Continued embolization now prunes the remaining branches, with the contrast now easily revealing the more proximal origin of the lingual artery *(large arrow).* This vessel is to be embolized because of the large descending branch to the tumor mass *(small arrows).* There is minimal supply to the tongue (not seen on this injection).

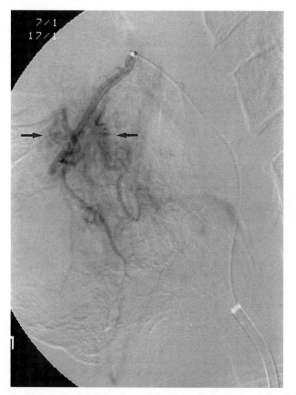

Figure 14-6 Selective injection of the large inferior branch of the lingual artery fills a more cephalad portion of the tumor *(arrows),* with another vessel seen to course inferiorly. These branches must also be occluded to eliminate any collateral supply to the abnormal capillary bed; this is accomplished by embolizing with 150- to 250-micron PVA particles.

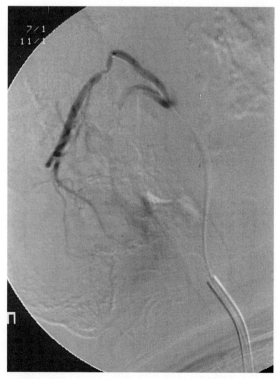

Figure 14-7 Partial embolization of this vessel has pruned the tree but left the branches. Continued embolization is performed to deter recanalization of the tumor via these remaining branches.

Case 1 continues

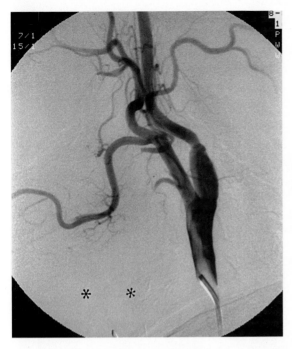

Figure 14-8 Final postembolization angiogram demonstrates an essentially avascular throat region *(asterisks)*. Not only did the bleeding stop, but the expected postembolization aching that can accompany a procedure such as this did not occur. The chronic recurrent bleeding episodes have now completely ceased.

the resistant case of Osler-Weber-Rendu syndrome discussed in Chapter 13. This particular case appeared to have developed existing collaterals to a far more extensive degree than the typical tumor, but not to an unusual degree for this disease. As opposed to cases of "typical" epistaxis, which are almost always permanently cured after one endovascular treatment, repeated therapy was necessary.

The use of small particles (150 to 250 microns or smaller) in an excessively proximal location (a large trunk) can result in devascularization of an area too broad to maintain viability; the collateral pathways to surrounding normal structures could all be blocked in too drastic a fashion. It is for this reason that true superselective catheterization and strategic embolization has to be employed. Simple random flooding of an area with very small microparticles is *unacceptable*. In addition, if any surgery becomes necessary, broad devascularization can adversely affect the surgical treatment and outcome. Incisions will not heal as well (or at all) and reconstruction attempts will not be as successful.

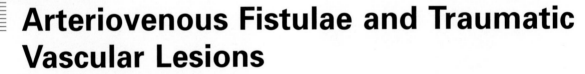

CHAPTER 15

Arteriovenous Fistulae and Traumatic Vascular Lesions

J.J. Connors III / J.C. Wojak

GENERAL CONSIDERATIONS

Arteriovenous (AV) fistulae are approached in many ways, depending on their location and characteristics. By definition, they are direct connections between the arterial tree and the venous system, without intervening capillaries and without the tangle of vessels (the nidus) of an arteriovenous malformation (AVM). The route of blood flow is short and usually direct. These entities can overlap; many AVMs contain fistulous components, and some apparent fistulae are far more complex than is typical of simple AV fistulae (e.g., intracranial dural fistulae).

Theoretically, the ideal solution for a simple AV fistula would be for the "channel" or vessel in question to vanish; a surgical ligature around the vessel would be the closest approximation to this. Determining the treatment strategy hinges on choosing between the ease and safety of surgery and that of endovascular therapy.

Specific Types of Arteriovenous Fistulae

Specific types of fistulae and their origins, patterns, and strategic approaches are presented here and in following chapters. These include typical spinal and paraspinal AV fistulae, vertebral AV fistulae, traumatic AV fistulae, dural AV fistulae, carotid-cavernous fistulae, and intracranial pial AV fistulae.

Clinical Presentation

Presenting symptoms of AV fistulae depend on their location, flow rate, and drainage pattern. Peripheral AV fistulae usually present with local pain, with or without cardiovascular effects. In AV fistulae of the head or neck, additional symptoms may be secondary to increased intracranial pressure or mass effect (headache or focal neurologic deficit), seizures, increased pressure of venous drainage of the cord with subsequent myelopathic changes, or steal from the intracranial supply. The size and location of an associated venous varix have as much influence on the patient's symptoms and age at presentation as does the pattern of venous drainage.[1]

Theory of Treatment

Obliteration of the actual *fistula,* not just of the feeding vessel or the draining vein, is necessary for cure of this pathologic entity. Occlusion of the arterial feeder or feeders proximal to the fistula site usually is ineffective and may worsen the situation (but would probably not be as predictable a failure as proximal embolization of an AVM).

The variable nature, location, and clinical circumstances of AV fistulae dictate the choice of approach and materials. A single long tapering feeder with a tight fistulous site is ideal; either a pile of coils or a single balloon can provide a complete cure. Preservation of both the feeding artery (if vital) and draining veins is ideal, but this is sometimes not possible. The fistulous connection is frequently short or nonexistent and the taper minimal. Fistulous formation often is possible because of the preexisting close association of a large artery and vein, rendering any connecting channel short or nonexistent. It is this situation that sometimes makes treatment a challenge.

Surgical treatment of a recently acquired traumatic AV fistula can be much more difficult than that of a mature sinus; the difference in the complexity of endovascular treatment may be more moderate. The approach to endovascular treatment of a recent traumatic AV fistula is generally similar to that of a mature fistula, but additional treatment may be necessary to eliminate the capillary "oozers" (see "Traumatic Arteriovenous Fistulae" below).

Materials for Arteriovenous Fistula Occlusion

The larger the shunt and more direct the venous communication with the central vasculature, the more necessary proximal flow control is to prevent migration of the balloon or coils until flow is totally stopped. Even after stasis is achieved, simple arterial pulse pressure (or even a cough) can force migration of the embolic mass. Friction is the only thing holding this mass in position.

Flow Control

Proximal flow control is possible in practically any situation (see "Flow Control Catheters" in Chapter 1) and for any embolic material. This not only renders any embolization safer but also decreases the pulse rate of the operator and is highly recommended for difficult cases. In addition, if sacrifice of the parent vessel is necessary and coils are utilized, absolute flow arrest is necessary to prevent antegrade thromboemboli to the brain.

Two types of occlusion balloon catheters are available: those designed for use in simple test occlusions, and those used as guide catheters. The latter allow placement of a detachable balloon through the lumen during the occlusion, whereas the former allow a microcatheter to be placed to a more distal location where appropriate occlusion can be performed using coils (see Chapter 35).

Strategic Choice of Embolic Agents

Detachable balloons are considered the most effective means for occluding short segments of large channels (see "How to Mount a Detachable Balloon," "Prepping a Balloon," and "Steering a Detachable Balloon" in Chapter 3). Using more than one balloon is safer than using a single balloon because a single one can deflate or migrate.

For tenuous locations, Amplatz vascular obstructing devices (Cook, Inc.) are useful in specific locations (see Chapter 1). These devices can anchor firmly in a short segment, and coils can be piled onto them for total occlusion. Alternatively, a balloon can be anchored by this device.

Coils are easier to deliver, but accurate placement and tight packing can be difficult, and they are not as effective in large vessels. With high flow, considerable patency can still be present even after a mass of coils has been placed. If this occurs, further packing with thinner (0.018″ or 0.010″) coils can be done. In addition, cessation of flow by proximal temporary occlusion can allow thrombus to form around the coil mass, completing the occlusion. When occlusion has been obtained by effective packing with coils, the channel does not usually re-open. (Even a vessel totally occluded with coils can reopen if fibrinolytics are used elsewhere in the body shortly thereafter.)

Liquid embolic agents, such as cyanoacrylates, are primarily used in the ancillary treatment of AV fistulae to prevent movement of the embolic mass, not as the primary agent. They may be used as the primary embolic agents in the treatment of dural fistulae. Significant complications can occur with the use of liquid embolic agents, and these agents only occasionally are indicated in the direct treatment of typical large-lumen AV fistulae. Hydrogels, although capable of filling the lumen, do not appear to be capable of remaining in place when exposed to pulsing arterial pressure.

TRAUMATIC HEAD AND NECK HEMORRHAGE

Bleeding from the head and neck that requires an endovascular approach is from a large vessel secondary to a penetrating wound (and inaccessible to the surgeon), from a primary nosebleed, or related to a tumor.

If a penetrating wound is the cause of head or neck bleeding, it should be controlled by external compression or repaired by a vascular surgeon. Angiography may be necessary for proper evaluation, however, and endovascular therapy may then be preferred. Lesions in the upper neck, zones 2 and 3, are frequently more amenable to endovascular approach than to surgical approach.

Traumatic hemorrhage in the head or neck originates from a branch of the external carotid artery, from the side of the common or internal carotid artery, or from the vertebral artery. Intracranial origins of bleeding are not considered specifically in this chapter, but bleeding from a meningeal vessel is treated the same as bleeding from an external carotid artery branch (i.e., embolized with resultant vessel sacrifice if necessary, as described later).

These situations, therefore, yield only three therapeutic challenges: bleeding from a branch vessel, from a hole in the side wall of a major vessel, or from a transected great vessel.

Branch Vessel Hemorrhage

Treatment of a bleeding branch vessel is relatively straightforward: the vessel is occluded just proximal to the site of injury, usually with one or more coils (Case 1, Fig. 15–1). Minor wound oozing can be controlled with local compression. Rarely is an external carotid artery branch truly vital, especially after it has already been transected! The wall of the vessel allows packing of embolic material and thus control of the occlusion.

Hole in the Side of a Great Brachiocephalic Vessel

A much more difficult task is endovascular repair of a hole in the side wall of a great vessel. Hemorrhage from this site requires open surgical repair unless sacrifice of the vessel is acceptable. Ongoing work involving covered stents, however, yields great promise for an alternative therapy of this pathology (see Chapter 37).

If the vertebral artery is bleeding, sacrifice is usually acceptable (depending on hemodynamics), although occlusion on the venous side (external to the arterial lumen) by a detachable balloon pressing against the hole in the artery is a more elegant maneuver. Alternatively, occlusion can be performed *immediately above and below* the hole (or exactly over it), initially at the distal limb (see Chapter 16). This also is acceptable treatment of a pseudoaneurysm.

Ongoing hemorrhage from a carotid artery usually is not encountered. By the time the patient gets

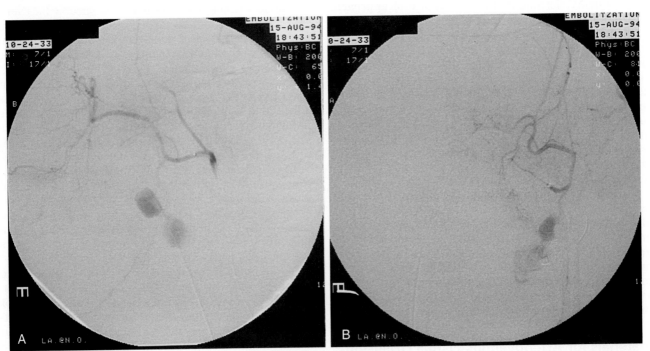

Figure 15-1 Case 1. *A* and *B,* Images obtained during embolization of hemorrhage resulting from surgical drainage of a submandibular abscess. A small branch of the internal maxillary artery was bleeding. Cessation of bleeding was achieved by particulate embolization (PVA, 250 to 350 microns). This allows the body to heal normally.

to the angiography suite, external compression has stopped the active bleeding, leaving either a pseudoaneurysm or an AV fistula. Each of these is difficult to resolve by endovascular means with preservation of the parent vessel.

If ongoing hemorrhage is present, temporary occlusion with a nondetachable temporary occlusion balloon is possible until definitive surgical or endovascular therapy is possible. This is mandatory before occlusion if antegrade flow to the intracranial contents remains. It is unacceptable to place a mass of coils in the vertebral or carotid system to occlude these vessels without proximal flow control. The mass of coils will release a shower of emboli before occlusion is complete, with consequences.

TRAUMATIC ARTERIOVENOUS FISTULAE

Traumatic AV fistulae can occur anywhere in the body, and depending on the location of the fistula and vascular origin, open surgery may be the treatment of choice. As stated earlier, a traumatic AV fistula can originate from a branch of the external carotid artery, from the side of the common or internal ca-

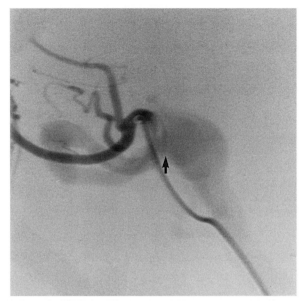

Figure 15-3 Catheterization of the internal maxillary artery has been performed, but the tip of the catheter is slightly past the arterial supply to the fistula. The densely filled arteries are of normal caliber, while the artery supplying the fistula is far too large and is washed out by the high flow of unopacified blood through it to the fistula. The entire loop is arterial; the site of the actual fistula is where the vascular channel suddenly enlarges *(arrow)*. If embolization is performed in the loop proximal to the actual fistula site, normal arterial collaterals will be recruited to fill the venous sump, and the problem will not be solved.
Case 2 continues

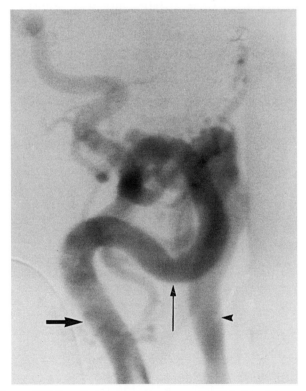

Figure 15-2 Case 2. A 4-year-old boy presented to the emergency room with a pulsatile mass in his left cheek. A left carotid angiogram was performed. Access to the vascular tree was achieved via the right common femoral artery using a micropuncture set (Cook, Inc.), and a 4-Fr. catheter was placed in the left common carotid artery. Note the huge size of the common carotid artery *(thick arrow)* and external carotid artery *(thin arrow)*, which is larger than the internal carotid artery. The large vascular structure on the right is the internal jugular vein descending from the fistula *(arrowhead)*. This fistula was thought to be acquired (either post-traumatic or postinfectious).

rotid artery or the vertebral artery, or from a transected artery.

Treatment of an AV fistula supplied by a branch of the external carotid system is the same as that for hemorrhage from a branch, that is, packing with coils or with a detachable balloon just proximal to the hole (coils usually suffice; Case 2, Figs. 15–2 to 15–8). Treatment of a traumatic AV fistula originating from the side of the carotid artery presents problems similar to those discussed later in "Pseudoaneurysms of Brachiocephalic Vessels." Because there is no true fistulous tract but rather a tunnel in the soft tissues, placing coils or a balloon in this tract usually does not completely solve the problem. Even when the fistulous flow is stopped, the hole in the side of the vessel usually remains (i.e., a pseudoaneurysm). For treatment of this situation, see below. The use of stent-grafts in the management of fistulae and pseudoaneurysms arising from the great vessels is described in Chapter 37.

A simple fistula that involves the vertebral artery is treated as described in Chapter 16. A traumatic AV fistula, however, can develop into a complex structure involving multiple large feeders, a myriad of capillary oozers, and multiple venous exits—a pathologic entity hemodynamically indistinguishable from dural AV fistulae. This is particularly true when the fistula is caused by a bullet that leaves a residual tract (Case 3, Figs. 15–9 to 15–27). Occlusion of the main arterial feeders, although adequate in most cases of fistulous flow from external carotid branches

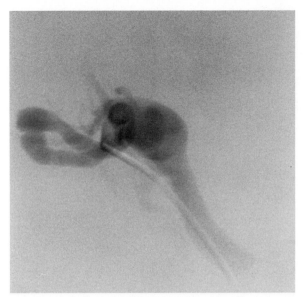

Figure 15-4 Selective injection of the arterial feeder reveals the high-flow status of the shunt and the huge venous receptacle. Care must be maintained not to allow any embolic material (coils) to be washed through the fistula into the venous side and thus into the lungs.

to veins, can still leave these small oozers. The more superselective and distal the embolization, the more recruitment of microcollaterals that occurs. It may be impossible to eliminate all of these by direct arterial embolization.

Occlusion of the venous receptacle may therefore

be necessary. This is not as easy as it sounds. The venous access routes frequently are extremely tortuous and are not as direct as arterial pathways. Also, veins are typically not as easy to catheterize as arteries anywhere in the body; their walls seem to have more friction, their course is not direct, and they tend to "give" with pushing force rather than to transmit the force downstream. Even with hydrophilic-coated microcatheters and guidewires, accurate access to the specific area can be challenging and even impossible.

Occlusion of the venous drainage in too proximal a location can result in the recruitment of a myriad of alternative drainage pathways, most or all of which are even smaller and more difficult to access and treat. This creates a miserable situation: a multitude of small arteries draining into a multitude of small venules surrounded by an abundance of hypervascular tissue. Total venous occlusion on the initial approach is therefore the goal of this therapy.

An alternative approach is to puncture the venous pouch percutaneously and then to fill this pouch with coils or other embolic material. This approach usually is not considered by interventional neuroradiologists because percutaneous access typically is not possible intracranially; the technique more commonly is employed by peripheral interventionists. Puncturing the venous pouch may be technically difficult, but it is possible. Filling it with coils then effectively cures the abnormal venous sump (see Figs. 15–26 and 15–27). Chapter 18 contains further discussion of therapeutic options for this challenging entity.

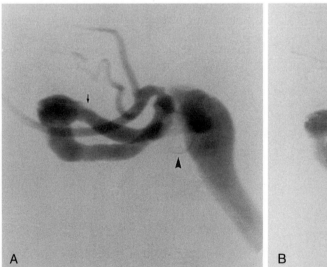
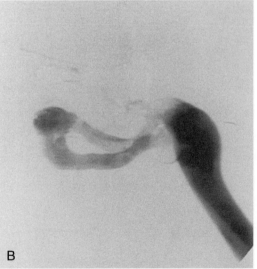

Figure 15-5 A and B, In A, an occlusion balloon *(arrowhead)* has been placed into the internal maxillary artery proximal to the origin of the artery that supplies the fistula. Note the normal distal vessel filling in addition to the large arterial loop. The balloon is used for flow control and to prevent the inadvertent displacement of any coil downstream through the fistula before full cessation of fistulous flow. Note also the small filling defect along the outer curve of the loop. This is due to a small artery, also supplying the fistula, which is providing unopacified wash-in now that flow is slowed proximally.

In B, later in the same injection, the antegrade flow in the normal branch has reversed, and wash-in is now coming from this source also. This is because the occlusion balloon is blocking the normal supply, and the fistulous sump is causing reversal of flow in the distal internal maxillary territory, thus yielding the wash-in.

Case 2 continues

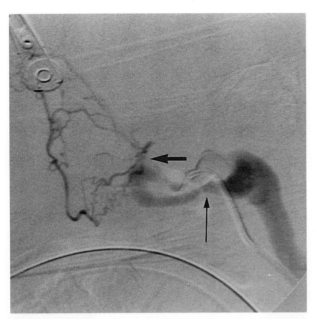

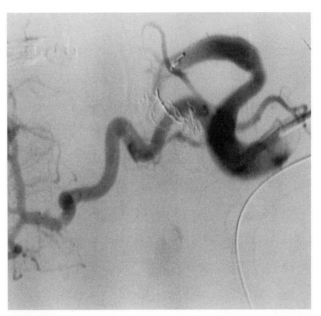

Figure 15-6 The occlusion balloon has been advanced into the arterial feeder of the fistula but cannot be advanced further. Injection now reveals the vessel producing the filling defect noted in the previous series and supplying the distal loop of the arterial feeder *(thick arrow)*. This confirms that occlusion at this point (the location of the catheter tip) will be ineffective; these small arteries will enlarge and continue to supply the venous sump. Therefore, occlusion has to be achieved distal to this point but proximal to the artery/vein confluence *(thin arrow)*.

Figure 15-7 Multiple coils have now been deposited, using the temporary occlusion balloon catheter to provide proximal flow control. Note the coils extending around the curve of the arterial feeding trunk and the lack of venous filling.

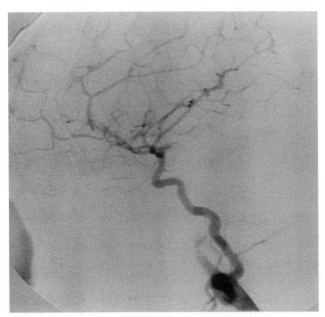

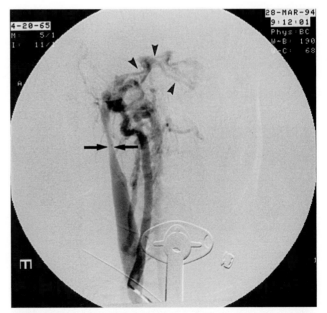

Figure 15-8 Final control angiogram during left common carotid artery injection. Again, note the huge common carotid artery and normal internal carotid artery. Also note the small (normal) occipital, posterior auricular, lingual, and other branches of the external carotid artery, and the tremendous discrepancy in size between these vessels and the occluded internal maxillary artery feeder (the transverse facial artery).

Figure 15-9 Case 3. This female patient was shot through the mouth. The right internal carotid artery was nicked and developed a pseudoaneurysm. The posteroanterior (PA) angiographic view of the right vertebral artery reveals abrupt cessation of antegrade flow at the C1 level with massive arteriovenous shunting and venous drainage into the jugular and paraspinal systems. Note the mass effect on the jugular vein *(arrows)*, presumably from soft tissue swelling. Note also, because of the limited normal venous drainage, the retrograde filling of the ipsilateral inferior petrosal sinus, with flow across the cavernous sinus and down the opposite inferior petrosal sinus *(arrowheads)*.

Case 3 continues

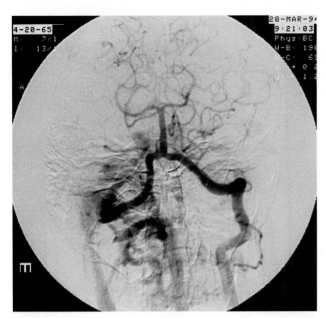

Figure 15-10 Left vertebral artery injection reveals some continued antegrade flow supplying the basilar artery but significant retrograde flow down the distal opposite (right) vertebral artery to the arteriovenous fistula site. On the lateral angiogram, there was a 3-cm absent segment of the right vertebral artery. This long segment of destruction by the bullet rendered this vessel unsalvageable.

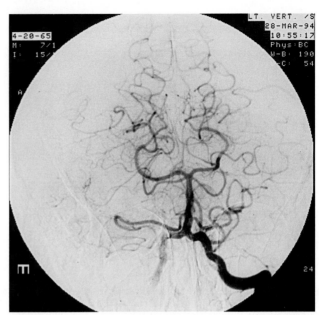

Figure 15-11 After attempted occlusion of the arteriovenous fistula on the venous side by a detachable balloon, occlusion of the distal vertebral segment proximal to the posterior inferior cerebellar artery and just distal to the site of transection was performed via a left vertebral artery approach. This was followed by occlusion of the proximal segment of the right vertebral artery, just proximal to the fistula, via a right vertebral artery approach. The left vertebral angiogram now reveals good intracranial perfusion with no further fistulous flow.

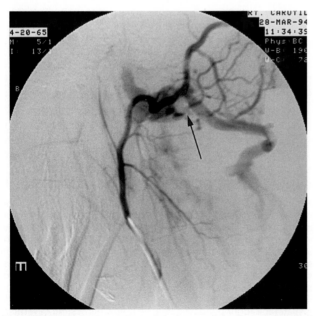

Figure 15-12 Selective right occipital artery injection now reveals arteriovenous shunting, however. Note the previously placed balloon *(arrow)*.

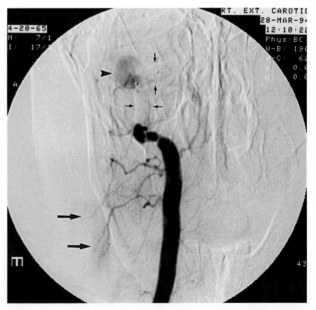

Figure 15-13 Repeat angiogram of the occluded right vertebral artery now reveals filling of a venous pouch (probably the bullet tract) *(arrowhead)* even though the feeders are not well seen. The rapidity of filling is indicated by the fact that the muscular branches are just entering their capillary phase *(large arrows)*. Note the balloon just distal to the pouch (inside the vertebral artery just distal to the transection) as well as the balloon in the vertebral artery just proximal to the transection *(small arrows)*.

Case 3 continues

PSEUDOANEURYSMS OF BRACHIOCEPHALIC VESSELS

In simple terms, a true aneurysm is a ballooning out of a portion of the wall of the vessel, whereas a pseudoaneurysm is an actual hole in the vessel wall. Depending on location, a pseudoaneurysm can be contained by adventitia or by perivascular tissues, such as muscle. However, there is no true aneurysm per se. In an acute post-traumatic situation, these perivascular tissues determine whether the patient immediately exsanguinates or stabilizes with formation of an extravascular pocket of blood or clot. After a period of stabilization (days or weeks), this pocket can become lined with organized thrombus or fibrin and then eventually with endothelial cells.

In interventional neuroradiology, pseudoaneurysms are of primary consideration in the neck and are mostly post-traumatic and secondary to penetrating wounds. They may, however, be chronic or related to repeated vascular stress. While a ruptured intracranial aneurysm (or AVM) may acquire an associated pseudoaneurysm, this entity is dealt with in the same manner as an unruptured intracranial aneurysm or AVM, albeit with a degree of increased urgency or care by the neurosurgeon or interventional neuroradiologist (the pseudoaneurysm is much more fragile than the true aneurysm and therefore subject to potential intraprocedural hemorrhage; see Chapters 20 and 24).

A pseudoaneurysm is not always life-threatening;

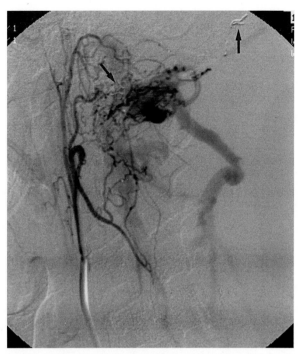

Figure 15-15 The patient underwent attempted surgical repair of the pseudoaneurysm of the right internal carotid artery. Unfortunately, this vessel occluded postoperatively, leaving only the left carotid and left vertebral arteries to supply the intracranial contents. Several months later, she began to experience symptoms referable to the posterior fossa, and there was concern that residual or recurrent arteriovenous shunting could be stealing what little vascular reserve she might have left. Angiography revealed reperfusion of the previously identified venous pouch by the previously embolized ascending pharyngeal artery. Note the embolic agents (coils) placed during the previous procedure *(arrows)*. The angiographic appearance is now reminiscent of a dural AV fistula. Note the multitude of small feeders to the large venous receptacle.

Case 3 continues

this depends on its size, location, and stability (primarily determined by its age). Pseudoaneurysms found around dialysis shunts as a result of repeated punctures are usually of only minor consequence. A post-traumatic pseudoaneurysm of a great vessel of the neck, however, can be an expanding mass that can compress the airway to a critical, life-threatening extent in a short time. It can dissect down into the mediastinum or into the retropharyngeal space. In addition, these entities can transform over time into larger or smaller masses, or evolve into true arteriovenous fistulae (Case 4, Figs. 15–28 to 15–40).

If the hole from a penetrating wound to the neck becomes an AV fistula, the impetus to be an expanding mass and thus cause airway compression subsides to some degree; the AV fistula provides pressure relief. This can allow time for more appropriate definitive treatment.

Direct surgical repair is possible if the lesion is in an accessible location, and this gives the most elegant and direct solution. Otherwise, treatment of a pseudoaneurysm in the neck involves a multidisciplinary approach.

Simple manual compression of the aneurysm with or without ultrasound guidance has not been widely

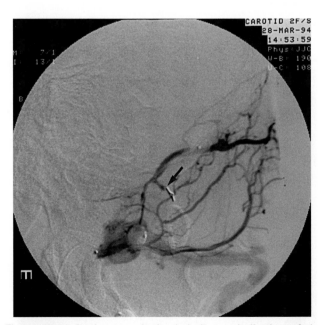

Figure 15-14 Angiogram obtained during embolization of the right occipital artery. A side branch to the fistula has been embolized with 150- to 250-micron PVA particles, followed by two coils *(arrow)*. The injection reveals good downstream normal perfusion but continuing arteriovenous shunting. Further embolization was performed at this session (occipital artery, posterior auricular artery, posterior and ascending cervical arteries, and the ascending pharyngeal artery) until no further significant shunting was seen and maximal therapeutic benefit was considered to have been achieved.

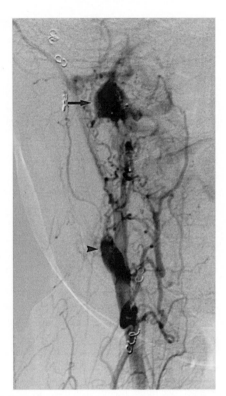

Figure 15-16 Right common carotid angiogram shows the stump of the internal carotid artery *(arrowhead)* and numerous abnormal external carotid branches recruited to supply the fistula. Note the densely opacified venous pouch *(arrow)*.

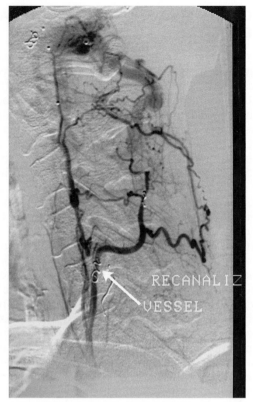

Figure 15-17 Selective injection of the previously embolized ascending cervical artery now reveals not only recanalization through the coil *(arrow)*, but also recruitment by the venous sump of numerous indirect and highly tortuous collaterals. To eliminate each of these at the site of the fistula is effectively impossible.

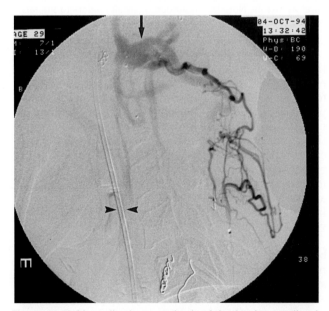

Figure 15-18 More distal superselective injection is revealing in that the terminal branches of the ascending cervical artery are noted to fill another vessel via capillary collaterals in a retrograde manner. This appears to supply the fistula and shows the venous receptacle well *(arrow)*. Since it was previously determined that transarterial therapy would be impossible, a venous catheter has been placed *(arrowheads)*.

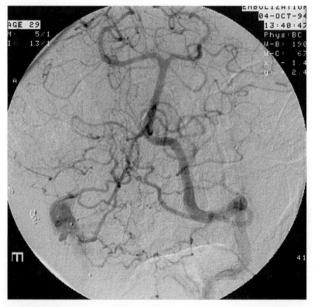

Figure 15-19 Even the left vertebral artery is now seen to supply the pouch across the midline via numerous small tortuous vessels (some of which appear to be pial or meningeal collaterals).
Case 3 continues

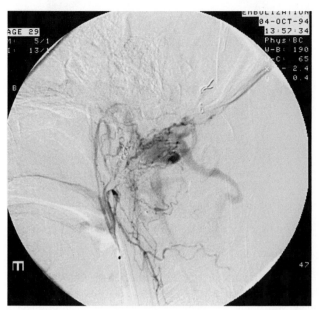

Figure 15-20 Superselective injection of the posterior division of the ascending pharyngeal artery (previously embolized) reveals the massive recruitment this venous sump has achieved and confirms the impossibility of treatment from an arterial approach. Every one of these microvessels would need to be eliminated at the actual arteriovenous connection; even then, new ones would grow. The *sump itself* has to be eliminated.

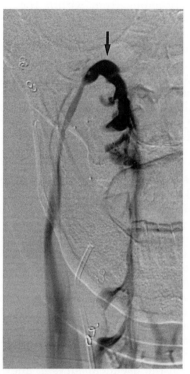

Figure 15-21 A transfemoral venous approach is now undertaken to attack the pathology from this direction. The microcatheter has been manipulated (with great difficulty) into the venous pouch *(arrow)*. Injection reveals both paraspinal and jugular drainage.

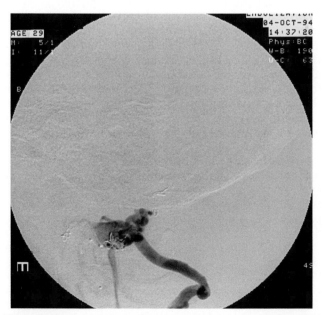

Figure 15-22 Lateral view of venous pouch injection after partial coil embolization (note coils in pouch). Injection reveals large venous receptacle and drainage routes.

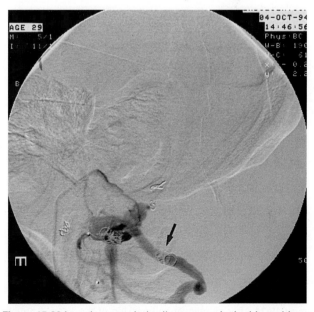

Figure 15-23 In order to occlude all venous exits in this multicompartmented "hole" (originally just the bullet tract), the main venous drainage is selectively and specifically occluded *(arrow)*. Remember, the pouch itself is not like a dural sinus with definite walls.

Case 3 continues

performed in the neck. There is always the risk of displacing thrombus from within the pseudoaneurysm pocket into the parent vessel, usually the internal carotid artery; this is an undesirable, but rare, event. Also, the pseudoaneurysm frequently is not in a convenient place to apply external pressure effectively. This technique is not considered appropriate for pseudoaneurysms in this location.

Direct filling of the pseudoaneurysm sac with either 0.018", 0.025", or 0.035" coils usually is not adequate because of the lack of true walls of the pseudoaneurysm and its ability to expand when filled. The flow into the hole is usually too great to allow the hole to seal or heal completely. Blood swirling around coils in this pocket renders the coils ineffective, and true "packing" is not usually possible because of the ability of the sac to expand as needed, especially with packing. It is probably worthwhile to try this, however, if the hole in the vessel is in a surgically difficult or inaccessible location. The pseudoaneurysm pocket can also be approached for coil embolization by a direct percutaneous puncture.

Attempts have been made to place a stent across the hole; success with this technique has been limited[2–4] (Case 5, Figs. 15–41 to 15–46). This is thought to work by changing the flow dynamics at the hole and thence in the pseudoaneurysm, allowing thrombus to form in the now partially stagnant pouch. If flow still fills the aneurysmal pocket after the stent is in place, it is possible to fill the pocket with platinum coils by catheterizing it through the lattice of the stent or, once again, *by direct percutaneous puncture.* Simply allowing some time for the blood within

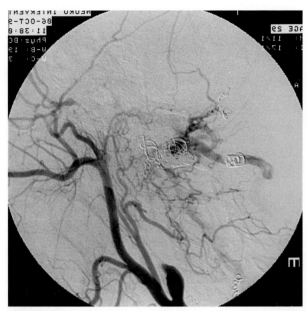

Figure 15-25 The decision to attack the pouch directly (percutaneously) was made; this option is usually unavailable for a typical intracranial dural AV fistula. The initial common carotid artery injection clearly reveals the shunt still to be present, with filling via numerous recanalized and bizarre recruited feeders from the external carotid artery. Note the mass of coils in the venous pouch and continued drainage through the coils in the main posteriorly draining vein. (The image is reversed to maintain consistent perspective for this example. Only the anteroposterior tube was used for performance of this procedure, thus reversing the perspective.)

Case 3 continues

the pocket to thrombose after stent placement also has been successful.[2]

The problem with waiting for the pocket to thrombose, however, is that the pseudoaneurysm is not cured, and there is the potential for further growth, sometimes precipitously and to the point of a life-threatening airway obstruction. The threat of sudden, precipitous growth makes an arterial injury in the neck an emergency (although this may be debatable). Inadequate or nondefinitive treatment, therefore, does not resolve the emergency situation. For this reason, the interventional neuroradiologist or vascular surgeon may believe that "watching and waiting" is inadvisable.

Some peace of mind for the surgeon, interventional neuroradiologist, and patient can be obtained if the patient is kept intubated while waiting for the aneurysm or pouch to clot. This removes the main potential for disaster from this pathologic process. The patient may have no desire to remain intubated for days, however.

Covered stents have been described for use in the treatment of brachiocephalic pseudoaneurysms (see Chapter 37). The covering can be a synthetic material (e.g., Gore-Tex), silicone, or autologous vein. This would be an ideal solution if the long-term effects of these devices were known. Short-term studies with silicone covering in animal models demonstrated an extreme intimal reaction at the two ends of the stent where the silicone ends. In a vital brachiocephalic

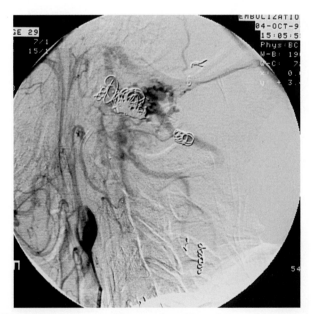

Figure 15-24 After significant coil packing of the venous pouch, an angiogram performed by injection through the arterial catheter, which had been left in place in the left common carotid artery, clearly demonstrates the inadequacy of treatment to this point. Note the mass of coils in the pouch and draining vein but continuing arteriovenous shunting. The procedure was terminated at this point owing to loss of ideal position of the transfemoral venous catheter while pushing a coil.

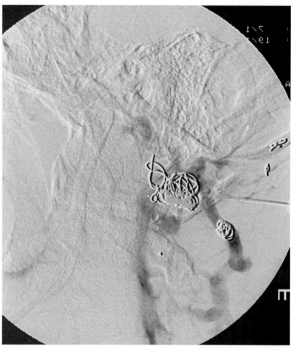

Figure 15-26 Percutaneous access to the venous pouch was achieved with a micropuncture set (Cook, Inc.). Contrast injection confirms correct position in the venous pouch. This set allows a choice of options. The microneedle itself can accept an 0.018″ wire, and thus permits direct deposition of microcoils. In addition, however, it is possible to place a soft sleeve over this (see Chapter 1) and establish a lumen that can accept a 0.038″ wire, allowing macrocoils to be placed. This is achieved while working with a system employing a needle only 7 cm long, which is much easier to work with than a typical Chiba-type system.

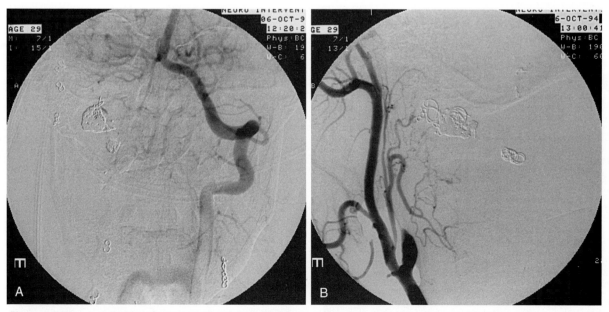

Figure 15-27 *A* and *B*, After further packing of this pouch (bullet tract) with coils, follow-up PA left vertebral artery and lateral common carotid artery angiograms reveal no further shunting. The fistula is cured.

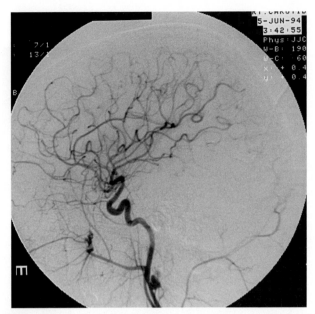

Figure 15-28 Case 4. Lateral projection of a right common carotid angiogram performed after this female patient was stabbed in the neck reveals a pseudoaneurysm arising from the high cervical internal carotid artery. The vessel had already been explored and the hole was too high to access easily.

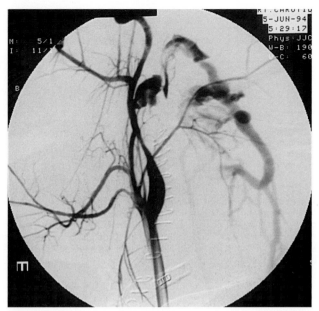

Figure 15-29 After a delay of 1 hour and 45 minutes until the attending surgeon could be contacted to discuss the management of this lesion, a repeat angiogram revealed evolution of the pseudoaneurysm into an arteriovenous fistula. The venous drainage is initially along a soft tissue tract until it ruptures into the venous system. Rapid flow is present; note the venous system filling proximally out of the field while the external carotid artery branches are filled to the arteriolar level. In addition, note the appearance of the damaged internal carotid artery.

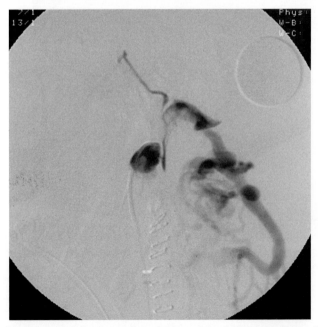

Figure 15-30 Selective catheterization of the hole in the internal carotid artery was next performed during the initial phase of coil embolization. Injection reveals the lumen of the pseudoaneurysm and the path of extravasation leading to the draining veins.

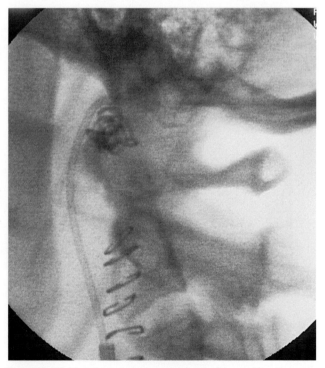

Figure 15-31 Unsubtracted view obtained after packing the pseudoaneurysm with 0.038″ Gianturco coils.

Case 4 continues

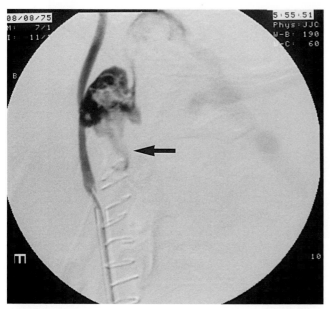

Figure 15-32 Follow-up injection of the internal carotid artery demonstrates the pseudoaneurysm to have grown in the interval and the fistulous flow still to be present. In addition, there appears to be new dissection extending inferiorly *(arrow)*. The pseudoaneurysm has no true walls and can continue to grow no matter how many coils are placed within it.

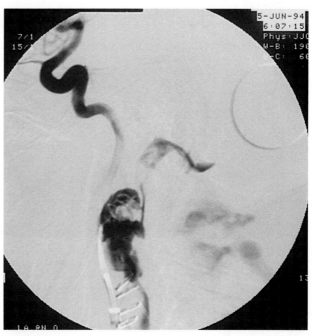

Figure 15-33 Ten minutes later, the inferior pouch of the pseudoaneurysm has grown considerably. Stent placement is now deemed appropriate.

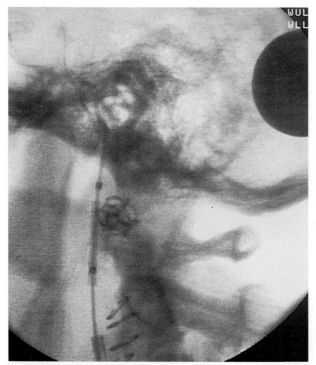

Figure 15-34 A Palmaz stent (Johnson & Johnson Interventional Systems) is in place before deployment; it is centered on the hole, not the coils.

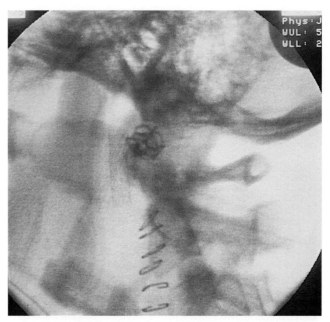

Figure 15-35 The stent is shown after deployment.

Case 4 continues

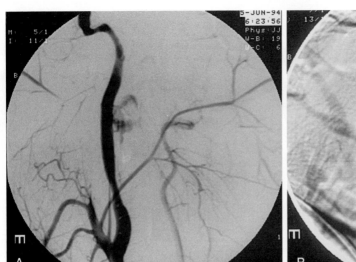
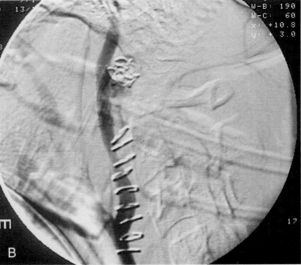

Figure 15-36 *A* and *B*, After stent placement, the fistulous flow appears to have ceased, but the pseudoaneurysm pouch remains. Good flow in the internal carotid artery is present.

vessel, the potential hazards of the covering are not known; any foreign body placed in the lumen could be dangerous. If the vessel can be electively occluded, this is the therapy of choice.

The potential long-term problems with a stent in the neck (i.e., in the cervical carotid artery) are distal embolization from a thrombogenic source and intimal hyperplasia with subsequent occlusion of the vessel, with or without preliminary embolic or hemodynamic events. In addition, the Palmaz stent is easily compressible and could undergo an accidental and abrupt occlusion. (See Chapters 43 and 47 for further discus-

sion of the use of stents in the great vessels of the neck.)

Temporary occlusion of the vessel with a balloon over the hole might allow the cavity to thrombose, but this requires anticoagulation for the temporarily occluded main vessel (the internal carotid artery) and thus may be inadvisable and ineffective. Perfusing through a temporary occlusion balloon, such as the Zeppelin (Medtronic/MIS), may obviate this problem distally but not proximally. A true perfusing occlusion balloon would be ideal in this situation but has yet to be developed.

A separate catheter (from the opposite femoral ar-

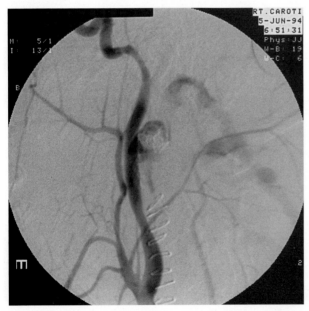

Figure 15-37 Fifteen minutes later, a repeat angiogram revealed fistulous flow again to be present. It was felt at this time that the patient was probably stable (she was intubated) and that there was no risk of airway compression. A period of watchful waiting was indicated.

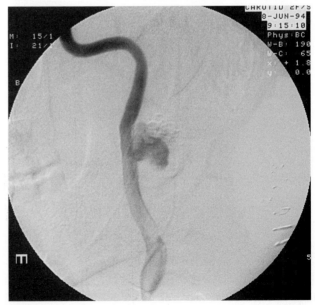

Figure 15-38 Three days later the patient was brought back for re-evaluation. The internal carotid artery now looks normal, but there is still a pseudoaneurysm. The inferior pouch has grown considerably.

Case 4 continues

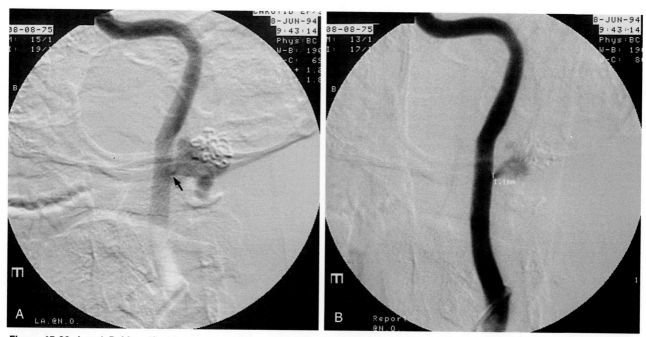

Figure 15-39 *A* and *B*, Magnified images reveal the exact hole *(small arrow)*. Even though this appears to measure more than 1 mm in diameter, it was not possible to access the lumen of the pseudoaneurysm from the internal carotid artery through the hole in the stent. Direct percutaneous puncture was a possibility at this point, but the attending physician wished to have the vessel permanently occluded above and below the pseudoaneurysm to guarantee no further growth.

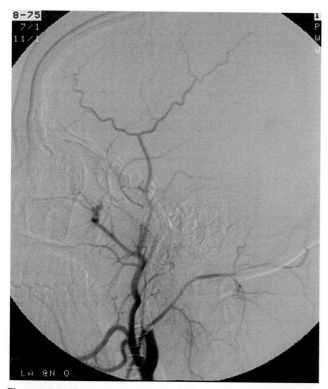

Figure 15-40 Examination obtained after occlusion of the vessel above and below the hole. Note the beads of the Gold Valve balloons. Permanent occlusion of the internal carotid artery is performed only after complete temporary test occlusion.

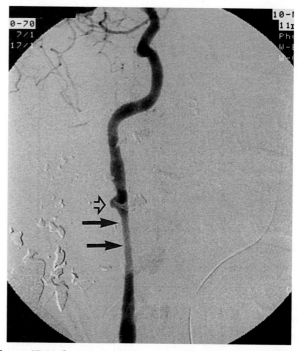

Figure 15-41 Case 5. A 26-year-old man was shot in the face, with resultant massive extravasation while he was in the emergency room. Immediate packing of the open maxillary sinus was performed, followed by ligation of the external carotid artery. An emergency angiogram revealed a pseudoaneurysm of the right internal carotid artery *(open arrow)*. Note the spasm *(arrows)* proximal to the hole in the vessel (practically speaking, indistinguishable from an intimal dissection). The hole is less than 3 cm from the skull base at the level of C1–C2, a very difficult operative site. Endovascular treatment was requested.

Case 5 continues

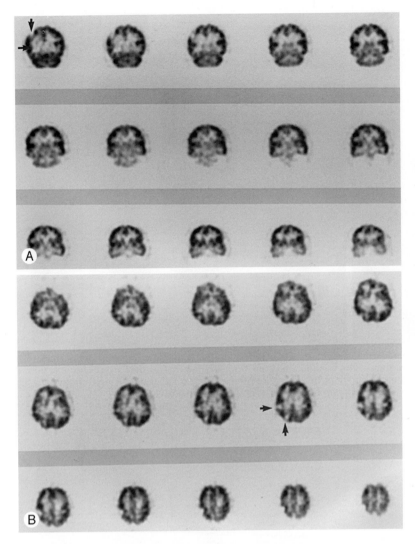

Figure 15-42 *A* and *B,* Because the patient was intubated and paralyzed with pancuronium (Pavulon), a standard test occlusion utilizing clinical criteria could not be performed. Therefore, a radionuclide single-photon emission computed tomography (SPECT) scan was performed with a temporary test occlusion balloon in place in the right internal carotid artery to evaluate the possibility of permanently occluding this vessel. This revealed at least two and possibly more defects *(arrows).* These probably represented sequelae from the original blast or the ligation process but could also represent some additional evidence of vascular insufficiency secondary to the test occlusion. It was decided that permanent occlusion was unwise and therefore to attempt to approximate the torn surfaces of the vessel by means of a stent. Obviously, a covered stent would be ideal, but none was commercially available. The decision was made not to try to custom fabricate one to be placed in this location owing to the bulk and potential thrombotic nature of this construction. A standard Palmaz stent was chosen.

Case 5 continues

tery) placed in the artery proximal to the occlusion balloon can wash out this segment, allowing a prolonged occlusion over the hole. We have not performed this maneuver, but it appears to be a viable option.

Definitive Endovascular Therapy for a Pseudoaneurysm

When all else fails and the surgical approach is not feasible, it is still possible to wait and see if the pseudoaneurysm heals on its own (which rarely happens and is dangerous, as noted earlier) or to perform a temporary test occlusion and then permanently occlude the vessel (if feasible) either endovascularly (with detachable balloons or coils) or surgically. Although this can be a definitive therapy, sacrifice of the parent vessel is not an ideal solution, particularly because many of these patients are relatively young. It is, however, a proven and safe means of therapy when performed by skilled personnel. It is also perhaps more advisable than placing a covered stent in the internal carotid artery of a young patient. Time will eventually answer this question.

Vertebral Artery Pseudoaneurysm

If the vascular hole is in a vertebral artery, the equation shifts. Direct open surgical access to the vertebral artery is severely limited because of the path of the vessel through the foramina of the cervical spine. This makes proximal control, distal control, and local surgical repair nearly impossible. For this reason, endovascular treatment is necessary. If the damage to the vessel is simply a pseudoaneurysm, occlusion of the vertebral artery over the hole (preferably external to the arterial lumen), or proximal and distal to the hole, as described earlier, resolves the problem. Either detachable balloons or coils can be used; however, proximal flow arrest is mandatory before coil occlusion of any vessel flowing to the brain.

If the hole in the artery has become an AV fistula, treatment is more complex. See Chapter 16 for the rationale and technique of therapy.

INTRACRANIAL PIAL ARTERIOVENOUS FISTULAE (NONGALENIC)

Direct simple fistulae within the cranium are rare. Unlike vein of Galen malformations, most of these

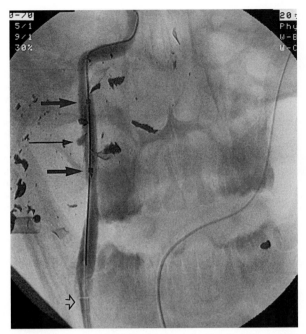

Figure 15-43 A 9-Fr. Brite-Tip catheter (Cordis Corp.) was placed directly through the skin, mounted over a 7-Fr. Berenstein catheter (USCI), as described in Chapter 1, and into the internal carotid artery (the tip of the guide catheter is indicated by a small open arrow). A Palmaz stent was then placed across the hole in the vessel and inflated with a 2 cm × 5 mm balloon *(thick arrows)*. There is excellent flow through the vessel but still some narrowing (spasm) proximal to the stent. The pseudoaneurysm is still seen lateral to the vessel wall *(thin arrow)*.

It had been hoped that there was a linear tear in the vessel and that the stent might approximate the two sides, thus allowing healing of the tear. This appearance after placement of the stent suggests that there was a true hole.

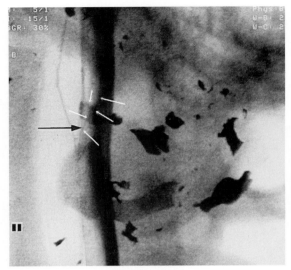

Figure 15-45 Follow-up angiography performed 2 days later revealed the pseudoaneurysm to be mostly occluded. Struts *(white arrows)* can be seen to cross directly over the hole, with the inferior anterior portion of the pseudoaneurysm no longer filling *(long black arrow)*. Continued watchful waiting was undertaken. The patient was still grossly sedated and therefore clinically untestable to determine the possibility of permanent occlusion.
Case 5 continues

present after the age of 2 years. Indeed, the range in age of presentation is wide, covering infancy, early childhood, adolescence, and adulthood.

Presenting symptoms relate to the mass (neurologic deficits, headache), congestive heart failure, seizures, and intracranial bleeding. Most patients (about 60%) in most age groups present with symptoms related to mass effect, and about one third have seizures.[5–7]

The typical radiographic sign of a pial AV fistula is a large superficial cerebral vein (usually a huge varix) seen on magnetic resonance imaging. The exact point of the fistula may be difficult to see because of the size of the varix. Typically, angiography reveals a single feeder with a huge draining vein that is enlarged, tortuous, and even looped back on itself. The arterial supply is directly related to its location, frontal lesions are supplied by the anterior cerebral artery, parietal lesions by the middle cerebral artery, and occipital lesions by the posterior cerebral artery. In watershed zones, there can be overlap from the adjacent vascular territories.

Surgical ligature has been the standard procedure and has worked effectively. It is possible, however, to place a clip in a slightly incorrect location, and thus to clip the vein, or clip the artery in a location so proximal that the fistula can recruit new supply.

Figure 15-44 Anteroposterior and lateral views confirm that there is a true round hole in the vessel *(arrows)*, not a slit. Measurement of the hole yielded a diameter of approximately 3 mm, with the pseudoaneurysm filling easily, and it was thought that the chance of this closing in the near future was small. One to three more stents (stacked) could yield more coverage of the hole by wire struts, possibly allowing thrombosis of the pocket, but might also potentially result in many stagnant pockets for thrombus formation. It was not known whether to keep the patient on heparin and risk another massive bleed or take him off heparin and risk thrombotic events secondary to the stent and the pseudoaneurysm. The use of ticlopidine (Ticlid) was decided upon.

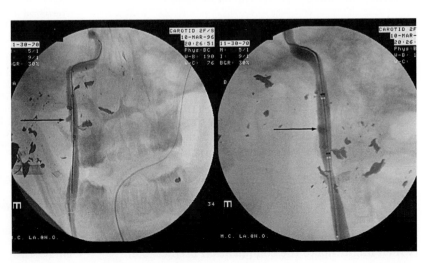

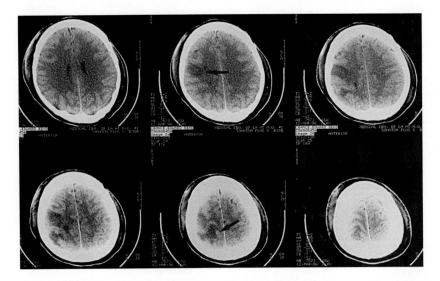

Figure 15-46 CT scan obtained 2 days after the injury and at the same time as the follow-up angiogram shows the two lesions *(arrows)* demonstrated on the SPECT scan previously. A temporary test occlusion, performed 2 weeks later, resulted in a clinical failure, confirming the previous uncertain SPECT findings, and therefore permanent occlusion was not performed. *Note*: a clinical failure in the presence of a recent embolic infarct may not be completely valid; any portion of the penumbra still recuperating from an ischemic event could perhaps demonstrate dysfunction if stressed.

Endovascular therapy of these lesions has been performed successfully using either detachable balloons (for large fistulae) or Guglielmi detachable coils (GDCs).

The use of coils can be dangerous if proximal flow control is not used because the coils can easily be blown through the hole into the large draining varix. Until there is cessation of flow, there is a tremendous current traversing the lesion. The platinum microcoils are easily displaced. Proximal flow control can be achieved using the Zeppelin or tandem catheters; one of the tandem catheters uses a nondetachable balloon, such as the Endeavor (ITC/Target Therapeutics). Proximal flow control can also be obtained by using the Grapevine microcatheter (Medtronic/MIS) in a more distal location.

GDC coils have been used for these lesions with success. Sacrifice of the vessel invariably occurs but does not necessarily result in a small infarct. Collateral supply frequently keeps the small area of parenchyma viable. Surgically, the same outcome results with use of a clip. Reconstructing a small cortical artery (about 1 mm) and maintaining patency of this vessel are extremely difficult. Sacrifice by surgical or endovascular means yields the same result.

POTENTIAL COMPLICATIONS OF THERAPY OF ARTERIOVENOUS FISTULAE

Complications of therapy related to this pathology can be surprising. Once the flow is cut off, there can be normal perfusion pressure breakthrough, as can be seen with AVMs[8] (see "Normal Perfusion Pressure Breakthrough" in Chapter 64). Contrary to the treatment of a large AVM, there is no practical way to stage the treatment of a large fistula to allow for intracranial hemodynamic adaptation. Once the lesion is occluded, either there is normal pressure breakthrough or there is not. Unfortunately, development of this complication does not appear to be directly related to the preexisting shunt gradient (which might make the complication predictable).[1]

An unusual complication of AV fistula treatment is thrombosis of the large draining varix with subsequent massive pulmonary emboli. In the case of large draining veins in the neck, it is difficult, if not impossible, to prevent the formation of thrombus in a large stagnant venous structure, whether the patient is anticoagulated or not. Time is the greatest ally for prevention of this problem (the vein eventually shrinks); however, if there is any question, it would be prudent to remove surgically or ligate this useless vein once the flow is stopped.

REFERENCES

1. Lownie SP, Duckwiler GR, Fox AJ, Drake CG. Endovascular therapy of nongalenic cerebral arteriovenous fistulas. In Vinuela F, Halbach VV, Dion JE (eds): Interventional Neuroradiology: Endovascular Therapy of the Central Nervous System. New York: Raven Press, 1992, pp 87–106.
2. Geremia G, Haklin M, Brennecke L. Embolization of experimentally created aneurysms with intravascular stent devices. *AJNR* 1994;15:1223–1231.
3. Marks MP, Drake MD, Steinberg GK, et al. Stent placement for arterial and venous cerebrovascular disease: preliminary experience. *Radiology* 1994;191:441–446.
4. Horowitz MB, Miller G III, Meyer Y, et al. Use of intravascular stents in the treatment of internal carotid and extracranial vertebral artery pseudoaneurysms. *AJNR* 1996;17:693–696.
5. Parkinson D, Bachers G. Arteriovenous malformations: summary of 100 consecutive supratentorial cases. *J Neurosurg* 1980;53:285–299.
6. Smith RR, Haerer AF, Russel WF. Vascular Malformations and Fistulas of the Brain. New York: Raven Press, 1982, p 50.
7. Patterson JH, McKissock W. A clinical survey of intracranial angiomas with special reference to their mode of progression and treatment: a report of 110 cases. *Brain* 1956;79:233–266.
8. Halbach VV, Higashida RT, Hieshima GB, Norman D. Normal perfusion pressure breakthrough occurring during treatment of carotid and vertebral fistulas. *AJNR* 1987;8:751–756.

ADDITIONAL READINGS

Arteriovenous Fistula

Berguer R, Feldman AJ, Wilner HI, Lazo A. Arteriovenous vertebral fistulae: cure by combination of operation and detachable intravascular balloon. *Ann Surg* 1990;196:65–68.

Colley DP. Vertebral arteriovenous fistula: an unusual complication of Swan-Ganz catheter insertion. *AJNR* 1985;6:103–104.

Fairman RM, Grossman RI, Goldberg HI, et al. A new approach to the treatment of vertebral arteriovenous fistulas. *Surgery* 1984;95:112–115.

Gabrielsen T, Deveikis J, Introcaso J, Coran AG. Congenital arteriovenous fistulas supplied by a single branch of the maxillary artery. *AJNR* 1994;15:653–658.

Goodman SJ, Hasso A, Kirkpatrick D. Treatment of vertebrojugular fistula by balloon occlusion. *J Neurosurg* 1975;43:362–367.

Guglielmi G, Guidetti G, Mori S, Silipo P. Therapeutic embolization of an ascending pharyngeal artery-internal jugular vein fistula. *J Neurosurg* 1988;69:132–133.

Haimov M, Baez A, Neff M, Slifkin R. Complications of arteriovenous fistulas for hemodialysis. *Arch Surg* 1975;110:708–712.

Kendall B. Results of treatment of arteriovenous fistulae with the Debrun technique. *AJNR* 1983;4:405–408.

Maroun FB, Mangan MA, Cornel G, Jacob JC. Balloon occlusion of traumatic vertebral arteriovenous fistula. *Surg Neurol* 1983;19:122–125.

Miller RE, Hieshima GB, Giannotta SL, et al. Acute traumatic vertebral arteriovenous fistula: balloon occlusion with the use of a contralateral approach. *Neurosurgery* 1984;14:255–259.

Pile-Spellman JM, Baker KF, Liszczak TM, et al. High-flow angiopathy: cerebral blood vessel changes in experimental chronic arteriovenous fistula. *AJNR* 1986;7:811–815.

Pritz MB, Pribam HFW. Intracerebral hemorrhage from a middle meningeal arteriovenous fistula with a giant venous varix. *Surg Neurol* 1992;37:460–463.

Quatromoni JC, Johnson JM, Wood M. Vertebral arteriovenous fistulas. *Am J Surg* 1979;138:907–911.

Robinson PN, Jewkes DA, Kendall B. Vertebrovertebral arteriovenous fistula: a complication of internal jugular catheterisation. *Anaesthesia* 1984;39:46–47.

Smith M, Russell E, Levy R, Cromwell R. Transcatheter obliteration of a cerebellar arteriovenous fistula with platinum coils. *AJNR* 1990;11:1199–1202.

Takeshi K, Tamaki N, Takeda N, et al. Fatal intracranial hemorrhage after balloon occlusion of an extracranial vertebral arteriovenous fistula. *J Neurosurg* 1988;69:945–948.

Vinuela F, Fox AJ. Interventional neuroradiology and the management of arteriovenous malformations and fistulas. *Neurol Clin* 1983;1:131–154.

Yakes WF, Luethke JM, Merland JJ, et al. Ethanol embolization of arteriovenous fistulas: a primary mode of therapy. *J Vasc Interv Radiol* 1990;1:89–96.

Dissection

Anson J, Crowell J. Cervicocranial arterial dissection. *Neurosurgery* 1991;29:89–96.

Morgan M, Sekhon L. Extracranial-intracranial saphenous vein bypass for carotid or vertebral artery dissections: A report of six cases. *J Neurosurg* 1994;80:237–246.

Ringel S, Harrison S, Norenberg M, Austin J. Fibromuscular dysplasia: Multiple "spontaneous" dissecting aneurysms of the major cervical arteries. *Ann Neurol* 1997;1:301–304.

Schievink WI, Mokri B, Michels VV, Piepgras DG. Familial association of intracranial aneurysms and cervical artery dissections. *Stroke* 1991;22:1426–1430.

Schievink WI, Mokri B, O'Fallon W. Recurrent spontaneous cervical-artery dissection. *N Engl J Med* 1994;330:393–397.

Schievink WI, Mokri B, Piepgras DG. Angiographic frequency of saccular intracranial aneurysms in patients with spontaneous cervical artery dissection. *J Neurosurg* 1992;76:62–66.

Zuber M, Meary E, Meder J-F, Mas J-L. Magnetic resonance imaging and dynamic CT scan in cervical artery dissections. *Stroke* 1994;25:576–581.

Trauma

de Villiers JC, Grant AR. Stab wounds at the craniocervical junction. *Neurosurgery* 1985;17:930–936.

Friedman AH. Traumatic injury of neck and intracranial vessels. *Contemp Neurosurg* 1990;12:1–6.

Goodwin JR. Carotid injury secondary to blunt head trauma: case report. *J Trauma* 1994;37:119–122.

Halbach VV, Higashida RT, Dowd CF, et al. Endovascular treatment of vertebral artery dissections and pseudoaneurysms. *J Neurosurg* 1993;79:183–191.

Karlin RM, Marks C. Extracranial carotid artery injury: current surgical management. *Am J Surg* 1983;146:225–227.

Krysl J, Nöel de Tilly L, Armstrong D. Pseudoaneurysm of the internal carotid artery: complication of deep neck space infection. *AJNR* 1993;14:696–698.

Li MS, Smith BM, Espinosa J, Brown RA, et al. Nonpenetrating trauma to the carotid artery: seven cases and a literature review. *J Trauma* 1994;36:265–272.

Mehringer C, Hieshima GB, Grinnell VS, et al. Therapeutic embolization for vascular trauma of the head and neck. *AJNR* 1983;4:137–142.

Menawat SS, Dennis JW, Laneve LM, Frykberg ER. Are arteriograms necessary in penetrating zone II neck injuries? *J Vasc Surg* 1992;16:397–401.

Pearce WH, Whitehill TA. Carotid and vertebral arterial injuries. *Surg Clin* 1988;68:M705–723.

Prêtre R, Reverdin A, Kalonji T, Faidutti B. Blunt carotid artery injury: difficult therapeutic approaches for an underrecognized entity. *Surgery* 1994;115:375–381.

Reiber ME, Burkey J. Intracavernous carotid pseudoaneurysm after blunt trauma: case report and discussion. *Head Neck* 1994;16:253–258.

Watridge CB, Muhlbauer MS, Lowery RD. Traumatic carotid artery dissection: diagnosis and treatment. *J Neurosurg* 1989;71:854–857.

Endovascular Therapy for Vertebral Artery Arteriovenous Fistulae

A. Aymard / R. Chapot / E. Houdart / A.E. Casasco / H.S. Jhaveri / D. Reizine / J.-J. Merland

GENERAL CONSIDERATIONS

Vertebral arteriovenous fistulae (AVFs) are rare lesions defined by the presence of an abnormal communication between the extracranial vertebral artery (VA) or one of its branches and a neighboring vein. They can be high or low flow but are usually high flow and direct.

Etiology

Vertebral AVFs are spontaneous or post-traumatic lesions.

Spontaneous vertebral AVFs are presumed to be congenital, even if there is no proof that they existed at birth. They may be seen in young children.[1, 2] They are sometimes associated with diseases such as fibromuscular dysplasia,[3] neurofibromatosis,[4] or Ehlers-Danlos syndrome and thus may require a minimal event such as a slight trauma or sneezing to become manifest. They may also be associated with particular conditions that change the hemodynamic balance, such as pregnancy or arterial hypertension.[5] Some authors [6, 7] suggest that as the time between trauma and the onset of symptoms is variable, "spontaneous" vertebral AVFs are acquired, caused by some forgotten episode of trauma.

Post-traumatic vertebral AVFs may be due to neck injuries, usually knife wounds or gunshot injuries.[8–10] Iatrogenic causes include inadvertent vertebral puncture after internal jugular vein puncture for central venous line placement[11] or after direct puncture of the carotid artery for diagnostic angiography. Other uncommon iatrogenic causes include surgery in the neck,[12] complications of anterior interbody fusion,[13, 14] or blunt trauma in association with cervical spine fracture.[15, 16]

Anatomy

The fistulae can be on either side. In cases of iatrogenic fistulae, the affected side is related to the technique of central venous catheter placement.

The portion of the VA involved in the fistula is variable, according to the etiology. The proximal second portion of the VA is involved in most traumatic fistulae, while spontaneous vertebral AVFs affect the third portion of the VA, from the foramen of the atlas to the foramen magnum.[2, 5, 7, 8]

The absence of a surrounding sheath may explain why vertebral fistulae develop more frequently than carotido–jugular vein fistulae.

The venous drainage is variable but almost always involves the jugular system to some degree, although most may be by another route. In the series from Beaujeux et al,[2] 13% of the cases had venous drainage that was cephalad, a potentially dangerous situation with consequences similar to cortical venous drainage in cases of dural fistulae (although not nearly as serious). The epidural venous plexus is involved in about one quarter of cases, with possible implications concerning venous hypertension in the cord. Mass effect on the cord appears to be more common.

Clinical Presentation

Most vertebral AVFs have been reported in adults, but there have been a few reported cases in children and infants.[1, 2]

Suspicion should be raised in anyone with intracranial aneurysms and/or other signs of vessel wall weakness who develops a spontaneous AVF; this may be a manifestation of Ehlers-Danlos syndrome. This may result in a potentially fatal situation during any attempt at intra-arterial therapy (even diagnostic angiography carries increased risks in patients with this disorder).[17]

Vertebral AVFs are mostly a benign condition. They may be asymptomatic, discovered incidentally at routine auscultation in 30%.[2] When present, symptoms are related to flow rate, age of the shunt, and the venous drainage pattern. Clinical symptoms related to high turbulent flow are seen in 60%[2] and include tinnitus, bruit in the cervical region, and vertigo. There may also be neurologic symptoms related to mechanical compression, arterial steal, or venous hypertension in 10%. Mechanical compression symptoms include cervical radiculopathy or Brown-Séquard syndrome[18] due to radicular or medullary compression by dilated veins or an epidural hematoma.[7] Asymptomatic fistulae can gradually become symptomatic secondary to intracranial steal. This steal can affect the brainstem, resulting in vertebrobasilar insufficiency. Venous hypertension may affect the normal venous drainage of the spinal cord, generating paraparesis or tetraparesis in the same way that dural fistulae with medullary venous drainage do.[19] Finally, cardiac insufficiency is a rare clinical presentation of vertebral AVF in children.

Diagnosis

Definite diagnosis relies on angiography, even if duplex color Doppler ultrasound shows a flow increase in the VA and large arterialized venous plexus. An abnormal number of vascular structures can be seen on computed tomography or magnetic resonance imaging in the posterior cervical region.

Angiography will show the characteristics of the vertebral AVF. Initial injection of the subclavian artery is critical to show the main feeders and the location of the fistula. It must be followed by selective catheterization of the involved VA, the contralateral VA, and all arteries that may feed the fistula (mainly the ascending cervical, deep cervical, and occipital arteries). The precise location and size of the fistula, the number of AV shunts, and their relation to normal branches such as a posterior inferior cerebellar artery (PICA) or a radiculomedullary artery may be better seen by injection of indirect feeders in cases of large-flow fistulae. The most appropriate oblique view must be found to avoid superimposition of the fistula with the VA and to better understand the precise anatomy of the point of the shunt. The morphology of the parent artery must also be assessed, to look for an associated lesion such as a transection if the vertebral AVF is of a traumatic origin, or to determine whether the diameter and tortuosity of the artery are suitable for endovascular access.

Injection of the involved VA will show the significance of arterial steal. The vascular supply of the basilar trunk must be demonstrated; it often arises solely from the contralateral VA in cases of significant steal.

Another point is to localize cervical radiculomedullary arteries (if possible) before occlusion of the fistula or during balloon test occlusion at various levels of the VA.

Angiography must include a careful analysis of the venous drainage, which is often primarily responsible for the clinical symptoms. The involved vessels are mostly the vertebral veins but can also be epidural veins. In rare cases, the drainage recruits perimedullary or intracranial veins.[2]

THERAPEUTIC APPROACH

Indication

Vertebral AVFs are in most cases benign conditions that do not require emergent therapy. Furthermore, treatment is not always indicated; a simple clinical follow-up may be proposed in an asymptomatic elderly patient.

Treatment is indicated in cases of low tolerance of functional symptoms, if neurologic symptoms due to arterial steal occur, or in cases of potentially dangerous venous drainage via the epidural and perimedullary veins.

Treatment

The "Gold Standard"

The goal of therapy is to eliminate the fistulous flow. Treatment consists of selective occlusion of the fistula with preservation of the VA; the "gold standard" is endovascular occlusion with a detachable balloon.

In a simple situation, with a small fistula and easy antegrade arterial access (Case 1, Fig. 16–1), endovascular navigation will result in balloon placement on the venous side, after easy advancement of the microcatheter in the VA. The inflated balloon is detached by gentle traction on the microcatheter after positioning to allow perfect VA preservation without protrusion of the balloon into the artery and without any residual false aneurysm on the most appropriate oblique view. The detachable balloon has to be directly against the hole, because if it is not and the draining vein alone is simply occluded, it may allow recruitment of a myriad of new venous exits for the still patent fistula.

The patient is kept awake under slight neuroleptanalgesia, which allows continuous neurologic monitoring. Anticoagulation is achieved by an initial bolus of 2000 units of heparin and continuous flush through the catheters at a rate of 2500 U/hr in a 70-kg patient.

Bifemoral access is needed for balloon placement and angiographic control during placement and detachment in case of VA occlusion. A 6- or 7-Fr. guide catheter with a lumen sufficient for the balloon to progress is placed in the subclavian or vertebral artery. The coaxial system is continuously flushed with saline through a sidearm attachment. A three-way stopcock is placed between the flush and hemostatic valve for contrast media injection.

The usual occlusive devices are latex balloons: BAL 1 or 2 (Balt) according to the size of the fistula; alternatively, balloons from Nycomed (Paris, France) can be used (No. 9 for a large-sized, No. L1 or L2 for a middle-sized, and No. 17 for a small-sized fistula). Balloons are mounted on a coaxial 3-Fr./2-Fr. detachment catheter (Nycomed) or on a single Mini-Torquer catheter (Nycomed), according to the desired floppiness. Balloons are filled with a mixture of saline and nonionic iso-osmolar contrast agent at a ratio of one third saline and two thirds contrast.

Special Situations

There are more complex situations in which some difficulties may be encountered. If occlusion on the venous side directly at the arterial input site is not possible, occlusion of the VA itself may be necessary, either directly over the hole or *both distal and proximal to* the hole. This is particularly true in the case of a transected VA with no clear venous structure as an outlet. A proximal surgical suture ligation is not satisfactory and should be avoided. In the case of a large fistula, there may be a pseudoaneurysm that cannot be treated selectively. Inflation of a balloon in the pseudoaneurysm causes expansion of the aneurysm without closure of the fistula. Complete treat-

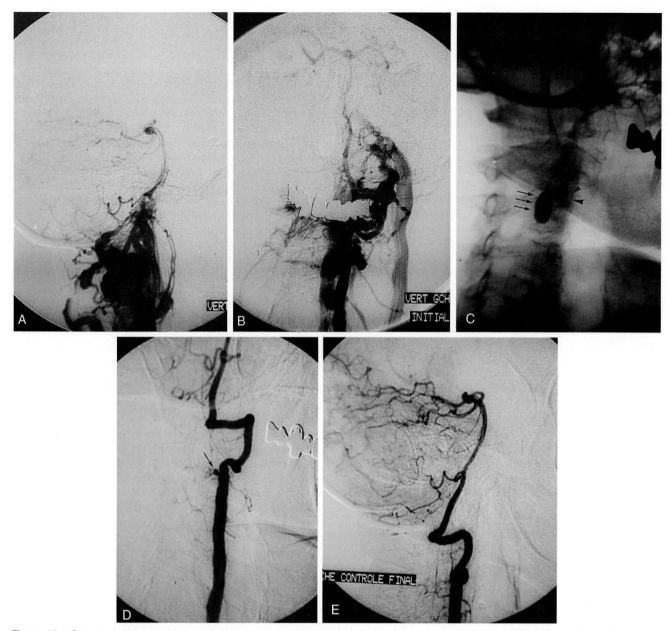

Figure 16-1 Case 1. A 65-year-old patient who complained of cervical bruit for 6 months. *A,* Lateral view of the left vertebral artery (VA) reveals a vertebral arteriovenous fistula (AVF) located at the V2 segment. *B,* The anteroposterior (AP) view shows drainage in the left vertebral vein and through occipital veins into the internal jugular vein. *C,* Selective treatment is obtained with two detachable balloons: the first is placed in the venous portion *(arrows)* and the second in the arteriovenous shunt *(arrowheads). D,* The fistula is excluded and the left VA remains patent *(arrow). E,* AP view of the left VA shows a small remaining dysplastic arterial segment.

ment can be obtained only with definite sacrifice of the parent VA. In rare cases, there may be multiple fistulous shunts requiring more than one balloon; the only effective treatment is an arterial occlusion. In the future, the development of covered stents should offer the possibility of preserving the patency of the VA in such cases.

If occlusion is to be performed at the fistulous site, the definitive occlusion is preceded by an occlusion test that lasts 20 minutes. During this balloon test occlusion, clinical and angiographic evaluation must be performed, including evaluation of the contralateral VA and bilateral internal and external carotid arteries. There is usually good tolerance of the occlu-

sion test as the flow of the injured VA is diverted toward the fistula and the posterior circulation is fed by the contralateral VA. The other important reason for the angiographic evaluation during the occlusion test is to assess the adequacy of occlusion of the fistula itself. If the occlusion of the VA is too proximal, the fistula remains patent by retrograde filling through the contralateral VA.

If no adequate placement of the balloon can be found, trapping of the fistula must be performed (Case 2, Fig. 16–2). The first balloon is placed distal to the fistula in the VA and the second one proximally; this ensures permanent occlusion without recanalization of the fistula. If only the proximal side is occluded

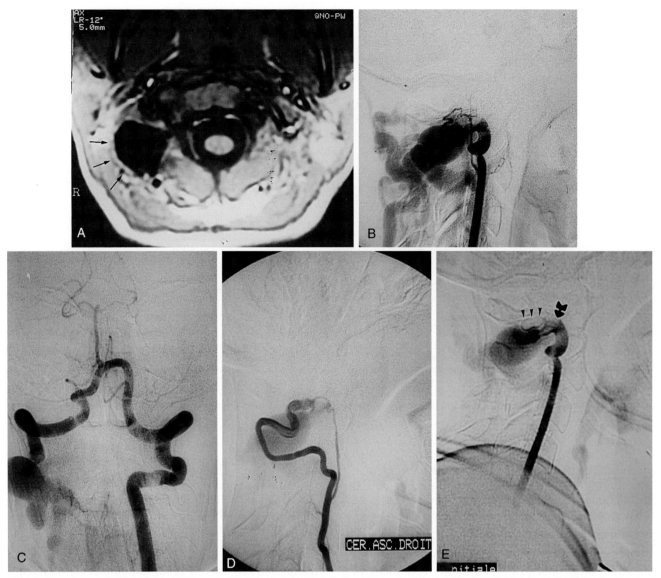

Figure 16-2 Case 2. This patient with a spontaneous vertebral AVF presented with debilitating tinnitus and bruit in the cervical region. *A,* A T1-weighted magnetic resonance axial view at the C3 level shows a large hypointense vascular pouch *(arrows),* related to the high flow. *B,* Angiography reveals a large AVF of the right VA with flow completely diverted to the fistula. *C,* The left VA is feeding the posterior cerebral circulation and the fistula through the contralateral distal VA. *D,* Lateral view of the ascending cervical artery, feeding the vertebral AVF through another shunt. *E,* After exclusion of the posterior portion of the fistula by placement of a balloon *(arrowheads)* introduced via the cervical artery, the anterior shunt *(arrow)* remains, fed by both VAs.

Illustration continued on following page

(currently the only supply to the fistula if there is flow past the lesion in the VA), the fistula will recruit additional new supply from the distal limb of the VA at the least, possibly inducing or worsening a clinically significant intracranial steal with uncertain but potentially acute and dire consequences. Therefore, it is important to occlude the *distal limb of the vertebral artery first,* even if both are to be done at the same sitting. This is particularly true if there is to be any delay between occlusion of the two limbs.

In dealing with a VA that continues to have antegrade flow past the fistula, the risk of inadvertent embolization to the brain still exists. A flow control guide catheter will allow safe deployment of a detachable balloon without this risk. If there is *retrograde*

flow in the distal segment of the VA, the brain is protected from embolic consequences and the procedure is safer.

In certain cases of transection or high flow, it may be difficult to reach the distal part of the VA with the balloon in an antegrade fashion. Advancing the guide catheter beyond the fistula allows easier placement of the balloon in the distal limb of the VA. If one cannot reach the distal limb with the guide catheter, one may try with a microcatheter and guidewire, performing coil occlusion distally followed by proximal balloon occlusion.

A transected VA is difficult or impossible to occlude in its distal portion from a direct antegrade approach. This is because either a balloon catheter or

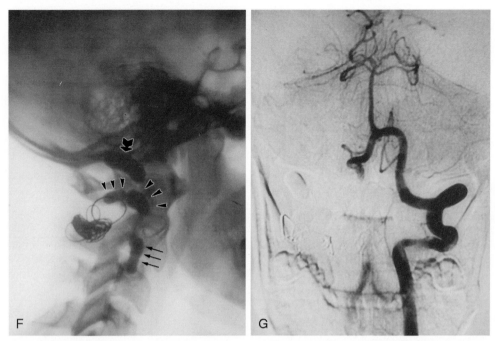

Figure 16-2 *Continued. F,* Definite exclusion of the vertebral AVF is obtained by trapping after failure of selective treatment with a balloon or with coils (very large communication): a first balloon is placed in the right VA above the fistula *(thick arrow),* a second balloon below the fistula *(large arrowheads),* and a third security balloon more proximal *(thin arrows).* Note the balloon *(small arrowheads)* occluding the posterior fistula. *G,* A final AP view of the left VA shows that the fistula is occluded; the basilar artery is normally filled and the right posterior inferior cerebellar artery preserved.

plain guidewire-directable catheter will tend to get sucked into the hole or will be unable to find the lumen distal to the transection without a vessel wall for the wire or catheter to follow.

In case of failure of the antegrade approach, contralateral access can be attempted by cross-over technique. This is generally not difficult since there is usually a large shunt in this direction, resulting in a large lumen for the entire route (and a small basilar artery) in addition to the high flow. Either a balloon, placed just distal to the hole in the VA, or a pile of coils will function to occlude the flow at this site. A balloon can be navigated in a retrograde manner after catheterization of the contralateral VA, or a microcatheter/microguidewire system can be used for coil placement. In any case, as discussed above, the distal vertebral limb must be occluded before the proximal. If not, primary proximal occlusion may divert the flow of the contralateral VA from the posterior cerebral circulation to the fistula, increasing the arterial steal and inducing vertebrobasilar insufficiency.

In exceptional cases, direct puncture of the fistula can be achieved in case of failure of approach via the arterial route or previous surgical arterial ligation. Retrograde venous navigation can be proposed in cases of primary vertebral vein drainage. If access to the venous side directly at the fistula is possible, packing with coils can successfully cure the problem.

Other occlusive devices have been proposed in rare instances; in small fistulae where it may not be possible to advance the balloon into the venous portion of the fistula, easier microcatheter navigation allows coil placement. The best choice is a retrievable system such as GDC platinum coils (Target Therapeutics) or MDS tungsten coils (Balt).

Some fistulae may also occlude "spontaneously" after angiography. This may be related to the viscosity of contrast media or to hemodynamic variations due to local manipulation with the catheter.

Postembolization Care

Immobilization of the cervical spine with a soft cervical collar during the next 3 days is necessary to avoid any premature balloon deflation due to the neighboring bone, and to prevent any mobilization of potential thrombus.

Low-molecular-weight heparin is maintained for 2 to 3 days to avoid thrombus formation and/or migration.

OUTCOME
Results

Complete occlusion has been obtained in more than 90% of cases.[2] Clinical improvement is always obtained after total or subtotal occlusion.

Delayed balloon migration with latex balloons has not been observed. Some recurrences have been due to early balloon deflation or to underlying arterial wall weakness in cases of selective treatment and preservation of VA patency.[2, 8]

Delayed false aneurysm formation at the fistula site after selective obliteration, encountered in carotid-cavernous fistulae, has not been seen in vertebral AVFs.

Technical Problems, Complications, and Solutions

With adequate technique, complications are exceptional. Potential complications previously reported with endovascular therapy include contrast media–related reactions, emboli, dissection, and vascular spasm.[2, 8]

One case has been reported of Wallenberg's syndrome due to secondary occlusion of the PICA; the vessel origin was near the fistula.[8]

In the case of a large, long-standing AVF, gradual occlusion or staged occlusion can avoid the so-called normal perfusion pressure breakthrough.[8] For a long-standing fistula with a chronic intracranial steal, abrupt occlusion of the fistula has been reported to cause intracranial hemorrhage.[20] In cases such as this, the chronic hypoperfusion state induced in the posterior fossa can apparently cause loss of autoregulatory response of the arterioles with a rebound hyperperfusion state similar to normal pressure breakthrough after surgery for intracranial arteriovenous malformations. The abrupt return of full pulse pressure from the VA to the posterior fossa is of concern. Some means of achieving a graduated occlusion of the shunt is preferable but possibly difficult, if not impossible. Perhaps a graduated means such as a Selverstone clamp may be of use.

If the vertebral (or other) AVF is of long standing, the vein (and arterial feeder) may be huge and the vein may be used *only* for drainage of the fistula (it has been "high pressure" long enough to prevent usage by other veins). Once the fistula is closed, this vein becomes simply a large reservoir of stagnant blood. This will then thrombose and the mass can potentially embolize to the lungs with disastrous results. The operator should beware. Simply turning the head may produce enough force to mash this thrombus of "toothpaste" consistency downstream toward the lungs. In cases of huge residual venous structures, postocclusion distal surgical ligation should be performed if it is possible. If not, it is believed that the vein will eventually return to a more normal size once the high-flow pressure head has been removed. In these cases, a soft cervical collar is left in place for several days to try to allow venous adaptation (i.e., shrinkage) and prevent any movement of potential thrombus, as well as to permit any thrombus to organize better. It is not known whether this collar is necessary (or for how long) or even if it actually works, but it is simply used on an empirical basis (it seems reasonable). This maneuver is performed in view of the observation of serious embolic consequences (death) associated with a large stagnant draining vein.

In addition, continued heparinization may be maintained in an effort to prevent too rapid thrombosis of the draining vein and allow shrinkage. Low-molecular-weight heparin can also be used for this purpose.

CONCLUSION

Endovascular occlusion of vertebral AVFs is safe, effective, and definitive. It must be considered primarily in this condition. Balloon occlusion remains the best tool to achieve adequate treatment.

REFERENCES

1. Sadasivan B, Mehta B, Dujovny M, et al. Balloon embolization of nontraumatic vertebral arteriovenous fistulae in children. *Surg Neurol* 1989;32:126–130.
2. Beaujeux RL, Reizine DC, Casasco A, et al. Endovascular treatment of vertebral arteriovenous fistula. *Radiology* 1992;183:361–367.
3. Bahar S, Chiras J, Carpena JP, et al. Spontaneous vertebro-vertebral arterio-venous fistula associated with fibro-muscular dysplasia. *Neuroradiology* 1984;26:45–49.
4. Parkinson D, Rankin H. Neurofibromatosis. *Surg Neurol* 1986;25:109–113.
5. De Bray JM, Bertrand P, Bertrand F, Jeanvoine H. Les fistules artérioveineuses spontanées de l'artère vertébrale: à propos d'un cas, revue de la littérature. *Rev Med Interne* 1986;7:133–139.
6. Debrun G, Legre I, Kasbarian M, et al. Endovascular occlusion of vertebral fistulae by detachable balloons with conservation of vertebral blood flow. *Radiology* 1979;130:141–147.
7. Nagashima C, Iwasaki T, Kawanuma S, et al. Traumatic arteriovenous fistula of the vertebral artery with spinal cord symptoms. *J Neurosurg* 1977;46:681–687.
8. Halbach VV, Higashida RT, Hieshima GB. Treatment of vertebral arteriovenous fistulas. *AJNR* 1987;8:1121–1128.
9. Sherk HH, Giri N, Nicholson JT. Gunshot wound with fracture of the atlas and arteriovenous fistula of the vertebral artery. *J Bone Joint Surg* 1974;56A:1738–1740.
10. Roper PR, Guinto FC, Wolma FJ. Posttraumatic vertebral artery aneurysm and arteriovenous fistula: a case report. *Surgery* 1984;96:556–559
11. Verrières D, Bernard C, Dacheux J, et al. Fistules artério-veineuses cervicales après cathétérisme jugulaire interne. *Ann Fr Anesth Reanim* 1986;5;162–164.
12. Cosgrove GR, Theron J. Vertebral arterio-venous fistula following anterior cervical spine surgery. *J Neurosurg* 1987;66:297–299.
13. Weinberg PE, Flom RA. Traumatic vertebral arteriovenous fistula. *Surg Neurol* 1973;1:162–167.
14. Cosgrove GR, Theron J. Vertebral arteriovenous fistula following anterior cervical spine surgery. *J Neurosurg* 1987;66:297–299.
15. Hayes P, Gerlock AJ Jr, Cobb CA. Cervical spine trauma: a cause of vertebral artery injury. *J Trauma* 1980;20:904–905.
16. Avellanosa AM, Glasauer FE, Oh YS. Traumatic vertebral arteriovenous fistula associated with cervical spine fracture. *J Trauma* 1977;17:885–888.
17. Weir B. Intracranial aneurysms and subarachnoid hemorrhage: an overview. In Wilkins RH, Rengachary SS (eds): Neurosurgery. New York: McGraw Hill, 1985, pp 1308–1329.
18. Freitag H-J, Grzyska U, Zeumer H. The use of the "cross over technique" in the management of a traumatic vertebro-vertebral fistula. *Neuroradiology* 1997;31:174–176.
19. Woimant F, Merland JJ, Riche MC. Syndrome bulbo-medullaire en rapport avec une fistule artério-veineuse méningée du sinus latéral à drainage veineux médullaire. *Rev Neurol* 1982;138:559–566.
20. Kondoh T, Tamaki N, Takeda N, et al. Fatal intracranial hemorrhage after balloon occlusion of an extracranial vertebral arteriovenous fistula. *J Neurosurg* 1988;69:945–948.

Embolization of Spinal Vascular Malformations

A.E. Casasco / E. Houdart / H.S. Jhaveri / A. Aymard / D. Herbreteau / J.-P. Guichard / D. Reizine / K.L. Mourier / J.-J. Merland

GENERAL CONCEPTS

Since the mid-1980s, rapid advances in neuroimaging and improvements in neuroangiography have led to better understanding of spinal cord vascular malformations. Significant technical improvements in catheters and delivery systems, as well as in various embolic materials, have led to marked technical improvement in endovascular therapy for spinal cord vascular malformations. These malformations are best managed in specialized medical centers where a dedicated team with refined techniques and skills is available.

CLASSIFICATION

The clinical presentation is usually directly influenced by the location as well as the angioarchitecture of the spinal canal and the cord vascular malformation. The vertebral body–spinal cord complex may participate in many types of vascular malformations. Various vascular lesions will be discussed in the order they are listed in Table 17–1—from the inside of the spinal cord to the outside (paravertebral region), including associated syndromes.

GENERAL APPROACH TO TREATMENT

Vascular malformations can be broadly grouped into two groups: arteriovenous fistulae (AVFs), where a direct shunt between an artery and vein is identified, and arteriovenous malformations (AVMs), where there is an intervening nidus between the artery and vein.

The specifics of endovascular therapy depend on the type of vascular malformations, but there are some common technical ground rules.

Critical Anatomic Considerations

Three longitudinal arterial axes supply the spinal cord, which include a single, midline, anterior spinal artery (ASA) and two posterior spinal arteries. These axes are fed primarily by anterior or posterior radiculomedullary arteries, which usually accompany a root as it joins the spinal cord. The radiculomedullary arteries in the cervical region arise from branches of both subclavian arteries: the vertebral arteries; and the ascending and deep (posterior) cervical arteries.

Blood supply in the thoracic and thoracolumbar regions arises from dorsospinal branches of intercostal and lumbar arteries.

The anterior two thirds of the spinal cord is supplied by the ASA, whereas the remaining posterior one third is supplied by the two posterior spinal arteries. Accidental embolization of a posterior radiculomedullary artery usually has no major clinical consequences. However, untoward embolization of an anterior radiculomedullary artery may lead to major neurologic complications, including injury to pyramidal tracts and severe motor deficit.

These lesions are supplied by the ASA, the posterior spinal arteries, or both. They may be on the surface of the cord, intramedullary, or both. They typically have vessels in the 100- to 700-micron diameter range and are thus difficult to image angio-

---

T A B L E 1 7 – 1   Classification of Spinal Vascular Malformations

A. Simple
  A1: Spinal canal vascular malformation
    a. Intramedullary vascular lesions
        i. AVM
       ii. AVF
      iii. Cavernoma
       iv. Telangiectasia
    b. Perimedullary arteriovenous fistulae
        i. Type I
       ii. Type II
      iii. Type III
    c. Spinal dural AVF with perimedullary venous drainage
    d. Intracranial dural malformation with perimedullary venous drainage (type V of intracranial dural AV fistulae)
    e. Epidural AVF and AVM
        i. Single shunt
       ii. Multiple shunts
  A2: Perivertebral malformations
    a. Paraspinal
    b. Costovertebral angle
    c. Nerve root foramina
  A3: Vertebral angiomas
    a. Nonevolutive vertebral angiomas
    b. Active evolutive vertebral angiomas
B. Complex
    a. AVMs in Cobb's syndrome
    b. Disseminated angiomatosis (Osler-Weber-Rendu syndrome)

AVM, arteriovenous malformation; AVF, arteriovenous fistula.

graphically.[1] The key to the therapeutic challenge is the location of the feeder. If the supply is all from the posterior spinal artery(ies), a surgeon could treat the lesion with no difficulty. Anterior spinal arteries are extremely difficult to reach surgically, however. This is what necessitates endovascular therapy.

Cardinal rules to be strictly observed before any anterior radiculomedullary artery embolization include a number of anatomic and hemodynamic considerations:

1. One should identify arterial anastomoses with the ASA above and below the vascular malformation, which will supply blood to normal cord in case of accidental occlusion of the ASA during embolization.
2. Any arterial stenosis of the ASA should be identified, since embolic agents may prove to be occlusive at such a point.
3. Flow dominance to the vascular malformation should be identified, since greater blood flow to the vascular malformation than to upper and lower normal branches prevents migration of emboli to normal vessels.
4. Embolization in a radiculospinal artery should never be performed with the catheter in a wedged position when the tip of the catheter is distant from the embolization target. The ASA and posterior spinal arteries anastomose via the pia mater perispinal network. These anastomoses can open when injection is performed with high pressure.

Selection of Embolic Agents

See Table 17–2 for a list of embolization materials.

Embolization with Particles

Gelfoam

Gelfoam is a nonpermanent embolic agent that is resorbable within 8 to 10 days. It may be cut into small fragments of desired size and shape, but this is difficult to do for use with a microcatheter. Soaking of small fragments of Gelfoam in alcohol enhances their thrombogenicity.

Polyvinyl Alcohol Particles

Polyvinyl alcohol (PVA) particles are available in many sizes ranging from 45 to 2000 microns. PVA particles are flow directed and slowly injected into an arterial pedicle under fluoroscopic control. Injection of PVA particles is stopped if venous drainage is no longer seen, or if the blood flow is significantly slowed. The technique of injecting PVA should change according to the region to be embolized.

When the radiculospinal artery is arising from a deep cervical branch, the tip of the catheter is left in the common trunk of the deep cervical artery. However, if a radiculospinal artery is arising from the vertebral artery, two methods of approach are possible: (1) one can superselectively catheterize the

TABLE 17–2   List of Material for Embolization of Spinal Vascular Malformations

1. 5-Fr. Terumo introducer (Terumo, Japan)
2. 5-Fr. Cobra catheter (Terumo)
3. 0.035″-guidewire (Terumo)
4. Jetstream-10 microcatheter (Medtronic/MicroInterventional Systems)
5. Dasher-14 microguidewire (Target Therapeutics)
6. Contour Emboli PVA particles (ITC/Target Therapeutics)
7. Histoacryl (Braun)
8. FasTRACKER-10 (Target Therapeutics)
9. Dasher-10 (Target Therapeutics)
10. Lipiodol (Guerbet, France)
11. Tantalum (Nycomed, France)
12. Syringes, 1 cc, 3 cc, 5 cc
13. Gelfoam (Laboratoire Houdé, Paris, France and Upjohn)
14. Terumo 10 guidewire
15. Magic catheter (Balt Extrusion)
16. TRACKER-18 (Target Therapeutics)
17. Latex balloon (Nycomed)
18. Latex balloon (Balt Extrusion)
19. Omnipaque: nonionic contrast medium
20. GDC coils (Target Therapeutics)
21. MDS coils (Balt Extrusion)
22. Embospheres (Guerbet, France)

feeder using a TRACKER-10 microcatheter, or (2) one can perform temporary balloon occlusion of the vertebral artery distal to the arterial feeders supplying the AVM using a 1.8-Fr. Magic catheter with a balloon mounted on it, and then catheterize the vertebral artery proximally and inject flow-directed PVA particles in the trunk of the vertebral artery.

If the second technique is chosen, one must aspirate several times before deflating the balloon to avoid possible inadvertent migration of embolic material into the posterior intracranial circulation. Also, 4000 units of heparin should be injected intravenously as soon as the balloon is inflated to temporarily occlude the vertebral artery and avoid possible clot formation and eventual distal migration.

However, this maneuver is very risky owing to the possibility of a few particles remaining in the vertebral artery at the end of the procedure and embolizing to the brain after the occlusion balloon is deflated.

Below the cervical region, PVA particles are injected into the trunk of the lumbar or intercostal arteries giving origin to the involved radiculospinal arteries. A small piece of Gelfoam, a small coil, or a small drop of dilute *N*-butyl-2-cyanoacrylate (NBCA) (Histoacryl, Braun) is used for occlusion of the distal trunk, to protect the involved intercostal and lumbar territories and to direct the PVA particles to the involved dorsospinal arteries.

Detachable Balloons

This technique is applied only in the case of a large arteriovenous fistulous shunt. The detachable balloon is secured either by hand ligature or by a mechanical valve (installed at the time of manufacture).

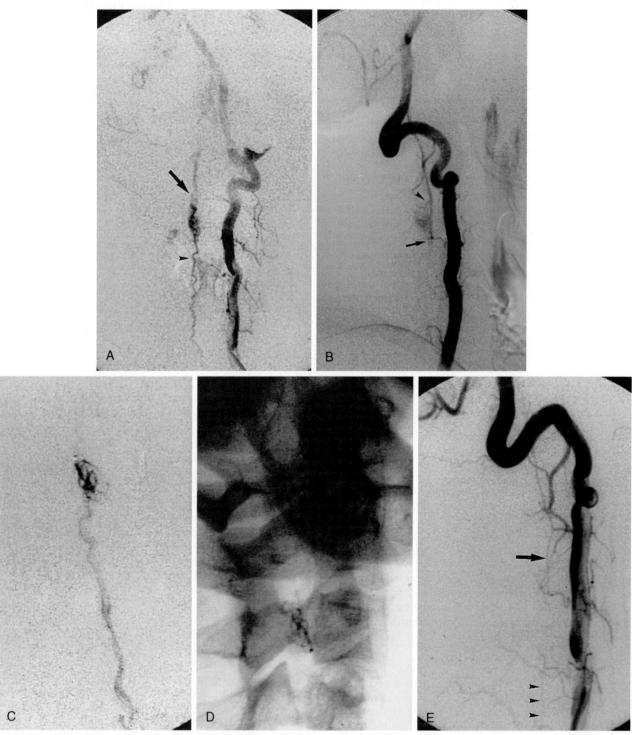

Figure 17-1 Case 1. *A,* An anteroposterior (AP) view of a left vertebral arteriogram reveals an intramedullary arteriovenous malformation (AVM) of the cervical region supplied by the anterior spinal artery (ASA) *(arrow),* with descending venous drainage *(arrowhead). B,* On a lateral view of the left vertebral artery, the dilated ASA is opacified and the sulcocommissural artery is perfusing the malformation *(arrowhead).* Note the hemodynamic arrest of the ASA beyond the malformation *(arrow). C,* Superselective catheterization of the nidus of malformation and injection of contrast media opacifies multiple shunts and venous drainage without opacification of normal spinal artery. This is an ideal position for injection of *N*-butyl-2-cyanoacrylate (Histoacryl).

   D, A postembolization oblique plain film shows the Histoacryl cast in the malformation. *E,* A postembolization lateral view of the left vertebral artery shows total occlusion of the AVM with preservation of the ASA *(arrow).* Reappearance of the distal territory of the ASA is seen *(arrowheads).*

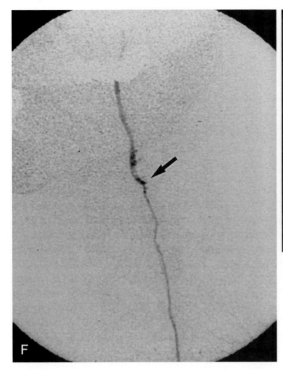

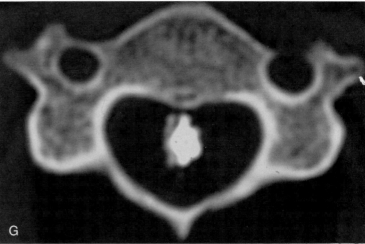

Figure 17-1 *Continued. F,* An AP view shows a dorsal radiculomedullary artery supplying the ASA in the cervical region over its entire extent. The change of caliber of the ASA corresponds with the point of the AVM *(arrow).* G, A postembolization computed tomographic (CT) scan reveals Histoacryl in the malformation.

Coils

Mechanical or electrically detachable coils may be used to embolize direct AVFs.

Liquid Embolic Agent

Histoacryl is a liquid polymerizing agent and is used most frequently in our department. As discussed in Chapter 1, Histoacryl polymerizes when it comes in contact with an ionic medium, such as blood. The speed of polymerization depends on how close the tip of the microcatheter is to the nidus of AVM and how fast the flow is in the AVM. The polymerizing time can be effectively prolonged by mixing Histoacryl with iodized oil (Lipiodol). Tantalum powder is added to enhance the radiographic opacification of the embolic agent. Normally, we inject very small quantities of NBCA (0.1 to 0.2 ml) to avoid or to reduce occlusion of the arterial pedicle as well as to avoid migration of Histoacryl into draining veins.

SPINAL CORD ARTERIOVENOUS MALFORMATIONS

Anatomy

The angioarchitecture of a spinal cord AVM is similar to that of a cerebral AVM (Fig. 17–1). The nidus is formed by arteriolar-venular fistulae.[2] Spinal cord AVMs usually extend over one or more spinal segments. The nidus may be purely intraparenchymal (pure intramedullary AVM), on the surface of the spinal cord (pure pial), or mixed.

Anterior and posterior radiculomedullary arteries always participate in the blood supply of a spinal cord AVM. If a median anterior branch taking off from an anterior radiculomedullary artery is present, this suggests an intraparenchymal location of the lesion. However, if a posterior radiculomedullary branch is exclusively supplying the AVM, this indicates a pial location of the AVM. Usually, AVMs are multipedicular lesions, and most often anterior radiculomedullary arteries participate in their vascularization.

The nidus is made up of a tangle of abnormal vessels, with arteriovenous shunts of different types and sizes. A single AVF is usually found in extramedullary AVMs (pial AVMs). The existence of an aneurysm either on the ASA or on the posterior spinal artery that supplies an intramedullary AVM carries a high risk of bleeding.[3, 4] The presence of a true aneurysm on the arterial side may be flow related. A false aneurysm due to a previous hemorrhagic event may be discovered. Venous stenosis with venous ectasia presents a risk factor for hemorrhage.

Intramedullary AVMs are generally drained by ascending and descending perimedullary veins. The perimedullary vein joins a radiculomedullary vein, which leaves the dural sheath at the level of the intervertebral foramen and drains into epidural or foraminal veins. The draining vein leaves the spinal canal at a neural foraminal level close to the AVM.

Clinical Presentation

Intramedullary AVMs are congenital in origin and present in the 2nd or 3rd decade of life.[5–8] These lesions are relatively rare. They may present with subarachnoid hemorrhage and an acute medullary syndrome.

Most patients with high-flow lesions present with hemorrhage; patients with slow-flow lesions may present with myelopathic symptoms related to venous hypertension. The most common initial symptom is nerve root or back pain (15% to 20%). Decreased strength eventually occurs in almost all patients, accompanied by sensory loss. Many of these patients will have already bled by this time. Approximately 80% of patients have additional bleeds with clinical deterioration. Interestingly, increased intra-abdominal pressure associated with bowel movements can aggravate the symptoms. Children are frequently weak or paralyzed at the time of presentation with this entity.

Clinical symptoms may progress rapidly or there may be partial remissions. The prognosis of intramedullary vascular malformation is poor. Because of the long-term poor outcome of hemorrhagic events, we prefer to treat a spinal cord AVM, even if it is clinically asymptomatic.[6, 7, 9]

Diagnosis

Myelography may be performed when state-of-the-art magnetic resonance imaging (MRI) is not available. It typically reveals a "bag of worms" appearance and widening of the spinal cord. MRI is currently the diagnostic tool of choice, however.

The postmyelography computed tomographic (CT) scan is valuable for localizing the vascular malformation inside or outside the spinal cord and for evaluating the local bony changes associated with prolonged pressure by the large tangle of dilated vessels.

Modern MRI has revolutionized pretherapeutic assessment. It is noninvasive and offers accurate diagnosis of intramedullary vascular malformations as well as evaluation of the cord surrounding the lesion. It may also reveal an acute hematomyelia.

Spinal angiography is an indispensable pretherapeutic diagnostic procedure. It not only confirms the suspected diagnosis but also offers exact localization as well as clear definition of the angioarchitectural characteristics of the lesion. An initial aortogram offers an overall view of the vascular malformation. Selective angiography provides information about the angioarchitecture. Selective angiograms are performed in anteroposterior and lateral projections.

Treatment

At our institution, all patients with spinal cord AVMs, once diagnosed, are offered therapy even if asymptomatic at the time. The aim of therapy is to suppress the risk of hemorrhage and arrest the progression of neurologic deficit.[5, 6, 9] Maximal suppression of arterial steal may reverse a progressive neurologic deficit.

The exact supply is usually difficult to see, and it may appear that there are numerous indirect feeders; these are the collateral supply to the remaining spinal vessels. Therefore, occlusion of the direct supply may not help at all when the collateral vessels take up the slack; they are typically more tortuous and, with present technique and technology, are impossible to treat correctly. These collateral vessels may not even be evident until occlusion of the primary supply has been accomplished (indicative of occlusion in too proximal a location; unfortunately, very easy to do with these lesions). Even when the AVM appears to get supply from various arteries, there is usually only one draining vein, suggesting that the AVM occupies only one compartment.

Surgery versus Endovascular Therapy

Surgical eradication of intramedullary AVMs is accompanied by significant major complications. We believe endovascular therapy should be the method of choice for spinal cord AVMs, even if the lesion is suitable for a surgical approach.[6, 8] One of the largest series[5] reveals that the risks of embolization are three to five times lower than those from surgery (5.7% incidence of irreversible deficit after embolization versus 15% to 28% incidence of irreversible deficit after surgery).

The angiographic criteria for endovascular therapy of intramedullary AVMs are:

- Enlarged prominent ASA
- Relatively short distance between feeders and the nidus
- Multiple commissural branches participating in the AVM
- Normal ASA above or below the AVM

Particulate PVA Embolization

Particulate embolization with PVA reduces arterial steal safely. Unfortunately, there is arterial recanalization, and these patients must be followed every year by angiography, during which time complementary embolization can be performed if necessary.

Histoacryl Embolization

Histoacryl is used in very specific situations.[5, 6] In vascular malformations solely perfused by a posterior spinal artery, use of liquid acrylic agents is associated with few complications, making them the embolic agents of first choice. However, if the malformation is predominantly perfused by the ASA, the criteria for use of Histoacryl as an embolic agent are more complex[6]:

1. The presence of normal anterior radiculomedullary arteries supplying the anterior spinal axis above as well as below the malformation.
2. The possibility of superselective catheterization close to the nidus of the vascular malformation. For superselective catheterization of the ASA, we use a FasTRACKER-10 microcatheter and Terumo 10 guidewire.

PERIMEDULLARY ARTERIOVENOUS FISTULAE
Location

In most cases, perimedullary fistulae are characterized by a single hole between one or more radiculomedullary arteries and perimedullary vein(s) on the surface of the spinal cord.[6, 8] Often, these are located near the cauda equina; however, they may rarely be in the lower cervical and upper thoracic regions.

Classification

The classification of these lesions used by us is as follows:

Type I: These AVFs are of small caliber, between the anterior or posterior spinal artery and a medullary vein. The fistula is at the point where there is change in vascular caliber. The venous drainage is minimally dilated (Fig. 17–2).

Type II: The anterior or posterior spinal artery is almost always dilated. There is a markedly dilated draining vein (Fig. 17–3).

Type III: This is a giant AVF with multiple feeders. The main arterial pedicle is the ASA. The proximal venous segment is ectatic (Fig. 17–4).

In AVFs of type I and II, radiculospinal draining veins leave the spinal cord away from the zone of shunt (e.g., an AVF located at the T12 level draining at the cervical level). However, in giant AVFs (type III), the draining veins leave the spinal canal close to the site of the fistula (similar to the venous drainage of intramedullary AVMs). Impaired venous return and the long intradural course of the venous drainage may be responsible for ascending myelopathy and spinal cord ischemia.

Clinical Manifestations

These lesions typically present in young adults (14 to 44 years), with no sex predilection. Progressive asymmetric myeloradicular deficit may be encountered. There is progressive paraplegia without remission. The progressively devastating clinical evolution can be arrested only by early diagnosis and appropriate treatment.[8] This is why we prefer to offer therapy, even when the lesion is clinically silent.

Diagnosis

Usually, plain films of the spine are unremarkable except in the case of a giant AVF, which may produce bone erosion. MRI may show vascular dilation on the surface of the spinal cord. Arteriography is indispensable, not only for precise diagnosis, but also to differentiate between types of fistulae.

Treatment

Surgery

If the AVF is of type I or II and is located posterior to the spinal cord, surgery may be of value.[7, 9] If the AVF is anterior to the spinal cord, excisional surgery may be associated with a high risk of damage to the spinal cord. In type III fistulae, surgery is indicated if endovascular therapy does not succeed.

Endovascular Therapy

Type I

These lesions are the most difficult to treat by embolization because of the difficulty of navigating the microcatheter in the ASA to the point of shunt.[8, 10] In this situation, one can use particulate, free-flow embolization with PVA of 55 to 150 microns in size.

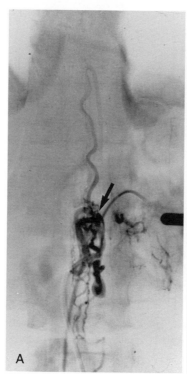 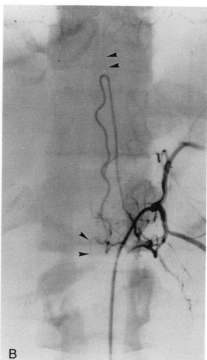

Figure 17-2 Case 2. *A*, An AP view of the left 12th intercostal artery demonstrates a perimedullary fistula (type I) perfused by the artery of Adamkiewicz. The anterior spinal artery is dilated. An arteriovenous shunt is found at the conus level *(arrow)*. *B*, The postembolization status after use of Embospheres as an embolic agent is shown in the same projection. There is total occlusion of the shunt and reappearance of the distal territory of the ASA beyond the malformation and its ascending branch *(arrowheads)*.

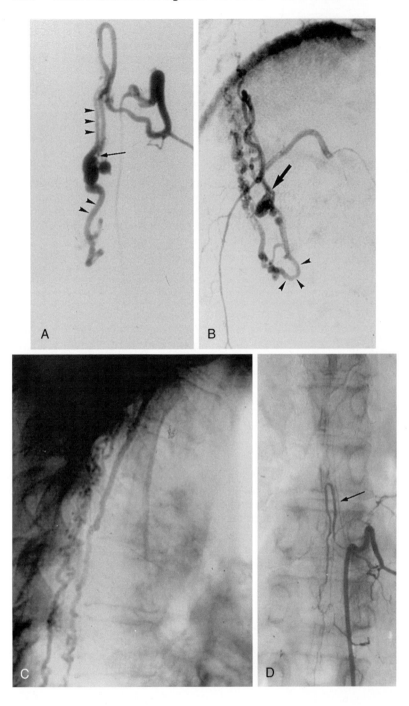

Figure 17-3 Case 3. *A,* An AP view of the left 11th intercostal artery shows the anterior spinal artery perfusing a perimedullary fistula (type II). The shunt is found at the level of the conus *(arrow)* and has ascending as well as descending venous drainage *(arrowheads). B,* Another view of the same artery demonstrates the shunt as well as venous dilation *(arrow).* Note the venous drainage around the conus medullaris, making a venous loop *(arrowheads). C,* A lateral view reveals venous drainage along the thoracic cord (final venous drainage is seen far away from the malformation). *D,* Angiographic follow-up was performed 6 months after particulate embolization. The shunt is obliterated. Note the decrease in caliber of the ASA; a posterior radiculomedullary artery arising from the same pedicle is seen *(arrow).*

This is rarely efficient therapy, but it helps to stabilize the symptoms (Fig. 17–2).

Type II

Arterial pedicles are dilated enough to facilitate navigation of a microcatheter (we use a FasTRACKER-10 microcatheter and Terumo 10 guidewire) to the point of shunt. We prefer to catheterize the radiculopial artery (this pedicle has minimal risk) and use Histoacryl as the embolic agent of choice.[1, 6] The aim is to block the first 1 to 2 cm of vein to occlude all the fistulous sites by a single injection. If Histoacryl cannot be used as an embolic agent, small fragments of Gelfoam soaked in a mixture of 3 ml absolute alcohol plus 2 ml contrast media are employed. More recently, Embospheres, which are well calibrated and can block into the shunt, have been used (Fig. 17–3).

Type III

If this is a single pedicle lesion, we prefer to use a latex balloon, inflated with dilute contrast media, to occlude the fistulous site. If there are multiple feeders to the fistula, the largest shunt is occluded with a detachable latex balloon, while the rest of the fistula is embolized with Histoacryl or Embospheres. The direct shunt can also be occluded with Guglielmi detachable coils (GDC) (Fig. 17–4).

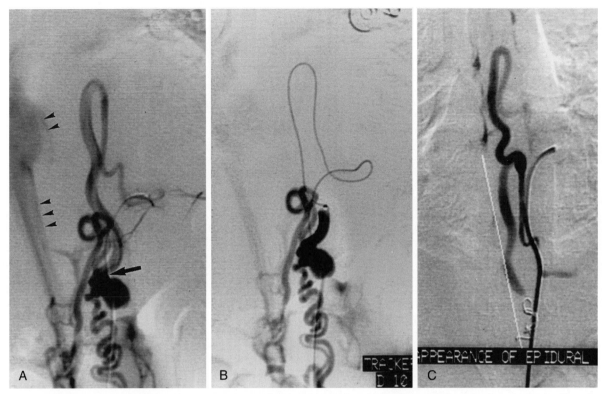

Figure 17-4 Case 4. *A*, AP view of a perimedullary fistula (type III) in a child. The anterior spinal artery is significantly dilated and there is a direct arteriovenous fistula with venous dilation *(arrow)*. Because of the very rapid flow in the malformation, it is possible to see the inferior vena cava as well as the right atrium during this relatively early-phase image *(arrowheads)*. *B*, Superselective catheterization of the ASA was performed using a TRACKER-18 catheter. There is excellent visualization of the shunt site. *C*, The appearance after embolization with Guglielmi detachable platinum coils at the level of the artery and vein. There is total occlusion of the fistula.

SPINAL DURAL ARTERIOVENOUS FISTULAE WITH PERIMEDULLARY VENOUS DRAINAGE

Anatomy

Even though the location of these may be intimately related to the dura, they are distinctly different from the intracranial dural-type AVFs. These are usually single pedicle (150- to 200-micron), small AVFs involving nonradicular branches of spinal arteries.[11] The arterial feeders are small, tortuous arterioles originating from the dura mater. The radicular draining vein is at the level of a spinal nerve root foramen, in contact with the bony pedicle. The shunt is inside the dura matter, usually on the posterolateral aspect.[6, 7, 9]

Clinical Presentation

There is a significant male predominance (5:1) and these patients are usually elderly. The pathophysiology is related to the induced venous hypertension in the cord, with slow, progressive mixed sensory and motor myelopathy. Leg weakness is usually the presenting symptom, followed by sensory disturbances. This may lead to paraplegia within 2 to 4 years if the patient is not treated. Clinical recovery depends on early therapy. Once loss of sphincter control and sexual dysfunction occur, they rarely regress. The sensory deficit is almost never above the T10 level.

Spinal dural fistulas never bleed. The anterior or posterior spinal artery never participates in dural fistulae.[6, 11]

Diagnosis

These AVFs are usually discovered in the midthoracic (T5–T7) and thoracolumbar (T12–L3) regions. Hyperintensity in the conus is seen on T2-weighted MRI sequences.[7, 8, 12] Spinal angiography must document the AVF, the ASA, and the venous drainage of the normal spinal cord. Usually, the point of shunt is below or medial to the pedicle of the corresponding vertebra. The draining vein is almost 10 times larger than the feeding artery. The dilated ascending radicular vein joins the anterior or posterior perimedullary venous system. Ascending venous drainage causes a conus syndrome, while descending drainage causes a cauda equina syndrome.[6] The arterial blood flow is slow and the normal ASA venous drainage is never seen; however, the postembolization reappearance of normal venous drainage is suggestive of successful treatment.

Treatment

The aim of therapy is to isolate the vein draining the fistula from perimedullary veins. This is accomplished by occluding the AVF *and the first 1 to 2 cm of draining vein.*[6]

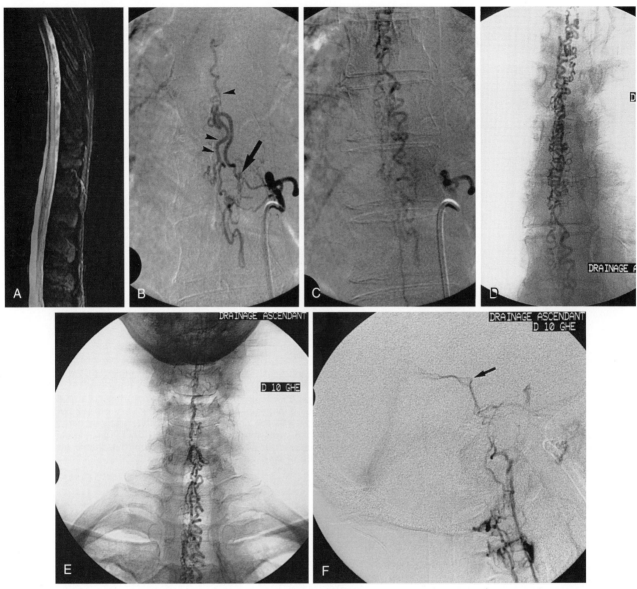

Figure 17-5 Case 5. *A,* A T2-weighted, sagittal view magnetic resonance image (MRI) in a 70-year-old patient with progressive paraparesis reveals increased signal in the spinal cord associated with perimedullary vascularity. These findings suggest a dural fistula with perimedullary venous drainage. *B,* An AP angiographic view reveals a dural fistula with perimedullary venous drainage *(arrowheads)* supplied by the 11th left intercostal artery. The shunt in the dura is seen as a change of caliber between the feeding artery and the venous drainage *(arrow). C,* A delayed image of the same injection reveals a dilated perimedullary venous plexus draining the fistula. *D,* Ascending venous drainage continues to be seen up to the high thoracic level. However, note the absence of radiculomedullary venous drainage all along the thoracic spine. *E,* Venous drainage continues in the cervical region. No lateral venous drainage is seen. *F,* The venous drainage of the T10 dural fistula joins the vein of Rosenthal intracranially *(arrow).*

Surgery

The definitive treatment for a spinal AVF is surgical eradication of the fistulous connection itself, best performed by suture ligation of the arterial vessel(s) and venous vessel(s). As is typical for most interventional neuroradiologic cases, the surgical approach is the problem, or the surgeons would not be seeking help. The role of the interventional neuroradiologist should be to aid the surgeon in accurate identification of the appropriate location to attack and to help control operative bleeding. Typically, the actual AVF

site is microscopic and thus difficult for the surgeon to identify. Eradication of the arterial supply and the venous drainage gives the best chance of a true cure, from either an endovascular or open surgical approach.

Surgery can be offered after failure of endovascular therapy. Selective clipping of the fistula and draining vein in its first 1 to 2 cm is performed.[11]

Embolization

The above-described vascular abnormality may appear relatively straightforward to treat, but this is

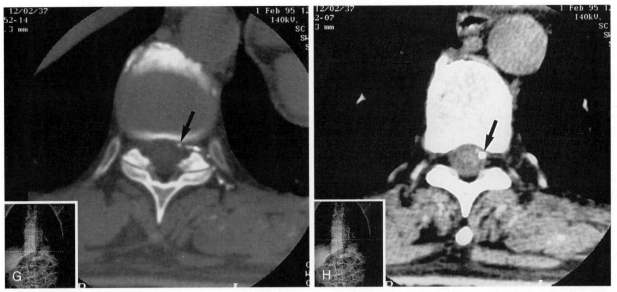

Figure 17-5 *Continued. G,* A postembolization CT scan shows the Histoacryl cast at the level of the fistula *(arrow). H,* A postembolization CT scan at a higher level shows the Histoacryl in the vein *(arrow).* This image confirms a good result of endovascular treatment.

not the case. Any approach is usually extremely tortuous and through very small vessels that branch and reform on their way to the true arterial feeder. Emboli are therefore potentially filtered by more distal branching arterial structures. In addition, these vascular pedicles may supply the cord or other vital structures. Proximal occlusion will not cure the problem and, depending on the embolic agent, may injure the arterial supply to a nerve root or other structure. However, a decrease in arterial input can decrease the venous hypertension causing the neurologic symptoms, help the patient (at least temporarily), and make surgery easier.

Histoacryl is the embolic agent of choice[6]: a mixture of 0.5 ml of Histoacryl plus 1.2 ml Lipiodol plus enough tantalum powder to allow adequate visualization, injected through a TRACKER-18 microcatheter after superselective catheterization. The goal of endovascular therapy is occlusion of the arterial feeder, the actual fistulous communication, and the venous outflow, just as with surgery. Therefore, timing of polymerization is crucial. If the glue hardens in the venous side, worsening of the venous hypertension will occur at a minimum; cord infarction and/or hemorrhage is possible. Embolization is contraindicated if an anterior radiculospinal artery arises from the dorsospinal artery that feeds the fistula (Fig. 17–5).

Venous Thrombosis

If, after embolization or surgery, there is thrombosis of the perimedullary vein, the clinical symptoms may worsen. This may include delayed radiculalgias (1 or 2 days after the procedure). Heparin must be rapidly instituted (2000 units in an intravenous bolus) and maintenance anticoagulation continued for 3 months.

EPIDURAL VASCULAR MALFORMATIONS

Anatomy and Presentation

Epidural vascular malformations are rare lesions, usually seen as part of a metameric syndrome complex. However, occasionally they may be found as isolated lesions. An epidural vascular malformation may be either a single AVF or an AVM nidus located in the epidural compartment. Clinical symptoms are related to venous drainage. If the veins in the intervertebral foramina are prominent, this may cause radicular compression.[7, 8]

Diagnosis

CT may show a tangle of vessels in the epidural space that take up contrast media. MRI both confirms the diagnosis and identifies the location and extent of the lesion.

Spinal angiography reveals the fistula or AVM, fed by either intercostal arteries or lumbar arteries. Venous drainage is to a perimedullary vein.

Treatment

When this vascular malformation is symptomatic, embolization or embolization followed by surgery can be performed.

Embolization

A single, large, high-flow AVF is usually treated by detachable balloon occlusion. If the AVF is very small, it can be effectively treated by Histoacryl as definitive therapy, or with particles preoperatively.

Surgery

After embolization, surgery is performed when flow through a high-flow fistula has considerably reduced.

As stated above, removal of the actual fistulous site itself is necessary, with a small length of arterial side and venous side eradicated.

PARASPINAL VASCULAR MALFORMATIONS

These are uncommon vascular malformations more often found in women. The lesions may be in the spinous process, costovertebral angles, and intercostal spaces.

Diagnosis

CT and MRI offer information about the extent of the lesion, but angiography is indispensable. Aortography provides an overall view of the vascular malformation and its arterial feeders, which may include intercostal, lumbar, or iliolumbar arteries. Angiography also discloses extension of the vascular malformation through nerve root foramina. Venous drainage is to the paraspinal venous plexus, including the azygous and hemiazygous veins. Venous reflux via intraforaminal veins may eventually reach perimedullary veins. The structure of this type of lesion may include a single-hole fistula, a well-defined AVM nidus, or a combination of both.

Treatment

Conservative therapy is offered to patients with clinically asymptomatic lesions. If intervention is deemed necessary, the selection of embolic material depends on the angioarchitecture of the vascular malformation. Embolization with acrylic material may be curative. If embolization is performed preoperatively, PVA particles may be used.

COBB'S SYNDROME

This syndrome consists of metameric AVMs of the spinal canal. These lesions, first described by Cobb, demonstrate varying involvement of dura, vertebrae, muscle, and skin.[6–9]

Clinical Presentation

Superficial angiomatosis is a part of this syndrome and may present as cutaneous angiomas with the typical port-wine stain appearance. These are capillary malformations that present as pink lesions in infancy and gradually darken with age. Discovery of cutaneous angiomas should trigger a search for spinal cord involvement as part of a metameric syndrome. Neurologic symptoms depend on the type, extent, and location of the lesion. Occasionally, spinal subarachnoid hemorrhage has been found, associated with evolution of limb angiomatosis.

Diagnosis

It is important to evaluate all components of the vascular malformation, because they each cause different clinical symptoms.

CT and MRI are the best noninvasive diagnostic tools for evaluation of the extent of the lesion. Angiography confirms the diagnosis and offers details of the angioarchitecture. An aortogram is followed by selective angiography to evaluate each component of the vascular malformation.

Treatment

Complete cure is very difficult. The aim of therapy is symptomatic relief. Embolization, surgery, and percutaneous vertebroplasty may be combined to stabilize or improve the patient's clinical condition.

VERTEBRAL HEMANGIOMAS

Classification and Diagnosis

Vertebral hemangiomas are found in 10% to 15% of autopsies. There are three types[6, 13]:

1. Evolutive or active vertebral hemangiomas
2. Nonevolutive vertebral hemangiomas
3. Intermediate types

Active Hemangiomas

These are often found in young patients and are similar to capillary malformations. They can cause progressive spinal cord compression and are often found at the T3–T9 levels.

On plain films, a prominent trabecular pattern is noted in the vertebral body. Lytic zones are evident. On CT, contrast enhancement of the lesion is seen. The lytic zone is noted to contain soft tissue that extends from the vertebral body to perivertebral tissue and the epidural space. Spinal angiography reveals dilation of the feeding arteries with diffuse contrast opacification of the lesion; however, no early venous drainage is seen.

Nonevolutive Vertebral Hemangiomas

Histologically, these are pure venous malformations with lipid content. Most often, they are in the lumbar region. Prominence of the trabecular pattern in the affected vertebral body is seen on plain films of the spine. CT and MRI show the hemangioma to be localized to the vertebral body, with preservation of the cortical margin. Little enhancement is seen on postcontrast CT scans. The lesion demonstrates predominantly lipid signal characteristics on MRI sequences.

Angiography reveals a normal feeding artery, delayed hypervascularity of the vertebral body, and no early venous drainage.

Intermediate Forms

These are a capillary venous type of hemangioma. Percutaneous biopsy reveals the pathologic diagnosis.

Treatment

Vertebroplasty

This is a procedure to reinforce the involved vertebral body with acrylic cement.[13] It is performed under biplane fluoroscopic control. The patient is generally positioned prone. After local anesthesia is administered, the pedicle is punctured using a 12-gauge needle via a posterior route to enter the vertebral body. Contrast media are injected to judge the speed of flow in the hemangioma. The process is repeated through the other pedicle of the same vertebra. After contrast injection, methacrylate cement is injected. For the cervical region, the patient is in the supine position and the vertebral body is approached via an anterolateral route. See also Chapter 29.

Surgery

Decompressive procedures such as laminectomy and excision of the intracanalicular angiomatous mass can be performed. Presurgical embolization with particles can also be performed to assist the surgeon.

SPINAL CORD TUMORS

Embolization plays a critical role in the overall therapeutic management of spinal neurinomas, meningiomas, and hemangioblastomas. These lesions may present with clinical signs of spinal cord compression. They receive blood supply from the dorsoscapular trunk, radicular arteries, and arteries of the spinal cord.[6, 14]

Neurinomas

These tumors are well demonstrated by MRI. Angiography reveals radicular artery supply, and selective injection shows a vascular blush. Preoperative embolization is useful.

Meningiomas

CT and MRI are diagnostic. Embolization plays an important role if the tumor is in a surgically inaccessible location but otherwise is seldom useful.

Hemangioblastomas

Presurgical embolization is very useful for these. One can usually reach the feeding arteries (anterior or posterior spinal arteries) superselectively with a microcatheter (FasTRACKER-10) and microguidewire (Terumo 10), and the tumor can be embolized using PVA particles.

CONCLUSION

Thanks to constantly improving, safer, and more flexible microcatheters and microguidewires, endovascular therapy for spinal cord vascular malformations has a positive role to play in the overall therapeutic management of these patients, with a direct impact on anatomic and clinical results. Endovascular embolization of some of these lesions has already significantly changed their poor natural history and

offered complete anatomic, as well as clinical, cure. Each case must be reviewed with a multidisciplinary team involving at least neurosurgery, interventional neuroradiology, and neurology.

Further developments in delivery systems, liquid embolic agents, and angiographic resolution will undoubtedly continue to improve the capabilities of endovascular therapy for all types of spinal vascular lesions.

REFERENCES

1. Berenstein A, Lasjaunias P. Surgical Neuroangiography, Vol 5: Endovascular Treatment of Spine and Spinal Cord Lesions. New York: Springer-Verlag, 1992.
2. Houdart E, Gobin YP, Casasco A, et al. A proposed angiographic classification of intracranial arteriovenous fistulae and malformations. *Neuroradiology* 1993;35:381–385.
3. Biondi A, Merland JJ, Hodges JE, et al. Aneurysms of spinal arteries associated with intramedullary arteriovenous malformations. I. Angiographic and clinical aspects. *AJNR* 1992;13:913–322.
4. Biondi A, Merland JJ, Hodges JE, et al. Aneurysms of spinal arteries associated with intramedullary arteriovenous malformations. II. Results of AVM endovascular treatment and hemodynamic considerations. *AJNR* 1992;13:923–931.
5. Biondi A, Merland JJ, Reizine D, et al. Embolization with particles in thoracic intramedullary arteriovenous malformations: long term angiographic and clinical results. *Radiology* 1990;177:651–658.
6. Casasco A, Houdart E, Gobin YP, et al. Embolization of spinal vascular malformations. *Neuroimaging Clin* 1992;2.
7. Hodges JE, Merland JJ, Casasco A, et al. Spinal vascular malformations: endovascular therapy. Published endovascular approach to central nervous system disease. *Neurosurg Clin* 1994;5.
8. Merland JJ, Reizine D, Laurent A, et al. Embolization of spinal cord vascular lesions. In Vinuela F, Halbach VV, Dion JE (eds): Interventional Neuroradiology: Endovascular Therapy of the Central Nervous System. New York: Raven Press, 1992.
9. Anson JA, Khayata MH, Merland JJ. Spinal arteriovenous malformations. Intravascular techniques. In Carter LP, Spetzler RF (eds): Neurovascular Surgery. New York: McGraw-Hill, 1995.
10. Riche MC, Melki JP, Merland JJ. Embolization of spinal cord vascular malformations via the anterior spinal artery. *AJNR* 1983;4:378–381.
11. Mourier KL, Gelbert F, Rey A, et al. Spinal dural arteriovenous malformations with perimedullary drainage. Indications and results of surgery in 30 cases. *Acta Neurochir (Wien)* 100:136–141.
12. Casasco A, Lylyk P, Hodges JE, et al. Percutaneous transvenous catheterization and embolization of vein of Galen aneurysms. *Neurosurgery* 1991;28:260–266.
13. Deramond H, De Buische, Pruvo JP. La vertébroplastie. *Feuillets Radiol* 1990;30:262–268.
14. Aminoff MJ. Spinal Angiomas. Oxford: Blackwell Scientific, 1976.

ADDITIONAL READINGS

Cosgrove GR, Bertrand G, Fontaine S, et al. Cavernous angiomas of the spinal cord. *J Neurosurg* 1988;68:31–36.
Djindjian R, Cophignon J, Rey A, et al. Superselective arteriography embolization by femoral route in neuroradiology: study of 60 cases. *Neuroradiology* 1993;6:132.
Djindjian R, Houdart R, Hurth M. L'Angiographie de la Moelle Epinière, Vol 1. Paris: Masson, 1970.
Fontaine S, Melanson D, Cosgrove R, Bertrand G. Cavernous

hemangiomas of the spinal cord: MR imaging. *Radiology* 1988;166:839–841.

Merland JJ, Reizine D. Malformations vasculaires vertebromédullaires. *Encyl Med Chir* Paris: Radiodiagnostic, 1987.

Merland JJ, Reizine D. Treatment of arteriovenous spinal-cord malformations. *Semin Intervent Radiol* 1987;4:281–290.

Merland JJ, Riche MC, Chiras J. Les fistules artérioveineuses intracanalaires extramédullaires à drainage veineux médullaires. *J Neuroradiol* 1980;7:271–320.

Rees G, Bertrand G, Fontaine S, et al. Cavernous angiomas of the spinal cord. *J Neurosurg* 1988;68:31–36.

Riche MC, Reizine D, Melki JP, Merland JJ. Classification of spinal cord vascular malformations. *Radiat Med* 1985;3:17–24.

Spetzler R, Zabramski J, Fiom R. Management of juvenile spinal AVM's by embolization and operative excision: case report. *J Neurosurg* 1989;70:628–632.

Touho H, Karasawa J, Ohnishi H, et al. Superselective embolization of spinal arteriovenous malformations using the Tracker catheter. *Surg Neurol* 1992;38:85–94.

Willinsky R, terBrugge K, Montanera W, et al. Spinal epidural arteriovenous fistulas: arterial and venous approaches to embolization. *AJNR* 1993;14:812–817.

CHAPTER 18

Endovascular Therapy and Long-Term Results for Intracranial Dural Arteriovenous Fistulae

C. Cognard / E. Houdart / A.E. Casasco / H.S. Jhaveri / R. Chapot / J.-J. Merland

Intracranial dural arteriovenous fistulae (IC-DAVFs) are acquired arteriovenous shunts located inside the dura mater. They account for 10% to 15% of all intracranial arteriovenous lesions. Their arterial supply arises from any and all meningeal branches of the external and internal carotid and vertebral arteries, and rarely from cortical branches. Their presentation and prognosis are highly variable. Almost all symptoms are due to arterialization of the venous system, either dural sinuses (tinnitus, intracranial hypertension), ophthalmic veins (ocular symptoms), or cortical veins (neurologic deficits, seizures, hemorrhages).

Endovascular treatment is particularly tricky. The choice of treatment depends on the natural risk of the disease, which may be estimated for each patient according to the type of venous drainage. The possibilities include abstaining from treatment, manual compression, arterial embolization with particles or glue, sinus occlusion with coils, or even cortical vein embolization. Surgery may be required alone or in combination with endovascular therapy. The therapeutic decision must take into account the potential evolution of the disease, either naturally or after embolization. All interventional neuroradiologists should keep in mind that the venous thrombosis most often at the origin of the fistula may have compromised the permeability of the dural sinuses; cerebral venous drainage must be carefully studied.

ETIOLOGY

Before the mid-1970s, dural arteriovenous fistulae (DAVFs) were considered to be congenital in origin.[1-3]

Occurrences in young children[4,5] and asymptomatic autopsy findings were cited to confirm this idea.[6,7] The higher frequency of DAVFs at the level of the skull base and the tentorium was thought to be due to delay in the development of the external carotid artery territory and to the numerous emissary veins present.[2,8] In 1976 and 1977, respectively, Castaigne et al and Djindjian et al reported cases secondary to cranial trauma, intracranial surgery, and intracranial venous thrombosis.[9,10] Many cases clearly related to various etiologic factors were published thereafter.[11-14] In our 1994 series, we were able to find an undoubted etiologic factor in only 26% of cases.[15] We considered etiologic factors to include angiographically proved thrombophlebitis, neurosurgical procedures, cranial trauma within the year before the onset of symptoms of the DAVF, otitis, sinusitis, phlebitis of the lower extremity, or general surgery (particularly gynecologic) in the week before the onset of symptoms. In some cases of DAVFs due to intracranial thrombophlebitis, however, the first symptoms of the DAVFs occurred a long time after the initial event (in one case, 9 years after the initial thrombophlebitis). In addition, it is well known that venous thrombosis (particularly at the level of the transverse sinus) may be clinically silent or associated with minimal headaches and that the incidence is certainly underestimated.

Thus, it seems clear that DAVFs are acquired lesions related to insult to the dural sinuses, particularly thrombophlebitis. Lasjaunias and Berenstein postulated that since DAVFs are relatively rare and the causative factors are more common, another factor ("underlying dural vascular weakness") should be implicated in the development of DAVFs in addition to the venous obstruction.[16] In summary, the pathophysiology of DAVFs is not fully understood, but they must be considered as a complex disease associating the arteriovenous shunt itself and other sequelae of thrombophlebitis such as dural sinus stenosis or occlusion.

PATHOPHYSIOLOGY

DAVFs have long been regarded as a benign disease compared with brain arteriovenous malformations. However, the first descriptions of intracranial hemorrhage from DAVFs modified this idea and led to the belief that all patients with DAVFs were potentially at risk. First, intracranial hemorrhage was attributed to a pial component. The idea that clinical symptoms could be related to the pattern of venous drainage appeared in the literature in 1972, when Houser et al. correlated angiographic features and clinical symptoms in 28 patients.[8] They concluded that intracranial hemorrhage occurred when the venous drainage was limited to the pial veins and particularly when there was an associated dilated arteriovenous pouch. In their review of 96 previously published cases, Obrador et al. concluded that "involvement of the pial venous system may produce subarachnoid hemorrhages" but also that "increased venous pressure at the torcular region induces headaches and papilledema."[4]

In 1976, Castaigne et al. placed the DAVFs draining into cortical veins into a separate group with a higher risk of intracranial bleeding.[9] A general classification of DAVFs correlating their pattern of venous drainage with the symptoms was then elaborated by Djindjian et al.[10] They assumed that DAVFs draining freely into a sinus produced benign symptoms only, while cortical venous drainage might produce aggressive neurologic symptoms and hemorrhage.

During the 1980s, many papers reported the particular risk of hemorrhage from DAVFs located at the floor of the anterior cranial fossa and at the tentorium cerebelli. Three comprehensive reviews of the literature have been compiled. In 1984, Malik et al. studied 223 previously reported cases and concluded that "lesions related to large dural sinuses are less likely to bleed than lesions with restricted dural outflow."[17] They did not, however, pay attention to other angiographic features, particularly the *pattern* of venous drainage. In 1986, Lasjaunias et al. presented a meta-analysis of 191 cases.[18] They analyzed the mechanism of neurologic manifestations and concluded that "apart from the peripheral cranial nerves palsy due to arterial steal phenomenon, central nervous system symptoms appear to be related to passive venous hypertension."

Finally, in 1990, Awad et al. reviewed 360 cases reported in the literature and 17 of their own cases to compare the angiographic features of 100 aggressive cases with 277 benign ones (they defined aggressive cases as those with hemorrhage or focal neurologic

T A B L E 1 8 - 1	Classification of Djindjian and Merland According to Venous Drainage
Types	**Patterns of Venous Drainage**
Type I	Drainage into a sinus, with a normal antegrade flow direction
Type II	Drainage into a sinus with insufficient antegrade venous drainage and reflux into other sinuses: IIa: into sinus(es) only IIb: into cortical vein(s) only IIa + b: into sinus(es) and cortical vein(s)
Type III	Direct drainage into a cortical vein without venous ectasia
Type IV	Drainage into a cortical vein with a venous ectasia
Type V	Drainage into spinal perimedullary veins

deficit and benign cases as others, even those with papilledema and increased intracranial pressure).[19] They concluded that leptomeningeal venous drainage, variceal or aneurysmal venous dilation, and galenic drainage correlated significantly with aggressive neurologic signs. They further stated that no location of DAVF was immune to aggressive neurologic behavior.

CLASSIFICATION ACCORDING TO THE TYPE OF VENOUS DRAINAGE AND IMPLICATIONS

We have published a series of 205 consecutive patients with DAVFs who were seen at our institutions within an 18-year period. Our purpose was to complete and validate the Djindjian and Merland classification of DAVFs as proposed in 1977.[10] The revisited classification of Djindjian and Merland is given in Table 18–1. The aim of this classification is to be able to predict the risk of any DAVF in order to make a better-informed decision regarding treatment. Because our series was quite large, we were able to statistically correlate our classification with aggressive neurologic behavior (Table 18–2). The therapeu-

| T A B L E   1 8 - 2 | Frequency of Symptoms According to Type of Venous Drainage |

	I	IIa	IIb	IIa + b	III	IV	V
Hemorrhage			2	1	10	19	5
Intracranial hypertension	1	8	1	2		4	
Deficit				6	8	2	1
Seizure		1		2	1	3	
Cardiac deficiency		1		1			
Myelopathy							
Nonaggressive symptoms	83	17	7	6	6	1	6
Total	84	27	10	18	25	29	12

T A B L E 1 8 - 3 **Clinical Risks and Therapeutic Plans Depending on Types of Venous Drainage**

Types	Clinical Risk	Treatment
I	Functional symptoms No neurologic risk	Goal: reduction of flow No treatment Vascular compression Arterial embolizations (particles or glue)
IIa	Intracranial hypertension (visual prognostic) 20% Lumbar puncture and lumboperitoneal shunts contraindicated	Goal: reduction of flow Arterial embolizations (particles or glue) Sinus occlusion
IIb, IIa + b	Bleeding risk 10% Focal neurologic deficits	Goal: complete cure Sinus occlusion
III–V	Bleeding risk 40% in type III, 65% in type IV Focal neurologic deficits Myelopathy	Goal: complete cure Endovascular treatment, arterial or venous (catheterization of cortical veins) Neurosurgery

tic implications of the classification are summarized in Table 18–3.

Type I

These DAVFs drain into a sinus with a normal, antegrade flow direction (Figs. 18–1 and 18–2). These fistulae always have "benign" behavior and present with functional symptoms such as tinnitus, retroauricular pain, or ocular symptoms. Nevertheless, the status of the other main dural sinuses and the cerebral venous drainage pattern have to be carefully studied. In one of our cases, a type I DAVF of the transverse sinus produced symptoms of intracranial hypertension because it was draining via the only functional sinus. Treatment in these DAVFs is justified by the functional symptoms, which may be very disturbing to the patient. Because of the total absence of neurologic risk related to these fistulae, the treatment itself has to be risk free.

Type IIa

Type IIa DAVFs drain into a sinus with insufficient or absent antegrade venous drainage and reflux into other sinuses (Figs. 18–3 and 18–4). The reflux is most often due to stenosis or thrombosis downstream to the fistula (Fig. 18–3) but may be due to an extremely high-flow fistula associated with a normal, patent sinus (Fig. 18–4). Symptoms of intracranial hypertension, such as headaches, transient visual disturbances, decreased visual acuity, and diplopia (due to cranial nerve VI palsy), were present in 20% of the type IIa fistulae in our series, along with either bilateral papilledema or optic disc atrophy seen on funduscopic examination.

Pathophysiology of Intracranial Hypertension

Kuhner et al. and Tomsick et al. postulated that the mechanism of intracranial hypertension in dural fistulae is increased pressure in the dural sinuses, leading to decreased cerebrospinal fluid (CSF) resorption.[20, 21] Lamas et al. showed that increased pressure in the superior sagittal sinus is directly related to the flow rate through the fistula into the sinus; in one patient, decreasing the flow rate by embolization normalized the pressure within the sinus.[22]

CSF resorption is a passive phenomenon, roughly depending on the following equation:

$$\text{CSF resorption} \cong \text{CSF pressure} - \text{superior sagittal sinus pressure/resistance to outflow}$$

Thus, an increase in sinus pressure lowers CSF resorption, which in turn leads to increased intracranial pressure. The increase in intracranial pressure restores the gradient across the villi.

Dangers of Lumbar Puncture or Shunting

Five cases in our series were particularly illustrative of the consequences of the pressure gradient between the sinus and the CSF. The altered equilibrium may be further modified by arterial embolization (for the better) or by lumbar puncture or shunting (for the worse). In two of the patients, asymptomatic chronic tonsillar herniation improved after embolization. The herniation was observed over a period of 15 and 16 years, respectively. After endovascular treatment, the lowered arterial (and thus sinus) pressure resulted in decreased intracranial pressure and a decreased degree of herniation.

Three patients, on the other hand, experienced acute clinical deterioration. Two of these had high-flow fistulae, followed for 3 and 8 years, respectively. The fistulae were complex, with multiple feeders. Arterial embolization in these cases resulted in a temporary clinical improvement (approximately 1 month in each case). Lumbar shunting was performed in these cases because of acute loss of visual acuity. After the shunting procedure, one patient died because of acute tonsillar herniation and resultant brainstem compression and respiratory compromise. The other became comatose shortly after the shunt procedure. Removal of the shunt resulted in the patient regaining consciousness. The third patient acutely deteriorated after a diagnostic lumbar puncture, experiencing profound confusion, hallucinations, and mild aphasia. One week later, after three sessions of endovascular treatment, the patient was asymptomatic.

The mechanism of the deterioration in these cases is believed to be that the rapid decrease in intraspinal CSF pressure induces acute herniation.

Angiographic Evaluation

DAVFs secondary to sinus thrombosis may involve not only the parent sinus but also other sinuses. The fistula itself and arterialization of the sinus(es) may

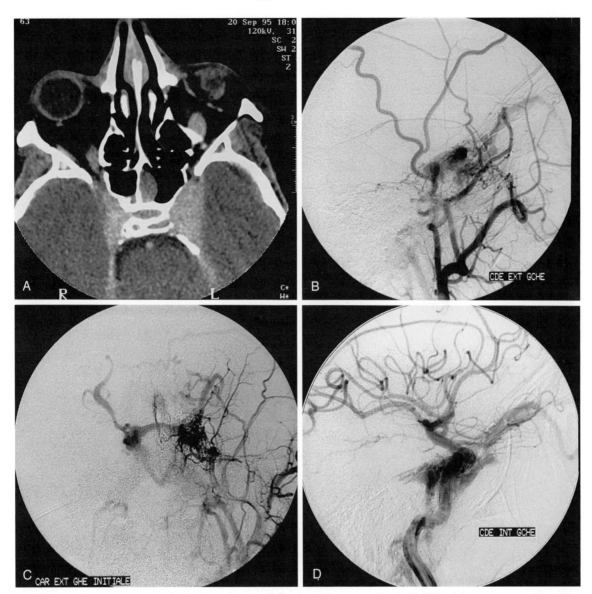

Figure 18-1 Case 1. Venous embolization of a type I dural arteriovenous fistula (DAVF) of the cavernous sinus. The patient presented with a 6-month history of sphenoid sinusitis and an acute onset of ocular symptoms, including bilateral chemosis, left oculomotor palsy, and proptosis. *A*, Computed tomographic (CT) scan shows an enlarged left cavernous sinus and left superior ophthalmic vein dilation. External carotid artery (ECA) *(B, C)* and internal carotid artery (ICA) *(D)* injections reveal a left cavernous sinus DAVF fed by numerous meningeal branches arising from the ECA and the ICA siphon. The venous drainage is ipsilateral, anteriorly in the left superior ophthalmic vein and in the inferior petrosal sinus. The contralateral venous drainage passes through the circular sinus into the right superior ophthalmic vein and in the right inferior petrosal sinus. The best treatment is venous embolization with coils. Embolization was performed through the left internal jugular vein and inferior petrosal sinus.

Illustration continued on following page

induce secondary lesions in the sinus wall.[23-27] Thus, three main factors influence venous drainage: (1) the initial thrombophlebitis and resultant sinus wall lesion, (2) arterialization of the sinus due to the fistula, and (3) secondary sinus wall lesions due to the increased flow. The best demonstration of these hemodynamic changes in the venous pathways is angiographic evaluation of cerebral venous drainage. Angiographic examination, with contrast injection into the contralateral internal carotid and vertebral arteries, is obligatory in order to accurately assess cerebral venous drainage. In all of our patients with intracranial hypertension, the cerebral venous drainage was abnormal, with prolongation of both the parenchymal and venous outflow phases. In our opinion, type IIa fistulae can be defined as fistulae with abnormal venous drainage, predisposing to intracranial hypertension and its complications.

Indications for Treatment

The decision to treat type IIa DAVFs is based not on the presence of disturbing functional symptoms, but on the risk of visual impairment. Long-term type IIa DAVFs may result in dramatic visual loss. The goal

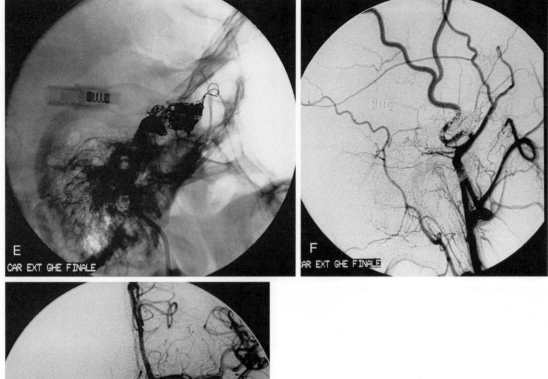

Figure 18-1 *Continued.* Dense packing of coils was achieved in the cavernous sinus *(E)*, leading to a complete angiographic cure *(F, G)* and rapid improvement of ocular symptoms.

of treatment is to reduce the flow through the fistula enough to allow normalization of cerebral venous drainage and intracranial pressure. Thus, a complete cure of the fistula is not mandated if treatment is too risky. Arterial embolization of the external carotid artery feeders, reducing the flow, may be sufficient. More aggressive treatment, with sinus occlusion, is not frequently required and must be performed very carefully.

Type IIb or IIa + IIb

DAVFs of types IIb to IV drain into cortical veins and thus are associated with a higher risk of hemorrhage; this risk increases from type IIb to type IV. Fistulae of type IIb or type IIa + IIb drain into a sinus with insufficient or absent antegrade flow and thus reflux into cortical veins as well as other sinuses. Intracranial hemorrhage was observed in 10% of the patients in our series with these types of fistulae; focal neurologic symptoms were observed in 29%. The risk of

hemorrhage or progressive neurologic dysfunction requires a complete and durable cure of the fistula in these cases. In most such cases, the best treatment is occlusion of the sinus with coils.

Types III and IV

These DAVFs drain directly into cortical vein(s) without (type III) or with (type IV) venous ectasia. These lesions are usually located at the tentorium cerebelli or the anterior cranial fossa but can also involve major sinuses. In these cases, the DAVF lies in the dura of the sinus. However, instead of draining into the sinus, it drains into a cortical vein. The sinus itself is often patent and may or may not secondarily drain the DAVF.[24] In our cases, the presence of an ectatic venous segment (>5 mm in diameter) increased the risk of bleeding from 40% to 65%. Neurologic symptoms were observed in 76% and 96% of cases, respectively. A complete and durable cure of the fistula is required; subtotal occlusion may produce rebleeding.

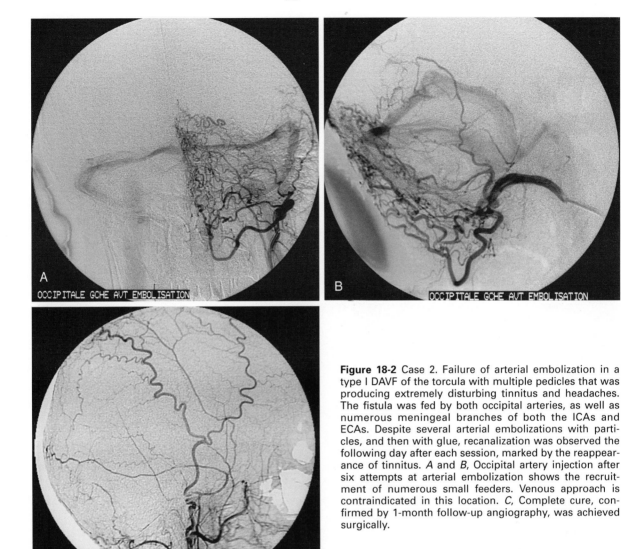

Figure 18-2 Case 2. Failure of arterial embolization in a type I DAVF of the torcula with multiple pedicles that was producing extremely disturbing tinnitus and headaches. The fistula was fed by both occipital arteries, as well as numerous meningeal branches of both the ICAs and ECAs. Despite several arterial embolizations with particles, and then with glue, recanalization was observed the following day after each session, marked by the reappearance of tinnitus. *A* and *B*, Occipital artery injection after six attempts at arterial embolization shows the recruitment of numerous small feeders. Venous approach is contraindicated in this location. *C*, Complete cure, confirmed by 1-month follow-up angiography, was achieved surgically.

Type V

These fistulae drain into spinal veins.[28–33] The pathophysiologic mechanism of the spinal symptoms is spinal cord venous hypertension. In fact, in our series of 12 patients with type V DAVFs, the six who presented with a myelopathy had extensive, slow-flow spinal perimedullary venous drainage descending to the thoracic cord. The other six, who presented without myelopathy (five with hemorrhages and one with a focal neurologic deficit), had spinal venous drainage limited to the cervical cord; a cervical radiculomedullary vein drained the arterialized flow from the DAVF into the epidural space, thus preventing spinal cord hypertension and myelopathy. This type of fistula has the same risk of neurologic deficit and hemorrhage as a type III or IV fistula, and must be treated the same way. This type of fistula has been placed in a separate category because the neuroradiologist looking for a spinal dural AVF in a patient with progressive myelopathy must keep in mind

these peculiar intracranial DAVFs and perform cerebral angiography if the spinal angiogram is normal.

LOCATION

The most common locations of DAVFs in our large series were the transverse sinus (50%), the cavernous sinus (16%), the tentorium cerebelli (12%), and the superior sagittal sinus (8%). Many reports in the literature have noted the high frequency of neurologic symptoms and bleeding when these lesions are located at the tentorium cerebelli, the anterior cranial fossa, or the superior sagittal sinus.[17, 19, 34–37] This was particularly evident in our study; the bleeding risk was 62% for DAVFs of the anterior cranial fossa, 58% for those at the tentorium, 44% for those in the torcular region, and only 24% for those at the transverse sinus (Table 18–4). However, if only types III and IV DAVFs are considered, there was no statistical difference in the frequency of bleeding according to the location. This may be because benign symp-

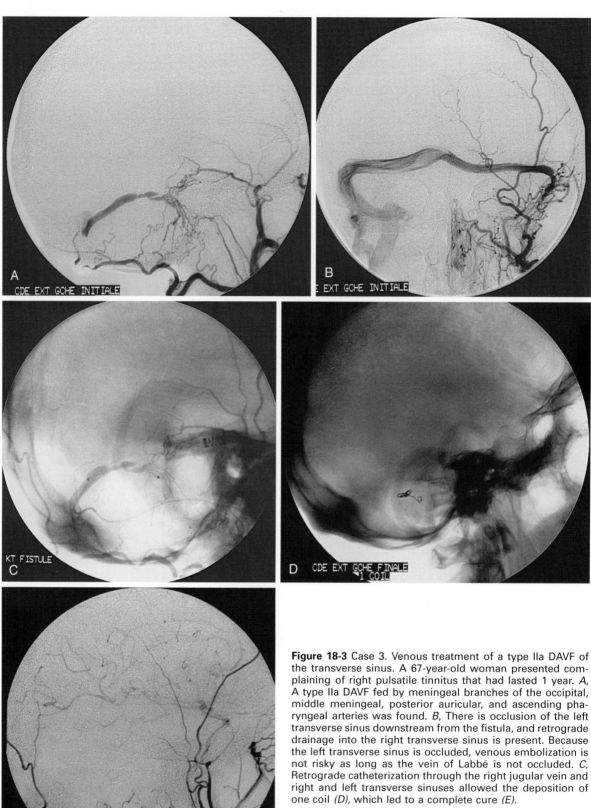

Figure 18-3 Case 3. Venous treatment of a type IIa DAVF of the transverse sinus. A 67-year-old woman presented complaining of right pulsatile tinnitus that had lasted 1 year. *A,* A type IIa DAVF fed by meningeal branches of the occipital, middle meningeal, posterior auricular, and ascending pharyngeal arteries was found. *B,* There is occlusion of the left transverse sinus downstream from the fistula, and retrograde drainage into the right transverse sinus is present. Because the left transverse sinus is occluded, venous embolization is not risky as long as the vein of Labbé is not occluded. *C,* Retrograde catheterization through the right jugular vein and right and left transverse sinuses allowed the deposition of one coil *(D),* which led to a complete cure *(E).*

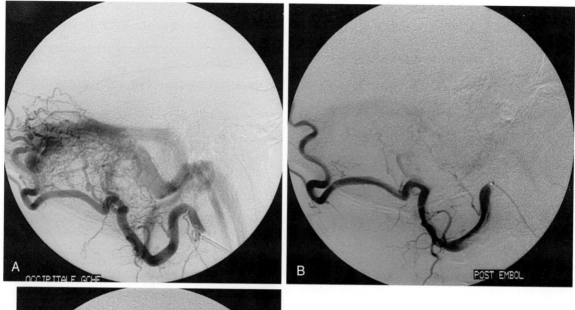

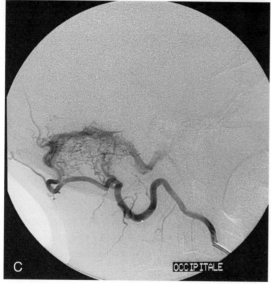

Figure 18-4 Case 4. Failure of particulate embolization in a type IIa DAVF of the transverse sinus. This patient presented with a moderately disturbing left pulsatile tinnitus. Doppler examination revealed increased left ECA velocity. *A,* Angiography reveals a left type IIa DAVF, fed mostly by the left occipital artery. Venous drainage was antegrade through the ipsilateral jugular vein and retrograde into the right transverse sinus. *B,* Embolization of the occipital artery with particles resulted in an incomplete cure, with moderate improvement of the functional symptoms. The fistula was still fed by a few small feeders from the ECA meningeal branches. *C,* The tinnitus reappeared 2 weeks later owing to reopening of the shunts. A venous approach was not undertaken because the left transverse sinus was patent and used by the normal cerebral drainage, and because the tinnitus was only moderately disturbing.

T A B L E 1 8 - 4   Frequency of Symptoms According to Location

	Hemorrhages	ICH*	Focal Deficit or Seizure	Myelopathy	Nonaggressive Symptoms
Transverse sinus	6	9	9	1	74
Torcular	4	2	3		
Superior sagittal sinus	4	2	5		6
Anterior cranial fossa	5		2		1
Deep venous system		1			
Tentorium cerebelli	14	2	4	2	2
Cavernous sinus					33
Superior petrosal sinus	1		1	3	2
Foramen jugulare					4
Foramen magnum	3				
Total	37	16	24	6	122

*Intracranial hypertension.

T A B L E 1 8 - 5   Type of Venous Drainage Encountered in Each Location

	I	IIa	IIb	IIa + b	III	IV	V
Transverse sinus	48	24	4	11	7	4	1
Torcular		1	1	2	1	3	1
Superior sagittal sinus	3	2	2	2	4	4	
Anterior cranial fossa					3	5	
Deep venous system						1	
Tentorium cerebelli					9	10	5
Cavernous sinus	29		3	1			
Superior petrosal sinus				2	1	1	3
Foramen jugulare	4						
Foramen magnum						1	2
Total	84	27	10	18	25	29	12

toms such as tinnitus or retroauricular pain herald the presence of DAVFs of the transverse sinus before they behave aggressively (Table 18–5).

The presence or absence of aggressive symptoms varies with the location of the DAVF because anatomy dictates the type of venous drainage most often encountered in each location. However, it is important to note that in comparing DAVFs of the same type, location does not influence the risk of hemorrhage.

THERAPEUTIC APPROACHES

Abstinence

Type I fistulae may not need treatment if the functional symptoms are not disturbing and if the cerebral venous drainage is normal. However, the patient must be made aware that any change in symptoms such as increased or decreased tinnitus, headaches, retroauricular pain, vertigo, or visual disturbance requires a new evaluation. Repeat angiography or Doppler evaluation of flow velocity should be performed.

Arterial Compression

This approach is not frequently proposed today but may be useful in the treatment of type I or IIa asymptomatic fistulae. Compression of the carotid artery (or even occipital artery) must be performed with the contralateral hand with increasing duration (from 10 to 30 seconds) and frequency (four to six times an hour). Compressions are performed by the patient while lying down or sitting to avoid possible trauma secondary to a vagal episode. Ocular compressions may be performed for DAVFs of the cavernous sinus. The treatment is safe and may occasionally occlude the fistula or improve the symptoms. Halbach et al reported a complete cure in 22% of their cases and clinical improvement in 33%.[38] The

presence of severe atherosclerotic disease is a contraindication to this technique.

Arterial Embolization with Particles

Indications for and Aim of Particulate Embolization

In treating types I and IIa fistulae, the aim is to achieve a complete cure. If this is not possible, therapy should be aimed at reducing the flow and thus decreasing or eliminating functional symptoms. With type IIa lesions, disappearance of the reflux into adjacent sinuses and decrease in symptoms of intracranial hypertension are the goals. Treatment can be repeated if needed. In the treatment of type IIb or IIa + b fistulae, arterial embolization with particles should be attempted before any consideration of occlusion of the sinus (which should be considered only when arterial embolization is unsuccessful). Embolization is frequently employed before surgical management of a DAVF; the goal is to decrease the intraoperative blood loss from the numerous arterial feeders and arterialized draining veins.

General Technique

We perform embolization with particles with the patient under general anesthesia, if possible, to allow better control during injection of particles and better visualization of reflux and potentially dangerous anastomoses. A 5- or 6-Fr. guide catheter is placed in the distal common carotid artery. Selective catheterization of the external carotid artery with the guide catheter is not necessary; it may decrease the flow in the feeding arteries of the DAVF and may induce spasm in the artery.

Microcatheterization of the external carotid artery feeders is performed with the help of roadmapping. The microcatheter is placed at the origin of the artery (middle meningeal, occipital, ascending pharyngeal, posterior auricular, or superficial temporal artery) to maintain good flow in the pedicle and avoid spasm induced by distal catheterization. We use a MAG 3-Fr.-2-Fr. catheter (Balt Extrusion) shaped with steam and a 0.016″ microguidewire (Terumo 16, Terumo Corp., Tokyo, Japan). Polyvinyl alcohol particles are used and injected under fluoroscopic observation. We use Contour Emboli (ITC/Target Therapeutics), generally in the 150- to 250-micron size.

If possible, all external carotid artery feeders are embolized to obtain the most complete devascularization. The more complete the embolization, the greater is the probability of a durable cure. It is not necessary to embolize the meningeal feeders arising from the internal carotid artery or vertebral artery. This is dangerous and the expected benefit does not justify the risk.

Important Procedural Considerations

Careful assessment for anatomic variants and thorough assessment of overall ophthalmic vascularization must be made before embolization of the middle meningeal artery. Checks for potentially dangerous arterial anastomoses must be made before and during embolization. Anastomoses between the occipital and vertebral arteries may appear and enlarge rapidly during embolization. The presence of anastomoses between the ascending pharyngeal, middle meningeal, and/or internal maxillary artery and the internal carotid artery must be excluded before embolization of these branches.

It is most important to maintain a good flow and particularly to avoid spasm in the feeding pedicle. Injection should not be performed when there is stasis within the pedicle. Cranial nerve palsies are extremely rare after embolization with particles greater than 150 microns in size.

Postoperative Management

Corticosteroids are given for 48 hours (dexamethasone, 4 mg every 4 hours). Analgesics are administered as needed for pain. A thorough clinical assessment is made after the procedure to document improvement in symptoms such as decrease in tinnitus, ptosis, or chemosis. Patients must be aware that any recurrence of symptoms mandates immediate clinical assessment (and usually angiographic evaluation). A control angiogram is generally obtained 2 to 3 months after the procedure.

Variability of Response to Therapy

The natural history and response to therapy of DAVFs are highly variable. In rare cases, they may disappear spontaneously (in one case in our series, during an airplane flight) or after carotid compression. In some cases, thorough embolization effects a definitive cure. On the other hand, some DAVFs are extremely difficult to treat; rapid reappearance of tinnitus and recanalization may be observed on angiography despite very efficient embolization (Figs. 18–2 and 18–4). The pathophysiology of DAVFs is not fully understood, but it appears that some are in a quiescent or even regressive phase, while others are in an evolving phase. Poor prognosis is associated with multiple pedicles (sometimes bilateral), large feeders arising from the internal carotid artery or vertebral artery, and incomplete embolization. Partial arterial occlusion frequently leads to recruitment of other feeding arteries or recanalization of embolized vessels.

Arterial Embolization with Glue

Indications for and Aim of Embolization with Glue

The ideal setting for embolization with glue is a type III to V fistula with few feeding pedicles (Figs. 18–5 and 18–6). The aim of treatment is to obtain a complete, definitive cure. In these cases, it is acceptable to perform embolization of the internal carotid artery and vertebral artery feeders. Type I or IIa fistulae that are not amenable to treatment with particles may be treated with glue if the tinnitus is extremely disturbing (Fig. 18–2) or in cases of intracranial hypertension.

It is sometimes difficult to choose between arterial embolization with glue and sinus occlusion in the setting of failure of arterial embolization with particles. Arterial embolization with glue may be extremely difficult to perform in cases of fistulae with multiple pedicles. Several procedures may be required, each associated with a not insignificant risk. Sinus occlusion, on the other hand, does achieve significant flow reduction, if not a cure, in one session.

General Technique

General anesthesia is required, as in embolization with particles. The guide catheter is again positioned in the common carotid artery during embolization of external carotid artery branches; it is positioned proximally in the vertebral artery or internal carotid artery during embolization of feeders arising from these vessels.

The microcatheter we use most often is a TRACKER-10 or TRACKER-18 (Target Therapeutics). If hydrophilic coating is required, the Fas-TRACKER (Target Therapeutics) or Slipstream (Medtronic/MIS) is used. A flow-directed catheter is sometimes advantageous; we use the Magic 1.8-Fr. (Balt Extrusion) or Ultralite (Medtronic/MIS), with a 0.010″ Terumo wire.

The microcatheter must be advanced as far distally as possible. Glue should be injected only if catheterization is distal enough to allow good control of flow (Figs. 18–5 and 18–6). The aim of the injection is to reach the shunt itself and the origin of the draining vein. Proximal injection in the feeding pedicle that does not reach the shunt and veins is absolutely to be avoided; it invariably results in recanalization and makes further treatment extremely difficult.

Injection of glue must be performed under high-resolution fluoroscopic guidance, very slowly and with minimal injection pressure. We use N-butyl-2-cyanoacrylate (NBCA) (Histoacryl, B. Braun Melsungen A.G.) diluted with Lipiodol (Andre Guerbert, Aulnay sous Bois, France). Our usual mixture is one third Histoacryl and two-thirds Lipiodol, but this may vary with the degree of flow control obtained by the microcatheterization. The glue is delivered via a 3-cc Luer-Lok syringe. At the end of the injection, it is important to aspirate slowly before rapidly withdrawing the guide catheter and microcatheter together.

Technical Considerations

The interventionist must keep in mind that glue injection is more dangerous than particulate injection. The main risk lies in forcing glue into an anastomosis between the internal and external carotid arteries, most of which are not visible on preembolization angiograms. Thus, one must know the anatomy and potentially dangerous anastomoses of the vessel in which one is working. Injection of glue must be slow and pressureless to avoid opening these anastomoses. It is also important not to allow glue to reflux, thereby gluing the catheter in place.

In most cases, treatment is performed under gen-

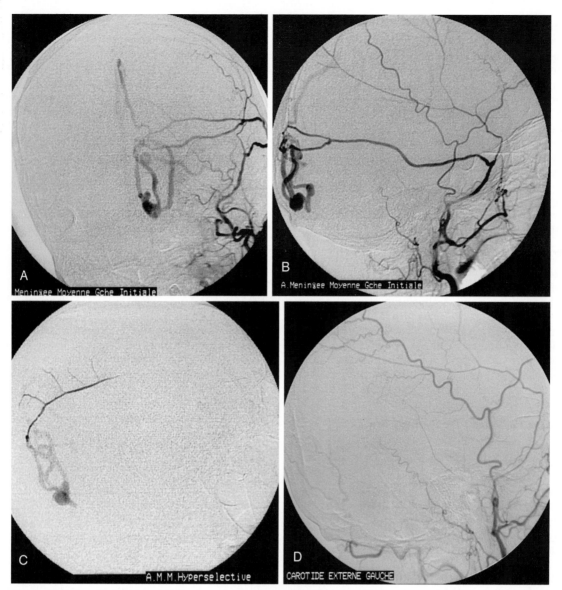

Figure 18-5 Case 5. Arterial embolization of a type III DAVF with glue. The presence of a type III DAVF of the superior sagittal sinus was heralded by subarachnoid hemorrhage in this patient. *A* and *B*, The fistula was fed mainly by the middle meningeal artery. It drained into a cortical vein with some ectasia, then into two veins joining the superior sagittal sinus. *C*, Catheterization of the middle meningeal artery resulted in good control of flow. *D*, Injection of *N*-butyl-2-cyanoacrylate (NBCA) yielded penetration of the fistula and a complete cure.

eral anesthesia, so provocative testing with lidocaine is not performed (this may yield false-positive or false-negative results).

External carotid artery feeders may be extremely difficult to catheterize because of tortuosity (especially involving the occipital artery). Most of the time, navigation of these tortuous feeders is easier with a flow-directed catheter.

Postoperative Management

Corticosteroids are given for 48 hours, as described previously. Analgesics are administered if needed.

Sinus Occlusion with Coils

Indications for Sinus Occlusion

The best indication for this procedure is a type IIb fistula with occlusion of the sinus on both sides of

the fistula and reflux into cortical veins. These fistulae are tricky and require complete treatment. The sinus and cortical veins are hemodynamically excluded and occlusion is safe. However, sinus catheterization may be very tricky.

Type IIa high-flow fistulae may produce devastating intracranial hypertension. It may be impossible to reduce the flow enough with arterial embolization in cases of fistulae with multiple pedicles. Sinus occlusion may definitively occlude the fistula or produce a dramatic decrease in the flow and reflux in the main sinuses, with consequent clinical improvement.

General Technique

The aim of venous embolization is to occlude the draining sinus with coils (Figs. 18–1 and 18–3). This usually allows a complete cure of the fistula or at

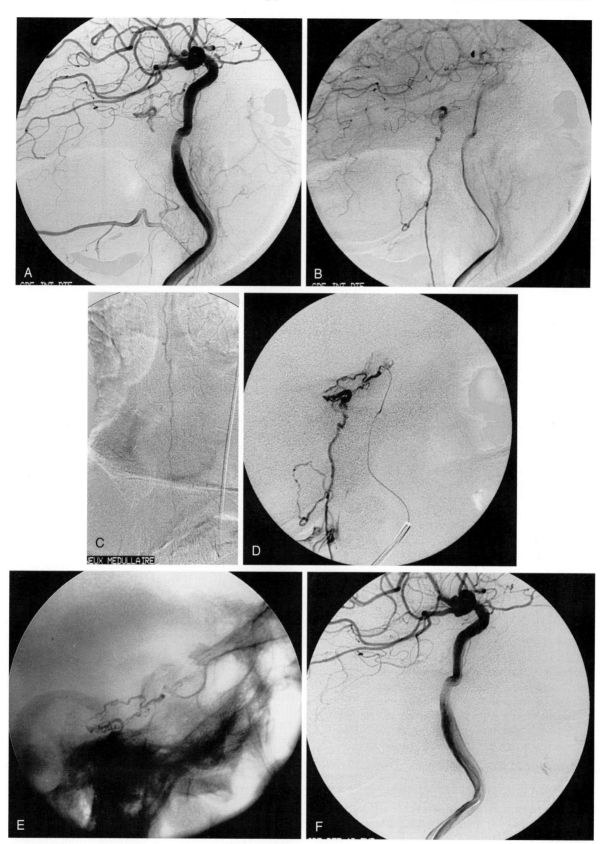

Figure 18-6 Case 6. Arterial embolization of a type V DAVF with glue. A 75-year-old man presented with a progressive history of lower limb weakness associated with sphincter disturbance. Magnetic resonance imaging revealed mildly increased signal intensity in the conus on T2-weighted images. Spinal angiography was normal except for delayed venous drainage of the artery of Adamkiewicz. *A* to *C,* Right ICA injection demonstrated a type V DAVF fed by the meningohypophyseal trunk, draining into a lateral mesencephalic and medullary descending vein. *D,* Superselective catheterization of the meningohypophyseal trunk yielded good flow control. *E,* Injection of NBCA resulted in a complete cure (*F*) and clinical improvement.

least a significant decrease in flow.[39–41] The interventional neuroradiologist faces two main challenges: to reach the sinus, which may be extremely tricky, and to ensure that sinus occlusion is safe.

A complete angiogram must be obtained to analyze the precise extension of the fistula along the sinus and to determine the site at which the sinus must be occluded. A 5-Fr. diagnostic catheter is left in the common carotid artery to facilitate roadmapping during venous catheterization and deposition of coils, and to evaluate the progress of the embolization. The procedure may be performed via a femoral or internal jugular venous approach. The femoral approach is more comfortable for the operator, and it allows approach through the contralateral internal jugular vein when the fistula cannot be reached via the ipsilateral vein. The main disadvantage is that catheterization of the sigmoid sinus may be difficult because of looping of the catheter in the right atrium. A 5- or 6-Fr. rigid guide catheter with a floppy tip must be used in these cases (FasGUIDE). Microcatheterization of the site of the fistula is then performed, and the sinus is occluded with coils. It is better to use detachable coils than pushable coils when they must be deposited precisely, for example, close to the origin of a cortical vein (vein of Labbé). Mechanically detachable coils (Target Therapeutics, Balt Extrusion) may be used, which are cheaper than GDC coils (Target Therapeutics). Standard coils may be used when the sinus is occluded on one or both sides and when embolization is safe. A large number of coils is often required to obtain a dense packing and to completely occlude the sinus. Sometimes, occlusion may be completed with Histoacryl and Lipiodol (50%/50% mixture). This must be injected very carefully to avoid reflux into the cortical veins or adjacent sinus.

When there is thrombosis of the sinus downstream to the fistula, the site can be reached either by recanalization of the sinus or by contralateral jugular vein catheterization (Fig. 18–3). Recanalization of thrombosed sinuses is often possible. It may be achieved either with the 5-Fr. guide catheter and a hydrophilic-coated 0.035″ guidewire or with the microcatheter. Sometimes, it is not possible to reach the sinus because it is occluded on both sides of the fistula with organized clot. The sinus may be approached by direct puncture either through a burr hole placed previously or at the time of the procedure. A 16-gauge intravenous-type catheter is used, through which the microcatheter is advanced.

Technical Considerations

The venous drainage of the fistula and the venous drainage of the brain must be carefully studied and compared. Occlusion of the sinus may have several consequences:

1. One of the main paths of drainage of the brain may be occluded. *It must be established whether the brain uses this sinus before occlusion.* In type I fistulae, occlusion should not be performed if the brain uses this sinus for drainage

(Fig. 18–4). In high-flow fistulae, when the arterialized sinus is hemodynamically excluded, occlusion may be performed.

2. Occlusion of the sinus may have terrible consequences when cortical veins drain into the sinus near the fistula. Common carotid artery injection allows precise analysis of the venous drainage of the fistula during the early phase and the cerebral venous drainage during the late phase. *When a cortical vein drains into the sinus, occlusion must not be performed or (in the case of partial treatment) performed beyond the origin of the vein.* An occlusion test with a nondetachable balloon may be performed to evaluate clinical tolerance of vein occlusion or to precisely locate the entrance of the vein into the sinus (cortical veins may run along the sinus for a distance before opening into it). In one patient with a superior sagittal sinus fistula, a transient hemiplegia occurred, indicating that occlusion was not possible. The accuracy of balloon test occlusion in predicting the occurrence of postprocedural deficits is not known.

3. If embolization of a sinus involves the jugular bulb, transient (or permanent) lower cranial nerve deficits can occur. There may be persistent cochlear or labyrinthine abnormalities due to endolymphatic hydrops. This is particularly true if the cavernous and inferior petrosal sinuses are compromised because of preexisting pathology involving these structures. This yields a very limited range of drainage paths for the brainstem, pons, and inner ear structures.

In addition to careful analysis of the cortical venous drainage into the transverse sinus (particularly the vein of Labbé), it should be remembered that the cerebellum also drains into the transverse sinuses. There may be nowhere else for the cerebellar hemispheres to drain if there is compromise of the cavernous sinus. It may be very difficult to identify accurately the normal venous drainage from the cerebellum because of abundant filling from supratentorial structures (from the posterior cerebral arteries) and the low total volume of flow from the cerebellar hemispheres. Before occlusion of a transverse sinus is considered, normal drainage of the posterior fossa into the sinus must be ruled out.

Test occlusion of a transverse sinus is technically difficult and potentially unrewarding. If test occlusion of the sinus is performed, the distal lumen of the catheter can be connected to a pressure transducer. If a "sawtooth" pattern is seen, this is predictive of venous hypertension (the sawtooth pattern is evidence of pulsatile pressure). Clinically, the patient may describe a feeling of "fullness" during the test occlusion, also indicative of developing intrasinus venous hypertension. The exact meaning of these findings is not clear, but early experience has indicated them to be possibly ominous.

Postoperative Management

Corticosteroids are given for 48 hours, as discussed previously, along with analgesic if needed. Intravenous heparin is administered for 48 hours, to keep the activated clotting time two to three times above control. Low-molecular-weight heparinoids are then administered for 5 days (Fraxiparine, 0.3 ml twice a day).

Venous Embolization with Glue

Retrograde catheterization and embolization with glue have been performed in a few cases.[42] Catheterization of the draining sinus is performed with a 5-Fr. guide catheter, and the vein in question is catheterized in a retrograde fashion from its entrance into the sinus to the point of the fistula with a flow-directed microcatheter. The aim is to occlude the source of the draining vein, yielding complete cure of the fistula. Unfortunately, this approach is rarely possible. It may be performed in single-shunt types III and IV fistulae when a large, not too tortuous draining vein allows access to the fistulous site.

SPECIFIC TREATMENT CONSIDERATIONS RELATING TO LOCATION OF THE FISTULA

Anterior Cranial Fossa Dural Arteriovenous Fistulae

These fistulae are rare and are always type III or IV. They are fed by the ipsilateral ethmoidal artery, and in some cases by the contralateral ethmoidal artery or distal branches of the internal maxillary or middle meningeal artery. They always drain through a frontal cortical vein or olfactory vein. The frequency of venous dilation seems to be higher than in other locations. The main presenting symptom is frontal hematoma (or subarachnoid hemorrhage). The goal of treatment is complete cure, which is most often achieved by surgical clipping of the draining vein. Surgery is safe and associated with a low rate of morbidity. Sometimes, a dilated ophthalmic artery will allow distal catheterization of the ethmoidal artery with good flow control, and injection of glue can be safely performed. Rarely, catheterization of the draining vein can be achieved to allow injection of glue at the site of fistulous drainage. Endovascular therapy is rarely proposed (when surgery is contraindicated or when the angiographic anatomy is favorable for an endovascular approach). Treatment is almost always surgical.

Tentorial Dural Arteriovenous Fistulae

These were observed in 12% of patients in our series. Owing to the anatomy, they are all types III to V. They almost always present with hemorrhage, neurologic deficit, seizure, or myelopathy. The goal of treatment is a complete cure. The indications for treatment depend on the architecture of the fistula. Endovascular therapy may sometimes result in a complete cure (when there are few feeders) when glue reaches the venous compartment.

The main feeder is frequently the meningohypo-physeal (via the artery of Bernasconi and Casanari) or inferolateral trunk. Embolization of these pedicles must be done very carefully and only if the conditions are optimal (good flow control, no reflux along the catheter). The use of a flow control balloon in the carotid siphon is not indicated and may be dangerous. By reversing the flow, it may facilitate the reflux of glue into other pedicles arising from the siphon. The risk of bleeding from these fistulae is high and one must not attempt too many embolizations before sending the patient to surgery. If arterial embolization with glue does not reach the venous compartment, the patient must undergo surgical clipping of the draining vein. In certain very tricky cases, radiosurgery may be useful to achieve complete cure of the fistula.

Cavernous Sinus Dural Arteriovenous Fistulae

These occur most frequently in postmenopausal women (70% of cases) or in association with pregnancy. A history of trauma is less often encountered than a history of sphenoid sinusitis.

The symptoms depend on the venous drainage pattern, with ocular symptoms (80% of cases) such as proptosis, chemosis, or diplopia (cranial nerve III or VI palsy) due to superior and inferior ophthalmic vein drainage (Fig. 18–1). Loss of visual acuity is common and highly variable in degree. Almost all of these findings resolve after closure of the fistula except severe visual loss (light perception only), which rarely improves. Pulsatile tinnitus is observed in 30% to 50% of cases due to petrosal sinus drainage.

Cortical venous drainage is rarely encountered (four of 33 cases in our series). Neurologic symptoms are rarely observed (zero of 33 cases). Drainage may be anterior (ophthalmic veins) or posterior (petrosal sinuses, pterygoid plexus). It may be contralateral (through the circular sinus), producing contralateral ocular symptoms. Sinus or vein thrombosis may occur as the cause or consequence of the fistula. Thrombosis of the ophthalmic venous drainage may produce acute ocular symptoms and cure of the fistula.

The results of carotid-jugular or ocular compression are much better than for fistulae in other locations, with complete cure achieved in 34% of patients.[43]

Aspirin (325 mg/day) may be given, particularly in patients with signs of sinus thrombosis. Aspirin should not be given when compression is being performed, since the goal of compression is cure of the fistula by sinus thrombosis, whereas the goal of aspirin is to induce recanalization of the thrombosed sinus with disappearance of the fistula.

Particulate embolization may result in cure of the fistula in up to 50% of cases.[43] Treatment is effective mainly when the fistula is fed only by meningeal branches of the external carotid artery; delayed recanalization may be observed. This approach is very safe and may be tried as the initial therapy.

Arterial embolization with glue must be performed only in cases of simple fistulae with a single pedicle or a few dilated pedicles. Glue should be injected only if distal catheterization allows good flow control, enabling glue to reach the venous side. In these cases, complete cure of the fistula may be achieved. Arterial embolization without penetration to the venous side must be absolutely avoided. If glue is not injected into the nidus itself, it may result in reflux into the siphon, entrance into anastomoses, and cranial nerve palsies. In addition, proximal embolization invariably results in recanalization.

Venous embolization is the most frequently performed treatment at present (Fig. 18–1). The goal is to reach the cavernous sinus and occlude it with coils. Generally, the procedure may be performed through the femoral vein and inferior petrosal sinus. When the inferior petrosal sinus is not opacified, an attempt at catheterization must be made anyway. It may be impossible because of inferior petrosal sinus thrombosis, absence of connection with the jugular vein, or a plexiform inferior petrosal sinus. In these cases, catheterization of the superior ophthalmic vein should be attempted through the facial and angular veins. This may be very difficult owing to the tortuosity of the vein. In a few cases, surgical exposure of the vein may be required. A microcatheter is placed through an intravenous-type catheter, allowing deposition of coils. Venous catheterization must be done with roadmapping. Injection of contrast through the microcatheter must be performed to ensure that the coils will be deposited in the initial compartment of the venous drainage. It is sometimes impossible to reach the site of the fistula in cases with trabeculation of the cavernous sinus.

The cerebral venous drainage must be carefully studied; the arterialized cavernous sinus is mostly hemodynamically excluded and occlusion is not dangerous. The aim must be a complete cure of the fistula. A dense packing is needed, and when it is not possible to deliver enough coils, the embolization may be completed with injection of glue. This must be performed very carefully, to avoid injection in the venous side or reflux into the arterial side (the siphon).

SPONTANEOUS OR POST-TREATMENT MODIFICATION OF VENOUS DRAINAGE

In 1997 we published seven cases of long-term worsening of the type of venous drainage DAVFs, with development of cortical venous drainage in five cases.[23] Some authors have related the clinical evolution to the worsening of the venous drainage,[8, 11, 14, 27] but to our knowledge, no angiographic proof of such evolution has ever been published. This reflects the fact that this pathologic entity occurs with great rarity. From the findings of our large series,[15] it seems that there is no natural progression from one type to another. From our last study, it seems difficult to draw any firm conclusions about the frequency of evolution into higher grades, since the time between the initial angiogram and the diagnosis of evolution ranged from 1 month to 20 years, with a mean of 7

years. This indicates the necessity of very-long-term follow-up of incompletely treated cases.[23] Three different mechanisms may explain worsened venous drainage patterns:

1. *Stenosis or thrombosis of the venous outflow.* Thrombosis at the site of the venous drainage led to worsening of the type in four patients. The thrombotic disease underlying the formation of the fistula may explain the progressive thrombosis of the sinus(es). On the other hand, the role of the fistula itself in sinus stenosis or occlusion remains unclear. Piton et al proposed that the different types of venous drainage most likely correspond to stages in the course of the disease.[27] They presumed that distention of mural vessels progressively reduces the venous lumen and may result in complete obstruction, with subsequent drainage through the contralateral sinus. Nishijima et al postulated that stenosis of the sinus lumen was mainly due to the marked thickening of its intima and the development of an abnormal vascular network within its wall.[26] In their study concerning grading of venous restrictive disease in DAVFs, Lalwani et al proposed that DAVFs are a dynamic disease that can progress at a variable rate from a minimal venous restrictive disease to a more serious outflow impairment.[25] Besides the role of the fistula in creating a thickened sinus wall, it may be assumed that the high arterial flow can produce lesions in the sinus wall at a distance from the shunt itself. Occlusion upstream from the fistula may be explained by the impaired venous drainage and stagnation where the normal venous drainage of the brain and the fistula drainage are in competition.

   Three reports in the literature have proved the role of fistulae in the formation of sinus thrombosis.[24, 44, 45] However, in these cases, occlusion of the sinus resulted in spontaneous disappearance of the fistula. Thus, even if the supposition that the hemodynamics of DAVFs can be modified by venous stenosis or occlusion is generally accepted, such modifications have never been shown angiographically. Consequently, it seems difficult to consider a progression from one stage to another as a natural course of a DAVF.

   The role of postembolization reduced arterial flow in the development of stenosis or occlusion of the sinus may be questioned. A high flow could maintain sufficient pressure in the sinus to avoid the formation of thrombus. Thus, embolization without complete obliteration of the fistula might favor the development of thrombosis and worsened venous drainage. Alternatively, high-flow arterialized drainage may stimulate "arterialized" stenosis.

2. *Increased arterial flow.* In two patients the drainage worsened from type I and type IIa without any change in the sinuses. Doppler

evaluation revealed increased arterial flow on long-term follow-up. It seems reasonable to believe that in these two cases the evolution in type of venous drainage was due to the increase in arterial flow.

3. *Appearance of new fistulae or extension of the initial shunt.* In two patients we observed the development of new fistulae. It is difficult to determine whether the same pathologic mechanism at the origin of the initial fistula created the other shunts, or whether the hemodynamic changes created by the first fistula resulted in the other fistulae. Barnwell et al. reported seven cases of multiple DAVFs.[46] They postulated that a state of hypercoagulability may lead to thrombosis and thus to fistulae at different sites. They also stated that impaired venous drainage into the main sinuses, causing stagnation, could give rise to a second fistula.

Management Implications

On the initial angiogram, at the time of diagnosis, the venous outflow must be analyzed with caution, and any stenosis of the venous drainage must be considered a potential risk factor for evolution into a worse grade. After the initial diagnosis and treatment, patients with type I or IIa fistulae who are not completely cured must be informed that any change in their symptoms, for better or worse, is an absolute indication for re-evaluation. Furthermore, in our institutions, we systematically perform an annual Doppler examination to screen for an increase in arterial flow rate.

REFERENCES

1. Newton T, Greitz T. Arteriovenous communication between the occipital artery and the transverse sinus. *Radiology* 1966;87:824–828.
2. Takekawa S, Holman C. Roentgenologic diagnosis of anomalous communications between the external carotid artery and intracranial veins. *J Roentgenol* 1965;95:822–825.
3. Aminoff M. Vascular anomalies in the intracranial dura mater. *Brain* 1973;96:601–612.
4. Obrador S, Soto M, Silvela R. Clinical syndromes of arteriovenous malformations of the transverse sigmoid sinus. *J Neurol Neurosurg Psychiatry* 1975;38:436–451.
5. Verf A. Sur un cas d'anéurysme artério-veineux intradural bilatéral de la fosse posterieur chez un enfant. *Neurochirurgie* 1964;10:140–144.
6. Cormick WM, Boutler T. Vascular malformations ("angiomas") of the dura mater. *J Neurosurg* 1966;25:309–311.
7. Aminoff M, Kendall B. Asymptomatic dural vascular anomalies. *Br J Radiol* 1973;46:662–667.
8. Houser O, Baker H, Rhoton A, Okazaki H. Intracranial dural arteriovenous malformations. *Radiology* 1972;105:55–64.
9. Castaigne P, Bories J, Brunet P, et al. Les fistules artério-veineuses méningées pures à drainage veineux cortical. *Rev Neurol* 1976;132:169–181.
10. Djindjian R, Merland J, Theron J. Superselective Arteriography of the External Carotid Artery. New York: Springer-Verlag, 1977, pp 606–628.
11. Chaudhary M, Sachdev V, Cho S, et al. Dural arteriovenous malformations of the major venous sinuses: an acquired lesion. *AJNR* 1982;3:13–19.
12. Brainin M, Samec P. Venous hemodynamics of arteriovenous meningeal fistulas in the posterior cranial fossa. *Neuroradiology* 1983;25:161–169.
13. Graeh D, Dolman C. Radiological and pathological aspects of dural arteriovenous fistulas. *J Neurosurg* 1986;64:962–967.
14. Watanabe A, Takahara Y, Ibuchi Y, Miukami K. Two cases of dural arteriovenous malformation occurring after intracranial surgery. *Neuroradiology* 1984;26:375–380.
15. Cognard C, Gobin Y, Pierot L, et al. Neurological symptoms of intracranial dural arteriovenous fistulas: clinical and angiographic correlation in 205 cases. A revisited classification of the venous drainage. *Radiology* 1994;194:671–680.
16. Lasjaunias P, Berenstein A. Surgical Neuroangiography, Vol 2: Endovascular Treatment of Craniofacial Lesions. New York: Springer-Verlag, 1987.
17. Malik G, Pearce J, Ausman J, Mehta B. Dural arteriovenous malformations and intracranial hemorrhage. *Neurosurgery* 1984;15:332–339.
18. Lasjaunias P, Chiu M, Terbrugge KT, et al. Neurological manifestations of intracranial dural sinus arteriovenous malformations. *J Neurosurg* 1986;64:724–730.
19. Awad I, Little J, Akrawi W, Ahl J. Intracranial dural arteriovenous malformations: factors predisposing to an aggressive neurological course. *J Neurosurg* 1990;72:839–850.
20. Kühner A, Krastel A, Stoll W. Arteriovenous malformations of the transverse dural sinus. *J Neurosurg* 1974;45:12–19.
21. Tomsick T, Tew J, Lukin R. Intracranial arteriovenous malformations with increased intracranial pressure: response to embolization. In Smith RR, Haerer AF, Russel WF (eds): Vascular Malformations and Fistulas of the Brain. New York: Raven Press, 1982, pp 119–127.
22. Lamas E, Lobato R, Esperza J, Escudero L. Dural posterior fossa AVM producing raised sagittal sinus pressure. Case report. *J Neurosurg* 1977;46:804–810.
23. Cognard C, Houdart E, Casasco A, et al. Long term modification of intracranial dural arteriovenous fistulas leading to a worsening in the type of venous drainage. *Neuroradiology* 1997;39:59–66.
24. Barnwell S, Halbach V, Dowd C, et al. A variant of arteriovenous fistulas within the wall of dural sinuses. *J Neurosurg* 1991;74:199–204.
25. Lalwani A, Dowd C, Halbach VV. Grading venous restrictive disease in patients with dural arterio-venous fistulas of the transverse/sigmoid sinus. *J Neurosurg* 1993;79:11–15.
26. Nishijima M, Takaku A, Endo S, et al. Etiological evaluation of dural arteriovenous malformations of the lateral and sigmoid sinuses based on histopathological examinations. *J Neurosurg* 1992;76:600–606.
27. Piton J, Guilleux H, Guibert-Tranier F, Caille J. Fistules du sinus latéral. *J Neuroradiol* 1984;11:143–159.
28. Gobin Y, Rogopoulos A, Aymard A, et al. Endovascular treatment of intra-cranial dural arterio-venous fistulas with perimedullary venous drainage. *J Neurosurg* 1992;77:718–723.
29. Woimant F, Merland J, Riche M, et al. Syndrome bulbo-médullaire en rapport avec une fistule artério-veineuse méningée que sinus latéral à drainage veineux médullaire. *Rev Neurol* 1982;138:559–566.
30. Gaensler E, Jackson D, Halbach VV. Arteriovenous fistulas of the cervicomedullary junction as a cause of myelopathy: radiographic findings in two cases. *AJNR* 1990;11:518–521.
31. Willinsky R, TerBrugge K, Lasjaunias P, Montanera W. The variable presentation of the craniocervical and cervical dural arteriovenous malformations. *Surg Neurol* 1990;34:118–123.
32. Wrobel C, Oldfield E, Chiro GD, et al. Myelopathy due to intracranial dural arteriovenous fistulas draining into spinal medullary veins. Report of three cases. *J Neurosurg* 1988;69:934–939.
33. Rivierez M, Gazengel J, Chiras J, et al. Les fistules artério-veineuses vértebro-durales du trou occipital à drainage médullaire. Deux observations. *Neurochirurgie* 1991;37:179–184.
34. Gaston A, Chiras J, Bourbotte G, et al. Fistules artério-veineuses méningées à drainage veineux cortical. *J Neuroradiol* 1984;11:161–177.
35. Picard L, Bracard S, Islak C, et al. Fistules durales de la tente du cervelet. *J Neuroradiol* 1990;17:161–181.
36. Pierot L, Chiras J, Meder J, et al. Dural arteriovenous fistulas

of the posterior fossa draining into subarachnoid veins. *AJNR* 1992;13:315–323.

37. Martin N, King W, Wilson C, et al. Management of dural arteriovenous malformations of the anterior cranial fossa. *J Neurosurg* 1990;72:692–697.
38. Halbach V, Higashida R, Hieshima G, et al. Dural fistulas involving the transverse and sigmoid sinuses: results of treatment in 28 patients. *Radiology* 1987;163:443–447.
39. Urtasun F, Biondi A, Casasco A, et al. Cerebral dural arteriovenous fistulas: percutaneous transvenous embolization. *Radiology* 1996;199:209–217.
40. Halbach V, Higashida R, Hieshima G, et al. Transvenous embolization of dural fistulas involving the transverse and sigmoid sinuses. *AJNR* 1989;10:385–392.
41. Gobin Y, Rogopoulos A, Aymard A, et al. Percutaneous transvenous embolization through the thrombosed sinus in two transverse sinus dural fistulas. *AJNR* 1993;14:1102–1105.
42. Casasco A. Endovascular pial transvenous approach to dural and pial AVMs. Paper presented at the IVth International Symposium of Interventional Neuroradiology, Mexico City, 1993.
43. Halbach V, Higashida R, Hieshima G, et al. Dural fistulas involving the cavernous sinus: results of treatment in 30 patients. *Radiology* 1987;163:437–442.
44. Rohr J, Gautier G. Regression spontanée d'une fistule artério-veineuse dure-mèrienne de la fosse postérieure. *Rev Neurol* 1985;141:240–244.
45. Bitho S, Onishi T, Takimoto N, et al. Dural arteriovenous fistula after removal of a meningioma: a case report. *Neurol Surg* 1978;6:397–400.
46. Barnwell S, Halbach V, Higashida R, et al. Complex dural arteriovenous fistulas. *J Neurosurg* 1989;71:352–358.

ADDITIONAL READINGS

Albright AL, Latchaw RE, Price RA. Posterior dural arteriovenous malformations in infancy. *Neurosurgery* 1983;13:129–135.
Barnwell SL, Halbach VV, Dowd CF, et al. Dural arteriovenous fistulas involving the inferior petrosal sinus: angiographic findings in six patients. *AJNR* 1990;11:511–516.
Barnwell SL, Halbach VV, Dowd CF, et al. Multiple dural arteriovenous fistulas of the cranium and spine. *AJNR* 1991;12:441–445.
Chaloupka JC, Goller D, Goldberg RA, et al. True anatomical compartmentalization of the cavernous sinus in a patient with bilateral cavernous dural arteriovenous fistulae. *J Neurosurg* 1993;79:592–595.
Chen J-C, Tsuruda JS, Halbach VV. Suspected dural arteriovenous fistulas: results with screening MR angiography in seven patients. *Radiology* 1992;183:265–271.
De Marco JK, Dillon WP, Halbach VV, Tsuruda JS. Dural arteriovenous fistulas: evaluation with MR imaging. *Radiology* 1990;175:193–199.
Djindjian R, Cophignon J, Theron J, et al. Embolization by superselective arteriography from the femoral route; review of 60 cases; technique, indications, complications. *Neuroradiology* 1973;6:20–26.

Findlay JM, Mielke BW. Fatal rebleeding from a dural arteriovenous malformation of the posterior fossa: case report with pathological examination. *Can J Neurol Sci* 1994;21:67–71.
Gensburg RS, Radford LR. Embolization of a dural sinus fistula by direct puncture of the occipital arteries. *AJR* 1993;160:1265–1266.
Halbach VV, Higashida RT, Hieshima GB, Cahan L. Treatment of dural arteriovenous malformations involving the superior sagittal sinus. *AJNR* 1988;9:337–343.
Halbach VV, Higashida RT, Hieshima GB, David CF. Endovascular therapy of dural fistulas. In Vinuela F, Halbach VV, Dion JE (eds): Interventional Neuroradiology: Endovascular Therapy of the Central Nervous System. New York: Raven Press, 1992, pp 29–50.
Halbach VV, Higashida RT, Hieshima GB, et al. Dural arteriovenous fistulas supplied by ethmoidal arteries. *Neurosurgery* 1990;26:816–823.
Halbach VV, Higashida RT, Hieshima GB, et al. Treatment of dural fistulas involving the deep cerebral venous system. *AJNR* 1989;10:393–399.
Kataoka K, Taneda M. Angiographic disappearance of multiple dural arteriovenous malformations. *J Neurosurg* 1984;60:1275–1278.
Kuwayama N, Akai T, Horie Y, et al. Dural arteriovenous fistulae involving the transverse-sigmoid sinus and foramen magnum. *Surg Neurol* 1994;41:389–395.
Magidson MA, Weinberg PE. Spontaneous closure of a dural arteriovenous malformation. *Surg Neurol* 1976;6:107–110.
McDermott VG, Sellar RJ. Case report: thyrocervical arterial supply to an intracranial dural arteriovenous malformation. *Clin Radiol* 1993;47:362–363.
Mourier KL, Gobin YP, George B, et al. Intradural perimedullary arteriovenous fistulae: results of surgical and endovascular treatment in a series of 35 cases. *Neurosurgery* 1993;32:885–891.
Nakada T, Kwee IL, Ellis WG, St John JN. Subacute diencephalic necrosis and dural arteriovenous malformation. *Neurosurgery* 1985;17:653–656.
Nakagawa H, Kubo S, Nakajima Y, et al. Shifting of dural arteriovenous malformation from the cavernous sinus to the sigmoid sinus to the transverse sinus after transvenous embolization. *Surg Neurol* 1992;37:30–38.
Ott D, Bien S, Krasznai L. Embolization of a tentorial dural arterio-venous fistula presenting as atypical trigeminal neuralgia. *Headache* 1993;33:503–508.
Partington MD, Rufenacht DA, Marsh WR, Piepgras DG. Cranial and sacral dural arteriovenous fistulas as a cause of myelopathy. *J Neurosurg* 1992;76:615–622.
Picard L, Bracard S, Mallet J, et al. Spontaneous dural arteriovenous fistulas. *Semin Intervent Radiol* 1987;4:219–240.
Sergott RC, Grossman RI, Savino P, et al. The syndrome of paradoxical worsening of dural-cavernous sinus arteriovenous malformations. *Ophthalmology* 1987;94:205–212.
Sundt TM Jr, Piepgras DG. The surgical approach to arteriovenous malformations of the lateral and sigmoid dural sinuses. *J Neurosurg* 1983;59:32–39.
Vinuela F, Fox AJ, Pelz DM, Drake CG. Unusual clinical manifestations of dural arteriovenous malformations. *J Neurosurg* 1986;64:554–558.

CHAPTER 19

Treatment of Carotid-Cavernous Sinus Fistulae

Donald Larsen / Randall T. Higashida / J. J. Connors III

Carotid-cavernous fistulae are spontaneous or acquired connections between the carotid artery and the cavernous sinus and can be classified as direct or indirect. Direct carotid-cavernous fistulae represent direct connections between the internal carotid artery (ICA) and the cavernous sinus and may occur as a result of a ruptured intracavernous carotid artery aneurysm (Fig. 19–1), trauma (Figs. 19–2 to 19–4), collagen deficiency syndromes (Fig. 19–5), fibromuscular dysplasia, arterial dissection, or direct surgical trauma.[1–13] Indirect carotid-cavernous fistulae are usually supplied by dural branches of the external carotid artery but can be supplied by dural branches of the ICA. The exact cause of indirect carotid-cavernous fistulae is unknown; however, factors associated with their development include pregnancy, sinusitis, trauma, surgical procedures, and cavernous sinus thrombosis.

ETIOLOGY

Trauma

Motor vehicle accidents represent the most common cause of traumatic carotid-cavernous fistulae (Fig. 19–2). Trauma from falls and penetrating injuries is less frequent. Closed head trauma associated with basal skull fracture or penetrating trauma to the head and orbit may result in a post-traumatic carotid-cavernous fistula (Fig. 19–3). The ICA is fixed by a dural attachment between the foramen lacerum and the anterior clinoid process. The shearing forces of severe head trauma, often accompanied by penetrating injury from bony spicules, can cause the ICA to be torn between its points of dural attachment. The laceration of the ICA is usually single, large (2 to 5 mm), and unilateral. The unusual bilateral traumatic carotid-cavernous fistula is generally associated with more severe head trauma, is more commonly fatal, and therefore is less frequent.[14] Rarely, a unilateral carotid-cavernous fistula may present with bilateral orbital symptoms by supplying the contralateral cavernous sinus with arterialized blood via the circular sinus, thus creating free intercavernous communication.

Collagen Deficiency Syndromes

Spontaneous direct carotid-cavernous fistulae can arise from conditions that predispose the wall of the ICA to weakening in approximately 60% of cases.[15, 16] Specific disorders resulting in a defect in the arterial wall media include aneurysms of the cavernous ICA, Ehlers-Danlos syndrome,[17–19] fibromuscular dysplasia,[20] and pseudoxanthoma elasticum.[21]

An inherited group of disorders of connective tissue, all of which have abnormalities of collagen composition, make up the Ehlers-Danlos syndrome. At least 10 different subtypes have been described on the basis of clinical and genetic differences.[17, 19, 22] Those patients with a type IV disorder (also known as ecchymotic or arterial type) have a deficiency in type III collagen[17, 22, 23] (Fig. 19–5). These patients are also particularly prone to developing spontaneous direct carotid-cavernous fistulae[24–28] and commonly die at an early age as a result of aortic dissection, arterial or myocardial rupture, or bowel perforations.

Iatrogenic Injury

Less common are iatrogenic causes of direct carotid-cavernous fistulae. These include injury to the ICA during Fogarty catheter manipulation for carotid angioplasty,[29] transsphenoidal hypophysectomy,[13] thromboendarterectomy,[5, 30] trigeminal rhizotomy, and nasopharyngeal biopsy.

CLASSIFICATION

Various categorizations have been used to describe carotid-cavernous fistulae.[31–34] Specific questions need to be answered when studying any fistula. Is the fistula actually a ruptured aneurysm? Is it a hole in the ICA caused by unsuspected (or unremembered) trauma? Is it idiopathic? Is it both indirect and direct? Peeters and Kroger[35] and Barrow et al.[36] classified carotid-cavernous fistulae as follows:

A. Intracavernous ICA to cavernous sinus.
B. Dural ICA branches to cavernous sinus.
C. Dural external carotid artery (ECA) branches to cavernous sinus.
D. Dural ICA and ECA branches to cavernous sinus.

Carotid-cavernous fistulae can also be considered as three different pathologies, based on the structural situation and etiology, which have direct implications concerning therapy:

Type 1. A traumatically acquired direct arteriovenous fistula. A fracture or shear injury

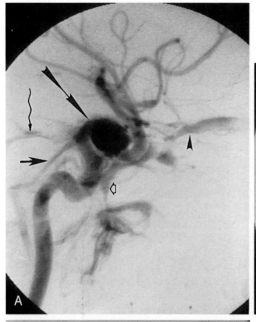

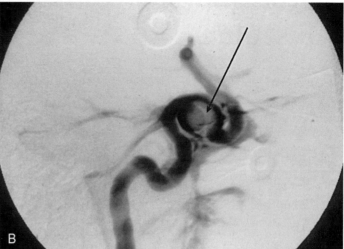

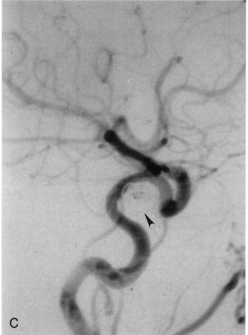

Figure 19-1 Case 1. A 68-year-old man with a spontaneous direct carotid-cavernous fistula secondary to a ruptured cavernous carotid aneurysm. *A,* A right internal carotid cerebral angiogram, lateral view, demonstrates the level of the neck of a carotid cavernous aneurysm *(long arrow).* Venous outflow from the fistula via the superior ophthalmic vein *(arrowhead),* the superior petrosal sinus *(curly arrow),* the inferior petrosal sinus *(short arrow),* and pterygoid venous plexus *(open arrow)* is well shown. *B,* A right internal carotid cerebral angiogram, lateral view, after placement of a single detachable silicone balloon *(arrow).* Although the fistula demonstrates slightly decreased flow, it still remains predominantly patent. *C,* Right internal carotid cerebral angiogram, lateral view. Utilizing the Guglielmi detachable coil (GDC) system, detachable coils were placed alongside the detachable silicone balloon within the cavernous aneurysm *(arrowhead),* with subsequent complete closure of the carotid-cavernous fistula and occlusion of the cavernous carotid aneurysm.

causes rupture of the wall of the ICA just as it exits the petrous bone, with resultant direct flow into the cavernous sinus. Alternatively, an acquired direct fistula can be present in patients with intrinsic vascular abnormality, typically forms of Ehlers-Danlos syndrome. These appear the same as a traumatic type and are treated in a similar fashion, albeit with a heightened degree of care and concern. Reports have shown that even simple angiography may carry up to 20% to 30% mortality in these patients (Ehlers-Danlos).[37]

Type 2. These fistulae are caused by rupture of a preexisting intracavernous aneurysm into the cavernous sinus, leaving a walled pouch of aneurysm within the cavernous sinus as a separate structure. There are therefore two separate holes: one from the ICA into the aneurysm (which can be of any size, even huge), and the other from the aneurysm into the cavernous sinus (also of varying size).

Type 3. A typical dural-type arteriovenous fistula involving the cavernous sinus with indirect supply to the sinus from ECA branches or meningeal perforators arising from the ICA. The difficulty of treatment varies with the origins of the feeding vessels.

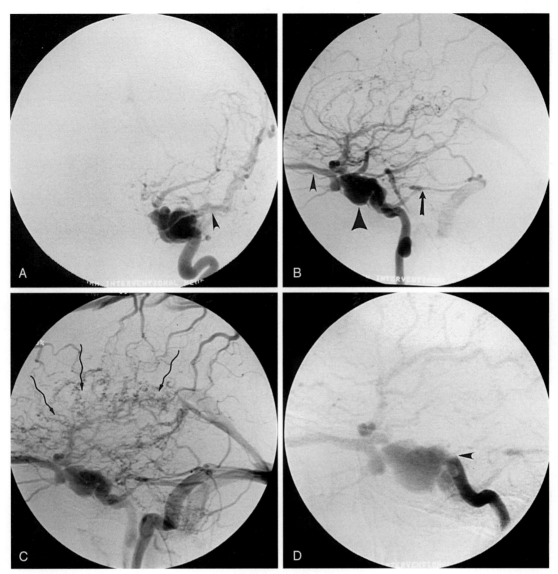

Figure 19-2 Case 2. A 30-year-old male motor vehicle accident victim with blunt head trauma. *A*, A left internal carotid cerebral angiogram, anteroposterior view, demonstrates a large cavernous sinus varix and evidence of cortical venous drainage *(arrowhead)* as demonstrated by retrograde flow through the sphenoparietal sinus and superficial middle cerebral veins. *B*, A left internal carotid cerebral angiogram, lateral view, demonstrates the large cavernous sinus varix *(large arrowhead)* and retrograde flow through an enlarged superior ophthalmic vein *(small arrowhead)*. There is also an enlarged superior petrosal sinus draining into the left transverse sigmoid sinus *(arrow)*. *C*, A left internal carotid cerebral angiogram, venous phase, shows marked reflux into cortical veins of the superficial middle cerebral system *(arrows)*. *D*, A left internal carotid cerebral angiogram, high-magnification lateral view, demonstrates abrupt angiographic cutoff at the site of the fistula *(arrowhead)*. It is unclear from this sequence alone if the carotid artery is transected or if this merely represents a single-hole fistula.

Illustration continued on following page

Type 4. A combination of a direct and indirect fistula (e.g., a type 3 fistula with either a type 1 or 2 fistula).

PATHOPHYSIOLOGY AND CLINICAL PRESENTATION

The clinical presentation of carotid-cavernous fistulae is related to their size, duration, location, and adequacy and route of venous drainage and to the presence of arterial and venous collateral vessels.

The superior and inferior ophthalmic veins provide normal venous drainage from the orbit to the cavernous sinus. The superficial middle cerebral veins drain the brain through the sphenoparietal sinus to the cavernous sinus. The cavernous sinus normally drains through the superior and inferior petrosal sinuses to the jugular bulb and via emissary veins to the pterygoid plexus.

Reversal of direction of flow through the ophthalmic veins and/or sphenoparietal sinus is possible if an arteriovenous connection develops in the caver-

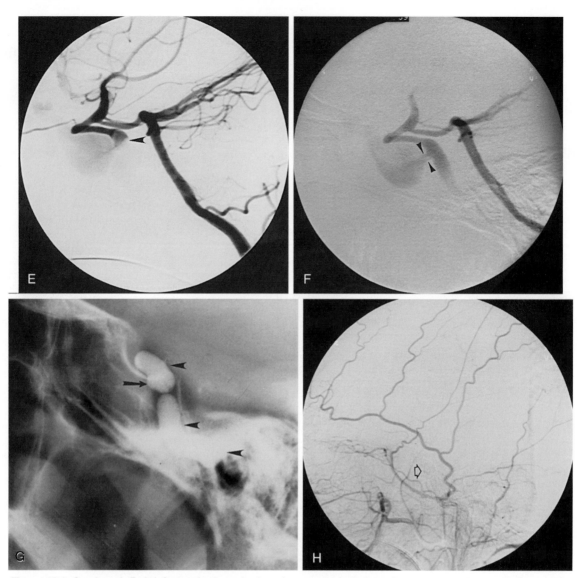

Figure 19-2 *Continued. E*, A left vertebral cerebral angiogram, lateral view, demonstrates retrograde flow to the level of the fistula via the posterior communicating artery *(arrowhead)*. Again, the exact site of the fistula is not clearly delineated. *F*, A left vertebral angiogram with left carotid compression, lateral view, shows the contrast jet created by the laceration and ventral wall of the left internal carotid artery (ICA) *(arrowheads)* to best advantage. *G*, A lateral skull radiograph demonstrates placement of three contrast-filled detachable silicone balloons *(arrowheads)*. A slight bulge in the distal balloon demonstrates the site of the fistula *(arrow)*. It was necessary to treat this fistula with carotid occlusion, as it was not possible to navigate a detachable silicone balloon through the ostium of the fistula itself. *H*, A left common carotid cerebral angiogram, lateral view, shows no residual filling of the fistula. The left ICA is occluded by the three detachable silicone balloons, subtracted out on this digital subtraction angiogram *(arrow)*.

nous sinus, especially if normal routes of venous drainage of the cavernous sinus are occluded. Elevated venous pressure in veins draining the orbit may produce orbital venous congestion, transudation of interstitial fluid into the orbit with resultant proptosis, increased intraocular pressure due to impaired drainage of aqueous humor, and secondary glaucoma.[38, 39] Elevated venous pressure and increased intraocular pressure can compromise retinal perfusion and result in severely diminished visual acuity.[39] "Steal" away from the ophthalmic artery into the fistula via reversal of flow in the supraclinoid carotid artery can cause diminished arterial pressure

to the orbit. Mild decreases in visual acuity can be reversed with definitive closure of the fistula. If severe compromise of visual acuity has developed, with loss of light perception, the chances of visual recovery are unlikely. All patients with carotid-cavernous fistulae should undergo frequent ophthalmologic examinations to document intraocular pressure and to identify early visual decline, which would necessitate immediate treatment. In patients with severe proptosis, markedly elevated intraocular pressure, and rapidly declining visual acuity, a lateral canthotomy may be necessary as a temporizing measure until the fistula can be closed. If the intraocular pressure rises

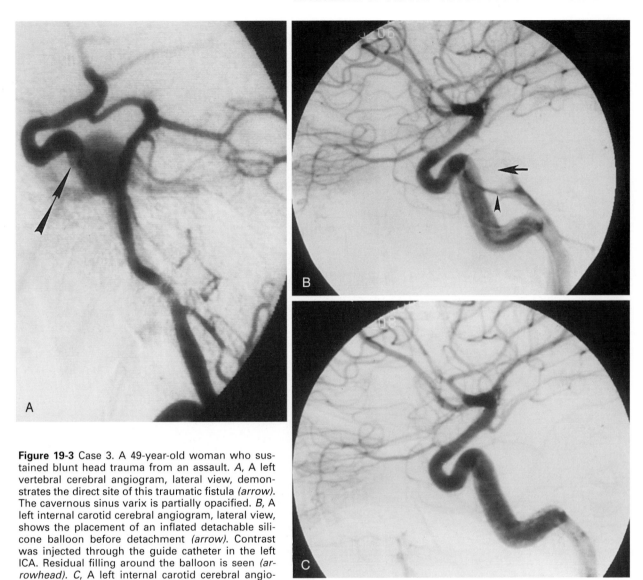

Figure 19-3 Case 3. A 49-year-old woman who sustained blunt head trauma from an assault. *A*, A left vertebral cerebral angiogram, lateral view, demonstrates the direct site of this traumatic fistula *(arrow)*. The cavernous sinus varix is partially opacified. *B*, A left internal carotid cerebral angiogram, lateral view, shows the placement of an inflated detachable silicone balloon before detachment *(arrow)*. Contrast was injected through the guide catheter in the left ICA. Residual filling around the balloon is seen *(arrowhead)*. *C*, A left internal carotid cerebral angiogram, lateral view, after additional inflation of the balloon and detachment from its delivery catheter. Complete occlusion of the fistula is demonstrated.

above 40 mm Hg, emergency treatment should be instituted to prevent permanent loss of vision. Pharmacologic management with topical β-adrenergic blockers and acetazolamide (Diamox) in an attempt to lower intraocular pressure should be considered as adjunctive therapy, and definitive treatment should be directed toward closure of the fistula.[40] Edema of orbital contents due to impaired orbital venous drainage can result in mechanical limitation of extraocular muscle movement and can contribute to the development of diplopia. Diplopia, however, may be a direct result of ophthalmoplegia secondary to a cavernous sinus syndrome caused by mass effect on the cavernous sinus from the fistula.

Less frequently, there is reversal of venous drainage into the sphenoparietal sinus, with resultant cerebral cortical venous hypertension. These patients are at risk of intracerebral hemorrhage and should also receive emergent therapy.

Halbach et al[40] identified high-risk features of direct and indirect carotid-cavernous fistulae representing indications for urgent treatment. These are summarized in Table 19–1.

The clinical presentation may not accurately reflect the pathology. There are numerous cases of total transection of the carotid artery with intracranial steal, extremely high pressure, and massive venous drainage that did not present until months after the accident and then only with minimal symptoms. Conversely, there are numerous cases of ruptured intracavernous aneurysms that presented with acute orbital decompensation and only minimal arteriovenous shunting.

Orbital symptoms are frequently related not only to the degree of shunt but also to the adequacy of external drainage of the superior ophthalmic vein. Very-slow-flow shunts have caused severe proptosis and chemosis because of poor or nonexistent external

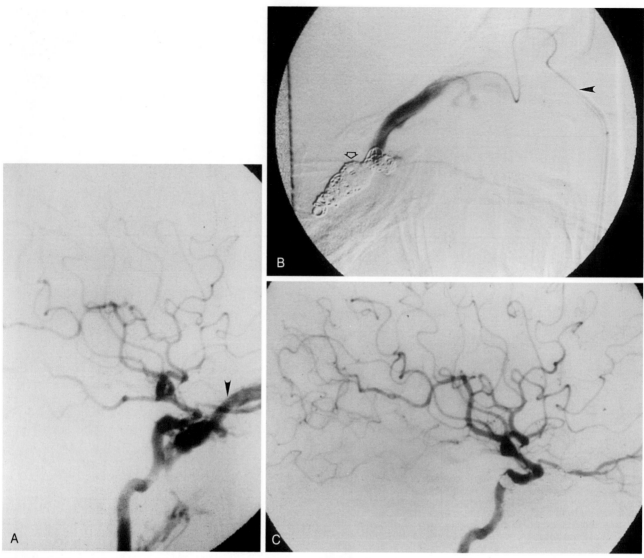

Figure 19-4 Case 4. A 17-year-old man with direct head trauma. *A,* A right internal carotid angiogram, lateral view, demonstrates a direct carotid-cavernous fistula with primary drainage via the superior ophthalmic vein *(arrowhead)* in a retrograde fashion, as well as drainage via the pterygoid venous plexus. The inferior petrosal sinus does not demonstrate spontaneous filling. Multiple attempts to reach the cavernous sinus via the inferior petrosal sinus were unsuccessful. Efforts to achieve transarterial access to the fistula with a detachable balloon (or microcatheter of any sort) were also unsuccessful. *B,* A right superior ophthalmic venogram, lateral view, demonstrates the tip of the guide catheter at the level of the angular vein via the right facial vein approach *(arrowhead)*. A microcatheter has traversed the superior ophthalmic vein, with subsequent placement of multiple-fibered microcoils in the cavernous sinus and posterior aspect of the superior ophthalmic vein *(open arrow)*, resulting in closure of the fistula. *C,* A postembolization right internal carotid cerebral angiogram, lateral view, shows complete closure of the fistula with fibered microcoils alone, deposited transvenously.

drainage; conversely, huge shunts that drained via equally huge facial veins and the inferior petrosal sinus have presented with minimal symptoms.

HISTORY

The first reported case of hemorrhage as a complication of carotid-cavernous fistulae was 1908 by de Schweinitz and Holloway.[41] In 1920 Sattler,[42] in a review of 322 cases of carotid-cavernous fistulae, reported the incidence of fatal epistaxis to be 1.5% and intracerebral hematomas 0.9%. In the more recent study by Halbach et al. mentioned previously, a review of 155 cases of carotid-cavernous fistulae re-

vealed 13 patients (8.4%) with associated hemorrhage. Four (2.6%) of these patients had fatal subarachnoid hemorrhage and three of the four had a varix of the cavernous sinus. We treat urgently those patients with angiographic evidence of a cavernous sinus varix or pseudoaneurysm. Eleven patients in Halbach et al.'s series, all of whom had cortical venous drainage, were symptomatic, with signs and symptoms suggestive of increased intracranial pressure. Four of these 11 also suffered intracerebral hemorrhage. All of these patients had hypoplasia or occlusion of normal cavernous sinus outflow pathways, with diversion of outflow into cortical veins, and all had symptoms that abated after clo-

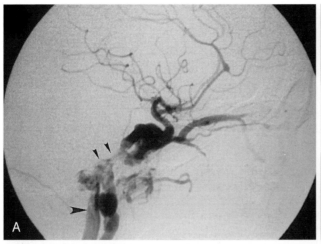
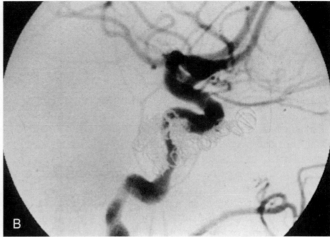

Figure 19-5 Case 5. A 38-year-old woman presented with a history of Ehlers-Danlos syndrome type IV, with spontaneous direct carotid cavernous fistula. *A,* A right internal carotid cerebral angiogram, lateral view, demonstrates a direct carotid-cavernous fistula with drainage via the inferior petrosal sinus *(small arrowheads)* into the jugular vein *(large arrowhead)* and superior ophthalmic vein. Incidentally noted are arteriopathic changes in the petrous and cavernous carotid artery and a small aneurysm in the pericallosal artery. *B,* A right internal carotid cerebral angiogram, lateral postembolization view after transvenous access to the cavernous sinus via the inferior petrosal sinus. Multiple-fibered microcoils were placed within the cavernous sinus and proximal superior ophthalmic vein for complete occlusion of this fistula.

sure of the fistula.[40] Patients with cortical venous drainage are at risk of intracerebral hemorrhage and should be given emergent therapy.

RADIOGRAPHIC EVALUATION

The "gold standard" diagnostic imaging study is selective cerebral angiography. Although the diagnosis is essentially a clinical one, magnetic resonance imaging (MRI) and computed tomography (CT) can be useful in establishing the degree of brain injury. CT is especially useful to identify skull fractures that may compromise the carotid artery lumen and create bony encroachment on the optic canal.

High-resolution digital subtraction angiography equipment with rapid filming and roadmapping capability is necessary for optimal angiographic assessment. The initial angiographic evaluation should be tailored to obtain the following information:

1. Size and location of the fistula in the ICA
2. Identification of any associated cavernous carotid aneurysm that may have ruptured
3. Differentiation of a direct carotid-cavernous fistula from an indirect lesion (dural arteriovenous fistula)
4. Identification and confirmation of patency of outflow pathways of the cavernous sinus
5. Identification of high-risk features such as cortical venous drainage, pseudoaneurysm, and cavernous sinus varix
6. Identification of associated vascular injuries in traumatic carotid-cavernous fistulae

In high-flow direct carotid-cavernous fistulae, it may not be possible to identify the morphology of the fistula on selective ICA angiograms without specific maneuvers to slow flow through the fistula. The Mehringer-Hieshima maneuver consists of a gentle ipsilateral selective ICA injection and manual compression of the ipsilateral carotid artery while filming at a slower frame rate. By eliminating the high-flow arterial input from the ipsilateral carotid artery, the fistula fills at a slower rate, which allows for better delineation of the fistula site. The Heuber maneuver is a similar technique that opacifies the fistula through a patent posterior communicating artery (if one exists) during injection of the dominant vertebral artery while manually compressing the ipsilateral carotid artery. These techniques may also demon-

TABLE 19-1 High-Risk Features of Carotid-Cavernous Fistulae

Complication	Type of Fistula		Total
	Direct	*Indirect*	
No. of cases	127	28	155
Hemorrhage			
Intracerebral	4 (3.1%)	0	4 (2.6%)
Epistaxis	4 (3.1%)	0	4 (2.6%)
Otorrhagia	1 (0.8%)	0	1 (0.6%)
Subarachnoid	4 (3.1%)	0	4 (2.6%)
Total	13 (10.2%)	0	13 (8.4%)
Increased intraocular pressure	11 (8.7%)	1 (3.6%)	12 (7.7%)
Decreased visual acuity	41 (32.3%)	7 (25.0%)	48 (31.0%)
Blindness	4 (3.1%)	3 (10.7%)	7 (4.5%)
Rapidly progressive proptosis	2 (1.6%)	0	2 (1.3%)
Cerebral ischemia	1 (0.8%)	0	1 (0.6%)
Fatalities	5 (3.9%)	0	5 (3.2%)

From Halbach VV, Hieshima GB, Higashida RT, et al. Carotid cavernous fistulae: indications for urgent therapy. *AJNR* 1987;8:627–633.

strate the unusual case of a carotid-cavernous fistula with more than one tear or complete transection of the ICA. With complete transection of the cavernous ICA, no intracranial opacification of vessels is identified. Ipsilateral external carotid arteriography is usually normal in acute direct carotid-cavernous fistula but may be helpful for surgical planning if a bypass procedure is necessary or to exclude associated vascular injuries in traumatic cases. In the case of traumatic carotid-cavernous fistulae, arteriography may demonstrate associated vascular injuries, including pseudoaneurysm proximal or distal to the fistula or in the contralateral ICA.

The venous phase of the angiogram demonstrates the pattern of venous outflow from the cavernous sinus. Anterior drainage to the ophthalmic venous system leads to proptosis, chemosis, conjunctival injection, venous retinopathy, secondary glaucoma, decline in vision, and increased intraocular pressure. Reversed flow in the ophthalmic venous system may drain anteriorly into the facial veins and subsequently into the external jugular vein. This route may be necessary for transvenous coil embolization if conventional routes are not available. Patients with posterior drainage of the cavernous sinus through the superior and inferior petrosal sinuses may present with complaints of pulsatile tinnitus or may have some dysfunction of cranial nerve III, IV, V_1, or VI. Superior drainage to the sphenoparietal sinus places the patient at risk of cortical venous drainage and associated intracerebral hemorrhage. Most frequently, a mixed drainage pattern is encountered with clinical manifestations corresponding to the predominant venous drainage pathway. The venous phase of the angiogram also allows identification of a cavernous sinus varix. Either of these can place the patient at higher risk of hemorrhage. The patency of the inferior petrosal sinus may also be assessed if transvenous embolization is required.

Evaluation with CT and MRI is useful in the diagnostic work-up of traumatic carotid-cavernous fistulae to identify associated traumatic injuries. As mentioned, cranial nerves III, IV, V_1, and VI may be impaired as a result of the fistula, because of compression of the nerve by the dilated cavernous sinus, but may also be injured at the time of trauma. Delayed onset of symptoms suggests the presence of a carotid-cavernous fistula, while acute onset of deficits suggests direct traumatic nerve injury and may herald a poorer prognosis. An arterial steal phenomenon of blood supply to the cranial nerves (due to the fistula) may contribute to nerve dysfunction as well as to venous hypertensive changes. CT is more sensitive and more useful than MRI in the acute setting to identify skull fractures and intracranial hemorrhage. Direct coronal CT or axial CT with coronal reformatted images through the cavernous sinus, with bone windows, is helpful to identify fractures of the floor of the sella turcica, which, if associated with an ICA pseudoaneurysm, can result in fatal hemorrhage. However, MRI is more sensitive in identifying non-

acute intracerebral hemorrhage and ischemic brain injury.

TREATMENT OPTIONS
General Considerations

After a thorough evaluation of the patient's condition from a clinical, anatomic, and hemodynamic standpoint, and with a full understanding of the therapeutic options available, taking into account the risks and benefits, a treatment plan may be formulated. When there is rapid visual decline, increasing intracranial pressure, or cortical venous drainage, treatment should be initiated urgently. In the specific instance of acute traumatic carotid-cavernous fistulae, more critical injuries may require medical attention before the fistula is treated.

The treatment of direct carotid-cavernous fistulae has evolved since the mid-1950s. The early treatment of proximal occlusion or trapping has fallen out of use because of the high incidence of stroke and blindness associated with these therapies, often without complete closure of the fistula.[28, 39, 43] Prolo and Hanbery[44] described the use of a fixed balloon to close both the fistula and the carotid artery. Serbinenko[45] and Debrun et al[46] described techniques to close fistulae with detachable balloons, often with preservation of the ICA. Large series have proved the effectiveness of transarterial balloon embolization,[46–49] which is currently the treatment of choice for this disease (Figs. 19–1 to 19–3). When transarterial routes are unsuccessful, transvenous embolization[45, 48] often succeeds (Figs. 19–4 and 19–5). Direct surgical exposure and embolization with copper wire or balloons has been performed.

Balloon Occlusion

Transarterial balloon embolization is the treatment of choice for symptomatic direct carotid-cavernous fistulae, and most can be obliterated in this fashion. Detachable balloons can be flow directed through the fistula. The balloon can be inflated to a volume larger than the fistula orifice to prevent balloon migration back into the carotid artery. Rarely, transarterial balloon occlusion is unsuccessful—the fistula orifice may be too small to allow entry, the venous compartment may be too small to allow balloon inflation, or sharp objects (bone fragments, foreign objects) may puncture the balloon during the inflation. In some patients who have had previous balloon embolization with subtotal occlusion, navigation of additional balloons into the fistula is often unsuccessful owing to the presence of balloons partially blocking the fistula orifice. For these patients, transvenous or transarterial occlusion of the fistula with platinum microcoils may be necessary. It is rarely necessary to occlude the carotid artery to treat a carotid-cavernous fistula.

If occlusion is necessary, however, a temporary test occlusion (see Chapters 34 and 36) should be performed unless there is direct evidence that the ipsilateral carotid artery is no longer needed for cerebral perfusion. This evidence is present if there is consistent reversal of flow distal to the fistula (eliminating the fistula would only improve the intracranial hemodynamics in this situation).

Occlusion of the ICA almost always does not cause ischemic injury to the eye owing to abundant supply from the external carotid artery. Resolution of pain caused by the fistula occurs quickly after carotid occlusion, and eye movement improves or returns to normal in approximately 80% of patients.[45] The duration of symptoms does not predict the degree or speed of improvement, but total ophthalmoplegia is almost uniformly associated with a worse prognosis.

Proximal suture ligation of the ICA by a surgical approach has been shown to be minimally effective, with up to 67% of patients having little or no improvement in the cranial neuropathy.[47] In addition, this blocks endovascular access for a true cure and may induce a severe steal, with life-threatening results. This maneuver should therefore be avoided.

Endovascular therapy has several advantages. These procedures can be performed under local anesthesia, allowing continuous neurologic monitoring of the patient. This is particularly important in the unlikely event of parent vessel occlusion. In the acutely injured patient, time is of the essence; if life-threatening hemorrhage, airway compromise, or cerebral ischemia has developed, therapy can be rendered immediately after adequate diagnostic angiography. Recovery time is faster and there is less trauma to adjacent cranial nerves and vessels.

Complications associated with endovascular embolization are rare and include (1) thromboembolic and ischemic events due to catheter and balloon manipulation injury to the parent vessel or inadvertent balloon detachment; (2) pseudoaneurysm formation due to balloon deflation or migration; and (3) alteration of arterial flow resulting in hemorrhage, edema, or worsening of ocular symptoms.

We prefer the use of detachable silicone balloons (ITC/Target Therapeutics) filled with the polymerizing agent and a water-soluble curing system. Most detachable balloons rely on a valve mechanism to prevent early deflation, but the reliability of this mechanism varies from balloon to balloon. Even if the valve mechanism functions properly, balloon deflation may be delayed. Late deflation of latex balloons may be caused by biodegradation of the balloon shell. While not biodegradable, silicone balloons may eventually deflate because of fatigue of the balloon shell. Deflation of balloons is undesirable when treating a carotid-cavernous fistula while preserving the parent artery, because this can result in thromboembolism or recanalization of the fistula. Balloon deflation can lead to the development of a pseudoaneurysm, which can produce cranial nerve palsies. After successful placement of the balloon in the fistula and after filling the balloon with metrizamide contrast medium, arteriography is performed to confirm closure of the fistula before detachment of the balloon.

If the fistula remains closed, the contrast medium can be replaced with a equivalent volume of an activated HEMA mixture; the polymerization takes 40 to 60 minutes at body temperature, after which time the delivery catheter is detached from the balloon and control angiography is performed to confirm persistent closure of the fistula. Currently, silicone detachable balloons are not approved by the Food and Drug Administration (FDA) and are available only when an FDA-approved Investigational Device Exemption (IDE) has been established. Used in this scenario, detachable balloons are not polymerized with HEMA, since silicone is currently not FDA approved either. Instead, the balloons are inflated with iso-osmolar contrast after final positioning has been achieved, and detached (see Chapter 35).

A flow-control guide catheter can be used to increase the safety of detachable balloon occlusion of the ICA. If any antegrade flow is present past the fistula, errant detachment of the balloon can result in embolization to the brain. Partial occlusion of the proximal ICA by means of a flow-control guide catheter can reverse the flow distal to the lesion, providing a margin of safety. In addition, if the fistula is to be trapped, after the balloon is detached distal to the fistula the flow-control catheter can be fully inflated, thus stopping any tendency for the balloon to migrate distally before further balloons can be placed (see Chapter 35).

If any difficulty is encountered when trying to deflate a detachable balloon, it should not be moved; any attempt at withdrawal of a partially inflated balloon may result in errant detachment. A guidewire can be placed through the catheter into the balloon, thus stenting the lumen and allowing aspiration and possible deflation. If this is not possible, the balloon should be overinflated and ruptured where it sits. The catheter can then be withdrawn.

Transcatheter Coil Embolization

If placement of balloons by the intra-arterial approach is not possible, coil embolization of the fistula via an arterial or a venous route may be attempted. We have found that platinum microcoils with attached Dacron fibers may be delivered through a microcatheter directly into the cavernous sinus by a transfemoral venous approach, with successful occlusion of the fistula. Care should be taken with this technique, especially in the case of long-standing fistulae that may be quite dilated and variable in dimensions. The fistula can immediately communicate with a wide variety of venous drainage pathways, including the superior petrosal sinuses, sphenoparietal sphenobasal sinuses, and midline connections to the contralateral cavernous sinus. Occlusion of one venous outflow can redirect the flow into the remaining pathways, causing aggravation of ocular symptoms (superior ophthalmic vein) or hemorrhage (cortical drainage). Transarterial coil embolization with fibered platinum microcoils has the associated risk of having the coil deposited into the ICA if the microcatheter recoils into the parent artery during placement. Transarterial coil embolization with detachable, retrievable platinum alloy coils from the Guglielmi detachable coil (GDC) system (Target Therapeutics) may reduce this risk, but at this time these are not as thrombogenic as pushable, fibered microcoils.

For transvenous occlusion of the cavernous sinus, it is necessary to catheterize the inferior petrosal sinus (if present) and then the cavernous sinus. Care should be maintained, because drainage of the pons and brainstem may be via the inferior petrosal sinus, and any damage to these veins may result in fatal venous thrombosis (see Chapter 38 for the technique of catheterization of the inferior petrosal sinus). Conversely, if the inferior petrosal sinus is involved in the pathology, it may be necessary to gain access to the cavernous sinus via the facial vein, periorbital vein, and superior ophthalmic vein. This technique is possible only with hydrophilic-coated microcatheters. Previously, it was necessary to directly access the superior ophthalmic vein either by a cutdown or through the draining facial vein over the nose; this may still be necessary, depending on the specific situation.

Once access to the cavernous sinus has been gained, occlusion with a mass of coils is possible. However, as stated previously, occlusion at the wrong site can worsen the situation. The outflow of the cavernous sinus is normally via the inferior petrosal sinus, but with the abnormally increased flow secondary to the fistula, the superior ophthalmic vein is recruited for drainage. Symptoms related to the change in flow and pressure in this vein are the usual proximate cause for clinical presentation. More ominous is the recruitment of cortical veins for drainage. Proximal occlusion of the usual drainage of the cavernous sinus with coils (i.e., the inferior petrosal sinus) can significantly worsen the transocular venous drainage or induce cortical venous drainage, with potentially dire results (venous infarct, hemorrhage, death).

If transvenous occlusion is to be performed, the most dangerous visualized veins should be occluded first, making sure the actual fistulous site is occluded. Typically, this means starting on the superior ophthalmic vein side of the cavernous sinus and working back toward the inferior petrosal sinus. Care must be taken not to occlude the inferior petrosal sinus first, before any cortical draining vein is occluded. If there is a cortical vein draining the sinus, occlusion on the side of the cavernous sinus at the origin of this vessel must be performed first. Completion of packing of the cavernous sinus where the actual fistula is located is then necessary and is usually curative.

Beware of an errant coil exiting the fistula into the carotid artery. If the fistula is large and this circumstance is possible, a Solstice balloon catheter (Medtronic/MIS) can be placed across the fistula from the arterial side (inside the ICA) during coil packing.

INDIRECT CAROTID-CAVERNOUS FISTULAE

An excellent discussion of this subject is presented in Chapter 18. Indirect carotid-cavernous fistulae (dural fistula involving the cavernous sinus) affect females more frequently than males, and the appearance of the lesion may be associated with pregnancy or menopause.[40, 47] They are also associated with sphenoid sinusitis and previous embolization of the cavernous sinus for treatment of a direct carotid-cavernous fistula.

These fistulae do not appear to act as malignantly as dural fistulae of the transverse and sigmoid regions, apart from the dramatic symptoms related to the eye. The cavernous sinus is circumscribed and small with limited drainage, as opposed to the posterior (transverse) sinus complex, which is large and interconnected. Posterior (transverse) sinus dural arteriovenous fistulae can and do progress to death.

Evaluation of these lesions should be as thorough as for any other vascular pathology. Even though it may be clinically apparent where the problem is, accurate analysis of the intracranial hemodynamics is always necessary. An injection of the affected common carotid artery may not show how the usual intracranial distribution of this vessel is being supplied (although this problem is more frequently the case with direct traumatic fistulae).

It is frequently possible to achieve a complete cure of an indirect carotid-cavernous fistula with transarterial embolization alone if the supply arises solely from the external carotid artery, because of the limited potential abnormal supply to this area. Selective embolization of the external carotid artery branches supplying the fistula with polyvinyl alcohol (PVA) particles in the 150- to 250-micron range is performed. Even if only 60% to 80% of the flow is eliminated, it is still possible to achieve a cure by simply waiting or utilizing the carotid compression maneuver (below). The danger of any of these therapies is that supply to cranial nerves III, IV, V, VI, VII, IX, X, XI, and XII can arise from branches that supply cavernous dural arteriovenous fistulae.

CAROTID COMPRESSION MANEUVER

This technique is discussed in Chapter 3. The carotid compression technique of carotid-cavernous fistula treatment is performed by having the patient use the hand opposite the side to be compressed to hold firm pressure on the carotid artery for 1 minute about every 30 minutes. This can be done for weeks and may result in a cure. While this seems to be an innocuous procedure, complications have occurred. The rationale for this maneuver is that if there is any vascular compromise because of this compression, it will cause weakness in the arm opposite the compression site and thus stop the occlusion.

In addition, not only is the carotid artery occluded, but the jugular vein should be also, potentially causing cessation of flow in the carotid-cavernous fistula for two reasons: arterial occlusion and venous occlusion. This may allow thrombus formation in the cavernous sinus, potentially curing the fistula. Unfortunately, this maneuver has resulted in at least one reported inadvertent death, but that was thought to be an aberration, and the technique has been employed successfully for years.[48]

CONCLUSIONS

Direct carotid-cavernous fistulae associated with acute visual decline or hemorrhage should be treated urgently. The endovascular occlusion of the fistula with detachable silicone balloons, or alternatively by transvenous coil embolization, is safe and effective in experienced hands. These procedures should be performed in medical centers in which interventional neuroradiologists, neurosurgeons, and neuro-ophthalmologists have developed a cooperative team effort to offer the best array of treatment services for these patients.

REFERENCES

1. Dandy WE. Carotid-cavernous aneurysms (pulsating exophthalmos). *Zentralbl Neurochir* 1937;2:77–113.
2. Dany F, Fraysse A, Priollet P, et al. Syndrome dysmorphique et dysplasie vasculaire: une forme atypique d'Ehlers-Danlos type IV. *J Mal Vasc* 1986;11:263–269.
3. Davie JC, Richardson R. Distal internal carotid thrombo-embolectomy using a Fogarty catheter in total occlusion. Technical note. *J Neurosurg* 1967;27:171–177.
4. Delens E. De la communication de la carotide interne et du sinus caverneux (anevrysme arterioveineux) (thesis). Paris: A Parent, 1870.
5. Eggers F, Lukin R, Chambers AA, et al. Iatrogenic carotid-cavernous fistula following Fogarty catheter thromboendarterectomy. Case report. *J Neurosurg* 1979;51:543–545.
6. Hamby WB. Carotid Cavernous Fistula. Springfield, IL: Charles C Thomas, 1966.
7. Lister JR, Sypert GW. Traumatic false aneurysm and carotid-cavernous fistula: a complication of sphenoidotomy. *Neurosurgery* 1979;5:473–475.
8. Motarjeme A, Keifer JW. Carotid-cavernous sinus fistula as a complication of carotid endarterectomy. A case report. *Radiology* 1973;108:83–84.
9. Pedersen RA, Troost BT, Schramm VL. Carotid cavernous sinus fistula after external ethmoid-sphenoid surgery. Clinical course and management. *Arch Otolaryngol* 1981;107:307–309.
10. Song IC, Bromberg BE. Carotid cavernous sinus fistula occurring after a rhinoplasty. Case report. *Plast Reconstr Surg* 1975;55:92–96.
11. Spetzler RF, Selman WR. Pathophysiology of cerebral ischemia accompanying arteriovenous malformations. In Wilson CB, Stein BM (eds): Intracranial Arteriovenous Malformations. Baltimore: Williams & Wilkins, 1984, pp 24–31.
12. Spetzler RF, Wilson CB, Winstein P, et al. Normal perfusion pressure breakthrough theory. *Clin Neurosurg* 1978;25:651–672.
13. Takahashi M, Killeffer F, Wilson G. Iatrogenic carotid cavernous fistula. Case report. *J Neurosurg* 1969;30:498–500.
14. Wilms G. Unilateral double carotid cavernous fistula treated with detachable balloons. *AJNR* 1990;11:517.
15. Kupersmith MJ, Berenstein A, Choi IS, et al. Management of nontraumatic vascular shunts involving the cavernous sinus. *Ophthalmology* 1988;95:121–130.
16. Lasjaunias P, Berenstein A. Surgical Neuroangiography, Vol 2: Endovascular Treatment of Craniofacial Lesions. New York: Springer-Verlag, 1987, pp 176–211.
17. Farley MK, Clark RD, Fallor MK, et al. Spontaneous carotid-
cavernous fistula and the Ehlers-Danlos syndrome. *Ophthalmology* 1983;90:1337–1342.
18. Graf CJ. Spontaneous carotid-cavernous fistula. Ehlers-Danlos syndrome and related conditions. *Arch Neurol* 1965;13:662–672.
19. Hollister DW. Heritable disorders of connective tissue: Ehlers-Danlos syndrome. *Pediatr Clin North Am* 1978;25:575–591.
20. Kaufman HH, Lind TA, Mullin S. Spontaneous carotid cavernous fistula with fibromuscular dysplasia. *Acta Neurochir* 1978;40:123–129.
21. Koo AH, Newton TH. Pseudoxanthoma elasticum associated with carotid rete mirabile. Case report. *AJR* 1972;116:16–22.
22. McKusick VA. Heritable Disorders of Connective Tissue, 4th ed. St. Louis: CV Mosby, 1972, pp 292–371.
23. Lach B, Nair SG, Russell NA, et al. Spontaneous carotid-cavernous fistula and multiple arterial dissections in type IV Ehlers-Danlos syndrome. Case report. *J Neurosurg* 1987;66:462–467.
24. Beylot C, Bioulac P, Doutre MS. Les manifestations artérielles du syndrome d'Ehlers-Danlos. *Ann Med Interne (Paris)* 1983;134:451–457.
25. Fox R, Pope FM, Narcisi P, et al. Spontaneous carotid cavernous fistula in Ehlers-Danlos syndrome. *J Neurol Neurosurg Psychiatry* 1988;51:984–986.
26. Guiolet M, Jouhaud F, Malbrel C, et al. Maladie D'Ehlers-Danlos—fistule artèrio-veineuse. *Bull Soc Ophthalmol Fr* 1984;84:267–268.
27. Halbach VV, Higashida RT, Dowd CF, et al. Treatment of carotid-cavernous fistulas associated with Ehlers-Danlos syndrome. *Neurosurgery* 1990;26:1021–1027.
28. Halbach VV, Higashida RT, Hieshima GB, et al. Transvenous embolization of direct carotid cavernous fistulas. *AJNR* 1988;9:741–749.
29. Flandroy P, Lenelle J, Collignon J. Carotid cavernous fistula associated with Fogarty catheter angioplasty. *AJNR* 1988;9:1242.
30. Barker WF, Stern WE, Krayenbuhl H, et al. Carotid endarterectomy complicated by carotid cavernous sinus fistula. *Ann Surg* 1968;167:568–572.
31. Dandy WE, Follis RH Jr. On pathology of carotid-cavernous aneurysms (pulsating exophthalmos). *Am J Ophthalmol* 1941;24:365.
32. Katsiotis P, Kiriakopoulos C, Taptas J. Carotid-cavernous sinus fistulae and dural arteriovenous shunts. *J Vasc Surg* 1974;8:60–69.
33. Newton TH, Hoyt WF. Dural arteriovenous shunts in the region of the cavernous sinus. *Neuroradiology* 1970;1:71–78.
34. Debrun GM, Vinuela F, Fox AJ, et al. Indications for treatment and classification of 132 carotid-cavernous fistulas. *Neurosurgery* 1988;22:285–289.
35. Peeters FLM, Kroger R. Dural and direct cavernous sinus fistulas. *AJR* 1979;132:599–606.
36. Barrow DL, Spector RH, Braun IF, et al. Classification and treatment of spontaneous carotid-cavernous fistulas. *J Neurosurg* 1985;62:248–256.
37. Weir B. Intracranial aneurysms and subarachnoid hemorrhage: An overview. In Wilkins RH, Rengachary SS (eds): Neurosurgery. New York: McGraw-Hill, 1985, pp 1308–1329.
38. Jorgensen JS, Guthoff R. Ophthalmoscopic findings in spontaneous carotid cavernous fistula: an analysis of 20 patients. *Graefes Arch Clin Exp Ophthalmol* 1988;226:34–36.
39. Sanders MD, Hoyt WF. Hypoxic ocular sequelae of carotid-cavernous fistulae. Study of the causes of visual failure before and after neurosurgical treatment in a series of 25 cases. *Br J Ophthalmol* 1969;53:82–97.
40. Halbach VV, Hieshima GB, Higashida RT, et al. Carotid cavernous fistulae: indications for urgent therapy. *AJNR* 1987;8:627–633.
41. de Schweinitz GE, Holloway TP. Pulsating Exophthalmos: Its Etiology, Symptomatology, Pathogenesis and Treatment. Philadelphia: WB Saunders, 1908.
42. Sattler CH. Handbuch der Gesamten Augenheilkunde. Berlin: Springer-Verlag, 1920.
43. Halbach VV, Higashida RT, Hieshima GB, Hardin CW. Direct puncture of the proximally occluded internal carotid artery

for treatment of carotid cavernous fistulas. *AJNR* 1989; 10:151–154.

44. Prolo DJ, Hanbery JW. Intraluminal occlusion of the carotid-cavernous sinus fistula with a balloon catheter. Technical note. *J Neurosurg* 1971;35:237–242.

45. Serbinenko FA. Balloon catheterization and occlusion of major cerebral vessels. *J Neurosurg* 1974;41:125–145.

46. Debrun GB, Lacour P, Vinuela F, et al. Treatment of 54 traumatic carotid-cavernous fistulas. *J Neurosurg* 1981;55:678–692.

47. Debrun GB, Lacour P, Fox AJ, et al. Traumatic carotid cavernous fistulas: etiology, clinical presentation, diagnosis, treatment, results. *Semin Intervent Radiol* 1987;4:242–248.

48. Higashida RT, Halbach VV, Tsai FY, et al. Interventional neurovascular treatment of traumatic carotid and vertebral artery lesions. Results in 234 cases. *AJR* 1986;153:577–582.

49. Norman D, Newton TH, Edwards MS, et al. Carotid-cavernous fistula: closure with detachable silicone balloons. *Radiology* 1983;149:149–159.

ADDITIONAL READINGS

Batjer H II, Purdy PD, Neiman M, Samson DS. Subtemporal transdural use of detachable balloons for traumatic carotid-cavernous fistulas. *Neurosurgery* 1988;22:290–297.

Brismar G, Brismar J. Spontaneous carotid-cavernous fistulas: phlebographic appearance and relation to thrombosis. *Acta Radiol Diagn* 1975;17:180–192.

Courtheoux P, Labbe D, Hamel C, et al. Treatment of bilateral spontaneous dural carotid-cavernous fistulas by coils and sclerotherapy. *J Neurosurg* 1987;66:468–470.

Francis PM, Zabramski JM, Spetzler RF, et al. Treatment of carotid cavernous fistulas: Part II. Surgical interventions. *Barrow Neurological Institute (BNI) Q* 1991;7:7–15.

Golnik KC, Miller NR. Diagnosis of cavernous sinus arteriovenous fistula by measurement of ocular pulse amplitude. *Ophthalmology* 1992;99:1146–1152.

Gotto K, Halbach VV, Hardin CW, et al. Permanent inflation of detachable balloons with a low-viscosity hydrophilic polymerizing system. *Radiology* 1988;169:787–790.

Guglielmi G, Vinuela F, Briganti F, Duckwiler G. Carotid-cavernous fistula caused by a ruptured intracavernous aneurysm: endovascular treatment by electrothrombosis with detachable coils. *Neurosurgery* 1992;31:591–597.

Halbach VV, Higashida RT, Barnwell SL, et al. Transarterial platinum coil embolization of carotid-cavernous fistulas. *AJNR* 1991;12:429–433.

Halbach VV, Higashida RT, Hieshima GB, et al. Normal perfusion pressure breakthrough occurring during treatment of carotid and vertebral fistulas. *AJNR* 1987a;8:751–756.

Halbach VV, Higashida RT, Hieshima GB, et al. Transvenous embolization of aural fistulas involving the cavernous sinus. *AJNR* 1989;10:377–383.

Halbach VV, Higashida RT, Hieshima GB, et al. Dural fistulas involving the cavernous sinus: results in treatment of 30 patients. *Radiology* 1987b;163:437–442.

Higashida RT, Hieshima GB, Halbach VV, et al. Closure of carotid cavernous sinus fistulae by external compression of the artery and jugular vein. *Acta Radiol* 1986;369(Suppl):580.

Hirabuki N, Fujita N, Hashimoto T, et al. Follow-up MRI in aural arteriovenous malformations involving the cavernous sinus: emphasis on detection of venous thrombosis. *Neuroradiology* 1992;34:423–427.

Hosobuchi Y. Electrothrombosis of carotid cavernous fistulas. In Wilson C, Stein BM (eds): Intercranial Arteriovenous Malformations. Baltimore: Williams & Wilkins, 1984, pp 246–258.

Hosobuchi Y. Electrothrombosis of carotid cavernous fistulas. *J Neurosurg* 1975;42:76–85.

Isamat F, Ferrer E, Twose J. Direct intracavernous obliteration of high-flow carotid-cavernous fistulas. *J Neurosurg* 1986;65:770–775.

Keltner JL, Satterfield D, Dublin AB, Lee BCP. Dural and carotid cavernous sinus fistulas: diagnosis, management and complications. *Ophthalmology* 1987;94:1585–1600.

King WA, Hieshima GB, Martin NA. Venous rupture during transvenous approach to a carotid-cavernous fistula. *J Neurosurg* 1989;71:133–137.

Kupersmith MJ, Berenstein A. Neurovascular Neuro-ophthalmology. Berlin: Springer-Verlag, 1993, pp 70–108.

Kupersmith MJ, Berenstein A, Choi IS, et al. Percutaneous transvascular treatment of giant carotid aneurysms: neuro-ophthalmologic findings. *Neurology* 1984;34:328–336.

Leipzig TJ, Mullan SF. Deflation of metrizamide-filled balloon used to occlude a carotid-cavernous fistula. Case report. *J Neurosurg* 1983;59:524–528.

Lewis AI, Tomsick TA, Tew JM Jr. Management of 100 consecutive direct carotid-cavernous fistulas: results of treatment with detachable balloons. *Neurosurgery* 1995;36:239–245.

Manelfe C, Berenstein A. Traitement des fistules carotido-caverneuses par voie veineuse. A propos d'un cas. *J Neuroradiol* 1980;7:13–21.

Mehringer CM, Hieshima GB, Ginnell VS, et al. Therapeutic embolization for vascular trauma of the head and neck. *AJNR* 1983;4:137–142.

Miyasaka Y, Tokiwa K, Irikura K, et al. The effects of a carotid-jugular fistula on cerebral blood flow in the cat: an experimental study in the acute period. *Surg Neurol* 1994;1:396–398.

Morley TP, Barr HWK. Giant intracranial aneurysms: diagnosis, course, and management. *Clin Neurosurg* 1968;16:73–93.

Mullan S. Treatment of carotid-cavernous fistulas by cavernous sinus occlusion. *J Neurosurg* 1979;50:131–144.

Nishijima M, Kamiyama K, Oka N, et al. Electrothrombosis of spontaneous carotid-cavernous fistula by copper needle insertion. *Neurosurgery* 1984;14:400–405.

Pierot L, Poisson M, Jason M, et al. Treatment of type D aural carotid-cavernous fistula by embolization followed by irradiation. *Neuroradiology* 1992;34:77–80.

Sadato A, Taki W, Yamashita K, et al. Treatment of a spontaneous carotid cavernous fistula using an electrodetachable microcoil. *AJNR* 1993;14:334–336.

Santhosh J, Rao VRK, Ravi Mandalam K, et al. Endovascular management of carotid cavernous fistulae: observation on angiographic and clinical results. *Acta Neurol Scand* 1993;88:320–326.

Scialfa G, Vaghi A, Valsecchi F, et al. Neuroradiological treatment of carotid and vertebral fistulas and intracavernous aneurysm. Technical problems and results. *Neuroradiology* 1982;24:13–25.

Taki W, Handa H, Yamagata S, et al. Balloon embolization of a giant aneurysm using a newly developed catheter. *Surg Neurol* 1979;12:363–365.

Taki W, Handa H, Yamagata S, et al. Radiopaque solidifying liquids for releasable balloon technique: a technical note. *Surg Neurol* 1980;13:140–142.

Teng MMH, Guo W-Y, Huang C-L, et al. Occlusion of arteriovenous malformations of the cavernous sinus via the superior ophthalmic vein. *AJNR* 1988; 9:539–546.

Toya S, Shiobara R, Izumi J, et al. Spontaneous carotid-cavernous fistula during pregnancy or in the postpartum stage. *J Neurosurg* 1981;54:252–256.

Tress BM, Thomson KR, ApSimon TH, et al. Treatment of caroticocavernous fistulae with detachable balloons introduced by percutaneous catheterization. *Med J Aust* 1983;1:373–377.

Tsai FY, Hieshima GB, Mehringer M, et al. Delayed effects in the treatment of carotid-cavernous fistulas. *AJNR* 1983;4:357–361.

Wessbecher F, Hartling RP, Nieves M, et al. Treatment of carotid cavernous fistulas: a new balloon delivery system. *AJNR* 1992;13:331–332.

Yamashita K, Taki W, Nishi S, et al. Transvenous embolization of aural caroticocavernous fistulae: technical considerations. *Neuroradiology* 1993;35:475–479.

Yang PJ, Halbach W, Higashida RT, et al. Platinum wire: a new transvascular embolic agent. *AJNR* 1988;9:547–550.

CHAPTER 20

Intracranial Arteriovenous Malformations: General Considerations

J.J. Connors III / J.C. Wojak

Arteriovenous malformations (AVMs) are the most common intracranial vascular malformation (but not the most common vascular *pathology*). The incidence of AVMs is one-seventh to one-tenth that of aneurysms, and AVMs occur in about 0.02% to 0.05% of the population. Ninety percent of intracranial AVMs are supratentorial.[1] They consist of a tangle of vessels of different wall thicknesses and diameters with associated arteriovenous shunting. Varying degrees of thrombosis and calcification can be seen. Atrophy of the surrounding parenchyma caused by steal may be seen.

Presenting symptoms can include seizures, progressive neurologic deficit, intractable headache, intracranial hemorrhage, and hydrocephalus. About 64% of cases present by 40 years of age[1]; 30% to 50% present secondary to hemorrhage. The risk of death from bleeding in a patient with an AVM is about 29%; an additional 20% to 30% of patients suffer neurologic deficits. The incidence of bleeding from an unruptured AVM is about 2% to 4% per year; the risk of rebleeding is 6% in the first year and then decreases to 2% to 4% per year. Each bleeding episode carries a 10% to 15% mortality rate.[2–5]

Hemorrhage from an AVM is usually related to 1) an associated aneurysm, 2) outflow restriction, or 3) pure deep venous drainage.

SPETZLER AND MARTIN GRADING SYSTEM

Spetzler and Martin[6] proposed a grading scale that assigns points based on the size of the AVM, the eloquence of the surrounding brain, and the pattern of venous drainage. This is outlined in Table 20–1.

Deep drainage is considered present if *any* drainage is into the deep system (e.g., internal cerebral veins, basal veins, precentral cerebellar vein). Eloquent brain regions are defined as those that, when disrupted, yield a readily identifiable neurologic deficit. Specific eloquent areas include the sensorimotor, language, and visual cortex; the hypothalamus and thalamus; the internal capsule; the brainstem; the cerebellar peduncles; and the deep cerebellar nuclei. Even if lesions are not directly within these territories, retraction of normal structures nearby can cause postoperative deficits. Noneloquent areas, such as the anterior pole of the frontal or temporal lobe and the cerebellar cortex, are thought to give rise to minimal symptoms. Electrophysiologic testing is not necessary for localization of these lesions, but it can be used along with superselective Wada testing.

When the points are totaled, a number from 1 to 5 is generated. This is the grade of the AVM (grade I is the mildest, grade V the most severe). Inoperable lesions are considered to be grade VI. The risk of morbidity and mortality rises steadily with increasing grade.

Surgical results are available for the treatment of the various grades of AVM. Figures are presented here to give the reader some idea of the morbidity and mortality associated with surgery performed by an excellent surgical team. In Spetzler and Martin's paper presenting the grading system for these lesions, data were given concerning the relation between grade and outcome.[6] These results are listed in Table 20–2.

An interesting note is made: no deaths occurred in 100 patients who underwent surgery for AVMs of any grade.

TABLE 20-1 Grading of Arteriovenous Malformations

Graded Feature	Points Assigned
Size of arteriovenous malformation	
Small (<3 cm)	1
Medium (3–6 cm)	2
Large (>6 cm)	3
Eloquence of surrounding brain	
Noneloquent	0
Eloquent	1
Pattern of venous drainage	
Superficial only	0
Deep	1

From Spetzler RF, Martin NA. A proposed grading system for arteriovenous malformations. *J Neurosurg* 1986;65:476–483.

TABLE 20-2 Incidence of Postoperative Deficit in Relation to Arteriovenous Malformation Grade

Grade	Minor Deficit (%)	Major Deficit (%)
I	0	0
II	5	0
III	12	4
IV	20	7
V	19	12

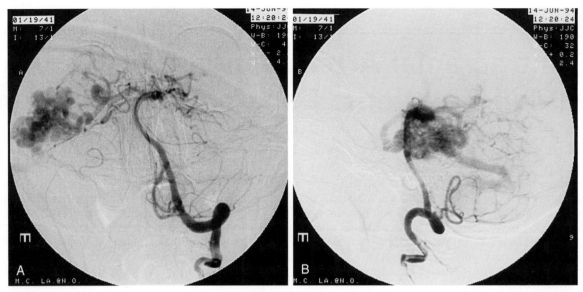

Figure 20-1 Case 1. *A* and *B*, Posteroanterior (PA) and lateral vertebral angiogram revealing a large, high-flow, posterior temporal arteriovenous malformation (AVM) being fed by the right posterior cerebral artery in this 53-year-old woman. Additional evaluation revealed minimal supply from the right middle cerebral artery also. The patient refused surgery but desired treatment.

GENERAL PHILOSOPHY OF THERAPY

In treating AVMs, the nidus of the lesion must be removed or obliterated. Only when the surgical approach or actual removal of the AVM is difficult or risky is endovascular therapy contemplated. Because the endovascular cure rate for AVMs is only 5% to 10%, endovascular therapy usually is used for preoperative assistance or to shrink the mass as much as possible before radiotherapy. In our experience, a total cure is rare, but it appears that at least one of our patients has been cured (Figs. 20–1 to 20–8).

Preoperative embolization using glue or alcohol may be performed to shrink a lesion before radiotherapy. There is no clear proof, however, that this form of therapy provides a better outcome than that seen with the natural history of the disease.

A possible reason for primary endovascular therapy may be when surgery is inadvisable or refused by the patient, but some relief from symptoms (mass effect or intracranial hypertension or hydrocephalus) is desired. In this case, partial occlusion may be indicated and effective. Partial embolization for symptomatic relief has been performed with success (Figs. 20–9 to 20–15).

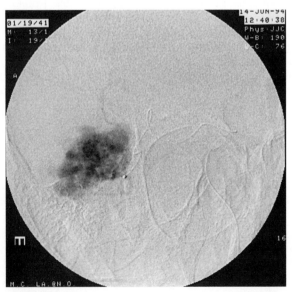

Figure 20-2 Initial microcatheter injection poorly opacifies the lesion owing to high flow. The catheter tip appears to be within the nidus, and pharmacologic testing was (predictably) uneventful.

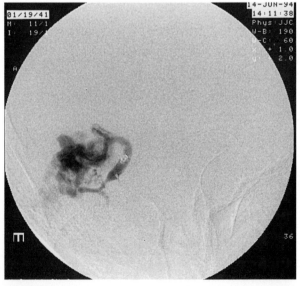

Figure 20-3 Initial embolization was performed utilizing polyvinyl alcohol (PVA) particles and alcohol followed by a coil to slow the flow in the huge residual channel and enable the alcohol to work. Note the absence of a large portion of the nidus, but not the fistula.

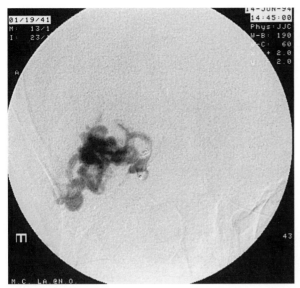

Figure 20-4 After additional embolization with PVA particles and alcohol, more of the nidus is gone, but the shunt is still open.

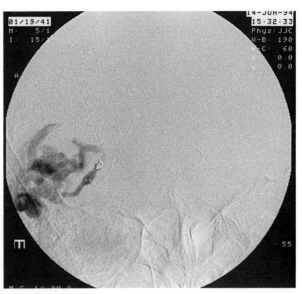

Figure 20-6 To our consternation, the large arteriovenous shunt is now noted to be open again, as is a previously occluded channel. Maximal therapeutic effort was thought to have been achieved, and the procedure was terminated at this time, with this fistula still open even after additional ethanol embolization.

Most interventional neuroradiologists believe that cyanoacrylates can yield a higher cure rate than particles, but still only a small percentage of patients can be totally cured. Only about 40% of practitioners who routinely use cyanoacrylates for embolization of AVMs claim to have achieved a true cure of any AVM. Ethanol embolization may yield somewhat better results but with possibly increased long-term danger. See Chapter 22 for further details concerning this therapy.

THEORY OF AVM EMBOLIZATION

The aim of providing aid to the surgeon determines the strategy of this procedure and should be similar to that of preoperative tumor embolization. Occlusion of problematic feeders to the AVM should be the goal, but only at their entry into the mass. Occlusion of

feeders even millimeters proximal to the AVM can render surgery *more* complicated by causing recruitment (or enlargement) of a myriad of small vessels that otherwise would not have been significant. In addition, proximal occlusion may damage normal structures. A discussion of current strategies for preoperative AVM embolization is presented below.

Goal of Embolization

It is useless to perform a procedure without a clear goal in mind. Even with the best technique, permanent cure of an AVM by any endovascular means is unusual. For this reason, most procedures are preoperative.

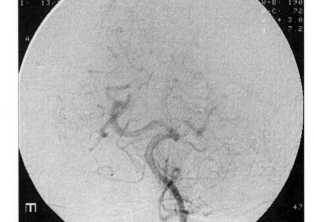

Figure 20-5 The AVM *appears* to be cured, but waiting for further evaluation is deemed appropriate.

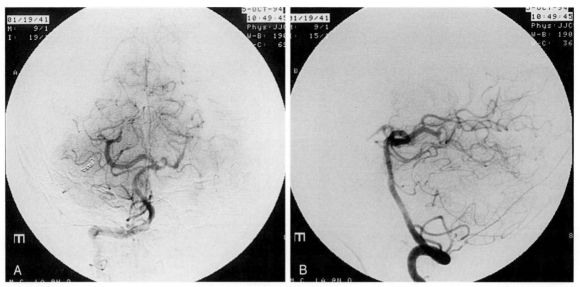

Figure 20-7 *A* and *B,* Four months later the patient was brought back for further evaluation and possible treatment. Not only is the AVM no longer filling from the posterior cerebral artery, but it appears to be totally gone.

With this in mind, what is the purpose of the procedure? It is to render surgery safer and more accurate. Essentially no increase in surgical morbidity and mortality related to the procedure is therefore imperative, and some benefit should be expected for the trouble of the procedure. This is rendered by drying the surgical field. Drying of the surgical field is achieved by blocking the direct arterial feeders as well as the collateral supply that will develop.

The more the nidus of the AVM is occluded, the less collateral supply will develop and the longer it will take. An initial good result of embolization can

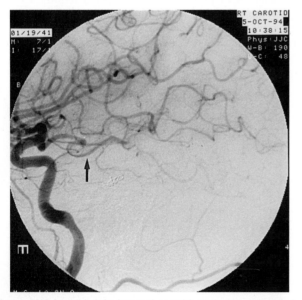

Figure 20-8 Lateral right internal carotid angiogram obtained at the same time demonstrating lack of visualization of the embolized AVM. Note the residual large posterior communicating artery but only minimal flow into the P2 segment of the posterior cerebral artery itself (*arrow*) owing to lack of flow to the downstream AVM.

be achieved but there may be an amazing rebound by the time the procedure is over (Figs. 20–16 to 20–18). This pattern demands true intranidal occlusion so that revascularization (which almost inevitably occurs) takes as long as can be managed.

For this reason, a combination of intranidal occlusion and rapid postprocedure surgery is indicated. The sooner the surgery, the better. Some particulate embolizations persist for days or months, but others last only hours.

Vessel Selection

Frequently, the easiest vessel for the endovascular operator to occlude is also the easiest for the surgeon to reach. The goal of therapy must be kept in mind, and the endovascular procedure should not add risk to an already risky situation. The targets of endovascular therapy should be the vessels that are potentially dangerous to the patient and the surgeon, that is, difficult to control at surgery.

In addition, some vessels are intrinsically dangerous from either an embolization or a surgical standpoint. Specifically, if the AVM has previously hemorrhaged, a pseudoaneurysm often is associated with the mass. The feeder to this pseudoaneurysm should be occluded first; it has already bled once. If occlusion of other feeders is performed first, there is an increased risk of rebleeding because of increasing flow in the remaining feeders, including the supply to the pseudoaneurysm.[7]

A true aneurysm may be present in the vessel leading to an AVM because of the high flow rate within this vessel. Embolization of the AVM distal to the aneurysm may increase the mean pressure within the proximal vessel (and thus the aneurysm), causing a rupture of this aneurysm with potentially devastating results.

Pre-embolization clipping of proximal aneurysms,

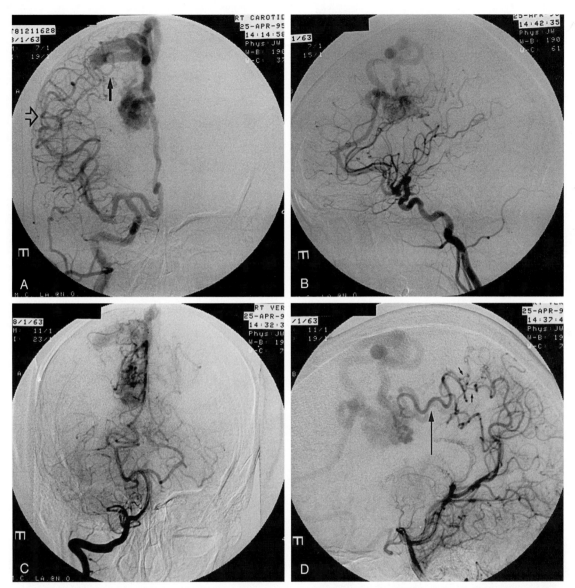

Figure 20-9 Case 2. A 32-year-old HIV-positive woman with increasing headaches, visual disturbances, and "blackout" spells or seizures. A computed tomography scan and angiography revealed a large, very-high-flow AVM in the deep right posterior frontal lobe. This was supplied by the anterior, middle, and posterior cerebral arteries, with a massive amount of drainage through the extremely enlarged superficial veins. PA and lateral views of the right common carotid artery *(A and B)* and right vertebral artery *(C and D)* demonstrate these findings. Surgical excision was thought to be inadvisable, and endovascular treatment was requested for potential symptomatic relief of the increased intracranial pressure secondary to the high-flow AVM (symptomatic relief is not a well-recognized clinical indication or common therapeutic option).

Note the direct approach to the huge anterior cerebral feeder *(A and B)*. Although no direct evidence of supply from the middle cerebral artery is seen, suspicion should be aroused by the size of at least one branch *(open arrow, A)* and the suggestion on the PA view of a very long medial course *(arrow, A)*. There does not appear to be any access to the portion supplied by the posterior circulation *(C and D)*. The posterior supply has been recruited by the sump of the AVM utilizing pial collaterals *(small arrows, D)*, which normally connect the posterior cerebral circulation to the anterior cerebral artery distribution. Note the large artery *(thin arrow, D)*, which has the typical appearance of a marginal callosal branch but is now flowing retrograde from the posterior circulation to the AVM. Also note the sump effect of the AVM through the posterior communicating artery on the vertebral artery injection. On this injection, the posterior pericallosal artery does not appear to supply the lesion (the vessel is very small and does not reach the area).

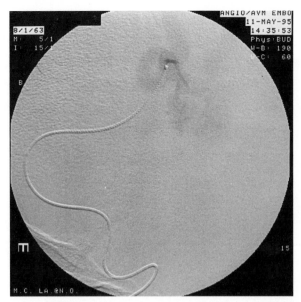

Figure 20-10 An approach to the AVM has been made through the pericallosal artery. Injected contrast is hardly seen owing to the extremely high flow and immediate washout.

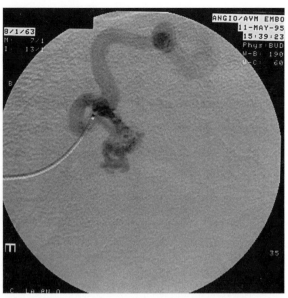

Figure 20-12 Further embolization now results in an appearance not infrequently seen. The once small microtubules seem to have enlarged and almost have the appearance of a "cavernous transformation." There is now massive direct flow through these fistulae without any apparent AVM nidus. This transformation in flow pattern is dramatic and potentially depressing. The particle size may need to be changed (increased), or a change to an Avitene sludge or an alcohol, PVA, and Avitene cocktail can be made. Cyanoacrylate could deal with this situation well.

when feasible, or even coil occlusion (Guglielmi detachable coil, GDC), should be considered. Current opinion among interventional neuroradiologists is divided. Spetzler believes that ignoring any proximal aneurysm is a poor choice (verbal communication).

Deep perforators (such as thalamostriates and lenticulostriates) frequently are the most difficult for surgeons to control during open excision but also can be some of the most difficult to treat preoperatively using an endovascular approach. For example, embolization of the anterior choroidal artery has a complication rate of about 15% to 20% (i.e., a significant stroke).

During a procedure, it may be necessary to test a vessel before occlusion to avoid inducing a neurologic deficit. This can be performed by direct superselective administration of amobarbital or methohexital (see "How to Test a Vessel Prior to Embolization [Provocative Testing]" in Chapter 3) (Figs. 20–19 to 20–21).

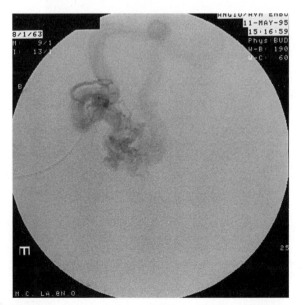

Figure 20-11 After partial embolization with 150- to 250-micron PVA particles, there is some slowing of flow. Note the now visible microfeeders. The bulk of the AVM is still unseen from this injection.

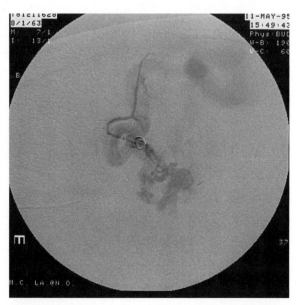

Figure 20-13 After the use of an Avitene, alcohol, and PVA sludge, the flow dynamics changed again, now revealing a small cortical branch. Because of its appearance, a switch to coils has already been made.

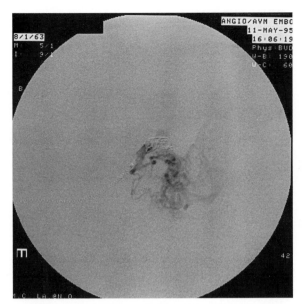

Figure 20-14 After further occlusion with coils, the large main trunk is now seen to supply an inferior portion of the nidus through small branches. Note the coils placed slightly distally. Particles followed by coils were used to occlude this portion of the vessel.

Most practitioners believe that embolization of more than two pedicles during one procedure increases the risk of hemodynamic alteration and subsequent complications. In other words, a severe reduction in antegrade flow through the lesion may induce venous thrombosis, a severe consequence. (See Chapter 64 for a further discussion of this problem.)

Pre-embolization Functional Testing

When there is any doubt concerning the danger of occlusion of the vessel that the catheter is in, functional testing can be performed. This technique is described in detail in Chapter 3. Testing is performed primarily when the catheter tip is not truly within the abnormality where occlusion would, by definition, be safe. This situation was formerly common because of the inability to obtain accurate positioning of the catheter tip. With newer catheters, this problem is not as common; there is confidence that accurate distal positioning of the catheter tip can be obtained. Indeed, many practitioners now perform procedures with the patient under general anesthesia, precluding functional testing.

TECHNIQUES OF THERAPY

This topic is covered further in Chapters 21 and 22. The basic theory of embolization and its application to specific areas is covered in the introduction to this chapter. The lack of a capillary bed complicates embolization of AVMs. Particulate embolization invariably results in some degree of pulmonary embolization; this should be kept to a minimum. Because of the varying size of arteriovenous shunts, appropriate selection of the size of particles is difficult. Attempts have been made to quantify when to change particle size during embolization, but with minimal success.[8, 9]

Many AVMs contain large arteriovenous shunts, and alternative particulate embolization methods may be necessary. A slurry of Avitene and polyvinyl alcohol (PVA) particles can occlude large channels. The addition of a small amount of alcohol (about 30% in the final solution) can render the transient occlusion of the slurry more permanent (i.e., cause endothelial damage).

Care should be taken to avoid overinjection of particles or coils. When flow has slowed, the possibility of rupture of the AVM or the arterial feeder increases (see Chapter 65). Wedging of the catheter during particulate embolization is discouraged because of the possibility of overinjection in a closed system, with the chance of rupture.

Preoperative Embolization

When undertaking preoperative embolization of AVMs, care must be taken to avoid occluding too much of the high-flow vascular supply at once. This can result in an increased incidence of normal perfusion pressure breakthrough and possible frank hemorrhage, owing to changing hemodynamics in regions of chronic ischemia secondary to steal by the AVM[10] (see Chapter 64). This situation necessitates the use

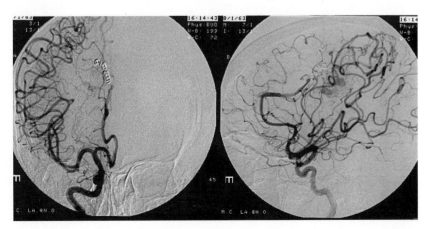

Figure 20-15 The final postembolization appearance is dramatically improved. The high flow has considerably decreased. Note, however, what appears to be incipient recruitment of middle cerebral artery branches. The AVM is obviously not cured (the posterior cerebral supply is unchanged), but the tremendous arteriovenous shunt has been greatly reduced. This patient was cured from the standpoint of intracranial hypertension and headache.

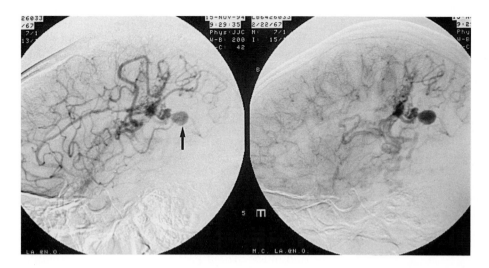

Figure 20-16 Case 3. A lateral right internal carotid angiogram demonstrates an AVM filling from the pericallosal artery as well as at least one large middle cerebral artery branch. Note the large venous varix (arrow). This 27-year-old patient presented with a seizure.

of *staged* procedures. The eventual goal is to occlude as much of the AVM as possible. It is sometimes necessary to allow the brain, arteries, arterioles, and capillaries to adapt to the change in vascular flow and pressure before continuing with the therapeutic procedure.

How long should the period be between procedures? No large, controlled series exist to answer this question, but interventional neuroradiologists generally believe that 1 week is barely long enough and 10 weeks is too long. The goal is to allow adaptation of the vessels that currently exist without allowing enough time for development of major new collateral supply to the AVM.

Surgeons also differ in their opinions on the best time to operate after embolization. Some believe that operating immediately after embolization is best, whereas others believe that waiting about 1 week is

better. This difference may be related to the type of embolization performed.

When only proximal pedicle embolization is performed, immediate surgery probably is the most beneficial. This allows a minimal amount of time for collateral vascular supply to form to the AVM. When true intranidal occlusion is performed, however, particularly with an inflammatory agent such as cyanoacrylate or ethanol, allowing a period of time for a decrease in the amount of surrounding inflammation is helpful. These are decisions that must be made jointly by the team of physicians involved in the patient's care.

MATERIALS FOR EMBOLIZATION
Cyanoacrylates

Although embolization of AVMs usually is performed preliminary to other therapy, permanent complete

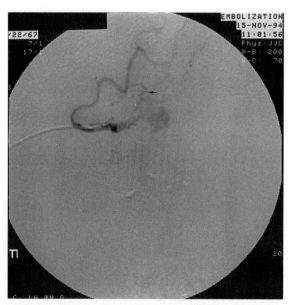

Figure 20-17 After partial embolization with PVA particles, injection shows poor flow through the AVM, with reflux back into a side branch. Early microcollaterals are visible arising from the callosomarginal branch (arrow).

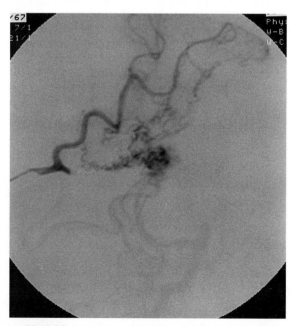

Figure 20-18 Minutes later, extensive recruitment of microcollaterals from the callosomarginal branch is seen, as well as failure of the PVA with recanalization of the nidus of the AVM.

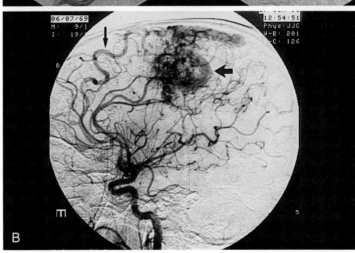

Figure 20-19 Case 4. *A* and *B*, APA and lateral right common carotid angiogram demonstrating a large AVM deep within the right parietal lobe in a 26-year-old man with seizures. The middle cerebral artery feeders should be simple for the surgeon to ligate at the time of surgery, along with the tortuous, large, superficial callosomarginal artery *(thin arrow, B)*. There appear to be two deep anterior cerebral branches (pericallosal), however, which could supply a portion of the tumor from below and may be difficult for the surgeon to reach. Embolization was requested for control of these. A large draining vein is also seen *(fat arrow, B)*.

cure is possible. Cyanoacrylates are capable of this, but the degree of permanency of this treatment is still unknown. Cyanoacrylates are usually diluted by at least half with a nonpermanent oil, such as Ethiodol (Savage Laboratories) or Pantopaque. Even so, the degree of permanency probably is high. Alternatively, polymerization of this glue can be slowed by the use of glacial acetic acid, resulting in deposition of nearly 100% glue; the exact parameters of this use have not been defined clinically and may be unpredictable.[11, 12] (See Chapter 21 for a definitive discussion of cyanoacrylate embolization of AVMs.)

Particles

Particles are used only in cases that are clearly presurgical. Although safer to use, they are not considered permanent. Typically, PVA is the agent used. Newer agents, such as cellulose microspheres, have been developed that show some promise of permanency.

The technique of particle use is similar to that of other embolization procedures, except that the location for this embolization is intracranial. Exacting technique is therefore necessary. Distal location of the catheter tip is vital, and cautious infusion of embolic material is also indicated. It is better to start with particles that are too small and too dilute than slightly too large or too concentrated. A mixture that

is too concentrated invites clumping, which can render fine control of infusion difficult.

Additionally, although dilute contrast is always used, if it is too dilute it is difficult to see, again making fine manual control of infusion difficult. Therefore, use of three fourths concentration with more dilute particles is preferred. This may require more syringes, but even 20 3-cc syringes of slightly dilute contrast yield only about 45 ml of contrast.

Particles that are 150 to 250 microns in size are sufficient to occlude a portion of most AVMs, but a fair number of particles go through larger channels, and thus a staged increase in particle size is necessary. Particles up to 1000 microns in size or even larger may be required. At this point, small coils become necessary.

Judging when to change to larger particles can be difficult. Measurement of back pressure in AVMs has been used as a guide, but in general, if a lack of slowing is apparent with embolization of a pedicle with two or three syringes (3 cc), then progression to the next size particle is warranted. Gradual increases in particle size accomplish the intended goal.

Once the flow is slowed significantly, no further particle embolization is performed. Final blockage is then performed with small microcoils. The goal is not total vascular stasis but rather filling of the nidus with embolic material to prevent recruitment before surgery and then blocking the feeding vessel supplying the lesion.

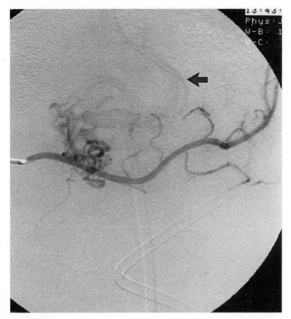

Figure 20-20 The pericallosal artery was catheterized but was seen to supply the AVM via small feeders in an en passant fashion. The distal portion of the pericallosal artery was seen to supply a large region of the posterior deep medial parietal lobe. After several injections with careful observation, it was believed that no significant collateral supply to the downstream territory was present. This was because (1) the flow from the pericallosal artery anterior to the AVM went *past* the AVM to this downstream territory (if any supply entered downstream, it would be expected to be drawn in a retrograde fashion toward the AVM); (2) no wash-in could be seen in any portion of the downstream distribution (to imply that another vessel entered); and (3) injection of the vessel beyond the AVM revealed very slow (typical) filling of arterioles and capillary bed. It was determined that this vessel could not be sacrificed, and the small feeders arising from it could not be accurately catheterized. This vessel was therefore not embolized. Again, note the large draining vein *(arrow)*.

Absolute Alcohol

Absolute alcohol can be used for complete obliteration of vascular channels, but its ability to penetrate to the capillary level with subsequent destruction of all cells touched renders this a dangerous tool. Extremely accurate placement of the catheter tip is necessary for its use. Infusion must be completely within the abnormality; "close" is not adequate. (See Chapter 22 for a discussion of this technique.)

Proximal Coil Occlusion of Feeders

Recent work has shown that more proximal occlusion by coils without any microparticulate embolization can have a beneficial effect on surgery without risk of ischemic damage to normal structures. The surgery should be performed as soon after embolization as possible (within 1 or 2 days, at most) to preclude recruitment of abundant new feeders, which invariably occurs rapidly. Even though the lesion is not dry, occlusion of the feeders apparently controls *major* hemorrhage and permits adequate surgical dissection. In addition, it appears that nearby normal structures remain viable without as much risk of

embolic consequences as from small particulate or liquid embolization. This approach necessitates an understanding of normal intracranial hemodynamics as well as close cooperation between the surgical team and the endovascular team. As stated earlier, if there is any delay between this type of embolization and surgery, a myriad of new feeders can grow, complicating the operative procedure significantly.

This approach has undergone no controlled evaluation, and it will be years before any judgment can be made concerning this strategy. The obvious advantage is that of simplicity for the operator; superficially, it may also be safer from the viewpoint of the interventional neuroradiologist. Some interventional neuroradiologists favor this technique, and some neurosurgeons find this technique acceptable. A large study is necessary to evaluate the incidence of ischemic complications from the less superselective placement of the coils as well as to evaluate the surgical benefit of this approach.

Extensive coil embolization may be necessary. Straight, 2-mm coils generally are adequate. These coils can be injected into the AVM nidus by saline bolus rather than pushed with a coil pusher. This tends to deposit them farther toward or actually in the nidus of the AVM rather than in a more proximal location. Many coils may be necessary to achieve the desired result.

Liquid Coils

Target Therapeutics manufactures platinum coils that are extremely flexible and capable of being carried by injection to a distal location. These are supplied in tubes with a porous cap that allows injection of saline to preload them for injection. The tube is then introduced into the hub of the microcatheter and the coil is gently injected into the proximal shaft. A 3-ml syringe filled with saline is then attached to the microcatheter and the coil is injected just as other microcoils can be.

These coils are supplied in various sizes, the smallest of which are capable of traversing a high-flow AVM and eventually lodging in the lungs. Some trial and error is necessary to be proficient at selection of sizes to achieve penetration of these coils to the nidus without traversing the AVM. They can also be difficult to see during fluoroscopy.

Other Agents

Early experimental work has been done evaluating additional agents, including hydrogels, oils, sclerosing agents, plastics, and boiling contrast, but consideration of their use is beyond the scope of this discussion.

ROLE OF EMBOLIZATION IN RADIOSURGERY

Preliminary embolization before radiosurgery has been a trend in certain medical centers. The original belief was that an AVM that is too large for primary

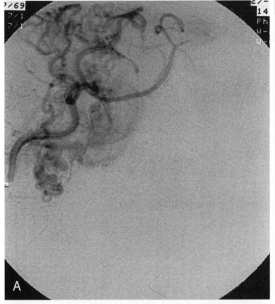

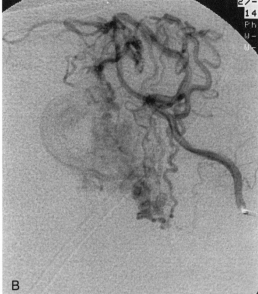

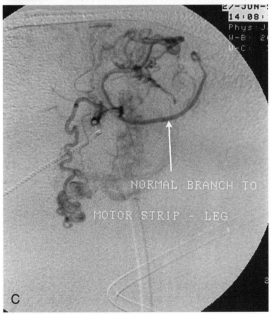

Figure 20-21 *A* to *C*, A large marginal branch arising from the pericallosal artery and leading to the AVM was then catheterized *(A and B)*. This flows toward the medial surface of the hemisphere near the central sulcus. It is seen to drape over the lesion and send supply to it from both the medial and inferior aspects as well as from the superior surface. In addition, however, a normal-appearing branch is seen to flow past the lesion toward the posterior parietal lobe. The catheter was advanced until it was almost directly at the point that several branches to the AVM arose *(C)*. An amobarbital test injection was made at this point (a 50-mg bolus). The patient immediately lost all motor function in his leg; sensory function was preserved. It was not considered appropriate to try to embolize any vessel from this location.

The information gained from this procedure is very useful for the neurosurgeon. It is now known that sacrifice of certain vessels is not possible, and careful observation for en passant supply has to be made.

therapy might be reduced to a size suitable for therapy; this is not the case in many instances. After supposedly permanent partial embolization and radiosurgery were performed, long-term follow-up revealed a black hole (the radiosurgically treated AVM) in the center of an apparently recurrent AVM. Interventional neuroradiologists generally agree that pre-radiosurgery embolization does not necessarily convert an AVM into a good candidate for radiosurgery. However, this is currently not uncommonly the best solution. (The role of radiosurgery is discussed further in Chapter 23.)

TECHNICAL PROBLEMS, COMPLICATIONS, AND SOLUTIONS IN AVM EMBOLIZATION

Even though the number and incidence of complications associated with embolization appear daunting,

the most diehard critics agree that the overall clinical outcome is better with than without embolization for most types of AVM.

Published data indicate a general range of major complications resulting from embolization of AVMs of 5% to 15%. Minor complications are widely underreported. Minor transient ischemic attacks are reported to occur in about 1% to 5% of cases, but a significant portion of skilled interventionalists think the rate is probably between 5% and 15% (verbal communications). These rates are presented, despite a lack of true scientific published data, to give the reader at least some idea of the current state of the art. Verbal communications from specific practitioners indicate that between 30% and 50% of patients have single-photon emission computed tomography or magnetic resonance imaging changes after embolization, most of which are asymptomatic. Certain other complications also are addressed in Chapter 64.

Retrograde Thrombosis

Retrograde thrombosis appears to be a common major problem. Retrograde thrombosis is seen when a large feeder is occluded successfully, leaving the huge trunk from which it arose to supply only a small normal branch or two (as described in Chapter 64). This may then thrombose, occluding the supply to these normal vessels. An additional compounding feature may be that the parent vessel can suffer endothelial damage from the catheter traversing it during the procedure; this could be a difference between endovascular occlusion and surgical ligation. Retrograde thrombosis, however, occurs even with surgical ligations. Spetzler often places patients on heparin within hours after craniotomy for AVM resection in an attempt to prevent thrombosis of these residual vessels (personal communication). Although heparinization sometimes is unsuccessful at keeping these vessels open, urokinase may succeed in reopening these channels, and the platelet cascade may then stop.

Nontarget Occlusion

Nontarget occlusion is probably more common than realized, and can be related to technique or changing hemodynamics during the procedure. This can be a major problem during extracranial work, when inadvertent intracranial migration of particles can be disastrous, but it also occurs with AVM treatment. Vessels previously unknown, unseen, and unrevealed during the provocative testing may become apparent after a portion of the steal from the AVM is removed. It is at this point that further embolization can be dangerous. Periodic amobarbital or methohexital testing is necessary during most embolizations of large AVMs.

Periembolic Inflammation

Periembolic inflammation can arise when using ethanol. The territory around the AVM may become intensely irritated to the point that significant swelling or shift becomes apparent, with or without neurologic change. This should be treated aggressively with steroids and usually is transient (only a small number of cases are reported in print; most have been reported verbally by Yakes). The cause of these changes is not known (i.e., does the ethanol ooze into adjacent territories, does the ethanol contact these territories directly, or are they just reacting to the nearby destruction?).

Normal Perfusion Pressure Breakthrough

Normal perfusion pressure breakthrough occurs when the high-flow shunt of the AVM is occluded and nearby normal brain and its capillary bed are exposed to normal perfusion pressure. These nearby structures have lost the ability of autoregulation as a result of chronic hypoperfusion and may be incapable of responding to the tremendous rise in local intracranial flow. This results in edema formation and possibly in hemorrhage. (This topic is discussed further in Chapter 64.) Normal perfusion pressure breakthrough can be of major significance and is difficult to treat. Strict control of blood pressure is necessary. Measures aimed at reducing edema (such as diuretic therapy) may be helpful.

Venous Thrombosis

Occlusion of major blood supply to an AVM may eliminate the supply to a large vein also draining normal structures. This vein may then occlude because of sluggish flow, resulting in a venous infarct in the normal territory. Although this can occur even when the patient is receiving heparin or aspirin, these agents may help prevent it. If a period of a few days or weeks can be passed successfully, the vein will shrink, the residual flow will increase in speed, and the threat of secondary thrombosis will lessen. This large thrombosed vein also can be the source of pulmonary emboli. Only if the venous pouch is huge will the embolic insult be of clinical significance, but this has occurred.

Vascular Perforation

Vascular perforation during an embolization has happened to about three fourths of skilled interventional neuroradiologists polled. Most of these events are inconsequential.[13] No large series has been published, but from verbal reports, perforations appear to be mostly produced by guidewires. As stated elsewhere, guidewires are small (about 30 gauge), and perforation with a guidewire usually is not evident clinically, even if seen on angiography or follow-up computed tomography (see Chapter 65). If bleeding is persistent, the assistance of the neurosurgeon should be sought. Perforation of almost any major intracranial arterial branch is easily repairable by a neurosurgeon; a touch of Avitene or, at most, a single microstitch can seal the hole.

Rupture of an AVM during embolization can be fatal. Typically, the hole is large and is in a vessel that may be abnormal. Intrinsic hemodynamic adaptation probably is nonexistent. Anticoagulation should be reversed rapidly and occlusion with coils achieved as quickly as possible (assuming the bleed is of significance). Occasionally, the rupture is discovered after the procedure. As stated earlier, the incidence of rupture appears to be slightly higher with intranidal glue use than with simple particle embolization (unpublished anecdotal results).

REFERENCES

1. Okazaki H. Fundamentals of neuropathology. New York: Ikagu-Shoin, 1983.

2. Wilkins RH. Natural history of intracranial vascular malformations: a review. *Neurosurgery* 1985;16:421–430.

3. Brown RD, Wiebers DO, Forbes G, et al. The natural history of unruptured intracranial arteriovenous malformations. *J Neurosurg* 1988;68:352–357.

4. Crawford PM, West CR, Chadwick DW. Arteriovenous malformations of the brain: natural history in unoperated patients. *J Neurol Neurosurg Psychiatry* 1986;49:1–10.

5. Graf CJ, Perret GE, Torner JC. Bleeding from cerebral arteriovenous malformations as part of their natural history. *J Neurosurg* 1983;58:331–337.

6. Spetzler RF, Martin NA. A proposed grading system for arteriovenous malformations. *J Neurosurg* 1986;65:476–483.

7. Garcia-Monaco R, Rodesch G, Alvarez H, et al. Pseudoaneurysms within ruptured intracranial arteriovenous malformations: diagnosis and early endovascular management. *AJNR* 1993;14:315–321.

8. Duckwiler GR, Dion JE, Vinuela F, et al. Intravascular microcatheter pressure monitoring: experimental work and early clinical evaluation [Abstract]. *AJNR* 1989;10:876.

9. Jungreis CA, Horton JA, Hecht ST. Hemodynamic changes in feeders to cerebral arteriovenous malformations during therapeutic embolization [Abstract]. *AJNR* 1989;10:876.

10. Batjer HH, Devous MD. The use of acetazolamide-enhanced regional cerebral blood flow measurement to predict risk for arteriovenous malformation patients. *Neurosurgery* 1992;31:213–217.

11. Cromwell LD, Kerber CW. Modification of cyanoacrylate for therapeutic embolization: preliminary experience. *AJR* 1979;132:799–801.

12. Spiegel SM, Vinuela F, Goldwasser MJ, et al. Adjusting polymerization time of isobutyl-2-cyanoacrylate. *AJNR* 1986;7:109–112.

13. Halbach VV, Higashida RT, Dowd CF, et al. Management of vascular perforations that occur during neurointerventional procedures. *AJNR* 1991;12:319–327.

ADDITIONAL READINGS

Al-Rodhan NRF, Sundt TM, Piepgras DG, et al. Occlusive hyperemia: a theory for the hemodynamic complications following resection of intracerebral arteriovenous malformations. *J Neurosurg* 1993;78:167–175.

Albert P, Salgado H, Polaina M, et al. A study on the venous drainage of 150 cerebral arteriovenous malformations as related to haemorrhagic risks and size of the lesion. *Acta Neurochir (Wien)* 1990;103:30–34.

Barnett GH, Little JR, Ebrahim ZY, et al. Cerebral circulation during arteriovenous malformation operation. *Neurosurgery* 1987;20:836–842.

Batjer HH, Devous MD, Seibert GB, et al. Intracranial arteriovenous malformation: relationships between clinical and radiographic factors and ipsilateral steal severity. *Neurosurgery* 1988;23:322–328.

Batjer HH, Purdy PD, Giller CA, Samson DS. Evidence of redistribution of cerebral blood flow during treatment for an intracranial arteriovenous malformation. *Neurosurgery* 1989;25:599–605.

Becker DH, Townsend JJ, Kramer RA, Newton TH. Occult cerebrovascular malformations: a series of 18 histological verified cases with negative angiography. *Brain* 1979;102:249–287.

Berenstein A. Technique of catheterization and embolization of the lenticulostriate arteries. *J Neurosurg* 1981;54:783–789.

Boulos R, Kricheff II, Chase N. Value of cerebral angiography in the embolization treatment of cerebral arteriovenous malformations. *Radiology* 1970;97:65–70.

Brown RD Jr, Wiebers DO, Forbes GS. Unruptured intracranial aneurysms and arteriovenous malformations: frequency of intracranial hemorrhage and relationship of lesions. *J Neurosurg* 1990;73:859–863.

Chioffi F, Pasqualin A, Beltramello A, Da Pian R. Hemodynamic effects of preoperative embolization in cerebral arteriovenous malformations: evaluation with transcranial Doppler sonography. *Neurosurgery* 1992;31:877–885.

Cunha e Sa MJ, Stein BM, Solomon RA, McCormick PC. The treatment of associated intracranial aneurysms and arteriovenous malformations. *J Neurosurg* 1992;77:853–859.

Dias MS, Sekhar LN. Intracranial hemorrhage from aneurysms and arteriovenous malformations during pregnancy and the puerperium. *Neurosurgery* 1990;27:855–866.

Dowd CF, Halbach VV, Barnwell SL, et al. Particulate embolization of the anterior choroidal artery in the treatment of cerebral arteriovenous malformations. *AJNR* 1991;12:1055–1061.

Ezura M, Takahashi A, Yoshimoto T. Successful treatment of an arteriovenous malformation by chemical embolization with estrogen followed by conventional radiotherapy. *Neurosurgery* 1992;31:1105–1107.

Fleischer LH, Young WL, Pile-Spellman J-P, et al. Relationship of transcranial Doppler flow velocities and arteriovenous malformation feeding artery pressures. *Stroke* 1993;24:1897–1902.

Goldberg RA, Garcia GH, Duckwiler GR. Combined embolization and surgical treatment of arteriovenous malformation of the orbit. *Am J Ophthalmol* 1993;116:17–25.

Hayashi S, Arimoto T, Itakura T, Fuji T, et al. The association of intracranial aneurysms and arteriovenous malformations of the brain. *J Neurosurg* 1981;55:971–975.

Hecht ST, Horton JA, Kerber CW. Hemodynamics of the central nervous system arteriovenous malformation nidus during particulate embolization. *Neuroradiology* 1991;33:62–64.

Hilal SK, Michelsen JW. Therapeutic percutaneous embolization for extra-axial vascular lesions of the head, neck, and spine. *J Neurosurg* 1975;43:275–287.

Horton JC, Chambers WA, Lyons SL, et al. Pregnancy and the risk of hemorrhage from cerebral arteriovenous malformations. *Neurosurgery* 1990;27:867–872.

Jungreis CA, Horton JA. Pressure changes in the arterial feeder to a cerebral AVM as a guide to monitoring therapeutic embolization. *AJNR* 1989;10:1057–1060.

Jungreis CA, Horton JA, Hecht ST. Blood pressure changes in feeders to cerebral arteriovenous malformations during therapeutic embolization. *AJNR* 1989;10:575–577.

Kikuchi K, Kowada M, Hiroyasu S. Vascular malformations of the brain in hereditary hemorrhagic telangiectasia (Rendu-Osler-Weber disease). *Surg Neurol* 1994;41:374–380.

Kondziolka D, Humphreys RP, Hoffman HJ, et al. Arteriovenous malformations of the brain in children: a forty year experience. *Can J Neurol Sci* 1992;19:40–45.

Kumar AJ, Vinuela F, Fox AJ, Rosenbaum AE. Unruptured intracranial arteriovenous malformations do cause mass effect. *AJNR* 1985;6:29–32.

Lindegaard K-F, Grolimund P, Aaslid R, Nornes H. Evaluation of cerebral AVM's using transcranial Doppler ultrasound. *J Neurosurg* 1986;65:335–344.

Marks MP, Pelc NJ, Ross MR, Enzmann DR. Determination of cerebral blood flow with a phase-contrast cine MR imaging technique: evaluation of normal subjects and patients with arteriovenous malformations. *Radiology* 1992;182:467–476.

Mason R. Arteriovenous aneurysm of mid-brain and retina, facial naevi and mental changes. *Brain* 1943;66:163–189.

Miyasaka Y, Yada K, Kurata A, et al. Correlation between intravascular pressure and risk of hemorrhage due to arteriovenous malformations. *Surg Neurol* 1993;39:370–373.

Mizoi K, Takahashi A, Yoshimoto T, et al. Surgical excision of giant hemispheric arteriovenous malformations following preoperative embolization. *J Neurosurg* 1992;76:1008–1011.

Morgan MK, Johnston I, Besser M, Baines D. Cerebral arteriovenous malformations, steal, and the hypertensive breakthrough threshold. *J Neurosurg* 1987;66:563–567.

Mullan S. Reflections upon the nature and management of intracranial and intraspinal vascular malformations and fistulae. *J Neurosurg* 1994;80:606–616.

Mullan S, Brown FD, Patronas NJ. Hyperemic and ischemic problems of surgical treatment of arteriovenous malformations. *J Neurosurg* 1979;51:757–764.

Okamoto S, Handa H, Hashimoto N. Location of intracranial aneurysms associated with cerebral arteriovenous malformation: statistical analysis. *Surg Neurol* 1984;22:335–340.

Pasqualin A, Barone G, Cioffi F, et al. The relevance of anatomic and hemodynamic factors to a classification of cerebral arteriovenous malformations. *Neurosurgery* 1991;28:370–379.

Pasqualin A, Scienza R, Cioffi F, et al. Treatment of cerebral arteriovenous malformations with a combination of preoperative embolization and surgery. *Neurosurgery* 1991;29:358–368.

Purdy PD, Batjer HH, Samson D. Management of hemorrhagic complications from preoperative embolization of arteriovenous malformations. *J Neurosurg* 1991;74:205–211.

Purdy PD, Samson D, Batjer HH, Risser RC. Preoperative embolization of cerebral arteriovenous malformations with polyvinyl alcohol particles: experience in 51 adults. *AJNR* 1990;11:501–510.

Rootman J, Kao SCS, Graeb DA. Multidisciplinary approaches to complicated vascular lesions of the orbit. *Ophthalmology* 1992;99:1440–1446.

Scialfa G, Scotti G. Superselective injection of polyvinyl alcohol microemboli for the treatment of cerebral arteriovenous malformations. *AJNR* 1985;6:957–960.

Sipos EP, Kirsch JR, Nauta HJW, et al. Intra-arterial urokinase for treatment of retrograde thrombosis following resection of an arteriovenous malformation. *J Neurosurg* 1992;76:1004–1007.

Sugiura K, Baba M. Total removal of an arteriovenous malformation embedded in the brain stem. *Surg Neurol* 1990;34:327–330.

Swanström S, Flodmark O, Lasjaunias P. Conditions for treatment of cerebral arteriovenous malformation associated with ectasia of the vein of Galen in the newborn. *Acta Paediatr* 1994;83:255–257.

Taneda M, Hayakawa T. The paradoxical blood pressure-flow relationship in the brain with an arteriovenous malformation. *Surg Neurol* 1993;40:390–394.

Tarr RW, Johnson DW, Horton JA, et al. Impaired cerebral vasoreactivity after embolization of arteriovenous malformations: assessment with serial acetazolamide challenge xenon CT. *AJNR* 1991;12:417–423.

Terada T, Nakamura Y, Nakai K, et al. Embolization of arteriovenous malformations with peripheral aneurysms using ethylene vinyl alcohol copolymer. *J Neurosurg* 1991;75:655–660.

Tomlinson FH, Houser OW, Scheithauer BW, et al. Angiographically occult vascular malformations: a correlative study of features on magnetic resonance imaging and histological examination. *Neurosurgery* 1994;34:792–800.

Vinters HV, Lundie MJ, Kaufmann JCE. Long-term pathological follow-up of cerebral arteriovenous malformations treated by embolization with bucrylate. *N Engl J Med* 1986;314:477–483.

Vinuela F, Fox AJ, Debrun G, Pelz D. Preembolization superselective angiography: role in the treatment of brain arteriovenous malformations with isobutyl-2 cyanoacrylate. *AJNR* 1984;5:765–769.

Wolpert SM, Barnett FJ, Prager RJ. Benefits of embolization without surgery for cerebral arteriovenous malformations. *AJNR* 1981;2:535–538.

Yeates A, Enzmann D. Cryptic vascular malformations involving the brainstem. *Radiology* 1983;146:71–75.

Yeh H-S, Tew JM, Gartner M. Seizure control after surgery on cerebral arteriovenous malformations. *J Neurosurg* 1993;78:12–18.

CHAPTER 21

Intracranial Arteriovenous Malformations:
The Approach and Technique of Cyanoacrylate Embolization

V.A. Aletich / G.M. Debrun

The materials needed in addition to a standard angiography set-up are listed in Table 21–1.

The combined incidence of all central nervous system vascular malformations in the general population is difficult to estimate, but in autopsy studies it has been reported to be approximately 6% for cerebral lesions.[1] Cerebral arteriovenous malformations (AVMs) are a subset of vascular malformations with an incidence of approximately 0.15% to 3%, or about one tenth that of cerebral aneurysms. Although the incidence of AVMs in the general population is small, patients with these lesions suffer major morbidity and mortality. This is primarily due to intracerebral hemorrhage, which occurs in approximately 34% of patients with AVMs over a 20-year period. In annual terms, hemorrhage occurs at a rate of approximately 2% to 3% per year, and death at a rate of 1% to 2% per year.[2]

The treatment goal for AVMs is complete obliteration of the anomalous arterial venous connection and restoration of normal cerebral blood flow. Therapeutic options include radiosurgery, conventional surgery, and endovascular embolization, either alone or in conjunction with radiosurgery or surgery. At the time of diagnosis, 30% of AVMs are less than 3 cm in size, 60% are between 3 and 6 cm, and 10% are greater than 6 cm.[3] Surgery is restricted to lesions that are relatively small, are located in noneloquent regions of the brain, and do not have complex deep venous drainage. Radiosurgery is limited to intracranial vascular lesions less than 3 cm. Even in AVMs less than 3 cm, radiosurgery is not our first choice of treatment if the patient has a history of hemorrhage (and therefore increased risk of subsequent hemorrhage) or if the patient is young, with an unknown risk of long-term side effects of irradiation. Therefore, a significant portion of patients with AVMs are not amenable to these two procedures

T A B L E 2 1 - 1   Materials Needed for Cyanoacrylate Embolization of Intracranial Arteriovenous Malformations

1. Sheath
   6- or 7-Fr.
   Dependent on guide catheter size
2. Stopcocks
   a. One-way: Total (3)
      Placed on hemostatic valve, Weinberg or H1H, sheath side arm if needed
   b. One-way (3 mm bored): Total (1)
      Placed on guide catheter, allows advancement of microcatheters
   c. Three-way: Total (4)
      Two per flush line from infusion pumps (guide catheter, microcatheter)
3. Flush
   a. Heparinized saline: 2000 units/500 ml
   b. Pressure bag to sheath
   c. Infusion pump: Total (2)
      One to guide catheter via rotating hemostatic valve (Target Therapeutics), one to microcatheter
4. Target Therapeutics rotating hemostatic valve (1)
   Flushes guide catheter and holds microcatheter
5. Wires
   a. Balt mandrel (enclosed with Magic catheter) (Target Therapeutics)
   b. Bentson 0.038″
   c. Cook 0.052″
      If needed for advancement of guide catheter
   d. Exchange Terumo 0.038″ angled Glidewire (Medi-Tech)
      If needed to perform an exchange
   e. Terumo 0.010″ (Medi-Tech)
      If needed to advance Magic

6. Catheters
   a. Guide catheter
      Usually 6- or 7-Fr. straight (Schneider, Cordis Corp., Medtronic/MIS)
      90 cm in length
      Large inner luminal diameter (minimum 0.042″)
      Formed to shape of access vessel
   b. Weinberg or H1H
      Used in diagnostic examination and as inner catheter with guide catheter for direct placement of guide instead of performing an exchange
   c. Balt Magic microcatheter (distributed by Target Therapeutics)
      155 or 165 cm
      Progressive taper 3 to 1.8- or 1.5-Fr.
      Mandrel comes with microcatheter to aid in advancing catheter into guide catheter
7. N-butyl-2-cyanoacrylate (NBCA) (Histoacryl)
   Mix with lipiodol (Ethiodol)
   Increasing Ethiodol proportion increases polymerization time
   Typical ratio 1 ml Histoacryl/3 ml Ethiodol (25% Histoacryl)
8. D5W (Dextrose)
   Used to flush catheter before cyanoacrylate injection
   Prevents polymerization in microcatheter
9. Syringes (for use with microcatheter)
   a. 1-cc Luer-Lok: (3)
   b. 3-cc Luer-Lok: (3) Contrast
   c. 5-cc Luer-Lok: (3) Flush
10. Bowls (Plastic): (2)
11. Normal saline
12. Contrast
13. Ceramic crucible
    For mixing Histoacryl and Ethiodol
14. Sterile tray
    Holds materials to be used with microcatheter

alone, and there are no alternative treatment options other than endovascular embolization.

The goal of embolization of AVMs is to permanently reduce the size and diminish the anomalous flow of the vascular malformation in an effort to reduce the risk of hemorrhage, so that the curative procedures of surgical resection or radiosurgery can be performed with minimal risk to the patient. Also, in 5% to 10% of AVMs, endovascular occlusion of the lesion may be curative.[4–7]

Endovascular embolization is not a new science and has been continually evolving since the early 1970s in conjunction with the development of new embolic agent formulations and advancement in guidewire and microcatheter technologies. Currently available embolic agents fall into two general categories: particulate agents (polyvinyl alcohol [PVA], balloons, coils, silk thread), and liquid agents (alcohol, Ethibloc, EVAL, N-butyl-2-cyanoacrylate [Histoacryl, Braun Melsungen, Germany]). All these agents have their particular place in interventional neuroradiology; however, with respect to central nervous system vascular malformations, only the cyanoacrylate glues have proved consistently useful. The cyanoacrylate compounds, particularly Histoacryl, are extensively used in Europe and Canada and have until recently

been used in the United States. Withdrawal of Tri-Point L.P.'s investigational device exemption for the use of Avacryl in 1992 has severely limited the U.S. use of Histoacryl (which we consider the best therapeutic option for patients with large AVMs that are not amenable to surgical resection or radiosurgery). Endovascular embolization of these AVMs with Histoacryl continues at a reduced scale at institutions that allow its use pending Food and Drug Administration approval, and with particulate agents elsewhere. However, the goals and risks of particulate embolization differ significantly from Histoacryl embolization:

1. We consider embolization with solid particles (PVA, silk, coils, balloons) as an adjunctive, preoperative procedure only, since these agents do not provide permanent occlusion. This disadvantage makes the use of radiosurgery after particulate embolization less attractive. The curative effects of radiosurgery may not be observed for up to 2 to 3 years and the attendant risks of hemorrhage remain unchanged from the natural history of the disease.

Evidence in the literature[5, 8–10] supports the permanence of Histoacryl occlusion of the vascular bed. Permanent occlusion allows radiosurgery to be performed on the remaining nidus without the possibility that recanalization in the previously embolized nidus may expose the patient to the renewed risk of hemorrhage from these portions.

2. Solid particles require larger delivery systems that are less flexible and require the use of guidewires for catheter placement, which significantly increases the risk of vascular damage compared with the flow-directed microcatheters used with liquid agents. Also, because of their larger size and increased stiffness, the catheters utilized in particulate embolization are difficult to place in close proximity to the AVM nidus, thereby increasing the risk of the embolic agent refluxing into normal cerebral vasculature, with resultant parenchymal damage.

The goal of this chapter is to set out our approach to the treatment of AVMs and to describe in detail our technique of single-column, flow-controlled nidus embolization with Histoacryl.

INITIAL EVALUATION

All brain AVMs referred to our institution, including those that have not bled, are considered for treatment with cyanoacrylate glue embolization. The final goal of treatment is permanent cure, with or without additional therapy such as surgical resection or radiosurgery. Pretherapeutic assessment includes the following:

1. Comprehensive medical examination, including complete neurologic and cognitive assessment by staff neurosurgeons and neuroradiologists. If the vascular malformation involves vessels in or about the optic tracts, subspecialty evaluation by a neuro-ophthalmologist is also obtained.
2. Complete neuroradiologic evaluation, including computed tomography (CT), magnetic resonance imaging (MRI), and magnetic resonance angiography (MRA).
3. Angiography. After the angiographic examination, the lesion is graded according to Spetzler and Martin's grading system (see Table 20–1), which lists grades I to VI.[11] One grade is added in the presence of acute hemorrhage. A subclassification of A, B, or C is added as necessary:
   A. Constriction or stenosis of the venous drainage
   B. Presence of incidental, feeder, or intranidal aneurysms (single or multiple)
   C. Periventricular location

These subclassifications are added because it is well documented in the literature that the risks of hemorrhage of the AVM are increased when these conditions are present.[12–16]

After the above assessment, the case is presented during a daily neurovascular conference headed by neuroradiologists, neurosurgeons, and radiotherapists (when applicable). If warranted by a particular case, neuro-ophthalmologists and neurologists are also consulted. For each case the attendant risks and possible complications of all treatment options are discussed. Recommendations for a plan of treatment are agreed on by the specialists.

Upon the patient's acceptance of the treatment proposal, the interventional procedure is scheduled and the patient admitted under the care of the neurosurgical department. On the day of admission, which is 1 day before the embolization procedure, a full clinical and neurologic assessment is repeated. Laboratory evaluations include routine blood analysis, coagulation parameters, and urinalysis. A CT scan is obtained before embolization unless a recent one is available. Systemic steroid therapy is initiated, typically with dexamethasone, in an effort to minimize the expected inflammatory response to cyanoacrylate injection in the immediate postembolization period.

The diagnostic angiogram is reviewed. Any associated aneurysms, high-flow fistulae, venous ectasia, and draining vein stenosis are ascertained. The relative occurrence of associated aneurysms is 15% to 20%; of true intranidal fistulae, 22%; and of venous stenosis and marked venous ectasia, less than 10%. The presence of one or all of these findings is crucial in selecting the initial feeder vessels to be embolized. The approach to the initial embolization of AVMs is to first treat any associated aneurysms or true intranidal fistulae to prevent subsequent rupture (Fig. 21–1). In the case of incidental aneurysms, this treatment may require a separate procedure such as coiling or surgical clipping. In the case of flow-related feeder aneurysms in close proximity to the AVM nidus or intranidal aneurysms, the vessel harboring

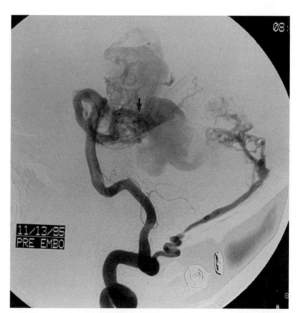

Figure 21-1 Lateral vertebral angiogram demonstrating a high-flow cerebral arteriovenous malformation (AVM) with an associated true intranidal fistula *(arrow)*. Initial embolization attempts should be to decrease or close the true fistula.

the aneurysm is the first vessel selected for embolization, in an attempt to include the aneurysm in the glue cast (Fig. 21–2). A feeder aneurysm that is not in close proximity to the AVM nidus poses a difficult dilemma (Fig. 21–3). Embolization in the proximal trunk of the feeder carries a high risk of embolizing normal parenchymal branches, which is unacceptable. In these situations, the feeder with the aneurysm is usually avoided if possible, and an attempt is made to diminish the shunt through the AVM via other feeders in the hope that the flow-related aneurysm will regress.

In AVMs associated with a marked venous ectasia or venous outflow obstruction, the initial embolization is aimed at diminishing the flow through the nidus compartment draining through the stenosed or ectatic vein (Fig. 21–4). In all other cases, the largest

feeding vessels are selected, as these are the easiest to catheterize and provide the best access to the AVM nidus. Collateral circulations should be avoided, because direct access to the AVM nidus is extremely difficult if not impossible (Fig. 21–5).

Once the feeders to be embolized are determined, the access vessel (carotid or vertebral artery) is evaluated for concomitant disease, such as arteriosclerotic changes, and for tortuosity, which determines the selection and shaping of the guide catheter to be used in the procedure.

TECHNIQUE

The embolization is performed in the angiographic suite after the patient has been placed under general anesthesia by an anesthesiologist. All monitoring of

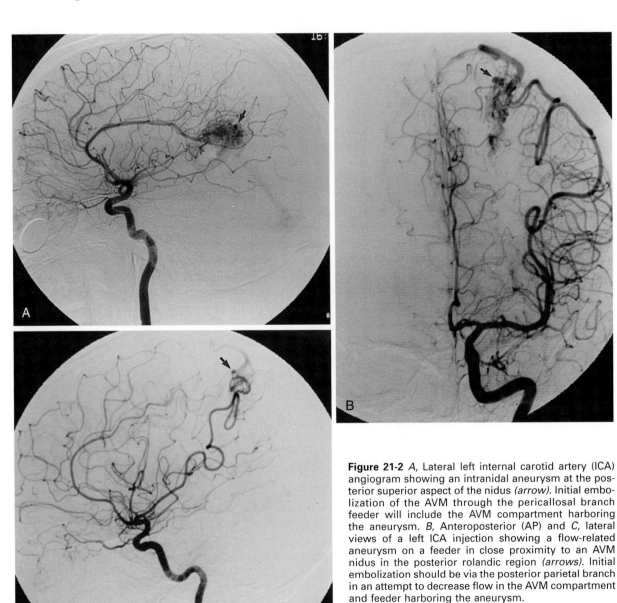

Figure 21-2 *A*, Lateral left internal carotid artery (ICA) angiogram showing an intranidal aneurysm at the posterior superior aspect of the nidus *(arrow)*. Initial embolization of the AVM through the pericallosal branch feeder will include the AVM compartment harboring the aneurysm. *B*, Anteroposterior (AP) and *C*, lateral views of a left ICA injection showing a flow-related aneurysm on a feeder in close proximity to an AVM nidus in the posterior rolandic region *(arrows)*. Initial embolization should be via the posterior parietal branch in an attempt to decrease flow in the AVM compartment and feeder harboring the aneurysm.

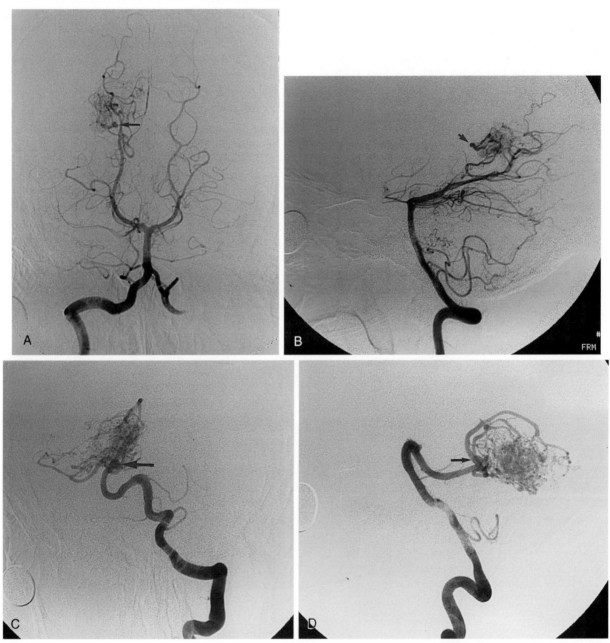

Figure 21-3 *A*, AP and *B*, lateral views of a right vertebral injection. A flow-related aneurysm is seen *(arrow and arrowhead)* arising from the lateral posterior choroidal artery at some distance from the AVM nidus. In this case (the same patient as in Fig. 21–2*A*), the AVM nidus also filled from feeders off the pericallosal artery. Initial embolization would be through the pericallosal artery. *C*, AP and *D*, lateral view of a left vertebral angiogram showing a feeder aneurysm at proximal branching of the right superior cerebellar artery *(arrows)*. As the AVM nidus fills primarily via the right superior cerebellar artery, it is not possible to avoid passing this aneurysm with the microcatheter in order to selectively catheterize the nidus to perform embolization. The presence of this aneurysm substantially increases the risks of the procedure.

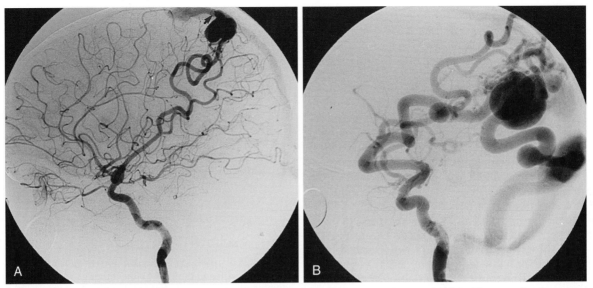

Figure 21-4 *A,* Lateral right ICA angiogram showing a small, high-flow posterior parietal AVM with a true fistula, venous stenosis *(arrow),* and associated venous ectasia. *B,* Lateral right ICA angiogram showing a true intranidal fistula, associated with venous stenosis and ectasia. Initial embolization should be to attempt to close the true fistula and decrease flow through the stenotic vein.

vital signs is performed by the anesthesiology team in the same way as they are monitored during any neurosurgical case performed in the operating room. Systemic heparinization (5000 units in an intravenous bolus, followed by 1000 U/hr throughout the procedure) is added to the treatment protocol when the nidus of the AVM is less than 3 cm in diameter and has few and relatively small feeders. Heparin,

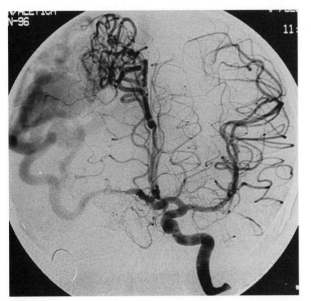

Figure 21-5 AP view of a left ICA injection in a patient with a high-flow right parietal AVM. The right pericallosal and callosomarginal vessels provide collateral filling of the AVM and fistula. Note that these collateral vessels are tortuous and relatively small, which would make microcatheter navigation extremely difficult and the nidus impossible to reach. An initial approach would be to embolize through the middle cerebral artery (MCA) branches, closing the fistula and filling the nidus, which would effectively disconnect the collateral circulation.

however, is not given in AVMs larger than 3 cm with multiple large feeders from two or three major intracranial vessels, as inadvertent emboli will most likely travel to the AVM because of the high-flow shunt. Also, in cases in which hemorrhagic complications are more likely to occur, because of either normal pressure breakthrough phenomena or multiple feeder aneurysms, heparin may potentiate the severity of bleeding; this is of particular concern in large high-flow AVMs. All catheters used during the procedure, including the guide catheter and microcatheter, are continuously flushed with heparinized saline (4000 U/L) via an infusion pump.

A 90-cm 6- or 7-Fr. guide catheter that resists kinking and has a large inner diameter (Schneider, Cordis Corp., Medtronic/MIS) is shaped in steam to approximate the curve of the access vessel, and positioned as close as technically feasible to the skull base, either directly using a coaxial system with an inner smaller catheter (such as a Weinberg) and wire (Bentson), or by exchange. This facilitates advancement of the microcatheter and allows for microcatheter exchange if required. Occasionally, during placement of the guide catheter, local vasospasm may develop secondarily to wire manipulation or mild straightening of the vessel by the guide catheter. Vasospasm can be alleviated with 30 to 60 mg papaverine, infused through the guide catheter over 5 to 10 minutes.

Once the guide catheter is in position and any secondary local vasospasm has been resolved, a preembolization baseline angiogram is performed to allow the interventionist to assess for interval change since the initial diagnostic angiogram, and to confirm the selected approach to the AVM. The guide catheter is then continuously flushed with heparinized saline via an infusion pump during preparation of the microcatheter.

The microcatheter most commonly used at our institution is the flow-directed Balt 1.8-Fr. Magic microcatheter (Target Therapeutics). The 1.5-Fr. Magic is rarely used at present because the Terumo 0.010″ Glidewire (Medi-Tech) is also employed to aid in catheter advancement, and this wire will not pass through the distal 15 cm of the 1.5-Fr. Magic owing to its smaller inner diameter. The QuickSilver microguidewire (Medtronic/MIS) is a hydrophilic-coated wire used by other interventionists in conjunction with the Magic microcatheter (personal communication), but our experience with this wire is limited, and comparisons with the Terumo wire cannot be made at the time of this writing.

The Magic is removed from its packaging, the mandrel removed, and the microcatheter examined for flaws and integrity. Evaluation for perforations is important and can be done easily by infusing the catheter with saline and gently pinching the tip. The mandrel is reinserted to the distal pink segment, and the tip of the microcatheter is steam shaped into a small question mark with a curve diameter of approximately 5.0 mm (Fig. 21–6). This curve provides some operator control in catheter migration of the distal cerebral vasculature. After shaping of the tip, the mandrel is carefully inserted for the remainder of its length and the microcatheter is placed in a rotating hemostatic valve (Target Therapeutics or equivalent) so that continuous flushing of the guiding catheter can be maintained during advancement of the microcatheter (Fig. 21–7). The Magic is then placed into the guide catheter and advanced until the proximal green portion of the microcatheter has entered the hemostatic valve, at which time the mandrel is removed. This procedure ensures ease of initial catheter advancement into the guide catheter and prevents the tip of the microcatheter with the mandrel in place from exiting the end of the guide catheter, risking damage to the wall of the access vessel. Continuous flushing of the microcatheter is

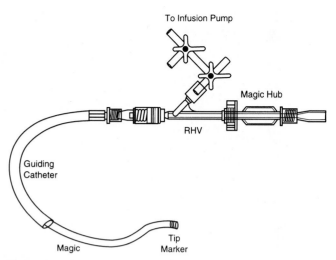

Figure 21-7 Schematic representation of our system to provide continuous flushing of the guide catheter while using the Magic microcatheter. The rotating hemostatic valve is labeled RHV.

provided by an assistant with a 5-cc syringe filled with heparinized saline, and the microcatheter is advanced through the cerebral vasculature and feeder of the AVM by flow control, augmented by raising the mean arterial blood pressure (using phenylephrine HCl [Neo-Synephrine]) to approximately 110 to 115 mm Hg. Visualization of the microcatheter and vessel being selected can be enhanced by the use of contrast injected with a 3-cc syringe. If the Magic catheter fails to progress to the nidus of the AVM or does not negotiate the tortuous AVM feeder, the hydrophilic Terumo 0.010″ Glidewire can be used to provide proximal stiffness and increased "pushability." The Terumo wire is not used to direct the microcatheter, as in standard microwire/microcatheter systems, and the technique of its use in this situation is different. The wire is not extended beyond the tip of the microcatheter, minimizing the risk of vessel perforation. Also, in view of the elasticity and flexibility of the Magic, one must be extremely cautious in advancing the wire through sharp angulations and loops of the cerebral vessels, to avoid catheter perforations. To traverse sharp turns and loops, the Terumo and Magic should be advanced cautiously as a unit until the wire is distal to the angulation, turn, or loop. The Magic may advance with wire advancement or with wire withdrawal as potential energy builds within it, and both techniques are used to reach the nidus (Fig. 21–8).

This technique should be considered only by interventionists who are extremely familiar with the use of flow-directed microcatheters and microguidewires; the technique is not the same as that used for standard, "geometry-guided" catheters and wires such as the TRACKER (Target Therapeutics).

Once the tip of the microcatheter is positioned within the nidus of the AVM or at the entrance of a fistula, a superselective angiogram is obtained with approximately 1 ml of water-soluble iodine contrast material, using biplane digital subtraction angiogra-

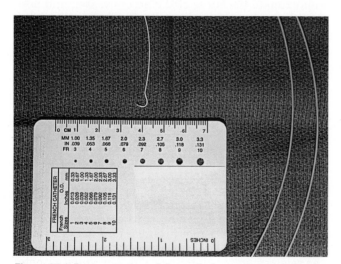

Figure 21-6 Demonstration of the typical curve we place on the Magic microcatheter by steam shaping. This curve provides some operator control of the Magic during advancement in the cerebral vasculature.

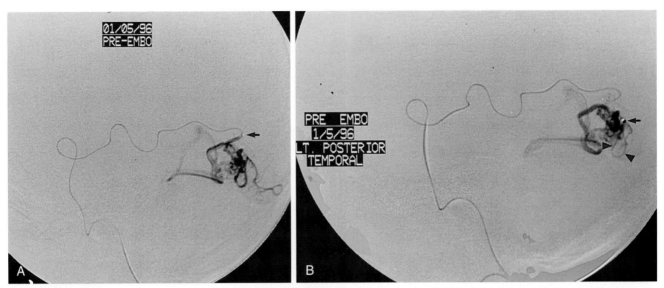

Figure 21-8 *A,* Lateral view of superselective injection through Magic microcatheter. The Magic tip is located at some distance from the AVM nidus *(arrow)* and would not advance farther with use of flow control. Embolization should not be performed with the microcatheter tip at this location. *B,* Lateral view of superselective injection through the Magic microcatheter after using the Terumo 0.010″ wire. Note the further advancement of the Magic tip to the AVM nidus *(arrow)* and the course of the Magic through the feeder *(arrowheads).* Use of the Terumo wire has consistently enhanced our success rate of obtaining a wedge position within the nidus of the AVM, improving penetration of glue in the nidus and minimizing the risk of embolic material entering normal parenchymal branches.

phy (DSA) at 3 frames/sec to evaluate the flow characteristics, angioarchitecture, and venous outflow of the vascular malformation. This angiogram is utilized to determine the mixture of Histoacryl in ethiodized oil (Ethiodol) appropriate for the particular AVM. The following criteria must be met before the embolization proceeds (Fig. 21–9):

1. The microcatheter tip is *wedged* in the AVM nidus or at the entrance of a fistula.
2. There is no reflux of contrast proximal to the tip of the microcatheter as determined by the preembolization superselective test injection.
3. A portion of the nidus or the fistula fills with contrast.
4. There is complete understanding of the circulation time through the AVM nidus or fistula.
5. No loops are identified along the course of the Magic microcatheter that might inhibit withdrawal of the microcatheter. This has to be checked with DSA at 1 frame/sec, centered to evaluate the entire microcatheter from its exit from the guide catheter to its tip.

One caveat is that occasionally the Magic catheter tip wedges in the distal aspect of the feeder and not directly within the nidus of the AVM; this occurs primarily in small feeders. If the feeding vessel and portion of AVM to be embolized are in a noneloquent area of the brain, it is considered that embolization with cyanoacrylate glue can be performed safely even a few centimeters away from the nidus of the AVM, provided that the catheter is in an absolute wedged position and no normal parenchymal vessels are opacified with the test injection (Fig. 21–10). If the AVM feeder is in an eloquent area of the brain, embo-

lization proceeds only if the tip of the Magic is wedged at the entrance to or within the nidus.

Embolization then proceeds with the patient hypotensive (mean arterial pressure 60 mm Hg, achieved by titrating a sodium nitroprusside drip) and under real-time biplane roadmapping using a 1024 × 1024 matrix. The progression of radiopaque glue should not be evaluated only in a single plane, or without DSA fluoroscopic imaging. The microcatheter is prepared by flushing it with a 5% dextrose solution before glue injection. A 25% mixture of Histoacryl in Ethiodol is prepared and a 3-cc syringe filled with the mixture. Injection is performed slowly, using full-column, flow-controlled technique, filling the interstices of the nidus up to the draining vein. If glue is observed to pass through the nidus and into the draining vein, the injection is halted for 2 or 3 seconds and then resumed. This technique continues until proximal reflux of glue begins to extend along the microcatheter, or until the nidus has filled and there is no more progression of glue. At this point, the syringe is aspirated, and the guide catheter and microcatheter are quickly removed as a unit and examined to ensure retrieval of the entire microcatheter. Typical injection volumes are between 0.4 and 0.8 ml and average injection time is 1 to 2 minutes, with the average volume and injection time increasing in direct correlation with the experience of the interventionist (see Fig. 21–9C).

Treatment of a true fistula, which is a direct communication between the feeding artery and draining vein without an interposed nidus, and is demonstrated by the passage of the Magic tip into the vein, is by injection of pure Histoacryl using a "sandwich" technique. The dead space of the microcatheter (0.2

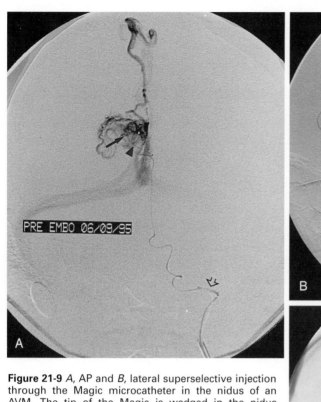

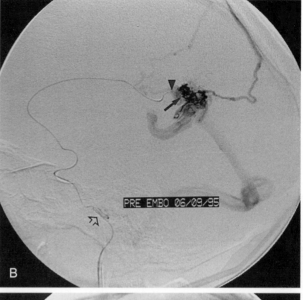

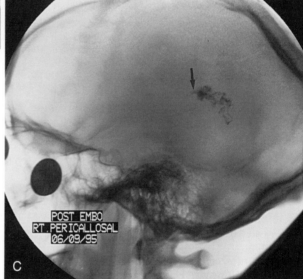

Figure 21-9 *A,* AP and *B,* lateral superselective injection through the Magic microcatheter in the nidus of an AVM. The tip of the Magic is wedged in the nidus *(arrows)* and no reflux along the Magic is seen *(arrowheads).* A large portion of the nidus fills during this injection, and the draining veins are well identified. Review of the entire sequence gives information of the flow characteristics. No fistulae are identified and the concentration of Histoacryl to Ethiodol to be selected for this embolization will be 1 to 3 ml (25% Histoacryl). A redundant loop of catheter in the petrous portion of the ICA *(open arrows)* needs to be removed before glue injection to minimize the potential risk of gluing the catheter tip. *C,* A glue cast is seen after injection of a 0.5 ml 25% Histoacryl/Ethiodol mixture with the microcatheter placed as shown in *A* and *B.* Note the presence of glue in the proximal aspect of a vein *(arrow)* and the correlation of the glue cast to the filled nidus as shown during superselective test injection before embolization.

ml) is flushed with 5% dextrose. A 3-cc syringe is then filled with 2.8 ml 5% dextrose. Histoacryl (0.2 ml) is then aspirated with the syringe held vertically, so that the Histoacryl layers at the bottom (Fig. 21–11). A total of 0.4 ml is then injected over 1 to 2 seconds, followed by immediate rapid retrieval of the guide catheter and microcatheter system (Fig. 21–12).

Depending on the size of the vascular malformation, one to three more injections may be performed as above in different feeders. In large AVMs, several sittings may be necessary to embolize all the available feeders. After occlusion of the larger feeders of an AVM, there is continued flow through smaller feeders that subsequently enlarge, allowing an easier catheterization at the second sitting. Also, in large AVMs, embolization of more than 30% of the AVM volume significantly alters the hemodynamics of flow

through the AVM and potentiates the risk of normal pressure breakthrough. Therefore, embolization of large AVMs is usually a series of staged procedures occurring approximately 4 weeks apart to allow stabilization of the flow hemodynamics of the remaining nidus, and to permit further thrombosis with subsequent regression of the recently occluded feeders.

After the embolization session, heparin (if given) is reversed with protamine sulfate (1 mg per 80 to 90 total units heparin given). The patient is awakened from general anesthesia and a complete neurologic examination is performed to assess any changes from baseline. The patient is then transferred to the neuro-intensive care unit for monitoring. Mean arterial blood pressure is maintained approximately 10% to 15% below baseline to minimize the controversial phenomenon of normal pressure breakthrough and to decrease the risk of postembolization

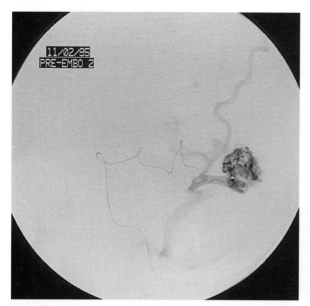

Figure 21-10 Lateral view superselective injection through a Magic microcatheter. The Magic tip is wedged within the feeder approximately 0.5 to 1 cm proximal to the AVM nidus in the posterior temporal region. In this instance we consider proceeding with embolization as the catheter tip is wedged, no reflux proximally along the feeder is demonstrated, and no normal parenchymal branches are seen.

delayed hemorrhage in cases in which partial venous outlet occlusion has occurred (considered the most significant cause of hemorrhage). The patient is usually discharged the following day on a tapering dose of dexamethasone, barring any complications. If the patient requires further embolization, this is scheduled before discharge; if not, a clinic visit is scheduled within 3 or 4 weeks to discuss and determine when the definitive therapy of surgery or radiosurgery is to be performed.

Some readers may note that the above technique does not utilize physiologic testing of the vascular territory supplied by the feeder to the AVM with amobarbital (Amytal) or methohexital (Brevital) before embolization. This issue remains controversial in interventional neuroradiology,[7, 17, 18] and a brief discussion of our reasons for not using preembolization physiologic testing is warranted. I (GMD) have embolized brain AVMs almost exclusively with cyanoacrylate glue since 1976, initially with IBCA (isobutyl-cyanoacrylate), and then with Histoacryl when this formulation became available. During this experience, amobarbital testing in the awake patient was performed in more than 300 different feeders to AVMs, and outcomes of the injections were consistently predicted, based on the distance of the microcatheter tip from the nidus of the AVM and the presence or absence of eloquent brain surrounding the AVM. It has been only since the mid 1990s that embolizations have been performed under general anesthesia without amobarbital testing. The decision to abandon the amobarbital test was not based solely on the opinion that similar information can be ob-

tained by accurate knowledge of the anatomy and location of the AVM (as there are medical legal issues at stake), but also on the need for an anesthetized patient.

For safety, nidus embolization must be performed under biplane DSA guidance, which is extremely sensitive to motion. Any movement of the patient during embolization results in loss of landmarks and image quality, increasing the risk and interrupting the embolization prematurely. Therefore, safe maximal embolization of the nidus cannot be performed without general anesthesia and a paralyzed patient.

Proponents of physiologic testing argue that if the feeder of the AVM is not tested before embolization, the risk of inadvertent embolization of normal parenchymal branches is increased. Nidus embolization requires that the tip of the microcatheter be wedged within the nidus, which minimizes the risk of reflux. The nidus of a AVM is nonfunctional tissue and there is little risk of neurologic complications if the glue is delivered strictly into the nidus. Also, we use a mixture of Histoacryl (25% Histoacryl, 75% Ethiodol) that is more dilute than has been used in the past. This increases polymerization time and allows embolizations to be performed very slowly, over 1 to 2 minutes, improving the control and accuracy of the injection (as compared with higher concentrations of Histoacryl, which need to be injected rapidly). The increased polymerization time also reduces the risk of permanently gluing the tip of the microcatheter,

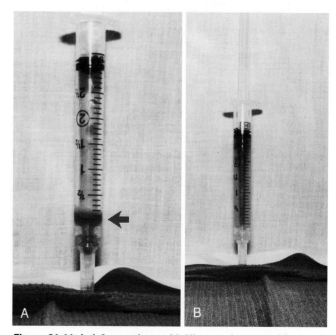

Figure 21-11 *A*, A 3-cc syringe with Histoacryl prepared for sandwich technique. The Magic catheter is flushed with 5% dextrose and a 3-cc syringe is filled with 2.8 ml of dextrose. Pure Histoacryl (0.2 ml) is then aspirated into the vertically held syringe so that the Histoacryl layers at the bottom *(arrow)*. This is injected rapidly (over 1 to 2 seconds) through the preflushed Magic to close the fistula. Compare this with *B*, which shows a 3-cc syringe containing a 25% mixture of Histoacryl in Ethiodol for slow intranidal injection.

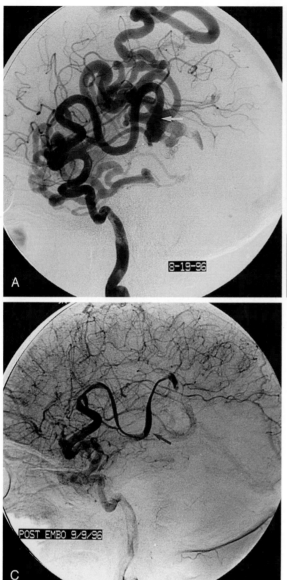

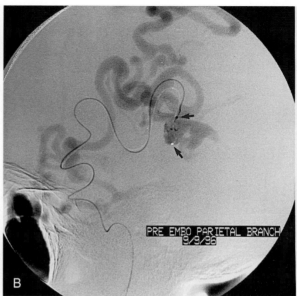

Figure 21-12 *A,* Diagnostic lateral right ICA angiogram showing a true fistula *(white arrow)*. *B,* Lateral superselective angiogram through a Magic microcatheter. The microcatheter tip is initially within the draining vein, but with injection recoils to the entrance of the fistula *(arrows)*. *C,* A lateral right ICA angiogram after embolization of the fistula using the sandwich technique demonstrates that the fistula is closed and there is stasis within the feeder *(arrow)*.

as reflux is readily visualized (which terminates the injection). Embolization in a vessel of passage can be done with this technique if the tip of the microcatheter is wedged in the feeder at least 5 mm distal to the branch point with the vessel of passage.

One criticism of our technique is that patients undergo the additional risk of general anesthesia for each embolization session, but there has not been one complication directly related to the anesthesia. We consider that the risks associated with patient motion during embolization far outweigh the risks associated with general anesthesia.

ILLUSTRATIVE CASES

Case 1. A 35-year-old man was found to have an incidental AVM during work-up for a prolactin-secreting adenoma. The neurologic examination results were normal and the lesion had never bled. The AVM

nidus was located in the left posterior parietal cortex and measured approximately 2 cm in diameter. There was a single large middle cerebral artery (MCA) branch feeder with superficial cortical venous drainage (Fig. 21–13A and B). This was an asymptomatic Spetzler grade II AVM without previous hemorrhage. Radiosurgery offers an 85% to 90% cure at 2 years. Surgery was considered, but with the AVM located within the dominant parietal cortex, the surgical risks were considered to be higher than those of embolization with cyanoacrylate glue. The patient subsequently underwent a single embolization with 0.8 ml 25% Histoacryl/Ethiodol (Fig. 21–13C to E). The immediate postembolization angiogram demonstrated absence of the AVM. The patient remained asymptomatic after embolization, and a 14-month follow-up angiogram showed complete cure of the AVM (Fig. 21–13F and G). No further therapy was necessary and the patient was to be followed with yearly MRI and MRA studies.

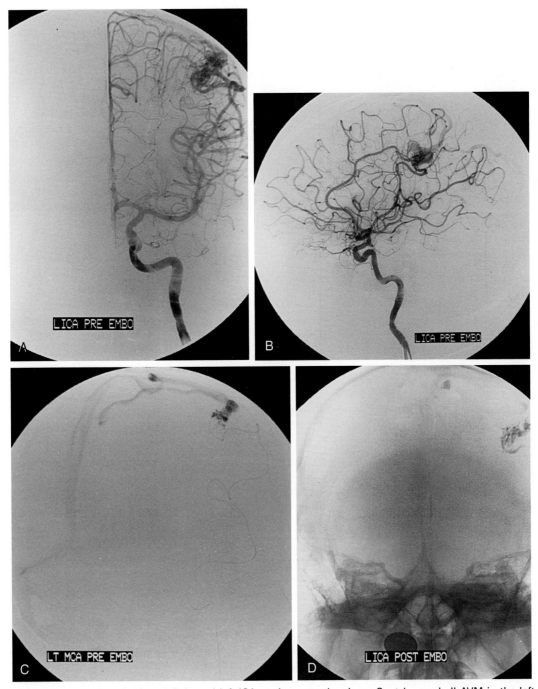

Figure 21-13 Case 1. *A,* AP and *B,* lateral left ICA angiograms showing a Spetzler grade II AVM in the left parietal region. Primary feeders include branches of the left MCA, with venous drainage being superficial. *C,* An oblique projection superselective injection through a 1.8-Fr. Magic microcatheter was obtained because this projection offered the best view of the microcatheter tip position to observe for reflux. Good wedge position is confirmed.

Case 1 continues

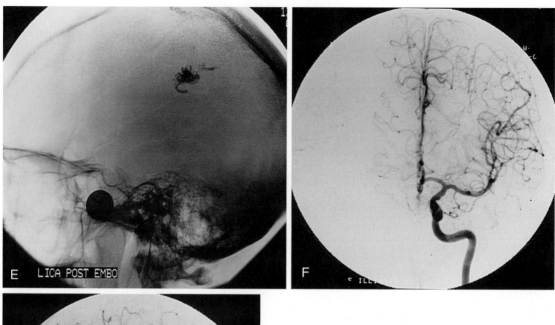

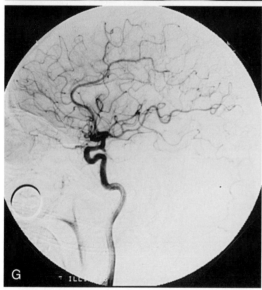

Figure 21-13 *D,* AP and *E,* lateral skull films show the glue cast after embolization with 0.8 ml of 25% Histoacryl. *F,* AP and *G,* lateral left ICA angiograms 14 months after embolization demonstrate complete cure.

Case 2. A 65-year-old man was found to have a right parietal AVM during evaluation of a single seizure episode. He was neurologically intact and had no history of hemorrhage. The pertinent clinical history included recurrent deep venous thrombosis (requiring two previous hospitalizations for anticoagulation), hypertension, and renal insufficiency. The diagnostic angiogram showed a Spetzler grade II AVM of the right parietal lobe within the motor cortex. Primary feeders included several branches of the MCA; venous drainage was by superficial cortical veins (Fig. 21–14*A* to *C*). This lesion could have been treated by radiosurgery alone with 80% to 85% chance of cure in 2 years; however, the recurrent deep venous thrombosis requiring anticoagulation and a history of hypertension placed the patient at increased risk of hemorrhage during the postirradiation period. Surgery in this case could also have been performed, but with the lesion in the right motor cortex and with concomitant medical problems, surgical risks would

be increased. We considered that, in this case, embolization coupled with radiosurgery offered the lowest risk. Embolization offers a 5% to 10% chance of cure but can also decrease the flow through the AVM and diminish the size of the nidus, improving the percentage of cure by radiosurgery and decreasing the risk of hemorrhage during the postirradiation period. This plan was adopted and the patient subsequently underwent a series of staged embolizations with a total of five separate feeder embolizations (Fig. 21–14*D* and *E*). The flow through the AVM was substantially reduced, and the remaining nidus after the last embolization was less than 1 cm (Fig. 21–14*F* and *G*). The patient underwent radiosurgery approximately 1 month after the last embolization. Throughout the treatment period he remained asymptomatic and awaits a 1-year follow-up.

Case 3. A 23-year-old man with a history of medically controlled seizures since age 11 years was found to

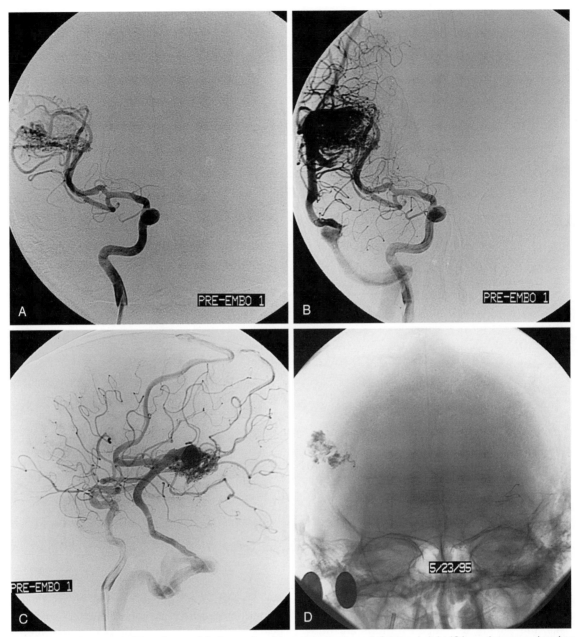

Figure 21-14 Case 2. *A*, AP early arterial phase, *B*, midarterial phase, and *C*, lateral right ICA angiograms showing a Spetzler grade II AVM. *D*, AP and *E*, lateral skull films after staged embolization of five feeders show glue casting of the nidus.

Case 2 continues

have minor weakness of the right hand, and psychoneurologic testing showed minor memory and cognitive deficits. There was no history of hemorrhage. The diagnostic angiogram showed a Spetzler grade III high-flow AVM of the posterior left frontal lobe. Feeders were derived from the right MCA and anterior cerebral artery, and venous drainage was superficial. Intranidal true fistulae and venous ectasia were also identified (Fig. 21–15*A* to *D*). The treatment plan for this patient included embolization, followed by radiosurgery or surgical resection, dependent on the final results of embolization. The size of the nidus (>3 cm) made radiosurgery alone unattractive, since the cure rates for this size of lesion are variable but less than 65% to 70%. Surgery can be performed, but

the presence of true fistulae and venous ectasia and the size of the nidus increase the surgical risks. The patient underwent a series of staged embolizations, and a total of 13 separate feeders were embolized (Fig. 21–15*E* and *F*). Two true fistulae were encountered and treated successfully with pure glue injection using the sandwich technique. At the end of embolization, there was a significant reduction of flow through the nidus. However, the overall size of the nidus was only slightly reduced, as the glue permeated the nidus in a "patchwork" fashion primarily within the center of the nidus (Fig. 21–15*G*). Surgical resection was the only option for complete cure, with the least long-term risk, and this was performed approximately 1 month after the last emboli-

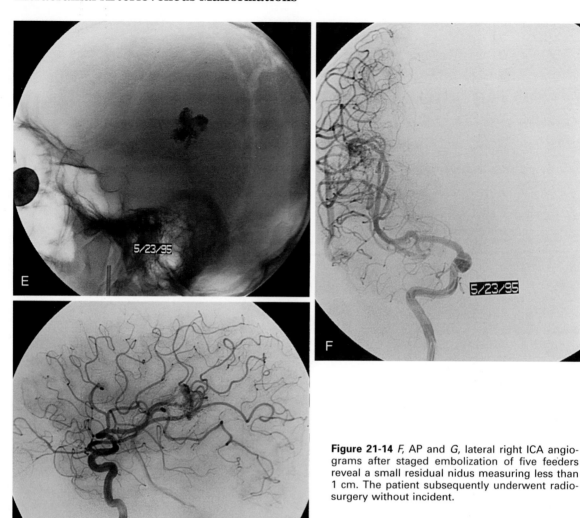

Figure 21-14 *F*, AP and *G*, lateral right ICA angiograms after staged embolization of five feeders reveal a small residual nidus measuring less than 1 cm. The patient subsequently underwent radiosurgery without incident.

zation. The postoperative angiogram showed complete resection of the AVM (Fig. 21–15*H* and *I*). Clinically, the patient developed a moderate right hemiparesis in the immediate postoperative period; over the subsequent 3 months, there was approximately 95% resolution, and he was left with only mild weakness of the right hand.

RISKS, POTENTIAL COMPLICATIONS, AND SOLUTIONS

The risks and potential complications associated with intracranial AVM embolization include all the attendant risks of cerebral angiography, and cerebral embolization in general, irrespective of the embolic material used. However, there are some risks and complications relatively specific to embolization with cyanoacrylate adhesives.

Intracranial Hemorrhage

Vessel perforation during microcatheter placement and delayed hemorrhage from the controversial nor-mal pressure breakthrough or venous outflow obstruction are the most significant causes of peri- and postembolization intracranial hemorrhage. The risk of intracranial hemorrhage from vessel perforation during microcatheter placement has been significantly reduced since the development of the flow-directed microcatheters, which are more flexible than "geometry-directed" microcatheters and have played a significant role in the success of AVM embolizations with cyanoacrylate glue. More important, the flow-directed microcatheters do not require a metal guidewire extended beyond the tip of the microcatheter for advancement and navigation in the feeder of an AVM, which is the most significant cause of vessel perforations.

The use of the Terumo 0.010″ Glidewire has consistently improved the success rate in navigating distal tortuous vessels and selectively catheterizing the nidus of AVMs. However, this wire reintroduces the potential risks of vessel perforation when used in the flow-directed Magic microcatheter. Extreme caution must be exercised when using this wire at sharp

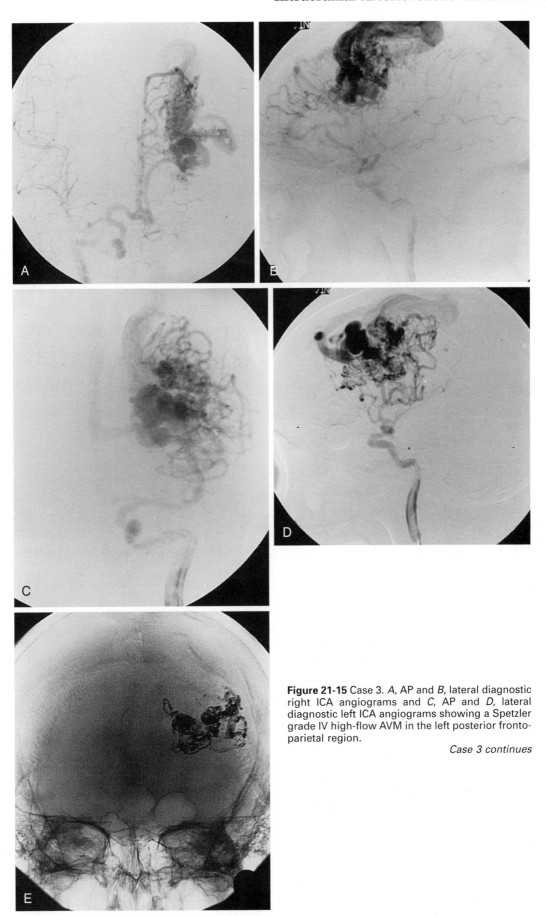

Figure 21-15 Case 3. *A*, AP and *B*, lateral diagnostic right ICA angiograms and *C*, AP and *D*, lateral diagnostic left ICA angiograms showing a Spetzler grade IV high-flow AVM in the left posterior fronto-parietal region.

Case 3 continues

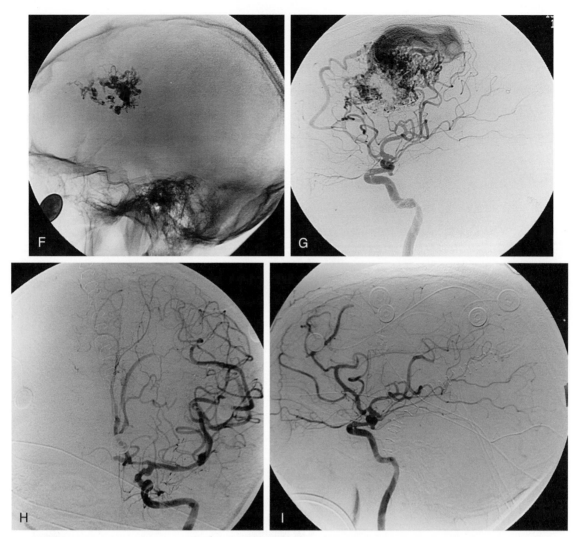

Figure 21-15 *Case 3 (continued). E,* AP and *F,* lateral plain skull films show the glue cast after staged embolization of 13 feeders, two of which demonstrated true fistulae. These were treated successfully with pure Histoacryl using the sandwich technique. *G,* A lateral left ICA angiogram obtained on the same date reveals that significant nidus remains. However, there has been a substantial reduction of flow through the AVM. *H,* AP and *I,* lateral left ICA angiograms obtained after surgical resection of the AVM demonstrate no residual nidus.

angulations, turns, and loops in the vessel, or in the presence of an aneurysm along the feeder to the AVM. The Terumo/Magic microcatheter system does not behave like the typical guidewire/microcatheter system: the wire is not used primarily to direct the microcatheter, but to increase the proximal stiffness of the Magic and increase its "pushability." As stated, only individuals familiar with the use of flow-directed microcatheters and microguidewires should utilize this technique. In over 180 superselective catheterizations using the Terumo wire in conjunction with the 1.8-Fr. Magic microcatheter, only one vessel perforation occurred, and no other complications were observed.

The incidences of normal pressure breakthrough and venous outflow occlusion with resultant postembolization intracranial hemorrhage are less than 5% and 1%, respectively. Normal pressure breakthrough tends to occur in patients with large high-flow AVMs and multiple large feeding vessels. To minimize the

risk of intracranial hemorrhage in these cases, embolization of the AVM nidus volume is limited to 30% per session, and the patient's mean arterial pressure is maintained at 15% to 20% below baseline during the first 24 hours after embolization. Subsequent embolizations are performed at approximately 3- to 4-week intervals. The rationale for this is to allow stabilization of the altered cerebral hemodynamics that occur after embolization.

Occlusion of the draining venous outlet during embolization of AVMs with cyanoacrylate adhesives can be devastating.[19, 20] As the goal of embolization is to fill the interstices of the AVM with embolic material up to the draining vein, prevention of venous occlusion becomes a significant concern. This risk is minimized by using a dilute Histoacryl/Ethiodol mixture (25% Histoacryl and 75% Ethiodol), injecting the mixture slowly, and employing the technique of pausing the injection for 2 or 3 seconds if glue passes into the draining vein, as described under "Technique." In experienced hands, the risk of venous occlusion will be minimal and may not be significantly different from the risks associated with PVA/ethanol mixture embolizations.[17, 21–25] In the unwanted instance of venous outflow occlusion during embolization, similar precautions are undertaken as for minimizing the risk of normal pressure breakthrough (reduction of mean arterial pressure). Subsequent embolizations can then be performed, if needed, at 3- to 4-week intervals.

Stroke

Cerebral ischemia may occur from catheter-induced thrombotic emboli or, more specific to embolization, reflux of embolic material into normal cerebral vessels. Systemic heparinization and continuous flush of all catheters and microcatheters with heparinized saline, as described under "Technique," are instrumental in minimizing the risk of catheter-induced thrombotic emboli. The incidences of heparin-induced platelet aggregation and subclinical coagulopathies are low and do not sufficiently outweigh the risk of catheter-induced thrombosis to warrant performing potentially prolonged embolization procedures without the use of heparin.

Reflux of embolic material into normal parenchymal branches during embolization is a real and potentially devastating complication. This has been addressed under "Technique" and will be only summarized here. The use of a state-of-the-art imaging system is crucial to the technique. Biplane digital capabilities, high detail, and high contrast resolution allow the interventionist to plan and execute embolization with minimal risk, which will then be related primarily to the limits of technique and experience.

Wedge positioning of the microcatheter at or within the nidus of the AVM, in conjunction with a more dilute mixture of Histoacryl and Ethiodol, allows for longer injection times and greater control of the injection. The presence of a vessel of passage is not a contraindication to the use of acrylic glue. However, one must maximize the margin of safety of embolization by having the maximal length of microcatheter within the branch feeder off the vessel of passage, and the tip wedged in the nidus of the AVM.

Finally, general anesthesia, which provides an absolutely motionless patient, allows maximal use of the imaging system and removes patient discomfort during a long procedure. Patient motion can severely degrade roadmapped images with loss of image detail and landmarks, causing premature interruption of embolization to avoid complications. General anesthesia precludes the use of physiologic testing, which remains controversial and has been discussed previously.

Microcatheter Retention

Gluing the tip of the microcatheter in the nidus of the AVM is a problem specific to the use of cyanoacrylate glue. This complication rarely has neurologic sequelae and occurs in less than 3% of all embolizations. The risk can be minimized by ensuring that the catheter tip is wedged, preventing glue reflux proximally along the microcatheter, removing any redundant loops in the microcatheter before embolization, using a dilute glue mixture (which prolongs glue polymerization time), and aspirating the injection syringe in conjunction with abrupt guide catheter and microcatheter withdrawal at the end point of the embolization. This last point is critical and requires an experienced assistant familiar with cyanoacrylate glue embolizations. The abrupt withdrawal of the guide catheter and Magic is mandatory, for if the microcatheter is glued within the nidus, abrupt withdrawal will break the microcatheter in its middle to distal segment and decrease the risk of rupture of the nidus. This is analogous to the behavior of "Silly Putty." Rapid pulling of "Silly Putty" results in snapping and breaking of the putty in its middle segment, but slow pulling results only in continued stretching and elongation of the substance.

If and when a Magic microcatheter is glued within the nidus, only the last 15 to 25 cm of the microcatheter are retained, with the proximal portion usually located within the distal cervical segment or petrous portion of the internal carotid artery. If a vertebral approach was used to catheterize the nidus, the proximal portion of the retained microcatheter will reside within the distal vertebral artery. Usually, there is no recoiling of the microcatheter if a 1.8-Fr. Magic is used; however, when a 1.5-Fr. microcatheter is retained, the proximal segment of the retained microcatheter may recoil distally and coil on itself within the major access vessel or within the feeder, markedly increasing the risk of thrombosis. When this complication occurs, same-day surgical resection of the AVM will allow retrieval of the retained catheter, as the microcatheter is easily seen within the cerebral vessel. Also, surgical resection performed weeks to months after gluing of a microcatheter will typically result in retrieval of the retained segment, as there is no apparent adhesion to the vessel wall. There is no reason not to take advantage of surgical retrieval when gluing of a microcatheter occurs, either acutely when coiling of the retained catheter occurs or remotely, during routine planned resection of the AVM. Retained microcatheters that remain straight and do not recoil do not appear to promote thrombosis.

Since the mid-1990s, when we began using the technique described in this chapter, we have glued eight microcatheters during a total of 403 separate vessel embolizations (2%). Only one microcatheter was removed emergently secondary to coiling within the basilar artery and in fear of potential thrombosis. The microcatheter was easily seen within the feeder at surgery and was removed without incident. No permanent postoperative neurologic sequelae were observed. A second microcatheter was removed 24 hours after embolization; however, surgery was performed secondarily to postembolization delayed hemorrhage from partial venous outflow occlusion and was not directly related to the retained microcatheter fragment. Three microcatheters were removed easily during routine AVM resection 3 to 6 months after the embolization procedure, and three microcatheters have not been removed to date. In our total experience in embolizing AVMs, including techniques that have since been modified, the longest time that a patient has harbored a retained catheter segment was 6 years. This patient underwent a series of staged embolizations followed by surgical resection. The AVM was successfully resected. However, at the time of surgery, the retained catheter fragment was not retrieved. To date, there have been no sequelae directly related to the retained microcatheter segment in these situations. Patients with retained microcatheter segments are anticoagulated for 3 to 6 months, after which the anticoagulation is stopped if there have been no complications.

The mandatory requirement for abrupt guide catheter and microcatheter withdrawal emphasizes the need for a neurointerventional team consisting not only of neurointerventionists but also of neurosurgeons, anesthesiologists, nurses, and technologists all familiar with the procedure.

CONCLUSION

We believe that cyanoacrylate glue formulations, specifically *N*-butyl-2-cyanoacrylate, represent the optimal embolic agent for the treatment of AVMs at the present time. Cyanoacrylate can be curative in a higher percentage of small AVMs (grades I and II) and can be used in conjunction with radiosurgery or surgery for lesions that are not amenable to these two procedures alone. The risks are great, but in experienced hands the morbidity and mortality rates of the procedure do not exceed those of more conventional therapy.

The technique of nidus embolization with *N*-butyl-2-cyanoacrylate glue presented in this chapter is not the only approach to AVM embolization, but it is considered to provide optimal results with minimal risk. This technique requires considerable experience in interventional procedures, and more specifically, complete familiarity with flow-directed microcatheters, microguidewires, and cyanoacrylate glue. It should not be attempted by the novice interventionalist.

Many controversies exist within the interventional community regarding the best approach to the embolization of AVMs. It is hoped that the material here explains our rationale for adopting this technique.

REFERENCES

1. Jellinger K. Vascular malformations of the ventral nervous system: a morphological review. *Neurosurg Rev* 1986;9:177–216.
2. Ondra SI, Troupp H, George ED, Schwab K. The natural history of symptomatic arteriovenous malformations of the brain: a 24 year follow up assessment. *J Neurosurg* 1990;73:387–391.
3. Valvanis A. Arteriovenous malformations of the brain. In Interventional Neuroradiology. Berlin: Springer-Verlag, 1993, pp 93–110.
4. Deruty R, Pelissou-Guyotat I, Mottolese C, et al. The combined management of cerebral arteriovenous malformations. Experience with 100 cases and review of the literature. *Acta Neurochir (Wien)* 1993;123:101–112.
5. Fournier D, TerBrugge KG, Willinsky R, et al. Endovascular treatment of intracerebral arteriovenous malformations: experience in 49 cases. *J Neurosurg* 1991;75:228–233.
6. Hurst RW, Berenstein A, Kupersmith MJ, et al. Deep central arteriovenous malformations of the brain: the role of endovascular treatment. *J Neurosurg* 1995;82:190–195.
7. Wilms G, Goffin J, Plets C, et al. Embolization of arteriovenous malformations of the brain: preliminary experience. *J Belge Radiol* 1993;76:299–303.
8. Brothers MF, Kaufmann JCE, Fox AJ, Deveikis JP. *N*-Butyl-2-cyanoacrylate—substitute for IBCA in interventional neuroradiology: histopathologic and polymerization time studies. *AJNR* 1989;10:777–786.
9. Fournier D, TerBrugge K, Rodesch G, Lasjaunias P. Revascularization of brain arteriovenous malformations after embolization with bucrylate. *Neuroradiology* 1990;32:497–501.
10. Marks MP, Lane B, Steinberg GK, et al. Endovascular treatment of cerebral arteriovenous malformations following radiosurgery. *AJNR* 1993;14:297–304.
11. Hamilton M, Spetzler R. The prospective application of a grading system for arteriovenous malformations. *Neurosurgery* 1994;34:2–6.
12. Miyasaka Y, Yada K, Ohwada T, et al. An analysis of the venous drainage system as a factor in hemorrhage from arteriovenous malformation. *J Neurosurg* 1992;76:239–243.
13. Marks KP, Lane B, Steinberg G, Chang P. Vascular characteristics of intracerebral arteriovenous malformations in patients with clinical steal. *AJNR* 1991;12:489–496.
14. Marks MP, Lane B, Steinberg GK, Chang PJ. Hemorrhage in intracerebral arteriovenous malformations: angiographic determinants. *Radiology* 1990;176:807–813.
15. Lasjaunias P, Piske R, TerBrugge K, Willinsky R. Cerebral arteriovenous malformations (C. AVM) and associated arteriovenous aneurysms (AA): analysis of 101 C. AVM cases, with 37 AA in 23 patients. *Acta Neurochir (Wien)* 1988;91:26–36.
16. Willinsky R, Lasjaunias P, TerBrugge K, Pruvost P. Brain arteriovenous malformations: analysis of the angio-architecture in relationship to hemorrhage (based on 152 patients explored and/or treated at the hôpital de Bicêtre between 1981 and 1986). *J Neuroradiol* 1988;15:225–237.
17. Khayata M, Aymard A, Guichard JP, Merland JJ. Interventional neuroradiology. *Curr Opin Radiol* 1992;4:71–78.
18. Peters KR, Quisling RG, Gilmore R, et al. Intraarterial use of sodium methohexital for provocative testing during brain embolotherapy. *AJNR* 1993;14:171–174.
19. Duckwiler GR, Dion JE, Vinuela F, Reichman A. Delayed venous occlusion following embolotherapy of vascular malformations in the brain. *AJNR* 1992;13:1571–1579.
20. Jafar JJ, Davis AJ, Berenstein A, et al. The effect of embolization with *N*-butyl cyanoacrylate prior to surgical resection of cerebral arteriovenous malformations. *J Neurosurg* 1993; 78:60–69.
21. Kline JN, Ryals TJ, Galvin JR, et al. Pulmonary embolization and infarction. An iatrogenic complication of transcatheter embolization of a cerebral arteriovenous malformation with polyvinyl alcohol sponge. *Chest* 1993;103:1293–1295.
22. Nakstad PH, Bakke SJ, Hald JK. Embolization of intracranial arteriovenous malformations and fistulas with polyvinyl alcohol particles and platinum fibre coils. *Neuroradiology* 1992;34:348–351.
23. Nakstad PH, Nornes H. Superselective angiography, embolisation and surgery in treatment of arteriovenous malformations of the brain. *Neuroradiology* 1994;36:410–413.
24. Pelz DM, Fox AJ, Vinuela F, et al. Preoperative embolization of brain AVMs with isobutyl-2 cyanoacrylate. *AJNR* 1988;9:757–764.
25. Schumacher M, Horton JA. Treatment of cerebral arteriovenous malformations with PVA. Results and analysis of complications. *Neuroradiology* 1991;33:101–105.

CHAPTER 22

Ethanol Endovascular Management of Brain Arteriovenous Malformation:
Initial Experience

W.F.J. Yakes

Since the introduction of embolization of cerebral arteriovenous malformations (AVMs) in 1960 by Luessenhop and Spence,[1, 2] later utilizing the transfemoral approach to embolize brain AVMs (as reported in 1972 by Kricheff et al.[3]), embolization of brain vascular pathology has grown slowly into a significant specialty. Because of collaboration among neurosurgery, neurology, and interventional neuroradiology, there has been an explosive growth in the use of cerebral endovascular procedures as a preoperative adjunct, and in select cases as a primary mode of therapy for many types of vascular lesions. First developed by Kerber in 1976, calibrated-leak balloon catheters were the first catheters used to navigate the intracranial vessels to embolize brain AVMs.[4–6] This required the use of liquid embolic agents such as isobutyl-2-cyanoacrylate (IBCA). Since the 1980s, there has been the development of multiple microcatheters that can gain access to the most distal cerebral circulation. Concurrently, a vast array of embolic agents have been developed that are now routinely used to perform embolization procedures through these microcatheters.

RATIONALE FOR USE

Ethanol Versus Other Embolic Agents

Many embolic agents have been utilized to treat brain AVMs. However, the dominant embolic materials are polyvinyl alcohol (PVA) of varying sizes, microcoils of varying sizes, and various tissue adhesives. It is known that PVA can cause an acute occlusion in a brain AVM, but recanalization is seen at follow-up. Coils cause a very proximal occlusion and do not occlude at the nidus. It was long thought that IBCA and *N*-butyl-cyanoacrylate (NBCA) had the potential for permanence. However, because of the dilution of the acrylic substance with Lipiodol/Ethiodol from a minimum of 1:1 up to a 1:4 dilution of the acrylic, recanalization is possible. With a too proximal NBCA polymerization resulting in occlusion proximal to the nidus, there occurs a neovascular stimulation recruitment phenomenon that can markedly worsen the condition and impair the ability to treat the malformation. Too distal an NBCA polymerization in the outflow vein can lead to a catastrophic AVM rupture, hemorrhage, and death. Many reports in the literature have documented recanalization and

the neovascular stimulation recruitment phenomenon.[7–14] Another issue with regard to tissue adhesives (acrylics) is the ease of surgical excision. With the use of acetic acid and of weaker dilutions with oily contrast to retard polymerization of the acrylic substance, hard casts can form that may create problems with surgical retraction, cutting, and coagulation.[14] Also, these tissue adhesives are not Food and Drug Administration (FDA) approved, which raises the question of medicolegal risks.

In a 1995 article, Frizzel and Fisher performed a retrospective review of 1246 patients in 32 reported clinical series over a 35-year period to evaluate endovascular procedures and the management of brain AVMs.[8] They observed that the AVM cure rate with embolization was 4% before 1990 and 5% after 1990. In this review article, multiple authors noted that embolization is largely a preoperative measure or pre-radiosurgical adjunct. The embolic agents reviewed included PVA, coils, Surgicel, silk suture, IBCA/NBCA, and a 30% ethanol mixture with PVA. A constant feature reported by many authors was a recanalization phenomenon that occurred with all these agents. Embolotherapy with these agents cannot be compared with surgical results since the endovascular cure rates of brain AVMs are so low. Our current cure rate with ethanol as an embolic agent is greater than 50%. If significantly higher cure rates are possible with the use of ethanol, endovascular results may then finally be directly compared with surgical results.

Permanence

As noted above, permanence is an important issue with regard to the embolic agents used to occlude these malformations, particularly when embolization is performed in conjunction with radiosurgery.

After significant experience and consistently successful cures of large peripheral AVMs with ethanol at long-term follow-up,[15–30] we proceeded to use ethanol in neurologically sensitive areas such as the pelvis, paraspinal area, and head and neck region. Cure of peripheral AVMs with embolic agents other than ethanol is unusual but is common with the use of ethanol, and so when we investigated its use, it was reviewed not only as a primary mode of therapy to treat brain AVMs but also to determine whether ethanol had advantages over current embolic materials as a preoperative and pre-radiosurgical adjunct. This is the first patient series utilizing undiluted absolute ethyl alcohol as a brain AVM embolic agent.[31]

Mechanism of Action

Ethanol embolization of normal tissues will lead to total tissue devitalization without collateral flow, progressing to necrosis. Ethanol, being a liquid agent, travels to the capillary bed level, thus excluding all collateral circulation. It is for this explicit reason that inadvertent embolization must be avoided. Ethanol in contact with blood causes denuding of the endothelial cells from the vascular wall and precipitates their protoplasm. There is fracturing of the blood vessel wall to the level of the internal elastic lamina. This phenomenon is well documented in the management of tumors and large peripheral AVMs that have undergone ethanol endovascular therapy. Angionecrosis does not appear to occur in peripheral AVMs or in brain AVMs. In the surgically resected specimens of three patients with brain AVMs in our series,[31] there was no histologic evidence of angionecrosis. The issue of necrosis is a problem of nontarget embolization to capillary beds that are normal. As the capillary beds occlude, the tissues fed by these capillary beds become devitalized, and then infarct and become necrotic. The kidney, which can be considered to have an end-organ vascular supply like that of the brain, is an excellent model for evaluating this phenomenon. Ethanol has been used extensively to treat angiomyelolipomas, renal cell carcinomas, and AVMs. One presenting complaint of patients with these conditions is intractable hematuria. After ethanol ablation of a renal cell cancer, an angiomyelolipoma, or an AVM, hematuria is abruptly controlled. All three conditions frequently have aneurysms causing erosions into the urinary collecting system. If angionecrosis is a factor, symptomatic hematuria should be a persistent problem after the procedure, rather than being controlled by this technique.

Technique of Use

Ethanol has many attractive properties for use in vascular malformation management. When required, ethanol is opacified with metrizamide powder (Amipaque). This does, however, decrease the efficacy of ethanol compared with pure unopacified ethanol. The mixture of ethanol and metrizamide also causes it to become more viscous. In high-flow lesions where reflux is not a problem, we often use unopacified ethanol and then switch to opacified ethanol to achieve greater control as the AVM slows down. Significantly, once ethanol passes through the AVM nidus and then enters an outflow vein, it is diluted and rendered ineffectual. Therefore, outflow vein occlusion, which

can result from mistakes in calculating the polymerization of NBCA, cannot occur. Thus, outflow vein occlusion with acute nidus rupture and hemorrhage has not been encountered. Another attractive property of ethanol is the progressive occlusion that occurs over time, even in weeks. In patients in whom embolization was not taken to completion and residual arteriovenous shunting was still identified angiographically, follow-up arteriograms demonstrated total AVM occlusion.

Dangers

Ethanol is the most dangerous intravascular substance that can be injected. Inadvertent embolization must be completely avoided by superselective positioning. If this is not possible, ethanol should not be used. Being a fluid agent, it will penetrate to the capillary bed level and totally devitalize normal tissues. Therefore, superselective positioning and experience with the use of ethanol is absolutely necessary to minimize the risks of its use. Only after significant experience with ethanol as an embolic agent can it be used appropriately in neurologically sensitive areas such as the head and neck, paraspinal regions, pelvis, and brain. A physician's first use of ethanol as an embolic agent should never be in the brain. Physicians are recommended to gain experience with the use of ethanol by working with their interventional radiology colleagues and embolizing renal cell carcinomas, which, because of the arteriovenous shunting and end-organ status, can simulate brain AVM pathology. Working with this agent in experimental dogs to achieve a level of proficiency is also recommended.

CONCEPTS IN PATIENT MANAGEMENT

Patient Selection

All patients continue to be classified according to the Spetzler-Martin grading system.[32, 33] Most patients treated in our series were grade III and above.[31]

Team Approach to Management

A collaborative effort with neurosurgery is extremely important to optimally manage patients with brain AVMs. Each specialist brings specific skills and knowledge to the table. As in all of medicine, multidisciplinary approaches usually yield the best results. At times, it may be determined that endovascular approaches are no longer possible. The roles of radiosurgery and traditional surgery then become very important if total cure is to be achieved. Ethanol has proved to be a permanent embolic agent; recanalization and neovascular stimulation recruitment phenomenon do not occur.[15–30] Therefore, its role as a pre-radiosurgical adjunct is extremely attractive.

Brain AVMs that were cured by ethanol embolization remain cured at long-term follow-up. It is hoped that the experience of our group with brain AVMs will equal their success in peripheral AVM management with ethanol endovascular therapy.[31]

Preprocedure Education

All patients are counseled extensively with regard to the anatomic location, grade, and published natural history of their particular AVM lesion. They are advised of the various management strategies, including radiosurgery, embolization and radiosurgery, surgery, embolization and surgery, the use of a non–FDA-approved embolic agent (IBCA/NBCA) and its published results, ethanol embolization, ethanol embolization and radiosurgery, and ethanol embolization and surgery. It was explained to all patients in our series that it was hoped that with serial ethanol embolotherapy, their AVM might be completely cured.[31] However, surgery and/or radiosurgery might ultimately be required to completely treat the AVM if it proved impossible to treat residual portions endovascularly. The expected outcome and permanence with other embolic agents were discussed. The vascular neurosurgery staff discussed the neurosurgical issues with the patients. Initially, because of what was presumed to be a technical inability to reach the nidus with current catheters, several patients were not deemed candidates for ethanol embolotherapy and were not offered this option. However, no patients who were offered ethanol endovascular therapy for their brain AVM refused this option.

Initial Aspects of the Procedure (Preparation for Embolization)

With intravascular ethanol, pain control is an issue. Anesthesiologists greatly aid in solving this problem, leaving interventional neuroradiologists free to concentrate on the case at hand. In all patients, Swan-Ganz catheter and arterial line placement for monitoring is performed. General anesthesia is used in pediatric patients. All catheterizations are performed via the transfemoral route using various guide catheters and microcatheter/guidewire systems. A direct carotid approach has not been required in any patient up to this time. In one patient, surgical resection of a redundant cervical loop of the internal carotid artery was performed to allow a more straightforward catheterization of the distal vasculature.

After microcatheter placement in the AVM nidus is achieved, provocative testing proceeds with amobarbital (Amytal). Usually, 50 to 150 mg is administered as a rapid bolus through a tuberculin syringe. The patient is then evaluated to determine whether any neurologic deficits have developed. In one patient with an occipital lobe AVM, provocative testing re-

vealed a total hemianopia. However, with distal advancement of the microcatheter by approximately 3 mm, a repeat provocative test was normal. After passing provocative testing, patients are placed under deep neuroleptic intravenous sedation. Ethanol embolotherapy can then proceed (Figs. 22–1 and 22–2).

Periprocedural Care

Before the procedure, patients are given 10 to 12 mg dexamethasone (Decadron) intravenously. All procedures are performed without systemic anticoagulation. In all patients thus far, ethanol has been the only intra-arterial embolic agent utilized. All patients are admitted to the intensive care unit (ICU) for overnight observation after the procedure and placed on intravenous dexamethasone, usually 4 to 6 mg every 6 to 8 hours. On the first postoperative day, all patients undergo magnetic resonance imaging (MRI) to evaluate any hemorrhage, thrombosis, or edema. Most patients are transferred from the ICU to the ward for 1 to 2 days and then discharged. After discharge, patients are placed on a tapering dose of dexamethasone for 10 to 15 days along with other medications as required. Follow-up studies consist of neurologic evaluation, MRI, and cerebral arteriography. It is unusual to cure a brain AVM totally in one sitting, although it has been accomplished. Serial endovascular therapy every 4 to 8 weeks is the usual scenario.

TECHNICAL PROBLEMS, COMPLICATIONS, AND SOLUTIONS

Complications

Complications are classified as transient and permanent. Transient complications in our series[31] included one woman with a grade II AVM who suffered a subarachnoid hemorrhage (SAH). Two days after the ethanol embolization procedure, this patient developed a minor headache, and an MRI scan was performed that showed no evidence of SAH, parenchymal hemorrhage, or stroke. On postoperative day 4, the patient underwent resection of the AVM, at which time the SAH was discovered. Of patients with grade III AVMs, one had a reading difficulty that resolved within 7 days and another had a right partial homonymous hemianopia that resolved in 2 months. A third patient suffered a right hemiparesis that completely resolved; a fourth had a right graphesthesia that completely resolved. Of patients with grade IV AVMs, one developed right lower extremity weakness that totally resolved, while two experienced right homonymous hemianopia that totally resolved. In patients with grade V AVMs, there was one episode of right hand numbness, one episode of right homonymous hemianopia, and one short-term memory loss, all of which totally resolved. One patient with a grade V AVM suffered a deep venous

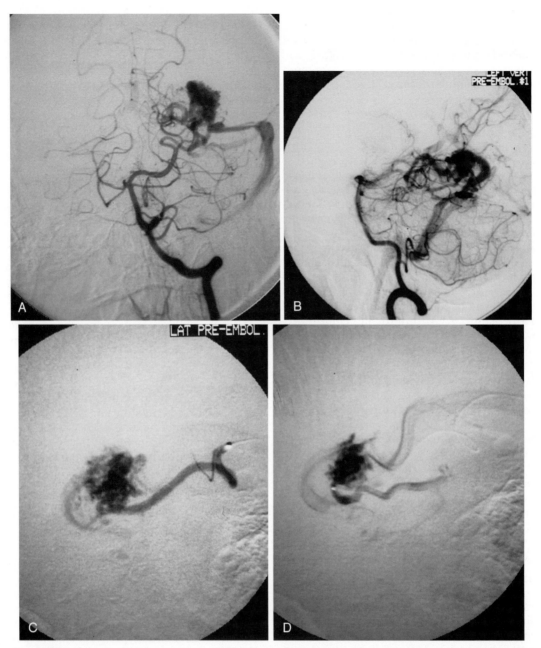

Figure 22–1 Case 1. *A,* Anteroposterior (AP) left vertebral arteriogram demonstrating an arteriovenous malformation (AVM) supplied by the left posterior cerebral artery. The patient refused radiosurgery. *B,* Lateral left vertebral digital subtraction arteriogram (DSA) demonstrating a brain AVM of the occipital lobe. *C,* Lateral left posterior cerebral artery preembolization DSA. *D,* Lateral view during injection of the AVM nidus. Note the filling of the AVM with multiple outflow veins. This is an intranidal injection.

Case 1 continues

thrombosis and pulmonary embolism that was treated with heparinization.

Of the group of patients with permanent complications, one patient with a grade III AVM (splenium) suffered short-term memory loss that improved slightly but appears to be permanent at 3-year follow-up. One patient with a grade IV AVM experienced a fatal SAH 14 months after partial therapy. A woman with a grade VI AVM within the thalamus and basal ganglia did well after two embolizations, with no complications. However, after a third embolization, she suffered a right third nerve palsy, worsen-

ing of the left hemiparesis, preferential inferior gaze, and development of dysarthria. This patient was then started on an aggressive rehabilitation program and progressed to where she was ambulating with assistance and communicating in an understandable manner. She was also alert, oriented, and fully cognizant of the situation. Unfortunately, 10 weeks after the third embolization, while undergoing rehabilitation, she suffered an SAH that resulted in a significant setback and worsened the neurologic deficits. Sixteen weeks after the third embolization (6 weeks after the previous SAH), the patient sustained a sec-

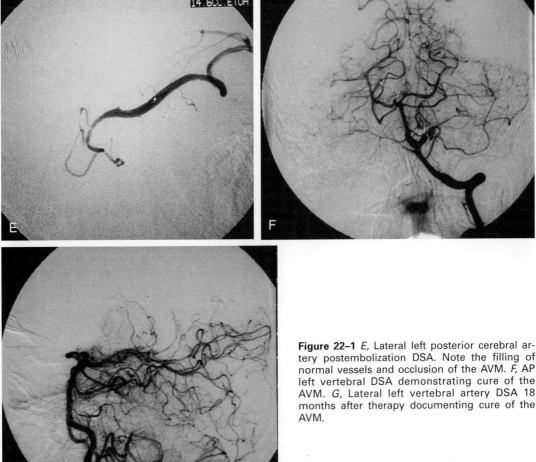

Figure 22–1 *E,* Lateral left posterior cerebral artery postembolization DSA. Note the filling of normal vessels and occlusion of the AVM. *F,* AP left vertebral DSA demonstrating cure of the AVM. *G,* Lateral left vertebral artery DSA 18 months after therapy documenting cure of the AVM.

ond SAH and died. In summary, five patients have had transient complications and three have had permanent complications, as described.

Heparin Use

Total systemic heparinization during interventional neuroradiologic procedures is an extremely controversial issue at this time. Some interventionists advocate its use; others do not. The rationale for total systemic heparinization is that heparin may decrease the risk of clot embolization from coaxially placed catheters. However, those who do not advocate its use counter that heparin increases the risks of significant or fatal hemorrhage during treatment of AVMs or aneurysms. The approach at our institution is not to heparinize patients undergoing brain AVM therapy. If there is to be an extremely tortuous catheterization, 1000 to 2000 units of heparin may be given on a case-by-case basis before the catheterization. This allows anticoagulation during the manipulation of a catheter but does not prolong the time of heparinization. The debate on this issue is ongoing.

Provocative Testing

Provocative testing is not completely foolproof. It must be repeated throughout a procedure, because hemodynamic changes can occur as progressive embolization causes AVM thrombosis and decreases the amount of shunting. Because of the high-flow state in AVMs, we prefer a higher dosage level and concentration of amobarbital, and inject with a 1-cc tuberculin syringe. In this fashion, we hope that the hemodynamic shunting will be overcome and better perfusion of any small vessels undergoing vascular steal will then occur. Provocative testing is not an infallible indicator of potential neural injury but is nonetheless useful in lessening the morbidity and mortality rates in interventional neuroradiologic procedures.

Postembolization Thrombosis and Edema

When ethanol is used, the edema related to postembolization thrombosis can cause transient neurologic

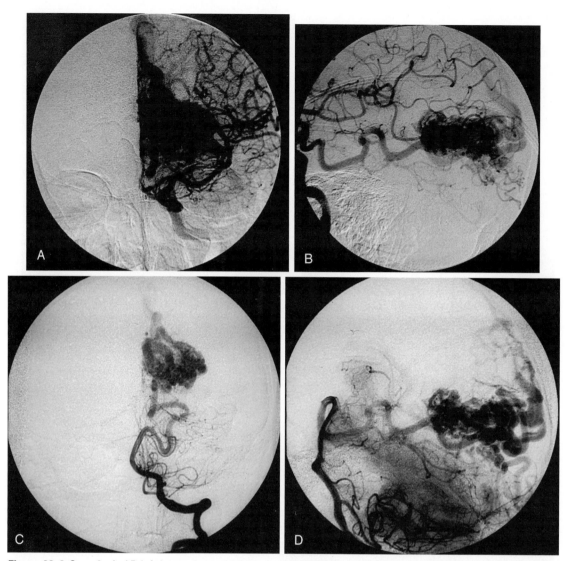

Figure 22–2 Case 2. *A,* AP left internal carotid DSA demonstrating a left occipital lobe grade IV AVM. *B,* Lateral left internal carotid DSA demonstrating a grade IV AVM supplied from the left posterior cerebral artery and middle cerebral artery branches. *C,* AP left vertebral artery DSA showing supply to the AVM from the left posterior cerebral artery. *D,* Lateral left vertebral artery DSA demonstrating left posterior cerebral artery supply to the AVM.
Case 2 continues

deficits. However, aggressive dexamethasone therapy can reverse these and resolve the edema.

Normal Perfusion Pressure Breakthrough

Normal perfusion pressure breakthrough phenomenon is an important concept in neurovascular procedures. This phenomenon has been observed after surgery and endovascular therapy for all or part of a vascular malformation or arteriovenous fistula.[34] With tissue adhesives and other embolic agents, rapid devascularization of an AVM can occur. This may contribute to the perfusion pressure breakthrough phenomenon, and because of decreased ability to autoregulate arterial flow, it can result in edema and even hemorrhage. Because of the slow progress of thrombosis in the AVM that occurs over time with the use of ethanol, it is hoped that the effect of this phenomenon may be lessened.

Cardiopulmonary Considerations

Anesthesiologists not only greatly aid in solving the pain problems, but are an invaluable asset in monitoring pulmonary artery pressures and arterial pressures during the procedure. Swan-Ganz (pulmonary pressure) and arterial monitoring are considered very important at our institution. Hemodynamic consequences such as cardiopulmonary collapse can occur as rare sequelae of ethanol embolization procedures. Despite this rarity, it is very real when it occurs. Swan-Ganz line and arterial line placement allow for total physiologic monitoring during the procedure. The physiologic sequence of events begins with a bolus of ethanol arriving at the pulmonary artery capillary bed and inducing precapillary spasm. This causes pulmonary artery pressures to rise, which in turn increases right ventricular afterload. This then decreases right ventricular con-

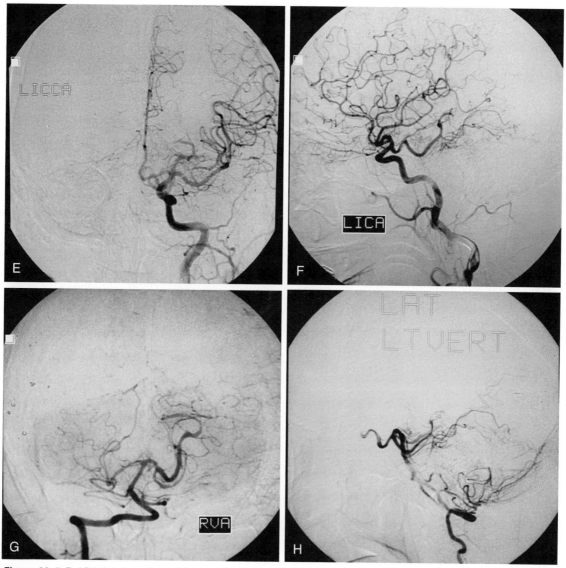

Figure 22–2 *E,* AP left internal carotid artery DSA 7 months after therapy. Note the absence of the AVM. *F,* Lateral left internal carotid DSA demonstrating a normal study without filling of the AVM. *G,* AP right vertebral artery DSA showing normal vascularity and absence of the AVM. *H,* Lateral left vertebral artery DSA demonstrating normal vessels and absence of the AVM.

tractility and right ventricular cardiac output. This results in decreased left heart filling, decreased left heart cardiac output, systemic hypotension, and decreased coronary artery perfusion. If severe enough, this can lead to cardiac arrhythmia and cardiopulmonary collapse. We have encountered this phenomenon during the treatment of peripheral vascular malformations. If pulmonary artery pressures start to rise during monitoring with the Swan-Ganz line, one should cease embolizing with ethanol. If necessary, nitroglycerin can be instilled through the Swan-Ganz line catheter to perfuse the pulmonary artery bed, which reverses this process. It is important for an anesthesiologist to monitor the patient physiologically during an interventional neuroradiologic procedure. In the event of an adverse occurrence such as hypertension, hypotension, cardiac arrhythmia, or elevated pulmonary artery pressures, and if intuba-

tion is required, the morbidity to the patient can be diminished. See Chapter 64 for further discussion of this problem.

DISCUSSION

Technological advances with regard to fluoroscopic equipment, C-arm designs, digital subtraction angiography (DSA), roadmapping capability, catheter and microcatheter system technology, a vast array of embolic materials, sophisticated angiographic techniques, provocative testing, and sensory evoked potentials, plus an increased knowledge and understanding of neurovascular anatomy and physiology, have led to ever-increasing applications of surgical neuroangiographic procedures. Since the mid-1980s, a mushrooming of procedures and clinical applications, directly related to the development of microcatheter systems, have led to improved care and better clinical outcomes in patients with complex neurovascular problems. Broader applications of current surgical neuroangiographic techniques and the unveiling of newer procedures will undoubtedly occur.

REFERENCES

1. Luessenhop AJ, Spence WT. Artificial embolization of cerebral arteries. Report of use in the case of arteriovenous malformation. *JAMA* 1960;172:1153–1155.
2. Luessenhop AJ, Kachmann R, Shevlin W, Ferrero AA. Clinical evaluation of artificial embolization in the management of large cerebral arteriovenous malformations. *J Neurosurg* 1965;23:400–417.
3. Kricheff II, Madayag M, Braunstein P. Transfemoral catheter embolization of cerebral and posterior fossa arteriovenous malformations. *Radiology* 1972;103:107–111.
4. Kerber C. Balloon with a calibrated leak. A new system for superselective angiography in occlusive catheter therapy. *Radiology* 1976;120:540–550.
5. Kerber CW. Flow-controlled therapeutic embolization: a physiologic and safe technique. *AJR* 1980;134:557–561.
6. Bank WO, Kerber CW, Cromwell LD. Treatment of intracerebral arteriovenous malformations with IBCA: initial clinical experience. *Radiology* 1981;139:609–616.
7. Fournier D, TerBrugge K, Rodesch G, Lasjaunias P. Revascularization of brain AVMs after embolization with bucrylate. *Neuroradiology* 1990;32:497–501.
8. Frizzel RT, Fisher WS. Cure, morbidity, and mortality associated with embolization of brain AVMs: a review of 1,246 patients in 32 series over a 35 year period. *Neurosurgery* 1995;37:1031–1040.
9. Nakstad PH, Hornes H. Superselective angiography, embolization and surgery in treatment of AVMs of the brain. *Neuroradiology* 1994;36:410–413.
10. Rao VRK, Mandalam KR, Gupta AK, et al. Dissolution of isobutyl 2-cyanoacrylate on long-term follow-up. *AJNR* 1989;10:135–141.
11. Schweitzer JS, Chang BS, Madsen P, et al. The pathology of AVMs of the brain treated by embolotherapy. II. Results of embolization with multiple agents. *Neuroradiology* 1993;35:468–474.
12. Vinuela F, Fox AJ, Pelz D, Debrun G. Angiographic followup of large cerebral AVMs incompletely embolized with IBCA. *AJNR* 1986;7:919–925.
13. Widlus DM, Murray RR, White RI Jr, et al. Congenital AVMs: tailored embolotherapy. *Radiology* 1988;169:511–516.
14. Purdy PD, Batjer HH, Risser RC, Samson D. Arteriovenous malformations of the brain: choosing embolic materials to enhance safety and ease of excision. *J Neurosurg* 1992;77:217–222.
15. Yakes WF, Pevsner PH, Reed MD, et al. Serial embolizations of an extremity AVM with alcohol via direct percutaneous puncture. *AJR* 1986;146:1038–1040.
16. Vinson AM, Rohrer DB, Willcox CW, et al. Absolute ethanol embolization for peripheral AVM: a report of two cures. *South Med J* 1988;81:1052–1055.
17. Takebayashi S, Hosaka M, Ishizuka E, et al. AVMs of the kidneys: ablation with alcohol. *AJR* 1988;150:587–590.
18. Yakes WF, Haas DK, Parker SH, et al. Symptomatic vascular malformations: ethanol embolotherapy. *Radiology* 1989;170:1059–1066.
19. Yakes WF, Haas DK, Parker SH, et al. Alcohol embolotherapy of vascular malformations. *Semin Intervent Radiol* 1989;6:146–161.
20. Yakes WF, Luethke JM, Parker SH, et al. Ethanol embolization of vascular malformations. *RadioGraphics* 1990;10:787–796.
21. Yakes WF, Luethke JM, Merland JJ, et al. Ethanol embolization of arteriovenous fistulas: a primary mode of therapy. *J Vasc Interv Radiol* 1990;1:89–96.
22. Mourao GS, Hodes JE, Gobin YP, et al. Curative treatment of scalp AV fistulas by direct puncture and embolization with absolute alcohol. *J Neurosurg* 1991;75:634–637.
23. Yakes WF. Extremity venous malformations: diagnosis and management. *Semin Intervent Radiol* 1994;11:332–339.
24. Yakes WF, Rossi P, Odink H. How I do it: arteriovenous malformation management. *Cardiovasc Intervent Radiol* 1996;19:65–71.
25. Yakes WF. Diagnosis and management of vascular anomalies. In Castaneda-Zuniga WR, Tadavarthy SM (eds): Interventional Radiology. Baltimore: Williams & Wilkins, 1992, pp 152–189.
26. Yakes WFJ, Dake MD. Angiographic and interventional procedures of the hand. In Gilula LA, Yin Y (eds): Imaging of the Wrist and Hand. Philadelphia: WB Saunders, 1996, pp 499–522.
27. Vogelzang RL, Yakes WF. Vascular malformations: effective treatment with absolute ethanol. In Yao JST, Pearce WH (eds): Arterial Surgery: Management of Challenging Problems. Stamford, CT: Appleton & Lange, 1996, pp 533–549.
28. Yakes WF. Diagnosis and management of venous malformations. In Savader SJ, Trerotola SO (eds): Venous Interventional Radiology with Clinical Perspectives. New York: Thieme, 1996, pp 139–150.
29. Yakes WF. Interventional neuroradiologic procedures in the head and neck: ENT perspective. In English GM (ed): Otolaryngology. New York: Lippincott-Raven, 1996, pp 1–26.
30. Yakes WF. Diagnosis and management of AVMs. In Haskal ZJ, Kerlan RK, Trerotola SO (eds): SCVIR Syllabus: Thoracic and Visceral Vascular Interventions. Fairfax, VA: Society of Cardiovascular and Interventional Radiology Publishers, 1996, pp 314–322.
31. Yakes WF, Krauth L, Ecklund J, et al. Ethanol endovascular management of brain arteriovenous malformations: initial results. *Neurosurgery* 1997;40:1145–1154.
32. Spetzler RF, Martin NA. A proposed grading system for AVMs. *J Neurosurg* 1986;65:476–483.
33. Hamilton MG, Spetzler RF. The prospective application of a grading system for AVMs. *Neurosurgery* 1994;34:2–7.
34. Spetzler RF, Wilson CB, Weinstein P, et al. Normal perfusion pressure breakthrough theory. *Clin Neurosurg* 1978;25:651–672.

CHAPTER 23

The Role of Embolization in Combination with Stereotactic Radiosurgery in the Management of Pial and Dural Arteriovenous Malformations

B.E. Pollock / L.D. Lunsford /
J.C. Flickinger / D. Kondziolka

Brain arteriovenous malformations (AVMs) are vascular anomalies that shunt blood abnormally from arteries to veins without an intervening capillary bed. There are two types of intracranial AVM (pial and dural) that differ in their etiology, presentation, and indications for treatment. Pial AVMs are congenital lesions that reside within the brain parenchyma and have an estimated incidence of 0.04% to 0.52%.[1, 2] Dural AVMs are thought to be acquired lesions and the nidus is located in the dura mater; the incidence of dural AVMs is unknown. Intracerebral hemorrhage is the most common presentation of pial AVMs,[3–12] whereas nonhemorrhagic symptoms (seizures, tinnitus, headaches) more commonly bring dural AVMs to clinical attention.[13–17] The indications for intervention in and management of pial and dural AVMs are also quite different. This chapter reviews the radiosurgical management of intracranial AVMs and the role that embolization can play in conjunction with radiosurgery in their treatment.

PIAL ARTERIOVENOUS MALFORMATIONS

Natural History and Factors Associated with Hemorrhage

Intracerebral hemorrhage represents the most devastating and potentially fatal complication of AVMs. Natural history studies of untreated AVMs have documented an overall 2% to 4% annual rate of hemorrhage.[3–8, 10, 11] Risk factors believed to predispose AVM patients to bleed include a history of a previous hemorrhage,[4–7, 11] small AVM size,[7, 9, 12] deep venous drainage,[9, 18] restricted venous outflow,[11, 18] intranidal aneurysms,[19–21] diffuse AVM morphology,[11] and higher feeding artery pressures.[9]

In analyzing AVM reports, it is important to determine whether the report is descriptive of a case series[9, 12] or based on the longitudinal follow-up of AVM patients.[3–8, 10, 11] Descriptive studies often confound factors associated with the clinical presentation of bleeding with factors that actually increase the an-

nual AVM hemorrhage rate. For example, several studies have stated that small or centrally located AVMs bleed more frequently than larger or hemispheric AVMs.[9, 12] However, smaller or deep AVMs are less likely to cause headaches or seizures and are diagnosed only after a significant intracerebral hemorrhage. Most natural history studies have found a history of hemorrhage to be the most significant factor predictive of further bleeding.[4–8, 11] The annual hemorrhage rate for the year after a bleed has been reported as 6% to 18%; this rate returns to 2% to 4% in subsequent years. Ondra et al. failed to find any correlation between presentation and further bleeding.[10] Despite the completeness and long follow-up of this study, hemorrhagic events were analyzed in 5-year periods. A transient increase in annual hemorrhage rate was most likely lost by this method of data analysis. Nonetheless, the cumulative lifetime risk for young patients is substantial,[22] and observation is indicated only for the elderly or for lesions that pose a high treatment risk.[23, 24]

Technique of AVM Radiosurgery

Stereotactic radiosurgery is single-fraction, high-dose irradiation of an imaging-defined target. The biologic effect of radiosurgery on tissues is approximately two to five times that of an equivalent radiation dose delivered in multiple fractions. Stereotactic radiosurgery can be performed with one of three devices: the Gamma knife, modified linear accelerators, or specially designed cyclotrons. Regardless of the technique, it is essential that the equipment is capable of a high level of mechanical accuracy (<1 mm) to ensure that the radiation is safely delivered to the patient.

The first step in AVM radiosurgery is proper patient selection. At our center, a weekly vascular conference is attended by neurosurgeons with expertise in radiosurgery and vascular neurosurgery, interventional neuroradiologists, and radiation oncologists. We review each AVM considered for treatment and all follow-up angiograms. If an AVM patient is considered a good candidate for radiosurgery, an outpatient office consultation is arranged and the potential risks and benefits of the patient's management options are discussed in detail. Patients who opt for radiosurgery require a minimum of preoperative studies (Fig. 23–1). Patients with lobar AVMs are placed on anticonvulsants preoperatively to minimize the risk of postoperative seizures. Patients without a seizure disorder are tapered off the medication in the week after surgery.

The patient is brought to the preoperative holding area, where nurses obtain vital signs and prepare the patient's head with alcohol. Local anesthesia is used, and a Leksell G stereotactic coordinate frame is secured by four-point pin fixation to the skull. Measurements of skull dimensions are taken, and the patient is then transported to the magnetic resonance imaging (MRI) suite. A stereotactic MRI and magnetic resonance angiogram (MRA) is then performed to delineate the three-dimensional shape of the nidus and to identify the relative position of any large draining veins that will be excluded from the radiosurgical dose plan.[25–27] Currently, the MRI sequence used for AVM dose planning is an axial, gadolinium-enhanced, T1-weighted volume acquisition study (512 × 256 pixels, two excitations), which requires less than 10 minutes to obtain. An MRA is then produced from the source images, and the studies are transferred to the computer workstation at the radiosurgical suite via Ethernet. The dose-planning software (GammaPlan, Version 4.01) is able to reconstruct sagittal and coronal studies from the axial MRI. This makes it possible to display the AVM in multiple views, thereby saving a great deal of time because MRI sequences do not have to be obtained in multiple planes.

After the MRI is completed, the patient is transferred to the angiography suite. If he or she has not previously undergone a complete angiogram (four-vessel and external carotid injections if the AVM is peripherally located), a full study is obtained at the time of radiosurgery. This study is designed to outline the arterial supply to the malformation, define the nidus and draining veins, and examine for the presence of associated aneurysms. Once the complete arterial supply to the AVM is determined, subtraction films are obtained of the AVM in the early, middle, and late arterial phases, as well as a film of the venous phase. Previous attempts to obtain stereotactic digital subtraction angiograms have been unsuc-

cessful because of unpredictable warping of images taken from the image intensifier. The angiographic films are then scanned into the dose-planning database using a high-resolution digital scanner.

Radiosurgical dose planning based on the stereotactic MRI/MRA and angiogram images is then undertaken at the computer work station in the radiosurgical unit. The dose-planning software allows rapid analysis of changes to the dose plan. The goal is to design a conformal dose plan that provides complete coverage of the AVM nidus without including feeding arteries or draining veins. By minimizing the target volume to be irradiated, a higher radiation dose can be delivered to the nidus with a steeper radiation falloff to the surrounding normal brain parenchyma. The radiation dose selected is based primarily on the integrated logistic model for prediction of complications after AVM radiosurgery.[28] After surgery, the stereotactic frame is removed and the patient is given intravenous methylprednisolone (40 mg). Patients with lesions in epileptogenic areas also receive additional anticonvulsant medication after radiosurgery (phenobarbital, 90 mg). Patients are observed overnight in the general neurosurgical ward and discharged home the following day.

Patients are requested to undergo MRI at 12, 24, and 36 months after radiosurgery to document nidus obliteration and/or the development of post-radiosurgical imaging changes (increased signal on long-TR MRI). Post-radiosurgical imaging changes are seen at a median of 12 months after radiosurgery (range, 1 to 23 months) in approximately 30% of patients.[29, 30] If the AVM is obliterated on post-radiosurgical MRI (absence of flow-void signal abnormalities) at 24 to 36 months, patients are asked to undergo follow-up angiography to document complete angiographic obliteration. If AVM nidus is still present on the 36-month follow-up MRI, repeat radiosurgery without follow-up angiography is generally recommended because the positive predictive value of post-radiosurgical MRI has been 100%.[31] With this protocol, it has been possible to substantially reduce the number of post-radiosurgical angiograms.

Results of AVM Radiosurgery

Stereotactic radiosurgery is an effective management strategy for properly selected AVM patients.[32–44] Three conditions are required for AVM radiosurgery to be considered a complete success. First, the AVM must be obliterated to eliminate the risk of AVM hemorrhage. Second, the patient must not sustain morbidity secondary to AVM bleeding before AVM obliteration. Third, radiation-associated complications must be avoided. Factors believed to be associated with successful AVM radiosurgery include AVM volume,[33, 34, 37, 38] AVM location,[29] and age of the patient.[45]

Radiosurgical reports have documented a 64% to 81% AVM obliteration rate[32–34, 40, 41] and a permanent radiation-induced complication rate of 1% to 5.1%.[29, 34, 40, 41] Patients continue to be at risk for AVM hemor-

1. Admit patient to same-day surgery—overnight
2. NPO after midnight except normal AM medications with a sip of water
3. D$_5$1/2 NS with 20 KCl/L at 100 ml/hr
4. Lorazepam, 1.0 mg PO on call to gamma unit
5. Lab—platelet count, PT/PTT, BUN/Cr, anticonvulsant level (for patients with AVMs in cortical regions)

Figure 23-1 Sample preoperative orders for arteriovenous malformation (AVM) radiosurgery.

rhage after radiosurgery during the 1- to 4-year latency interval before obliteration. The annual bleed rate for the first 3 years after radiosurgery has been reported as 3.7% to 16%.[32, 35, 40, 46, 47] The hemorrhage rate of incompletely obliterated AVMs beyond 3 years is 0% to 5%.[32, 40, 46] Thus, most studies support the concept that radiosurgery does not change the annual bleed rate of AVMs before obliteration. However, Karlsson et al. observed only 49 bleeds in a series of 1604 AVM patients with 2-year follow-up, which, when compared with the expected number of hemorrhages (assuming a 4% annual hemorrhage risk, n = 94), was significantly fewer.[44] They found that radiosurgery provided partial protection against bleeding within 6 months, and that low treatment doses and increased patient age were risk factors for post-radiosurgical AVM hemorrhage. Thus, radiosurgery may have a partial protective effect against AVM hemorrhage before obliteration. However, it is important to remember that patients continue to be at risk for AVM bleeding until there is complete nidus obliteration. Patients are believed to be free from the risk of hemorrhage once post-radiosurgical angiography confirms complete obliteration. Only one report to date has suggested an AVM hemorrhage after post-radiosurgical angiography was thought to have confirmed complete obliteration.[48] Retrospective review of that angiogram showed that the AVM was still patent.

From August 1987 to September 1996, we performed 612 AVM radiosurgical procedures at the University of Pittsburgh Center for Image-Guided Neurosurgery. The patient characteristics are outlined in Table 23–1. The mean age of the patients was 34 years (range, 2 to 79 years). In 77 patients (13%), resection of the AVM had previously been attempted, and 101 patients (17%) had undergone one or more earlier embolization procedures to reduce the size of the AVM before radiosurgery. The mean AVM volume at the time of radiosurgery was 3.7 cm³ (range, 0.1 to 24.1 cm³).

Fifty-nine patients (10%) underwent two radiosurgical procedures to eliminate the AVM. Of these, 49

T A B L E 2 3 - 2 Obliteration Rate of Arteriovenous Malformation Patients Eligible for 36-Month Follow-Up Angiography After Radiosurgical Management

AVM Volume (cm³)	No. of Patients	AVM Obliteration (%)
<1	41	88
1–4	91	87
4–10	59	78
>10	9	56

(83%) had repeat radiosurgery after the first procedure failed to obliterate the nidus, and 10 (17%) had the AVM irradiated in separate sessions (volume staging). The angiographic obliteration rates after one or two radiosurgical procedures are shown in Table 23–2. After radiosurgery, patients with vascular headache syndromes have a more than 50% decrease in symptoms as the malformation regresses.[49] Most patients with epilepsy (70%) have a reduction of seizure frequency, and approximately 25% are able to discontinue their anticonvulsant medication.[50, 51]

Factors Associated with Successful AVM Radiosurgery

For AVM radiosurgery to be considered a complete success, the AVM must be obliterated after radiosurgery and the patient must not develop any new neurologic deficits. A standard method for reporting patient outcomes after AVM radiosurgery has been proposed.[38] Patient outcomes after AVM radiosurgery include

1. Excellent: AVM obliteration without new neurologic deficit
2. Good: AVM obliteration with a new minor deficit that does not interfere with the patient's level of functioning
3. Fair: AVM obliteration with a new major deficit that causes a decline in the patient's level of functioning
4. Unchanged: Incomplete nidus obliteration without new neurologic deficit
5. Poor: Incomplete nidus obliteration with any new deficit
6. Death

By this method, any neurologic decline, regardless of its cause, is accounted for in relation to the obliteration status of the AVM. For example, two patients had complete obliteration of occipital AVMs after radiosurgery. Both developed partial quadrantanopias after radiosurgery; one sustained a post-radiosurgical hemorrhage, whereas the other developed symptomatic radiation-induced changes. Despite the causes of their neurologic deficits being different, both would be considered to have good outcomes after radiosurgery.

One important consideration in reporting radiosur-

T A B L E 2 3 - 1 Characteristics of 612 Arteriovenous Malformation Patients Managed by Stereotactic Radiosurgery from August 1987 to September 1996

Characteristic	No. of Patients (%)
AVM location	
Cerebral hemisphere	388 (63)
Deep (thalamus, basal ganglia, brainstem, corpus callosum)	183 (30)
Cerebellum	41 (7)
Presentation	
Hemorrhage	323 (53)
Seizure	194 (32)
Headache	58 (9)
Other	37 (6)

T A B L E   2 3 - 3   Pittsburgh Arteriovenous Malformation Radiosurgery (PAR) Grading Scale

Calculation of Predicted Outcome Score:

0.18 +
(0.02) (patient age; years) +
(0.10) (AVM volume; cm³) +
(0.63) (AVM location; cerebral hemisphere = 0, deep/cerebellar = 1) +
(0.35) (no. draining veins) +
(0.65) (previous embolization; no = 0, yes = 1)

PAR Grade	Predicted Outcome Score
I	<1.50
II	1.50–2.24
III	2.25–2.99
IV	>3.00

gical outcomes is the question of what is the appropriate neuroimaging end point: post-radiosurgical angiography or MRI? Traditionally, AVM obliteration has been defined as the absence of arteriovenous shunting, with complete normalization of the venous drainage on follow-up angiography.[37, 40] However, radiosurgical series have reported only a 72% to 83% rate of obtaining follow-up angiography 2 or more years after radiosurgery.[33, 34, 46] Pollock et al. compared post-radiosurgical MRI and angiography to determine the usefulness of follow-up MRI.[31] They found that post-radiosurgical MRI had a negative predictive value of 91% (the percentage of the time that MRI correctly predicted angiographic AVM obliteration) and a positive predictive value of 100% (the percentage of the time that MRI correctly predicted incomplete angiographic AVM obliteration). The overall accuracy of MRI in comparison with angiography was 95% (155 of 164 comparisons). These findings have two important implications. The first is that MRI accurately predicts angiographic outcome after radiosurgery and can be used in the reporting

of AVM radiosurgical series. Second, patients with flow-void abnormalities on 3-year follow-up MRI do not need an additional diagnostic angiogram to document AVM patency before repeat radiosurgery.

Although several AVM grading systems exist to predict patient outcomes after surgical resection,[52–55] none of these systems are appropriate for prediction of AVM radiosurgical outcomes. A multivariate analysis of clinical and angiographic factors associated with patient outcomes in 220 AVM patients managed before 1992 was performed.[38] Five factors significantly correlated with patient outcomes: (1) patient age, (2) AVM volume, (3) AVM location, (4) number of draining veins, and (5) previous embolization. An equation based on the regression coefficients of the significant variables was developed and a predicted outcome score was calculated for each AVM (Table 23–3). The Pittsburgh AVM Radiosurgery (PAR) grading scale correlated directly with patient outcomes after AVM radiosurgery (Fig. 23–2). Using this scale, we now have the ability to determine specific rates of success and failure for individual patients.

The development of the PAR grading scale was based on data from patients whose radiosurgical dose planning consisted only of conventional biplanar stereotactic angiography, which is limited in the ability to define the actual three-dimensional volume of the AVM nidus (Fig. 23–3).[25–27] We currently use both stereotactic MRI and complete cerebral angiography for AVM dose planning. This integrated method of AVM volume determination allows true conformal radiosurgical dose planning. Such dose planning is likely to increase the AVM obliteration rate and decrease the number of radiation-induced complications. A prospective application of the PAR grading scale is under way to determine its accuracy and reproducibility utilizing contemporary radiosurgical dose planning. It is likely that the use of stereotactic MRI will eliminate the number of draining veins as a significant factor in terms of successful AVM radiosurgery.

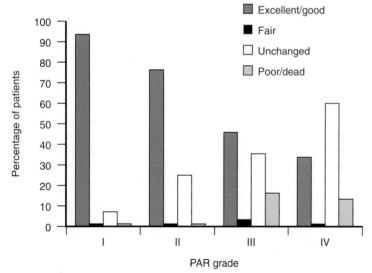

Figure 23-2 Correlation of the Pittsburgh AVM Radiosurgery (PAR) grading scale with patient outcomes after AVM radiosurgery.

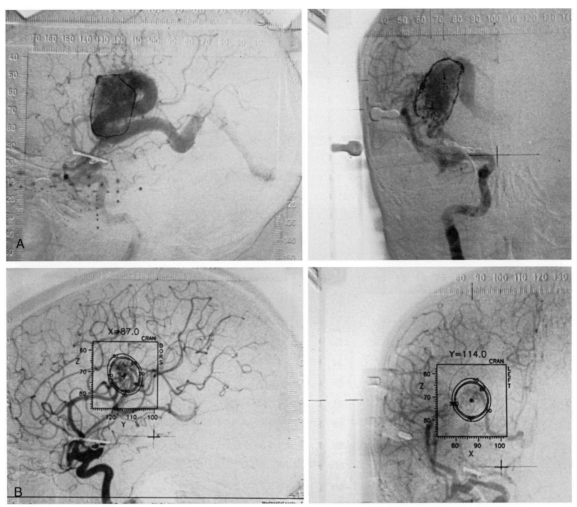

Figure 23-3 Case 1. Lateral *(left)* and anteroposterior *(right)* stereotactic angiograms of a 47-year-old man with a right frontal/basal ganglia AVM who sustained a subarachnoid hemorrhage 5 months before radiosurgery and had a clipping of two aneurysms (carotid bifurcation and middle cerebral artery aneurysms). *A,* Angiogram at the time of the initial radiosurgery. *B,* Angiogram 48 months later at the time of repeat radiosurgery. The posterosuperior residual component of the nidus was obscured by the large draining vein and was outside the original irradiated volume.

Role of Embolization in Combination with AVM Radiosurgery

Embolization is frequently used in combination with radiosurgery in the management of larger AVMs.[56–61] The goal of pre-radiosurgical embolization is clear: permanent volume reduction of the nidus. Mathis et al. reported their experience with radiosurgery after embolization for large AVMs.[59] Twelve of 24 patients (50%) treated with this management strategy had complete obliteration on post-radiosurgical angiography, and only one patient sustained a new neurologic deficit during the follow-up interval. Gobin et al. in 1996 published their management results in 96 patients undergoing radiosurgery after one or more embolizations to reduce the AVM volume to a size more suitable for radiosurgery.[57] In 53 of 90 (59%) evaluable patients there was complete AVM obliteration. However, 16 patients (12.8%) developed new neurologic deficits, and two died of intracerebral hemorrhages before radiosurgery. Twelve of 88 pa-

tients (13.6%) had recanalization of an embolized portion of the malformation after radiosurgery.

It was surprising that embolization before AVM radiosurgery was a negative predictor for patient outcomes after radiosurgery in our multivariate analysis.[38] In our review on the causes of incomplete obliteration after AVM radiosurgery, we found recanalization of a portion of the AVM in three of 19 patients (16%) who underwent pre-radiosurgical embolization (Fig. 23–4); repeat radiosurgery was required.[62] Recanalization of embolized AVMs has been reported after embolization with both polymers[63, 64] and polyvinyl alcohol.[65] Previously embolized AVMs may also make dose planning more difficult if the resultant shape of the AVM is irregular or has been divided into multiple compartments. In such cases, conformal dose planning becomes nearly impossible.

Recognition of the limitations of embolization as an adjunct to radiosurgery has led our group to begin treating some large AVMs with staged radiosurgery. Volume staging of AVMs into multiple radiosurgical

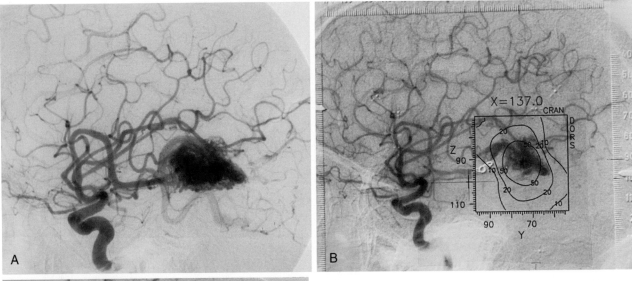

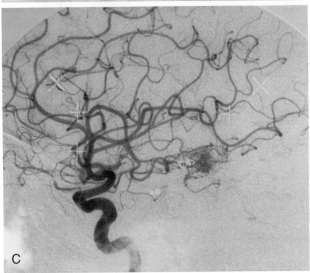

Figure 23-4 Case 2. Lateral cerebral angiograms of a 32-year-old man with a left temporal AVM who presented with headaches. *A,* Angiogram at the time of embolization. The AVM volume was estimated to be approximately 12 to 14 cm³. Embolization was performed with polyvinyl alcohol and coils. *B,* Stereotactic angiogram at the time of radiosurgery. The AVM volume was 5.7 cm³ after embolization, and the AVM was irradiated with a marginal dose of 17 Gy. *C,* Stereotactic angiogram 40 months later at the time of repeat radiosurgery. The previously embolized anterior component of the nidus recanalized and required further treatment. Note that the posterior nidus shows complete obliteration.

sessions separated by 6 months allows a higher radiation dose to be delivered to the entire AVM volume. This increases the likelihood that total obliteration will occur, while minimizing the number of radiation-induced complications after AVM radiosurgery. Although it is too early to present the results of this management strategy, to date 10 AVM patients have been managed by volume staging their AVMs with radiosurgery. The primary liability of this technique is the same as that of single-stage radiosurgery for AVMs: the patient remains at risk for AVM hemorrhage until the nidus obliterates. Several reports have documented that radiosurgery does not change the annual rate of AVM bleeding during the latency interval before obliteration[46, 47] and may provide partial protection before obliteration.[44] Assuming that patients managed by volume staging will need up to 5 years for their AVM to be completely obliterated, and that approximately 5% of patients will develop permanent radiation-induced complications, the risk of neurologic deficits or death in such patients is approximately 10% to 15%. This figure compares favorably with the results of embolization combined

with either surgical resection[23, 56] or radiosurgery[36, 57, 60, 61] for these difficult AVMs.

Comparison of AVM Management Strategies

What is the best management strategy for AVM patients? When comparing the results of AVM series, it is important to examine closely the composition of the AVMs treated. Although the percentage of AVMs of Spetzler-Martin grade III or higher is similar between radiosurgical and microsurgical studies (approximately 60%), the locations of the AVMs are quite different. In our series, 183 patients (30%) had AVMs in the basal ganglia, thalamus, corpus callosum, or brainstem. Hamilton and Spetzler operated on only eight of 120 patients (7%) with AVMs in either the thalamus or basal ganglia,[23] whereas Heros et al. resected 16 of 153 AVMs (11%) in these locations.[24] Furthermore, some surgical series include only those patients who underwent complete resection of their AVM, and not the surgeons' entire operative experience.[23, 55]

Complete occlusion of complex AVMs generally requires multiple procedures to eliminate the nidus, independent of the management strategy employed. In Hamilton and Spetzler's microsurgical series of 120 AVM patients, the mean number of procedures (including preoperative embolizations) increased with AVM grade: grade I, 1.0; grade II, 1.3; grade III, 1.7; grade IV, 2.9; and grade V, 4.4.[23] Gobin et al. required an average of 3.8 procedures per patient in their series of AVM patients who underwent embolization followed by radiosurgery.[57] Lawton et al. presented the results of multimodality treatment of 32 patients with AVMs located in the thalamus, basal ganglia, and brainstem.[36] In these 32 patients, 112 procedures were performed (average, 3.5 procedures per patient). Only six of 14 patients (43%) managed before the availability of radiosurgery with embolization, surgical resection, or both had complete resection of their AVM; in 13 of 18 patients (72%) managed after radiosurgery was available, the AVM was eliminated. Thus, the number of patients requiring repeat radiosurgery compares favorably with other management strategies for complex AVMs. Francel et al. presented 60 patients who underwent repeat radiosurgery after their AVM failed to be completely obliterated after single-session radiosurgery.[66] In 26 of 36 patients (72%) undergoing follow-up angiography, there was complete obliteration. One patient developed a radiation-induced complication. This parallels our experience in 49 patients undergoing repeat AVM radiosurgery: 10 of 16 patients (63%) eligible for follow-up angiography had complete nidus obliteration. Assuming that 60% to 70% of patients undergoing repeat radiosurgery achieve AVM obliteration without developing a new major neurologic deficit, more than 85% of patients in our AVM series will reach an excellent or good outcome after one- or two-stage radiosurgery.

DURAL ARTERIOVENOUS MALFORMATIONS

Natural History and Factors Associated with Hemorrhage

Dural AVMs are rare lesions that typically present in adulthood and are more common in women.[13–15] They are composed of one or more arteriovenous fistulae, and it has been suggested that they be called dural arteriovenous fistulous malformations (AVFMs).[14] Most are believed to be acquired lesions secondary to thrombosis of an adjacent venous sinus.[13] Patients with dural AVFMs often complain of pulsatile tinnitus, headaches, seizures, or ocular complaints. Intracranial hemorrhage is less common as the presenting symptom in patients with dural AVFMs than in those with pial AVMs. The most frequent sites of involvement are the transverse and sigmoid sinuses, but dural AVFMs occur at the cavernous sinus, the anterior cranial base, and the tentorium also. Brown et al. followed 52 patients with dural AVFMs for a mean of 6.6 years.[15] They observed five hemorrhages during this period for an annual bleeding rate of 1.6%. The presence of a varix on a draining vein correlated with an increased risk of hemorrhage in this series. Awad et al. performed a meta-analysis of the literature to determine factors predisposing dural AVFM patients to hemorrhage.[13] In the 377 cases cited, leptomeningeal venous drainage, venous dilation, and galenic drainage were significant factors for dural AVFM bleeding. Unfortunately, the results of this study were based on a univariate analysis of the data; multivariate analysis was not performed. Borden et al. proposed a classification of spinal and cranial dural AVFMs based on the type of venous drainage.[14] Type I dural AVFMs drain directly into a dural venous sinus or meningeal vein, type II drain into the venous sinus with retrograde flow into the subarachnoid veins, and type III drain directly into the subarachnoid veins. These authors recommended that symptomatic type I dural AVFMs and all type II and III AVFMs require treatment owing to their propensity to hemorrhage or become symptomatic secondary to venous hypertension.

Radiosurgery of Dural AVFMs

There have been several reports on the management of dural AVFMs with radiosurgery.[16, 17, 42, 67] Link et al. reported 29 patients with dural AVFMs who underwent radiosurgery[17]; 18 of the 29 (62%) had had previous particulate embolization because of cortical venous drainage, disabling bruit, or ophthalmoplegia. The mean nidus volume was 3.3 cm^3 and the average marginal dose to the fistulae was 19.2 Gy. In 15 patients (52%) the symptoms improved, and nine patients had stable symptoms. No postradiosurgical hemorrhages were noted. In 13 of 18 patients eligible for follow-up angiography, there was complete obliteration of the AVFM. Lewis et al. managed seven patients who had tentorial dural AVFMs with a combination of embolization and radiosurgery.[16] All patients showed improvement of the preoperative symptoms. Angiographic obliteration was seen on follow-up angiography in four patients.

Only four patients with dural AVFMs have received radiosurgery at our center. Three had AVFMs of the tentorium; the fourth patient's malformation involved both the tentorium and the cavernous sinus. Two patients had undergone previous embolization. At last follow-up, three patients were stable clinically, whereas one patient had recurrent headache and proptosis after a previously embolized portion of the AVFM was recanalized. Only two patients consented to follow-up angiography: one had angiographic obliteration and the other had recanalization. We have also identified seven more patients with mixed pial/dural AVMs who underwent radiosurgery. Most were discovered after the initial radiosurgery failed to completely obliterate the nidus because of additional arterial supply from the external carotid artery. Now all patients with peripherally located AVMs have external carotid artery injections either preoperatively or at the time of radiosurgery to ensure that there is no portion of the nidus not visualized by internal carotid artery injections.[62]

We agree with the rationale of radiosurgery *before* embolization in the management of dural AVFMs.[17] For dural AVFM patients who require intervention and who are considered poor candidates for surgical resection, radiosurgery and embolization provide an acceptable alternative management strategy. Radiosurgery performed before embolization enables all the fistulae of the malformation to be targeted and to undergo progressive occlusion. Embolization can then be performed to reduce the symptoms in an attempt to protect the patient to some degree from the future risk of hemorrhage.

REFERENCES

1. Courville CB. Pathology of the Central Nervous System: A Study Based Upon a Survey of Lesions Found in a Series of Forty Thousand Autopsies, 3rd ed. Mountain View, CA: Pacific Press, 1950, pp 142–152.
2. McCormick WF. Pathology of vascular malformations of the brain. In Wilson CB, Stein BM (eds): Intracranial Arteriovenous Malformations. Baltimore: Williams & Wilkins, 1984, pp 44–63.
3. Brown RD, Wiebers DO, Forbes G, et al. The natural history of unruptured intracranial arteriovenous malformations. *J Neurosurg* 1988;68:352–357.
4. Crawford PM, West CR, Chadwick DW, Shaw MDM. Arteriovenous malformations of the brain: natural history in unoperated patients. *J Neurol Neurosurg Psychiatry* 1986;49:1–10.
5. Forster DMC, Steiner L, Hakanson S. Arteriovenous malformations of the brain: a long-term clinical study. *J Neurosurg* 1972;37:562–570.
6. Fults D, Kelly DL Jr. Natural history of arteriovenous malformations of the brain: a clinical study. *Neurosurgery* 1984;15:658–662.
7. Graf CJ, Perret GE, Torner JC. Bleeding from cerebral arteriovenous malformations as part of their natural history. *J Neurosurg* 1983;58:331–337.
8. Itoyama Y, Uremura S, Ushio Y, et al. Natural course of unoperated intracranial arteriovenous malformations: study of 50 cases. *J Neurosurg* 1989;71:805–809.
9. Kader A, Young WL, Pile-Spellman J, et al. The influence of hemodynamic and anatomic factors on hemorrhage from arteriovenous malformations. *Neurosurgery* 1994;34:801–808.
10. Ondra SL, Troupp H, George ED, Schwab K. The natural history of symptomatic arteriovenous malformations of the brain: a 24-year follow-up assessment. *J Neurosurg* 1990;73:387–391.
11. Pollock BE, Flickinger JC, Lunsford LD, et al. Factors that predict the bleeding risk of cerebral arteriovenous malformations. *Stroke* 1996;27:1–6.
12. Spetzler RF, Hargraves RW, McCormick PW, et al. Relationship of perfusion pressure and size to the risk of hemorrhage from arteriovenous malformations. *J Neurosurg* 1992;76:918–923.
13. Awad IA, Little JR, Akrawi WP, Ahl J. Intracranial dural arteriovenous malformations: factors predisposing to an aggressive neurological course. *J Neurosurg* 1990;72:839–850.
14. Borden JA, Wu JK, Shucart WA. A proposed classification for spinal and cranial dural arteriovenous fistulous malformations and implications for treatment. *J Neurosurg* 1995; 82:166–179.
15. Brown RD, Wiebers DO, Nichols DA. Intracranial dural arteriovenous fistulae: angiographic predictors of intracranial hemorrhage and clinical outcome in nonsurgical patients. *J Neurosurg* 1994;81:531–538.
16. Lewis AI, Tomsick TA, Tew JM Jr. Management of tentorial arteriovenous malformations: transarterial embolization combined with stereotactic radiosurgery or surgery. *J Neurosurg* 1994;81:851–859.
17. Link MJ, Coffey RJ, Nichols DA, Gorman DA. The role of radiosurgery and particulate embolization in the treatment of arteriovenous fistulas. *J Neurosurg* 1996;84:804–809.
18. Miyasaka Y, Yada K, Ohwada T, et al. An analysis of the venous drainage system as a factor in the hemorrhage from arteriovenous malformations. *J Neurosurg* 1992;76:239–243.
19. Marks MP, Lane B, Steinberg GK, Chang PJ. Hemorrhage in intracranial arteriovenous malformations: angiographic determinants. *Radiology* 1990;176:807–813.
20. Marks MP, Lane B, Steinberg GK, Snipes GJ. Intranidal aneurysms in cerebral arteriovenous malformations: evaluation and endovascular treatment. *Radiology* 1992;183:355–360.
21. Turjman F, Massoud TF, Vinuela F, et al. Aneurysms related to cerebral arteriovenous malformations: superselective angiographic assessment in 58 patients. *AJNR* 1994;15:1601–1605.
22. Kondziolka D, McLaughlin MR, Kestle JRW. Simple risk predictions for arteriovenous malformation hemorrhage. *Neurosurgery* 1995;37:851–855.
23. Hamilton MG, Spetzler RF. The prospective application of a grading system for arteriovenous malformations. *Neurosurgery* 1994;34:2–7.
24. Heros RC, Korosue K, Diebold PM. Surgical excision of cerebral arteriovenous malformations: late results. *Neurosurgery* 1990;26:570–578.
25. Blatt DL, Friedman WA, Bova FJ. Modifications based on computed tomographic imaging in planning the radiosurgical treatment of arteriovenous malformations. *Neurosurgery* 1993;33:588–596.
26. Kondziolka D, Lunsford LD, Kanal E, Talagala L. Stereotactic magnetic resonance angiography for targeting in arteriovenous malformation radiosurgery. *Neurosurgery* 1994;35:585–591.
27. Petereit D, Mehta M, Turski P, et al. Treatment of arteriovenous malformations with stereotactic radiosurgery employing both magnetic resonance angiography and standard angiography as a database. *Int J Radiat Oncol Biol Phys* 1993;25:309–313.
28. Flickinger JC. An integrated logistic formula and prediction of complications from radiosurgery. *Int J Radiat Oncol Biol Phys* 1989;17:879–885.
29. Flickinger JC, Kondziolka D, Pollock BE, et al. Complications from arteriovenous malformation radiosurgery: multivariate analysis and risk modeling. *Int J Radiat Oncol Biol Phys* 1997;38:485–490.
30. Flickinger JC, Lunsford LD, Kondziolka D, et al. Radiosurgery and brain tolerance: an analysis of neurodiagnostic imaging changes after Gamma knife radiosurgery for arteriovenous malformations. *Int J Radiat Oncol Biol Phys* 1992;23:19–26.
31. Pollock BE, Kondziolka D, Flickinger JC, et al. Magnetic resonance imaging: an accurate method to evaluate arteriovenous malformations after stereotactic radiosurgery. *J Neurosurg* 1996;85:1044–1049.
32. Colombo F, Pozza F, Chierego G, et al. Linear accelerator radiosurgery of cerebral arteriovenous malformations: an update. *Neurosurgery* 1994;34:14–21.
33. Engenhart R, Wowra B, Debrus J, et al. The role of high-dose, single-fraction irradiation in small and large intracranial arteriovenous malformations. *Int J Radiat Oncol Biol Phys* 1994;30:521–529.
34. Friedman WA, Bova FJ, Mendenhall WM. Linear accelerator radiosurgery for arteriovenous malformations: the relationship of size to outcome. *J Neurosurg* 1995;82:180–189.
35. Kjellberg RN, Hanamura T, Davis KR, et al. Bragg-peak proton-beam therapy for arteriovenous malformations of the brain. *N Engl J Med* 1983;309:269–274.
36. Lawton MT, Hamilton MG, Spetzler RF. Multimodality treatment of deep arteriovenous malformations: thalamus, basal ganglia, and brain stem. *Neurosurgery* 1995;37:29–36.
37. Lunsford LD, Kondziolka D, Flickinger JC, et al. Stereotactic radiosurgery for arteriovenous malformations of the brain. *J Neurosurg* 1991;75:512–524.
38. Pollock BE, Flickinger JC, Lunsford LD, et al. The Pittsburgh AVM Radiosurgery (PAR) grading scale. *Radiosurgery* (in press).
39. Steinberg GK, Fabrikant JI, Marks MP, et al. Stereotactic

heavy-charged-particle Bragg-peak radiation for intracranial arteriovenous malformations. *N Engl J Med* 1990;323:96–101.

40. Steiner L, Lindquist C, Adler JR, et al. Clinical outcome of radiosurgery for cerebral arteriovenous malformations. *J Neurosurg* 1992;77:1–8.

41. Yamamoto Y, Coffey RJ, Nichols DA, Shaw EG. Interim report on the radiosurgical treatment of cerebral arteriovenous malformations. The influence of size, dose, time, and technical factors on obliteration rate. *J Neurosurg* 1995;83:832–837.

42. Steiner L, Prasad D, Lindquist C, et al. Gamma knife surgery in vascular lesions and tumors. In Schmidek HH, Sweet WH (eds): Operative Neurosurgical Techniques: Indications, Methods, and Results. Philadelphia: WB Saunders, 1995, pp 667–694.

43. Flickinger JC, Pollock BE, Kondziolka D, Lunsford LD. A dose-response analysis of arteriovenous malformation obliteration after radiosurgery. *Int J Radiat Oncol Biol Phys* 1996;36:873–879.

44. Karlsson B, Lindquist C, Steiner L. Effect of Gamma knife surgery on the risk of rupture prior to AVM obliteration. *Minim Invasive Neurosurg* 1996;39:21–27.

45. Kondziolka D, Lunsford LD, Flickinger JC. Stereotactic radiosurgery in children and adolescents. *Pediatr Neurosurg* 1991;16:219–221.

46. Pollock BE, Flickinger JC, Lunsford LD, et al. Hemorrhage risk after stereotactic radiosurgery of cerebral arteriovenous malformations. *Neurosurgery* 1996;38:652–661.

47. Friedman WA, Blatt DL, Bova FJ, et al. The risk of hemorrhage after radiosurgery for arteriovenous malformations. *J Neurosurg* 1996;84:912–919.

48. Yamamoto M, Jimbo M, Hara M, et al. Gamma knife radiosurgery for arteriovenous malformations: long-term follow-up results focusing on complications occurring more than 5 years after irradiation. *Neurosurgery* 1996;38:906–914.

49. Pollock BE, Lunsford LD, Kondziolka D, et al. Patient outcomes after stereotactic radiosurgery for "operable" arteriovenous malformations. *Neurosurgery* 1994;35:1–8.

50. Gerszten PC, Adelson PD, Kondziolka D, et al. Seizure outcome in children treated for arteriovenous malformations using Gamma knife radiosurgery. *Pediatr Neurosurg* 1996;24:139–144.

51. Huang C, Somaza S, Lunsford LD, et al. Radiosurgery in the management of epilepsy associated with arteriovenous malformations. In Kondziolka D (ed): Radiosurgery 1995. Basel: Karger, 1996, pp 195–200.

52. Garretson HD. Intracranial arteriovenous malformations. In Wilkins RH, Rengachary SS (eds): Neurosurgery. New York: McGraw-Hill, 1985, pp 1448–1458.

53. Luessenhop AJ, Gennarelli TA. Anatomical grading of supratentorial arteriovenous malformations for determining operability. *Neurosurgery* 1977;1:30–35.

54. Shi Y, Chen X. A proposed scheme for grading intracranial arteriovenous malformations. *J Neurosurg* 1986;65:484–489.

55. Spetzler RF, Martin NA. A proposed grading system for arteriovenous malformations. *J Neurosurg* 1986;65:476–483.

56. Deruty R, Pelissou-Guyotat I, Amat D, et al. Multidisciplinary treatment of cerebral arteriovenous malformations. *Neurol Res* 1995;17:169–177.

57. Gobin YP, Laurent A, Merienne L, et al. Treatment of brain arteriovenous malformations by embolization and radiosurgery. *J Neurosurg* 1996;85:19–28.

58. Hurst RW, Berenstein A, Kupersmith MJ, et al. Deep central arteriovenous malformations of the brain: the role of endovascular treatment. *J Neurosurg* 1995;82:190–195.

59. Mathis JA, Barr JD, Horton JA, et al. The efficacy of particulate embolization combined with stereotactic radiosurgery for treatment of large arteriovenous malformations of the brain. *AJNR* 1995;16:299–306.

60. Wikholm G, Lundqvist C, Svendsen P. Embolization of cerebral arteriovenous malformations: Part I. Technique, morphology, and complications. *Neurosurgery* 1996;39:448–459.

61. Wikholm G, Lundqvist C, Svendsen P. Embolization of cerebral arteriovenous malformations: Part II. Aspects of complications and late outcome. *Neurosurgery* 1996;39:460–469.

62. Pollock BE, Kondziolka D, Lunsford LD, et al. Repeat stereotactic radiosurgery of arteriovenous malformations: factors associated with incomplete obliteration. *Neurosurgery* 1996;38:318–324.

63. Debrun G, Vinuela FV, Fox AJ, Drake CG. Embolization of cerebral arteriovenous malformations with bucrylate: experience in 46 cases. *J Neurosurg* 1982;56:615–627.

64. Fournier D, TerBrugge KG, Willinsky R, et al. Endovascular treatment of intracerebral arteriovenous malformations: experience in 49 cases. *J Neurosurg* 1991;75:228–233.

65. Germano IM, Davis RL, Wilson CB, Hieshima GB. Histopathological follow-up study of 66 cerebral arteriovenous malformations after therapeutic embolization with polyvinyl alcohol. *J Neurosurg* 1992;76:607–614.

66. Francel PC, Steiner L, Steiner M, Lindquist C. Repeat radiosurgical treatment in arteriovenous malformations following unsatisfactory results of initial high-dose radiation (abstr). *J Neurosurg* 1991;74:351A.

67. Chandler HC Jr, Friedman WA. Successful radiosurgical treatment of a dural arteriovenous malformation: case report. *Neurosurgery* 1993;33:139–142.

ADDITIONAL READINGS

Alexander E III, Loeffler JS. Radiosurgery using a modified linear accelerator. *Neurosurg Clin* 1992;3:167–190.

Fabrikant JI, Levy RP, Steinberg GK, et al. Charged-particle radiosurgery for intracranial vascular malformations. *Neurosurg Clin* 1992;3:99–1139.

Flickinger JC, Schell MC, Larson DA. Estimation of complications for linear accelerator radiosurgery with the integrated logistic formula. *Int J Radiat Oncol Biol Phys* 1990;19:143–148.

Friedman WA, Bova FJ. Linear accelerator radiosurgery for arteriovenous malformations. *J Neurosurg* 1992;77:832–841.

Friedman WA, Bova FJ, Spiegelmann R. Linear accelerator radiosurgery at the University of Florida. *Neurosurg Clin* 1992;3:141–166.

Lunsford LD, Kondziolka D, Bissonette DJ, et al. Stereotactic radiosurgery of brain vascular malformations. *Neurosurg Clin* 1992;3:79–98.

Marks MP, Lane B, Steinberg GK, et al. Endovascular treatment of cerebral arteriovenous malformations following radiosurgery. *AJNR* 1993;14:397–403.

Phillips MH, Frankel KA, Lyman JT, et al. Comparison of different radiation types and irradiation geometries in stereotactic radiosurgery. *Int J Radiat Oncol Biol Phys* 1990;18:211–220.

Redekop GJ, Elisevich KV, Gaspar LE, et al. Conventional radiation therapy of intracranial arteriovenous malformations: long-term results. *J Neurosurg* 1993;78:413–422.

Yasanuga T, Takada C, Uozumi H, et al. Radiotherapy of spontaneous carotid-cavernous sinus fistulas. *Int J Radiat Oncol Biol Phys* 1987;13:1909–1913.

Intracranial Aneurysms: General Considerations

J.J. Connors III / J.C. Wojak

Intracranial aneurysms do not have a single cause. They are not truly congenital; rather, there are congenital disorders that affect vessel wall architecture and predispose to aneurysm formation. The more common causes of intracranial aneurysms include vessel degeneration from hematologic factors (the standard aneurysm at a bifurcation point where there is turbulent flow), atherosclerosis, high-flow states, and underlying vascular disorders. Other causes include trauma, infection (mycotic aneurysms), drug abuse (producing hemodynamic alteration and vasculitis), and neoplastic invasion. Disorders associated with an increased incidence of aneurysms include hypertension, aortic coarctation, adult polycystic kidney disease, fibromuscular dysplasia, connective tissue disorders (e.g., Marfan syndrome, Ehlers-Danlos syndrome), and moyamoya disease.[1] The relative incidence of aneurysms in various locations is given in Table 24–1.[1]

INCIDENCE AND NATURAL HISTORY

The incidence of intracranial aneurysms in the general population has been estimated to be between 1.5% and 8%.[2, 3] This percentage yields a huge number of patients with this disorder. The peak age for rupture is 40 to 70 years. The mean age of occurrence of fatal hemorrhage is 50.2 years.[4] Aneurysms less than 5 mm in diameter rarely bleed, whereas those 6 to 10 mm in diameter often present with a bleed.[5] Although giant aneurysms frequently simply grow, they also can bleed. Multiple aneurysms are present in 20% of patients. Females are affected more often than males (56% compared with 44%),[6] and aneurysms are rarely found in children. Giant aneurysms may not bleed as often as smaller aneurysms, but their long-term outlook is grim. In the posterior fossa

(typically basilar tip), the mortality rate for giant aneurysms approaches 100% at 5 years, whereas in the anterior circulation, the morbidity and mortality rates for giant aneurysms approach 80%.

Patients with aneurysms that are more distal in the intracranial vasculature (i.e., arising from the middle cerebral artery, the anterior cerebral artery, or the anterior communicating artery) have a greater chance of survival at the time of rupture (chance of death, 49% to 55%) than do those patients who have aneurysms on the internal carotid artery or arising in the posterior circulation (chance of death, 69% to 79%).

A national cooperative study of patients with acute subarachnoid hemorrhage secondary to aneurysm rupture revealed a 36.2% mortality rate and an additional 17.9% morbidity rate (serious neurologic sequelae); *only 46% of patients had a favorable outcome at 90 days.*[7] Ultimately, two thirds of patients succumb to their disease or are permanently disabled. Twenty percent of deaths occurred within 24 hours, 40% within the first week, and 66% within the first 3 weeks. Rebleeding reached a peak on day 7 at 4%.

These statistics do not directly address the morbidity and mortality associated with surgery for this condition. About one third of patients experience symptoms of postoperative vasospasm, which can complicate their recovery (although the treatment of this complication is improving; see Chapter 51). Vasospasm is defined as arterial narrowing of at least 50% and is demonstrated angiographically in up to 70% of posthemorrhage patients; only one third of patients have *symptomatic* vasospasm.

The classification proposed by Hunt and Hess[8] is used routinely to grade patients with acute aneurysmal subarachnoid hemorrhage (Table 24–2). This classification is used to determine the timing of intervention; whether surgical or endovascular, outcome is closely related to grade. This classification is also used in the assessment of new treatments for subarachnoid hemorrhage–associated vasospasm.

In 50% to 70% of patients, intracranial hemorrhage is caused by a ruptured aneurysm. About 15% of patients with subarachnoid hemorrhage die before reaching a hospital. Rebleeding occurs in 20% of the remainder within 2 weeks, in 30% within 1 month, and in 40% by 6 months. In addition, rebleeding is associated with a mortality rate of more than 40%. Most aneurysms rupture when they are 5 to 15 mm in diameter, with an average diameter of 10 mm.

Aneurysms do not stop bleeding because of some

T A B L E 2 4 - 1 Relative Incidence of Intracranial Aneurysms by Location

Location	Incidence (%)
Anterior communicating artery	30–35
Internal carotid artery or posterior communicating artery	30–35
Middle cerebral artery bifurcation	20
Posterior fossa	2–10
Distal basilar	5
Miscellaneous sites distal to circle of Willis	1–3

T A B L E 2 4 - 2 The Hunt and Hess Grading System for Subarachnoid Hemorrhage

Grade	Clinical Features
I	No symptoms or minimal headache and slight nuchal rigidity
II	Moderate to severe headache, nuchal rigidity, and no neurologic deficit other than cranial nerve palsy
III	Drowsiness, confusion, or a mild focal neurologic deficit
IV	Stupor, moderate to severe hemiparesis, possible decerebrate rigidity, and vegetative disturbances
V	Deep coma, decerebrate rigidity, and moribund appearance

From Hunt WE, Hess RM. Surgical risk as related to time of intervention in the repair of intracranial aneurysms. *J Neurosurg* 1968;28:14–20.

magical "cork." During a bleed, the intracranial pressure is raised to levels approaching systolic pressure, thus slowing flow secondary to tamponade. This causes decreased cerebral perfusion pressure and therefore decreased cerebral blood flow. This then allows a platelet plug to form, which during the next few hours is reinforced with fibrin.

The ideal solution for the treatment of an intracranial aneurysm is exclusion of this abnormality from the circulation. The gold standard for this therapy is open neurosurgical clipping of the neck of the aneurysm.

IMAGING

The computed tomography (CT) scan is positive in up to 90% of patients with intracranial aneurysm hemorrhages when performed within 1 day; it also yields diagnostic clues in about half of cases (Table 24–3).

Computed tomography can also yield important prognostic information. The grading system developed by Fisher et al. is based on retrospective and prospective studies demonstrating that the amount and location of intracranial blood in patients with aneurysmal bleeds correlated very strongly with the incidence, severity, and location of subsequent vasospasm.[9, 10] This grading system is summarized in Table 51–1 in Chapter 51.

For detection of an unruptured aneurysm or for screening purposes, high-resolution computed tomography with contrast enhancement accurately demonstrates most large aneurysms, but misses up to one third of all aneurysms less than 6 mm in diameter. High-resolution magnetic resonance angiography (MRA) can detect aneurysms as small as 3 to 4 mm. MRA has been shown to be suboptimal because of poor flow characteristics within aneurysms, rendering visualization dependent on flow characteristics rather than the size of the aneurysm. Spiral CT angiography, in contrast, is not dependent on flow *rate,* but rather on the presence or absence of nonclot-

ted blood (and thus contrast); it is also not susceptible to artifact due to pulsation. Three-dimensional reconstructions can be performed with either modality. Screening for unruptured aneurysms is indicated in a family with a history of aneurysms, but the choice of MRA, CT angiography, or traditional angiography should be made by the patient and attending physician.

HISTORY OF ENDOVASCULAR THERAPY

Before direct attack of aneurysms became popular, purposeful parent vessel occlusion was performed, in many cases with excellent results.[11, 12] This was performed by occluding the internal carotid artery with a detachable balloon just proximal to the aneurysm or by occluding *both* vertebral arteries if the aneurysm was in the posterior fossa. Test occlusions performed before the occlusion were of the clinical type. This procedure appeared to work well, and in certain circumstances is still considered a viable option.

The advantage of balloon occlusion over Selverstone clamping in cases of carotid sacrifice is the reduction in the dead space within the carotid artery above the clamp (see Chapters 34 and 35). This dead space may result in a large volume of thrombus in the long segment of stagnant vessel; this thrombus could be mashed cephalad from simple head motion. Therefore, embolic occlusion of an intracranial vessel is the primary problem with proximal ligation of the internal carotid artery, not flow dependent ischemia.[13–17]

In years past, numerous different approaches were tried for direct endovascular therapy of intracranial aneurysms. The most popular early attempts at treatment of intracranial aneurysms involved the use of detachable balloons within the aneurysm.[18–20] Em-

T A B L E 2 4 - 3 Computed Tomography Findings Associated with Aneurysm Location

Site of Aneurysm	Usual Findings
Middle cerebral artery	Sylvian fissure clot Basal ganglia hematoma Frontal or temporal lobe clot
Anterior communicating artery	Interhemispheric clot Paramedian frontal lobe clot Lateral or third ventricular blood
Posterior communicating artery	Suprasellar cistern clot Basilar cistern blood Infratemporal hematoma
Basilar tip	Third ventricular blood Basilar cistern blood
Posterior inferior cerebellar artery	Isolated fourth ventricular blood Cerebellopontine angle blood Vermian clot

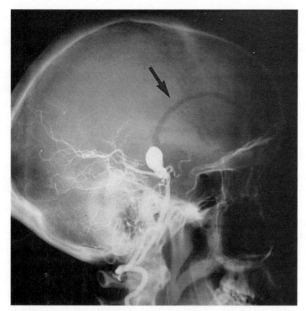

Figure 24-1 Case 1. A 59-year-old woman with a long history of worsening motor and sensory symptoms and a growing basilar tip aneurysm. She had been refused surgery by several neurosurgeons and had undergone two attempted surgical repairs (note the craniotomy, *arrow*). She was referred for a last-ditch attempt at treatment of the aneurysm by the (then) new detachable balloon method. Unfortunately, owing to her anatomy, the nonsteerable balloon could not be steered into the aneurysm (it kept going out into the left posterior cerebral artery). In desperation, the use of platinum microcoils was suggested to the neurosurgeon.

Case 1 continues

bolic coils were initially described by Hilal and colleagues.[21] More recently, the Guglielmi detachable coil (GDC) has been approved by the Food and Drug Administration.[22, 23] Polymerizing and other agents have also been employed for attempts at occlusion of aneurysms, either in practice or experimentally.[24] In Japan, EVAL, a form of hydrogel (see Chapter 1), has been used for aneurysm filling; another form of hydrogel has been used to fill an aneurysmal sac in experimental tubing.

There is considerable evidence that successful results have been achieved using detachable balloons with minimal risk and patient discomfort. Fox and colleagues[12] reported in 1987 on 68 patients with unclippable aneurysms treated by proximal carotid artery occlusion by means of detachable balloons. There was only a 13.2% incidence of delayed ischemia and only one case of permanent stroke. Other series have shown results in this same range, which is excellent for unclippable aneurysms.

Direct occlusion of aneurysms by detachable balloons with preservation of the parent vessel and without rupture of the aneurysm has a much worse track record. Results indicate a combined morbidity and mortality rate of 25% to 30%—not a stellar treatment modality. The problem with this therapy is that if the balloon is even a little too small, it will rattle around in the sac and the aneurysm will not be cured. If the balloon is slightly too big, it can either rupture the aneurysm or protrude into the vessel

lumen, with subsequent potential occlusion. Therefore, detachable balloons are no longer used for the treatment of aneurysms except for parent vessel occlusion.

CURRENT ENDOVASCULAR THERAPIES

Ongoing investigation is aimed primarily at platinum coil use but also at using other materials to fill the aneurysmal lumen.

Balloons may be a quick and easy means to fill a space, but as stated earlier, it is practically impossible to inflate a balloon to the exact size needed to fill the aneurysm. An incorrect amount of filling can have a worthless result or cause a catastrophe.

Coil embolization of aneurysms has been performed for many years. The original use involved the placement of a microcatheter within the aneurysm and then placement of coils within this volume by shoving them out the end of the catheter. This can be nerve-racking when the practitioner realizes that the tip of the microcatheter can easily become displaced in the middle of the coil extrusion process. We found that the early treatment of aneurysms by coil embolization (using normal, "push-them-out-the-end," nonretrievable coils) can be an emotionally stimulating event (Case 1, Figs. 24–1 and 24–2).

When using the GDC technique of coil embolization of aneurysms, the catheter should be placed accurately within the aneurysm in a stable location. The practitioner needs to have an extremely good

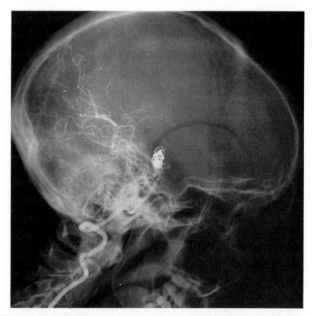

Figure 24-2 Follow-up image after placement of 33 platinum flower coils (Target Therapeutics), not GDC (which had not been invented yet). The aneurysm actually thrombosed but later redeveloped a neck owing to insufficient density of the coiling and subsequent packing of the coils. The patient's symptoms improved for a time, but as the aneurysm regrew, recoiling was necessary. The patient again did well, but the coils again packed and the aneurysm recurred. Further coil placement was undertaken, with a satisfactory result. She was doing well until lost to follow-up 3 years later.

feel for the resistance to pushing of the coil and should understand the tendency for recoil that a microcatheter might have under these circumstances. This technique is difficult to learn, difficult to practice in a laboratory, and cannot be explained simply. A combination of factors are involved—resistance to the shove of the wire, tension (pressure) on the microcatheter, visual registration of the adaptability and malleability of the coil within the vessel lumen, and cognitive understanding of the total amount of material that can be expected to fit within the designated space. See Chapter 25 for a thorough description of this procedure.

Proximal Parent Vessel Occlusion

Proximal parent vessel occlusion has been applied for many years to various aneurysms with some excellent results. The actual technique has been nearly perfected. A full discussion of this technique is given in Chapters 35 and 36. This therapy has been shown to be of positive benefit in some types of aneurysms, of questionable benefit in other types, and of no benefit in still other types.

Proximal parent vessel occlusion can be the treatment of choice for certain conditions. Previous therapeutic choices have centered on the exact means to occlude the vessel, but these disagreements appear to be disappearing. The occlusion can be made in the common carotid artery or the internal carotid artery, rapidly or slowly (Selverstone clamp), by means of a balloon, coils, or clamp, with or without distal trapping of the aneurysm, and with or without preoperative extracranial-intracranial artery bypass.

Currently, with adequate preocclusion testing and meticulous technique for occlusion (described in Chapters 35 and 36), the endovascular approach is the preferred method for permanent proximal occlusion of a parent vessel.

Preocclusion Testing

Preocclusion testing is mandatory for all carotid sacrifices. The technique of testing is described in Chapter 34.

For sacrifice of the vertebral artery the technique of testing is still hemodynamic but if there is an observed adequate contralateral vertebral artery, the chance of successful permanent occlusion of the vertebral artery in question is nearly 100%. Occlusion of the basilar artery by a surgical ligature is also possible, and this also can be tested. This can be done with the Drake maneuver (see "Basilar Tip Berry Aneurysms" below).

Allcock Maneuver

Injection of the vertebral artery while occluding each carotid artery in turn reveals the size of the posterior communicating artery. If the posterior communicating arteries are greater than 1 mm in diameter, blood supply to the posterior fossa is probably adequate for subsequent posterior fossa isolation by means of occlusion of supply from the vertebral arteries.

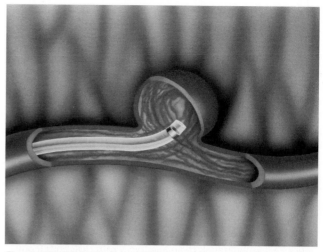

Figure 24-3 Embolization of an aneurysm with GDC coils. This illustration demonstrates the proper positioning of the TRACKER catheter within the neck of an aneurysm. Note that the tip of the catheter has been steam-shaped in a curve to facilitate this positioning. The catheter is not touching the walls of the aneurysm.

Guglielmi Detachable Coils

Platinum microcoils are the standard endovascular material used for aneurysm occlusion. The GDC is a platinum coil soldered to the end of an insulated stainless steel introducing guidewire, allowing repositioning of the coil as needed to achieve the optimal placement (Figs. 24–3 to 24–5). A low-voltage current employs electrolysis to detach the coil (dissolve the solder) when the coil is accurately positioned. This device is commercially available. GDC coils are not fibered and therefore are not as thrombogenic as typical fibered coils, but the ability to reposition these coils is a tremendous advantage to their use.

When coils were initially used for treatment of aneurysms, there was high hope for their complete

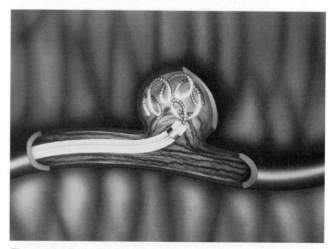

Figure 24-4 Embolization of an aneurysm with GDC coils (continued). The initial coil is being placed within the aneurysm. Ideally, there should be several loops of the coil across the neck of the aneurysm and it should form a framework for the placement of additional coils to occlude the aneurysm.

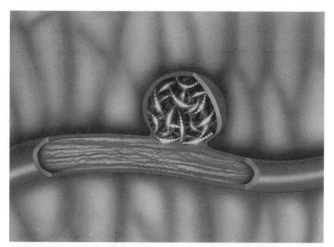

Figure 24-5 Embolization of an aneurysm with GDC coils (continued). After the placement of several additional coils, there is solid filling of the aneurysm. The dome has been adequately filled, as has the neck. No loops or ends of coils are protruding into the parent vessel to serve as a source of emboli.

trated one of the first examples of "coil packing" and reopening of the neck of the aneurysm. This initial coil packing was treated by additional placement of coils, which also were packed into the dome of the aneurysm, again exposing the neck. Another case of coil packing with recanalization of the aneurysm is shown in Figures 24–6 to 24–16.

This case was an early example of one problem associated with coil use for aneurysms. Other problems are continued growth of the neck or aneurysm around the coil mass, inability to occlude the neck of the aneurysm completely, perforation of the aneurysm during coil placement, and potential occlusion or compromise of the parent vessel. The lack of a truly effective permanent therapy mandates further research into the endovascular treatment of aneurysms.

Benefits of GDC Use

The inability of endovascular therapy to provide a permanent cure for this disease raises the question of what the role is of GDCs or other coils in the treatment of aneurysms. In fact, coils accomplish certain tasks, and GDCs perform far better than other available coils and embolic agents. They provide a permanent cure in many cases. In addition, it

success. Unfortunately, this has not been the case. One of the earlier cases of coil embolization of an aneurysm (basilar tip) in the United States was performed in 1989,[25] and the mid-term follow-up illus-

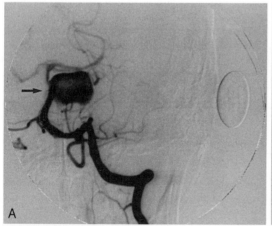
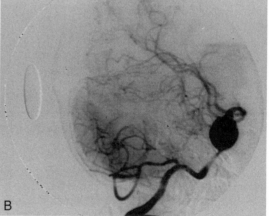

Figure 24-6 Case 2. *A* and *B*, A 34-year-old woman presented to the emergency room with a massive intracranial bleed. Within minutes she had become comatose. After a period of several days, she awakened and improved to the point of generalized weakness with a depressed state of consciousness.

A left vertebral angiogram reveals a large lobulated aneurysm arising from the midbasilar artery. Note the characteristic kink of the vessel at the point of aneurysm formation, typical for midshaft aneurysms. This kink is due to the mechanism of formation of these aneurysms. The side wall of the vessel where the aneurysm arises has a failure of wall strength (thought to be due to a breakdown in elastin); this leads to stretching of the wall as the aneurysm forms, making this side of the vessel longer than the other and thus causing bowing. At this point the aneurysm grows until it ruptures.

The visible chamber, which is filling with contrast, can be either entirely a true aneurysm or an aneurysm with some component of pseudoaneurysm (i.e., an extraluminal clot with a hole in it).

The right side of the vessel at the level of the aneurysm *(arrow)* may have a viable vessel wall, but there is no telling how much of the remainder of the vessel at this point is redeemable. Surgical repair may necessitate transection of the vessel with reanastomosis of the proximal and distal portions; alternatively, use of a clip might make it possible to reconstruct the side wall where the aneurysm is.

Reports have been made of coiling an aneurysm such as this with preservation of the lumen; there is the possibility of at least some portion of a coil protruding into the lumen of the vessel with potential constant downstream embolization or incomplete occlusion of the aneurysm lumen. Utilizing the remodeling technique with GDC, it might be possible to preserve the lumen and treat this aneurysm.

Note the incomplete filling of the posterior cerebral vessels. This might have been due to the early stage of the injection, but it was shown to be due to the presence of large posterior communicating arteries.

Case 2 continues

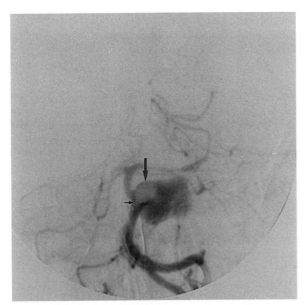

Figure 24-7 Endovascular therapy was recommended by the attending neurosurgeons. In the knowledge that coil embolization would probably occlude the basilar artery, a test occlusion was first performed.

After a thorough cerebral angiogram confirmed communication between the anterior and posterior circulations via adequately sized posterior communicating arteries, it was deemed feasible to attempt a test occlusion of the midbasilar artery. This was thought to be necessary if a realistic attempt at occlusion of the aneurysm was to be made from an endovascular approach. Although it would be wonderful to "occlude" the aneurysm with preservation of the parent vessel, it was thought that this result could not be counted on.

The patient was fully anticoagulated. An Endeavor balloon catheter (formerly called the NDSB, ITC/Target Therapeutics) was advanced into the aneurysm and inflated *(large arrow)*. Contrast injection reveals the balloon to be within the aneurysmal sac. Note the characteristic "stretching" appearance of the balloon on the end of the catheter *(small arrow)*. This is somewhat disturbing when first seen, but it always occurs, and this is a lesson that has to be learned as far as the strength of silicone is concerned.

The use of coils to protect the aneurysm from further immediate hemorrhage appears to be relatively safe and effective and ultimately may be one of the best uses for this device.

Intermediate Results of GDC Embolization

Overall Outcome

Malisch and colleagues have published the results of a prospective analysis of the first 100 patients with aneurysms treated by GDC embolization at UCLA.[27] These patients had a total of 104 aneurysms (4 were found incidentally during work-up of the presenting aneurysm). Although six patients were lost to follow-up, they were able to collect 2- to 6-year follow-up information on 94 patients.

Of these 94 patients, 6 died of unrelated causes. Another seven died from their initial hemorrhage (all Hunt and Hess grade IV or V). Twenty patients underwent subsequent surgical treatment or endovascular procedures (clipping or parent vessel occlu-

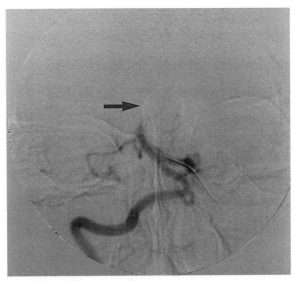

Figure 24-8 The inflated Endeavor has been withdrawn to the point that it fits snugly against the inlet side of the aneurysm *(arrow)*. The balloon should *not* be inflated to actually fill the aneurysm to occlude the vessel, or occlude the flow on the *downstream* side of the aneurysm.

Inflating the balloon to the point of filling the vessel could rupture the aneurysm: not a good thing. Occluding the vessel on the downstream side of the aneurysm could also rupture the aneurysm by *increasing the intraluminal pressure* within the aneurysm due to pulse pressure, and could yield a false result during test occlusion by allowing any perforators arising from *within the aneurysm* to continue to fill (they will be occluded when the aneurysm is embolized with coils).

Consider this problem, however. There are known pontine perforators arising all along the basilar artery; some of these may be involved in the aneurysmal section. Surgery (i.e., clipping) would exclude these from the circulation, just as coil occlusion would. If either of these would cause loss of a vital pontine perforator, should therapy of any kind be performed? To confuse the problem even more, if the perforator arose on the side of the vessel that is not diseased, could it be saved?

These are very difficult issues.

The patient tolerated occlusion of the basilar artery, which was maintained for 15 minutes.

Case 2 continues

is thought that they may provide a degree of protection from rebleeding, allowing a period of recovery for the patient until surgery can be performed. These coils can sometimes complicate surgical clipping, but this appears to be of only minor consequence.

Data indicate that the carotid ophthalmic and basilar tip aneurysms are the most frequently treated[26]; the most common reason for coil occlusion is the anticipated difficulty of surgery. Small aneurysms with small necks yield the best results, whereas large aneurysms with large necks have the worst results.

Parent vessel occlusion and cerebral embolization are the most common complications. Parent vessel occlusion occurs in about 1% to 3% of cases, hence the need for a test occlusion. Distal arterial embolization occurs subclinically in a significant percentage (about 30%) of cases, but hard data are lacking concerning symptomatic embolization. Recanalization occurs in about 30% of giant aneurysms.[26] An additional potential complication is that of aneurysm perforation. This appears to be relatively rare, occurring in less than 3% of cases.

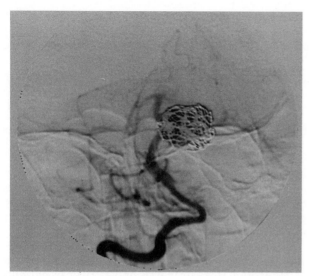

Figure 24-9 After partial packing of the aneurysm with complex helical coils, there is still significant filling of the lumen (indeed, almost complete!). More coil packing is necessary. Intracranial flow should not have been allowed through this coil mass; proximal flow arrest should have been used.

Case 2 continues

sion) for incomplete thrombosis of the aneurysm, mass effect, coil herniation into the parent vessel, or coil migration. These patients were excluded from most analyses, but none experienced aneurysmal hemorrhage following GDC embolization.

The remaining 61 patients were evaluated, using the Glasgow Outcome Score to classify outcome.[28] Forty-six patients (75%) had excellent outcomes, seven (11%) had good outcomes, three (5%) had fair outcomes, one (2%) had a poor outcome, and four (7%) were dead. Of the 57 surviving patients, 54 were neurologically improved or stable (89%) and 3 were worse (5%). Intraprocedural thromboembolic events were responsible for the cases of worsened neurologic status.

Outcome and Clinical Presentation

The effect of clinical presentation on outcome was analyzed. All patients except those dying of unrelated causes were considered. Of 20 patients with incidental aneurysms, 100% had excellent or good outcomes. The 32 patients presenting with Grade I or II subarachnoid hemorrhage had a 92% rate of excellent or good outcome. Of the three patients in this group with fair or poor outcome, one was a result of surgical misadventure and two were the result of thromboembolic procedural complications. There were seven patients with Grade III subarachnoid hemorrhage, of which six (86%) had excellent or good outcomes. The one patient with a fair result required surgery for mass effect produced by the coils.

On the other hand, of nine patients with Grade IV or V subarachnoid hemorrhage, seven died of their initial hemorrhage, one had a fair outcome, and one had a poor outcome.

Mass Effect. Nineteen patients available for follow-up presented with mass effect. Of these, 12 (63%) had an excellent or good outcome. The neurologic status was improved in ten (53%), unchanged in five (26%), and worsened in four (21%). All six patients with small or large aneurysms improved or were stable. Five patients with giant aneurysms were improved, four were stable, and four were worse. Subsequent surgery or endovascular therapy was required in 35% of these patients. Whereas six of nine patients presenting with mass effect on cranial nerves improved (67%), only four of ten patients presenting with mass effect on the brain did (40%).

Outcome and Aneurysm Size

The relationship of outcome to aneurysm size is summarized in Table 24–4. All four deaths in patients receiving definitive GDC therapy who were not Grade IV or V on presentation were in patients with inoperable, previously unruptured, partially thrombosed aneurysms that bled 12 to 20 months after coil embolization. Therefore, all aneurysm-related deaths in the series were in patients with giant aneurysms or Grade IV or V subarachnoid hemorrhage.

Lessons Learned

When these 100 patients were compared with the subsequent 100 patients treated at UCLA, the rate of complications with permanent sequelae declined from 2% to 1%, and the rate of complications with fatal outcomes dropped from 2% to 1%. Whereas 25% of the initial 100 patients had giant aneurysms, only 16% of the next 100 patients did. The number of patients requiring multiple embolization sessions declined from 27% to 10%, while the number of patients undergoing subsequent surgical or endovascular therapy declined from 20% to 6%.

GDC Embolization versus Surgery

Comparisons between the patients in this series with subarachnoid hemorrhage and a series of patients undergoing surgical therapy, such as the series presented in the International Cooperative Study on the Timing of Aneurysm Surgery,[29, 30] is difficult because of the differences in demographics. More posterior circulation aneurysms (66% to 8%), more giant aneurysms (11% to 2%), worse pretreatment neurologic status, longer clinical follow-up, and slightly longer interval between presentation and treatment were recorded in the GDC series. In addition, this series was accumulated a decade later than the surgical series, and the patients benefited from advances in the management of postsubarachnoid hemorrhage vasospasm. Therefore, the 68% rate of excellent or good outcome and the 22% rate of poor outcome or death in the surgical series cannot be compared directly with the GDC results. No matched, controlled series of surgically treated patients is available for comparison at this time.

An additional factor is that while patients undergoing GDC therapy were more likely to require multiple sessions than those undergoing surgical therapy, the morbidity of repeated embolization was 0%,

T A B L E   2 4 - 4   Relationship of Outcome to Aneurysm Size in Patients Undergoing GDC Embolization

Aneurysm Size	No. of Patients	Excellent or Good Outcome	Improved or Stable	Deaths	Post-GDC Hemorrhage
Small (<15 mm)	30	28 (93%)	29 (97%)	0	0
Large (15–25 mm)	21	20 (95%)	20 (95%)	0	1 (4%)
Giant (>25 mm)	10	5 (50%)	5 (50%)	4 (40%)	5 (50%)

From Malisch TW, Guglielmi G, Vinuela F, et al. Intracranial aneurysms treated with the Guglielmi detachable coil: Midterm clinical results in a consecutive series of 100 patients. *J Neurosurg* 1997;87:176–183.

whereas repeat surgery is felt to carry an increased risk of premature aneurysm rupture (25% vs. 14% in primary surgical cases) and approximately a 16% rate of moderate-to-severe disability.

Conclusions

GDC embolization of aneurysms is safe (2% overall morbidity, 0% if Grade IV and V patients were excluded). It is effective in small and large aneurysms, with only one post-GDC hemorrhage in a patient with a large aneurysm, and stabilization or improvement in symptoms of mass effect in six of six patients. Nearly all patients with small or large aneurysms had good or excellent outcomes and were improved or stable neurologically.

Giant aneurysms were more problematic. Good or excellent outcome was observed in 50% of patients, as was a stable or improved status, whereas 40% of patients died. Mass effect did not respond to treatment as well as in small or large aneurysms, and not infrequently worsened.

Patients presenting with Grade IV or V subarachnoid hemorrhage did poorly no matter what size the aneurysm was, even if treatment was effective (although there were seven deaths, there were no post-GDC hemorrhages).

MANAGEMENT OF THERAPEUTICALLY CHALLENGING ANEURYSMS

Fusiform Aneurysms

Tortuous elongation of diseased vascular walls is usually related to advanced atherosclerosis. These fusiform aneurysms can occur in any location but are most common in the distal vertebral artery, basilar artery, supraclinoid internal carotid artery, main trunk of the middle cerebral artery, and the P1 and P2 segments of the posterior cerebral arteries. A special type of fusiform aneurysm is a long serpentine aneurysm of the middle cerebral artery (usually a cortical branch).

Hemorrhage from these aneurysms is rare. Embolization and mass effect are the primary problems. Certain fusiform aneurysms are not treatable by any means, such as large fusiform aneurysms of the basilar artery.

Giant Aneurysms

General Considerations

The natural history of asymptomatic giant aneurysms is not known. It appears that their aggressiveness is related not only to their size but also to their

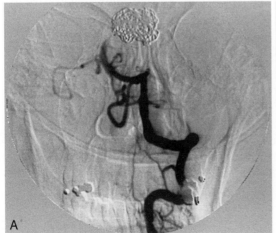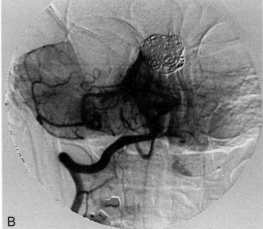

Figure 24-10 *A* and *B*, Left and right vertebral artery injections after occlusion of the aneurysm with multiple complex helical platinum coils. Total occlusion of the aneurysm has been obtained, and filling all the way to the coils is seen.

At this point, the patient became comatose. The initial worry was that the basilar tip had become occluded.

Case 2 continues

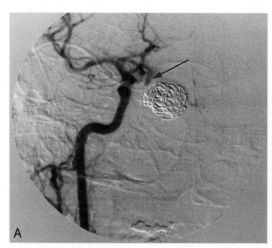
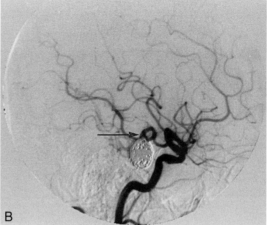

Figure 24-11 *A* and *B*, A right common carotid angiogram performed after coil occlusion of the basilar aneurysm reveals good filling of the posterior circulation and distal basilar artery *(long arrows)*. However, the patient remained comatose.

It was considered at this time that the goal of the therapy had been achieved, that no visible or correctable problem could be found, and that the clinical state was caused by the sudden thrombosis of the aneurysm, with subsequent swelling of the mass and compression of the brainstem.

Over a period of several days the patient recovered, and was discharged neurologically intact. She returned to work several weeks later.

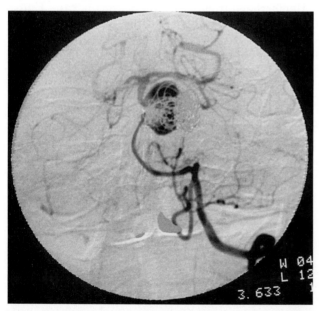

Figure 24-12 Over two years later, the patient began to experience unusual headaches. A repeat angiogram was performed, revealing recanalization of the aneurysm with some apparent enlargement of the base of the aneurysm. The apex of the aneurysm still appears to be thrombosed, with a dense mass of coils within it. Repeat treatment was thought to be indicated.

The recanalization of the basilar artery was a surprise. In a basilar tip aneurysm, where the force of blood flow is pounding on the coil mass, it is not a surprise that the base of the aneurysm should reopen and enlarge. However, at the end of a stagnant column, the reappearance of the lumen and enlargement of the aneurysm has to be blamed on clot retraction within the coil mass, with or without intrinsic fibrinolysis. Either way, the reappearance of the aneurysm caused much consternation.

Note the extreme angulation of the "kink" in the basilar artery now.

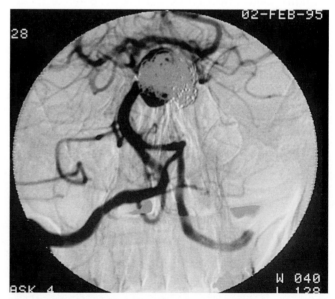

Figure 24-13 Partial filling of the neck has been performed. When coils are piled within the aneurysm, there is always the concern that old thrombus associated with the preexisting coils could be broken off. These are all complex helical coils (not GDC, unfortunately) and the mass they are forming is not filling the entire lumen of the aneurysm, complicating later placement. To further occlude the proximal lumen, a sharp curve in the catheter is necessary to reach this area. Again, flow arrest should be used, but this would require bilateral vertebral artery occlusion with a flow-control catheter not available at that time.

Case 2 continues

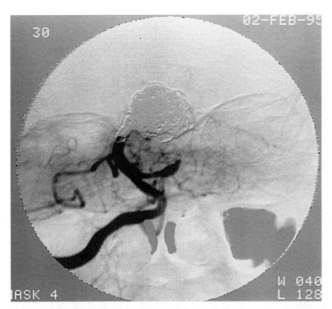

Figure 24-14 After final wadding of the coils in the aneurysm and reflux of the final Tornado coil (Cook Inc.) into the shaft of the basilar artery, the vertebral injection shows total occlusion of the basilar artery (again), with satisfactory packing of the aneurysm lumen with the coils.

These coils (non-GDC) are far more thrombogenic than GDCs and require less mass to achieve thrombosis and occlusion. In addition, the fibers are more inflammatory than the plain platinum of the GDC and more permanent.

location. In addition, the underlying health of the patient is a determinant of the prognosis of the aneurysm as well as the surgical outcome. These aneurysms are more likely to grow than smaller aneurysms. Just like a balloon, once they start to expand, it becomes easier for them to stretch. Treatment is usually easier in the initial stages because they become larger and more difficult to treat with time.

Giant aneurysms usually present about a decade later in life than smaller aneurysms. Only about one fourth to one third present with hemorrhage; the rest present with mass effect and resultant focal neurologic deficit. Headache is common. Women are about twice as likely to acquire these as men.

Symptomatic giant aneurysms have a grave prognosis. Within 5 years, about 80% of these patients are dead or incapacitated. The initial symptoms of presentation progress to complete neurologic dysfunction. When symptoms are related to compression of the optic tract, blindness occurs within a few years. If compression of the brainstem is present, paralysis or death occurs within months. The only exception to this grim prognosis is with giant intracavernous aneurysms.

Symptoms are dependent on aneurysmal location. A noteworthy point is that all anterior circulation giant intracranial aneurysms are near the visual pathways and can thus have symptoms related to sight. Giant cavernous internal carotid artery (ICA) aneurysms present with ophthalmoplegia (diplopia), retro-orbital headache, facial sensory loss, and occasionally massive epistaxis (see Fig. 24–17 for an additional unusual finding). Paraophthalmic (paracli-

noid) ICA aneurysms also present with retro-orbital headache and visual field cuts or decreased vision secondary to optic nerve or chiasm compression. Carotid bifurcation aneurysms also cause visual field defects, frequently homonymous hemianopia, but also can cause hemiparesis or seizures. Although giant aneurysms of the anterior communicating artery are rare, they too cause visual field deficits (bitemporal hemianopia) along with a frontal lobe syndrome.

In patients with rapidly progressing visual symptoms, endovascular therapy may not be adequate, and a more aggressive approach involving open surgery may be in order. Additionally, carotid occlusion is relatively contraindicated in patients with bilateral cavernous (or other ICA) aneurysms. Occluding one side simply worsens the other, with potentially catastrophic results.

In general, the more proximal the aneurysm, the more successful parent vessel occlusion is at producing subsequent thrombosis of the aneurysm. About 90% of petrous or intracavernous aneurysms eventually thrombose after parent vessel occlusion. This drops to about 75% for paraophthalmic aneurysms, which can get some retrograde flow from the ophthalmic artery. If the aneurysms are more distal in the ICA (e.g., paraclinoid, posterior communicating), they receive some flow from the posterior communicating artery; only about half of these will eventually thrombose.

If the aneurysm does not thrombose completely, the incidence of bleeding and continued growth is about the same as for an untreated aneurysm.

Analysis of Specific Giant Aneurysms from Proximal to Distal

Petrous Internal Carotid Artery Aneurysms

The cause of petrous aneurysms can be traumatic (e.g., skull base fracture), infectious (e.g., otitis me-

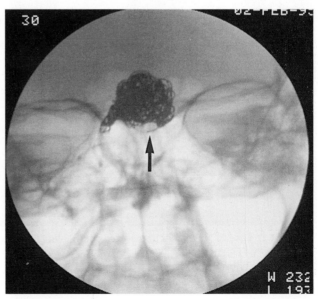

Figure 24-15 Unsubtracted image of the coil mass. Note the tip of one coil in the inferior portion of the aneurysm *(arrow)*. Where is this? Did the reader notice this on previous images?

Case 2 continues

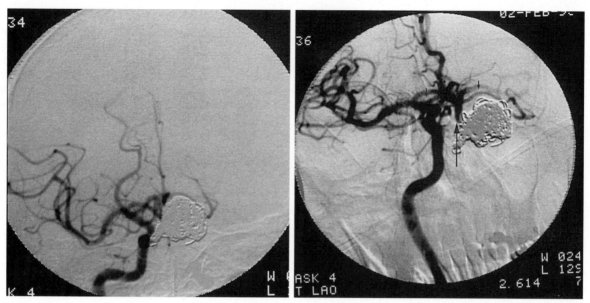

Figure 24-16 *A* and *B*, Final PA and slight oblique projections demonstrate the filling of the distal basilar artery *(long arrow)* and superior cerebellar arteries *(short arrows).*

The patient had been warned of possible recurrent coma after the aneurysm had been packed again, but this did not occur. However, after the case she did complain of visual disturbance. She was unable to describe the changes and was able to read fine print in a fashion similar to her preoperative status. Great concern was raised, however, over the possibility of emboli to the posterior cerebral artery territories, and heparinization was instituted. Follow-up magnetic resonance imaging the next day was totally unremarkable, and the patient's clinical status was now also unremarkable. She blamed the "funny vision" on all the drugs she had had during the procedure. She was discharged the next day neurologically intact. In all likelihood, she *did* suffer emboli to her posterior cerebral arteries, which rapidly (and luckily) dissolved.

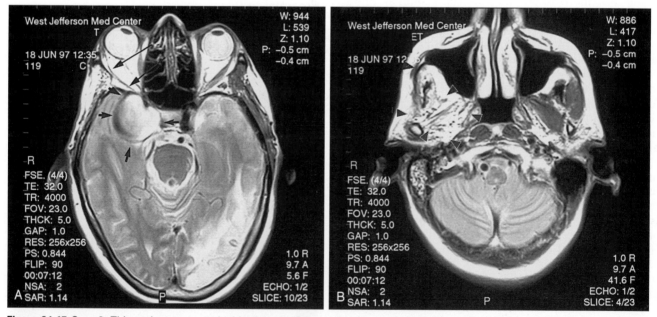

Figure 24-17 Case 3. This patient presented with diplopia. On examination, a sunken right temple was noted, originally thought to represent the sequela of a traumatic fracture. T2-weighted magnetic resonance imaging (MRI) revealed the true reason for this, however: atrophy of the masseters, pterygoid muscles, and temporal muscle *(arrowheads).* A huge aneurysm is seen in the right cavernous sinus *(short arrows).* Note also the atrophy of the lateral rectus *(long arrows).* This is due to the mass effect of the aneurysm and involvement of cranial nerves V3 and VI.

dia), or congenital. Surgical therapy is difficult because of the overlying bone and the inability to perform a direct vascular repair.

Endovascular therapy frequently is employed in this case using proximal balloon occlusion, with or without a distal balloon for trapping. The aneurysm usually thromboses in short order either way.

Intracavernous Internal Carotid Artery Aneurysms

As stated previously, visual deficits are the most frequent presentation of these aneurysms because the cavernous sinus harbors cranial nerves III, IV, V, and

VI. Inability to open the eye, along with other palsies, may be present. Retro-orbital pain, proptosis, and chemosis may be present, although these symptoms are more common with a true carotid-cavernous fistula. Massive epistaxis may be the initial and final presentation (Figs. 24–18 to 24–21).

Treatment of this condition is controversial. Some practitioners do not treat these aneurysms at all, whereas others attempt a direct surgical approach. Although possible with newer techniques, surgery is accompanied by significant morbidity and mortality. The primary problem, even with excision of the aneu-

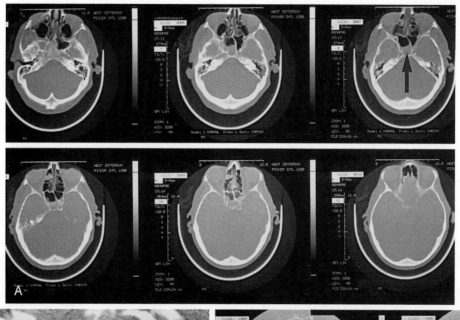

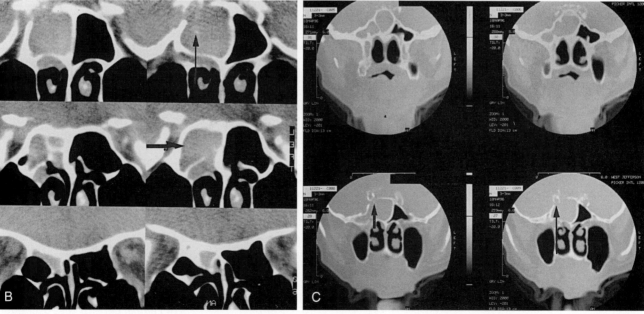

Figure 24-18 Case 4. This 72-year-old man presented to the emergency room with an episodic nose bleed. A computed tomographic (CT) scan *(A)* reveals an air-fluid level within the right sphenoid sinus *(arrow)*, thought to represent sinusitis. The patient was given antibiotics and referred to an otolaryngologist. Ten days later he reappeared in the emergency room, this time with massive nasal bleeding. An otolaryngologist saw him at that time and packed his nose but was convinced that this was more than a simple nosebleed. The CT scan obtained at that time *(B)* revealed an opacified sinus, with the hint of a mixed (higher) density within the sinus (not merely water) *(thick arrow)*, as well as a calcification *(thin arrow)*. *C,* In addition, the roof of the sinus was absent *(short arrow)*, and there was some discontinuity in the calcified rim of the carotid artery *(long arrow)*.

Case 4 continues

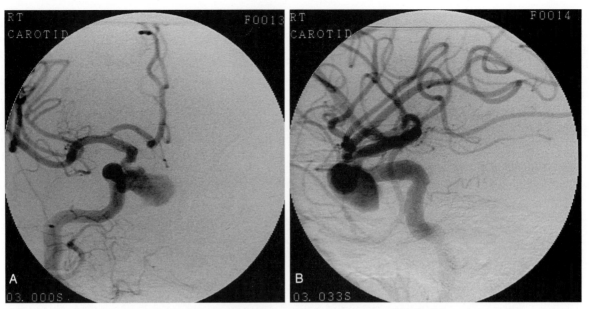

Figure 24-19 *A* and *B*, Posteroanterior (PA) and lateral view of right common carotid injection reveals a huge pseudoaneurysm, with blood filling the entire right side of the sphenoid sinus. The gap in the floor of the vessel was approximately 8 mm long, with a distal vessel lumen of 2 mm. It was determined that sacrifice of the vessel was necessary, but no detachable balloons were available at this outlying hospital, and thus coil occlusion was undertaken.

rysm and replacement with a short saphenous vein bypass graft, is the cranial nerve injury associated with the direct approach.

For aneurysms with a reasonable neck, GDC embolization is possible. This procedure is even more feasible with the use of a protective balloon in the ICA

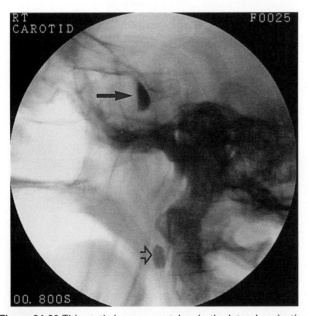

Figure 24-20 This static image was taken in the lateral projection, revealing the flow control guide catheter (Zeppelin, Medtronic/ MIS) in place in the internal carotid artery *(open arrow)*. This catheter can be used for the test occlusion as well as flow control during the occlusion procedure. Note the stagnant contrast-fluid level within the large pseudoaneurysm *(arrow)*. This balloon will be maintained in place during the coil occlusion procedure to eliminate the possibility of any embolic particles coursing in an intracranial direction from the coil mass during occlusion. This is very important!

Case 4 continues

for the purpose of maintaining the position of the coils during packing (the remodeling technique).

Alternatively, if the aneurysm cannot be directly occluded, endovascular therapy is aimed at isolation of the cavernous segment of the ICA by placement of a distal balloon past the cavernous sinus aneurysm, followed by occlusion of the proximal vessel in a fashion described later (Chapters 34, 35, and 36). If it is not possible to occlude the vessel distal to the aneurysm, proximal occlusion is performed first with the thought of returning at a later time, if necessary, to clip the intracranial segment distal to the aneurysm. Proximal occlusion of the ICA alone will result in cure of the aneurysm in the vast majority of cases, with failure occurring in those cases that have collateral supply from petrous or cavernous branches of the ICA that are keeping the aneurysm patent.

Coil occlusion of the distal site should not be performed just proximal to the ophthalmic artery because of the possibility of emboli originating from this location and coursing in an intracranial direction. If distal occlusion is necessary and the distance is limited, a surgical clip should be used.

Parent vessel occlusion of the ICA for treatment of an intracavernous aneurysm is a safe and effective therapy, yielding a cure in the vast majority of cases. Complications are essentially limited to ischemic events secondary to occlusion, not to the aneurysm, and occur in about 5% to 10% of patients; most are temporary, but permanent deficits occur in about 1% to 3% of patients.[11, 12] Therefore, careful test occlusion is necessary (see Chapters 34, 35, and 36).

Paraclinoid and Paraophthalmic Aneurysms

With proper modern surgical technique, clipping of a large portion of these aneurysms can be performed; GDC therapy can be performed in the bulk of the

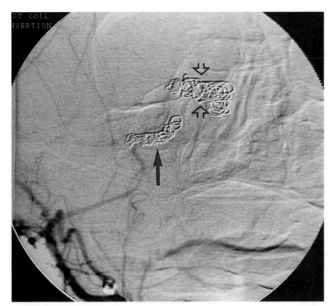

Figure 24-21 PA right common carotid angiogram after placement of microcoils. Note that even though the carotid artery was to be occluded, the aneurysm sac itself was first packed off *(open arrows)*. This was to prevent the possibility of rebleed into the sphenoid sinus due to retrograde flow from the distal internal carotid artery. The internal carotid artery was then further occluded in the stable intrapetrous portion *(arrow)*. Additional occlusion was then performed utilizing 0.038[11] Gianturco coils in the internal carotid artery just distal to the bulb of the carotid artery. Gianturco coils were used because of their extreme thrombogenicity and because they are much cheaper than platinum microcoils.

After complete packing of the aneurysm and petrous internal carotid artery, the heparin was reversed and the lumen of the guide catheter left open around the microcatheter to allow retrograde flow in the proximal internal carotid artery, in order to prevent overpressurization of the segment between the proximal occlusion balloon and the distal coil mass. It is very important not to pack additional coils into this closed segment without allowing some exit for the blood trapped in this location, so as not to force any material downstream from the distal coil mass. After complete packing was done as described above, the balloon was left in place for 1 hour to allow thorough thrombosis of the entire internal carotid artery. The final angiogram confirms total occlusion of the artery.

remainder. The aneurysms that are difficult to treat surgically, however, are the same that are difficult to treat with GDCs (i.e., those with large size, wide necks, and partial thrombosis or calcification). For this reason, parent vessel occlusion is still performed. Because of the inflow from the ophthalmic artery, these aneurysms do not thrombose at nearly the rate of cavernous aneurysms and thus occasionally require distal clipping. To facilitate thrombosis of the aneurysm, it is possible to occlude the origin of the ophthalmic artery, using a fibered coil in order to prevent retrograde flow from this vessel into the aneurysm.

The strategy is the same as for cavernous aneurysms, with distal surgical clipping performed when needed.

Supraclinoid Aneurysms

Supraclinoid aneurysms comprise posterior communicating artery aneurysms and anterior choroidal an-

eurysms, but it frequently is not possible to determine the origin of giant aneurysms in this location. Surgical clipping is the therapy of choice; carotid occlusion rarely is necessary. This is particularly true in light of the fact that blood supply from the ophthalmic artery or posterior communicating artery can maintain patency in the aneurysm.

Carotid Bifurcation, Anterior Cerebral Artery, and Middle Cerebral Artery Aneurysms

These giant aneurysms are typically treated surgically and rarely need proximal occlusion. When they do, it is most often done surgically, either with or without an attempt to bypass the vascular segment.

Vertebral Artery Aneurysms

Vertebral artery giant aneurysms commonly are fusiform and generally cannot be clipped. They can be the source of emboli and can result from dissection in the moving portion of the vertebral artery near C1 and C2. They can be restricted to the portion proximal to the posterior inferior cerebellar artery (PICA) or involve its origin. Rarely, they are true giant berry aneurysms originating at the PICA origin. If so, they occur at the distal crotch of the origin of the PICA from the vertebral artery.

The vertebral artery pierces the dura at the posterolateral edge of the foramen magnum and immediately enters the subarachnoid space, where it is adjacent to the medulla. Just past its origin, the PICA is adjacent to, or even splits, the hypoglossal nerve and then is encased by cranial nerves IX, X, and XI. Thus, surgery in this region is extremely difficult. Even retraction of these nerves can cause permanent palsy, with resultant swallowing difficulty, dysarthria, or aspiration.

Vertebral artery aneurysms can cause cerebellopontine angle syndrome. Most presentations are related to hemorrhage, just as with other aneurysms; even the dissecting aneurysms tend to bleed more than simply grow. Headache can be a sentinel event; classically, it is in the suboccipital region.

Treatment is most easily performed by vertebral artery occlusion. This can be done at first intent if the opposite vertebral artery is normal in size or robust. Otherwise, a test occlusion can be performed in the vertebral artery using either an Endeavor (ITC/Target Therapeutics) or a Grapevine or Solstice catheter (Medtronic/MIS) (see Chapter 1). Rarely should the vertebral artery be occluded if the support from the opposite vertebral artery is inadequate. This can still be possible if the Allcock test reveals robust supply from the anterior circulation or if a bypass to the posterior circulation is performed in addition (see Chapter 49).

Proximal occlusion of the vertebral artery should be all that is necessary for treatment of these lesions; it may be difficult to position a balloon in a stable position past the aneurysm and proximal to the PICA. Retrograde flow down the distal vertebral artery to the PICA keeps the PICA open, but the aneurysm will thrombose proximal to it. The only problem is the continued worry concerning embolic material coming from the stump, just as in the carotid artery. This danger decreases after the first several months.

If the aneurysm is between the PICA and the vertebrobasilar junction, trapping is indicated. There is usually about 15 mm between the origin of PICA and the vertebrobasilar junction; clips are the therapy of choice for isolating this segment. Proximal occlusion of the vertebral artery appears fruitless.

Fusiform Aneurysms of the Vertebrobasilar Junction

Fusiform aneurysms of the vertebrobasilar junction are extremely difficult to manage. The portion of the vertebral artery between the PICA and the vertebrobasilar junction contains no perforators; thus, aneurysms can grow in this location in an essentially symptom-free manner. These aneurysms, however, may involve both distal vertebral arteries and the basilar artery, a location not amenable to reconstruction. Efforts at therapy are directed at decreasing the pressure within these structures.

Occlusion of one vertebral artery appears capable of decreasing the pulse pressure within the aneurysm, but this is not necessarily true. Altering the flow dynamics may make the problem worse. Cases have occurred in which this type of aneurysm initially bled *after occlusion of one vertebral artery*. Therefore, occlusion of both vertebral arteries probably is the therapy of choice, if it can be accomplished. Each artery can be tested successively with temporary occlusion balloons; the second vertebral artery to be occluded is the exciting one.

Basilar Tip Berry Aneurysms

Basilar tip berry aneurysms are the most common aneurysms of the posterior fossa, constituting about half of all posterior circulation aneurysms. They can present either with hemorrhage or with mass effect. The symptoms from mass effect are dependent on the direction the aneurysm projects; if it projects posteriorly, it presents with pseudobulbar palsy, ataxia, and various degrees of weakness in all four extremities. If slightly asymmetric, the mass can compress the cerebral peduncle and compress the third nerve, with resultant Weber's syndrome (contralateral hemiparesis and ipsilateral oculomotor palsy). Bilateral sixth nerve palsies result in paralysis of lateral eye movement with preservation of medial movement.

The overall mortality rate secondary to a symptomatic basilar artery aneurysm is about 60% to 70%, with most deaths occurring within 3 years of presentation. In a series compiled by Peerless and Drake,[31] all 26 patients treated nonoperatively died within 3 years.

These lesions are difficult to treat surgically. The approach is extremely difficult, and once there, even placing a clip is nearly impossible. The top of the basilar artery is covered with valuable perforators, and the base of the aneurysm can cover a long distance over essentially rotting vessel.

Peerless and Drake[31] described 132 patients in whom they placed a tourniquet around the basilar artery without tightening it and then waited until the patient awoke for neurologic testing. Gradual tourniquet tightening was then performed while the patient was awake, and reversed if any problem occurred. Although a good or excellent outcome was obtained in 68% of these patients, about one third eventually had a poor outcome or died, with irreversible ischemic deficits. (These results are impressive but not necessarily good; performing an endovascular test occlusion is far simpler.) The patients who had one or two small (1 mm or less) posterior communicating arteries had poor outcomes. Eighty-six percent of patients tolerated unilateral vertebral artery occlusion, and 75% tolerated lower basilar artery occlusion; only 50% tolerated upper basilar artery occlusion.

Endovascular therapy is performed with GDCs. Various forms of parent vessel occlusion have been used, however, with varying degrees of success. Aymard and colleagues[32] reported on 21 patients with aneurysms of the vertebrobasilar circulation treated with unilateral or bilateral vertebral artery occlusion. Of the 21, 13 had good outcomes, with complete clinical and angiographic cure; an additional 6 patients had partial thrombosis. There was one death and one treatment failure (stroke).

In a report by Tomsick et al.,[33] a comparison of outcome was made between patients undergoing surgery and those treated with GDCs for basilar apex aneurysms. Over 4 years, 41 patients were treated; 20 of these underwent surgery and 21 received coil therapy. There were no significant differences in the dimensions or configurations of the aneurysms between the two groups. Sixty-six percent of the patients treated surgically after subarachnoid hemorrhage had a good outcome (Glasgow Outcome Score of 1–2), compared with 90% after endovascular therapy. One person in the surgical group died compared with none in the endovascular group. All of the electively treated GDC group had good outcomes, compared with 80% of the surgical group (there was one death—a 20% rate). In addition, the length of hospital stay of patients undergoing surgery was twice that of patients in the GDC group.

Although long-term follow-up is lacking, these results indicate that GDC therapy for basilar tip aneurysms is a safe alternative in this therapeutically challenging condition.

Fusiform Basilar Artery Aneurysms

Although not uncommon, fusiform basilar artery aneurysms are essentially untreatable. Multiple perforators arise from this vessel, the wall is frequently calcified, and the location for reconstruction is suboptimal. If the vessel thromboses, unforeseen results may occur. Proximal occlusion does not appear to be an option in this case.

HAZARDS OF ANEURYSM EMBOLIZATION

Aneurysm embolization is one of the more dangerous procedures performed by an interventional neuroradiologist (other than intracranial angioplasty); worse, any complication can be totally unpredictable and even unknown (at least for a time). When injecting glue, the danger is readily evident and immediately obvious. When dealing with a long procedure such as aneurysm embolization, however, some of the risk is simply from the length of the procedure (e.g., intracranial vascular damage, intrinsic thrombus formation, intimal damage to the parent vessel by the guide catheter). In addition, pushing coils into the aneurysm can dislodge indwelling thrombus from within the aneurysm; this may not be apparent nor even suspected until the follow-up postprocedure angiogram or MRI. Even then, the radiographic findings may be subtle, although significant.

Aneurysm Rupture

The most disastrous complication is rupture of the aneurysm (see Chapter 64). Because of the nature of the rupture (a linear tear, not a hole), occlusion of the perforation is difficult, and the rate of bleeding is extremely high. The wall of the aneurysm is incapable of aiding in cessation of flow, and thus this event often is terminal. A flow-control guide catheter can be life-saving. As stated in Chapter 64, rapid placement of small fibered coils (dipped in thrombin if possible) may be the best chance for rescue of this situation. Suggestions for use of cyanoacrylates or hydrogels have been made, but these have not undergone thorough clinical double-blind trials. If a flow-control catheter were employed as a guide catheter during the reported cases of rupture, bizarre emergency embolization techniques probably would not be as prominently suggested. A large percentage of these ruptures occurred in the posterior circulation, however, where a flow-control guide catheter may be of no use.

Of note is the use of a protective balloon in the remodeling technique described in Chapter 25. If this Solstice balloon (Medtronic/MIS) is in place, inflation can immediately stop the hemorrhage.

Coil Malposition

The inadvertent placement of a portion of coil in the parent vessel is more common than perforation but is not necessarily disastrous. Although cases have been reported of subsequent embolic events relative to a dangling intraluminal coil, many instances of inadvertent coil malposition have resulted in no untoward events. No statistics are available related to these complications because of the lack of published information concerning this subject, but they are reported as verbal communication from other practitioners in this field. If a coil has protruded into the lumen, anticoagulant therapy and platelet antiaggregant therapy are required for at least several days if not months. It should be realized that flowing blood will always and invariably be in contact with coils, however.

The remodeling technique is a method that is capable of greatly decreasing the incidence of coil fragments dangling into the parent vessel.

Guide Catheter Complications

Complications related to the guide catheter occur more often than would be presumed. Spasm or a small intimal tear may or may not be significant. A patient with a recent subarachnoid hemorrhage may be more prone to thrombus formation than usual, however, and any intimal damage to the parent vessel may be significant in that it may induce abundant thrombus in the internal carotid artery, vertebral artery, or wherever the catheter had been positioned. Normally, an embolic complication would not be a big problem because of the availability of vasodilators (e.g., nitroglycerin, amyl nitrate, papaverine) and fibrinolytics (e.g., urokinase); in the presence of a previously hemorrhagic intracranial aneurysm, however, treatment options are limited.

In addition, the vascular damage may be in the form of an intimal tear that becomes a downstream spiral dissection, with catastrophic results. Patients with aneurysms often have intrinsically pathologic vessels. The radiologic appearance of a spiral dissection sometimes can be difficult to distinguish from intraluminal thrombus, but when a long segment of abnormal vessel is seen that was not there previously, the possibility of a spiral dissection should be considered.

Some of these statements are hypothetical but must be considered by anyone performing this procedure. Considering all potential problems is perhaps more necessary in this field than in many others and allows the operator to avoid problems.

Distal Embolization

Reports have been made of embolic material displaced during the detachment process (i.e., the electrolytic process); the solder joint has fragmented and embolized distally.[34] This does not appear to be as much a clinical problem as a CT problem. Frequently, the small branch occlusion has no clinical or hemodynamic effect. This result appears to have been reduced considerably with the newer GDCs.

An additional complication of coil embolization of an intracranial aneurysm may be displacement of intra-aneurysmal thrombus into the parent vessel and thus downstream (as stated previously). Depending on where the thrombus goes and how large it is, this may or may not be a major problem. It is not known how old (or mature) this fragment may be, but there is a good possibility that this fragment may be considerably resistant to thrombolysis. It appears from anecdotal reports that the frequency of mature thrombus fragments being displaced downstream is relatively low.

In cases in which retreatment of an aneurysm that contains indwelling coils is necessary, there is probably thrombus surrounding these coils, but displacement of thrombus from these is uncommon. Unfortunately, just as in many areas of this specialty, exact numbers are not known at this time (see Figs. 24–6 to 24–16). Anecdotal reports indicate that there is far less thrombus around these coils than originally thought, thus decreasing the risk of embolic events, but also decreasing the cure rate.

An important point to remember is that the presence of an aneurysm remnant (generally the neck) means that the condition has not been cured.

Perhaps the greatest fear of embolic events occurs in situations in which the coil protrudes from the neck by a fraction of a millimeter or there is flow into the neck around some of the coils. No accurate statements can be made concerning the actual risk associated with this problem. Many interventionists routinely leave their patients on anticoagulants for the first 1 to 3 days following GDC use if there is any worry about this. This is particularly true regarding aneurysms at the middle cerebral artery or internal carotid artery bifurcation, or those carotid aneurysms with wide necks.

POTENTIAL ADVANCES IN INTRACRANIAL ANEURYSM TREATMENT
Enhancement of GDC Performance

Poor endothelialization of GDCs has been demonstrated in vivo and in vitro; attempts are being made to enhance this property. Ion implantation technology combined with protein coating of coils was performed and evaluated.[35] Various coatings, including segmental polyurethane and protein coating (fibrinogen or type I collagen), were tested in vitro for cell adhesion. In addition, in a chronic experimental study, 40 aneurysms in swine were either treated with normal GDCs or coated GDCs (fibrinectin, type I collagen, vitronectin, laminin, or fibrinogen; all ion-implanted preoperatively). The in vitro study demonstrated acceleration of cell adhesion and proliferation on the treated GDCs; both simple coating and ion-treated coating elicited this response. The strength of attachment was better on the ion-treated coating. In the in vivo study, the standard GDCs demonstrated poor, thin layer covering whereas the ion-implanted coated GDCs demonstrated well-organized fibrous tissue bridging the aneurysm neck.

The results of this study indicate that GDC performance can be enhanced by surface manipulation.

Other Advances

The ideal treatment of an aneurysm is total exclusion from the circulation. A surgical clip effectively does this. Endovascular attempts at treatment of this pathology have been less than ideal, but potential new therapies are on the horizon. These include filling the aneurysm with a more adaptable substance, such as a liquid agent (EVAL or a hydrogel), or an expandable metal mesh that is easier to place accurately and capable of packing the aneurysm more thoroughly. Lining the interior of the parent vessel with

an inner coat (e.g., a coated stent), effectively excluding the aneurysm from the circulation, could yield a perfect cure. This is theoretically ideal, but placement of this stent is technically extremely difficult and could be hazardous, considering the necessity of not occluding the orifice of any vital vessel nearby (which might be very small and nearly invisible).

A Potential Endovascular Cure

An alternative therapy would be to line the *inside of the aneurysm*, thus placing a coating over the mouth of the aneurysm, but from the inside, not the outside. This lining could be in the form of a sack, stuffed with embolic material such as fibers, coils, or particles. All of these would be effectively contained within this bag but would push the bag to the outside, against the wall and mouth of the aneurysm. The material of the bag could be formulated to induce endothelial growth, thus reconstituting the wall of the vessel and sealing the aneurysm from the circulation.

REFERENCES

1. Osborn A. Diagnostic Neuroradiology. St. Louis: CV Mosby, 1994, pp. 248–253.
2. Jellinger K. Pathology and aetiology of intracranial aneurysms. In Pia HW, Langmaid C, Zierski J (eds). Cerebral Aneurysms: Advances in Diagnosis and Therapy. New York: Springer, 1979, pp. 5–19.
3. Bannerman RM, Ingall GB, Graf CJ. The familial occurrence of intracranial aneurysms. *Neurology* 1970;20:283–292.
4. Stehbens WE. Aneurysm and anatomical variation of the cerebral arteries. *Arch Pathol* 1963;75:45–64.
5. Graf CJ. Prognosis for patients with nonsurgically-treated aneurysms: analysis of the cooperative study of intracranial aneurysms and subarachnoid hemorrhage. *J Neurosurg* 1971;35:438–443.
6. Fox JL. Intracranial Aneurysms, Vol 1. New York: Springer-Verlag, 1983.
7. Adams HP Jr, Kassell NF, Torner JC, et al. Early management of aneurysmal subarachnoid hemorrhage: a report of the cooperative aneurysm study. *J Neurosurg* 1981;54:141–145.
8. Hunt WE, Hess RM. Surgical risk as related to time of intervention in the repair of intracranial aneurysms. *J Neurosurg* 1968;28:14–20.
9. Fisher CM, Kistler JP, Davis JM. Relation of cerebral vasospasm to subarachnoid hemorrhage visualized by computerized tomographic scanning. *Neurosurgery* 1980;6:1–9.
10. Kistler JP, Crowell RM, Davis KR. The relation of cerebral vasospasm to the extent and location of subarachnoid blood visualized by CT scan: A prospective study. *Neurology* 1983;33:424–436.
11. Debrun G, Fox A, Drake C, et al. Giant unclippable aneurysms: treatment with detachable balloons. *AJNR* 1981;2:167–173.
12. Fox AJ, Vinuela F, Pelz DM, et al. Use of detachable balloons for proximal artery occlusion in the treatment of unclippable cerebral aneurysms. *J Neurosurg* 1987;66:40–46.
13. Barnett HJM, Peerless SJ, Kaufman JC. "Stump" of internal carotid: a source for further embolic ischemia. *Stroke* 1978;9:448–456.
14. Heros RC. Thromboembolic complications after combined internal carotid ligation and extra-to-intracranial bypass *Surg Neurol* 1984;21:175–179.
15. Landolt AM, Milliken CH. Pathogenesis of cerebral infarction secondary to mechanical carotid artery occlusion. *Stroke* 1970;1:52–62.
16. Miller JD, Jawad K, Jennett B. Safety of carotid ligation and

its role in the management of intracranial aneurysms. *J Neurol Neurosurg Psychiatry* 1977;40:64–72.

17. Roski RA, Spetzler RF, Nulsen FE. Late complications of carotid ligation in the treatment of intracranial aneurysms. *J Neurosurg* 1981;54:583–587.

18. Serbinenko FA. Balloon catheterization and occlusion of major cerebral vessels. *J Neurosurg* 1974;41:125–145.

19. Debrun G, Lacour P, Caron JP, et al. Detachable balloon and calibrated leak balloon technique in the treatment of cerebral vascular lesions. *J Neurosurg* 1978;49:635–639.

20. Hieshima GB, Grinnell VS, Mehringer CM. A detachable balloon for transcatheter occlusions. *Radiology* 1981;138:227–228.

21. Hilal SK, Khandji AG, Chi TL, et al. Synthetic fiber-coated platinum coils successfully used for endovascular treatment of arteriovenous malformations, aneurysm and direct arteriovenous fistulae of CNS [Abstract]. *AJNR* 1988;9:1026.

22. Guglielmi G, Vinuela F, Dion J, Duckwiler G. Electrothrombosis of saccular aneurysms via endovascular approach. Part 2: preliminary clinical experience. *J Neurosurg* 1991;75:8–14.

23. Guglielmi G, Vinuela F, Duckwiler G, et al. Endovascular treatment of posterior circulation aneurysms by electrothrombosis using electrically detachable coils. *J Neurosurg* 1992;77:515–524.

24. Kinugasa K, Mandai S, Terai Y, et al. Direct thrombosis of aneurysms with cellular acetate polymer. Part II: Preliminary clinical experience. *J Neurosurg* 1992;77:501–507.

25. Connors JJ, Neal JC, Smith RR. Percutaneous endovascular therapy for inoperable intracranial aneurysm. *J Miss State Med Assoc* 1990;21:369–371.

26. Vinuela F. Review of the USA multicenter GDC study group for treatment of intracranial aneurysms. Paper presented at the 1995 Course in Interventional Neuroradiology of the American Society of Interventional and Therapeutic Neuroradiology.

27. Malisch TW, Guglielmi G, Vinuela F, et al. Intracranial aneurysms treated with the Guglielmi detachable coil: Midterm clinical results in a consecutive series of 100 patients. *J Neurosurg* 1997;87:176–183.

28. Jennett B, Bond M. Assessment of outcome after severe brain damage. A practical scale. *Lancet* 1975;1:480–484.

29. Kassell NF, Torner JC, Haley EC, et al. The International Cooperative Study on the Timing of Aneurysm Surgery. Part 1: Overall management results. *J Neurosurg* 1990;73:18–36.

30. Kassell NF, Torner JC, Jane JA, et al. The International Cooperative Study on the Timing of Aneurysm Surgery. Part 2: Surgical results. *J Neurosurg* 1990;73:37–47.

31. Peerless SJ, Drake CG. Management of aneurysms of the posterior circulation. In Youmans JR (ed): Neurological Surgery: A Comprehensive Reference Guide to the Diagnosis and Management of Neurosurgical Problems, 3rd ed. Philadelphia: WB Saunders, 1990, pp. 1764–1806.

32. Aymard A, Gobin YP, Hodes JE, et al. Endovascular occlusion of vertebral arteries in the treatment of unclippable vertebrobasilar aneurysms. *J Neurosurg* 1991;74:393–398.

33. Tomsick TA, Zimmerman GA, Gruber DP, et al. A comparison between endovascular and surgical management of basilar apex aneurysms. Paper presented at the American Society of Therapeutic and Interventional Neuroradiology/World Federation of Therapeutic and Interventional Neuroradiology Scientific Conference. New York, September 1997.

34. Halbach V, Dowd CF, Higashida RT, et al. Metallic fragment emboli resulting from treatment with electrolytically detachable coils. Paper presented at the Western Neuroradiological Society Meeting, October 6–9, 1994.

35. Murayama Y, Vinuela F, Suzuki F. Cell adhesion control on GDC surface by ion implantation: In vitro and in vivo evaluation. Paper presented at the American Society of Therapeutic and Interventional Neuroradiology/World Federation of Therapeutic and Interventional Neuroradiology Scientific Conference. New York, September 1997.

ADDITIONAL READINGS

Aymard A, Hodes JE, Rufenacht D, Merland JJ. Endovascular treatment of a giant fusiform aneurysm of the entire basilar artery. *AJNR* 1992;13:1143–1146.

Berenstein A, Ransohoff J, Kupersmith M, et al. Transvascular treatment of giant aneurysms of the cavernous carotid and vertebral arteries. *Surg Neurol* 1984;21:3–12.

Chaloupka JC, Guglielmi G, Vinuela F. Direct thrombosis of aneurysms [Letter]. *J Neurosurg* 1993;78:1006–1007.

Duong H, Lycette C, Pile-Spellman J, et al. Guglielmi detachable coil treatment of a serpentine middle cerebral artery aneurysm. *J Neurovasc Dis* 1996;1:33–39.

Ebina K, Suzuki M, Andoh A, et al. Recurrence of cerebral aneurysm after initial neck clipping. *Neurosurgery* 1982;11:764–768.

Fernandez Zubillaga A, Guglielmi G, Vinuela F, Duckwiler GR. Endovascular occlusion of intracranial aneurysms with electrically detachable coils: correlation of aneurysm neck size and treatment results. *AJNR* 1994;15:815–820.

Fraser KW, Halbach VV, Teitelbaum GP, et al. Endovascular platinum coil embolization of incompletely surgically clipped cerebral aneurysms. *Surg Neurol* 1994;41:4–8.

Gelber BR, Sundt TM. Treatment of intracavernous and giant carotid aneurysms by combined internal carotid ligation and extra- to intracranial bypass. *J Neurosurg* 1980;52:1–10.

Graves V, Partington C, Rufenacht D, et al. Treatment of carotid artery aneurysms with platinum coils: an experimental study in dogs. *AJNR* 1990;11:249–252.

Graves VB, Strother CM, Rappe AH. Treatment of experimental canine carotid aneurysms with platinum coils. *AJNR* 1993;14:787–793.

Halbach V. The "current" status of aneurysm treatment? *AJNR* 1993;14:799–800.

Hieshima GB, Higashida TH, Wapenski J, et al. Balloon embolization of a large distal basilar artery aneurysm: case report. *J Neurosurg* 1986;64:413–416.

Higashida RT, Halbach VV, Dowd CF, et al. Intracranial aneurysms: interventional neurovascular treatment with detachable balloons. Results in 215 cases. *Radiology* 1991;178:663–670.

Hilal SK, Solomon RA. Endovascular treatment of aneurysms with coils [Letter]. *J Neurosurg* 1992;76:337–338.

Hodes JE, Aymard A, Gobin YP, et al. Endovascular occlusion of intracranial vessels for curative treatment of unclippable aneurysms: report of 16 cases. *J Neurosurg* 1991;75:694–701.

Hosoda K, Fujita S, Kawaguchi T, et al. Saccular aneurysms of the proximal (M1) segment of the middle cerebral artery. *Neurosurgery* 1995;36:441–446.

Huston J III, Rufenacht DA, Ehman RL, Wiebers DO. Intracranial aneurysms and vascular malformations: comparison of time-of-flight and phase-contrast MR angiography. *Radiology* 1991;181:721–730.

Khayata MH, Spetzler RF, Mooy JJA, et al. Combined surgical and endovascular treatment of a giant vertebral artery aneurysm in a child: case report. *J Neurosurg* 1994;81:304–307.

Kinoshita A. Detachable leak balloon with IBCA/NBCA for treatment of aneurysm [Letter]. *AJNR* 1992;13:1451–1452.

Kurokawa Y, Abiko S, Okamura T, Watanabe K. Direct surgery for giant aneurysm exhibiting progressive enlargement after intraaneurysmal balloon embolization. *Surg Neurol* 1992;38:19–25.

Kwan ES, Heilman CB, Roth PA. Endovascular packing of carotid bifurcation aneurysm with polyester fiber-coated platinum coils in a rabbit model. *AJNR* 1993;14:323–333.

Ladouceur DL. Transcranial clipping of recurrent cerebral aneurysms after endovascular treatment. *Stroke* 1993;24:1087–1089.

Larson JJ, Tew JM Jr, Tomsick TA, van Loveren HR. Treatment of aneurysms of the internal carotid artery by intravascular balloon occlusion: long-term follow-up of 58 patients. *Neurosurgery* 1995;36:23–30.

Linskey ME, Sekhar LN. Which cavernous sinus aneurysms should be treated? [Letter] *J Neurosurg* 1993;78:1008–1009.

Makita K, Tsuchiya K, Furui S, et al. Nondissecting vertebral fusiform aneurysm: embolization using wire-directed detachable balloons. *AJNR* 1993;13:340–342.

Mandai S, Kinugasa K, Ohmoto T. Direct thrombosis of aneurysms with cellulose acetate polymer. Part I: Results of thrombosis in experimental aneurysms. *J Neurosurg* 1992;77:497–500.

Mayberg MR, Batjer HH, Dacey R, et al. Guidelines for the management of aneurysmal subarachnoid hemorrhage: a statement for healthcare professionals from a special writing group of the Stroke Council, American Heart Association. *Circulation* 1994;90:2592–2605.

Nakahara I, Handa H, Nishikawa M, et al. Endovascular coil embolization of a recurrent giant internal carotid artery aneurysm via the posterior communicating artery after cervical carotid ligation: case report. *Surg Neurol* 1992;38:57–62.

Nichols DA. Endovascular treatment of the acutely ruptured intracranial aneurysm. *J Neurosurg* 1993;79:1–2.

Picard L, Roy D, Bracard S, et al. Aneurysm associated with a fenestrated basilar artery: report of two cases treated by endovascular detachable balloon embolization. *AJNR* 1993;14:591–594.

Sanchez LA, Faries PL, Marin ML, et al. A new model for the in vivo evaluation of intra-aneurysmal pressure following endovascular treatment [Abstract]. *J Endovasc Surg* 1996;3:97.

Scialfa G, Vaghi A, Valsecchi F, et al. Neuroradiological treatment of carotid and vertebral fistulas and intracavernous aneurysms. *Neuroradiology* 1982;24:13–25.

Scotti G, Righi C. The "hyperteloric happy face" sign: a misleading indicator of complete aneurysm closure with Guglielmi detachable coils [Letter]. *AJNR* 1994;15:795–796.

Solomon RA, Fink ME, Pile-Spellman J. Surgical management of

unruptured intracranial aneurysms. *J Neurosurg* 1994;80:440–446.

Spaziante R, De Chiara A, Lacaarino V, et al. Intracavernous giant fusiform aneurysm of the carotid artery treated with Gianturco coils. *Neurochirurgie* 1986;29:34–41.

Szikora I, Guterman LR, Wells KM, Hopkins LN. Combined use of stents and coils to treat experimental wide-necked carotid aneurysms: preliminary results. *AJNR* 1994;15:1091–1102.

Teng MMH, Chen CC, Chen SS, et al. N-butyl-2-cyanoacrylate for embolization of carotid aneurysm. *Neuroradiology* 1994;36:144–147.

Tsuruda JS, Servick J, Halbach VV. Three-dimensional time-of-flight MR angiography in the evaluation of intracranial aneurysms treated by endovascular balloon occlusion. *AJNR* 1992;13:1129–1136.

Turjman F, Acevedo G, Moll T, et al. Treatment of experimental carotid aneurysms by endoprosthesis implantation: preliminary report. *Neurol Res* 1993;15:181–184.

Turjman F, Massoud TF, Ji C, et al. Combined stent implantation and endovascular coil placement for treatment of experimental wide-necked aneurysms: a feasibility study in swine. *AJNR* 1994;15:1087–1090.

CHAPTER 25

Detachable Coil Embolization of Intracranial Aneurysms

M.E. Cronqvist / J. Moret

Interventional neuroradiology—mainly endovascular therapy of intracranial vascular diseases—has continuously progressed since the introduction of balloon embolization of intracranial aneurysms in the 1970s.[1–3] Even if the balloon occlusion technique was promising, it was often a difficult and time-consuming procedure fraught with risks and complications.[4–8] Further experiences and advances in endovascular technique, with development of new devices, led to the introduction of electrolytically detachable platinum coils (Guglielmi detachable coils [GDC], Target Therapeutics) in 1991.[9] The GDC coils offer a more controlled and safe filling of the aneurysmal sac than do balloons, and make it possible to obtain a total occlusion of the aneurysm lumen by a combination of electrothrombosis and dense packing.[10, 11]

Despite these advances, endovascular therapy for intracranial aneurysms is a difficult technique accompanied by certain risks of complications with sometimes disastrous consequences. As in any vascular procedure, a thorough knowledge of the anatomy, practical training, and experience are mandatory and crucial for all individuals aiming to devote themselves to interventional neuroradiology in general and treatment of aneurysms in particular.

PRETHERAPEUTIC EVALUATION AND INDICATIONS

Surgical clipping of intracranial aneurysms is still regarded as the "gold standard" method in most institutions. Timing of surgery and overall management protocols concerning aneurysmal subarachnoid hemorrhage (SAH) have differed remarkably among various neurosurgical centers in the 1980s and 1990s.[12–15] In recent years, the strategy has successively focused on early referral and immediate surgical intervention to minimize the risk of a rebleed and to optimize the possibilities for an aggressive pharmacologic approach to prevention of vasospasm and delayed deterioration due to ischemia.[16–20] However, early surgery (within 1 to 3 days from an SAH) or subacute surgery (within 4 to 14 days) is not always feasible and is strongly dependent on the clinical condition (graded according to Hunt and Hess[21]) of the patient upon admission, on angiographic and clinical evidence of vasospasm, and on surgical accessibility of the aneurysm to be treated.

The limitations and contraindications are often different in endovascular and surgical procedures. Endovascular therapy was initially restricted to aneurysms regarded as inoperable or surgically difficult to manage, predominantly within the posterior circulation (Fig. 25–1).[22–25] The development of GDC coils, together with the increased experience gained since the early 1990s, has widened these indications to include even aneurysms of the anterior circulation (Figs. 25–2 and 25–3).[26–29] Thus, endovascular treatment has become a true complement and alternative to surgery, especially when it enables an early and controlled obliteration of a recently ruptured aneu-

rysm, for example, in patients and aneurysms considered unsuitable for immediate craniotomy or surgical clipping. Consequently, a close collaboration between neuroradiologists and neurosurgeons is mandatory in all pretherapeutic evaluations concerning intracranial aneurysms, regardless of whether the aneurysm is an incidental finding, has recently bled, or is to be treated at a later stage.

The aim of both surgical and endovascular treat-

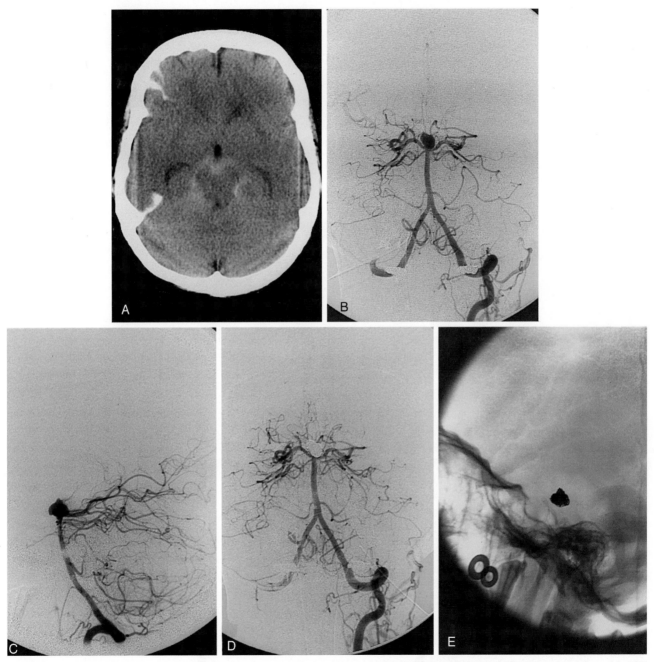

Figure 25-1. Case 1. This 54-year-old woman presented with a sudden onset of severe headache. *A,* Computed tomographic (CT) scan demonstrates blood within the subarachnoidal space and basal cisterns and around the mesencephalon.

B and *C,* Frontal and lateral projections of the left vertebral angiogram demonstrate a saccular aneurysm at the basilar tip with a favorable delineation of its origin in relation to the parent artery and adjacent branches.

D, Frontal projection after coil embolization. There is no opacification of the aneurysmal sac. Preserved filling of the P1 segments and distal branches is seen.

E, A nonsubtracted lateral projection demonstrates the coils densely packed within the aneurysmal sac.

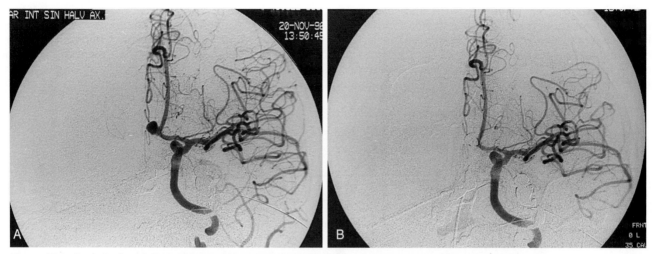

Figure 25-2. Case 2. *A* and *B,* A 46-year-old man who had a short episode of unconsciousness followed by severe headache. Multiple aneurysms were found on the subsequent angiogram (see Fig. 25–4). Frontal projections of a left internal carotid artery (ICA) angiogram show a small berry anterior communicating artery (ACoA) aneurysm before and after coiling.

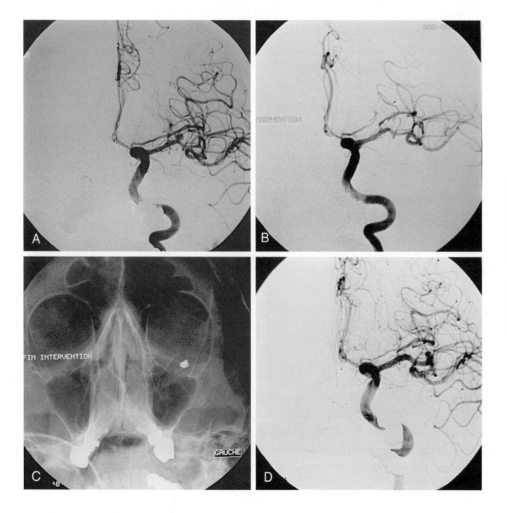

Figure 25-3. Case 3. Patient with a subarachnoid hemorrhage from a small aneurysm at the left middle cerebral artery (MCA) bifurcation. *A* and *B,* Frontal projection angiogram of the left ICA shows the aneurysm before and after treatment.
 C and *D,* A follow-up examination 2 years after the endovascular procedure demonstrates the coil configuration (nonsubtracted image) and a permanent aneurysmal occlusion.

ment is to achieve a permanent occlusion of the aneurysmal sac and a complete obliteration of its orifice. Before the appropriate therapeutic modality is selected, several factors have to be considered. These include the skill and experience of the individual physician, the patient's medical condition, and the natural history of the disease. Further, the benefits and risks associated with each approach have to be weighed, as well as the therapeutic accessibility.[30] The accessibility is based on vascular anatomy, aneurysm location and configuration, and the ratio between the diameter of the aneurysmal sac and its neck (ratio-sac-neck, or RSN).

Regardless of aneurysm location, GDC coiling is today applicable for most intracranial aneurysms.[29] Aneurysm size and the RSN are the main factors critical to the success of endovascular therapy.[31] The possibility of a complete, dense obliteration with coils is generally favorable in small berry aneurysms (<15 mm) and in large aneurysms (≥15 and <25 mm) with a good RSN (≥1.5). Whenever the RSN is moderate (>1.2 and <1.5) or poor (≤1.2), the chances of obtaining a dense filling and stable coil formation are reduced. However, since the introduction of the "remodeling technique" (see below), this limitation has been at least partly overcome.

Giant aneurysms (≥25 mm) and even larger aneurysms (>20 and <25 mm) are not good indications for coiling, since they carry the risk of a high percentage of recanalization and regrowth. The causes of this are probably multifold and combined; they include the size of the aneurysm, the delicate nature of the coils, the continuous flow-related stress upon these coils, and the possibility of preexisting thrombus formation within the aneurysmal pouch. The method of choice in such aneurysms is either permanent balloon occlusion of the parent artery or surgery. A test occlusion precedes the permanent balloon occlusion; if not tolerated, it is necessary to perform bypass surgery before sacrificing the artery.[3, 32]

A combination of coiling and clipping may occasionally be used in patients presenting with multiple aneurysms and SAH, specifically when it is unpredictable which aneurysm has bled (Fig. 25–4), or when the therapeutic access to the ruptured aneurysm is prohibited by the location of another aneurysm (Fig. 25–5).[33] Depending on their origin, it is sometimes preferable to treat multiple aneurysms in the same intervention; this may be carried out by either surgical clipping or endovascular occlusion alone (Fig. 25–5).[34] Furthermore, in rare cases of rerupture or regrowth of previously treated aneurysms (e.g., because of misclipping or coil compaction), coils may be used after clips, or vice versa (Fig. 25–6).[35]

LIMITATIONS IN AND CONTRAINDICATIONS TO ENDOVASCULAR THERAPY

Limitations

The limitations of endovascular therapy are basically related to vascular morphology; vascular disorders; and the location, size, and configuration of the aneurysm to be embolized. The most essential limitations that constitute the main reasons for failure during endovascular therapeutic attempts at our institutions are as follows[29]:

- Vessel tortuosity and moderate arteriosclerosis.
- Stenosis of various etiologies.
- Very tiny aneurysms (<2 to 3 mm). The rate of failure has decreased since the introduction of softer coils.
- Large or giant aneurysms. As noted previously in "Pretherapeutic Evaluation and Indications," experience has demonstrated an increased rate of a subtotal occlusion (initial and final) in these aneurysms because of recanalization, coil compaction, and regrowth. Partially, this may be dependent on flow-related stress and preexisting thrombus within the aneurysm.
- Broad-based aneurysms in which the remodeling technique has failed or is less feasible.
- An acute inverse direction of the aneurysmal neck and sac in relation to the parent artery (most evident in aneurysms of the anterior communicating artery [ACoA]).
- Very distally located aneurysms, i.e., beyond the A1/A2 junction of the anterior cerebral artery (ACA), M2 segment of the middle cerebral artery (MCA), and P1 segment of the posterior communicating artery (PCA).
- Vasospasm not responsive to superselective papaverine infusion.
- Coil compaction leading to recanalization and regrowth of the aneurysm. For this reason, short- and long-term follow-up angiograms are compulsory. A definitive cure by means of either further coiling or clipping will be necessary if the previous occlusion is impermanent.

Most likely, these limitations will be reduced to a large extent or overcome by further development of coils, other embolic agents, and the different devices used. In this context, we would like to stress a major limitation of all procedures in interventional neuroradiology. The endovascular procedures are often time consuming and render a high dose of radiation to each patient treated. Long-term follow-up of these patients is not only scientifically interesting with regard to the permanence of aneurysmal obliteration, but is mandatory in order to analyze the consequences of such radiation doses.

Contraindications

True contraindications are rare. They include

- Poor clinical condition (Hunt and Hess Grades IV and V).
- Coagulation disorders and known adverse reaction to heparin.
- History of anaphylactic or severe adverse reaction to contrast material.
- Renal failure and other conditions restricting use of contrast agents.
- Cases in which the access to the aneurysm is truly prohibited or dangerous owing to vascular tortuosity and/or advanced arteriosclerotic disorders.

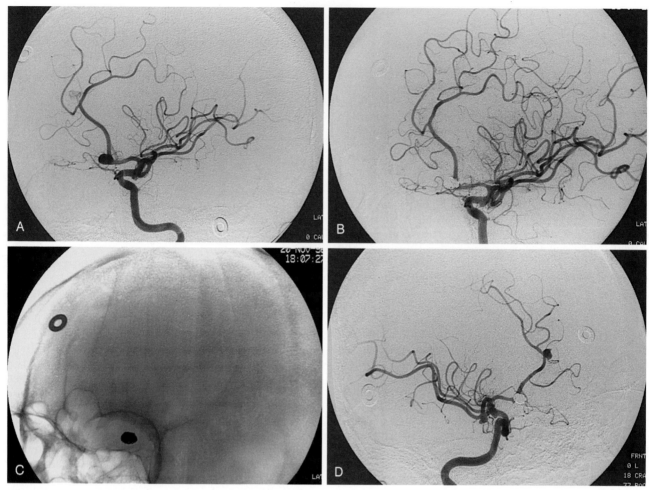

Figure 25-4. Same patient as in Figure 25-2. CT demonstrated a subarachnoid hemorrhage with a rather symmetric and bilateral distribution of the blood but with a slight predominance in the right sylvian fissure. Digital subtraction angiography showed multiple aneurysms. On the basis of the multiplicity, surgical accessibility, and uncertainty regarding which aneurysm had bled, a combination of endovascular and surgical therapy was proposed.

A to *C,* Lateral oblique projections of a left ICA angiogram demonstrate the ACoA aneurysm before and after coiling. (A faint opacification of a right-sided pericallosal artery aneurysm can be seen in (*A*).

D, Lateral oblique projection of the right ICA shows small berry aneurysms at the MCA bifurcation, at the pericallosal artery, and at the A1/A2 junction (just lateral to the coils). These additional aneurysms were successfully clipped by surgery 2 days after the endovascular procedure. The ACoA remained open.

- Diffuse and fusiform aneurysms (unless the intention is to occlude the parent artery[36]).
- Aneurysms in which it is impossible to distinguish the origin of the neck and its relation to adjacent branches (most common in MCA aneurysms).
- Severe vasospasm, either as a consequence of the SAH or induced by catheterization.

TECHNICAL DEVICES

Angiography Unit

Digital subtraction angiography (DSA) is necessary in interventional neuroradiology. A biplane angiographic unit is not mandatory but does facilitate the diagnostic and therapeutic procedures. Not only does it shorten the time spent to find the best projection for the endovascular procedure, it also allows a more exact morphologic evaluation and a safer packing of the aneurysm. The aim is to obtain an optimal visualization of the aneurysm sac, its configuration (size, direction), and its neck, in order to estimate the RSN. Fast subtraction rotational sequences are recommended whenever it is difficult to define the neck of the aneurysm and its relation to adjacent branches. High-quality fluoroscopy and roadmapping are crucial. Sufficient image-storing capacity is necessary for a true comparison of the angiograms taken before and after therapy as well as during the endovascular procedure. It is then possible to make continuous evaluation of the aneurysm packing, the relation of the coils to the parent artery, and the opacification of the more distal vascular tree, to avoid complications during the procedure.

GDC System

Guglielmi detachable coils are made of soft platinum alloy attached to a stainless steel delivery wire. All

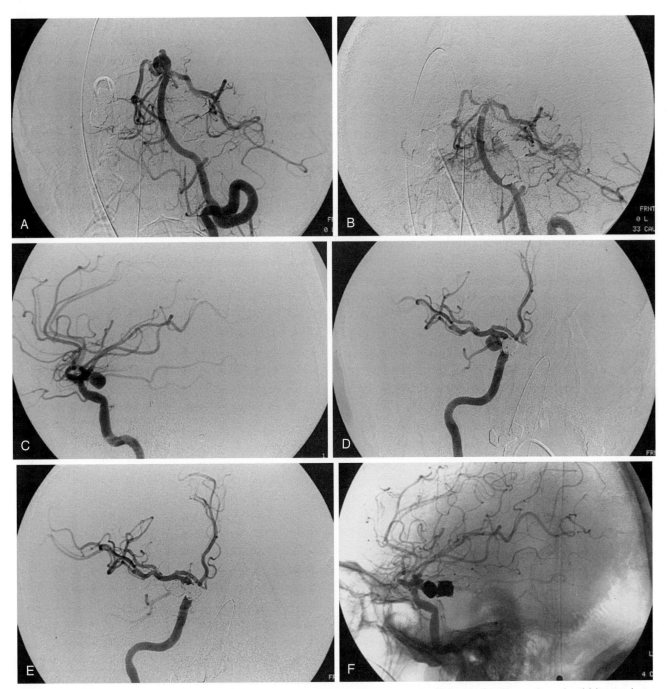

Figure 25-5. Case 4. Two closely related aneurysms were found on angiography in this patient with a subarachnoid hemorrhage. Surgical accessibility to the ruptured aneurysm was limited and regarded as hazardous because of the direction of the other aneurysm. Both aneurysms were treated by endovascular occlusion in the same procedure. *A* and *B,* Frontal projection of a left vertebral angiogram shows a basilar tip aneurysm before and after coiling. (Note the bleeding point at its dome in *A*).

C, An additional, closely related aneurysm was found at the origin of the posterior communicating artery (PCoA) on the right side (lateral ICA projection).

D and *E,* Frontal angiogram of the right ICA demonstrates the ICA aneurysm before and after treatment. (Coils within the basilar aneurysm are projected medially).

F, A nonsubtracted angiogram after therapy verifies the close aneurysmal location and the densely achieved packing of coils. Normal opacification of the PCoA was maintained.

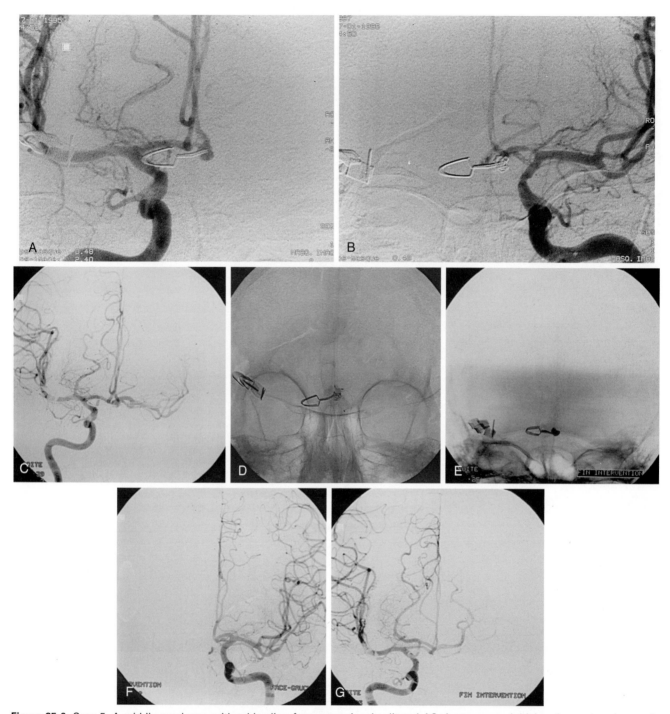

Figure 25-6. Case 5. A middle-aged man with rebleeding from a previously clipped ACoA aneurysm. Initial and repeat endovascular treatments were performed, with and without the remodeling technique (see Fig. 25-9). *A* and *B,* Frontal projections of a right and left ICA angiogram demonstrate a slipped clip and a small aneurysm. The remnant was occluded after coiling.
   C and *D,* A follow-up angiogram 6 months later showed aneurysmal regrowth, and a third treatment using the balloon protection technique was performed. The balloon is covering the aneurysmal ostium and protecting the left A1/A2 junction.
   E to *G,* Postprocedural images demonstrate a dense coil compaction, patent A1 and A2, and distal opacification within the anterior cerebral artery (ACA) circulation bilaterally.

coils are electrolytically detached by application of a low voltage current. Positioning or repositioning of the coils into the aneurysm has to be performed with utmost care and under direct fluoroscopic guidance.

Coils of various softness, helical diameter, and length are available. Appropriate sizes may be se-

lected for each individual aneurysm to be treated. Two types were initially manufactured (GDC-10 and GDC-18 standard coils), which varied in the diameter of the core wire and of the primary coil. To offer increased flexibility, new categories of softer coils have been developed, the GDC-10 Soft and GDC-18

Soft (coils with reduced diameter of the platinum core wire). Another generation of GDC is the two-diameter (2-D) coils, in which the first 1.5 loops of each coil have a smaller helical diameter, reduced to 75% of the stated coil diameter. The purpose of this design is to prevent the first edge of the coil from protruding into the parent artery. The 2-D coils are available in both coil sizes, GDC-10 and GDC-18.

Further coils are under development and clinical evaluation: the three-dimensional (GDC 3-D), with a more complex helical pattern, and the Vortx coils, with a progressively increased helical diameter. Both of these types of coils have been designed to achieve a more dense and complete obliteration of the aneurysmal sac. In the future, coils can probably be expected with incorporated fibers to increase their inherent thrombogenicity.

Guide Catheters

In the selection of the guide catheter, several factors have to be taken into consideration. Anatomic factors such as size, angulation, and tortuosity of the internal carotid artery (ICA) or vertebral artery (VA), as well as the conditions within the aortic arch, are all of great importance. It is often necessary to have the guide catheter placed fairly distally in the parent artery (ICA or VA) to obtain a stable position. Such a position facilitates microcatheterization and coil insertion and decreases the risks of mechanically induced vasospasm, dissection, and thromboembolic complications. The torqueability, stiffness, and coating are all factors that influence the maneuverability and behavior of the catheter.

Special care has to be taken in circumstances of small, narrow vessels and in situations of vasospasm induced during catheterization. In these conditions, catheters with a rigid tip should be avoided and replaced by others with a progressive and soft distal end or with a more smooth, hydrophilic coating.

One of the most crucial decisions to make is to select a catheter with a sufficiently large inner diameter. A large lumen facilitates microcatheterization, enables a continuous flush, and makes optimal roadmaps and control angiograms possible during the procedure. The 6-Fr. guide catheters generally comply with these requests and are the most commonly used. Several guide catheters are on the market with equal or almost comparable qualities, but the standard catheter by Balt and the Envoy (Cordis Corp.) are the most frequently used in our institutions. The Balt catheter is generally easy to handle and stable, especially in the situation of an acute angulation at the origin of the aortic arch. Owing to its rather rigid character, it is not convenient in tortuous, narrow, and spastic vessels. The Envoy is not quite as stable but is easily maneuvered and less traumatic because of its softer distal tip. During catheterization, the guide catheter should be connected to a hemostatic valve, and when it is positioned, a continuous flush of saline should be maintained to prevent retrograde

blood flow and reduce the risks of fibrin formation or clotting.

Microcatheters

A variety of different microcatheters have been designed to deliver the coils into the aneurysmal sac. The TRACKER-18 and TRACKER-10 microcatheters (Target Therapeutics) are made to be used together with the various GDC-18 and GDC-10 coils, respectively.

Resistance is not an uncommon problem during microcatheterization and is sometimes predictable. It is mainly a consequence of vascular morphology—tortuosity—or an inappropriate positioning of the guide catheter. Occasionally, it depends on the coating of the different catheters used. By repositioning the guide catheter, or by selecting a guide and/or microcatheter with a more hydrophilic coating, catheterization may be facilitated and friction avoided or reduced. Further, larger microcatheters such as the TRACKER-18, and especially the hydrophilic-coated FasTRACKER-18, are sometimes easier to maneuver than the smaller TRACKER-10 catheters of the same type. This is often the case in conditions of tortuous, dysplastic vessels and in patients with severe vasospasm.

In vessels with marked curvature, the TRACKER-18 microcatheter has a tendency to distort. This distortion deforms its inner lumen, results in persistent friction during coil passage, and makes the procedure more difficult. It may also lead to coil stretching and increased risk of coil breakage and migration. The TRACKER-10 microcatheters are more resistant to acute vessel angulation than the TRACKER-18. Most recently, we have used the Slipstream microcatheters (Medtronic/MIS) more regularly. These seem more easy to maneuver and are less vulnerable to deformation in tortuous vessels.

Regardless of the microcatheter chosen, it is usually preferable to make a small curve at its tip. This is done over steam while maintaining a continuous flow of saline through the microcatheter to prevent "kinking." Excessive steam shaping has to be avoided, since this may cause shrinkage of the catheter tip, lumen, and length. The shape of the curve has to be individually formed according to the origin of the neck, its direction, and the size of the aneurysmal sac. The intention is threefold. First, it facilitates access into the aneurysm. Second, it anchors the microcatheter in the aneurysmal sac, making it more stable. Third, it may prevent the first loop from bulging directly into the fragile wall or bleeding point.

Microwires

The choice of microwire follows to a certain extent the type of microcatheter chosen. A flexible, soft, shapeable, and atraumatic tip, together with low friction and reliable steerability, characterize the optimal guidewire, but the combination of these qualities is not easily provided. We prefer to use the Terumo

0.016″ and 0.010″ microwires (distributed in the United States by Medi-Tech, Inc.). This preference is based on the unique combination of excellent torqueability and a hydrophilic coating. On the other hand, these have a rather stiff, preformed tip that is impossible to reshape. These factors increase the risk of causing traumatic injuries to the vessel wall and aneurysmal sac. For these reasons, other wires with a formable and flexible tip of a less traumatic character, such as the Taper, Dasher, or Seeker Light (all from Target Therapeutics), or the Transcend (Medi-Tech, Inc.) can be used.

PROCEDURE

Anesthesia

All procedures are performed with the patient under general anesthesia. A fully cooperative patient throughout the treatment is rarely possible, since endovascular therapy is a time-consuming procedure, and is utterly dependent on the medical condition of the patient. Further, the endovascular technique requires exact, reproducible projections and roadmaps for the safety of the patient and the therapeutic process.

Editor's Note: The anesthesiologist/anesthetist must be aware of the need to avoid transient blood pressure spikes, especially when awakening and extubating a patient after GDC or AVM treatment. It is at this point that aberrations in blood pressure, which otherwise had been carefully controlled, may occur, with potentially disastrous results.

Anticoagulation

All endovascular treatment of intracranial aneurysms should be performed with the patient fully heparinized to minimize the risk of thromboembolic complications.[37] The timing and regimen of heparinization differ from one endovascular center to another. Some institutions prefer to delay heparin infusion until the first or the second coil has been placed within the aneurysmal sac. Heparin can be given either intravenously or intra-arterially (i.e., added to the continuous infusion of saline maintained in the guide and microcatheter).

In our institutions, heparin is given intravenously as soon as the decision to proceed with coil embolization is made, even in cases of recently ruptured aneurysms. Heparinization is begun with an intravenous bolus of 5000 U followed by a continuous infusion of 2500 to 3000 U/hr to achieve an activated clotting time (ACT) of two or three times the normal level. Postoperatively, heparinization is continued for 1 or 2 days, with an average dose of approximately 700 U/hr. Low-molecular-weight heparin is then given subcutaneously for 2 to 8 days, depending on whether the coils are protruding into or interfering with the parent artery, on whether there are thromboembolic complications, and on the location of the aneurysm treated. Thus, we tend to keep patients with MCA aneurysms on prolonged anticoagulation when the

aneurysm has a close relation with M2 branches. In addition, all patients, except those with recently ruptured aneurysms, are given aspirin intravenously, in a single dose of 250 mg, in the early phase of the procedure.

Editor's Note: Protamine (100 mg) should be kept on hand, drawn up and ready to inject when one is systemically anticoagulating a patient with an AVM or aneurysm. Other patients may be prone to clotting, particularly those who have just bled and those with posterior fossa abnormalities, so be prepared for these eventualities as well.

Preoperative Medication

Editor's Note: Premedication of unruptured or subacute ruptured aneurysms with nitropaste and aspirin should be considered.

The issue of heparinization during GDC use is far from resolved. Questions remain regarding points such as what protocols should be used for ruptured versus unruptured aneurysms and how long should the patient be kept heparinized after the procedure. A prospective study is needed to determine what is the greater risk—thromboembolic phenomena or hemorrhage.

For any procedure involving potential embolic and ischemic consequences, nimodipine (60 mg PO) is a good preoperative adjunct.

Giant Aneurysm Mass Effect

The mass effect and swelling seen after aneurysm coiling may respond to steroids and mannitol. It has been shown experimentally that a thrombosed aneurysm can swell 10% to 15%. This is particularly true with basilar tip aneurysms, which can have profound mass effect. Cranial nerve deficits may be caused by this swelling and mass effect rather than by occlusion of perforators. Therefore, when treating giant aneurysms, premedication with steroids is indicated (100 mg methylprednisolone sodium succinate bolus IV every 8 hours), with continuation of therapy for up to 2 weeks, depending on symptoms.

Microcatheterization and Positioning

The microwire should precede the tip of the microcatheter when entering the aneurysm. It is crucial to make sure that the tension within the catheter is eliminated as soon as it is in place. For this reason, withdrawal of the microwire from the distal part of the microcatheter has to be done with utmost caution and under fluoroscopic guidance.

The best position of the microcatheter depends on the diameter of the aneurysm. In most situations, it is suitable to have the tip placed in the proximal portion or in the middle of the sac. In smaller aneurysms (<3 mm in diameter) we tend to deploy the coils with the microcatheter positioned at the very origin of the aneurysm neck to reduce resistance and facilitate the formation of the coils.

The tension of the microcatheter varies during the procedure, especially during coil maneuvering. This tension is often more severe in smaller aneurysms, in aneurysms with a sharp angle at the origin, and in aneurysms directed in an opposite direction to the parent artery (retrograde to the flow and the microcatheter). Normally, this tension tends to build toward the end of the procedure, when most of the aneurysm is packed with coils and when the remaining part is in close relation to the aneurysm neck. Tension may also be induced in cases in which the neck has an eccentric location in relation to the sac and the direction of the parent artery. In such aneurysms, the positioning of the microcatheter is limited, and the spontaneous and flexible movements of its tip (repositioning) are restricted during coil delivery. Increased counterpressure, resistance, and an unequal distribution of the coils will follow (denser around the tip).

Tension not only increases the risks of the procedure, it also creates microcatheter instability, with increased risk of the catheter refluxing out of the aneurysmal sac or perforation. The stored tension may be removed by a slight withdrawal of the microcatheter and coil simultaneously, or of the catheter alone. It is occasionally beneficial to exit out of the neck with the microcatheter while keeping the coil extruded into the sac. The coil can then be used as a "guide" device to navigate the microcatheter into a new position. The same technique applies when there is an involuntary reflux of the microcatheter. The changed location allows for less tension and contributes to a more complete filling of the aneurysm.

Coil Characteristics and Selection

The choice of coils needs to be based on their individual character and the configuration of the aneurysm.

GDC-18 Standard Coils

These coils are meant to be used for large or giant aneurysms and are more stable and rigid than the GDC-10 coils. Owing to their larger coil wire dimension and primary coil diameter, GDC-18 coils are likely to be more resistant to further stresses caused by pulsatile blood flow directed toward the region of the aneurysm neck. However, the rigidity of GDC-18 coils in combination with vessel tortuosity, acute angles, and gradually increased aneurysmal coil compaction sometimes causes severe resistance during coil manipulation. Occasionally, these difficulties can be overcome either by deploying a coil of the same helical diameter but of a shorter length, or by exchange of the microcatheter used. Sometimes, it is advantageous to select softer coils at the end of the procedure to reduce the friction and facilitate final closure of the aneurysm.

GDC-18 Soft Coils

These are 59% softer than GDC-18 standard coils and almost as soft as GDC-10 standard coils. They are supposed to be used as the primary coil for smaller or large aneurysms, or in combination with GDC-18 standard coils in large and giant aneurysms. Because of their softness, they are less traumatic to the aneurysmal wall and are consequently more appropriate in certain cases of recently ruptured aneurysms. Use of GDC-18 Soft coils may avoid the many of the disadvantages associated with GDC-18 standard coils. So far, we have preferred to work with GDC-10 coils whenever possible.

GDC-10 Standard Coils

These are meant to be used in small or medium-sized aneurysms (<15 mm in diameter). Owing to the use of smaller-diameter coil wire and smaller primary coil diameter, GDC-10 coils are softer and less rigid than GDC-18 coils. For these reasons, GDC-10 coils are favored by us whenever we treat recently ruptured aneurysms and whenever the remodeling technique is used to treat an aneurysm (ruptured or unruptured). The combination of a TRACKER-10 and the GDC-10 coils should always be considered in situations when there is persistent friction during insertion of GDC-18 coils through a TRACKER-18 microcatheter.

GDC-10 Soft Coils

These were developed to be used in small, recently ruptured aneurysms, but they are also recommended in cases of smaller aneurysms (≤2 to 3 mm) in which three or fewer coils are needed. These coils may be combined with GDC-10 standard coils to obtain a dense coil compaction. However, the soft coils are more fragile and vulnerable to stretching during manipulation; specific precautions must be taken when they are delivered into an aneurysm previously filled with GDC-10 standard coils.

GDC-18 and GDC-10 Two-Diameter (2-D) Coils

These are designed to decrease the risks of having the leading edge of the coil return into the parent artery. An additional advantage is that they may be used in acutely ruptured aneurysms whenever the leading edge of the standcard coils tends to direct toward the point of rupture.

Editor's Note: These are the coils of choice for forming the "basket." They do not tend to exit the aneurysm or puncture the wall as readily as standard coils do. Once these have been placed, the center of the basket can be filled with smaller-size coils.

General Strategy of Coil Placement

The purpose of the first coil is twofold: (1) to create a supporting framework for the subsequent coils and (2) to bridge the aneurysm neck in order to prevent coil migration (Fig. 25–7). The helical size and length of the first coil to be delivered into the aneurysm have to be selected with regard to the configuration of the aneurysm. The first coil has to be as large and long as possible. Its size should correspond to the largest diameter of the aneurysmal sac and should not be less than the width of the ostium. On the other hand, it is fundamental to balance this with the need to keep the tension on the fragile wall to a minimum. An exchange from a standard coil to a 2-D coil can be made if the leading edge of the first coil has a tendency to dislodge into the parent artery.

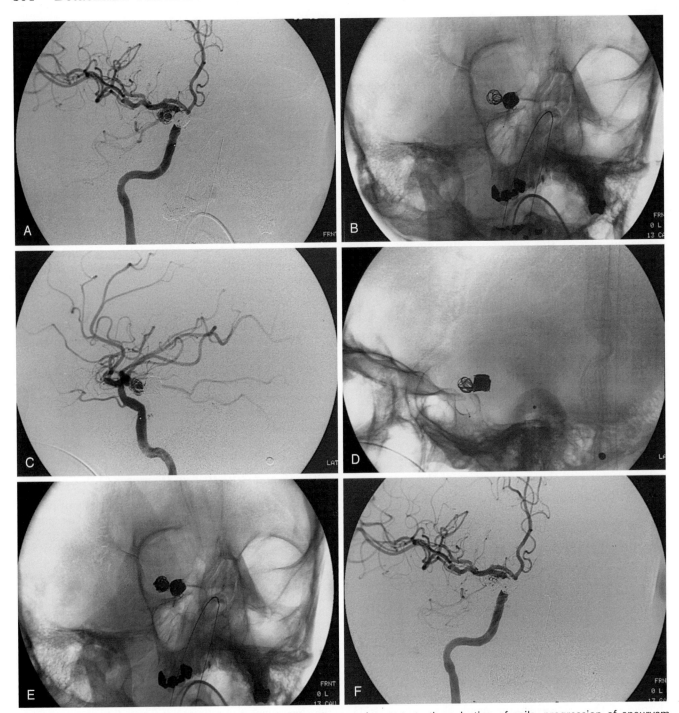

Figure 25-7. Same patient as in Figs. 25-2 and 25-4. These images demonstrate the selection of coils, progression of aneurysm obliteration, and coil compaction. *A to D,* Frontal and lateral projection. Two GDC-10 standard coils are positioned in the aneurysm. The helical diameter is adjusted to the diameter of the aneurysmal sac. Coils are bridging the aneurysm neck.
   E and *F,* Further coils are placed in the aneurysm with a reduced opacification and an increased coil compaction toward its origin.

To achieve an optimal covering of the entire inner surface of the aneurysm, it is usually preferable for the second coil delivered to be of the same helical diameter, but not necessarily of the same length. However, this is not always possible and is utterly dependent on the size of the aneurysm. It is important to have a smooth coil delivery, and a coil of smaller helical diameter should be considered whenever a persistent resistance develops.

A progressive and dense angiographic obliteration of the aneurysm is then achieved by additional coils of successively reduced helical diameter and length. In this manner, the filling is intentionally generated from the periphery toward the center and base of the aneurysmal pouch. A combination of standard and soft coils is sometimes beneficial in order to achieve a tight coil compaction. This strategy is generally applied in small (<15 mm) and large (≥15 and <25

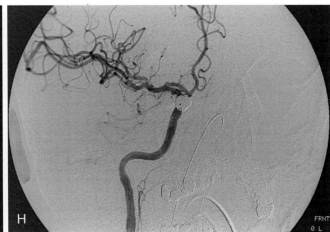

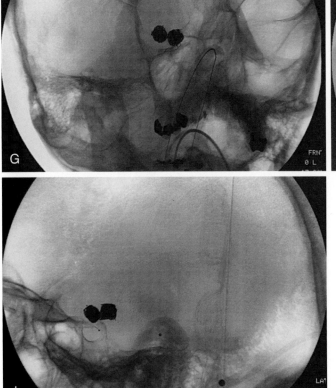

Figure 25-7 *Continued. G* to *I,* The aneurysm is finally totally occluded, its orifice angiographically covered and a dense coil compaction obtained.

mm) aneurysms, but occasionally it must be modified according to the circumstances present. If the aneurysmal sac has a narrow and elliptic "sausage-like" appearance, the principles guiding the selection of coils are entirely different. In such aneurysms, the helical size of the first coil has to be adjusted to the smaller sac diameter, and it is consequently almost impossible to bridge the neck with this coil. The subsequent coils need to be of similar or almost similar size and length to obtain a progressive obliteration of the aneurysm, accomplished from its dome toward the neck. Specific precautions with regard to the last coil have to be stressed, as this coil generally emerges in close relation to the aneurysm orifice, predominantly in smaller aneurysms. The choice of helical diameter of this coil must be based on the arrangement of the previous coils, and if necessary the diameter should exceed the size of the ostium to bridge the neck. An inappropriate selection of coil renders a potential risk of peri- or post-procedural dislodgment, which may lead to coil migration and further complications.

Since the introduction of the Magnet Exchange Device (Medi-Tech, Inc.), a combination of GDC-18 and GDC-10 coils may be considered for large aneurysms. In such cases, the GDC-18 coils are the initial coils to be deployed. Owing to their rigidity, they form a more solid nest with a larger resistance against the stress created by pulsatile blood flow. A Transcend-EX microwire (Medi-Tech, Inc.) is then placed into the aneurysm and kept in this position while it is connected to the magnet. This system allows an exchange to a microcatheter applicable to the GDC-10 coils without losing access to the aneurysmal sac.

GDC-10 coils are softer than GDC-18 coils; they are usually easier to pack and create less tension within the microcatheter and aneurysm during positioning. These qualities make them easier to compress, and thus the expansile forces against the aneurysmal wall are kept to a minimum. Moreover, these inherent characteristics facilitate the obtaining of a dense packing of the aneurysmal sac.

Before detachment of each coil, a control angiogram should be obtained to ensure a stable and appropriate coil formation and maintenance of the parent artery, and to observe the distal vascular tree. Movement of the coils may indicate the potential for migration once detached.

Precautions Related to Coil and Microcatheter Manipulation

Stretching is always an potential risk because of the delicate character of GDC coils and may be a precursor to breakage and coil migration. Generally, this is caused by factors creating tension, friction, or resistance during coil deployment. To avoid these problems, the main issue is to analyze and understand when, why, and how resistance and tension occur. Most of the predisposing factors have already been mentioned; these include tortuosity, acute curvature, and an adverse direction of the aneurysm in relation to the parent artery. Other major causes are acute orientation of the coil in relation to the microcatheter tip during coil maneuvering, inappropriate guide catheter or microcatheter positioning, and excessive coil manipulations (advancement or retraction). In addition to stretching, coil breakage or migration may result from premature coil detachment due to excessive manipulation and rotation of the delivery wire.

GDC-10 coils are more vulnerable to stretching, especially if used with a catheter of incompatible size (e.g., when the inner diameter is too large compared with the coil diameter). Prevention and management of stored tension and resistance will be made easier if the technical advice given above concerning coil and microcatheter manipulations is followed. Nevertheless, before coil retraction, withdrawal of the microcatheter within the sac is often necessary to ensure that the alignment of the tip and coil is accurate. If resistance or stretching persists, the microcatheter and coil should be removed as a unit. A simultaneous withdrawal of the guide catheter is sometimes necessary.

An additional important factor is clot or fibrin formation within the microcatheter or around the coil. Clotting not only increases the risk of thromboembolic complications, but also induces resistance during coil maneuvering. To reduce the possibility of clotting or fibrin formation, a continuous flush should be maintained through the microcatheter.

Considerations for Specific Circumstances

The Balloon Protection Technique: Remodeling of the Parent Vessel Wall

Indications

The remodeling or balloon protection technique was first presented by the author (JM) at the 20th Congress of the European Society of Neuroradiology (ESNR) in Nancy, France in 1994. The technique was developed to overcome the difficulties and limitations of the endovascular therapeutic approach in broad-based aneurysms (poor RSN) (Fig. 25–8A). In aneurysms with a poor RSN, it is usually impossible to form a stable coil nest, maintain the coils within the aneurysmal sac, and/or obtain a dense coil compaction without the risk of sacrificing the parent artery. Coils may protrude or dislodge into the parent artery, and there is an increased risk of clot formation.

The advantages of the balloon protection method are that it offers the possibility of achieving a stable coil formation and a more dense obliteration of the

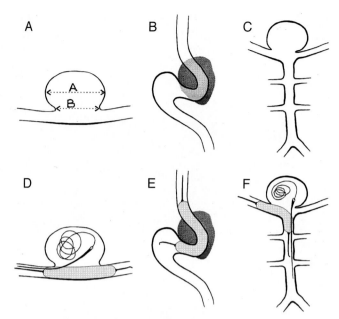

Figure 25-8. Schematic drawings illustrating three indications for the remodeling technique. *A,* Broad-necked aneurysm. There is a poor ratio between the aneurysmal (A) and neck (B) diameter. *B,* Poor visualization of the aneurysm neck and its relation to the parent artery (the aneurysm is illustrated in gray). *C,* A rather broad-based basilar artery (BA) aneurysm with its neck extending out to the right P1 segment (adjacent branch). *D* to *F,* Corresponding illustrations with a Solstice balloon inflated in the parent artery. The balloon is covering the aneurysm orifice, and the microcatheter with a coil is positioned in the aneurysm.

sac in such aneurysms, while maintaining the patency of the parent artery. It also minimizes the risk of coil migration and thromboembolic complications.

The remodeling technique may also be used in other situations, such as in aneurysms in which a true delineation of the neck and its relation to the parent artery is unclear (Fig. 25–8B) and in conditions where the neck of the aneurysm extends out into the proximal segment of an adjacent branch, creating a risk of having the coils obliterate this branch (Fig. 25–8C). The latter situation is not uncommon when dealing with basilar tip aneurysms with their close relation to the P1 segments of the PCAs (Fig. 25–8C).

Initially, this technique was restricted to aneurysms within larger vessels such as the supraclinoid portion of the ICA, the VA, and the basilar artery (BA) trunk or tip. However, with the Solstice occlusion balloon microcatheter (Medtronic/MIS), it is now possible to use this technique in smaller vessels distal to the circle of Willis. The Solstice catheter has an over-the-wire design that facilitates microcatheterization, renders better access to distal vessels, and offers a more stable and precise positioning of the balloon

We once used a latex balloon (BAL1, nonradiopaque), which we mounted and glued on a flow-guided, single-lumen, Magic 3F/1.8F microcatheter (both manufactured by Balt Extrusion). This device has now more or less been abandoned (Fig. 25–9).

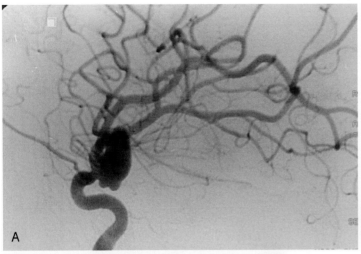

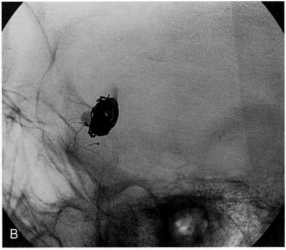

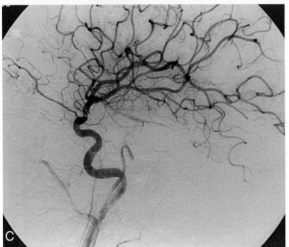

Figure 25-9. Case 6. The balloon protection technique (old variant) *A,* A lateral projection of a right ICA angiogram shows a large aneurysm with a vague delineation of its orifice.

B and *C,* A latex balloon glued on a Magic microcatheter is temporarily inflated in the parent ICA artery at the level of the aneurysm neck. Several GDC-10 coils have been positioned through a TRACKER-10 microcatheter placed in the aneurysm. A final angiogram after the procedure demonstrates a complete occlusion of the aneurysm with preservation of the parent artery.

Initial Approach

A bifemoral approach is necessary. Through the 6-Fr. introducer sheaths, two 6-Fr. guide catheters are inserted and positioned within the common carotid artery (CCA) and ICA or in both VAs, depending on the location of the aneurysm to be treated. In cases of one dominant and one small or abnormal (hypogenetic) VA, one of the guide catheters may be positioned in the ipsilateral subclavian artery close to the origin of the VA. Generally, the guide catheter for the microcatheter delivering the coils has to be positioned most distally in the ICA or VA. The guidewire used with the Solstice catheter is then navigated distally (i.e., beyond the location of the aneurysm neck) in order to "anchor" the balloon at its correct position (Fig. 25–10). Thus, the balloon catheter can be safely placed in such a position that it overlaps the ostium of the aneurysm.

How to Use a Solstice Catheter

The introduction of the Solstice microangioplasty balloon catheter has made it much easier to utilize the protection technique. Proper use of this balloon, however, requires meticulous technique.

The balloon microcatheter is flushed with a two-

thirds solution of contrast in normal saline. A Y-connector is placed on the hub of the catheter. A 3-foot or 6-foot microextension tube is attached to the Y-connector, and a 20-cc syringe filled with two-thirds contrast in normal saline is connected to the tubing. The uncurved Quicksilver-10 wire (Medtronic/MIS) is placed through the Y-connector and advanced into the balloon catheter to a point about 5 cm from the end. The 20-cc syringe is used to flush all bubbles out of the Y-connector, and then the valve is tightened around the wire. The infusion is continued until all bubbles are out of the catheter and thus the entire system.

One should allow a minute for the fluid to exit the top of the catheter; it takes time for the system pressure to equalize. Once this has occurred, it is possible to advance the wire out of the tip of the catheter and then to place a curve on it. The wire should then be withdrawn inside the microcatheter so that the tip of the wire is just within the tip of the catheter; this allows the catheter to be placed through the Y-connector of the guide catheter.

Because this balloon is *not* pressure dependent but rather volume dependent, accurate control of volume is indicated. *This can best be performed using a 1-cc syringe filled with the same two-thirds contrast in*

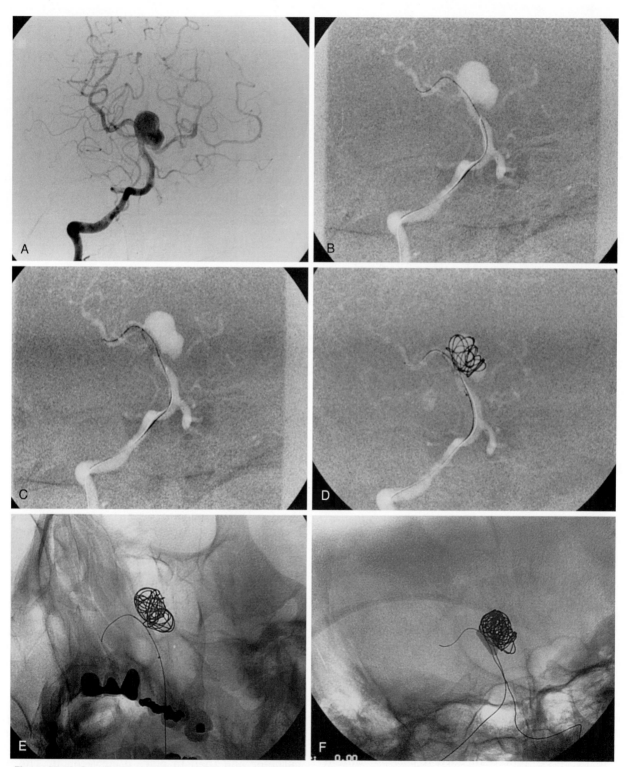

Figure 25-10. Case 7. Aneurysmal occlusion using the balloon protection or remodeling technique. *A* to *C*, Large and broad-based BA tip aneurysm. The Solstice catheter is advanced through the right vertebral artery, with the microwire anchored in the right P1 segment. The balloon is inflated and bridging the aneurysm neck.

D and *E*, The first coils have been delivered into the aneurysm with the balloon inflated. The balloon is then deflated to ensure patency of the parent artery and coil nest stability.

F and *G*, Further coils have been detached in the aneurysm. The balloon is inflated and a coil is positioned in the aneurysm via the left vertebral artery. A subtotal occlusion with a noteworthy flow reduction was obtained.

Case 7 continues

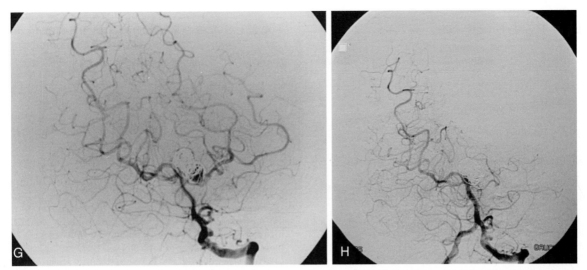

Figure 25-10 *H,* A follow-up angiogram and repeat treatment were scheduled some months afterward, but the aneurysm had spontaneously thrombosed. The left P1 segment was occluded, but the posterior cerebral artery (PCA) was fed by the left PCoA. No neurologic deficits were noted.

normal saline solution attached to the end of the microextension tubing.

The Occlusion Procedure

The Solstice catheter is advanced through its guide catheter to a position distal to the aneurysm.

The other microcatheter (with two tip markers) is then brought into the aneurysmal sac. The Solstice balloon is positioned over the aneurysm neck and inflated. The balloon follows the contour of the parent artery, covers the origin of the neck, and may be regarded as a "pseudowall" of the aneurysm, exerting counterpressure when the coils are delivered into the aneurysmal sac. Thus, it is possible to bridge the neck and create a basket/framework of the first coil within the aneurysmal sac. Further, because of the counterpressure, the helices of the coil will maintain a tight contact against the true aneurysmal wall. Altogether, these factors, in combination with the induced tension between the coil and aneurysmal wall, will make the framework stable, with a reduced tendency to be repositioned or dislodged out of the aneurysmal sac.

The balloon occlusion should not last more than 2 to 4 minutes. As soon as a coil is inserted, the balloon is slowly deflated while one observes for coil movement, to avoid ischemic events. This is followed by an angiogram to assess the position and configuration of the coil before detachment is initiated. If these are satisfactory, the coil is detached. The balloon is reinflated before withdrawal of the delivery wire of the detached coil, then deflated slightly. The next coil is advanced into the aneurysm, and the balloon is inflated fully. The coil is then positioned and deployed in the same manner as the first coil.

The same procedure is followed before and after each coil is delivered into the aneurysm. Once the first few coils have been placed, it may be possible to withdraw the delivery wire with the balloon only partially inflated. The balloon should be partially deflated and the wire slowly withdrawn. If there is no coil movement, the wire can be withdrawn fully. The coils bridging the aneurysm neck will generally follow the side of the balloon, parallel to the parent artery. When the balloon is removed, the coils will form the wall of the parent artery; this vessel remains open without any coils obliterating adjacent branches (see Fig. 25–6 *C* to *G*). Removal of the microcatheter from the aneurysm should be performed with the balloon inflated or partially inflated to prevent dislodgment of the coils out of the sac.

Generally, GDC-10 standard coils are preferable because of their softer, less rigid qualities. However, since the introduction of the Magnet Exchange Device, a combination of the GDC-18 and GDC-10 coils may be considered for large aneurysms.

Results

Our results using this technique are promising and are presented in Tables 25–1 to 25–8.[38] To analyze the results of the remodeling technique, these results were compared with those of a series of 236 berry aneurysms (<1.5 cm) in 208 patients treated with GDC coils ("normal" GDC treatment) from November 1992 to November 1996.

So far, we have had no post-procedural events of coil migration on either a short- or long-term basis. With this technique, the rate of complications is similar to the overall rate of complications for endovascular coiling of aneurysms. The remodeling technique, however, is more difficult to perform than "normal" GDC therapy and is associated with certain risks; it is therefore recommended only for those practitioners with extensive experience in neurointerventional procedures.

Recently Ruptured Aneurysm

The endovascular approach to a recently ruptured aneurysm is not much different from our routine strategy. However, since there may be an increased

T A B L E 2 5 - 1   Final Results

Occlusion Rate	Remodeling Technique	Normal GDC Treatment
Total	40 (77%)	157 (77%)
Subtotal	9 (17%)	35 (17%)
Incomplete	3 (6%)	12 (6%)
Total	52	205

The occlusion rate was classified as

- 100%, or total occlusion, when the sac and neck were angiographically observed to be densely packed with no contrast visible.
- 95% to 99%, or subtotal occlusion, when the sac was occluded but had an obvious but very small neck remnant or possible neck remnant.
- <95%, or incomplete occlusion, when loose packing and persistent opacification of the sac or neck remnant were angiographically observed.

*Last follow-up angiography or post-procedural results for the patients not yet controlled. Comparison between the remodeling technique and normal GDC treatment.

risk of perforation and rebleeding, specific precautions have to be taken. Tension within the microcatheter and during coil positioning has to be kept to a minimum. In a recently ruptured aneurysm, it may occasionally be preferable to start with a 2-D coil because of the smaller helical diameter of its first 1.5 loops. This type of coil usually exits into the sac without sliding along the inside of the aneurysmal wall. Consequently, the risk of having the leading tip directed toward the bleeding point may be avoided. Whenever the helical diameter of the initial coil chosen appears to be one size too small, the strategy has to be evaluated with regard to the preexisting RSN. If the ratio is good (≥1.5), it is sometimes better to detach and leave the coil in place in order to avoid a rebleed, which may result from a sudden increase of flow and pressure within the aneurysm during coil removal. The procedure is then continued with a new coil of the same size or, if possible, one size larger. However, if the ratio is poor (<1.2), one is obliged to make a coil exchange to reduce the risk of coil migration out of the sac.

Editor's Note: Treatment of an acutely ruptured aneurysm by GDC for protection purposes is successful only if the aneurysm actually thromboses. The coil packing must be tight enough to prevent swirling of blood within the cavity.

Anticoagulation during these procedures is even more of a controversy than during a routine procedure. A rational approach may be to begin heparin only after placement of

T A B L E 2 5 - 2   Final Results Depending on the Size of the Aneurysmal Neck

Occlusion Rate	Neck ≤4 mm	Neck >4 mm	Total
Total	24 (92%)	16 (61%)	40 (77%)
Subtotal	1 (4%)	8 (31%)	9 (17%)
Incomplete	1 (4%)	2 (8%)	3 (6%)
Total	26	26	52

T A B L E 2 5 - 3   Final Results Depending on the Size of the Aneurysmal Sac

Occlusion Rate	Sac <5 mm	Sac 5–10 mm	Sac 10–15 mm	Sac >15 mm
Total	17 (100%)	14 (82%)	7 (50%)	2 (50%)
Subtotal	–	3 (18%)	5 (35%)	1 (25%)
Incomplete	–	—	2 (15%)	1 (25%)
Total	17	17	14	4

the first coil and to use a slightly lowered bolus (3000 to 5000 units rather than 5000 to 10,000 units). Alternatively, some practitioners prefer to simply run their heparinized saline flush at a very high rate to achieve a local anticoagulation effect. Of course, this local effect is in exactly the location that is of greatest concern, the intracranial vasculature. The previously described bolus dose of protamine, already drawn up and ready to use if needed, is recommended.

Multiple Aneurysms

Patients presenting with multiple aneurysms may be treated by surgery, endovascular therapy alone, or a combination of both. Only one aneurysm should be treated by endovascular means during a single procedure if the aneurysms are located within the same artery or vascular region. However, if the aneurysms are distributed in different regions, such as within the anterior and posterior circulation or supratentorially but bilaterally, one may consider treating multiple aneurysms during the same intervention.

Vasospasm

Vasospasm is a known complication and one of the major attributes to delayed ischemia that may follow an SAH. Clinical and/or angiographically verified vasospasm is to some degree a limiting factor for both surgical and endovascular treatment of intracranial aneurysms in the subacute phase. This limitation is generally less important in regard to the endovascular approach. Microcatheterization with access to the aneurysm is often possible despite vasospasm. Nevertheless, microcatheterization may be difficult, and the presence of the catheter within the narrow lumen may further compromise the already stressed cerebral perfusion, especially in cases of severe vasoconstriction. However, a superselective, intra-arterial infusion of a spasmolytic drug, such as papaverine, may be performed through the microcatheter.[39, 40] Papaverine induces a temporary vasodilation, thus si-

T A B L E 2 5 - 4   Size of the Aneurysmal Neck Depending on the Size of the Sac

Aneurysmal Neck	Sac >5 mm	Sac 5–10 mm	Sac 10–15 mm	Sac >15 mm
≤4 mm	16*	9	1	0
>4 mm	1	8	13	4
Total	17	17	14	4

*These figures represent the number of aneurysms with the particular combination of aneurysm and neck size.

T A B L E 2 5 - 5 Final Results Depending on the Ratio Between the Aneurysmal Sac Diameter and the Size of the Neck (RSN)

Occlusion Rate	RSN <1.5	RSN >1.5	Total
Total	30 (94%)	10 (50%)	40 (77%)
Subtotal	2 (6%)	7 (35%)	9 (17%)
Incomplete	—	3 (15%)	3 (6%)
Total	32	20	52

T A B L E 2 5 - 7 Frequency of Perioperative Rupture and Clinical Outcome with the Remodeling Technique and Normal GDC Treatment

	Remodeling Technique	Normal GDC Treatment
Perioperative rupture	3/58 procedures (5%)	6/249 procedures (2.5%)
Clinical outcome	3 asymptomatic	4 asymptomatic 2 deaths (2/189 patients: 1%)

multaneously generating increased perfusion and a better availability to the aneurysm.

Our management strategy in circumstances of moderate or severe vasospasm is as follows: if catheterization is possible, one or two coils are initially positioned within the aneurysmal sac to reduce the flow and protect the dome from a rebleed (Fig. 25–11). The microcatheter is then withdrawn from the aneurysm, placed proximally within the constricted artery, and flushed with saline (to prevent crystal formation) before papaverine infusion is started. Papaverine (200 to 300 mg in 50 ml of normal saline) is then given by slow manual injection. The aneurysm is re-entered and obliteration is continued by placement of additional coils. To facilitate catheterization, a papaverine infusion may occasionally be considered before coil protection. However, this should be avoided and, if absolutely necessary, restricted to those patients with severe vasoconstriction and an urgent need for aneurysm occlusion.

When the aneurysm is densely packed and protected from a rebleed, a more aggressive postoperative management of vasospasm and delayed ischemia may be initiated in the intensive care unit. It is not always possible to achieve a complete aneurysmal occlusion in these extreme situations, and a subtotal obliteration may be acceptable in rare cases, as long as the dome is satisfactorily protected. Definitive treatment, surgical or endovascular, has to follow as soon as permitted by the medical condition of the patient.

COMPLICATIONS AND THEIR MANAGEMENT

The causes of complications are multifactorial; the experience and skill of the physician, the different kinds of devices used, and the duration of the endovascular procedure are some critical factors. However, aneurysm location is probably the most important individual factor, whereas the size of the aneurysm appears to be of less importance. Other essential factors are the maintenance of continuous flush through the various catheters used and the regimen of heparinization.

Thromboembolism

Thromboembolic events are the most common complications during the endovascular treatment of aneurysms and are by far the most important cause of permanent morbidity in those patients treated. Most thromboembolic complications are reported to occur in patients with aneurysms in the anterior circulation (most frequently within the MCA and its branches). In spite of systemic heparinization, this may happen during any part of the procedure, such as when the guide catheter is inserted into the main artery, at microcatheterization, when coils are placed into or withdrawn from the aneurysmal sac, and in cases of coil protrusion or migration.[41]

Editor's Note: The intended action of GDC (thrombosis) treatment, combined with the desire to avoid thrombosis during placement, is somewhat contradictory. While the

T A B L E 2 5 - 6 Frequency of Angiographic Clotting, Post-procedural Deficits, and Permanent Deficits with the Remodeling Technique Compared to the Normal GDC Treatment

Finding	Remodeling Technique	Normal GDC Treatment
Total clotting	3/58 procedures (5%)	27/249 procedures (11%)
Post-procedural deficits	1/50 patients (2%)	16/189 patients (8%)
Permanent deficits	1/50 patients (2%)	7/189 patients (4%)

T A B L E 2 5 - 8 Morbidity and Mortality due to the Remodeling Technique and Normal GDC Treatment

	Remodeling Technique	Normal GDC Treatment
Morbidity	1/50 patients (2%, Glasgow Outcome Scale [GOS] 2)	7/189 patients (4%, all GOS 2)
Mortality	0.50 patients (0%)	4/189 patients (2%) • 2 preoperative ruptures • 1 hematoma after urokinase • 1 hematoma under excessive anticoagulation

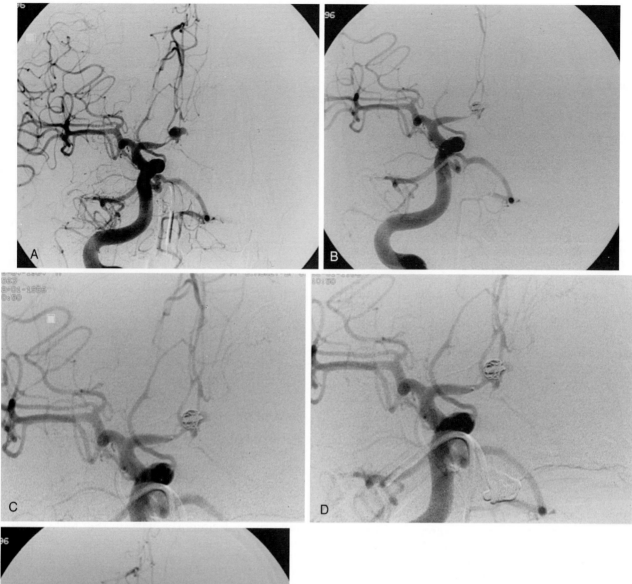

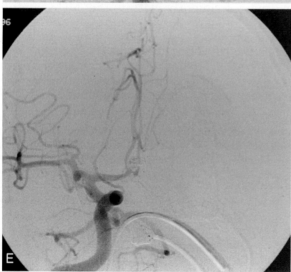

Figure 25-11. Case 8. Management strategy in a recently ruptured aneurysm complicated by severe vasospasm. *A* and *B,* Frontal projection of a right ICA angiogram demonstrates an ACoA aneurysm with spasm in the right A1 and the A2 segments bilaterally. A microcatheter was advanced and two coils were positioned in the aneurysm.

C and *D,* The microcatheter was withdrawn from the "protected" aneurysm and a superselective infusion of papaverine was performed proximally in the A1 segment. Vasodilation with increased flow was noted in the A1 and A2 segments bilaterally.

E, The aneurysm was re-entered and an almost complete obliteration of the aneurysm achieved. (Treatment was completed some months later.)

morbidity and mortality of GDC therapy have been reported to be very low, it would seem to be obvious that there would be a risk of a thrombus forming and being dislodged. The goal of tight packing of the aneurysm would seem to invite areas of stasis of flow with potential clot formation. In a report by Pelz et al. (presented at the American Society of Interventional and Therapeutic Neuroradiology Meeting, New York, September 1997), the rate of symptomatic thromboembolic events was 27.5%; the stroke rate was 15.5%, with permanent deficits occurring in 3.4%.

The use of heparin during coil placement would seem to

be mandatory, but it is somewhat ineffective. Heparin has essentially no effect on platelet aggregation. While no large series has been performed to evaluate the prevention of these events, institution of abciximab therapy may be useful. This drug should be used with the knowledge that the blockade of platelet aggregation is very strong and long acting (90% effective for a variable time, up to days after administration).

Treatment of Thromboembolism: Fibrinolysis

When a thromboembolic complication occurs, repeat angiograms have to be obtained bilaterally and sometimes in both the anterior and posterior circulation. The purpose is to evaluate the flow (i.e., if there is a mere reduction of flow or if a total occlusion has developed) and to examine the pattern of collateral blood supply. The decision to start thrombolytic therapy has to be made with utmost care because of the associated risks.[42] Thrombolysis is contraindicated in recently ruptured aneurysms as long as they are untreated or insufficiently packed with coils.

Thrombolysis may be avoided when clotting produces a mere reduction of flow without any tendency to propagate, if the occlusion involves a minor vessel feeding an area of less neurologic importance, and if a good collateral supply is observed. Patients should then be kept on intensified heparinization combined with a slight elevation of systolic blood pressure in order to obtain optimal perfusion within the region affected. However, when a large clot is formed or whenever a persistent vascular occlusion is noted, especially within an area of major neurologic eloquence, thrombolysis must be initiated.

Fibrinolysis is initiated either superselectively (with the tip of the microcatheter positioned distal to the thrombus) or, if not possible, selectively (within or just proximal to the thrombus). Disruption of the thrombus may be performed prior to thrombolysis by a combination of mechanical and chemical clot fragmentation. Flow may then be established, permitting the fibrinolytic drug to reach more distally, while at the same time the surface of the clot accessible to the drug is increased. Urokinase (15,000–20,000 U/ml or 1 million units in 50 ml normal saline) is then administrated either by a continuous manual injection or through an infusion pump. The infusion is repeatedly interrupted to obtain repeat angiograms.

Once reperfusion is established, or when the maximum dose of 1,500,000 U of urokinase has been given, thrombolysis is stopped. A final angiogram demonstrating the entire intracranial circulation must then be performed to evaluate and document the final vascular anatomy. The combined use of superselective catheter positioning and clot fragmentation has led to permanent revascularization in an increased number of patients, reducing morbidity in these patients.[41]

Editor's Note: The use of urokinase to treat parent vessel occlusion in the presence of a perforated vessel or previously ruptured aneurysm is hazardous at best and disastrous at worst; this should be avoided if at all possible.

(This is not the same situation as parent vessel occlusion during an angioplasty.) The recently ruptured aneurysm (or vascular perforation) is almost guaranteed to bleed if urokinase is used. If there is risk of parent vessel thrombosis, intraprocedural abciximab may be helpful, but its use is as risky as or more risky than simple heparinization during the procedure.

Fibrinolytic therapy is contraindicated in the presence of recently ruptured aneurysm or vascular perforation, even in the presence of parent vessel occlusion. Even though a stroke may be the price to pay, intracranial hemorrhage under these circumstances would very likely be fatal.

Rupture of the Aneurysmal Sac

A rupture or rebleeding may occur in any aneurysm during angiographic evaluation or endovascular therapy, but it is more common in recently ruptured aneurysms. It may be a spontaneous burst due to the delicate nature of the aneurysm or may be iatrogenically induced. Perforation is a rare complication during endovascular treatment and may be related to poor technique, microcatheter instability, inappropriate coil selection or deployment, or counterpressure created when the balloon protection technique is used. The bleeding causes a sudden increase of pressure within the subarachnoid space, which may be followed by dire consequences such as instant death or aggravation of later complications related to the disease (e.g., vasospasm, ischemia). When perforation occurs in the earlier phases of the procedure, it is more or less comparable with a burst from a nontreated, unruptured, or recently ruptured aneurysm. However, if perforation happens in the later phases of treatment, it seldom results in a devastating hemorrhage because the dome is often protected and the aneurysmal sac is to a certain extent eliminated from the circulation.

Detection of a rupture during GDC embolization of an intracranial aneurysm is the first step in managing this complication. Rupture is best recognized by careful monitoring of the patient's blood pressure; any significant rise should immediately raise suspicion.

If a rupture is suspected, it may or may not be revealed by a cerebral angiogram. The blood pressure should be immediately lowered (by pharmaceutical means). In all cases of rupture or rebleed due to perforation, it is mandatory to reverse heparinization totally or at least partially (protamine should always be drawn up and ready in a syringe during a GDC case).

Endovascular obliteration of the aneurysmal sac should then proceed. Additional GDCs should be placed as expeditiously as possible. It is hoped that this will result in thrombosis and cessation of hemorrhage. The success of this strategy can be evaluated by observing the cerebral circulation time. When the aneurysm is occluded and the treatment finished, heparinization can be maintained according to postoperative routine.

Editor's Note: If during deployment of a coil it is noted that the coil is protruding past the confines of the aneurysm, **it should not be withdrawn.** Rather, it should be further deployed and detached. Additional coils should then be expeditiously placed to prevent any further bleeding from the perforated aneurysm.

Coil Stretching, Breakage, and Migration

Specific endovascular foreign body retriever devices (snares), adapted to the specific anatomy of the cerebral vessel, have been developed for use in cases of premature coil detachment, breakage, or migration and in situations of persistent stretching during coil retraction. The design and characteristics of these retrieving devices are based on experiences with currently used microcatheters.[43] A variety of snares and sizes are available. The most commonly used device, the Retriever (Target Therapeutics), consists of a single wire in a specific microcatheter (see Chapter 1).

According to the circumstances, the size and type of snare has to be individually selected. If possible, it is advantageous to keep the coil within its microcatheter and to navigate the Retriever device through a 5- or 6-Fr. guide catheter introduced via the opposite groin. The guide catheter should be positioned as close as possible to the coil to facilitate manipulation of the snare device. The Retriever lacks a guidewire; the catheter is maneuvered by using the snare as a guide. The snare has some torqueability, which makes it possible to direct the catheter through tortuous segments. The loop of the snare is very soft and adapts to the configuration of the vessel wall.

When some part of the coil remains in its microcatheter, this catheter may be advanced or pushed to create a loop of the emerged portion of the coil. This loop can then be easily captured by the snare (Fig.

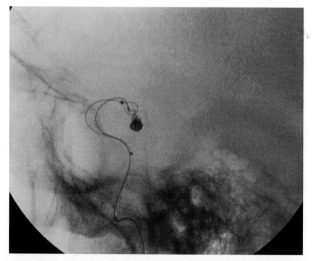

Figure 25-12. Case 9. A lateral projection demonstrates the use of a microsnare. A mechanically detachable spiral (MDS, Balt Extrusion) was prematurely detached within the microcatheter. Part of the spiral is outside the catheter and positioned in the aneurysm. The microcatheter was advanced to create a loop of the spiral, and it could then be captured by the snare. (The same strategy is applicable to GDC coils.)

25–12). Once the coil is grasped, the Retriever may be withdrawn and, together with the coil, removed from the guide catheter.

When the coil is undetached and stretched, it is generally difficult to visualize the unwound wire at fluoroscopy. In such circumstances, the coil must be snared at its nonstretched portion, ordinarily close to the origin of the aneurysm.

If the coil is detached outside the microcatheter or if it has migrated out of the aneurysmal sac, it may be even more difficult to grasp the coil, and success may be utterly dependent on the direction of its distal end. It is sometimes necessary to push the coil with the snare to create a loop that may be captured.

Withdrawal of a coil when some part of it remains in the aneurysm has to be done under fluoroscopic guidance. If the coil is stuck in the aneurysm, stretching may occur or, even worse, the nest of coils may protrude into the parent artery. Protrusion of the coils has to be avoided. If there is any sign of movement, removal should be abandoned, the coil released from the snare, and the patient put on intensified heparinization. It may be necessary to anchor the coil outside the vessel by a surgical incision of the CCA in the neck or, if possible, by advancing and releasing its stretched portion in the external carotid artery or in the descending aorta. The risks of having this coil segment within these main arteries are probably less than having the nest of coils obliterate the parent artery, especially if the patient is placed on prolonged anticoagulant therapy.

Editor's Note: In all cases of GDC use, there is contact of flowing blood with platinum coil. Only with packing behind a protective balloon will there not be extensive intra-aneurysmal swirling during the procedure. It is recognized, however, that some situations are worse than others. The question of how to manage a coil protruding into the parent vessel is also far from resolved. Possibilities include short-term anticoagulation, benign neglect, long-term anticoagulation, an attempt to push the coil into the aneurysm, an attempt to snare the coil, use of antiplatelet agents, and surgical removal.

An Endeavor balloon catheter (formerly NDSB, Target Therapeutics) can be advanced past the site of the protruding coil and withdrawn while inflated, in an attempt to push the errant loop of GDC coil back into the aneurysm. If the attempt is successful, coiling can be continued with the balloon in place, and the balloon may potentially hold the errant loop in position. This is most likely to be unsuccessful, however.

In general, pushing a loop back into an aneurysm with a balloon is ineffective. Pushing of a coil is most effectively performed with a partially deployed, very small GDC coil.

If a coil loop is seen to extend to an excessive degree into the lumen of the parent vessel, anticoagulation should be maintained. There are no controlled trials that clarify the implications of this circumstance, but the consensus of most interventional neuroradiologists is that antiplatelet agents should be maintained for life, and anticoagulation should be maintained for about 2 to 6 weeks. We use ticlopidine for 3 months after 3 days of heparinization, then maintain the patient on aspirin for life.

The solution to coil protrusion into the parent vessel may be to use 2-D coils for the beginning of the procedure (during basket building).

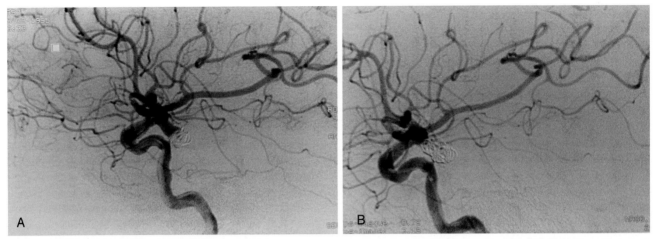

Figure 25-13. Case 10. Patient previously treated with GDC coils because of a ruptured ICA aneurysm. A follow-up angiogram 6 months after the initial therapy shows aneurysmal recanalization and regrowth. A repeat endovascular procedure was undertaken. (These images demonstrate the need for follow-up interval angiography.)

Pre-procedure Considerations of Complications and Patient Education

There are three fundamental precautions for all individuals performing neurointerventions such as treatment of aneurysms:

- Whenever possible, patients and their relatives must be given thorough information before endovascular therapy is initiated. This information should include the natural history of the disease, the aim of the treatment, and its potential risks. Even if this is obvious to most physicians, it must be stressed to everyone practicing interventional neuroradiology. In comparison with surgery, endovascular therapy is performed without a craniotomy and is generally less traumatic to the cerebral parenchyma. Consequently, patients often return to their work and social life after a shorter period of rehabilitation. These are the major advantages of this technique. However, in reality, these factors are also the most common reasons why patients and outsiders have trouble understanding the inherent difficulties of the technique, and accepting failures of treatment and post-procedural morbidity. Awareness and understanding of the existing circumstances through the given information makes everyone more prepared, not least the physician.
- Every incident and complication related to the technique, peri- or post-procedural, has to be thoroughly evaluated and analyzed before any endovascular corrective action is undertaken. Further manipulations, such as coil repositioning or retraction and thrombolysis, may be even more traumatic and may worsen the situation for the patient. Consequently, the relative advantages and risks of endovascular therapy as opposed to a more conservative attitude have to be estimated to determine the best option for a good clinical outcome.
- Immediate angiography and/or computed tomography has to be performed whenever any post-proce-

dural deterioration, explicable or inexplicable, occurs.

INTERVAL ANGIOGRAPHY AND FOLLOW-UP

Every patient who has had an aneurysm treated by the endovascular approach must be followed by regular, periodic clinical and angiographic examinations.

Post-procedural angiograms are methodically obtained at our institutions within 2 months after treatment of ruptured aneurysms and 4 to 6 months after therapy for unruptured aneurysms. Further studies are scheduled for 1 and 3 years after the initial treatment in order to follow the evolution of aneurysmal occlusion and the medical condition of the patient, and to compare anatomic results and clinical outcome. Additional treatment is performed whenever needed (Fig. 25–13). The follow-ups are also important for their impact on management strategy, understanding of the technique, and its future development.

REFERENCES

1. Serbinenko FA. Balloon catheterization and occlusion of major cerebral vessels. *J Neurosurg* 1974;41:125–145.
2. Romodanov AP, Shcheglov I. Intravascular occlusion of saccular aneurysms of the cerebral arteries by means of a detachable balloon catheter. *Adv Neurosurg* 1982;9:25–49.
3. Debrun G, Fox AJ, Drake C, et al. Giant unclippable aneurysms: treatment with detachable balloons. *AJNR* 1981;2:167–173.
4. George B, Aymard A, Gobin P, et al. Endovascular treatment of intracranial aneurysms: value and prospect based on a series of 92 cases. *Neurochirurgie* 1990;36:273–278.
5. Higashida R, Halbach V, Hieshima G, et al. Endovascular detachable balloon embolization therapy of cavernous carotid artery aneurysms: results in 87 cases. *J Neurosurg* 1990;72:857–863.
6. Moret J. Endovascular treatment of berry aneurysms by endosaccular occlusion. *Acta Neurochir (Wien)* 1991;53(Suppl):48–49.
7. Higashida R, Halbach V, Barnwell SL, et al. Intracranial

aneurysms: interventional neurovascular treatment with detachable balloon: results in 215 cases. *Radiology* 1991; 178:663–670.

8. Hodes JE, Fox AJ, Peerless SJ. Rupture of aneurysms following balloon embolization. *J Neurosurg* 1990;72:567–571.

9. Guglielmi G, Vinuela F, Sepetka I, et al. Electrothrombosis of saccular aneurysms via endovascular approach. Part 1: Electrochemical basis, technique and experimental results. *J Neurosurg* 1991;75:1–7.

10. Guglielmi G, Vinuela F, Dion J, et al. Electrothrombosis of saccular aneurysms via endovascular approach. Part 2: Preliminary clinical experience. *J Neurosurg* 1991;75:8–14.

11. Guglielmi G. Embolization of intracranial aneurysms with detachable coils and electrothrombosis. In Vinuela F, Halbach VV, Dion JE (eds): Interventional Neuroradiology: Endovascular Therapy of the Central Nervous System. New York: Raven Press, 1992, pp 63–75.

12. Ljunggren B, Säveland H, Brandt L, et al. Early operation and overall outcome in aneurysmal subarachnoidal hemorrhage. *J Neurosurg* 1985;62:547–551.

13. Adams HP Jr, Kassel NF, Kongable GA, et al. Intracranial operation within seven days of aneurysmal subarachnoidal hemorrhage. Results in 150 patients. *Arch Neurol* 1988; 45:1065–1069.

14. Kassell NF, Torner JC, Haley C, et al. The International Cooperative Study on the timing of aneurysmal surgery. Part 1. Overall management results. *J Neurosurg* 1990;73:18–36.

15. Kassel NF, Torner JC, Jane JA, et al. The International Cooperative Study on the timing of aneurysmal surgery. Part 2. Surgical results. *J Neurosurg* 1990;73:37–47.

16. Edner G. Early aneurysm surgery combined with normovolemic/hypervolemic hemodilution (abstr). *Acta Neurochir* 1986;79:161.

17. Awad IA, Carter LP, Spetzler RF, et al. Clinical vasospasm after subarachnoidal hemorrhage: response to hypervolemic hemodilution and arterial hypertension. *Stroke* 1987;18:365–372.

18. Säveland H, Ljunggren B, Brandt L, et al. Delayed ischemic deterioration in patients with early aneurysmal operation and intravenous nimodipine. *Neurosurgery* 1986;18:146–150.

19. Öhman J, Servo A., Heskanen O. Long-term effects of nimodipine on cerebral infarcts and outcome after aneurysmal subarachnoidal hemorrhage and surgery. *J Neurosurg* 1991;74:8–13.

20. Säveland H, Hillman J, Brandt L, et al. Overall outcome in aneurysmal subarachnoidal hemorrhage. *J Neurosurg* 1992;76:729–734.

21. Hunt WE, Hess RM. Surgical risk as related to time of intervention in the repair of intracranial aneurysms. *J Neurosurg* 1968;28:14–20.

22. Guglielmi G, Vinuela F, Duckwiler G, et al. Endovascular treatment of posterior circulation aneurysms by electrothrombosis using electrically detachable coils. *J Neurosurg* 1992;77:515–524.

23. McDougall C, Halbach V, Dowd C, et al. Endovascular treatment of basilar tip aneurysms using electrolytically detachable coils. *J Neurosurg* 1996;84:393–399.

24. Bavinzski G, Richling B, Gruber A, et al. Endosaccular occlusion of basilar artery bifurcation aneurysms using electrically detachable coils. *Acta Neurochir* 1995;134:184–189.

25. Graves VB, Strother CM, Weir B, et al. Vertebrobasilar junc-

tion aneurysms associated with fenestration: treatment with Guglielmi detachable coils. *AJNR* 1996;17:25–40.

26. Casasco A, Arnaud O, Gobin P, et al. Selective endovascular treatment of 71 intracranial aneurysms with platinum coils. *J Neurosurg* 1993;79:3–10.

27. Moret J, Pierot L, Boulin A, et al. Endovascular treatment of anterior communicating artery aneurysms using Guglielmi detachable coils. *Neuroradiology* 1996;38:800–805.

28. Halbach V, Higashida R, Dowd C, et al. The efficacy of endosaccular aneurysm occlusion in alleviating neurological deficits produced by mass effect. *J Neurosurg* 1994;80:659–666.

29. Cognard C, Weil A, Castaings L, et al. Endovascular occlusion of intracranial aneurysms. Angiographic and clinical results. Accepted for publication in *Radiology* 1997.

30. Richling B, Bavinzski G, Gross C, et al. Early clinical outcome of patients with ruptured cerebral aneurysms treated by endovascular (GDC) or microsurgical techniques. *Intervent Neuroradiol* 1995;1:19–27.

31. Zubilaga A, Guglielmi G, Vinuela F, et al. Endovascular occlusion of intracranial aneurysms with electrically detachable coils: correlation of aneurysmal neck size and treatment results. *AJNR* 1994;15:815–820.

32. Fox AJ, Vinuela F, Pelz DM, et al. Use of detachable balloons for proximal artery occlusion in the treatment of unclippable cerebral aneurysms. *J Neurosurg* 1987;66:40–46.

33. Marks MP, Lane B. Combined use of endovascular coils and surgical clipping for intracranial aneurysms. *AJNR* 1995;16:15–18.

34. Massoud TF, Guglielmi G, Vinuela F, Duckwiler GR. Endovascular treatment of multiple aneurysms involving the posterior intracranial circulation. *AJNR* 1996;17:549–554.

35. Gurian JH, Neil MA, Wesley R, et al. Neurosurgical management of cerebral aneurysms following unsuccessful or incomplete endovascular embolization. *J Neurosurg* 1995;83:843–853.

36. Gobin P, Vinuela F, Gurian JH, et al. Treatment of large and giant fusiform intracranial aneurysms with Guglielmi detachable coils. *J Neurosurg* 1996;84:54–62.

37. Debrun G, Vinuela F, Fox AJ. Aspirin and systemic heparinization in diagnostic and interventional neuroradiology. *AJNR* 1982;3:337–340.

38. Moret J, Cognard C, Weil A, et al. The "remodelling" technique in the treatment of wide neck intracranial aneurysms. *Interventional Neuroradiology* 1977; 3:21–35.

39. Kassell NF, Helm G, Simmons N, et al. Treatment of cerebral vasospasm with intra-arterial papaverine. *J Neurosurg* 1992;77:848–852.

40. Marks MP, Steinberg GK, Lane B. Intra-arterial papaverine for the treatment of vasospasm. *AJNR* 1993;14:822–826.

41. Cronqvist M, Cognard C, Moret J, et al. Local intra-arterial fibrinolysis of thromboemboli occurring during endovascular treatment of intracerebral aneurysms: comparison of anatomical result and clinical outcome. Accepted for publication in *AJNR* 1998.

42. Barnwell SL, Clark WM, Nguyen TT, et al. Safety and efficacy of delayed intraarterial urokinase therapy with mechanical clot disruption of thromboembolic stroke. *AJNR* 1994; 15:1817–1822.

43. Graves VB, Rappe AH, Strother CM, et al. An endovascular retrieving device for the use in small vessels. *AJNR* 1993;14:804–808.

PART III

MISCELLANEOUS INTERVENTIONAL NEURORADIOLOGIC PROCEDURES

CHAPTER 26

Current Management of Cervicofacial Superficial Vascular Malformations and Hemangiomas

D. Herbreteau / A. Aymard / H.S. Jhaveri / R. Chapot / A.E. Casasco / S. Slaba / E. Houdart / J.-J. Merland

Various terms have been used in the literature to characterize vascular abnormalities. The classification that has emerged is the one used by the international society for the study of superficial vascular malformations. This classification is based on clinical and vascular features, hemodynamic characteristics, and biologic and histopathologic features.

The two major types of superficial vascular abnormalities are hemangiomas and vascular malformations. Hemangiomas are benign tumors seen in children and characterized by phases of growth due to proliferation of endothelial cells and phases of involution with spontaneous slow regression.

Vascular malformations are composed of dysplastic vessels with a normal endothelial turnover. Depending on the type of the affected vascular compartment, flow characteristics, and the clinical symptoms, superficial vascular malformations can be divided into two categories: (1) slow-flow vascular malformations, which are further subdivided into capillary malformations, venous malformations, and lymphatic malformations, and (2) high-flow vascular malformations (arteriovenous vascular malformations, or AVVMs). There are also some complex combined types of vascular malformations.

HEMANGIOMAS

Hemangiomas are benign vascular endothelial tumors. They occur in about 10% of neonates and in-fants, with a significant female predominance (5:1). They grow during the first year of life and usually regress before 5 years of age. About 80% of hemangiomas do not need further work-up or therapy. These patients should be observed until lesion regression.

Ultrasound (color Doppler) and magnetic resonance imaging (MRI) are useful noninvasive examinations in patients in whom further evaluation is indicated to establish the diagnosis. MRI facilitates differentiation of a subcutaneous deep hemangioma from a dermoid cyst, a meningocele, or a lymphatic malformation. MRI may document associated lesions such as Dandy-Walker syndrome or a spinal cord malformation.

In about 20% of cases, hemangiomas grow enough to produce complications, such as compression or obstruction of important structures (e.g., eye, nose, mouth); even small lesions may obstruct the subglottic airway. The sole indication for more aggressive therapy is a large extending tumor that has failed medical treatment, including corticosteroids and interferon. In addition to compressing structures, these tumors may lead to heart failure and hemorrhage.

Angiography should not be performed in these cases, except before embolization. If performed, it shows a hypervascular tumor with an intense capillary blush and an early venous filling (Fig. 26–1). The lesion must not be mistaken for a vascular malformation. Embolization consists of occlusion of the

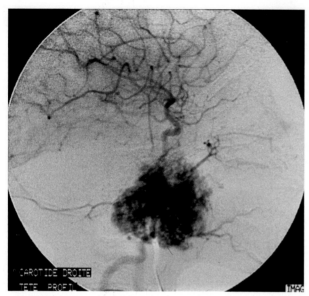

Figure 26-1 Case 1. Hemangioma of the parotid space. Angiogram of the common carotid artery showing an intense blush and early venous drainage, which must not be mistaken for an arteriovenous malformation. Angiography is not required for the diagnosis and should not be performed.

capillary tumor with calibrated microparticles after selective catheterization.

VASCULAR MALFORMATIONS

Venous Malformations

Venous malformations are spongy, bluish masses present at birth, which progressively enlarge throughout childhood and adolescence. There is no preferential localization. Cervicocephalic lesions are of particular interest because of their significant psychological impact. They have a wide spectrum of clinical presentation, extending from a limited cutaneous form to an extensive soft tissue–invading lesion. Such widely extensive venous malformations distort the bones and soft tissues, leading to functional impairment and dental malocclusion. The blue color is due to ectatic venous channels in the dermis.

Diagnosis

The diagnosis of a venous malformation is based on the clinical examination. Venous malformations enlarge when venous pressure increases, such as in the Valsalva maneuver and in declivity. Phleboliths may be palpable, are due to thrombosis in a venous pouch, and are specific for venous malformations. Blood stagnation also may be responsible for associated intravascular coagulopathy. A coagulation profile must be obtained before surgical treatment.

Magnetic resonance imaging is the examination of choice to determine the location and extent of the venous malformation because the deep extent may be more significant than clinically suspected and in a dangerous location, such as the airway. Multiplanar T2-weighted images provide good delineation.

Angiography is not needed for the diagnosis and has been supplanted by MRI. A selective angiogram may reveal grape-bunch–like staining of dysplastic stagnant venous lakes. The only remaining indication for angiography is before arterial embolization in cases of huge venous malformations. Venous pouch opacification by direct puncture is now standard before percutaneous therapeutic procedures.

Indications

The three main criteria for treatment are cosmetic abnormalities, functional impairment, and social tolerance. Large venous malformations justify early treatment, even in an infant. The therapeutic strategy is based on a multidisciplinary approach, including a dermatologist; vascular, plastic, and otorhinolaryngologic surgeons; a hematologist; and a pathologist, in addition to the interventional radiologist.

Techniques for Percutaneous Embolization

Several different sclerosing agents can be used, depending on the setting and specific therapeutic strategy.

EthiblocÆ

A common sclerosing agent is EthiblocÆ, available in a 7.5-cc syringe ready to inject. EthiblocÆ contains a dilution of zein in alcohol at a concentration of 210 mg/ml. Zein is a protein provided from corn. It is mixed with sodium diatrizoate (162 mg/ml) to ensure radiopacity, oeillette oil, oleum papaveris, water, and propylene glycol. In contact with blood or any other aqueous substance, EthiblocÆ precipitates and generates a viscous, biodegradable substance that persists for about 4 to 6 weeks. This substance produces a giant cell inflammatory reaction.

A mixture of 3.0 ml of EthiblocÆ, 1.0 ml of lipiodol, and 1.0 ml alcohol is prepared at the beginning of the procedure. Lipiodol (Lipiodol Ultrafluide, Laboratoire Guerliet, France) is added to enhance opacity, and alcohol is added to enhance the sclerosing ability. The mixture is stirred before aspiration of 1.0 ml in a tuberculin syringe.

The procedure is performed under neuroleptic analgesia. The venous malformation is punctured with either a 23- or 21-gauge needle. Multiple successive punctures are achieved.

Nonionic contrast media is injected under fluoroscopic control to document the volume, morphology, extent, and connections of the venous lakes. An amount of EthiblocÆ equal to one third of the estimated volume is injected in the venous lakes. If the venous malformation drains rapidly into the neighboring veins despite local vessel compression, percutaneous sclerotherapy is not performed to avoid migration of EthiblocÆ and embolic complications.

Corticosteroids are indicated during the procedure to minimize the local swelling and sometimes the fever. Nonsteroidal anti-inflammatory and mild antalgic medications are added for 5 days.

One or more sessions are scheduled, depending on

the clinical outcome evaluated 6 weeks after the initial procedure.

Velum and deep pharyngolaryngeal venous malformations are treated under endoscopic guidance with a temporary tracheostomy.

Complications are rare (10% of procedures) and minor. These consist of drainage of Ethibloc∕E at the puncture site, which stops spontaneously. Sometimes inflammatory nodules are incised to drain a yellow aseptic jelly with a discrete residual scar.

Alcohol

Sclerosis with alcohol is performed under general anesthesia because it is painful. The injected amount must be about one tenth of the volume of the pouch. Alcohol induces endothelial necrosis and thrombosis inside the malformation. The action remains focused inside the pouch, with a low level of alcohol in the general circulation even after injection of 50 ml of absolute alcohol. Rapid drainage of the pouch into the general circulation must be avoided, however, because it can lead to serious complications, such as pulmonary edema, heart failure, or nerve palsies. Tantalum powder may be added to visualize the alcohol.

Polidocanol

Polidocanol (Aetoxisclerol) is available at different concentrations; the 3% concentration is the most useful. After puncture of the superficial pouch with a 0.030″ needle, polidocanol is injected until discoloration of the venous pouch occurs. This usually requires 0.2 to 1.0 ml. Several punctures may be needed depending on the size of the malformation. Anesthesia is not required. Mild pain during injection indicates extravasation; this requires an adequate repositioning of the needle.

Coils

Coils have been used more recently in extensive venous malformations. They are placed through a 16-gauge needle and usually are used with ethanol or polidocanol. Tungsten peripheral 0.035″ coils (Balt) of various length and diameter are used.

N-Butyl-2-Cyanoacrylate

N-butyl-2-cyanoacrylate (NBCA; Histoacryl) can be used for percutaneous embolization of large venous malformations in conjunction with arterial embolization as a preoperative measure.

Treatment Strategy

The goal and results of percutaneous embolization vary according to the size and location of the venous malformation. Small malformations can be cured in a few sessions (usually 1 to 3) with polidocanol 3% (Fig. 26–2).

Pain and functional disabilities must be addressed in medium-sized lesions (venous pouch >3 to 4 ml). Ethibloc∕E is employed for these lesions. When this is not adequate, we place alcohol and coils through a 16-gauge needle.

Large malformations need combined repeated sclerotherapy and surgery (Figs. 26–3 and 26–4). Two different approaches are combined:

1. Percutaneous embolization with glue (NBCA) is achieved under fluoroscopic control.
2. Particulate arterial embolization is performed.

The combination of percutaneous sclerosis with arterial embolization helps the surgeon achieve adequate resection with limited blood loss.

In cases of inoperable extensive venous malformations, alcohol generally is used in conjunction with coils. Psychological management is an important point, particularly for large venous malformations that cannot be completely cured.

Lymphatic Malformations

Lymphatic malformations belong to the category of hemodynamically inactive vascular malformations.

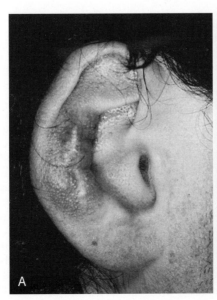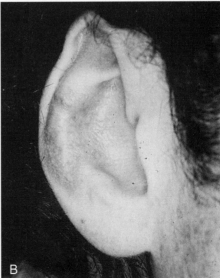

Figure 26-2 Case 2. Small venous malformation of the ear. *A,* Before infiltration with polidocanol. *B,* Discoloration and disappearance of swelling after sclerotherapy.

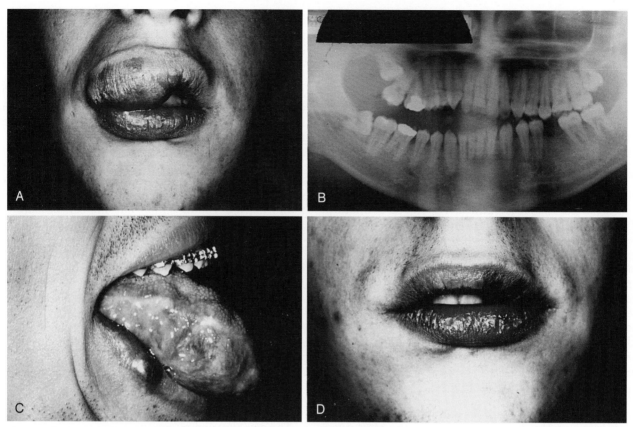

Figure 26-3 Case 3. Labial and lingual venous malformation. *A,* Failure of surgical removal, inducing extensive blood loss. *B,* Dental malocclusion due to mass effect. *C,* Orthodontic treatment. *D,* Final result after combined embolization and surgery.

Tissular lymphatic malformations are due to an abnormal development of the primitive lymphatic vessels. Lymphatic malformations usually are detected at birth but may be visualized prenatally on ultrasonography when large cysts are present. There are two main architectural types of lymphatic malformations that can be combined: the microscystic or tissular type and the macrocystic type.

Diagnosis

Lymphatic malformations are round, cold masses of overall soft consistency with focal hard spots. The volume of the lesion is not influenced by the patient's position or by exercise, but the size increases during inflammatory or infectious processes, such as rhinopharyngitis, otitis, or any inflammatory syndrome. Computed tomography and MRI are helpful in the evaluation of the deep extent of the malformation.

Fluoroscopic visualization of the lesion after direct percutaneous injection of contrast media is performed as the first stage of the therapeutic procedure. It demonstrates the size of the cysts, their morphology, and the different compartments as well as communications between the cysts and sometimes communications with veins.

Indications for Treatment

Indications for treatment include functional disability due to cosmetic impairment, inflammatory phases, progression, or intracystic bleeding. The microcystic or tissular lymphatic malformations cannot be treated by embolization and are difficult to remove surgically. Medical treatment combining antibiotics and corticosteroids can be given in the case of rapid progression. Treatment of these lesions with the yttrium-aluminum-garnet laser appears promising. The macrocystic type generally is suitable for percutaneous sclerotherapy (Fig. 26–5).

Procedure

The therapeutic procedure typically is performed under neuroleptic analgesia, except in neonates and infants, in whom general anesthesia is preferable.

A cyst is punctured using either a 19-gauge intramuscular needle or a 20-gauge Angiocath (Cathlon). If the embolization agent is viscous, a 16-gauge Angiocath is used. The serosanguinous fluid aspirated from the cyst is sent for pathologic analysis. Nonionic contrast media is injected through the same needle, under fluoroscopic control, to evaluate the volume and morphology of the lesion as well as the connections between the cysts and the venous drainage. A mixture of EthiblocÆ, lipiodol, and absolute alcohol is used for embolization. Lipiodol is added to enhance the radiologic visualization, and absolute alcohol is added to reduce the viscosity and to enhance the sclerosing ability. After reaspiration of the contrast media, the mixture is injected into the cyst.

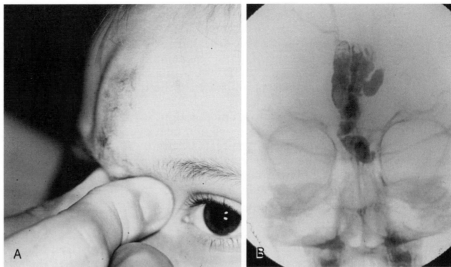

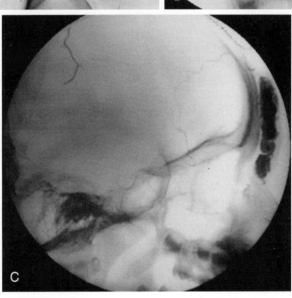

Figure 26-4 Case 4. Frontal venous malformation of the midline, which must not be mistaken for sinus pericranii. *A,* Injection of *N*-butyl-2-cyanoacrylate (NBCA, Histoacryl) and concomitant pressure on the inner canthus help to reduce drainage in the ophthalmic vein. NBCA was used as an immediate preoperative sclerosing agent. *B* and *C,* Cast of NBCA showing complete obliteration of the venous pouch.

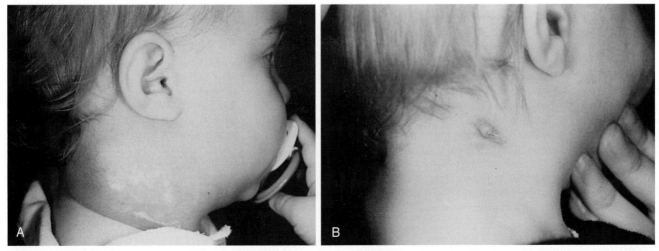

Figure 26-5 Case 5. Macrocystic lymphatic malformation of cervical localization. *A,* Recent size increase due to an inflammatory process. *B,* Six-month control after embolization reveals dramatic shrinkage; however, an inflammatory nodule with embolization material can be seen.

The volume of embolization material must not exceed 10% of the total volume of the cyst. These steps are repeated several times during the procedure, depending on the number and size of cysts. The amount of aspirated fluid varies from 5 to 150 ml. A maximum of 7.0 ml of the mixture is infiltrated to limit the inflammatory response.

Nonsteroidal anti-inflammatory medication is added for 5 days. The cysts become hard and firm in the following days. Regression of the cysts occurs in the subsequent 2 months, but it may take up to 6 months to complete. The best time for evaluation of the outcome is usually after 1 year. Another session is often required.

Results

Total regression of lymphatic malformations often can be achieved. Postsurgical recurrences also can be treated successfully. A residual component after the first sclerosing session with Ethibloc Æ is common and is treated with repeated sclerosing sessions. Failures may occur, mostly in the setting of a mixed histologic type. The initial aspect is that of a cystic lymphangioma. The macrocystic compartment is treated successfully, revealing the contiguous tissular compartment.

Complementary surgery may be required in the following situations:

- For aesthetic reasons, such as a facial reconstruction (e.g., labial, palpebral)
- In the case of insufficient regression, to remove the nonembolized part
- To incise and evacuate persistent inflammatory nodules, some yellowish liquid can be found corresponding to residual Ethibloc Æ
- In cases of lack of lymphocytes or unclear pathologic findings, in which the following underlying benign or malign cystic lesion must be sought: teratoma, hemangiopericytoma, branchial cyst, ganglioneuroma, or metastatic papillary carcinoma

Technical Problems and Complications

Minor complications occur more commonly (20%) in lymphatic than in venous malformations. Failure of resorption of Ethibloc Æ may lead to inflammatory nodules and fistulization to the skin. These leakages are treated by topical ointment and sometimes surgical approaches. Aseptic necrosis and nodules are removed with minor scars. In newborns, large cervical cystic lymphatic malformations may create respiratory distress. The volume increase due to inflammation after embolization usually is below the aspirated lymphatic volume. Children must be observed carefully because a lesion in a dangerous location may lead to an acute obstructive airway syndrome due to either inflammation or embolization.

Conclusion

Percutaneous embolization procedures are technically simple and of short duration (30 minutes). They can be repeated easily. The results appear good and reproducible as long as the cysts are well defined. Surgery should be performed for aesthetic reasons or to equilibrate a facial disproportion. Reconstructive surgery is especially useful in cases of mixed lymphatic malformations. This therapy is feasible in newborns and is the treatment of choice in those with superficial lymphatic cystic malformations.

Capillary Malformations: Port-Wine Stains and Telangiectasias

Capillary malformations are cosmetic problems usually treated by laser therapy.

Port-Wine Stains

Port-wine stains are reddish lesions obvious at birth. They consist of ectatic capillaries in the superficial dermis. An underlying extension must not be missed; if the port-wine stain is located in the dermatome of the trigeminal nerve, Sturge-Weber-Krabbe disease must be considered. The treatment of true port wine-stain lesions is well defined: several sessions of laser therapy produce good permanent decoloration.

Other superficial malformations must not be mistaken for port-wine stains. The false port-wine stain is warm, unlike the true port-wine stain, which is always cold. The false port-wine stain is a cutaneous extension of an underlying AVVM or a dermal AVVM, which is actually a mixture of a true AVVM and a capillary malformation. Angiography reveals a significant capillary blush and early venous drainage without real arteriovenous shunts. This dermal AVVM has a better prognosis than the usual AVVM, but it may spontaneously necrose. No treatment should be performed except surgical removal. Embolization may induce cutaneous necrosis. Treatment by laser must be avoided in false port-wine stains because it can lead to an expansion of the AVVM.

Cutaneous Telangiectasias

In case of resistance to laser or electrocoagulation, percutaneous treatment can be achieved using a sclerosing agent such as polidocanol similarly to its use for small venous malformations.

Osler-Weber-Rendu Disease

Osler-Weber-Rendu disease is congenital with an autosomal dominant inheritance pattern. It consists of a diffuse capillary malformation that often is associated with numerous AVMs (e.g., lung; central nervous system). Nasal and gastric mucosal lesions induce serious complications in up to 20% of patients.

The indication for intervention is repeated and incapacitating nasal bleeding. Epistaxis is treated in the acute phase by embolization of the facial and sphenopalatine arteries with microparticles, and sometimes by ligature of the ethmoidal arteries. Endovascular embolization is a palliative therapy of short duration because particles calibrated from 150 to 250 microns do not reach the telangiectasias but rather induce a proximal occlusion of the feeders, leading to the further development of collaterals.

Smaller particles (<150 microns) are not used because they induce mucosal and cutaneous necrosis.

The treatment of choice is devascularization by direct puncture of the telangiectasia and in situ injection of a sclerosing agent like Ethibloc. The procedure is performed under general anesthesia. Each telangiectasia is punctured under visual control, and 0.1 ml is infiltrated. A larger amount is not recommended to avoid inadvertent embolization of the ophthalmic artery. The procedure can be performed even in the presence of mucosal atrophy or infection and usually lasts less than 1 hour. Therapy may be repeated according to the symptoms, usually after about 1 year. An alternative to this treatment is laser sclerotherapy.

Arteriovenous Vascular Malformations

Natural History and Evaluation

Arteriovenous vascular malformations are the most dangerous vascular malformations because they are hemodynamically active and evolve in two phases: latent and evolutive phases.

These malformations generally are only a cosmetic disease, like a pseudo–port-wine stain, at initial clinical presentation, but they can evolve into a life-threatening problem. The factors leading to such a progression are not completely determined, but some are known to be related to an evolutive phase:

- Pregnancy, puberty, and hormonal variations
- Repeated minor trauma
- Iatrogenic trauma: inadequate proximal arterial li-

gation or partial proximal embolization without occluding the arteriovenous shunt
- Specific angioarchitectural factors: ill-defined outlines of the lesion, diffuse hypervascularity without defined macroscopic arteriovenous fistula (AVF), or local deep extension seen on MRI and angiography

The clinical presentation indicates the phase of the lesion. Quiescent AVVMs can be asymptomatic or present as a warm reddish pulsatile mass (Figs. 26–6 and 26–7). Indications for treatment include significant cosmetic impairment and a clearly defined AVF on angiography. In the case of a diffuse, ill-defined presentation, follow-up examination with comparative Doppler evaluation of both common carotid arteries should be performed, but therapy is not indicated.

Aggressive AVVMs can present with local ulcerations, leading to infection, local hemorrhage (Fig. 26–8), or progressive necrosis. Doppler examination is useful and shows an increase in the carotid flow; it also helps to identify a macroscopic AVF to be treated electively. MRI depicts the local, regional, and deep extension, even to osseous structures. Orthodontic evaluation includes clinical and radiologic workup.

The angioarchitecture must be analyzed before treatment because two groups must be distinguished: AVFs and AVMs. The differences between AVFs and AVMs are important to recognize to plan treatment and follow-up. Three types of angioarchitecture are recognized:

1. AVFs are large, direct shunts, congenital or

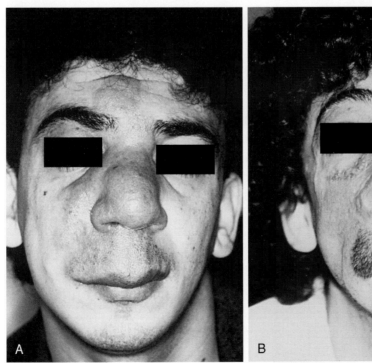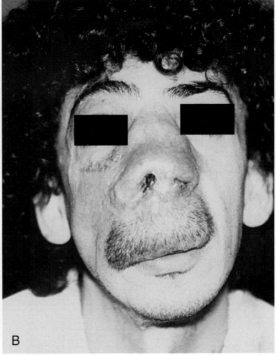

Figure 26-6 Case 6. False port-wine stain (Blanc Bonnet Dechaume syndrome). *A,* Clinical examination reveals a warm, reddish pulsatile mass. *B,* Five years after unsuccessful surgical attempts, the arteriovenous malformation has expanded, showing a marked evolution.

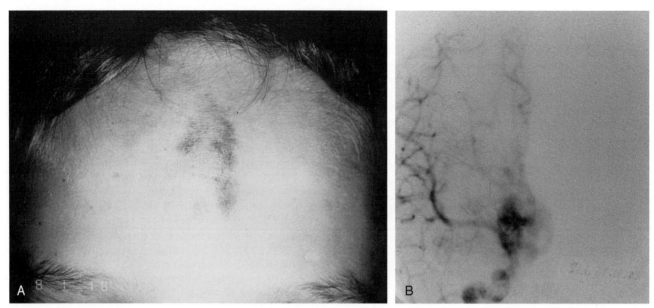

Figure 26-7 Case 7. Wyburn-Mason's syndrome, also called Blanc Bonnet Dechaume syndrome. *A,* The warm reddish and pulsatile frontal mass is an arteriovenous malformation. *B,* Injection of the internal carotid artery showing the intracranial extension of the malformation.

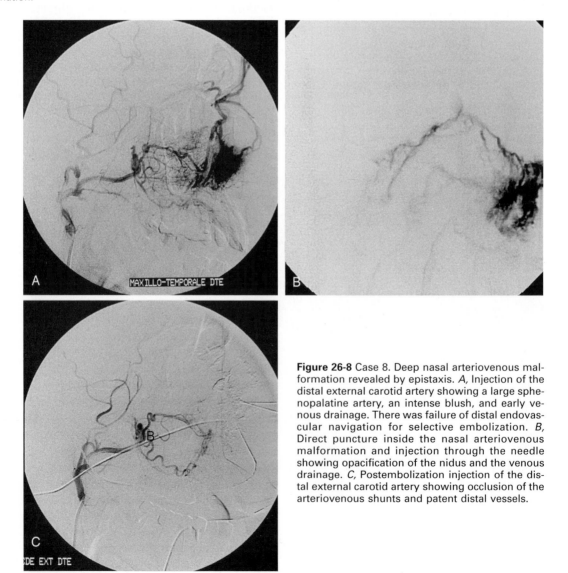

Figure 26-8 Case 8. Deep nasal arteriovenous malformation revealed by epistaxis. *A,* Injection of the distal external carotid artery showing a large sphenopalatine artery, an intense blush, and early venous drainage. There was failure of distal endovascular navigation for selective embolization. *B,* Direct puncture inside the nasal arteriovenous malformation and injection through the needle showing opacification of the nidus and the venous drainage. *C,* Postembolization injection of the distal external carotid artery showing occlusion of the arteriovenous shunts and patent distal vessels.

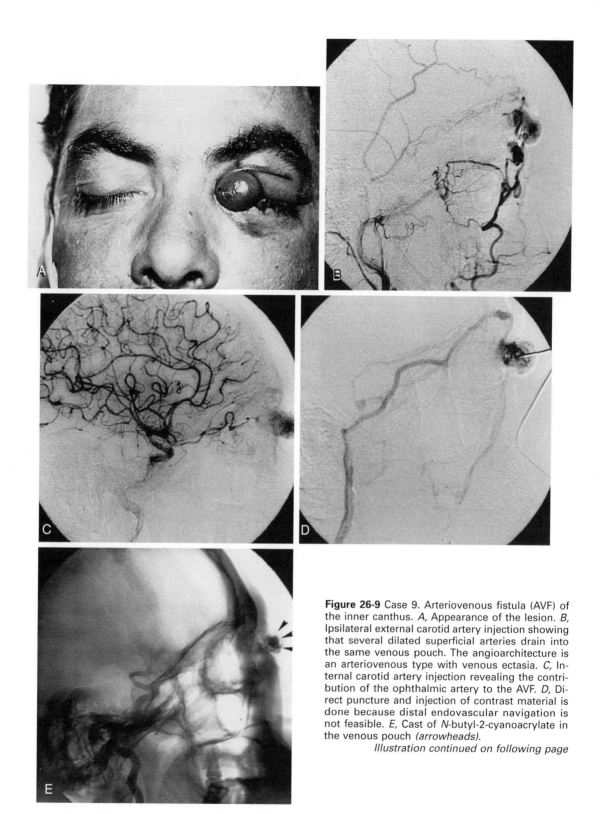

Figure 26-9 Case 9. Arteriovenous fistula (AVF) of the inner canthus. *A,* Appearance of the lesion. *B,* Ipsilateral external carotid artery injection showing that several dilated superficial arteries drain into the same venous pouch. The angioarchitecture is an arteriovenous type with venous ectasia. *C,* Internal carotid artery injection revealing the contribution of the ophthalmic artery to the AVF. *D,* Direct puncture and injection of contrast material is done because distal endovascular navigation is not feasible. *E,* Cast of *N*-butyl-2-cyanoacrylate in the venous pouch *(arrowheads).*
Illustration continued on following page

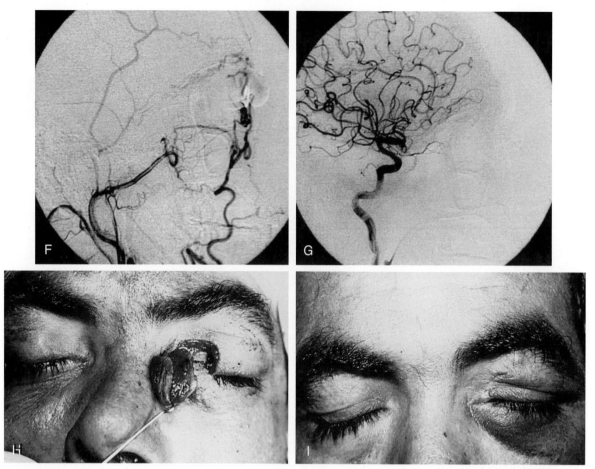

Figure 26-9 *Continued. F* and *G,* Postembolization injection of the external carotid artery revealing angiographic cure with complete occlusion of the AVF. *H,* Easy surgical removal for cosmetic cure without blood loss. *I,* One-week follow-up.

traumatic, between an artery and vein. One, two, or three feeders are possible.

2. AVMs are composed of congenital microfistulae called the *nidus;* this is the true AVVM. It is the most important type clinically because it has a high angiogenic (evolutive) tendency.

3. Arteriolovenous fistulae consist of multiple arteries entering a vein or a venous lake. These arteriolovenous fistulae appear to evolve like AVFs, and we include this type in the AVF group rather than with the AVMs.

The three types are sometimes mixed.

Treatment

A multidisciplinary approach to the management of these patients must be stressed. Decisions regarding treatment must be made with consideration of clinical progression, social and functional impairment, and hemodynamic and angioarchitectural criteria as studied by Doppler, MRI, and angiography.

Before making a therapeutic decision, proximal arterial occlusion by surgical or endovascular means must be prohibited because it can induce angiographic changes and development while compromising further adequate embolization.

We usually refuse to treat patients with asymptomatic AVMs, except when complete cure is possible.

We treat patients with asymptomatic AVFs because the stability of the result is usually good with appropriate therapy (Fig. 26–9). Selective angiography must focus on well-defined AVFs within the hypervascular area, which are the targets for treatment. The first step should be occlusion of the clearly defined AVFs to decrease the flow. This is done by superselective catheterization or direct puncture using liquid embolic agents (e.g., *N*-butyl-2-cyanoacrylate, Ethibloc/E, ethanol). The use of particles must be avoided because they can induce progression of the AVM.

In cases of persistent clinical progression despite a good angiographic result, combined treatment must be considered; this includes embolization preceding surgical resection with skin coverage. Multiple techniques of skin coverage are used, including skin expansion. Surgical resection is facilitated by previous embolization and is usually partial. Even with partial resection, adequate skin coverage gives a good functional and morphologic result; however, recurrences can occur in the nontreated portion.

ADDITIONAL READINGS

Boukobza M, Enjolras O, Guichard JP, et al. Cerebral developmental venous anomalies associated with head and neck venous malformations. *AJNR* 1996;17:987–994.

Enjolras O, Mulliken JB. The current management of vascular birthmarks. *Pediatr Dermatol* 1993;10:311–333.

Enjolras O, Riche MC, Mulliken JB, Merland JJ. Atlas des Hemangiomes et Malformations Vasculaires Superficielles. Paris: Medsi McGraw Hill, 1991.

Herbreteau D, Borsik M, Enjolras O, Riche MC. Arteriovenous malformations. *Rev Prat* (Paris) 1992;42:2031–2040.

Herbreteau D, Enjolras O, Gelbert F, et al. The current management of cervico-cephalic venous malformations. *Pediatr Surg Int* 1996;11:304–307.

Herbreteau D, Riche MC, Enjolras O, et al. Percutaneous embolization with Ethibloc of lymphatic cystic malformation with a review of the experience in 70 patients. *Int Angiol* 1993;12:34–39.

Houdart E, Gobin YP, Casasco A, et al. A proposed angiographic classification of intracranial arteriovenous fistulae and malformations. *Neuroradiology* 1993;35:381–385.

Lasjaunias P, Berenstein A. Surgical Neuroangiography, Vol 2: Endovascular Treatment of Craniofacial Lesions. Berlin: Springer Verlag, 1987.

Mulliken JB, Glowack J. Hemangiomas and vascular malformations in infants and children: a classification based on endothelial characteristics. *Plast Reconstr Surg* 1982;64:412–420.

Mulliken JB, Young AE. Vascular Birthmarks: Hemangiomas and Malformations. Philadelphia: WB Saunders, 1988.

Riche MC, Hadjean E, Tran Ba Huy P, et al. The treatment of capillarovenous malformations using a new fibrosing agent. *Plast Reconstr Surg* 1983;71:607–612.

Yakes W, Haas DK, Parker SH, et al. Symptomatic vascular malformations: Ethanol embolotherapy. *Radiology* 1989;170:1059–1066.

CHAPTER 27

Management of Extracranial Head and Neck and Paraspinal Vascular Malformations

W.F.J. Yakes

Interventional radiology and interventional neuroradiology have pioneered a minimally invasive therapeutic specialty to treat a wide variety of vascular and nonvascular lesions of the body, brain, spine, spinal cord, and head and neck. Interventional procedures routinely use minimally invasive, direct puncture, and transcatheter techniques to treat various conditions. In the head, neck, and paraspinal areas, most entities treated are of vascular origin. The extensive array of catheters, guidewires, embolic agents, digital imaging systems, and pharmaceutical products commonly used are a tribute to the hard work, insight, and imagination of the many dedicated investigators in this area. Because of significant laboratory and clinical research and extensive clinical experience, the judicious use of endovascular therapy is now commonplace in modern clinical practice. Now that it is firmly established as an essential therapeutic tool, its role will continue to grow. In the head, neck, and paraspinal regions, embolotherapy procedures have become an essential therapeutic tool that has assisted the interventionists' colleagues in otolaryngology, plastic and reconstructive surgery, neurosurgery, ophthalmology, vascular surgery, and various pediatric surgical specialties. Vascular malformations in the head and neck and paraspinal regions are discussed here.

Vascular malformations are rare lesions with a myriad of clinical presentations. They constitute some of the most difficult diagnostic and therapeutic enigmas encountered in the practice of medicine. The clinical presentations are extremely protean and can range from an asymptomatic birthmark to fulminant, life-threatening congestive heart failure. Attributing any of the extremely varied presenting symptoms to a vascular malformation can be challenging to the most experienced clinician. Compounding this problem is the extreme rarity of these vascular lesions. If a clinician sees a patient every several years, it is difficult to learn to diagnose and optimally manage the lesions. Typically, patients with vascular malformations bounce from clinician to clinician only to experience disappointing outcomes, complications, and recurrence or worsening of their presenting symptoms.

GENERAL CONCEPTS OF THERAPY

Surgical Therapy

Vascular malformations were first treated by surgeons. The early rationale of proximal arterial ligation of arteriovenous malformations (AVMs) proved totally futile as the phenomenon of neovascular recruitment reconstituted arterial inflow to the AVM nidus. Microfistulous connections became macrofistulous feeders. Complete extirpation of an AVM nidus proved very difficult and extremely hazardous, necessitating suboptimal partial resections. Partial resections could initially yield a good clinical result; however, with time the patient's presenting symptoms usually recurred or worsened. Because of the significant blood loss that frequently accompanied surgery, the skills of interventional radiologists were eventually employed to embolize these vascular lesions as a preoperative measure in the hope that it would allow a surgeon to do a more complete resection. However, complete extirpation of AVMs was still extremely difficult and rarely possible, particularly in the head and neck and paraspinal regions.[1, 2]

Recent Advances in Embolotherapy

With the improvement of catheter delivery systems and embolic agents, embolotherapy has emerged as a primary mode of therapy for vascular malformations. In many cases, these lesions are anatomically and surgically difficult to approach or in inaccessible areas. This has led to increased reliance on the sophisticated endosurgical skills of interventional radiologists and interventional neuroradiologists to manage these problematic patients.

CLASSIFICATION OF HEMANGIOMAS AND VASCULAR MALFORMATIONS

Historical Aspects

Because the clinical and angiographic manifestations can be extremely varied, hemangiomas and vascular malformations are difficult to classify. Moreover, a vast array of descriptive terms have been given to impressive clinical examples in the hope of distinguishing them as distinct syndromes. This has resulted in significant confusion in the categorization and treatment of these complex vascular lesions. Some of the confusing terms include congenital arteriovenous aneurysm, intraosseous arteriovenous malformation, cirsoid aneurysm, serpentine aneurysm, capillary telangiectasia, angioma telangiectaticum, angioma arteriale racemosum, angioma simplex, angioma serpiginosum, nevus angiectoides, hemangioma simplex, lymphangioma, hemangiolymphangioma, nevus flammeus, verrucous hemangioma, capillary hemangioma, cavernous hemangioma, and venous angioma.

Current Classification

A rational classification of hemangioma and vascular malformations has evolved, based on the landmark research of Mulliken et al, that should be incorporated into modern clinical practice.[3–8] This classification system, based on endothelial cell characteristics, has removed much of the confusion in terminology that is rampant in the literature today. Once all clinicians understand and use this important classification system, ambiguity and confusion will be removed as they will all speak a common language.

Hemangiomas

Hemangiomas are pediatric vascular lesions that are usually not present at birth, are clinically manifested within the first month of life, and exhibit a rapid growth phase in the first year. Their reported inci-

dence is 1.0% to 2.6%. More than 90% of hemangiomas spontaneously regress to near-complete resolution by 5 to 7 years of age. They are characterized by a proliferative phase whereby there is rapid growth, significant endothelial cell hyperplasia forming syncytial masses, thickening of endothelial basement membrane, ready incorporation of tritiated thymidine into the endothelial cells, and the presence of large numbers of mast cells. After this period of rapid expansion in the proliferative phase, hemangiomas can stabilize and grow commensurately with the child. Because of the complex nature of hemangiomas, the proliferative phase may continue as the involutive phase slowly begins to dominate. Involuting hemangiomas show diminished endothelial cellularity and replacement with fibrofatty deposits, exhibit a unilamellar basement membrane, demonstrate no uptake of tritiated thymidine into endothelial cells, and have normal mast cell counts.[3–5]

Most pediatric hemangiomas should not be treated; the natural history of involution should be allowed to occur. For hemangiomas that ulcerate or occasionally bleed, local compression and dressings usually suffice in combination with antibiotic therapy. Some rare conditions may warrant treatment. Upper eyelid hemangioma can cause refractive errors and amblyopia. Subglottic hemangioma may be a cause of chronic respiratory stridor. The presence of hepatic hemangiomas and isolated giant dermal hemangiomas may cause congestive heart failure or systemic coagulopathy. Systemic steroid therapy and direct injection of steroids have proved successful in medically inducing involution of pediatric hemangioma in approximately 30% of cases. If the hemangioma fails to respond to steroid therapy, alpha-interferon therapy can be instituted, whereupon the response rate may rise to approximately 50%. Other reported forms of medical therapy include cyclophosphamide and aminocaproic acid with cryoprecipitate (Fig. 27–1).[9–14]

Endovascular embolization may be necessary in hemangiomas for various reasons. Embolization can help control a high-output shunt until the natural involution of the hemangioma occurs. The Kasabach-Merritt syndrome is (usually) a self-limiting condition of consumptive coagulopathy with low platelet counts secondary to platelet trapping that may or may not require therapy. If medical management fails, embolization followed by platelet transfusions

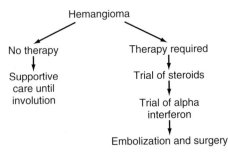

Figure 27-1 Clinical algorithm for management of pediatric hemangioma.

can help elevate platelet counts.[11, 15, 16] In patients in whom high-output failure is a problem, embolization can be used to minimize the shunting and decrease the cardiac consequences. In lesions that cause airway obstruction or are associated with chronic ulcerations and infections, embolization before surgery may be required. *Again, it is emphasized that most hemangiomas require no treatment.*

Congenital Vascular Malformations

Congenital vascular malformations are vascular lesions that are present at birth and grow commensurately with the child. There are also acquired vascular lesions that occur in the head and neck and spinal area and are related to trauma, venous thrombosis, mastoiditis, venous outflow stenosis, or other etiologies. Direct penetrating trauma can cause an abnormal connection between arteries and veins and in the healing process produce a fistula. Venous thrombosis, venous stenosis, venous outflow occlusion, mastoiditis, and blunt trauma can result in the formation of dural arteriovenous fistula (AVF).

Congenital vascular malformations histologically demonstrate no endothelial cell proliferation, contain large vascular channels lined by flat endothelium, have a unilamellar basement membrane, do not incorporate tritiated thymidine into endothelial cells, and have normal mast cell counts.[3–5] They may be formed from any combination of primitive arterial, capillary, venous, or lymphatic elements with or without direct arteriovenous shunts. Vascular malformations are true structural anomalies resulting from inborn errors of vascular morphogenesis and resorption. Congenital vascular malformations are categorized into arterial, capillary, venous, and lymphatic elements. The term *hemangioma* should be solely reserved for the previously described pediatric lesions that are usually not present at birth, become manifest within the first month of life, exhibit a rapid growth phase, and slowly involute to resolution by 5 to 7 years of age.

We classify vascular malformations as either high- or low-flow lesions. High-flow lesions (Figs. 27–2 to 27–4) are shunting malformations such as AVMs and congenital or acquired AVFs. Low-flow lesions (Fig. 27–5) include venous malformations, lymphatic malformations, and mixed lesions. The arteriography of these lesions demonstrates normal arteries and normal capillary beds. The malformation is truly a postcapillary lesion. The terms *cavernous hemangioma, vertebral body hemangioma,* and *hepatic hemangioma* should be replaced with the term *venous malformation.* If they were truly hemangiomas, they would not be present in the adult population.

RATIONALE FOR THERAPY

Surgical Experience

According to D. Emerick Szilagyi, MD, former editor of the *Journal of Vascular Surgery,* ". . . with few exceptions, their [AVMs] cure by surgical means is impossible. We intuitively thought that the only answer of a surgeon to the problem of disfiguring, often

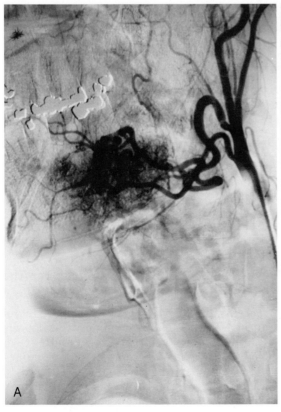

A

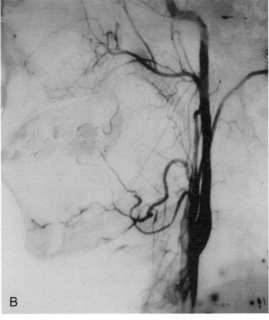

B

Figure 27-2 Case 1. *A,* Left facial arteriovenous malformation (AVM). *B,* Arteriogram 18 months after ethanol endovascular management of facial AVM. Note the filling of normal branches only. No residual AVM is present.

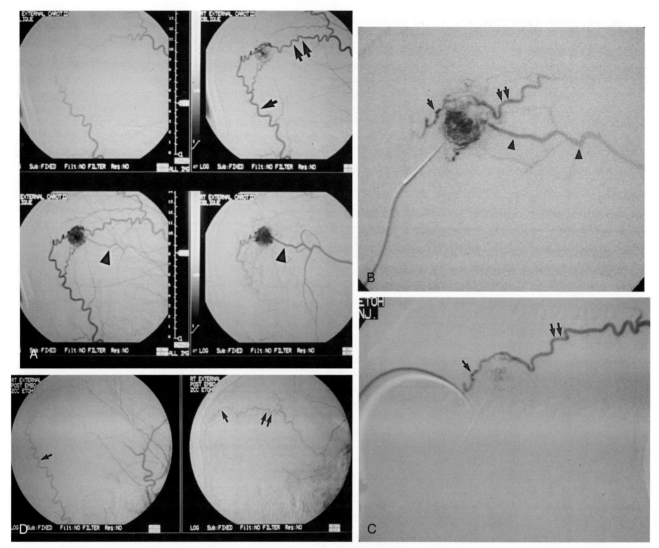

Figure 27-3 Case 2. *A,* Right scalp AVM supplied from the right occipital artery *(arrow)* and superficial temporal artery *(double arrows).* Note the outflow vein *(arrowheads). B,* Direct puncture of the scalp AVM demonstrating filling of the AVM nidus with reflux into the right occipital artery *(arrow),* right superficial temporal artery *(double arrows),* and outflow vein *(arrowheads). C,* Direct puncture angiogram after ethanol embolization. Note the nonfilling of the AVM and outflow vein. Note the reflux into the right occipital artery *(arrow)* and right superficial temporal artery *(double arrows). D,* Right external carotid digital subtraction angiogram after ethanol embolization. Note the filling of the right occipital artery *(arrow)* and right superficial temporal artery *(double arrows)* and nonfilling of the AVM or outflow vein.

noisome, and occasionally disabling blemishes and masses, prone to cause bleeding, pain, or other unpleasantness, was to attack them with vigor and with the determination of eradicating them. The results of this attempt at radical treatment were disappointing." Indeed, of 82 patients seen in this series, only 18 patients were even deemed operable. Of the 18 operated upon, 10 improved, two remained unchanged, and six were worse at follow-up.[1]

Complete extirpation of an AVM nidus is difficult and extremely hazardous, necessitating suboptimal partial resections that can be disfiguring. As noted, partial resections can result in an initial good clinical response, but with time the presenting symptoms recur or are worsened.[17–21] Although preoperative embolization by interventionists allowed more complete resections, complete extirpation of the AVM was still

complicated and rarely possible because of difficult or inaccessible anatomical areas.[2, 17–21] Indeed, it has been stated that ". . . while it is wrong to believe that AVMs are best treated by primary surgery, careful selection will enable up to 20% of patients to be cured or their lesions well controlled by this means."[20]

The Growing Role of Endovascular Therapy

As noted earlier, improvement in catheter delivery systems and embolic agents has led to increased reliance on the sophisticated endosurgical skills of interventional radiologists and interventional neuroradiologists and the emergence of endovascular occlusion procedures as a primary mode of therapy to manage and control peripheral vascular malformations.[22–38]

Vascular malformations are best treated when pa-

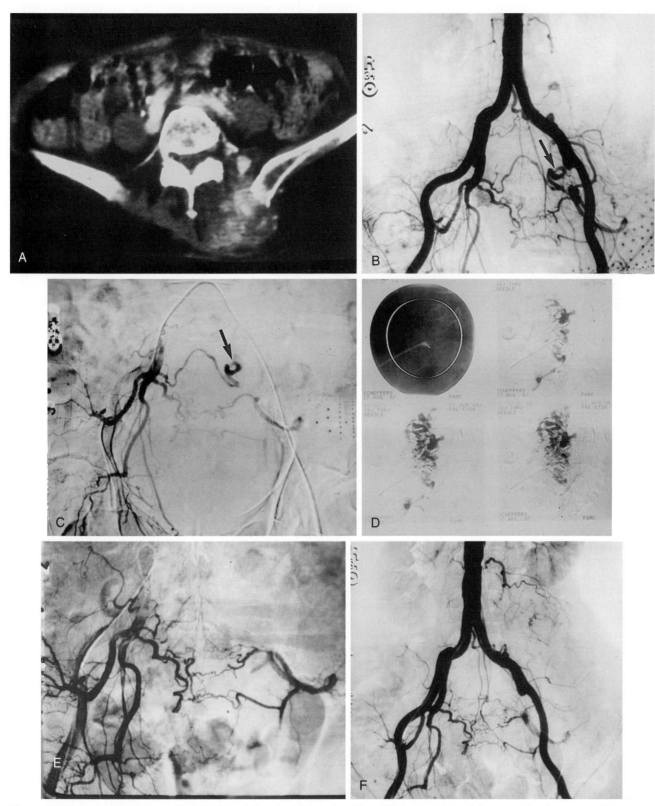

Figure 27-4 Case 3. *A,* Left paraspinal AVM involving the L4-5 region. Note the hypertrophy of the muscular tissues on this contrast computed tomographic scan with enhancement of the AVM. (From Yakes WF, Luethke JM, Merland JJ, et al: Ethanol embolization of arteriovenous fistulas: a primary mode of therapy. *J Vasc Inter Radiol* 1990; 1:89–96.) *B,* Anteroposterior (AP) abdominal aortogram. Note the transpelvic collateral coursing from the right internal iliac artery branch to the ligated stump of the left internal iliac artery. Note the reconstitution of flow to the branch supplying the AVM *(arrow). C,* Right internal iliac artery injection showing the middle sacral artery collateral to the branch supplying the AVM from the left internal iliac artery *(arrow). D,* Direct puncture angiogram and needle placement showing AVM opacification. *E,* Right internal iliac arteriogram 1 year after therapy. Note the nonopacification of the branch to the AVM. *F,* AP abdominal aortogram 1 year after therapy. Note the nonfilling of the AVM.

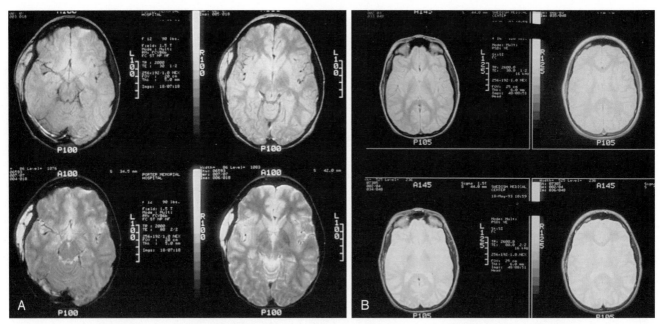

Figure 27-5 Case 4. *A,* Axial T1- and T2-weighted magnetic resonance image (MRI) through the scalp documenting a large venous malformation involving the subcutaneous tissues and right temporalis muscle. Note the increased signal, particularly on the T2-weighted sequences. This is consistent with a venous malformation. *B,* Axial T1- and T2-weighted MRI 2 years after therapy. Note the absence of the vascular mass and absence of the increased signal previously demonstrated on T2. This is consistent with total ablation of malformation.

tients are seen on a regular basis. The interventional radiologist or interventional neuroradiologist who occasionally evaluates these patients will never gain enough experience or knowledge to manage these challenging lesions effectively. All too frequently, the patient ultimately pays for the interventionalist's initial enthusiasm, inexperience, folly, and lack of necessary clinician back-up. To optimally manage these patients, a dedicated team should be in place. Interventionalists should combine with the various surgical and medical subspecialties to function together, much like the tumor board team of specialists. When patients are seen and treated regularly, experience can be gained, rational decisions made, complications appropriately managed, and patient care optimized. As a group, vascular malformations pose one of the most difficult challenges in the practice of medicine. A cavalier approach to their management will always lead to significant complications and dismal outcomes.

EMBOLIC AGENTS

Many endovascular embolic agents are used for various clinical scenarios. The choice of agent depends on several factors: the vascular territory to be treated, the type of abnormality, the possibility of superselective delivery, the goal of the procedure, and the permanence of occlusion required. The following occlusive agents have been used in the extracranial circulation and head and neck and paraspinal regions:

Gelfoam
Gelfoam powder
Avitene
Polyvinyl alcohol (PVA) particles
Coils
Detachable balloons
Tissue adhesives

Gelfoam, Gelfoam powder, Avitene, and PVA particles are considered temporary agents. I prefer Avitene to Gelfoam because of its ease of use and superior thrombogenicity. Gelfoam powder must be used with caution in the head, neck, and paraspinal regions owing to its ability to penetrate to the capillary bed; it can produce denervation and cranial nerve palsies due to occlusion of the vasa nervorum.[39]

Although cyanoacrylates were considered permanent agents initially, it is now well documented that recanalizations do occur.[24, 40–42] Cyanoacrylates have not received Food and Drug Administration approval (although clinical evaluation is proceeding), which raises medicolegal issues when they are used. Detachable balloons are thought to have a limited role to play in current management of vascular malformations.

Ethyl Alcohol

Ethanol (dehydrated ethyl alcohol injection USP, Abbott Laboratories) is a well-known sclerosing agent that induces significant thrombosis from the capillary bed backward. This results in total tissue devitalization. Ethanol induces thrombosis by denaturing blood proteins, dehydrating vascular endothelial cells and precipitating their protoplasm, denuding the vascular wall of endothelial cells, and segmentally fracturing the arterial wall to the level of the internal elastic lamina. Ethanol can induce significant pain when injected intravascularly, and so proper anesthesia is needed beforehand to control patient discomfort. Extreme caution must be taken when ethanol is used to minimize the possibility of nontarget embolization of normal tissues, thus preventing tissue necrosis and neuropathy.

Ethanol is an outstanding agent that has consistently demonstrated its curative potential in the management of vascular malformations.[22, 23, 25–38] Further, because it penetrates to capillary bed levels, ethanol is excellent for hypervascular tumors. The reason for the permanence routinely seen in vascular malformation management with ethanol is thought to be the fact that it destroys the endothelial cell and precipitates its protoplasm. The endothelial cell mediates the recanalization process encountered with all embolic agents. It is theorized that the endothelial cell also produces angiogenesis factors to promote the neovascular stimulation and neovascular recruitment phenomenon. When the endothelial cell is destroyed with ethanol, the problems of recanalization and neovascular stimulation are noticeably absent.

INITIAL EVALUATION

Clinical Evaluation

A thorough clinical examination and history can usually establish the diagnosis of pediatric hemangioma or vascular malformation. Hemangiomas are generally not present at birth and have a bright scarlet color that gradually deepens. Vascular malformations have a persistent color, depending on the dominant arterial, capillary, venous, or lymphatic component, and are present at birth. Evaluation for skeletal abnormalities, abnormal veins, arterial abnormalities, pulsatility or nonpulsatility of a lesion, dependent swelling and flattening upon elevation, disparity of limb size, the Nicoladoni-Branham test, and whether the lesion is warm or normal to the touch, along with neurologic evaluation and good history taking, can frequently enable diagnosis and even categorization of a vascular malformation. If reflex bradycardia occurs in the Nicoladoni-Branham test, the AVM shunting is of such high flow that it is truly causing cardiac consequences. In such patients, elevated cardiac output, elevated cardiac index, and abnormally lower systemic resistance can be demonstrated.

Bleeding

Bleeding is an uncommon complication of vascular malformations, unlike those of the brain and spinal cord, whose propensity to bleed is their main presenting symptom. Vascular malformations cause bleeding only if they involve the alimentary canal or in high-flow lesions that may cause superficial tissue ulceration. In these situations, the malformation requires primary treatment. Only then will the tissues become normal, heal, and discontinue the hemorrhagic or necrotic process. Attempts at skin grafting without treating the underlying malformation are doomed to failure.

Doppler Evaluation of Blood Flow

Color Doppler imaging (CDI) is an essential tool in the diagnostic work-up of AVMs. Accurate measurements of flow volumes (a calculated physiologic parameter) and resistive indexes can be helpful in the initial evaluation and are also important noninvasive parameters for follow-up after therapy. Documentation of decreased arterial flow volumes and normalization of the resistive indexes are specific and may obviate the need for repetitive follow-up arteriography.[43]

Magnetic Resonance Imaging

Magnetic resonance imaging (MRI) has replaced computed tomography (CT) in the evaluation of vascular malformation. It has proved to be a mainstay in the initial diagnostic evaluation as well as for assessing the efficacy of endovascular therapy. MRI can accurately distinguish between high- and low-flow malformations and also the relationship to adjacent anatomic structures such as muscles, nerves, and organs. CT is much less helpful than MRI in imaging vascular malformations and hemangiomas. The role of CT is more important when there is significant intraosseous involvement. Unlike CT, MRI easily distinguishes between high- and low-flow lesions. MRI is an excellent noninvasive imaging modality to determine the efficacy of therapy, many times obviating the need for more invasive vascular procedures. In high-flow lesions, the T1-weighted and gradient echo sequences are the most effective means for determining residual areas of the vascular lesion, the presence of thrombosis, and shrinkage of the lesion. In low-flow malformations, fast spin-echo T2-weighted fat-suppressed images best delineate the extent of the lesion. Further, decrease in signal in these lesions delineates the areas successfully treated compared with the remaining untreated areas demonstrating the increased T2 signal.[44]

CONCEPTS IN PATIENT MANAGEMENT

Team Approach

After the diagnosis has been established, the next major decision is to determine whether therapy is warranted. The interventional radiologist or interventional neuroradiologist should plan and direct the patient's care with surgical specialists who are familiar with the management of hemangiomas and vascular malformations and the problems they present. It is extremely important that appropriate surgical, medical, pediatric, and anesthesiologic specialists be involved for optimal patient care. They should function much like a tumor board team in the management of cancer.

The Role of Anesthesiology

As noted in Chapter 22, pain control is an issue with the use of intravascular ethanol. Anesthesiologists can greatly aid in solving this problem and determining whether general anesthesia or intravenous sedation is required for the proposed procedure. This leaves interventional radiologists and interventional neuroradiologists free to concentrate on the case in hand. For children, general anesthesia is required. In patients with large vascular malformations, Swan-Ganz and arterial line monitoring are also performed. The maximal volume of ethanol used to treat patients with vascular malformations rarely exceeds 0.5 ml/kg body weight total dose. In some unusual instances, up to 1 ml/kg body weight total is used. Most patients tolerate these total ethanol volumes very well; exceeding these doses can lead to ethanol toxicity.[22]

Cardiopulmonary collapse is a rare but dreaded sequela. Pulmonary artery Swan-Ganz line and arterial line monitoring is essential to minimize this possibility. Once pulmonary artery pressures begin to rise, it is best to wait and not inject any more ethanol until the pulmonary pressures begin to normalize. Further management of this situation is described below under "Complications."

Vascular Access to Precapillary Lesions

The area of vascular access, whether it be the groin, the arm, or other points of percutaneous catheter access, is prepared and draped in sterile fashion, as is the area of the malformation that is to be treated percutaneously. Fluoroscopy and/or CDI techniques are used in patients requiring percutaneous access. Detailed arteriography is performed to determine the angioarchitecture of normal and abnormal arteries. In high-flow lesions, in which the patient may have had previous therapy (e.g., surgical ligations, partial resections, coil placement, glue embolization), direct puncture techniques may be required to circumvent catheterization obstacles. Superselective placement of the catheter tip or needletip is necessary. Only then can ethanol be injected into the malformation and all normal vascular structures be spared. To achieve superselectivity, coaxial and even triaxial systems may be required. In some instances, a long 6- or 7-Fr. sheath may be placed from the groin into the abdominal aorta. Through this sheath, which provides support, a 5- or 6-Fr. catheter can be placed distally. Then, through this catheter, a microcatheter can be triaxially placed even more distally. Multiple arterial punctures may even be required to place additional catheters for distal embolization, or if necessary to place occlusion balloon catheters to achieve some element of vascular stasis.

At times, even these complex maneuvers may fail and direct puncture of the malformation may be required. The area of percutaneous puncture is prepared and draped in sterile fashion. The needle, usually in the 18- to 20-gauge range, is advanced under real-time ultrasound guidance or by means of arterial contrast injections and fluoroscopic guidance. Once correct placement has been achieved with the direct puncture needle, contrast injections as well as ethanol injections may be performed through that needle. Proximal in-flow occlusion may be necessary. Occlusion balloon catheters may be needed to achieve vascular stasis.

Bleeding is rarely a problem after removal of the direct puncture needle. However, if there is concern, Avitene, a topical hemostatic agent, can be injected (mixed with contrast) as the needle is retracted. This may be necessary in the direct puncture treatment of high-flow malformations but is not usually required in the direct puncture of low-flow malformations.

After ethanol injection, a wait of 10 to 15 minutes is customary before another direct puncture angiogram or catheter angiogram is obtained. Frequently, additional compartments of the vascular malformation fill as others become thrombosed. The procedure is terminated when the maximal amount of ethanol is reached, if a significant amount of malformation is successfully treated, or if a complication occurs requiring termination of the procedure.

TECHNIQUE OF DIRECT PERCUTANEOUS ETHANOL ABLATION OF POSTCAPILLARY LESIONS

This procedure should not be performed by anyone without extensive experience in the use of ethanol; the procedure is fraught with danger.

We use small (18- to 25-gauge) "butterfly" needles, flushed before use. These are placed directly into the mass, and observation is made for backbleeding. Once backbleeding is seen, contrast is injected very slowly under fluoroscopic observation to confirm intravascular location. The appearance of channels may be unusual and confusing. Backflow of lymph fluid can also be seen, but injection will still reveal a reticular network.

Contrast injection should be performed extremely slowly to allow flow into the channel without extravasation, which would confuse interpretation and also allow nontarget embolization. After contrast injection, the short tubing of the butterfly should be flushed slightly to allow infusion of ethanol without contrast precipitation. Depending on the size of the channels, 0.5 to 5 ml of ethanol can be infused.

After ethanol infusion, the butterfly tubing is laid aside; it is *not* removed from the skin. Immediate removal will allow extravasation not only of the current injection but also of any subsequent infusion, which can leak out the same hole rather than flow into the vascular channels that need therapy. A different butterfly is then used to puncture an additional site.

The spacing of these puncture sites depends on the nature of the lesion. If the vascular channels are very small and only about 1 ml of ethanol can be infused, the spacing of the punctures will need to be close (1 to 3 cm). The amount of ethanol that can be infused depends on observation of the contrast injection and on the "feel" of the injection. If the contrast flows easily into distal channels and there is no increasing resistance during injection, a larger amount of ethanol can be infused. Conversely, if the intraluminal space easily reaches capacity, it can be felt in the syringe and vaguely observed by blurring of the outline of the channels.

If the channels are large and a large amount of ethanol can be directly infused, the spacing of punctures can be expanded to 2 to 5 cm. Each subsequent puncture can result in aspiration of fresh blood, ethanol, or lysed and coagulated cellular products (confirming intercommunication of these channels).

Venous channels appear to be more linear and larger than lymphatic channels. Lymphatic channels are typically very reticular, angular, and microscopic. They, too, can be ablated with ethanol, however.

At the end of the procedure, all needles are pulled out of the skin and compression applied where necessary. Typically, the fluid extravasating from these punctures is watery and not initially thrombogenic. The lack of any real pressure within these structures allows hemostasis to occur easily.

Postoperative Management

After the procedure, patients are revived from anesthesia and sent to the recovery room for observation. From there, they are usually placed in a routine hospital ward for overnight observation. It is unusual for patients to require placement in the intensive care unit (ICU). Postoperative management consists of intravenous dexamethasone (Decadron), intravenous fluids, and intravenous droperidol (Inapsine) injection as needed to control nausea. Oral or intramuscular ketorolac tromethamine (Toradol) is helpful for controlling pain and swelling in adult patients. Pain after a vascular malformation treatment is unusual, but oral and intravenous pain medications may also be given if needed. Patients with gastrointestinal sensitivity to steroids can also be placed on ranitidine hydrochloride (Zantac) to protect against gastric and duodenal ulcer development. If no complications have occurred that require management, patients can be discharged the day after treatment. Discharge medications usually include a tapering dose of steroids over 7 days, Zantac management to prevent ulcer development, and pain medications if required. All patients are seen in follow-up 7 to 10 days after discharge or sooner if any problems develop.

Follow-Up

Patients always develop focal swelling in the area of malformation that is treated. In most, this swelling resolves within 2 weeks. Usually, all swelling is resolved after 4 weeks and patients, now at their new baseline, are ready for follow-up and further therapy

as required. After serial ethanol endovascular therapy, MRI and CDI can be used to document the efficacy of therapy. CDI spectral analysis gives accurate information in treated and untreated high-flow AVMs. AVMs demonstrate high-velocity and low-resistance waveforms that amplify the closer the transducer gets to the high-flow lesion. As the high-flow malformation serially becomes ablated, the waveform normalizes and the resistive indexes and flow volumes also become normalized.

MRI is also an important follow-up tool, being excellent for evaluating high- and low-flow lesions as well as pediatric hemangiomas. After serial ablation of a high- or low-flow lesion, alteration in the MRI signal characteristics becomes obvious. In high-flow lesions, flow voids on T1-weighted sequences become absent and thrombosed vessels are identified. Gradient echo sequences demonstrate decreased arterial vascularity because of the AVM thrombosis. In low-flow lesions, the T2-weighted fast spin-echo fat-suppressed imaging sequence is most important. Residual venous malformations will demonstrate markedly increased signal. Thrombosed and treated malformations have a much diminished signal. Patients are evaluated with noninvasive and angiographic studies annually. After several years of persistent closure, noninvasive imaging modalities are usually sufficient for continued follow-up.

COMPLICATIONS
General Considerations

Various complications can occur with any interventional procedure. Because vascular malformations are historically one of the most problematic lesions to be treated by any branch of medicine, complications must be expected. Our initial series reported a total complication rate of 30% (10% major, 20% minor).[23] With more experience, the complication rate has dropped to less than 10% overall.[22] Complications are related to the tissues being embolized. Nontarget embolization with ethanol leads to tissue necrosis as capillary beds of normal arteries are totally destroyed. The tissues being fed by these capillary beds will be devitalized and necrotic. Therefore, it is essential that superselective catheter positioning and superselective needle positioning be achieved before ethanol injection can be considered.

Involvement of the appropriate clinical specialists in the management of complications is essential to minimize the morbidity of the complication. A multidisciplinary team of specialists is required to treat vascular malformations. Each specialist brings important knowledge and experience to the management of these problematic lesions. It is important for this team of physicians to be involved routinely with patients who have vascular malformations so that when a complication occurs, the team is familiar with the underlying pathology and the complications that can result from treating it, and can manage the complication appropriately to minimize its morbidity.

Cardiopulmonary Collapse

If pulmonary artery pressures become pathologically high, the infusion of nitroglycerin, adenosine, or prostaglandin E_1 through the Swan-Ganz line can lower the intrapulmonary pressures; nitroglycerin is preferred. In some patients, increased pulmonary artery pressures related to ethanol injection reaching the pulmonary artery capillary bed may cause precapillary spasm, which is a transient phenomenon. However, in patients in whom pulmonary artery pressures remain elevated for a prolonged time or continue to elevate, nitroglycerin infusion through the Swan-Ganz line helps reduce these pressures to normal.[45]

The treatment of this complication must be first through recognition of the problem (via the indwelling Swan-Ganz catheter) and then by either watchful waiting or active intervention. The Swan-Ganz catheter should be in the main pulmonary outflow tract (the main pulmonary artery) and not in a peripheral subsegmental branch where only a small amount of pulmonary vascular bed would receive any infusion. The small lumen of the Swan-Ganz means that a forceful injection of fluid is necessary, with the concentration of nitroglycerin being relatively high (typically 200 µg/ml). In addition, an infusion of nitroglycerin should be ready to administer through a peripheral venous line, so that it can be added to the dose administered through the Swan-Ganz catheter, if necessary, to bring the pulmonary artery pressure down.

The only limiting factor to the rapid infusion of nitroglycerin is the systemic arterial pressure, which cannot be allowed to drop to an abnormally low level. Therefore, an arterial line is necessary for monitoring purposes, and it is placed at the beginning of the procedure.

Thrombosis, Edema, and Neural Injury

Vascular spasm, edematous tissues, and venous thrombosis can lead to complications. Localized skin blisters may occur, usually a minor annoyance that heals uneventfully. Injury to adjacent muscles, organs, or other tissues is possible. Motor or sensory nerve injuries can occur. Most neural injuries have been related to postprocedure swelling, with resultant nerve compression, rather than nontarget embolization of the vasa nervorum. Aggressive dexamethasone therapy is essential to minimize the effects of the swelling and allow the nerve to recover more quickly. It is unusual for nerve injuries to be permanent. For example, a 63-year-old woman underwent direct puncture embolization of a massive paraspinal AVM (see Fig. 27–4). Previously, the patient had undergone multiple surgeries and arterial ligations, and after these failed, had received radiation therapy. This exacerbated the problems. During the second ethanol embolization session, the patient developed paraspinal swelling and lost the function of the quadriceps femoris muscle group (iliofemoral nerve injury).[23] This developed into acute neuropraxia of the quadriceps femoris muscle group. Within 6 months, however, the patient was climbing stairs, riding bicycles, and dancing, thus documenting total nerve recovery. In the facial area, cranial nerve VII can be injured. One patient who had extensive venous malformation involving the left facial and tongue area suffered an acute postprocedure left seventh nerve neuropraxia not once, but twice. In both instances the nerve recovered completely within 2 months. Again, in this case an arterial embolization was not performed. It was the swelling from the venous malformation in the area of the parotid gland that caused this acute neuropraxia. Intense venous thrombosis can cause sufficient edema to initiate arterial thrombosis. The arterial thrombosis, coupled with the venogenic edema, can lead to extensive tissue necrosis. If this is suspected, arteriography and urokinase infusion must be performed to revascularize the tissues.

REFERENCES

1. Szilagyi DE, Smith RF, Elliott JP, Hageman JH. Congenital arteriovenous anomalies of the limbs. *Arch Surg* 1976;111:423–429.
2. Tanner NSB, Pickford MA. Preliminary report: intratumoural ligation as a salvage procedure for the management of life threatening AVMs. *Br J Plast Surg* 1993;46:694–702.
3. Mulliken JB, Glowacki J. Hemangiomas and vascular malformations in infants and children: a classification based on endothelial characteristics. *Plast Reconstr Surg* 1982;69:412–420.
4. Mulliken JB, Zetter BR, Folkman J. In vitro characteristics of endothelium from hemangiomas in vascular malformations. *Surgery* 1982;92:348–353.
5. Glowacki J, Mulliken JB. Mast cells in hemangiomas and vascular malformations. *Pediatrics* 1982;70:48–51.
6. Finn MC, Glowacki J, Mulliken JB. Congenital vascular lesions: clinical application of a new classification. *J Pediatr Surg* 1983;18:894–900.
7. Upton J, Mulliken JB, Murray JE. Classification and rationale for management for vascular anomalies in the upper extremity. *J Hand Surg (Am)* 1985;10:970–975.
8. Mulliken JB, Young AE (eds): Vascular Birthmarks: Hemangiomas and Malformations. Philadelphia: WB Saunders, 1988.
9. Stigmar G, Crawford JS, Ward CM, Thomson HG. Ophthalmic sequelae of infantile hemangiomas of the eyelids and orbit. *Am J Ophthalmol* 1978;85:806–813.
10. Overcash KE, Putney FJ. Subglottic hemangioma of the larynx treated with steroid therapy. *Laryngoscope* 1973;83:679–682.
11. Argenta LC, Bishop E, Cho KJ, et al. Complete resolution of life threatening hemangioma by embolization and cortical steroids. *Plast Reconstr Surg* 1982;760:739–742.
12. Bartoshesky LE, Bull M, Feingold M. Cortical steroid treatment of cutaneous hemangiomas: how effective? A report on twenty-four children. *Clin Pediatr* 1978;17:625–638.
13. Hurvitz CH, Alkalay AL, Slovinsky L, et al. Cyclophosphamide therapy in life threatening vascular tumors. *J Pediatr* 1986;109:360–363.
14. Warrell RP Jr, Kempin SJ. Treatment of severe coagulopathy in the Kasabach-Merritt syndrome with aminocaproic acid and cryoprecipitate. *N Engl J Med* 1985;313:309–312.
15. Bowles LJ. Perinatal hemorrhage associated with Kasabach-Merritt syndrome. *Clin Pediatr* 1981;20:428–429.
16. Esterly NG. Kasabach-Merritt syndrome in infants. *J Am Acad Dermatol* 1973;8:504–513.
17. Persky MS, Berenstein A. Combined treatment of head and neck vascular masses with preoperative embolization. *Laryngoscope* 1994;94:20–27.

18. Jackson IT, Carrion R, Potparic Z, Hussain K. Hemangiomas, vascular malformations and lymphovenous malformations: classification and methods of treatment. *Plast Reconstr Surg* 1993;91:1216–1230.

19. Halliday AW, Smith EJ, Jackson J, et al. Indications for surgery for AVMs. *Br J Surg* 1992;79:361–362.

20. Halliday AW, Mansfield AO. Congenital arteriovenous malformations. *Br J Surg* 1993;80:2–3.

21. Jackson IT, Jack CR, Aycock B, et al. The management of intraosseous AVMs in the head and neck area. *Plast Reconstr Surg* 1989;84:47–54.

22. Yakes WF, Rossi P, Odink H. How I do it: arteriovenous malformation management. *Cardiovasc Intervent Radiol* 1996;19:65–71.

23. Yakes WF, Haas DK, Parker SH, et al. Symptomatic vascular malformations: ethanol embolotherapy. *Radiology* 1989;170:1059–1066.

24. Widlus DM, Murray RR, White RI Jr, et al. Congenital arteriovenous malformations: tailored embolotherapy. *Radiology* 1988;169:511–516.

25. Yakes WF, Pevsner PH, Reed MD, et al. Serial embolizations of an extremity arteriovenous malformation with alcohol via direct percutaneous puncture. *AJR* 1986;146:1038–1040.

26. Takebayashi S, Hosaka M, Ishizuka E, et al. AVMs of the kidneys: ablation with alcohol. *AJR* 1988;150:587–590.

27. Vinson AM, Rohrer DB, Willcox CW, et al. Absolute ethanol embolization for peripheral AVM: a report of two cures. *South Med J* 1988;81:1052–1055.

28. Yakes WF, Haas DK, Parker SH, et al. Alcohol embolotherapy of vascular malformations. *Semin Intervent Radiol* 1989;6:146–161.

29. Yakes WF, Luethke JM, Parker SH, et al. Ethanol embolization of vascular malformations. *RadioGraphics* 1990;10:787–796.

30. Yakes WF, Luethke JM, Merland JJ, et al. Ethanol embolization of arteriovenous fistulas: a primary mode of therapy. *J Vasc Interv Radiol* 1990;1:89–96.

31. Mourao GS, Hodes JE, Gobin YP, et al. Curative treatment of scalp AV fistulas by direct puncture and embolization with absolute alcohol. *J Neurosurg* 1991;75:634–637.

32. Yakes WF. Extremity venous malformations: diagnosis and management. *Semin Intervent Radiol* 1994;11:332–339.

33. Yakes WF, Parker SH. Diagnosis and management of vascular anomalies. In Castaneda-Zuniga WR, Tadavarthy SM (eds): Interventional Radiology. Baltimore: Williams & Wilkins, 1992, pp 152–189.

34. Yakes WFJ, Dake MD. Angiographic and interventional procedures of the hand. In Gilula LA, Yin Y (eds): Imaging of the Wrist and Hand. Philadelphia: WB Saunders, 1996, pp 499–522.

35. Vogelzang RL, Yakes WF. Vascular malformations: effective treatment with absolute ethanol. In Yao JST, Pearce WH (eds): Arterial Surgery: Management of Challenging Problems. Stamford, CT: Appleton & Lange, 1996, pp 533–549.

36. Yakes WF. Diagnosis and management of venous malformations. In Savader SJ, Trerotola SO (eds): Venous Interventional Radiology with Clinical Perspectives. New York: Thieme, 1996, pp 139–150.

37. Yakes WF. Interventional neuroradiologic procedures in the head and neck: ENT perspective. In English GM (ed): Otolaryngology. New York: Lippincott-Raven, 1996, pp 1–26.

38. Yakes WF. Diagnosis and management of AVMs. In Haskal ZJ, Kerlan RK, Trerotola SO (eds): SCVIR Syllabus: Thoracic and Visceral Vascular Interventions. Fairfax, VA: Society of Cardiovascular and Interventional Radiology, 1996, pp 314–322.

39. Nakano H, Igawa M. Complication after embolization of internal iliac artery by gelatin sponge powder. *Hiroshima J Med Sci* 1986;35:21–25.

40. Vintner HV, Lundie MJ, Kaufmann JCE. Long-term pathological follow-up of cerebral arteriovenous malformations treated by embolization with bucrylate. *N Engl J Med* 1986;314:477–483.

41. Rao VRK, Mandalam KR, Gupta AK, et al. Dissolution of isobutyl 2-cyanoacrylate on long-term follow-up. *AJNR* 1989;10:135–141.

42. Schweitzer JS, Chang BS, Madsen P, et al. The pathology of arteriovenous malformations of the brain treated by embolotherapy. Results of embolization with multiple agents. *Neuroradiology* 1993;35:468–474.

43. Yakes WF, Stavros AT, Parker SH, et al. Color Doppler imaging of peripheral high-flow vascular malformations before and after embolotherapy (RSNA presentation). *Radiology* 1990;177(P):156.

44. Rak KM, Yakes WF, Ray RL, et al. MR imaging of symptomatic peripheral malformations. *AJR* 1992;159:107–112.

45. Yakes WF, Baker R. Cardiopulmonary collapse: A sequela of ethanol embolotherapy. *Radiology* 1993;189(P):145.

ADDITIONAL READINGS

Azzolini A, Bertani A, Riberti C. Superselective embolization and immediate surgical treatment: Our present approach to treatment of large vascular hemangiomas of the face. *Ann Plast Surg* 1982;9:42–62.

Baker LL, Dillon WP, Hieshima GB, et al. Hemangiomas and vascular malformations of the head and neck: MR characterization. *AJNR* 1993;14:307–314.

Bardach J, Panje W. Surgical management of the large cavernous hemangioma. *Otolaryngol Head Neck Surg* 1981;89:792–796.

Braun IF, Levy S, Hoffman JC. The use of transarterial microembolization in the management of hemangiomas of the perioral region. *J Oral Maxillofac Surg* 1985;239–248.

Cole IE. Haemangioendothelioma of the head and neck. *J Laryngol Otol* 1982;96:545–558.

Enjolras O, Mulliken JB. The current management of vascular birthmarks. *Pediatr Dermatol* 1993;10:311–333.

Fishman SJ, Mulliken JB. Hemangiomas and vascular malformations of infancy and childhood. *Pediatr Clin* 1993;40:1177–1200.

Wisnicki JL. Hemangiomas and vascular malformations. *Ann Plast Surg* 1984;12:41–59.

Yonetsu K, Nakayama E, Miwa K, et al. Magnetic resonance imaging of oral and maxillofacial angiomas. *Oral Surg Oral Med Oral Pathol* 1993;76:783–789.

Percutaneous Direct Embolization of Head and Neck Vascular Tumors

A.E. Casasco / E. Houdart / H.S. Jhaveri / D. Herbreteau / A. Aymard /
B. George / M. Wassef / P.T. Ba Huy / J.-J. Merland

Preoperative embolization of the arterial feeders of extracranial vascular neoplasms by superselective catheterization is a well-established procedure at major medical centers. Surgeons appreciate this technique, since it reduces intraoperative blood loss and facilitates tumor resection.

Most of these hypervascular tumors are supplied by multiple branches of the external carotid artery; these are accessible to superselective catheterization and embolization using polyvinyl alcohol particles (PVA) with minimal risk.[1-6] However, when these tumors invade the skull base, they recruit arterial supply from the ipsilateral internal carotid artery and/or vertebral artery, making embolization more difficult as well as riskier.[6, 7] For this specific reason, skull base tumors are often incompletely embolized and partially devascularized. This makes surgery more difficult.

In addition, the external carotid artery and/or its branches are occasionally ligated because of previous surgical therapy. In such situations, arterial catheterization can be performed by direct puncture of branches of the external carotid artery.[8] These embolizations can be effective but are not always complete, and this often leads to only partial devascularization of the tumor.

For all of these reasons, a percutaneous approach can be helpful.

GENERAL TECHNIQUE

Careful analysis of cross-sectional imaging of skull base tumors in both axial and coronal planes reveals that most are accessible with a needle via the nose, mouth, or precondylar region, or by directly puncturing the overlying skin if the lesion is subcutaneous.[9, 10]

We have developed a technique of direct intratumoral embolization using a polymerizing embolic agent such as *N*-butyl-2-cyanoacrylate (NBCA) (Histoacryl, Braun, Melsungen, Germany) or alcohol. After direct tumor puncture is performed, contrast gently injected directly into the tumor reveals the tumor capillary bed followed by draining tumor veins. A liquid embolic agent such as Histoacryl, when injected slowly under direct biplane fluoro-

scopic control, is well distributed throughout the tumor, and complete homogeneous devascularization is achieved. By this technique, one can reach areas of tumor that are supplied by pial branches or are difficult to reach via endovascular technique.[9, 10]

The materials required are listed in Table 28–1.

STRATEGY OF TREATMENT OF SPECIFIC TUMORS

Juvenile Nasopharyngeal Angiofibromas

Juvenile nasopharyngeal angiofibromas (JNAs) are highly vascular, benign tumors that occur in young males (Fig. 28–1). Common presenting symptoms include epistaxis, nasal discharge, and nasal obstruction.

Axial and coronal computed tomography (CT) usually shows a nasopharyngeal mass (Fig. 28–1*A*) with anterior bowing of the posterior wall of the maxillary antrum as well as a mass in the pterygopalatine fossa. Sometimes there is skull base erosion, intracranial extension, intraorbital extension, or extension across the midline. Multiplanar magnetic resonance imaging (MRI) with and without gadolinium may help evaluate intracranial extension of the tumor.

T A B L E   2 8 – 1   Materials for Percutaneous Embolization of Head and Neck Tumors

1. 5- and 6-Fr. sheath (Terumo, Japan)
2. 5-Fr. vertebral curve catheter (Terumo)
3. 0.035″ guidewire (Terumo)
4. Magic B1 microcatheter (Balt Extrusion, Montmorency, France)
5. 6-Fr. Casasco guide catheter (Nycomed, France)
6. 18- or 20-gauge spinal needles (3½″) or 0.7 × 9 cm
7. Polyethylene connecting tubing (1.0-mm diameter, 50-cm length)
8. Histoacryl
9. Tantalum powder (Nycomed)
10. Lipiodol (Guebert, France)
11. 16- or 18-gauge long lumbar puncture needles (for deep-seated tumors)
12. High-resolution biplane angiography unit with roadmapping

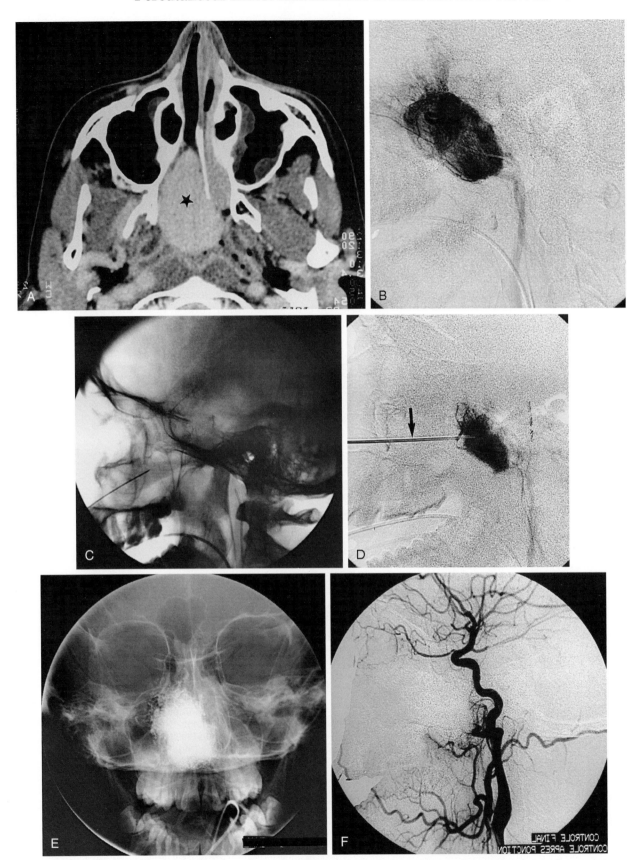

Figure 28-1 Case 1. *A,* A contrast-enhanced computed tomographic scan reveals a large soft tissue mass *(asterisk),* consistent with a right-sided juvenile nasopharyngeal angiofibroma. *B,* Superselective catheterization of the right sphenopalatine artery demonstrates a hypervascular tumor with posterior venous drainage on the lateral view. *C,* The tumor was approached transnasally, as shown in this lateral view. *D,* Intratumoral injection of contrast media (arrow indicates needle) reproduces the angiographic findings without extravasation of contrast. *E, N*-butyl-2-cyanoacrylate (Histoacryl) was then injected; the cast can be seen in this anteroposterior (AP) view. *F,* Total devascularization of the tumor is demonstrated on the postembolization angiogram.

The arterial supply to the tumor includes branches from the internal maxillary, ascending pharyngeal, and facial arteries.[5] Large tumors with intracranial extension may recruit from petrous or cavernous branches of the internal carotid artery. When the tumor is in contact with the orbit or the anterior compartment of the skull base, the ethmoidal branches of the ophthalmic artery may participate. This is discussed in Chapter 10.

Most of the arterial pedicles can be reached by endovascular techniques, and effective preoperative embolization can be performed utilizing PVA particles (Contour Emboli, ITC/Target Therapeutics) 150 to 250 and 255 to 355 microns in diameter.[5, 7, 11, 12] However, when there is erosion of the skull base by aggressive tumor, devascularization by an endovascular approach becomes more difficult, and even in experienced hands more than 20% of these pedicles cannot be embolized. Direct tumor puncture and injection of contrast to verify the position of the needletip, followed by injection of a polymerizing agent

(e.g., Histoacryl), allows embolization of the entire tumor capillary bed, regardless of its blood supply. This permits devascularization of areas difficult to reach by endovascular technique.

Paragangliomas

Paragangliomas are highly vascular benign neoplasms that are found most frequently in the jugular fossa, tympanic cavity, and carotid bifurcation and along the course of the vagus nerve. These tumors arise from neural crest cells; in about 5% of cases, they are known to secrete vasoactive substances such as catecholamines and serotonin, clinically manifesting as sustained or episodic hypertension, palpitations, and headache (Fig. 28–2).

Patients suspected of having a secreting tumor should undergo screening tests for catecholamines and serotonin (urinary VMA and 5-HIAA). Patients with vasoactive tumors are pretreated medically be-

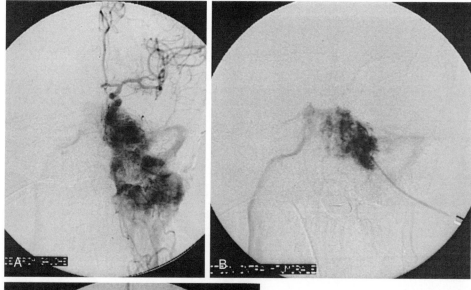

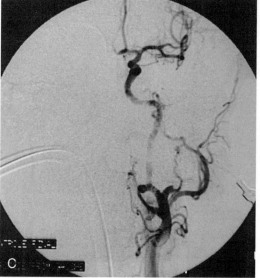

Figure 28-2 Case 2. *A,* An AP view of a left carotid angiogram reveals intra- and extracranial components of a glomus jugulare tumor. The tumoral venous drainage on the left side is via the transverse and sigmoid sinus, whereas on the right side it is via the inferior petrosal sinus. *B,* Direct percutaneous intratumoral injection of contrast allows visualization of the tumor vascular bed and venous drainage. The needle was introduced through the posterior portion of the left jugular foramen. *C,* An AP view of a left common carotid arteriogram performed after embolization shows total devascularization of the tumor.

fore any embolization or endovascular interventions (see Chapter 11).

Direct puncture of these tumors, followed by embolization with a liquid polymerizing agent (Histoacryl), can result in almost complete devascularization of the tumor. Postembolization reduction of mass effect and, in a few weeks, reduction of tumor volume by almost 50% on average has been observed. On long-term follow-up (3 to 24 months, mean of 12 months), Histoacryl-induced tumor necrosis was stable (Fig. 28–3).

Those paragangliomas restricted to the neck or with no obvious extension to the skull base are embolized by a percutaneous lateral cervical approach. Tumors with extension to the base of the skull and invading the posterior fossa are usually embolized by a retropetrosal approach, via the jugular foramen, which is generally enlarged.

Metastases

This technique of devascularization can slow or arrest the growth of secondary tumors. For hypervascu-

lar metastases presenting subcutaneously (e.g., metastases to the calvarium), alcohol is used as the embolic agent, since the necrotic tumor collapses and disappears after embolization. If Histoacryl is employed, the mass decreases in size, with a residual small, hard lump. This is palliative therapy only; tumor remissions last 4 to 6 months after treatment.

Vascular Tumors of the Skull Base

This technique can be applied to all hypervascular neoplasms reached by needle puncture. However, there is one cardinal rule: *the needle must not cross through any vital structure before puncturing the tumor.*[9] Postoperative recurrent tumor, or tumor adjacent to the jugular foramen, can be treated by direct needle puncture. We treated one case of ethmoidofrontal meningioma via a transnasal approach. On superselective angiography, if a tumor vascular blush is not found, it is preferable not to embolize by direct puncture and intratumoral injection of Histoacryl.

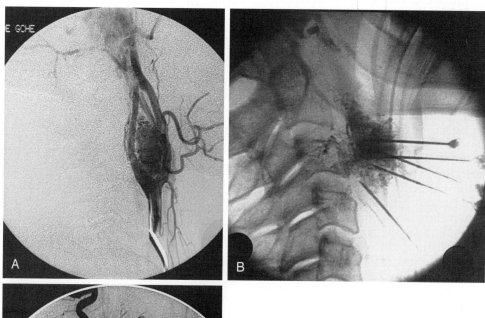

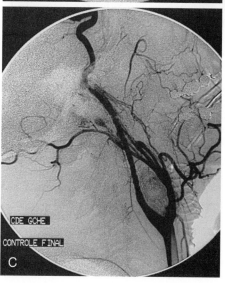

Figure 28-3 Case 3. *A,* A left common carotid angiogram reveals a hypervascular, bilobed vagal paraganglioma. *B,* This was embolized percutaneously with Histoacryl, using multiple needles. *C,* A postembolization left common carotid arteriogram shows total devascularization of the inferior lobe and about 80% devascularization of the superior lobe.

PRE-EMBOLIZATION PATIENT PREPARATION AND PERCUTANEOUS PUNCTURE TECHNIQUES

All patients are evaluated by axial and coronal CT, multiplanar MRI, or both (before and after contrast administration). These examinations provide critical information about the size, shape, location, and extent of the tumor and also help in deciding the most appropriate route for tumor puncture. This baseline cross-sectional imaging is crucial for future follow-up. Patients are premedicated with corticosteroids (24 mg dexamethasone) one day before embolization and receive a second dose after embolization.

Pre-embolization diagnostic angiography of the carotid and vertebral arteries is performed. The tip of the catheter is left in the appropriate vessel and connected to a continuous flush of heparinized saline. This allows angiographic verification of tumor devascularization during the embolization. Bony landmarks around the tumor are identified with the help of CT and/or MRI. General anesthesia is used for percutaneous tumor puncture and injection of embolic agents, since injection of alcohol or liquid polymerizing agents is painful.

Precautions and Relative Contraindications

The pre-embolization angiogram is carefully inspected for arterial supply to the tumor by feeders from the internal carotid or vertebral artery. If arterial supply to the tumor from the internal carotid artery below the origin of the ophthalmic artery is discovered, a standard Magic 1.8-Fr. catheter with a mounted balloon is used and the balloon gently inflated (with a mixture of two thirds contrast and one third normal saline) against the origin of the arterial blood supply to the tumor while Histoacryl is injected into the tumor under fluoroscopic monitoring. This is to prevent retrograde entry of Histoacryl into the internal carotid artery. Similar precautions are taken if a branch of the vertebral artery is found to be participating in the arterial blood supply to the tumor.

However, if the supraopthalmic portion of the internal carotid artery is found to be contributing to the arterial supply of the tumor, balloon protection is not used. In this situation, it is considered that direct puncture embolization of the tumor is relatively contraindicated. The feeders are surgically clipped, and that part of the tumor is not directly embolized.

If some of the ethmoidal branches of the ophthalmic artery are found to be contributing to the arterial blood supply of the tumor, those small branches are also surgically clipped, and that part of the tumor is not embolized by direct puncture technique.

Needles and Approach

For all superficial tumors, 19- or 21-gauge Butterfly-type needles are used. However, when the tumor is deep, biplane fluoroscopy is employed and the shortest and most direct route chosen. The puncture site and needle choice depend up the tumor site.

Transnasal Route

This route is selected to reach almost all JNAs as well as anterior skull base tumors. Most often, 18- or 20-gauge lumbar puncture needles (B.D. Yale, Princeton, NJ) are used; however, a 21-gauge Chiba needle can be used for more deeply located tumors.

The needle is introduced into the nostril under the inferior turbinate, parallel to the hard palate, and directed toward the desired location in the tumor (see Fig. 28–1).

Precondylar Route

This approach is preferred for tumors in the pterygomaxillary region. The needle is inserted anterior to the mandibular condyle via a lateral approach. A 16-gauge sheath needle (Jelco type) is chosen for this approach, using coaxial technique. Once the needle touches the tumor, the stylet of the needle is removed, and the sheath is used as a guide to introduce other 18- or 20-gauge needles and to avoid multiple skin punctures.

Retropetrosal Route

This approach is used mainly for glomus tumors and neuromas, and occasionally for meningiomas. Because of the slow-growing tumors, the jugular foramen is usually eroded and enlarged.

The patient's neck is placed in a hyperextended position and biplane fluoroscopy used. The lateral image is chosen to check the craniovertebral junction and second cervical vertebra.

The needle is introduced between the tip of the ipsilateral mastoid and mandibular ramus and directed superiorly, medially, and posteriorly. On the lateral view, the needle is parallel to the posterior wall of the second cervical vertebra.

Transbuccal Route

This approach is useful for laterally located juvenile angiofibromas. The needle is introduced anterior to the ramus of the ipsilateral mandible and behind the maxilla, piercing through the masseter muscle.

Intratumoral Injection

Once the needle is in the tumor, reflux of blood is noticed upon withdrawing the stylet. However, if the needletip is either in the tumor capsule or outside the tumor, blood return is not seen. Once blood return is seen, an extension tube is connected to the needle. A small amount of contrast is injected only if there is reflux of blood. If contrast is injected in the absence of blood egress from the needle hub, it may mask the subsequent intratumoral injections. Intratumoral contrast injection reveals tumor parenchymography (i.e., tumor stain along with venous return), and also verifies the needle location. Sometimes, it also reveals retrograde opacification of some arterial pedicles and helps to predict potential problems that may ensue if embolic agents are injected with as much or greater force.

Embolization

Most often, Histoacryl is the embolic agent used. The standard preparation is 0.5 ml Histoacryl, 0.5 ml iodized oil (Lipiodol), and tantalum powder. Because of the tantalum powder, the tumor retains a black color. Polymerization of the embolic material occurs in the tumor bed. The extension tube and needle are rinsed carefully with 5% dextrose solution before injecting the liquid embolic agent. Histoacryl injection is performed slowly, under constant fluoroscopic monitoring. If the embolic agent is seen entering the venous structures, the injection is immediately stopped for a few seconds before continuing. However, if the embolic agent is seen entering the arterial pedicle in retrograde fashion, the injection is stopped immediately, which prevents further progression of the agent in the pedicle, owing to countercurrent circulation. Five to ten needle punctures may be necessary; leaving the needle in the site helps guide the next needle (see Fig. 28–2). The devascularization of the tumor is verified by arteriography.

For malignant tumors or inoperable metastases, 96% alcohol (absolute ethanol) is used as *palliative* therapy. The alcohol is mixed with tantalum powder and injected very slowly and in very small volumes; progress is frequently checked by arteriography. In this way, good embolization results can be achieved.

POSTEMBOLIZATION CARE AND FOLLOW-UP

Patients are routinely given dexamethasone (16 mg/ day) for 48 hours after the embolization. For local pain, major analgesics are administered for 1 or 2 days after embolization. Immediately after the embolization, we obtain a CT scan to verify the location of the embolic agent. For patients undergoing surgery, MRI and CT scans are obtained to check for residual tumor or complete resection. These scans also act as a baseline to monitor for future tumor recurrence. For patients who undergo embolization as sole therapy, CT and MRI are performed every 3 months, along with clinical follow-up.

RESULTS

Over a period of 3 years, we treated 56 hypervascular tumors using this technique, including 29 JNAs, 22 glomus tumors (of which four were at the carotid bifurcation and six were jugular), four metastases to the calvarium with erosion of bone, and one ethmoidofrontal meningioma with skull base erosion.

Either complete or greater than 80% devascularization of tumor was observed in all patients, regardless of the arterial blood supply. Postembolization axial and coronal CT scans revealed tumor casts composed of embolic agent (Histoacryl mixed with tantalum).

Follow-up for Preoperative Embolization

In the patients who underwent surgery, the tumors were totally excised. Blood loss during surgery was significantly reduced and no blood transfusion was necessary. There was generally a good plane of cleavage and, thanks to the black discoloration caused by the tantalum, the tumors were easily identified. Follow-up of the patients with JNAs (3 months to 36 months, mean 16 months) revealed no recurrences.

Pathology of Tumors Embolized by Direct Puncture

On gross examination, embolized tumors are stained brown and black by the combination of Histoacryl and tantalum powder (Fig. 28–4A). Histologically, Histoacryl appears in the tissues as an irregularly shaped, translucent, intravascular mass. Embolized vessels are more widely dilated than after particulate embolization, and the number of occluded vessels within the lesion is higher than after intra-arterial embolization with either PVA or calibrated microspheres.[13] In the case of nasopharyngeal angiofibromas, the Histoacryl casts often occupy a significant portion of the tumor (Fig. 28–4B). All embolized lesions demonstrate degenerative changes, and in some cases (especially in paragangliomas), extensive necrosis may be present. In paragangliomas, the intra- or extravascular location of Histoacryl is often difficult to assess, owing to necrosis and disappearance of the thin walls of most of the vessels. In some places, however, the Histoacryl does appear to be clearly intravascular (Fig. 28–4C). Mild to moderate inflammation (polymorphonucleocytes and a few lymphocytes) is observed at the periphery of embolized areas, as in cases of transarterial Histoacryl embolization.[14] In rare cases, Histoacryl and metallic powder can be found outside the embolized lesion, in the peritumoral fibrosis or the nasopharyngeal mucosa, probably because of retrograde embolization of feeding arteries (Fig. 28–4D). These emboli are associated with focal necrosis and moderate inflammatory changes.

Embolization Without Surgery

The patients who were treated by this technique and did not undergo surgery were followed clinically as well as by MRI and CT. There was significant reduction or total disappearance of mass effect in every case. Clinical improvement was observed almost immediately, within 24 hours after embolization.

The maximal reduction in tumor volume was seen in the first 2 weeks and remained unchanged on subsequent follow-ups. However, the metastases that were embolized with alcohol showed recurrence in 6 months and were retreated by the same technique. The long-term outcome of the treatment of glomus

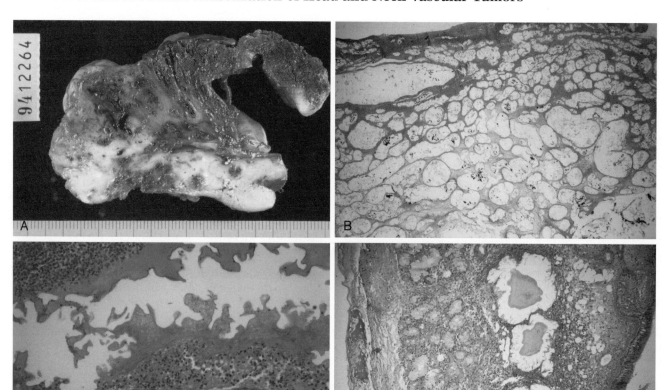

Figure 28-4 Case 4. *A,* A gross view of a transected nasopharyngeal angiofibroma embolized by direct puncture demonstrates the staining of the heavily embolized areas. White areas are not embolized or less well embolized. *B,* A low-power view of the tumor reveals the vessels to be dilated and to contain large amounts of translucent Histoacryl and some black tantalum particles. The dark border at the top of the specimen corresponds to the peripheral inflammatory infiltrate (H&E/saffron stain, 4× magnification). *C,* Intravascular location of Histoacryl in a paraganglioma is demonstrated (H&E/saffron stain, 50× magnification). The translucent embolic material is found in the lumen of the vessel, associated with clot and a few polymorphonucleocytes. *D,* Histoacryl is seen in an extratumoral location (nasal mucosa). Some vessels in the mucosa contain translucent Histoacryl and are surrounded by mild inflammatory changes (H&E/saffron stain, 12× magnification).

tumors remains unknown at this time. However, on short-term follow-up, this embolization technique has resulted in either clinical improvement or freedom from tumor-associated symptoms.

This technique of embolization either slows or arrests tumor growth. Long-term follow-up is essential. This method of embolization could be considered as an alternative to surgery in elderly and debilitated patients. If the long-term results in our series confirm our current observations, this technique may perhaps be considered as a sole therapy for glomus tumors involving the skull base.

TECHNICAL PROBLEMS, COMPLICATIONS, AND SOLUTIONS

Mostly minor complications have been experienced. After embolization, local pain is common and responds to analgesics. One patient with a glomus tumor developed a Horner's syndrome that lasted for 4 weeks, followed by complete recovery. Another patient, with a jugular glomus tumor, developed an

ipsilateral hypoglossal nerve paralysis that resolved in 2 weeks.

Two major complications were encountered during use of this technique. In our early experience, we were treating a patient with a JNA via a right transnasal approach. Toward the end of the procedure, while we were embolizing the portion of the tumor close to the base of the skull, the dense opacity of the already embolized tumor obscured the tip of the needle. The skull base was already eroded because of the large nasopharyngeal angiofibroma. When the Histoacryl was injected, a small amount entered the right internal carotid artery. Histoacryl injection was immediately halted. However, a small amount polymerized in the right middle cerebral artery. The patient developed an acute right middle cerebral artery infarction and died after 3 days. Since then, no matter which route we choose to introduce the needle, we obtain both anteroposterior and lateral views every time we inject contrast before embolization, and check carefully in both anteroposterior and lateral views while injecting Histoacryl. Also, the mixture being used at the time was 0.5 ml Histoacryl + 1.5 ml Lipiodol + 1.5 gm tantalum powder. The mixture has now been changed to 0.5 ml Histoacryl + 0.5 ml Lipiodol + 0.5 to 1 gm powder.

In another patient with a left-side JNA, the tumor involved the floor of the left orbit. Toward the end of the procedure, we were treating the tumor that had eroded the orbit floor. After contrast injection and verification of the needle position in both planes, we started slowly injecting the standard embolic agent mixture. A small collateral vessel to the ophthalmic artery, not seen on the pre-embolization injection, opened up, and a small amount of Histoacryl entered the ophthalmic artery in a retrograde fashion. The embolic agent injection was immediately stopped. However, a drop of Histoacryl occluded the left ophthalmic artery, and the patient developed acute loss of vision in the left eye.

Lessons Learned

During the final stages of embolization, unforeseen potential collateral communications may result in reflux of embolic agent into an arterial pedicle. If this is seen, the procedure must be stopped immediately to avoid complications. Biplane fluoroscopic equipment of excellent quality, with high resolution, is essential. Filling of tumor veins must not extend beyond the limits of the tumor (i.e., one must stop injecting embolic agent upon identifying tumor veins) to avoid complications.

CONCLUSION

Devascularization of skull base tumors by direct tumor puncture is a safe technique that can be performed by most interventional neuroradiologists, provided that they follow the proper guidelines. This is a very good technique for high-risk tumors or for tumors difficult to reach via an endovascular route.

Considering our preliminary long-term results, this method deserves to be considered as an alternative exclusive therapy in very elderly, debilitated patients or patients with high surgical risk.

REFERENCES

1. Berenstein A, Kricheff I. Microembolization techniques of vascular occlusion: etiology, pathologic and clinical correlation. *AJNR* 1981;2:261–267.
2. Davis KR, Debrun GM. Embolization of juvenile nasopharyngeal fibromas. *Semin Intervent Radiol* 1987;4:309–320.
3. Djindjian R, Merland JJ. Superselective Arteriography of the External Carotid Artery. Berlin: Springer-Verlag, 1978.
4. Forbes G, Earnest F IV, Jackson IT, et al. Therapeutic embolization angiography for extra-axial lesions in the head. *Mayo Clin Proc* 1986;61:427–441.
5. Halbach V, Hieshima G, Higashida R, David C. Endovascular therapy for head and neck tumors. In Vinuela F, Halbach VV, Dion JE (eds): Interventional Neuroradiology: Endovascular Therapy of the Central Nervous System. New York: Raven Press, 1992, pp 17–28.
6. Lasjaunias P. Nasopharyngeal angiofibroma: hazards of embolization. *Radiology* 1980;136:119–123.
7. Lasjaunias P, Berenstein A. Surgical Neuroangiography, Vol 2: Endovascular Treatment of Craniofacial Lesions. New York: Springer-Verlag, 1987, pp 101–126.
8. Gobin YP, Pasco A, Merland JJ, et al. Percutaneous puncture of the external carotid artery or its branches after surgical ligation. *AJNR* 1994;15:79–82.
9. Casasco A, Herbreteau D, Houdart E, et al. Devascularization of craniofacial tumor by percutaneous tumor puncture. *AJNR* 1994;15:1233–1239.
10. Tran Ba Huy P, Borsik M, Herman P, et al. Direct intratumoral embolization of juvenile angiofibromas. *Am J Otolaryngol* 1994;15:429–435.
11. Valvanis A. Preoperative embolization of head and neck: indications, patient selection, goals and precautions. *AJNR* 1986;7:943–952.
12. Davis KR. Embolization of juvenile nasopharyngeal angiofibroma. *AJR* 1979;133:657–663.
13. Beaujeux R, Laurent A, Hodes JE, et al. Calibrated sphere embolization of craniofacial tumors and arteriovenous malformations. *Neuroradiology* 1991;33(Suppl):562–564.
14. Vinters HV, Galil KA, Lundie MJ, Kaufmann JCE. The histotoxicity of cyanoacrylates. A selective review. *Neuroradiology* 1985;27:279–291.

Percutaneous Vertebroplasty:
Indications, Technique, and Complications

C. Depriester / H. Deramond / P. Toussaint / H.S. Jhaveri / P. Galibert

Many lesions of vertebrae may be treated by a percutaneous approach. The main application for percutaneous vertebroplasty with methylmethacrylate (MM) is seen in pathologic conditions that increase the fragility of the vertebral body. Vertebral pain is the major clinical indication for percutaneous vertebroplasty. This treatment can be curative as well as palliative.

We have performed percutaneous vertebroplasty since 1984. Initially, the major clinical indication was for aggressive spinal hemangiomas, but with more experience it was found that two other major clinical indications were osteoporotic vertebral crush fracture syndrome and spinal tumors.[1–9]

Other biomaterials such as alcohol or glue (N-butyl-2-cyanoacrylate [NBCA, Histoacryl], B. Braun Melsungen, Germany) may be injected into other types of vertebral lesions using the percutaneous approach; the common denominator is the percutaneous approach to the vertebral body.[6, 10–12]

PATHOLOGIES AMENABLE TO TREATMENT

The indication for vertebroplasty is any pathology that weakens the vertebral body, with or without resultant spinal pain (rachialgia, from the Greek *rhachis* for spine). Percutaneous vertebroplasty has two objectives: analgesia and solidification. As noted earlier, there are three major pathologic indications: vertebral hemangiomas, osteoporotic vertebral crush fracture syndrome, and malignant tumors of the spine.

Vertebral Hemangiomas

Vertebral hemangiomas are common and benign lesions of the spinal column. The incidence in the population is estimated to be 10% to 12%.[13] These (usually) asymptomatic lesions produce characteristic radiologic findings, including vertical thick trabeculations on plain films, decreased density on computed tomography (CT), and hyperintensity on T1-weighted magnetic resonance imaging (MRI) images due to the presence of abundant fat in the lesion.

Rarely, vertebral hemangiomas can be aggressive by clinical or radiologic criteria. The radiologic criteria of aggressivity are growth of the lesion, bone destruction, vertebral collapse, absence of fat in the vertebral body (isodensity on CT and iso- or hypointensity on T1-weighted MRI), and an active vascular component as demonstrated by hyperdensity on CT and hyperintensity on T1-weighted MRI after intravenous injection of contrast media. Lesions at the thoracic level are the most frequently aggressive ones.[12, 13]

The clinical criteria of aggressivity are intense localized spinal pain and/or neurologic signs related to compression of nerve roots or the spinal cord. Clinically aggressive spinal hemangiomas are frequently aggressive radiologically, especially when there are neurologic signs. Rarely, they may be benign radiologically, especially when clinical signs are limited to intense chronic spinal pain.

Indications

The indications for vertebroplasty are limited to hemangiomas that are aggressive clinically and/or radiologically. Treatment of aggressive vertebral hemangiomas has several objectives:

1. To obtain an antalgic effect
2. To obtain radiculomedullary decompression
3. To obtain spinal stabilization to avoid secondary deformity
4. To halt the evolution of these pseudotumoral vascular malformations

Several situations can be encountered:

- Intense and focalized spinal bone pain related to a spinal hemangioma involving only the vertebral body. In this situation, vertebroplasty has to be performed even if there is no radiologic indication of aggressivity. A rapid and permanent antalgic effect is obtained in more than 90% of cases. When the whole vertebral body is invaded by the vertebral hemangioma, it is often necessary to perform two vertebral punctures. The first allows injection of one hemivertebra; the second allows injection of the remaining hemivertebra. Sometimes, it is possible to obtain injection of the whole angiomatous vertebral body with only one puncture. This situation occasionally occurs at the cervical level (Fig. 29–1).
- Neurologic signs with or without rachialgias related to a radiologically aggressive form of spinal

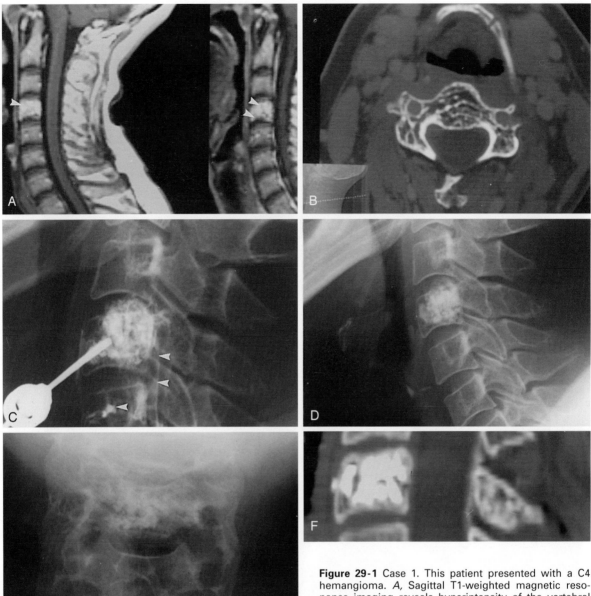

Figure 29-1 Case 1. This patient presented with a C4 hemangioma. *A,* Sagittal T1-weighted magnetic resonance imaging reveals hyperintensity of the vertebral body *(arrowheads). B,* Axial computed tomographic (CT) scan demonstrates trabeculation of the vertebral body and posterior arch involvement by the hemangioma. *C,* After an anterolateral approach, transosseous phlebography shows the draining veins *(arrowheads). D* and *E,* After vertebroplasty, sagittal and frontal plain film views were obtained. *F,* A CT scan with sagittal reconstruction was obtained after vertebroplasty and posterior *N*-butyl-2-cyanoacrylate (NBCA) injection.

hemangioma; there is an epidural invasion with nerve root and/or spinal cord compression. CT, MRI, or both after intravenous injection of contrast media reveals epidural invasion, the "buttock sign" (Fig. 29–2). In this situation, we perform vertebroplasty as a first step. This procedure consists of the injection of MM in the vertebral body, requiring two punctures in most cases. Care must be taken not to inject the epidural ("buttock-like") component with MM. Consequently, it is necessary to carefully observe the MM injection under excellent lateral fluoroscopic control, and to stop the injection before passage of MM beyond the projection of the posterior wall of the vertebral body. The 10-gauge

needles are not completely pulled back after the injection, and their tips remain in the isthmic part of the posterior neural arch.

During the procedure and after the MM injection, a puncture of a site in the vertebral body not injected with MM is performed. This site is often an inferior and posterolateral area of the vertebral body. An 18-gauge needle is used and placed via a posterolateral approach (at the thoracic and lumbar level). Reflux of blood when the stylet is pulled back indicates satisfactory positioning of the needle. Serial images of the remaining vertebral hemangioma and its epidural component by means of local injection of contrast media are then per-

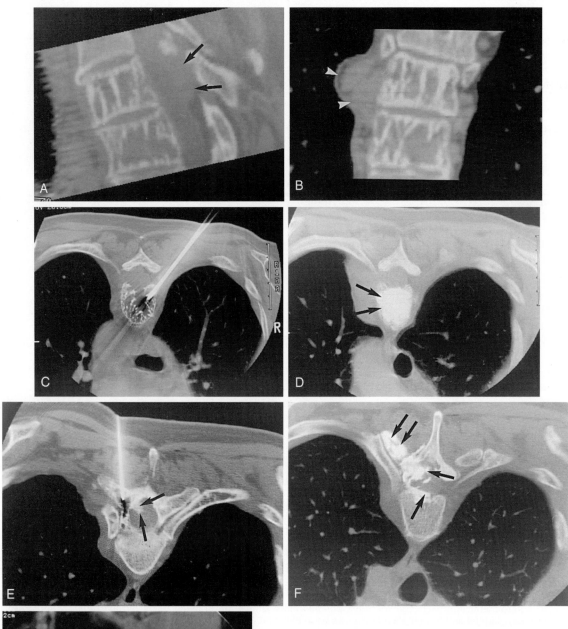

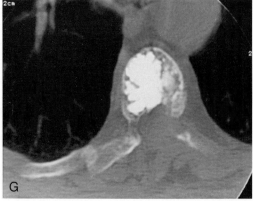

Figure 29-2 Case 2. A T4 and T5 aggressive spinal hemangioma with paraparesis. *A* and *B,* The hemangioma invades the whole of both vertebrae with an epidural component *(arrows)* and an extravertebral extension *(arrowheads). C,* A CT-guided right posterolateral approach is performed with a 10-gauge needle. *D,* The vertebral body is filled with cement *(arrows). E,* The posterior arch is then punctured with an 18-gauge needle, and contrast media is injected into the posterior arch and the epidural component *(arrows). F,* Glue (NBCA) is injected into the posterior arch, epidural component, and posterior component of the hemangioma *(arrows).* The subsequent surgery was easier and bloodless. *G,* Axial CT scan after posterior laminectomy.

formed. After this documentation of the epidural component of the hemangioma, 1 to 5 ml of absolute ethanol is injected very slowly, or a few milliliters of glue (NBCA) (Fig. 29–2).[6, 11]

If necessary, a contralateral puncture and injection of absolute ethanol or glue (NBCA) can be performed when the contrast injection shows only unilateral visualization of the epidural part of the hemangioma. It is also possible to inject the posterior neural arch with absolute ethanol if it is extensively involved by the hemangioma.[3]

Surgery is performed as a second step if necessary. The surgical excision of the hemangioma is easy and bloodless (Fig. 29–2). We have never observed an aggravation of the clinical status after vertebroplasty; in cases with progressive neurologic signs, there has been a quick and significant disappearance of the neurologic signs after vertebroplasty and sclerosis, perhaps because of diminution of the pulsatility of the hemangioma or because of the disappearance of the vascular shunt.

Finally, with our progressive experience in percutaneous treatment of aggressive vertebral hemangiomas over a period of 10 years, the following additional guidelines for the treatment of such a pathologic condition have suggested themselves:

- In patients with acute or subacute compression of the spinal cord, percutaneous vertebroplasty with acrylic cement is performed in association with percutaneous injection of NBCA or alcohol, followed by a decompressive laminectomy.
- In patients with progressive compression of neurologic elements or with intense spinal pain *only*, and when there is an aggressive radiologic appearance of the vertebral hemangioma with an epidural component, percutaneous vertebroplasty with acrylic cement is performed together with percutaneous injection of absolute ethanol in the same procedure, without subsequent surgery.

Osteoporotic Vertebral Crush Fracture Syndrome

Spontaneous vertebral fractures and those induced by minor trauma are complications of osteoporosis. They are the result of mechanical failure of demineralized vertebrae. The most common sites of osteoporotic fractures are the hip, the distal radius, and the vertebrae of the thoracolumbar junction. These fractures occur most frequently in postmenopausal women aged 60 years or older. These vertebral fractures are often highly painful and their clinical management consists of immobilization, analgesic drugs, and specific treatment of osteoporosis. However, immobilization increases demineralization and is potentially harmful, leading to complications, especially in the elderly. In spite of prolonged medical treatment, patients sometimes have incapacitating and persistent back pain. The medical treatment of osteoporosis consists of prevention of fracture, use of antiresorptive drugs (estrogen and calcitonin), and use of bone

formation–stimulating substances (fluoride). The initial symptoms tend to disappear after 4 to 6 weeks.

Recurrent episodes of fracture are usual and cause serious morbidity. Later consequences of vertebral fracture are reduced height, kyphosis, and chronic back pain. In these cases, vertebroplasty alleviates symptoms and reduces the duration of immobilization.[2, 4, 6, 11, 14–16]

We have treated many patients between 49 and 86 years of age by this method. In 75% of cases, the treated level was at the thoracolumbar junction; two vertebrae were treated in 35% of cases and three vertebrae in four cases. All patients had one or more collapsed vertebrae and incapacitating and persistent pain despite medical treatment and immobilization. Percutaneous vertebroplasty was performed 3 weeks to 5 months after the onset of the initial symptoms. In all cases, a bone biopsy was also performed during the same procedure, immediately before vertebroplasty (Figs. 29–3 and 29–4).

The results were excellent in all cases, with quick and complete relief of pain. Patients were capable of standing up and walking 24 to 48 hours after the procedure. This effect is prolonged and the follow-up result is excellent.

No complications have been found when treating patients for this condition. In some cases, an increase of rachialgia was noted immediately after vertebroplasty, but this pain is usually relieved in 2 days with anti-inflammatory drugs (intravenous ketoprofen, 100 to 300 mg/day).[2, 6]

Collapse of the adjacent vertebrae in contact with the one injected with cement is a potential risk. This happened in one patient, and we performed another vertebroplasty.

When the patient has only early collapse and back pain, a vertebroplasty may be performed to avoid the onset or aggravation of kyphosis and secondary collapse. Vertebroplasty must be associated with medical treatment of osteoporosis and sometimes an orthopedic corset to stabilize the spine.[2, 6]

Spinal Tumors

Many malignant spinal tumors, such as metastases, lymphomas, and myelomas, may be treated. These tumors are often painful. Medical pain therapy, radiotherapy, chemotherapy, embolization, and chemoembolization can be employed but are associated with failure and complications.

In the case of a previously untreated painful vertebral metastasis, radiotherapy is useful in 70% of cases to alleviate spinal pain, but this effect is delayed and may take 2 to 6 weeks.[17, 18] Radiotherapy does not prevent vertebral crush, because of tumoral necrosis and secondary deformity of the spine. The aim of vertebroplasty is to obtain an antalgic effect by solidification of the osteolytic lesion. It is only a palliative treatment. With vertebroplasty, disappearance of pain is quick (1 to 3 days), and vertebral consolidation and spinal stability are obtained.[6, 19]

The result is good if spinal pain was the major

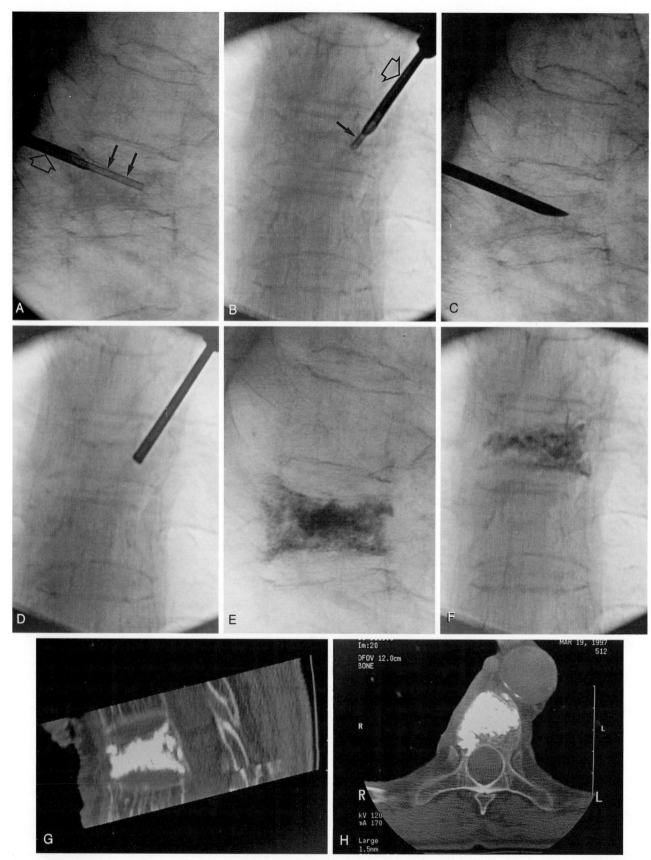

Figure 29-3 Case 3. A T6 osteoporotic crush fracture. *A* and *B,* Sagittal and frontal views demonstrate a right transpedicular approach with a 10-gauge needle *(open arrows)*; a 15-gauge biopsy needle is placed through the vertebroplasty needle *(arrows).* *C* and *D,* After bone biopsy, the vertebroplasty needle is placed into the vertebral body in a lateral position. *E* and *F,* Cement is injected by a right transpedicular approach, allowing a good injection of the whole vertebral body. It is sufficient to obtain a good vertebral consolidation for this pathology. *G* and *H,* Sagittal and axial views demonstrate a satisfactory injection in the vertebra without extravertebral leakage.

symptom, with significant relief of the pain and return to activities of normal living in more than 70% of patients.[20–22]

Indications and Contraindications

Theoretically, the best case would be an osteolytic lesion of the vertebral body, without rupture of the posterior wall, with or without vertebral collapse, and with intense pain. The reality is often very different, and each case is unique; the therapeutic decision must be reached via a multidisciplinary approach (clinical and radiologic).[6, 7, 20] Patients are often seen when there is an extensive osteolytic lesion with vertebral collapse and osteolysis of a part of the posterior vertebral wall. In these cases, vertebroplasty can be performed if there is no epidural invasion by the tumoral process.

From a technical point of view, it is important to inject both the osteolytic and the nonosteolytic parts of the vertebral body with MM. Consequently, two punctures by a transpedicular approach are necessary when this is possible.

As stated above, vertebroplasty is a palliative treatment and not curative (Fig. 29–5). Other therapies have to be undertaken. In the case of malignant lesions, radiotherapy and vertebroplasty should be coordinated. It is logical to perform vertebroplasty before radiotherapy because the analgesic effect is immediate after vertebroplasty and delayed after radiotherapy.[23] No modification of the radiotherapy protocols is necessary after cementation.[24]

When there are neurologic symptoms, percutaneous vertebroplasty can be an adjunct to surgery. It can precede or follow surgery in order to bring about a consolidation of the tumorous level, limiting orthopedic devices, and avoiding surgical anterior corporectomy. Corporectomy is major surgery when there are many metastases or when the patient's health is poor.[7, 16, 25] In cases with rupture of the posterior wall and extension to the spinal canal, the cement injection must be performed very carefully to avoid extravertebral cementation.

If the osteolytic lesion is situated in the posterior arch or if there is a significant extravertebral extension, percutaneous vertebroplasty is not performed. Other substances may be injected into tumoral lesions. Sometimes it is of value to obtain sclerosis; in such cases it is possible to inject alcohol or Ethibloc (Ethicon).[6, 26]

The excellent analgesic effect of vertebroplasty encourages the treatment of other metastatic lesions outside the spine, especially hip metastases, by a percutaneous approach.[6, 27]

MATERIALS AND DEVICES

Large trocars (Société Escoffier Frères SA, Thonon les Bains, France) are used for cement injection. These are 7 to 15 cm long and 10 to 15 gauge. In the lumbar region, a 15-cm, 10-gauge needle is used; a shorter (7- to 10-cm) and sometimes narrower (15-gauge) needle is used in the cervical or high thoracic region. These are specific trocars, with a mandrel, a large bevel, nickeled brass construction, and a Luer-Lok hub. The internal diameter is 2.5 mm and the external diameter 3.3 mm (10 gauge).

Strong (polycarbonate) 2.5- and 3-cc syringes with Luer-Lok hubs (Merit Medical) are needed for MM injection. Injection of a bone cement of high viscosity requires the use of syringes of small cross-sectional area that develop greater pressure; 2.5- to 3-cc syringes represent the best compromise between capacity and area. A syringe handle facilitates injection. We use a home-made device: a rectangular piece of metal with a hole corresponding to the syringe diameter drilled in it.

Acrylic bone cement (Surgical Simplex P, Howmedica International, Inc., Limerick, Ireland) consists of a powder component and a liquid component. The liquid component is composed of MM and an activator to promote polymerization. The powder is composed of polymethylmethacrylate and a radiopaque powder (usually barium sulfate). Tantalum powder (Merck, Inc.) must be added to the bone cement powder to increase the radiopacity so that the cement can be easily seen during fluoroscopic monitoring.

The glue to be injected in selected situations as described above is NBCA (Histoacryl). Ethibloc, also used in selected circumstances, is described in Chapter 1.

PREPROCEDURE ORDERS

Usually, vertebroplasty is performed with the patient under neuroleptanalgesia and local anesthesia. Sometimes, general anesthesia is needed because of the poor condition of the patient or when two or three levels have to be treated. Consequently, a preanesthetic consultation is needed.

Normal coagulation function is necessary, as for all percutaneous procedures. Appropriate laboratory work should be obtained, including prothrombin time and activated partial thromboplastin time.

Plain films of the spine and a CT scan localized on the lesion are always necessary before the procedure to enable it to be planned and to determine whether the posterior wall of the vertebra is intact, the location of the osteolytic part of the lesion, and what obliquity in the transpedicular approach should be given to the needle. MRI gives complementary information on the epidural component of the lesion in hemangiomas and malignant tumors.

DESCRIPTION OF PROCEDURE

The percutaneous approach to the vertebral body depends on the spinal level. An anterolateral approach is used for the cervical spine (Figs. 29–1 and 29–5), while a posterolateral (Fig. 29–6) or transpedicular (Figs. 29–3 and 29–4) approach is used at the thoracic and lumbar levels. When the pedicle is perfectly visualized under fluoroscopic control, the transpedicular approach is the best method because

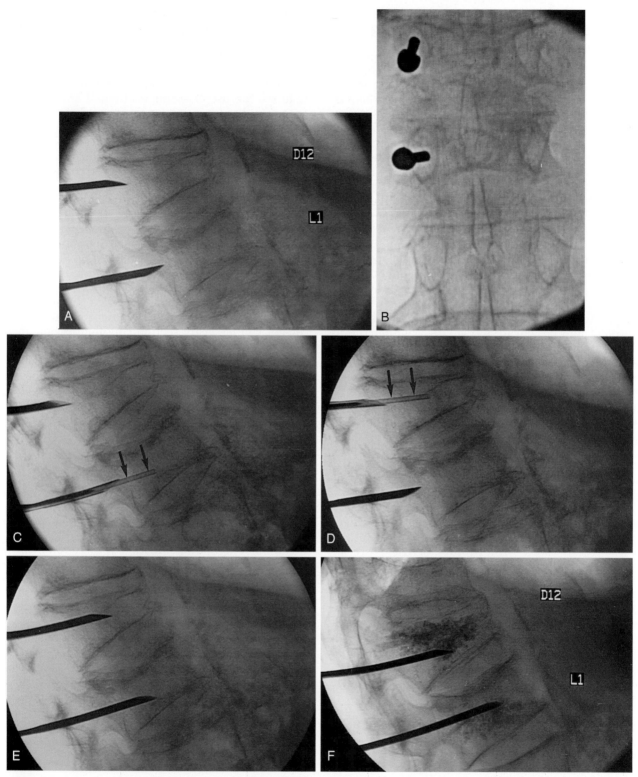

Figure 29-4 Case 4. T12 and L1 osteoporotic fractured vertebrae. First, a left transpedicular approach is performed at the two levels. *A* and *B,* Sagittal and frontal views. *C* and *D,* A bone biopsy is performed with a 15-gauge needle *(arrows)* at the two levels. *E,* After the biopsy, 10-gauge needles are placed into the vertebral bodies for cement injection. *F* and *G,* After the first puncture, a right transpedicular approach is performed at the two levels. *H* and *I,* An axial CT view and coronal reconstruction show good injection in the two vertebrae. *J,* Sagittal reconstructions show the cement injection into the two pedicles via the transpedicular route, with withdrawal of the 10-gauge needles *(arrowheads).*

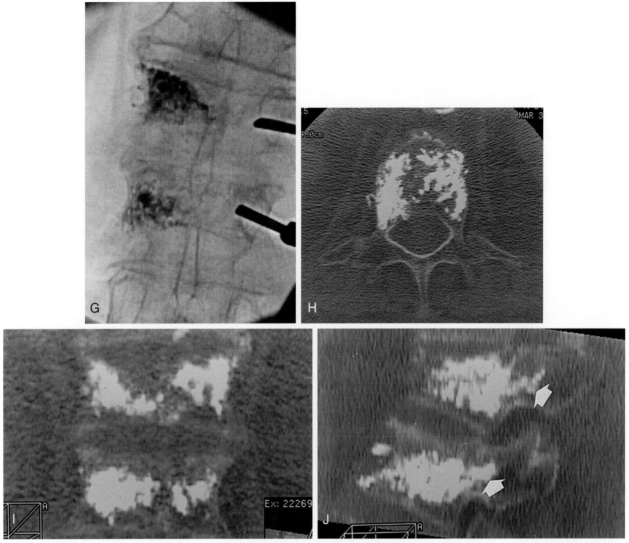

Figure 29-4 *See legend on opposite page*

it is easy to perform, is safe, and avoids leakage of cement near the nerve route, which is possible in the posterolateral approach. The needle is introduced under fluoroscopic control. Fluoroscopic C-arm or biplane guidance is essential (see Figs. 29–3 and 29–4). Sometimes, to treat complex lesions or lesions at the cervicothoracic junction, puncture may be performed under CT control (Fig. 29–2).[28, 29]

Once the periosteum is reached, penetration of the vertebra is best achieved with a hammer; the trajectory of the needle is straight and it avoids fragmentation of bone at the entry of the needle. It is possible to use the orientation of the bevel of the needle to adjust the trajectory and to guide the trocar along its course inside the pedicle and vertebral body.[6] A biopsy can precede the cement injection, using a trephine or a 15- to 18-gauge biopsy needle placed through the vertebroplasty needle (Figs. 29–3, 29–4, and 29–6).[5, 30]

In vertebral hemangiomas, transosseous phlebography (Fig. 29–1) may be performed to identify the perivertebral venous drainage. However, even if

there is early perivertebral venous drainage, cement injection is not contraindicated, because the viscosity of cement is very different from that of contrast media.[3, 5]

Once the needle is in good position, it is time for cement injection. Before mixing, the different components must be at room temperature. Polymethacrylate powder is supplied in a 20-cc syringe. The powder is emptied into a suitable clean, dry, and sterile mixing bowl; 1 mg of tantalum powder is added to improve the radiopacity. *One must add the liquid to the powder and not the opposite.* All mixing bowls and spatulas should be made of inert materials. Liquid methylmethacrylate (5 ml) is added and the preparation mixed until it becomes like toothpaste. The mixture is then transferred into a 10-cc syringe and from that into two 3-cc Luer-Lok syringes. It is then injected manually into the vertebral body under continuous lateral fluoroscopic control, to avoid undesirable passage of MM into the spinal canal. When CT guidance is used for the puncture, a coupled C-arm fluoroscopic unit allows good control during the injec-

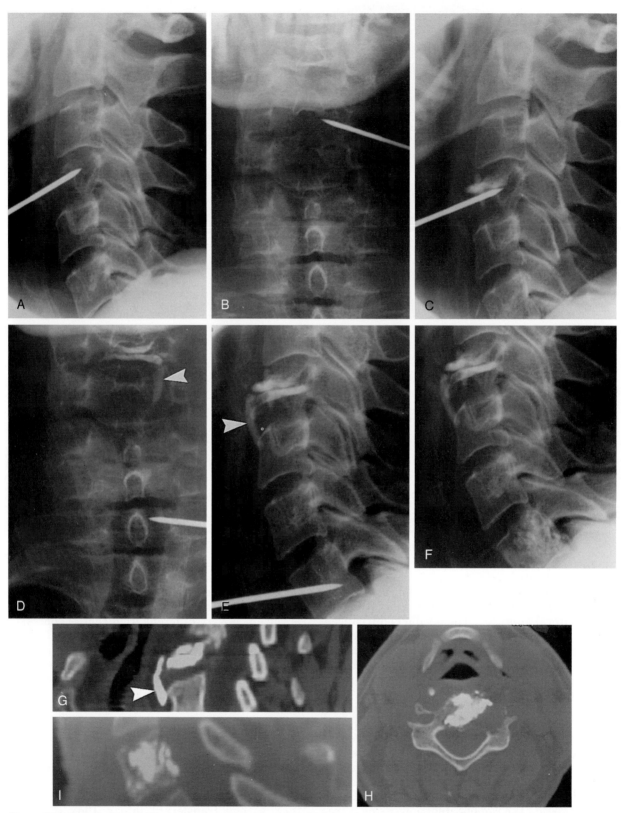

Figure 29-5 Case 5. C4 and C7 renal metastases. *A* and *B,* A C4 left anterolateral approach is made with a 15-gauge needle. The first injection was along the upper vertebral plate; a second puncture is performed. *C,* During the second cement injection, there is left anterolateral cement leakage without any clinical consequences (arrowheads in *D, E,* and *G*). *D* and *E,* A C7 left anterolateral approach is made with a 15-gauge needle. Note the leakage of cement in front of C4 from the second injection *(arrowheads). F,* A lateral plain film shows the two injections of cement. *G,* Sagittal CT scan of C4 obtained as a postvertebroplasty control shows the anterolateral leakage of cement *(arrowhead). H* and *I,* Axial and sagittal CT reconstruction of C7 after cement injection.

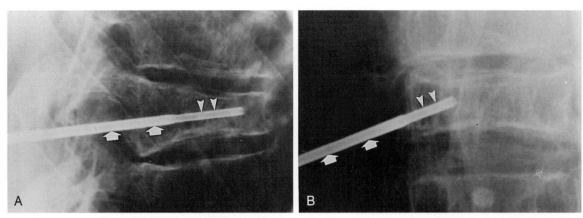

Figure 29-6 Case 6. *A,* Sagittal and *B,* frontal views of the posterolateral approach with a 10-gauge needle *(arrows)* and a 15-gauge biopsy needle *(arrowheads).*

tion. Because of the viscosity of the cement, syringes of small diameter (small cross-sectional area) and with a syringe handle (as described above) are used to inject the cement efficiently.

At the end of the injection, the mandrel of the needle is reinserted carefully while the needle is removed; to avoid adherence of the needle to the cement, it should be rotated for a few minutes until there is consolidation of the cement. The polymerization of the cement induces a local exothermic reaction.[31] Frequently a single puncture allows injection of a hemivertebra, and a contralateral puncture and injection is necessary to fill the whole vertebral body (see Fig. 29–4).

The injection is stopped immediately in cases of suspected perivertebral extravasation. Injection of anterior or lateral veins or discs induces no clinical consequences, but injection of epidural veins can be a source of complications.[32] It is absolutely necessary to have continuous, good lateral fluoroscopic monitoring during the injection of cement in order to be able to stop the injection before cement is seen beyond the posterior wall of the vertebral body.

The injection of insufficient amounts of cement, caused by an advanced state of polymerization or by stoppage of the injection related to an undesired leakage of cement, necessitates a new puncture of a part of the vertebra not yet injected and a new injection. Two or three vertebrae may be treated during the same procedure.

POSTPROCEDURE ORDERS

After the procedure, the patient is kept on bedrest for 24 hours. Sitting and standing up are allowed the morning after the procedure. The most spectacular effect on bone pain is seen in treatment of osteoporotic lesions. Several days after the vertebroplasty, plain films and a noncontrast CT scan with axial views and sagittal and coronal reconstructions are obtained to evaluate the intraosseous cement injection. In patients with intense spinal pain before vertebroplasty requiring morphine therapy, the analgesic drugs are progressively decreased.

All patients are examined 6 weeks after vertebroplasty, and plain films are obtained to examine the treated level. The same examination is performed 6 months later and annually thereafter.

TECHNICAL INCIDENTS AND COMPLICATIONS

Technical Incidents

Puncture Incidents

The risk of the transpedicular approach is a possible fracture of the internal cortex of the pedicle. This can be avoided by rigorous fluoroscopic control during the procedure and knowledge of how to use the bevel of the needle. For upper thoracic levels, this risk diminishes when the diameter of the needle is adapted to the smaller diameter of the pedicle (i.e., when a smaller needle is used).[32]

For the posterolateral approach, the major risk at the thoracic level is pneumothorax; at the lumbar level, the risk is of a psoas hematoma. We have never encountered such complications.

The leakage of cement along the needle course may cause nerve root compression and radicular pain. To avoid this problem, a transpedicular approach is recommended whenever possible. *If a puncture is performed, but the needle is not in good position and another puncture is needed, it is important to leave this first needle in place to avoid leakage of cement through the hole puncture during the injection.*

Extravertebral Cement Leakage

Perivertebral venous injection is possible. This never causes clinical complications if the injection is stopped rapidly in order to avoid passage into the inferior vena cava and the risk of pulmonary embolization. We have never seen this last complication. The use of cement with high viscosity will help avoid such a complication. When a perivertebral injection of cement is detected under fluoroscopic control, the injection must be stopped; it is possible to wait 10 seconds or more and then continue the injection—the venous leakage will not increase.

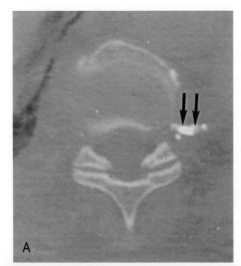

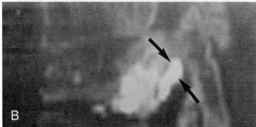

Figure 29-7 Case 7. *A,* Axial and *B,* sagittal CT images showing left-sided leakage of cement *(arrows)* around the nerve root course after a posterolateral approach.

The injection of epidural and/or foraminal veins is a different problem. It can lead to radicular compression, inducing pain (Fig. 29–7). To avoid such a complication, care must be taken not to inject cement beyond the projection of the posterior wall of the vertebral body under lateral fluoroscopy.

Injection of the disc with cement never leads to clinical complications. It is important to avoid the puncture of an intravertebral disc herniation, especially in osteoporotic vertebral crush syndrome or vertebral collapse due to malignant tumor, when a lateral placement of the needle in the vertebral body is used.

As noted previously, perivertebral leakage of cement along the needle track can lead to nerve root compression after a posterolateral approach at the thoracic or lumbar level, and to transient dysphagia after an anterolateral approach at the cervical level (see Fig. 29–5). This can be avoided by a transpedicular approach at the thoracic and lumbar levels.

Leakage into perivertebral tumoral extension is possible and does not lead to clinical complications.

Epidural and foraminal leakage of cement is a dreaded complication, especially when there is partial osteolysis of the posterior wall of the vertebral body. This leakage leads to the risk of spinal cord or nerve root compression.

Clinical Complications

The main risks of vertebroplasty are infection, cord compression, and the onset or aggravation of radicu-

lar pain. Clinical complications are mostly observed in the group of malignant spinal tumors (a 10% rate). They are rare and cured by medical treatment in the two other groups (a 2% rate in patients with hemangiomas and 1% in cases of osteoporotic vertebral crush syndrome).

General Complications

Hemodynamic alterations during or after cement injection have not been seen; in the case of vertebroplasty, the injected quantities of cement are lower than during orthopedic surgery of the hip, and there is no general toxicity.[33–35]

Local Complications

Temporary Increase of Rachialgia

This is more frequent in cases of osteoporotic or metastatic vertebral collapse. These rachialgias disappear quickly in 1 or 2 days with the use of anti-inflammatory drugs (intravenous ketoprofen, 100 to 300 mg/day).[27, 32]

Radicular Compression

Nerve root compression is more common in cases of metastatic vertebral involvement, because of the risk of an osteolytic lesion of the posterior vertebral wall.[3, 4, 6, 7, 16, 29, 32] This complication was noted in 2% of patients with vertebral hemangiomas. In these cases, systemic antalgic treatment or local infiltration (bupivacaine or absolute ethanol) always stops the pain. Accentuation or onset of radicular pain was noted in 8% of patients, and required surgical excision of the cement in the radicular canal in 1.5% of patients.

Cord Compression

Only one of our patients experienced this complication. This patient had aggravation of preexisting cord compression due to epidural spread of a vertebral metastasis. Vertebroplasty was indicated before surgery to facilitate stabilization of the spine. The surgical decompression led to a good neurologic outcome.

Infectious Complications

It is essential to maintain rigorously aseptic conditions to avoid infection, especially in the case of malignant spinal tumors, when chemotherapy frequently suppresses the immune system. We had one case of infection in our series; it was cured by a 3-month course of antibiotics.[7, 32]

REFERENCES

1. Darrason F. Place de la vertébroplastie percutanée acrylique dans le traitement des hémangiomes vertébraux agressifs. Thesis for Doctorat en Médecine. Université de Picardie, U.E.R. de Médecine d'Amiens, October 1988.
2. Debussche-Depriester C, Deramond H, Fardellone P, et al. Percutaneous vertebroplasty with acrylic cement in the treatment of osteoporotic vertebral crush fracture syndrome. *Neuroradiology* 1991;33:149–152.
3. Deramond H, Darrason R, Galibert P. La vertébroplastie percutanée acrylique dans le traitement des hémangiomes vertébraux agressifs. *Rachis* 1989;1:143–153.

4. Deramond H, Galibert P, Debussche C, et al. Percutaneous vertebroplasty with methylmethacrylate: technique, method, results (abstr). *Radiology* 1990;177(P):352.
5. Deramond H, Debussche C, Pruvo JP, Galibert P. La vertébroplastie. *Feuillets Radiol* 1990;30:262–268.
6. Deramond H, Depriester C, Galibert P. Percutaneous vertebroplasty. In Wilson D (ed): Interventional Radiology of the Musculoskeletal System. London, Edward Arnold, 1995, pp 133–142.
7. Deramond H, Depriester C, Toussaint P. Vertébroplastie et radiologie interventionnelle percutanée dans les métastases osseuses: technique, indications, contre-indications. *Bull Cancer* 1996;83:277–282.
8. Galibert P, Deramond H, Rosat P, Le Gars D. Note préliminaire sur le traitement des angiomes vertébraux par vertébroplastie acrylique percutanée. *Neurochirurgie* 1987; 233:166–168.
9. Galibert P, Deramond H. La vertébroplastie acrylique percutanée comme traitement des angiomes vertébraux et des affections dolorigènes et fragilisantes du rachis. *Chirurgie* 1990;116:326–335.
10. Cotten A, Deramond H, Cortet B, et al. Preoperative percutaneous injection of methylmethacrylate and *n*-butyl cyanoacrylate in vertebral hemangiomas. *AJNR* 1996;17:137–142.
11. Heiss JD, Doppman JL, Oldfield EH. Brief report: relief of spinal cord compression from vertebral hemangioma by intralesional injection of absolute ethanol. *N Engl J Med* 1994;331:508–511.
12. Laredo JD, Bellaiche L, Hubault A, Deramond H. Le traitement des hémangiomes vertébraux. L'Actualité Rhumatologique. Paris: Expansion Scientifique Française, 1993, pp 332–346.
13. Fox MW, Onofrio BM. The natural history and management of symptomatic and asymptomatic vertebral hemangiomas. *J Neurosurg* 1993;78:36–45.
14. Bascoulergue Y, Duquesnel J, Leclercq R, et al. Percutaneous injection of methylmethacrylate in the vertebral body for the treatment of various diseases. Percutaneous vertebroplasty (abstr). *Radiology* 1988;169(P):372.
15. Chiras J, Sola-Martinez MT, Weill A, et al. Vertébroplasties percutanées. *Rev Med Interne* 1995;16:854–859.
16. Lapras C, Mottolese C, Deruty R, et al. Injection percutanée de méthylméthacrylate dans le traitement de l'ostéoporose et ostéolyse vertébrale grave. *Ann Chir* 1989;43:371–376.
17. Shepherd S. Radiotherapy and the management of metastatic bone pain. *Clin Radiol* 1988;39:547–550.
18. Simon JM. Radiothérapie des métastases osseuses. Revue de la littérature. *Bull Cancer* 1996;83:290–298.
19. Weil A, Chiras J, Simon JM, et al. Spinal metastases: indications for and results of percutaneous injection of acrylic surgical cement. *Radiology* 1996;199:241–247.
20. Kaemmerlen P, Thiesse P, Bouvard H, et al. Vertébroplastie percutanée dans le traitement des métastases. *J Radiol* 1989;70:557–562.
21. Kaemmerlen P, Thiesse P, Jonas P, et al. Injection percutanée de ciment dans les vertèbres métastatiques. *Presse Med* 1989;18:983–984.
22. Kaemmerlen P, Thiesse P, Jonas P, et al. Percutaneous injection of orthopedic cement in metastatic vertebral lesions. *N Engl J Med* 1989;321:121.
23. Garmatis CJ, Chu F. The effectiveness of radiation therapy in the treatment of bone metastases from breast cancer. *Radiology* 1978;126:235–237.
24. Murray JA, Bruels MC, Lindberg R. Irradiation of polymethylmethacrylate. *J Bone Joint Surg (Am)* 1974;56:311–312.
25. Griffet J, Lacour C, Perraud M, et al. Utilisation du ciment acrylique armé dans les tumeurs malignes rachidiennes. *Lyon Chir* 1988;84:62–64.
26. Cotten A, Dewatre F, Cortet B, et al. Percutaneous vertebroplasty for osteolytic metastases and myeloma: effects of the percentage of lesion filling and the leakage of methylmethacrylate at clinical follow-up. *Radiology* 1996;200:525–530.
27. Cotten A, Deprez X, Migaud H, et al. Malignant acetabular osteolysis: percutaneous injection of acrylic bone cement. *Radiology* 1995;197:307–310.
28. Gangi A, Kastler B, Dietemann JL. Radiologie interventionnelle sous guidage scanographique. *Rev Im Med* 1992;1:231.
29. Gangi A, Kastler B, Dietemann JL. Percutaneous vertebroplasty guided by a combination of CT and fluoroscopy. *AJNR* 1994;15:83–86.
30. Ottolenghi CE, Schajowicz F, Deschant FA. Aspiration biopsy of the cervical spine. Technique and results in thirty-four cases. *J Bone Joint Surg (Am)* 1964;46:715–733.
31. Jefferis CD, Lee AJC, Ling RSM. Thermal aspects of self-curing polymethylmethacrylate. *J Bone Joint Surg (Br)* 1975;57:511–518.
32. Chiras J, Deramond H. Complications des vertebroplasties. In Saillant G, Laville C (eds): Echecs et Complications de la Chirurgie du Rachis. Chirurgie de Reprise. Paris: Sauramps Médical, 1995, pp 149–153.
33. Convery FR, Gunn D, Hugues D, Martin WE. The relative safety of polymethylmethacrylate. *J Bone Joint Surg (Am)* 1975;57:57–64.
34. Mallory TH, Stone W, St. Pierre R. Potential toxic effects of methylmethacrylate. *J Bone Joint Surg (Am)* 1972;54:1356.
35. Phillips H Cole PV, Lettin AW. Cardiovascular effects of implanted acrylic bone cement. *Br Med J* 1971;3:460–461.

ADDITIONAL REFERENCES

Chiras J, Cognard C, Rose M, et al. Percutaneous injection of an alcoholic embolizing emulsion as an alternative preoperative embolization for spine tumor. *AJNR* 1993;14:1113–1117.

Cortet B, Cotten A, Deprez X, Deramond H. Vertebroplasty with surgical decompression for the treatment of aggressive vertebral hemangiomas. *Rev Rhum* (Engl edition) 1994;61:14–21.

Harrington KD. The use of methylmethacrylate for vertebral body replacement and anterior stabilization of pathological fracture-dislocations of the spine due to metastatic malignant disease. *J Bone Joint Surg (Am)* 1981;63:36–46.

Laredo JD, Bard M, Leblanc G, et al. Technique et résultats de la ponction-biopsie transcutanée radioguidée du rachis dorsal. *Rev Rhum* 1985;52:283–287.

McCollister M, Evarts C. Diagnostic techniques: closed biopsy of bone. *Clin Orthop* 1975;107:100–111.

Vallee C, Rousselin B, L'huillier F, et al. Biopsies disco-vertébrales sous contrôle télévisé. *Feuillets Radiol* 1990;30:255–261.

CHAPTER 30

A Treatment for Head and Neck Cancer by Direct Arterial Infusion

C.W. Kerber / W.H.M. Wong / K.T. Robbins

BACKGROUND AND HISTORY

Head and neck cancers, most commonly squamous cell carcinomas, are difficult lesions to treat; the long-term survival rate remains 15% to 40%. Moreover, the personal cost of a cure is high, as cure may require the surgical removal of critical speech and swallowing organs; a serious and dramatic lessening of the quality of life is then inevitable. To make matters worse, the surgery takes place in a cosmetically sensitive area, and patients suffer further loss of self-esteem when looking at their postoperative deformity.

Those who were involved in attempts to treat head and neck cancers by intra-arterial chemotherapy infusions in the late 1970s were discouraged by the poor results and excessive complication rates. Long infusion times with indwelling catheters were generally attempted. However, more recent developments suggest that it is time to re-evaluate selective arterial infusion strategies. We were encouraged by Lee et al's[1, 2] excellent work and have developed a treatment plan that appears to offer promise.

In 1988 we began our first cohort of patients using a dose-escalating plan to determine the maximal amount of cisplatin (CDDP) we could infuse, having no idea about how the body would react to an unusually high dose of CDDP delivered intra-arterially. We began with 120 mg/m² given four times at 4-week intervals, and gradually increased the dose to 200 mg/m² given times but at weekly intervals. At this last dosage, we found that the toxic systemic effects were unacceptably high, and dropped back to 150 mg/m² per week, given four times. For comparison, a single treatment approximates a 1-week intravenous dose, but delivered in approximately 3 minutes.

In this first cohort of patients, we worked out the necessary physician/technician/nursing coordination that is needed to deliver the drug safely in a short time and simultaneously to infuse its antagonist. After analyzing the results of this first cohort, we added local radiation, 180 to 200 Gy/day (35 treatments), as there was literature evidence to indicate that CDDP was a potent radiation enhancer (or vice versa). All patients in the second cohort had untreated stage III or IV disease.

After analyzing the results in Cohort 2, we proceeded to evaluate (and are still evaluating) the effects of other simultaneous treatment modalities, such as the addition of tamoxifen. Our study continues to evolve to the present day.

THEORY

The basis of this approach is to deliver an extremely high concentration of the anticancer drug directly into the artery supplying the tumor, while circulating the drug's antagonist in the venous system. Thus, other sensitive organs, such as the bone marrow, gut, and kidneys, will be protected from the effect of the drug.

The advantage of delivering a drug by selective arterial infusion can be shown by the following equation:

$$R_t = 1 + \frac{\text{plasma clearance of the drug}}{\text{tumor plasma flow}}$$

where R_t is the relative advantage of arterial infusion. One would like to have R_t close to 20 to offset the hazards and costs of an intra-arterial infusion. From the equation, it can be seen that increasing the plasma clearance of CDDP is advantageous. This can be accomplished by presenting the tumor with an unusually high dose of the anticancer drug. An even more profound effect can be caused by making the denominator approach zero. This could be done either by balloon occlusion of the vessel (which would further add to the cost and risk) or by another strategy described below. In our study, the tumor was exposed to a CDDP concentration some 250 times that achievable by intravenous dosing (S. Howell, personal communication).

The essence of this strategy is that CDDP has an antagonist, thiosulfate. Thiosulfate forms a chelate with CDDP almost instantaneously, and this chelate is biologically inactive. Thus, if one were to circulate thiosulfate intravenously, CDDP, having passed through the tumor, would become chelated and then pass out through the kidneys without further activity. However, this presents a problem to the angiographer. How can one prevent this CDDP from chelating with the circulating thiosulfate before the CDDP reaches the tumor?

The slipstreams of blood are coherent; slipstreams cannot cross each other. Most angiographers have noticed streaming of contrast agent into vessels more selectively than they would desire when a slow intra-arterial infusion has been carried out. Many authors[3-5] have analyzed this phenomenon and have commented upon adverse effects when this factor is not taken into consideration.

Arterial Acceptance Test

We chose to solve these problems by performing what we have termed the *arterial acceptance test.* Having gently catheterized the artery perfusing the tumor, we connect the catheter to the pressure injector and begin infusing contrast agent at a rate that will completely fill the artery, excluding any blood ingress. Since flow in the external carotid artery varies with the pulse cycle, we choose a rate that will cause slight reflux into adjacent arteries during the heart's peak systolic output. We can thus see on live fluoroscopy that the contrast agent fills the vessel, preventing ingress of blood during the infusion. Completely excluding the blood from the feeding artery by this technique solves three problems for the angiographer. First, the tumor is presented with the highest possible concentration of CDDP in the shortest time. Second, complete filling of the artery precludes any chance of streaming of the CDDP more selectively than desired. Third, infusion at the maximal rate that the artery will accept excludes circulating thiosulfate from the CDDP, preventing its premature chelation.

This arterial acceptance test is easily and rapidly performed through the infusion catheter. With practice, a small hand injection of contrast agent gives some indication of the probable first infusion rate to test.

GENERAL APPROACH TO EVALUATION AND TREATMENT

Cohort 1

Patients entering the first cohort had far advanced head and neck cancer. They received a careful multidisciplinary evaluation that included a general physical examination and laboratory testing. Many underwent direct endoscopic evaluation, and then computed tomography (CT) or magnetic resonance imaging (MRI). As about half of this first cohort had undergone previous surgery and radiation therapy, it was common to find the absence of critical arteries that would have supplied the recurrent tumor.

Cohort 2

The second cohort was evaluated as was the first, but all patients in this cohort had untreated stage III or IV disease, and most had N2 or N3 local nodal disease.

Procedural Overview

After evaluation of the physical findings, the scans were analyzed to determine actual tumor extent and whether it crossed the midline. We then proceeded with diagnostic angiography, evaluating both common carotid arteries, especially the lateral views, to search for aberrant proximal vessels, and if surgical absence of vessels was found, to determine whether potential anastomotic channels could be utilized. The evaluation began with local anesthesia at the groin puncture site, plus occasional supplemental intravenous fentanyl and midazolam.

As most of the patients were elderly, and essentially all had extensive atherosclerosis, we began with a 5-Fr. polyethylene compound curve catheter (Cook, Inc.) to engage the orifice of the appropriate brachiocephalic vessel. We then introduced a 260-cm exchange guidewire into the common carotid artery, removed the first catheter, and replaced it with a 5-Fr. uncurved polyethylene catheter. We did not permit that second catheter or guidewire to pass beyond the carotid bifurcation, positioning its tip finally 2 to 4 cm proximal to the bulb. The first angiographic images were then obtained and evaluated. We next gently entered the proximal external carotid artery, leading the catheter with a curved 0.038″ hydrophilic guidewire. We did not permit either the catheter or guidewire to pass beyond the origin of the occipital, lingual, or facial arteries, having found that it was difficult to relieve spasm once it had occurred, but a simple matter to prevent it. Selective external carotid images were then obtained.

It was usually impossible to determine the actual tumor blood supply by angiographic criteria, since essentially all the primary squamous cell carcinomas were avascular. On the other hand, nodal disease was more vascular, and it was possible to infuse the nodal disease more selectively when such was present. In general, the lateral angiographic images were found to be the most valuable in determining infusion strategy; the frontal view was almost never found to be helpful.

At this point, the next decision point was reached. If the tumor was extensive (e.g., involving the pharynx, skull base, and tongue), we positioned the catheter proximally and performed the arterial acceptance test there, infusing the entire external carotid system (Fig. 30–1). At times, the lesion was nourished primarily by a single small vessel. In those circumstances, particularly in patients with laryngeal tumors and tongue base tumors, the superior thyroid or the lingual artery, respectively, was catheterized. A microcatheter was advanced through the 5-Fr. catheter, and the arterial acceptance test was performed (Fig. 30–2).

If the tumor had crossed the midline, we catheterized both carotid systems, estimated relative tumor bulk, and delivered most of the CDDP into the side with the larger part of the tumor (Figs. 30–3 and 30–4). Simultaneous bilateral injections were carried out until the chosen dose had been introduced into the side of the smaller tumor. Then, that side was excluded from the injection, and the injection continued to deliver the remainder of the dose into the side with the larger tumor, quickly and without delay, as

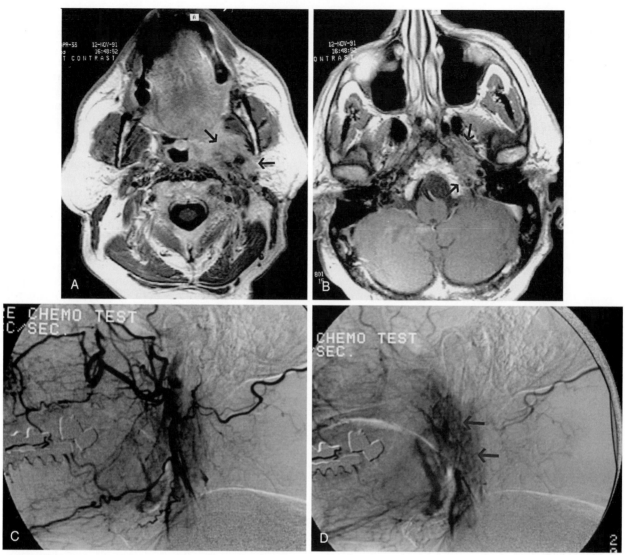

Figure 30-1 Case 1. A squamous cell carcinoma of the tonsillar fossa treated by infusion of the entire external carotid artery. *A,* A T1-weighted postgadolinium magnetic resonance imaging (MRI) scan demonstrates a mass arising from the tonsillar fossa *(arrows)*. *B,* The mass extends along the parapharyngeal and carotid spaces to the left skull base *(arrows)*. *C,* The angiogram shows that numerous arteries cover the entire extent of the tumor. In this patient, we chose to infuse the entire external carotid artery. *D,* In the capillary phase of the angiogram the tumor blush *(arrows)* helps confirm the adequacy of the infusion. The arterial acceptance test showed the artery accepted 3.5 ml/sec.

the thiosulfate continued to infuse into the venous circulation.

In the early patients, attempts were made to exclude the internal maxillary artery and the occipital arteries from the CDDP effects by the placement of coils into those vessels. This had the undesirable side effect of significantly increasing the cost of the procedure, and later some patients who experienced recurrence had it in the vascular distributions where coils had been placed. Coil occlusion was subsequently abandoned and in the last 85 patients we have not deliberately blocked the adjacent or distal vessels that did not pass directly into the tumor.

The infusion rate of the CDDP was that found by using contrast agent during the arterial acceptance test. This test, discussed in theory above, was extremely simple. Normal external carotid arteries generally carry 2 to 4 ml of blood per second. With only a little practice, it was possible to estimate the artery's acceptance rate when small hand injections of contrast agent were used during catheter positioning. If, for example, the operator chose 3 ml/sec, the catheter was connected to the pressure injector and set at 3 ml/sec for 2.5 seconds' total injection, and an angiographic run then performed to document that this was the maximal rate the artery would accept. It was desirable to find a small amount of reflux into more proximal vessels during peak systole. If no reflux was visible, the injection rate was increased by 0.5 ml/sec until such a reflux was evident. It was generally possible to deliver up to 1.5 ml/sec through microcatheters, although that rate is double what most manufacturers give as the injection limit.

We next attempted to have the patient dislodge

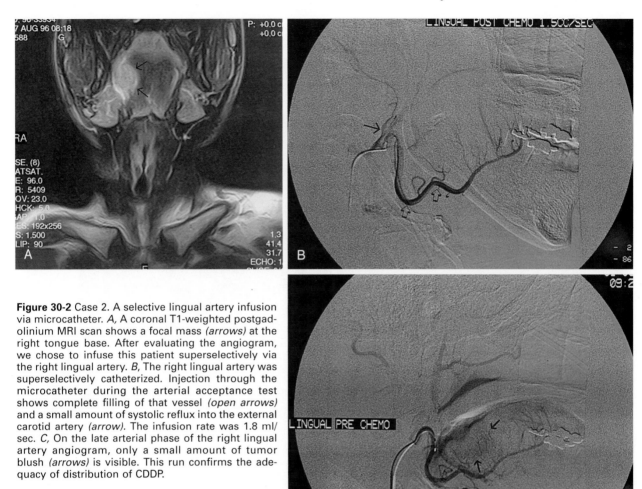

Figure 30-2 Case 2. A selective lingual artery infusion via microcatheter. *A,* A coronal T1-weighted postgadolinium MRI scan shows a focal mass *(arrows)* at the right tongue base. After evaluating the angiogram, we chose to infuse this patient superselectively via the right lingual artery. *B,* The right lingual artery was superselectively catheterized. Injection through the microcatheter during the arterial acceptance test shows complete filling of that vessel *(open arrows)* and a small amount of systolic reflux into the external carotid artery *(arrow).* The infusion rate was 1.8 ml/sec. *C,* On the late arterial phase of the right lingual artery angiogram, only a small amount of tumor blush *(arrows)* is visible. This run confirms the adequacy of distribution of CDDP.

the 5-Fr. catheter by repeated swallowing. If this occurred, we brought the catheter back to the distal common carotid artery and directed a microcatheter through the 5-Fr. catheter into the appropriate vessel.

TECHNIQUE

General Concepts

Standard techniques of cerebral angiography are known to practitioners in this field. It is emphasized, however, that prevention of spasm in the external carotid artery is one of the key factors in the success of the procedure and in the ability to repeat therapy at weekly intervals.

In general, a catheter is not pushed into the external carotid artery unless it is led by a soft-tipped guidewire. Even then, passage of the guidewire is not permitted beyond the more distal of the three or four proximal branches, (e.g., the lingual, occipital, or facial artery). It has been found that, since many of the patients have advanced atherosclerosis and their blood vessels are extremely tortuous, an uncurved catheter remains in the artery best. We do begin with a shaped catheter, generally one with a

compound curve, to engage the orifice of the brachiocephalic vessel; this is never the catheter that is allowed to enter or rest within the external carotid artery. It has been found that by placing an exchange guidewire into the common carotid artery, and performing an immediate exchange with the final placement of an uncurved catheter into the external carotid artery, spasm can be avoided. In the most recent 90 patients, no spasm had been produced when this technique has been employed. If a more distal placement of a catheter is necessary, a softer microcatheter is introduced through the 5-Fr. catheter.

The position of the catheter tip is important for several reasons. First, if it does not lie within the external carotid artery deeply enough, patient swallowing—which is inevitable when the CDDP infusion begins—will allow the catheter to fall back into the internal carotid artery. In this case, even a 1-cm more distal position will improve purchase, as long as the catheter does not lie distal to the arteries one needs to infuse. If there is any doubt, the 5-Fr. catheter is pulled back into the common carotid artery and a microcatheter is placed into the portion of the external carotid artery it is desired to infuse.

Double flushing of catheters remains a significant basic principle for the neurointerventionalist. This is

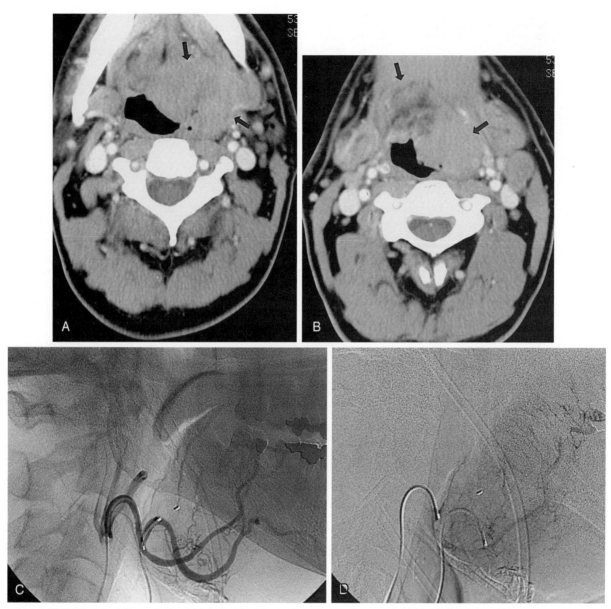

Figure 30-3 Case 3. Bilateral simultaneous treatment. *A,* computed tomographic (CT) scan shows a biopsy-proven squamous cell carcinoma arising from the left tongue base *(arrows),* crossing the median raphe to involve a small portion of the right tongue base. *B,* The cancer also extends inferiorly to the pre-epiglottic space but not into the hypopharynx. We chose to deliver 20% of the dose to the right and 80% to the left. *C,* Microcatheters were introduced superselectively into each lingual artery. After the arterial acceptance test, 40% of the CDDP dosage (20% to the right and 20% to the left) was infused simultaneously through a Y connector at a rate of 3 ml/sec. The right flow switch was then turned off, and the remaining 60% was infused unilaterally into the left lingual artery at 1.5 ml/sec. Total infusion time was less than 4 minutes. *D,* The capillary phase of this angiogram shows the tumor blush and the microvasculature of the remaining portions of the tongue.

particularly important when bilateral simultaneous infusions are performed. It is all too easy to allow blood to reflux back into one or both catheters during the hook-up procedure.

Arterial Acceptance Test

This seemingly simple test solves many problems for the angiographer—but only if it is performed correctly. It is impossible for us to quantitate what we mean by "a small amount of reflux into more proximal vessels during peak systole." However, in an attempt to quantify this, it is estimated that about 1% to 2% of the contrast agent (and also the CDDP dose) will pass to areas other than the tumor's primary blood supply. The chief problem is not too much reflux into adjacent arteries, but rather an infusion rate that is not high enough, allowing circulating thiosulfate to enter into the tumor's bed during the CDDP infusion process. It has been found that it is better to err on the high side than the low side of infusion rates. In actual practice, the slight reflux described is easy to perceive during the arterial test injection.

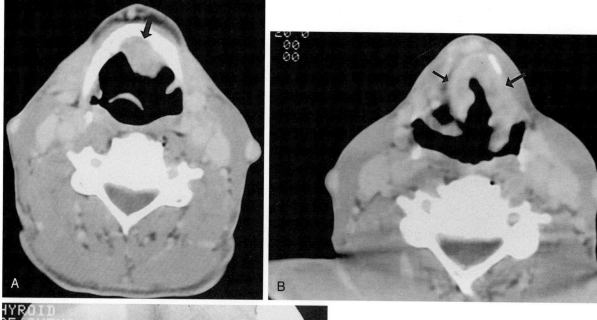

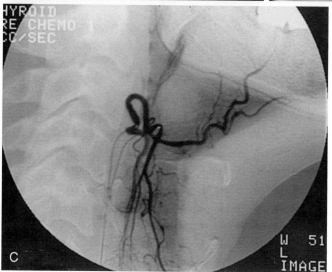

Figure 30-4 Case 4. Selective bilateral superior thyroid artery injections. *A,* A CT scan at the level of the thyroid bone demonstrates a tumor extending into the pre-epiglottic space *(arrow). B,* The tumor also extends inferiorly along the aryepiglottic folds into the hypopharynx and larynx *(arrows). C,* Both superior thyroid arteries were superselectively catheterized, and an arterial acceptance test was performed bilaterally. The arteries accepted 2.5 ml/sec. The right superior thyroidal artery had an anomalous connection with the lingual artery, which was considered to be an advantage in infusing this tumor.

Infusion Technique

Having determined the artery's optimal acceptance rate with the arterial acceptance test, the syringe containing the contrast agent is removed from the pressure injector and replaced with a prefilled syringe containing the CDDP. The CDDP is mixed by the pharmacy about 1 hour before the procedure begins. Next, the catheter is double-flushed with heparinized saline. A 10-cc syringe containing contrast agent is connected to a three-way stopcock, the male end of the stopcock is connected to the flow switch, bubbles are purged from the system, and the catheter is filled to its tip with contrast agent (Fig. 30–5). Now the pressure injector tubing is attached to the remaining female port of the three-way stopcock, and the contrast agent syringe is removed and replaced with a 20-cc empty syringe (Fig. 30–6). The stopcock arm is turned forward, and the system is again purged of bubbles by forward flushing the CDDP into the 20-cc syringe. This syringe is removed and

reserved, the three-way stopcock arm is placed in a position to allow infusion of the CDDP, and infusion is begun. At this point, the catheter's dead space will be filled with contrast agent, a most important point.

During these minutes, communication among the team is essential. Several minutes before the infusion of CDDP osmotic diuretics are begun, and 30 seconds before CDDP infusion the thiosulfate infusion is begun. If there is any doubt about arm circulation or arm venous dead space (which can be surprisingly large), a venous catheter can be placed more centrally to ensure good venous dispersion and mixing of the thiosulfate.

At this point, using the lateral projection with as much magnification as possible, the tip of the catheter is visualized and CDDP infusion begun. As the catheter contains contrast agent, it is possible to watch the first second or so of infusion with contrast agent, showing that the catheter tip has not moved.

The catheter tip is visualized repeatedly and frequently throughout the procedure, to ensure that

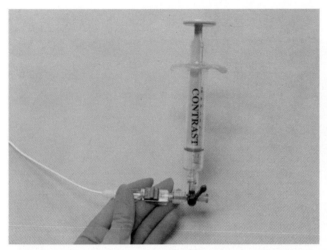

Figure 30-5 The arterial acceptance test has been completed and the power injector is programmed. The 5-Fr. straight polyethylene catheter lies in the vessel to be treated and has not been dislodged by the force of the injection. A flow switch leads to a three-way stopcock. This system is double flushed with heparinized saline, the contrast agent syringe is connected and de-bubbled, and the system is filled with contrast agent.

patient swallowing or the jet effect from the CDDP exiting the tip does not dislodge the catheter; 1 second of fluoroscopic evaluation every 10 seconds is usually adequate. At the completion of the infusion, follow-up angiography is performed through the same catheter to check that the catheter is still in an appropriate position and that there has been no change in the artery. The catheter is then removed,

and meticulous attention to groin care ensues, so that it is rarely necessary to enter the opposite groin on subsequent weeks.

Finally, a protocol sheet is filled out for use during the next treatment. The sheet details every single technique move made during the procedure. An actual full-sized drawing of the patient's arterial anatomy is made, and the catheter tip position is superimposed upon this drawing. These data have saved a remarkable amount of time during subsequent treatments.

Bilateral Infusion

Bilateral simultaneous treatments are more complex, and meticulous technique is called for. A 5-Fr. catheter is introduced via each groin and appropriately positioned as outlined above, and an appropriate rate is chosen using the arterial acceptance test. A Y adapter (Cook, Inc.) connects the two 5-Fr. catheters to the three-way stopcock, and de-bubbling and hook-up proceed as with one catheter. When the calculated simultaneous dose (the dose calculated for the side with the smaller tumor bulk) has been delivered, the infusion stops, the flow switch attached to the catheter on the side receiving the lower dose is turned off, the injector program is reset, and CDDP infusion continues. This step takes less than 30 seconds. The remainder of the dose calculated for the side with the larger tumor bulk is then delivered to that side.

Microcatheters

When microcatheters are used, the steps are similar, but one cannot depend on blood flowing back to ensure that no bubbles are present. Figure 30–7 shows the set-up. Because of the higher pressures needed, the three-way stopcock is dispensed with. The cathe-

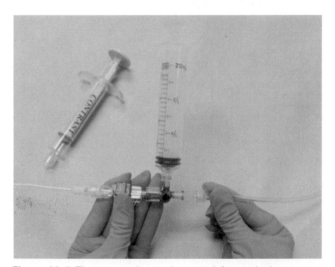

Figure 30-6 The stopcock arm is turned forward, the contrast agent syringe is removed, and an empty 20-cc syringe is connected to the stopcock. The pressure injector delivery tube now containing the CDDP is connected to the horizontal arm of the three-way stopcock, and the pressure injector is de-bubbled into the 20-cc syringe. The syringe is removed, the flow switch and stopcock are opened to the pressure injector, and, with the thiosulfate well circulating throughout the venous system, CDDP infusion is begun at the rate determined by the arterial acceptance test. The catheter tip is watched as the infusion begins. The contrast agent in the dead space will show the tip position and the runoff.

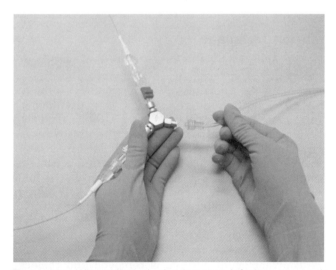

Figure 30-7 When bilateral, simultaneous infusions are made through microcatheters, the principles described for Fig. 30–6 are used, but the stopcock is deleted. Pressure at the catheter hub is so high that standard stopcocks frequently leak CDDP during the pressure infusion.

ters do contain contrast agent so that it is possible to watch these first critical seconds of CDDP infusion.

RESULTS
Cohort 1: CDDP Alone

Response

Most of the patients in cohort 1 were desperate individuals with recurrences after conventional previous treatments.[6, 7]

Some definitions are in order. Response was determined by physical examination, endoscopy (if needed), and comparison CT or MRI. *Complete response* was defined as disappearance of all tumor, *partial response* was a 50% to 99% decrease in size, and *no response* reflected a tumor that decreased less than 50% or actually increased in size. As noted above, in this cohort we began by giving CDDP, 120 mg/m² at 4-week intervals, and gradually increased the dose to 200 mg/m² while decreasing the time interval between treatments to 1 week. We finally settled on 150 mg/m² given weekly for a total of four treatments.

This first cohort contained 42 patients; of these, four could not be assessed. One of those four refused further therapy after the first treatment, one developed unrelieved spasm, and two had abnormal or absent vessels from previous surgery. Thirty-eight evaluable patients remained. Of the 22 who had no previous treatment, nine (41%) had a complete response and 10 (45%) had a partial response. Of the 10 patients previously treated by surgery or radiation, four (25%) had a complete response and six (38%) had a partial response.

Toxicity

Most of the patients tolerated the CDDP well until it was given at 200 mg/m². There were nine instances of severe toxicity among the 17 patients in this highest dose group. When the dose was dropped back to 150 mg/m² at weekly intervals, nine patients received 32 infusions; there was no severe toxicity and only infrequent mild toxicity.

Angiographic Complications and Problems

The first 42 patients underwent 140 transfemoral catheterizations. There were two failures to infuse, one because of toxicity and one because an atherosclerotic plaque occluded the nutrient artery to the tumor. Two patients had transient cardiac arrhythmias that needed no treatment. One patient seen early in the study had a transient retinitis and visual disturbance. We had accidentally infused the entire dose of CDDP into his internal carotid artery and almost immediately thereafter he developed the retinitis. We subsequently modified our monitoring, and have had no further dose delivery problems when we monitor the catheter tip frequently. One patient developed an 8 × 8 cm groin hematoma that needed no treatment, and one developed a 5 × 5 mm region

of cutaneous necrosis. No surgical treatment was required and the necrosis healed.

Cohort 2: CDDP Plus Local Irradiation

Response

In this phase, 85 patients were treated. All patients in this cohort had unresectable stage III or IV squamous cell carcinoma; 62% had N2 to N3 nodal disease. None had undergone previous treatments.

Seven patients in this cohort could not be evaluated. One of those died from pulmonary embolus during the course of therapy (but not while undergoing a treatment), two died from myocardial infarction after therapy was finished but before they could be re-evaluated, two did not complete therapy, and two never returned. Thus, 78 evaluable patients remained, of whom 72 (92%) had a complete response, five (6%) had a partial response, and one (1%) had no response.

Toxicity

Among the 84 patients, who received 323 arterial treatments, there were 17 severe toxic events. Nine of these involved the gastrointestinal tract; seven were hematologic. There were also six instances of neurologic problems (see below), and one patient died secondarily to pulmonary embolus (mentioned above).

Angiographic Complications and Problems

During the 323 infusions, only three times could a patient not be treated. Two patients in this group had atherosclerosis preventing superselective catheterization, and one had hypotension. Six patients had postinfusion decrease in neurologic function. Three of those were transient, but three remained permanently (0.9%).[8]

TECHNICAL PITFALLS, COMPLICATIONS, AND SOLUTIONS
Catheter Placement

Aside from the usual need for catheter hygiene, there are other areas of concern for the angiographic therapist. It has been found that a lateral view of the common carotid artery taken as the first angiographic run best allows the development of an accurate and complete map of the extracranial circulation (see Fig. 30–1). This set of images is then correlated with axial CT and MR images.

It is essential to know the vascular territories that each artery supplies; only then can a rational plan of therapy be made. In general, we treat the superior thyroid artery for laryngeal tumors, the lingual artery for tongue base lesions, and the entire external carotid system for pharyngeal and nasopharyngeal extensive tumors, but we cannot generalize beyond that. It is always the arterial anatomy that ultimately determines the infusion strategy. When the tumor extends across midline, bilateral simultaneous injections are carried out, with CDDP going proportionally to the side containing the largest part of the tumor, as described above (see Figs. 30–3 and 30–4).

Arterial Acceptance Test

Next, the arterial acceptance test gives a rapid and reliable indication of how fast CDDP can be infused. We use the same infusion equipment that will deliver the CDDP, injecting a nonionic contrast agent into the vessel supplying the tumor. This arterial acceptance test is repeated, increasing flow volumes until slight reflux is visible into more proximal vessels. Most external carotid artery systems accept 3 to 4 ml/sec through an uncurved 5-Fr. catheter. Injections through microcatheters give rates of 1.0 to 1.8 ml/sec.

Thiosulfate Administration

The next critical part of this strategy is that the antagonist must be infused and circulating throughout the venous system during the intra-arterial treatment. Thus, after CDDP passes through the tumor bed, it can be quickly chelated with thiosulfate. The chief problem is failing to appreciate the large dead space potentially present in the arm, especially if a distal (in the hand) needle placement is used. Needle placement into a hand vein should alert the angiographer that as much as 100 ml of thiosulfate could fill arm veins before passing centrally and being mixed in the pulmonary circulation. If there is any doubt about poor circulation time or a large venous reservoir in the arm, a small catheter can be placed into the opposite femoral vein and the thiosulfate infused by that route.

Spasm

In the first several patients, development of significant spasm of external carotid artery branches was a problem, and the spasm occasionally delayed or prevented the examination and treatment. Despite reports in the literature on the efficacy of nitrates in relieving spasm, we have found nitrates to be of little value. It is much easier to avoid spasm simply by keeping both the polyethylene catheter and the guidewire from entering any distal portion of the external carotid artery, and by always leading the catheter with a flexible or hydrophilic guidewire. It has also been found that whatever the patient's vascular state (and almost all of these patients had extensive atherosclerosis), a catheter with no curve stays in the vessel better during the infusion and does not cause spasm. The angiogram is begun with a catheter having a complicated enough curve to engage the proximal brachiocephalic origin, which is then immediately exchanged for an uncurved catheter using a 260-cm exchange wire, as noted above.

Swallowing

Infusion of CDDP, especially into the larynx, inevitably provokes swallowing. Swallowing and coughing should be expected, and after positioning of the catheter and before the arterial acceptance test, the patient is instructed to swallow and cough in an attempt to dislodge the catheter. A final adjustment is then made. If the catheter will not stay in the appropriate vessel, it is pulled back to a straighter portion of the common carotid artery, and a microcatheter is placed into the vessel to be infused.

Wrong Basic Diagnosis

We have treated a number of patients off this protocol for compassionate reasons. One who did not meet selection criteria had what was diagnosed by the pathologists as a squamous cell carcinoma. Her treatment was completely unsuccessful. Final diagnosis at postmortem examination was an esthesioneuroblastoma. Not all patients respond to this therapy; many tumors are CDDP resistant.

Previous Surgery

It is an unfortunate concept in surgery that proximal ligations of arteries are good technique. It is usually found, as with unsuccessful arteriovenous malformation surgery, that proximal ligations block endovascular access to recurrent tumors and preclude a good result. We have been only partially successful in treating recurrent tumors by perfusing them via collateral pathways.

Poor Groin Care

Clinicians have been surprised that the same groin can be re-entered on a weekly basis. Some patients, treated off protocol, have had eight full courses of treatment, usually through the same groin. When patients have extensive atherosclerosis, we begin by picking the femoral access route with the best pulse. However, if a large hematoma is allowed to develop, subsequent access is seriously hampered. It pays to be meticulously careful about groin care after catheter removal. As none of these patients receive heparin (except in the dead space flushing solution), groin care should be simple. The development of a hematoma is regarded as a serious technical failure.

Inadequate CDDP Infusion Rate

After the first several patient infusions and the development of the arterial acceptance test, there have been no problems with inadequate infusion rates. An inadequate infusion rate allows ingress of thiosulfate into the tumor bed during the treatment, thus lowering the concentration of active CDDP presented to the tumor, and allows streaming of the CDDP into areas more selectively than desired.

Artery Change Since Previous Treatment

As the tumor begins to get smaller through the action of the therapy, the *arterial acceptance rate* will

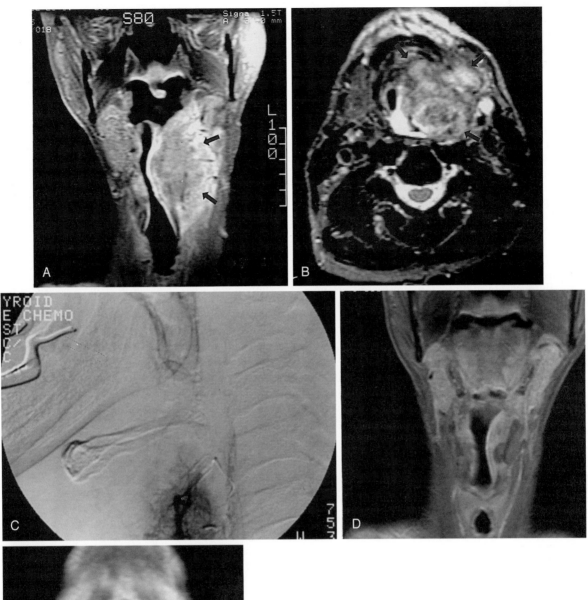

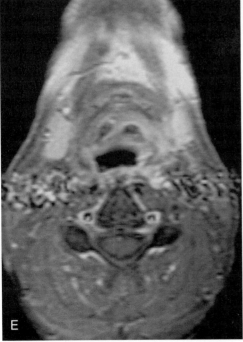

Figure 30-8 Case 5. A large tumor with a good result. *A,* MRI scan shows a large transglottic squamous cell carcinoma of the larynx that nearly occludes the airway *(arrows). B,* The mass extends into the paralaryngeal tissue and the carotid space *(arrows). C,* Superselective infusion of the left superior thyroid artery demonstrates the tumor blush. *D* and *E,* at 6 months, MRI shows complete disappearance of all tumor. Multiple random biopsies of the bed reveal no tumor.

change. Because an artery accepted 4 ml/sec on the last treatment does not mean that it will accept the same amount during the subsequent treatment. An arterial acceptance test is essential each time.

SUMMARY

Patients who present with squamous cell carcinoma of the head and neck are difficult to treat. They are often elderly, almost invariably have extensive atherosclerosis with vessel tortuosity, and often have other concomitant systemic disease. They are a sorrowful and pitiable group. Caring for them presents psychological, angiographic, and physiologic challenges to the therapist.

On the other hand, these patients, often in pain when they first present, usually stop asking for narcotics within the first week. By the third treatment, it is generally possible to discern a significant change in the size of the tumor. What a gratifying event for both patient and therapy team (Fig. 30–8).

We do not know whether this infusion strategy will stand the test of time. Many other promising strategies to treat this terrible disease have been tried in the past but have not been efficacious on long-term follow-up. The longest complete remission is now more than 2 years. Most important, though,

the infusion strategy outlined here does not preclude later standard surgical ablative treatment (with its concomitant deformities). As follow-up continues, patients can continue to live: without pain; without a lessened quality of life; and with their tongue, jaw, larynx, and face unchanged.

REFERENCES

1. Lee YY, Wallace S, Goepfert H, et al. Intra-arterial chemotherapy of head and neck tumors. *AJNR* 1986;7:343–348.
2. Lee YY, Dimery IW, Van Tassel P, et al. Superselective intra-arterial chemotherapy of advanced paranasal sinus tumors. *Arch Otolaryngol Head Neck Surg* 1989;115:503–511.
3. Silbergleit R, Steffey DJ, DeFilipp R, et al. Cerebral distribution of contrast medium during slow intracarotid infusion. *AJNR* 1989;10:1061–1064.
4. Blacklock JB, Wright DC, Dedrick RL, et al. Drug streaming during intra-arterial chemotherapy. *J Neurosurg* 1986;64:284–291.
5. Lutz RJ, Dedvick RL, Boretos JW, et al. Mixing studies during intracarotid artery infusions in an in vitro model. *J Neurosurg* 1986;64:277–283.
6. Robbins KT, Storniolo AM, Kerber CW, et al. Rapid superselective high dose cisplatin infusion for advanced head and neck malignancies. *Head Neck* 1992;14:364–371.
7. Robbins KT, Storniolo AM, Kerber CW, et al. Phase I study of highly selective supradose cisplatin infusions for advanced head and neck cancer. *J Clin Oncol* 1994;12:2113–2120.
8. Robbins KT, Vicario D, Seagren S, et al. A targeted supradose cisplatin chemoradiation protocol for advanced head and neck cancer. *Am J Surg* 1994;168:419–422.

CHAPTER 31

Intra-Arterial Chemotherapy for Central Nervous System Tumors

Jacques Chiras

BACKGROUND

Treatment of brain neoplasms remains controversial, although many therapeutic modalities have been employed, including radiotherapy, chemotherapy, immunotherapy, brachytherapy, surgery, and gene therapy. In the clinical setting, the "gold standard" remains complete removal of the lesion followed by radiotherapy and chemotherapy.

Intra-arterial chemotherapy has been developed as a way of administering antineoplastic agents that significantly increases their effect while reducing side effects as compared with systemic administration.

PHARMACOLOGIC AND EXPERIMENTAL DATA

Pharmacokinetic and experimental studies have demonstrated clearly that uptake of agents by tumor

cells depends on the pharmacologic properties of the agent, which determine whether it can pass through the blood-brain barrier,[1–4] as well as the intravascular concentration of the drug and arterial flow. In comparison, the role of exposure time to the drug appears to be accessory except for low-grade malignancies. Experimental and clinical studies have shown that, under the appropriate conditions, tumoral uptake is nearly 50 times higher when agents are administered intra-arterially than when they are given intravenously.[5–7]

Pharmacologic Properties

Lipid solubility and molecular size are important factors in determining the ability of an agent to cross the blood-brain barrier by transcapillary diffusion.[8, 9] Temporary blood-brain barrier disruption by osmotic or pharmacologic agents can increase this diffusion.

In addition, high first-pass circulation concentration increases uptake of drugs with short half-lives.[8]

Vascular Bed Considerations

Drug uptake by tumor cells is greatly increased when flow in the feeding artery(ies) is slow or when their effective diameter is reduced[8, 10, 11]; these conditions are realized with superselective chemoperfusion. However, the position of the tip of the catheter can induce flow disturbances that have been considered responsible for inadequate infusion of the drug. It is also important to infuse the complete tumor bed, because Kelly et al. have shown that tumor cells exist in the 3-cm margins surrounding the area of contrast enhancement on computed tomography.[12] It is necessary to include this surrounding margin in the infused vascular territory (Fig. 31–1).

Antimitotic Drugs

Many antimitotic drugs have been used over the past two decades, alone or in combination (Table 31–1). Among these, nitrosoureas and platinum derivatives are recognized as the most effective.[13] Many trials have been undertaken using BCNU; some more recent trials have used ACNU. Trials using carboplatin have also shown its efficacy in the treatment of brain neoplasms.

TECHNIQUES OF INFUSION

Three main techniques have been developed for intra-arterial infusion of chemotherapeutic agents in

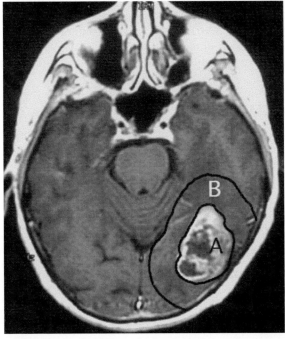

Figure 31-1 Evaluation of the tumor vascular bed on magnetic resonance imaging. A and B, tumor bed; A, contrast enhancement area; B, surrounding margin. The margin is up to 3 cm beyond the area of enhancement.

TABLE 31-1 Pharmacologic Properties of Chemotherapeutic Agents

Drug	Molecular Weight	Lipid Solubility	Ability to Cross BBB
BCNU	214	1.53	+ + +
ACNU	309	0.92	+ +
Cisplatin	300	−	+
Carboplatin	371	−	+
Vincristine	923	2.5	+
VM26	657	2.8	+

BBB, blood-brain barrier.

order to improve efficacy and/or reduce toxicity: (1) infusion after blood-brain barrier disruption, (2) selective infusion, and (3) superselective infusion.

Infusion After Temporary Blood-Brain Barrier Disruption

This technique was first reported by Neuwelt et al in relation to the treatment of primary cerebral lymphomas.[14] Blood-brain barrier disruption facilitates the intratumoral penetration of drugs that do not normally cross the barrier. This is achieved by intra-arterial injection of 25% hyperosmolar mannitol. This is very painful and necessitates deep sedation or general anesthesia. In the internal carotid artery, 125 ml of 25% mannitol is infused by mechanical pump over 30 seconds.[14, 15] In the vertebrobasilar system, the volume of mannitol is reduced to 80 ml infused in 30 seconds.[15] The mannitol produces disruption of the barrier lasting approximately 1 hour; the chemotherapeutic agent should be infused within this time.

The injection of mannitol is usually responsible for immediate periorbital vasoconstriction and can result in adverse reactions such as seizures (3% of patients) and transient asystole (1.5%). For these reasons, when the site and extent of the lesion dictate that two arterial territories (both carotid arteries or one carotid and one vertebral artery) should be infused, it seems reasonable to treat these in two separate sessions (typically with a 1- to 2-day delay between).[15]

Selective Infusion

This technique was developed during the 1970s but was rapidly discontinued because of the high incidence of ocular complications.[16, 17] The development of new antimitotic agents (ACNU, carboplatin) better tolerated by the optic system,[18–21] combined with a better understanding of the pathogenesis of ocular complications,[21] has resulted in a resurgence of interest in this modality.[13]

Visual complications that occur during intracarotid infusion of antineoplastic agents are generally the result of endarteritis involving the choroidal and retinal vessels. This may be due to the drug itself (cisplatin, nitrosoureas) or to the solvent used with some agents (BCNU) to improve blood-brain barrier penetration. This toxicity is related to the concentration of the agent in the blood and to its cumulative dose. This explains the observation that, when low-toxicity agents are used, ocular complications occur only after several sessions of intra-arterial chemotherapy. Investigations have shown that the adverse effects can be reduced by pretreatment with heparin and corticosteroids; 24 hours before intra-arterial chemotherapy, low-molecular-weight heparinoids and high-dose corticosteroids are begun and continued until 48 hours after the procedure.[20–22]

Before infusion, a complete evaluation of intracranial circulation is necessary in order to decide which arteries should be infused, given the site and extent of the tumor and the distribution of the vascular territories in the individual patient. Particular attention should be paid to anatomic variants of the circle of Willis (Fig. 31–2).[13]

Carotid Artery Infusion

The tip of a diagnostic catheter is carefully placed in the cervical portion of the internal carotid artery below C2, with care taken to avoid vasospasm (spasm necessitates delaying infusion until this resolves completely). Orbital pain during infusion of low-toxicity drugs such as ACNU or carboplatin is unusual; if it occurs, it is necessary to verify the correct placement of the catheter and absence of vasospasm.

The time of infusion is usually 15 to 30 minutes. A longer time does not appear indicated, as the goal is to achieve a high arterial concentration of the agent.

The dose should be carefully selected. It is usually a compromise between the local toxic dose and the systemic toxic dose. Most authors do not infuse more than 100 to 200 mg BCNU; for carboplatin, the intracarotid dose should be 400 mg. The low toxicity of ACNU allows infusion of the complete systemic dose

$(100\ mg/m^2)$ in the carotid artery. The cumulative dose of ACNU should not exceed 500 to 600 mg, to avoid ophthalmic complications.

With the ease and safety of modern microcatheter use, infusion can be performed distal to the ophthalmic artery.

Vertebral Artery Infusion

The tip of the catheter is placed in the proximal portion of the dominant vertebral artery. Looking retrospectively at the justification for this technique, I did not observe a significant difference in response rate between patients who received treatment in the carotid versus the vertebrobasilar system.[18] The amount of drug infused should be reduced to half the carotid dose. Specific attention should be paid when infusing BCNU, as this agent can produce acute brainstem toxicity. Again, infusion can be performed in the distal basilar artery to avoid the brainstem to some degree.

Superselective Infusion

This technique was originally proposed to prevent ocular complications after intra-arterial chemotherapy with BCNU. Infusion is performed after catheterization of the vascular pedicle of the tumor. Unfortunately, this technique significantly increases the risk of neurologic complications due to the high blood concentration of the agent and/or the distribution of the agent to both tumor and normal brain.[23–25] The use of sidehole microcatheters may diminish the risk of toxicity, but this has not yet been evaluated. According to published results, a significant decrease in the amount of drug infused is recommended (50 mg BCNU compared with 100 to 200 mg for intracarotid infusion).[24, 25] Nevertheless, this technique has yielded good clinical results in terms of tumoral response, and it should be considered in the setting of relative drug resistance of the tumor or hematologic toxicity.

CONCLUSION

Although its use is controversial, intra-arterial chemotherapy can result in a good clinical response in patients with malignant gliomas. Especially in cases of large inoperable tumors, it can be helpful in conjunction with radiation therapy.[26]

REFERENCES

1. Eckman WW, Patlak CS, Fenstermacher JD. A critical evaluation of the principles governing the advantages of intra-arterial infusions. *J Pharmacokinet Biopharm* 1974;2:257–285.
2. Levin VA, Landahl HD, Freeman-Dove MA. The application of brain capillary permeability coefficient measurements to pathological conditions and the selection of agents which cross the blood-brain barrier. *J Pharmacokinet Biopharm* 1976; 4:499–519.
3. Bullard DE, Bigner SH, Bigner DD. Comparison of intravenous versus intracarotid therapy with 1,3 bis(2-chloroethyl)-1-nitrosourea in a rat brain tumor model. *Cancer Res* 1985;45:5240–5245.

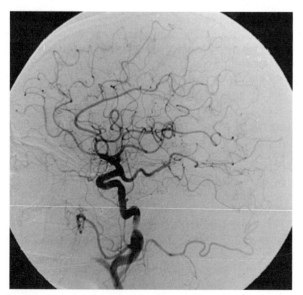

Figure 31-2 Variant of the circle of Willis (the posterior cerebral artery arises from the internal carotid artery).

4. Levin VA, Kabra PM. Brain and tumor pharmacokinetics of BCNU and CCNU following IV and intracarotid artery (ICA) administration. *Proc Am Assoc Cancer Res* 1975;16:19.

5. Levin VA, Kabra PM, Freeman-Dove MA. Pharmacokinetics of intracarotid artery ^{14}C-BCNU in the squirrel monkey. *J Neurosurg* 1978;48:487–493.

6. Tyler JL, Yamamoto L, Diksic M, et al. Pharmacokinetics of superselective intra-arterial and intravenous ^{11}C-BCNU evaluated by PET. *J Nucl Med* 1986;28:775–780.

7. Theron J, Villemure JG, Worthington E, et al. Superselective intra-cerebral chemotherapy of malignant tumors with BCNU. *Neuroradiology* 1986;28:118–125.

8. Poisson M, Pouillart P, Bataini JP, et al. Malignant gliomas treated after surgery by combination chemotherapy and delayed irradiation. *Acta Neurochir (Wien)* 1979;51:15–25.

9. Groothuis DR, Blasberg RG. Rational brain tumor chemotherapy: the interaction of drug and tumor. *Neurol Clin* 1985;3:801.

10. Fenstermacher JD, Cowles AL. Theoretic limitations of intracarotid infusions in brain tumor chemotherapy. *Cancer Treat Rep* 1977;61:519–526.

11. Blalock JB, Wright DC, Dedrick RL, et al. Drug streaming during intra-arterial chemotherapy. *J Neurosurg* 1986;64:284–291.

12. Kelly PJ, Daumas-Duport C, Scheithauer BW. Stereotactic histologic correlations of computed tomography– and magnetic resonance imaging–defined abnormalities in patients with glial neoplasms. *Mayo Clin Proc* 1987;62:450–459.

13. Chiras J, Chedid G, Debussche C. Intra-arterial chemotherapy of brain tumors. In Vinuela F, Halbach VV, Dion JE (eds): Interventional Neuroradiology: Endovascular Therapy of the Central Nervous System. New York: Raven Press, 1992.

14. Neuwelt EA, Diehl JT, Vu LH. Monitoring of methotrexate delivery in patients with malignant brain tumors after osmotic blood-brain barrier disruption. *Ann Intern Med* 1981;94:449–454.

15. Fauchon F, Chiras J, Poisson M, et al. Intra-arterial chemotherapy by cisplatin and cytarabine after temporary disruption of the blood-brain barrier for the treatment of malignant gliomas in adults. *J Neuroradiol* 1986;13:151–162.

16. Shapiro WR, Green SB. Reevaluating the efficacy of intra-arterial BCNU (letter). *Neurosurgery* 1987;66:313–315.

17. Miller DF, Bay JW, Lederman RJ, et al. Ocular and orbital toxicity following intra-carotid injection of BCNU (carmustine) and cisplatinum for malignant gliomas. *Ophthalmology* 1985;92:402–406.

18. Chiras J, Fauchon F, Poisson M, et al. Treatment of non-surgical gliomas by non-superselective intra-arterial chemotherapy followed by conventional radiotherapy. *Rev Neurol* 1989;145:829–837.

19. Fauchon F, Davila I, Chatellier G, et al. Treatment of malignant gliomas with surgery, intra-arterial infusions of 1-(2-hydroxyethyl)chloroethylnitrosourea and radiation therapy: A phase II study. *Neurosurgery* 1990;27:231–234.

20. Poisson M, Chiras J, Fauchon F, et al. Treatment of malignant recurrent glioma by intra-arterial infra-ophthalmic infusion of HECNU 1-(2-chloroethyl)-1-nitroso-3-(2-hydroxyethyl)urea. *J Neurooncol* 1989; 1–8.

21. Poisson M, Pereon Y, Chiras J, et al. Treatment of recurrent malignant supratentorial gliomas with carboplatin (CBDCA). *J Neurooncol* 1991;10:139–144.

22. Defer G, Fauchon F, Schiasson M, et al. Visual toxicity following intra-arterial chemotherapy with hydroxyethyl-CNU in patients with malignant gliomas: a prospective study with statistical analysis. *Neuroradiology* 1991;33:432–437.

23. Mahaley MS, Whaley RA, Blue M, et al. Central neurotoxicity following intracarotid BCNU chemotherapy for malignant gliomas. *J Neurooncol* 1986;3:297–314.

24. Burger PC, Kamenar E, Schold E, et al. Encephalomyelopathy following high-dose BCNU therapy. *Cancer* 1981;48:1318–1327.

25. Kapp JP, Vance RB. Supra-ophthalmic carotid infusion for recurrent gliomas. *J Neurooncol* 1985;3:5–11.

26. Chauvenic L, Sola-Martinez MT, Martin-Duverneuil N, et al. Intra-arterial chemotherapy with ACNU and radiotherapy in inoperable malignant gliomas. *J Neurooncol* 1996;27:141–147.

ADDITIONAL READINGS

Aoki S, Terada H, Kosuda S, et al. Supraophthalmic chemotherapy with long tapered catheter: Distribution evaluated with intraarterial and intravenous Tc-99m HMPAO. *Radiology* 1993;188:347–350.

Bonstelle CT, Kori SH, Rekate H. Intracarotid chemotherapy of glioblastoma after induced blood-brain barrier disruption. *AJNR* 1983;4:810–812.

Fujiwara T, Matsumoto Y, Honma Y, et al. A comparison of intraarterial carboplatin and ACNU for the treatment of glioma. *Surg Neurol* 1995;44:145–150.

Greenberg HS, Ensminger WD, Chandler WF, et al. Intra-arterial BCNU chemotherapy for treatment of malignant gliomas of the central nervous system. *J Neurosurg* 1984;61:423–429.

Greenberg HS, Ensminger WD, Seeger JF, et al. Intra-arterial BCNU chemotherapy for the treatment of malignant gliomas of the central nervous system: A preliminary report. *Cancer Treat Rep* 1981;65:803–810.

Kurpad SN, Friedman HS, Archer GE, et al. Intraarterial administration of melphalan for treatment of intracranial human glioma xenografts in athymic rats. *Cancer Res* 1995;55:3803–3809.

Monzen Y, Mori H, Matsumoto S, et al. Intraarterial infusion of cisplatin with and without preoperative concurrent radiation for urinary bladder cancer: A preliminary report. *Radiation Med* 1995;13:149–152.

Roman-Goldstein S, Mitchell P, Crossen JR, et al. MR and cognitive testing of patients undergoing osmotic blood-brain barrier disruption with intraarterial chemotherapy. *AJNR* 1995;16:543–553.

CHAPTER 32

Interventional Neuroradiologic Procedure for Wada Testing

J.J. Connors III / J.C. Wojak

Functional testing of cerebral structures has undergone periods of popular interest followed by disinterest. The development of sophisticated scanning techniques (e.g., positron emission tomography, single-photon emission computed tomography [SPECT], certain magnetic resonance imaging sequences) has reawakened interest in functional evaluation of the brain. There is only minimal need for intra-arterial evaluation of cerebral function other than for testing during endovascular embolization procedures. Depending on the neurosurgical team and their practice, however, conventional Wada testing may be requested, particularly in relation to surgery for seizures.

APPLICATIONS

Typically, Wada testing is done to evaluate which hemisphere is the dominant side for speech, memory implantation, and ingestion of new information. This knowledge is then used for planning neurosurgical procedures related to treatment of seizures. This is most often the case when surgery for epilepsy involving the temporal lobe is planned. Whenever surgery involving a potentially eloquent region is considered, however, this is important information. Intracarotid injection of amobarbital (Amytal) is employed for this purpose.[1, 2] Methohexital (Brevital) has also been used for this test,[3] as discussed previously (see "How to Test a Vessel Prior to Embolization [Provocative Testing]" in Chapter 3).

PROCEDURE

Initial Steps

An initial cerebral angiogram is performed, specifically to evaluate the distribution of the internal carotid artery. It is disconcerting to inject the internal carotid artery with amobarbital and have the patient suddenly become apneic because of a primitive connection (e.g., persistent trigeminal artery) between the anterior circulation and the basilar artery (and thus the posterior fossa structures; the pons and medulla affect respiratory as well as hemodynamic function).

Before beginning the procedure, a baseline neurologic examination is performed and a baseline electroencephalogram (EEG) obtained. The EEG leads are left in place. Once the absence of potentially dangerous anastomoses from the anterior circulation to the brainstem has been established, the catheter is positioned in the internal carotid artery to be tested. If both sides are to be tested, the side of interest is evaluated first, in case there is a problem and the examination must be terminated. This is also important because evaluation of the second side is less sensitive owing to residual circulating amobarbital from the first test.

Injection of Amobarbital

This test was originally performed by injecting the pharmaceutical agent into the common carotid artery.[1] This required sufficiently large doses of amobarbital (160 to 200 mg) such that testing of both hemispheres during one procedure was not feasible. The smaller doses used during selective injection into the internal carotid artery have made bilateral testing during the same procedure possible; a vast improvement for both the patient and the physicians.

Approximately 300 mg of amobarbital is premixed in 30 ml of normal saline. Two 12-ml syringes are filled and placed on the table. The first syringe is attached to the catheter. The patient is asked to raise the arms and begin counting loudly. After the patient has reached "20" (a predefined point at which everyone is ready), the amobarbital is injected in rapid bursts, 1 ml at a time, up to 7 ml (70 mg). If a slow infusion is performed, all the drug may flow out of the catheter in a laminar fashion and thus out the first side branch (e.g., ophthalmic artery, anterior cerebral artery). Therefore, many (about 4 to 8) rapid bursts are performed to mix the drug with the flowing blood.

In general, 60 to 90 mg of amobarbital is necessary to induce enough cerebral anesthesia for adequate testing of the brain. (Rarely, an additional 25 mg or so may be needed, so it is wise to have an extra amount prepared and ready to use; hence the second syringe.) Determination of adequate dose is made by having the patient raise both arms above the head and hold them there during the injection. When the amobarbital is injected, the appropriate arm becomes weak and falls. In addition, the patient can be made to talk continuously (e.g., by counting aloud) or can be quizzed when the arm falls. It is at this point that neurologic testing can be performed. It is not necessary to induce total paralysis of the arm; this can render testing difficult and inaccurate because of generalized cerebral dysfunction (poor comprehension or task performance) rather than specific focal neurologic dysfunction. It can also induce mutism, resulting in the inability to test memory, for example.

EEG monitoring is begun before administration of amobarbital and continued until return to baseline.

Neurologic Evaluation

The neurologic testing is discussed in depth in Chapter 33. Injection of amobarbital into the internal carotid artery supplying the dominant hemisphere for speech production results in mutism for 1 to 2 minutes, followed by dysnomia. Speech arrest is possible if a sufficiently large dose is injected into the contralateral hemisphere.[2] Dysnomia, however, is specific to the dominant hemisphere. Speech lateralization is therefore further evaluated by object-naming tasks. This commonly takes the form of asking the patient to remember an object or series of objects. The patient is then asked to perform another task, such as reading a sentence, after which the recall of the previous objects is tested. This is repeated throughout the period of effect of the drug. Speech dysfunction as demonstrated by this procedure has been shown to identify the dominant hemisphere correctly in up to 98.5% of cases.[2]

Memory function is assessed by the ability to recall the assigned objects during the period of drug effect and after the drug effect has ceased.[2] Prediction of postsurgical memory deficit is not as accurate as prediction of speech deficit.

Bilateral Examination

Once the testing has been performed, it is usually necessary to wait about 30 to 60 minutes for the drug to wear off before the other side can be tested. (The initial unilateral effects become systemic, thus confusing accurate evaluation of the second side.) The testing itself takes some of this time, and the opposite internal carotid artery can be selected after the testing, thus using a good portion of the time necessary for the drug to wear off.

Assessing Distribution of Amobarbital

It is possible to evaluate where the injected amobarbital goes. The amobarbital can be mixed with contrast material in a 30% mixture (any more can cause precipitation of the amobarbital). This can then be observed fluoroscopically or during a digital subtraction angiogram.

Alternatively, the amobarbital can be mixed with a radionuclide (technetium-99m hexamethylpropyleneamine oxime [^{99m}Tc HMPAO]) and injected. This mixture is taken up by the areas of the brain to which it flows and confirms adequate localization for the testing. A SPECT scan can then be performed after the Wada testing.

FALSE-POSITIVE WADA TEST

Because of hemodynamic or pharmacologic factors, some patients may fail standard Wada testing erro-

neously. This failure can manifest as overdose (obtundation), memory failure after injection of the ipsilateral internal carotid artery, or lack of findings after injection of the contralateral internal carotid artery. Most damning is true failure when injecting the ipsilateral internal carotid artery.

In a study performed by Hamberger and colleagues, selective injection (rather than global internal carotid artery injection) was performed to study the hippocampus and mesial temporal lobe accurately.[4] The vascular supply to this structure is presented in Chapter 33 and is seen to be from both the anterior and posterior choroidal arteries. The posterior choroidal artery arises from the posterior cerebral artery and can be selectively injected to evaluate this response further. However, simultaneously injecting the anterior and posterior choroidal arteries, as described below, is more definitive.

Technique of Selective Choroidal Artery Injection

Selective injection of the anterior choroidal artery can be performed by accurately occluding the internal carotid artery with either a Solstice balloon (Medtronic/MIS) or with an Endeavor (Target Therapeutics) (see Chapter 51 for a description of the preparation of these balloons). There are multiple sizes of Endeavors; the largest one should be used to occlude the carotid artery. This requires a large-lumen guide catheter; the 7-Fr. Lumax Neuroguide is preferred. Once occlusion has been performed just distal to the anterior choroidal artery (and thus just distal to the posterior communicating artery), amobarbital is infused through the guide catheter into the internal carotid artery. Amobarbital perfuses these two vascular territories and thus both choroidal artery territories, which effectively perfuses the entire hippocampus and mesial temporal lobe. Perfusion will also yield a homonymous hemianopsia.

Results of Selective Intra-Arterial Amobarbital Testing

In the evaluation performed by Hamberger and colleagues,[4] seven patients with left hemisphere language dominance and an ipsilateral seizure focus underwent selective evaluation. All patients underwent pre- and postoperative evaluation of cognitive function. Five of the seven patients passed testing after selective injection of the anterior and posterior choroidal arteries ipsilateral to their seizure focus. All five patients who passed the test underwent surgery and did well; two patients failed both tests and did not undergo surgery. No procedural complications or difficulties were encountered. The Hamberger study indicates that this procedure can be performed safely and can alter the ultimate therapy.[4]

REFERENCES

1. Wada JT, Rasmussen J. Intracarotid injection of sodium Amytal for the lateralization of cerebral speech dominance. *J Neurosurg* 1960;17:266–282.

2. Dodrill CB. Preoperative criteria for identifying eloquent brain: intracarotid Amytal for language and memory testing. *Neurosurg Clin* 1993;4:211–216.
3. Willmore LJ, Wilder BJ, Mayersdorf A, et al. Identification of speech lateralization by intracarotid injection of methohexital. *Ann Neurol* 1978;4:86–88.
4. Hamberger MJ, Duong H, Hacein-Bey L, et al. Utility of intraarterial amobarbital testing in candidates for temporal lobectomy. Paper presented at the American Society of Interventional and Therapeutic Neuroradiology/World Federation of Interventional and Therapeutic Neuroradiology Scientific Conference. New York, Sept 1997.

ADDITIONAL READINGS

Functional Neurologic Testing

Doppman JL, Girton M, Oldfield EH. Spinal Wada test. *Radiology* 1986;161:319–321.
Horton JA, Kerber CW. Lidocaine injection into external carotid branches: provocative test to preserve cranial nerve function in therapeutic embolization. *AJNR* 1986;7:105–108.

CHAPTER 33

Intracarotid Amobarbital (Wada) Test:
Neurology Perspective

Piotr Olejniczak / Bruce Fisch

The intracarotid amobarbital procedure (IAP), or Wada test, is used routinely in the presurgical evaluation of neurosurgery patients to localize cortical language function and to assess the bilateral distribution of memory function. Wada[1] originally described the IAP as a means of assessing laterality of language function and later adopted it for the presurgical localization of language at the Montreal Neurological Institute.[2] The IAP continues to be used for the localization of cortical language function, particularly in anticipation of epilepsy surgery involving the perisylvian area. In most cases in which resection of language areas is likely, however, language is also assessed by direct electrical cortical stimulation either during surgery or perioperatively using implanted intracranial subdural electrodes. Moreover, the most commonly performed epilepsy surgery, the anterior temporal lobectomy, rarely, if ever, produces a persistent aphasia.

A more important question for patients undergoing temporal lobectomy is whether the procedure will cause significant memory impairment. After the role of the temporal lobe in supporting memory function became apparent, Milner and others[3] modified the Wada test to assess memory. This is now the most important clinical application of the IAP. Normally, adequate memory function can be maintained after either the left or right mesial temporal–hippocampal structure is destroyed. In some patients who have undergone temporal lobectomy, however, unsuspected or preexisting damage to the contralateral temporal lobe resulted in complete and permanent anterograde amnesia. The Wada test is therefore used to predict whether the contralateral temporal lobe will be able to sustain adequate memory function after temporal lobectomy has been performed. More recently, IAP memory testing has been used to localize seizure onset. If only one hemisphere is found to contain poor memory function, then it is

highly likely that the epileptogenic zone involves that hemisphere.

PROCEDURE

The IAP test has not been standardized. Surveys of epilepsy centers[4] show that variations in protocols are the rule rather than the exception. In most centers, a cerebral angiogram is conducted before Wada testing to evaluate cerebral vasculature, assess hemispheric cross-flow, detect the presence of a patent posterior communicating artery or perfusion of the posterior cerebral artery, and document rare anomalous circulatory patterns that may influence amobarbital distribution.[5, 6] The amobarbital test is performed at the completion of the cerebral angiogram. The patient is asked to hold up the arms, perform continuous motions with the hands and feet, and verbalize. While the patient is performing these activities, a bolus injection of amobarbital solution is administered into the internal carotid artery through a transfemoral catheter as verified by fluoroscopy (the tip of the catheter is usually at the C3 to C4 vertebral level). Many centers use a set dosage of 125 or 150 mg of amobarbital delivered in 3 to 5 ml of solution. This regularly results in a period of global obtundation during which the patient is not responsive and cannot be tested reliably (although it has been reported that some patients may be able to recall material presented even while they are mute and apparently confused[7]). After 1 to 3 minutes, the patient becomes more alert, and the presentation of test materials begins. Evidence of unilateral hemispheric impairment is established by the presence of hemiparesis and other signs of unilateral dysfunction, such as homonymous hemianopia or dysphasia. The patient is then presented a list of pictures, written words, and objects to identify and memorize. Several minutes after complete recovery, the patient is asked to recall items presented during testing. If the patient cannot spontaneously recall the items, recall lists are used to test recognition memory. At some centers, spontaneous recall is not tested. Most centers test the second hemisphere 30 to 45 minutes after the injection of the first hemisphere. Fewer centers report testing each hemisphere on separate days. Electroencephalogram (EEG) testing and subjective assessment by patients suggest that the second hemisphere should not be tested sooner than 45 minutes after the first hemisphere injection. Testing each hemisphere on separate days is usually unnecessary and adds cost and potential risk.

At our center, the Wada test is conducted by a team that includes a neurologist-electrophysiologist, neuroradiologist, nurse anesthetist, nurse, EEG technologist, and radiology technologists. Cerebral angiography is performed immediately before testing. Both hemispheres are studied on the same day. The EEG is monitored continuously during the procedure. Although some centers do not perform simultaneous EEG monitoring, most do for the following reasons: (1) EEG monitoring provides another independent measure of unilateral hemispheric anesthesia that is probably more relevant for memory testing than other signs, such as hand strength[8]; (2) the EEG can be used to assess the timing of the testing in relation to the intensity of medication effects; and (3) EEG monitoring is useful for distinguishing unusual responses, such as seizures or vascular events, from abnormal testing results.

The examiner should stand on the side of the patient that is ipsilateral to the injection, to avoid being in the field of an amobarbital-induced homonymous hemianopia during testing. At our center, testing begins 1.5 minutes before the injection of amobarbital, when the patient is asked to name aloud and memorize a printed number. A printed color is then presented 1 minute before injection, with the same instructions. These test items allow for later testing of retrograde amnesia. The patient then is asked to hold up both arms, wiggle the fingers, and count aloud. When the patient reaches a count of 20, the neuroradiologist injects the amobarbital. The patient continues to count aloud and move the fingers until he or she cannot continue or is told by the examiner to stop. The amount of amobarbital used for each subject is typically between 80 and 120 mg. Unlike other centers where a standard dose is used, we titrate the dosage according to the patient's response, to avoid a prolonged confusional state. (For similar reasons, methohexital, which may be somewhat less sedating, has been proposed as an alternative to amobarbital.) The titration end point includes the appearance of continuous asymmetric or unilateral EEG delta activity and contralateral hemiparesis (the patient can no longer hold the arm up or make a fist). In most cases, the patient remains awake; although some degree of preservation of counting or of hand movements is common, there is usually a momentary delay in getting the patient's full attention for testing. The advantages of avoiding obtunda-

tion include the following: (1) a long period of confusion may result in a diminished unilaterality of the amobarbital effect by the time the patient is alert enough to cooperate with testing, (2) the end of the confusional state is better defined if the recovery time to alertness is brief, (3) it is likely that memory for test items presented as soon as the patient can cooperate is more predictive of surgical outcome,[9] and (4) using the lowest effective dosage facilitates same-day testing of both hemispheres.

Immediately after the patient becomes alert and attentive and while the EEG shows ipsilateral delta activity, three printed common nouns (e.g., house, truck, ball) are presented individually to be read. Even if the patient is unable to read the words, he or she is instructed to try to memorize them. Remarkably, patients who are mute are often able to recall parts of words or recognize them later from recall lists. Five easily recognizable objects (e.g., fork, toothbrush) are then presented to be named and memorized at 15- to 25-second intervals. Four minutes after the injection, the patient is asked to recall the number and color that were presented before the injection. Ten minutes after the injection, the patient is asked to recall the printed words and objects that were presented after amobarbital administration. If the patient is unable to recall the words or objects spontaneously, recall lists are used. Although a complete failure of spontaneous recognition alone does not constitute a failure of memory testing, testing both spontaneous recall and recognition allows for a greater range of scoring when comparing hemispheres.

APPLICATIONS
Language Assessment

The role of the Wada test in localizing language function has remained largely unchanged since it was described by Wada[1] and is the least controversial aspect of testing. Although estimates of left-hemisphere language dominance vary, it is generally accepted that 95% or more of right-handed individuals are left-hemisphere language dominant. In one series, only 2% of the right-handed patients developed aphasia after the occurrence of a right hemisphere lesion.[10] Twenty-four percent of the non–right-handed patients developed aphasia after right-hemisphere insult. Exclusive right-hemisphere language may be relatively rare, and language representation in patients with bilateral hemispheric representation may be regarded as a continuous rather than a dichotomous variable.[6, 11] Wada language results have been compared with detection of language areas during operative or extraoperative cortical electrical stimulation mapping, and there is generally agreement between techniques.[6, 12, 13] The Wada test has also served as a control for evaluating the efficacy of functional language localization using magnetic resonance imaging (MRI). Desmond and colleagues[14] reported that the two tests were concordant in each of seven studied patients.

Memory Assessment

The Wada test gradually has been adapted to predict degrees of postoperative memory decline in patients scheduled to undergo unilateral temporal lobectomy. The basis of this test rests on the assumption that transient pharmacologic ablation of dysfunctional mesial temporal structures in temporal lobe epilepsy patients should result in little compromise of memory function during Wada testing if the homologous structures in the opposite hemisphere are intact. The reliability of the Wada test to assess the risk of memory decline or complete anterograde amnesia remains controversial, however, in part because of the extremely rare occurrence of actual total anterograde amnesia after temporal lobectomy. In addition, it has been established that the posterior 75% of the hippocampus, the structure that ideally should be perfused by the amobarbital, is not supplied by the internal carotid circulation in most people[15, 16] (Fig. 33–1). This has raised the question of whether the hippocampus is affected directly during IAP testing.

Two separate studies of single-photon emission computed tomography using technetium-99m hexamethylpropyleneamine oxime suggest that mesial temporal structures are rarely perfused by amobarbital during intracarotid injection.[17, 18] These observations have led various investigators to develop selective angiographic techniques to ensure perfusion of the body of the hippocampus. Three main approaches have been used (see Fig. 33–1): (1) balloon occlusion distal to the origin of the anterior choroidal artery, with injection of amobarbital thereby forced into the vascular territories of the anterior choroidal, posterior communicating, and ophthalmic arteries; (2) selective catheterization of the anterior choroidal artery; and (3) selective catheterization of the posterior cerebral artery.[15, 19] These approaches have not been widely accepted, mainly because of the increased risk of morbidity and mortality compared with the internal carotid approach.

If much of the hippocampus is spared the direct infusion of amobarbital, it remains highly likely that the hippocampus is functionally interrupted by internal carotid artery administration. This conclusion is supported by EEG data obtained using temporal depth electrode recording during Wada testing.[20, 21] IAP memory testing results also appear to correlate with MRI volumetric analysis of the hippocampus and temporal lobe.[22] Greater memory impairment occurs when the hemisphere without atrophic changes is injected. In addition, in a case of post-temporal lobectomy amnesia, Loring and colleagues[9] found that the patient was unable to memorize objects presented early after amobarbital injection but could memorize materials presented later in the test. Finally, Wada memory asymmetries between ipsilateral and contralateral hemisphere injection appear to be predictive of verbal memory decline after left temporal lobectomy.[6, 23] Other methods for testing memory using neuroimaging techniques are in development, but the IAP continues to be the standard method for preoperative memory testing.

Lateralization of Seizure Onset

The IAP memory test has been established as an adjunctive diagnostic test for identifying which temporal lobe contains the epileptogenic zone[9, 13, 24, 25] and is similarly predictive of postoperative seizure control.[26] Thus, it is not surprising that IAP memory performance correlates with MRI temporal lobe or hippocampal atrophy.[22] It is also likely that recall for items presented shortly after injection is a better predictor of side of seizure onset than is recall of items presented later after injection.[9] Memory of real objects may be better than memory of line drawings for lateralizing seizure onset.[23]

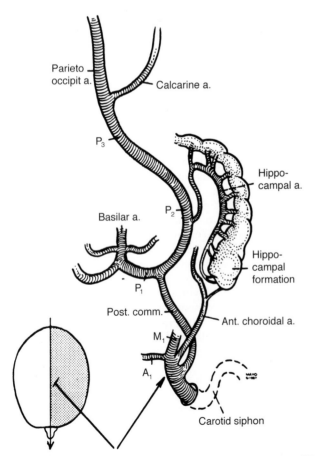

Figure 33-1 Arterial supply of the hippocampus. (From Jack CR Jr, Nichols DA, Sharbrough FW, et al. Selective posterior cerebral artery Amytal test for evaluating memory function before surgery for temporal lobe seizure. *Radiology* 1988;168:787–793.)

Labels in figure: Parieto occipit a.; Calcarine a.; P₃; Hippocampal a.; Basilar a.; P₂; Hippocampal formation; P₁; Post. comm.; Ant. choroidal a.; M₁; A₁; Carotid siphon

REFERENCES

1. Wada J. A new method for the determination of the side of cerebral speech dominance: a preliminary report on the intracarotid injection of sodium Amytal in man. *Igaku to Seibutsugaku* 1949;14:221–222.
2. Dodrill CB. Preoperative criteria for identifying eloquent brain: intracarotid Amytal for language and memory testing. *Neurosurg Clin* 1993;4:211–216.
3. Milner B, Branch C, Rasmussen T. Study of short-term mem-

ory after intracarotid injection of sodium Amytal. *Trans Am Neurol Assoc* 1962;87:224–226.

4. Rausch R, Langfitt JT. Memory evaluation during the intracarotid sodium amobarbital procedure. In Luders H (ed.): Epilepsy Surgery. New York: Raven Press, 1991, pp. 507–514.
5. Petersen RC, Sharbrough FW, Jack CR. Intracarotid amobarbital testing. In Wyllie E (ed): The Treatment of Epilepsy: Principles and Practice. Philadelphia: Lea & Febiger, 1993, pp. 1051–1061.
6. Trenerry MR, Loring DW. Intracarotid amobarbital procedure: the Wada test. *Neuroimaging Clin* 1995;5:721–728.
7. Lesser RP, Dinner DS, Luders H, Morris HH. Memory for objects presented soon after intracarotid amobarbital sodium injections in patients with medically intractable complex partial seizures. *Neurology* 1986;36:895–899.
8. Bouwer MS, Jones-Gotman M, Gotman J. Duration of sodium Amytal effect: behavior and EEG measures. *Epilepsia* 1993;34:61–68.
9. Loring DW, Meador KJ, King DW, et al. Stimulus timing effects on Wada memory testing. *Arch Neurol* 1994;51:806–810.
10. Benson DF. Language in the left hemisphere. In Mesulam MM (ed): Principles of Behavioral Neurology. Philadelphia: FA Davis, 1985, pp. 193–203.
11. Loring DW, Meador KJ, Lee GP, et al. Cerebral language lateralization: evidence from intracarotid amobarbital testing. *Neuropsychologia* 1990;28:831–838.
12. Hinz AC, Berger MS, Ojemann GA, Dodrill C. The utility of the intracarotid Amytal procedure in determining hemispheric speech lateralization in pediatric epilepsy patients undergoing surgery. *Childs Nerv Syst* 1994;10:239–243.
13. Wyllie E, Luders H, Murphy D, et al. Intracarotid amobarbital (Wada) test for language dominance: correlation with results of cortical stimulation. *Epilepsia* 1990;31:156–161.
14. Desmond JE, Sum JM, Wagner AD, et al. Functional MRI measurement of language lateralization in Wada-tested patients. *Brain* 1995;118:1411–1419.
15. Jack CR Jr, Nichols DA, Sharbrough FW, et al. Selective

posterior cerebral artery Amytal test for evaluating memory function before surgery for temporal lobe seizure. *Radiology* 1988;168:787–793.
16. Jack CR Jr, Nichols DA, Sharbrough FW, et al. Selective posterior cerebral artery injection of Amytal: new method of preoperative memory testing. *Mayo Clin Proc* 1989;64:965–975.
17. Jeffrey PJ, Monsein LH, Szabo Z, et al. Mapping the distribution of amobarbital sodium in the intracarotid Wada test by use of Tc-99m HMPAO with SPECT. *Radiology* 1991;178:847–850.
18. Hart J Jr, Lewis PJ, Lesser RP, et al. Anatomic correlates of memory from intracarotid amobarbital injections with technetium Tc 99m hexamethylpropyleneamine oxime SPECT. *Arch Neurol* 1993;50:745–750.
19. Wieser HG. Anterior cerebral artery amobarbital test. In Luders H (ed): Epilepsy Surgery. New York: Raven Press, 1991, pp. 515–523.
20. Gotman J, Bouwer MS, Jones-Gotman M. Intracranial EEG study of brain structures affected by internal carotid injection of amobarbital. *Neurology* 1992;42:2136–2143.
21. Ahern GL, Herring AM, Tackenberg JN, et al. Affective self-report during the intracarotid sodium amobarbital test. *J Clin Exp Neuropsychol* 1994;16:372–376.
22. Loring DW, Murro AM, Meador KJ, et al. Wada memory testing and hippocampal volume measurements in evaluation for temporal lobectomy. *Neurology* 1993;43:1789–1793.
23. Loring DW, Meador KJ, Lee GP, et al. Wada memory asymmetries predict verbal memory decline after anterior temporal lobectomy. *Neurology* 1995;45:1329–1333.
24. Engel J Jr, Rausch R, Lieb JP, et al. Correlation of criteria used for localizing epileptic foci in patients considered for surgical therapy of epilepsy. *Ann Neurol* 1981;9:215–224.
25. Perrine K, Westerveld M, Sass KJ, et al. Wada memory disparities predict seizure laterality and postoperative seizure control. *Epilepsia* 1995;36:851–856.
26. Sperling MR, Saykin AJ, Glosser G, et al. Predictors of outcome after anterior temporal lobectomy: the intracarotid amobarbital test. *Neurology* 1994;44:2325–2330.

CHAPTER 34

Temporary Test Occlusion of the Internal Carotid Artery

J.J. Connors III

Sacrifice of the internal carotid artery (the usual vessel of concern) can sometimes lead to a major, permanent neurologic deficit (stroke). Over the years, attempts have been made to try to determine which patients (or which internal carotid arteries) could be safely sacrificed without the threat of this disaster.

Abrupt internal carotid occlusion can result in neurologic deficit in up to one half of cases.[1, 2] Even with a clinically tolerated temporary balloon occlusion test, the failure rate of later permanent occlusion is 5% to 20%. Not only is there a potential problem with the temporary occlusion test, there is also a problem with interpretation of the results. This chapter attempts to address both these issues.

The performance of the temporary occlusion test is

under the direct control of the interventional neuroradiologist and should be performed with a reliable and high degree of safety. The interpretation of the results and the various methods used to obtain information concerning these results are still not perfect.

INDICATIONS

A test occlusion can be performed in almost any vessel but is mainly performed on the internal carotid artery when a permanent occlusion is desired. The following are common indications for test occlusion of the internal carotid artery:

- Traumatic injury to the internal carotid artery not amenable to open surgical repair

- Cavernous carotid aneurysm or carotid-cavernous fistula
- Possible sacrifice of the carotid (or other) artery during an interventional neuroradiologic procedure or surgery (usually for a head or neck tumor)
- Possible need to clamp a vessel for a prolonged period of time
- Permanent occlusion of the internal carotid artery for prophylaxis against continuing embolic events in a nonoperative candidate
- Other unusual complex vascular problems requiring internal carotid artery sacrifice

TOOLS

The two types of temporary balloon occlusion catheters suitable for test occlusions are an end-hole catheter (guidewire-directable) and a non–end-hole catheter. The end-hole guidewire-directable catheters were suboptimal in quality in the past, but improvements have been made in their design (see Chapter 1). The Zeppelin (Medtronic/MIS) is the most elegant design but is costly and slightly too stiff. A new, more reasonably priced model designed specifically for test occlusions is being developed. Medi-Tech, Inc. has introduced an updated model of its temporary test occlusion balloon and is working on further refinements (see Chapter 1). In addition, certain practitioners prefer to use Swan-Ganz occlusion balloons because of their softness. These are technically difficult to use, however, because they are floppy and most models lack guidewire directability. With the new model, a guidewire can be used and, with good technique, it can be exchanged over the proper exchange wire for correct placement. We have not used this type, but the concept of having a guidewire-directable catheter that is soft and atraumatic is appealing.

An additional difference between test occlusion balloons is the material the balloon is made of (silicone or latex). Latex has a much greater expansion range than silicone but develops a higher pressure (radial force) before expansion. This can result in true angioplasty of the vessel and possibly even dissection. Inflation of these balloons to the point of balloon deformation is therefore contraindicated. Because of the lesser force needed to expand silicone balloons, they are less likely to cause vascular damage.

Some practitioners use the ITC/Target Therapeutics Endeavor (formerly NDSB or nondetachable silicone balloon) for these procedures (see Chapter 1). The advantage of this balloon is its soft, atraumatic nature. The disadvantages are that a guide catheter is necessary because of its lack of guidewire directability. In addition, during occlusion, there is no way to maintain a downstream flush (the primary problem). For these reasons, most temporary test occlusions are performed with guidewire-directable balloon catheters, allowing downstream flushing with heparinized saline during the occlusion.

Of the three sizes of temporary test occlusion balloons made by Medi-Tech, two require a 7-Fr. sheath (producing a 9-Fr. hole in the access vessel, usually the common femoral artery). If a sheath is to be used, a neuro sheath is recommended. The third size is a new 5-Fr. design accepting an 0.035″ guidewire. This is suitable for most applications but does not fit through a 5-Fr. or a 6-Fr. sheath, and therefore a 7-Fr. sheath is still needed.

The Zeppelin occlusion balloon catheter can be introduced directly through the skin and has an excellent balloon and tip, requires a smaller hole in the access artery, and is potentially less traumatic to the carotid artery (although we use it through a neuro sheath). It is 5.4-Fr. and has to follow an exchange wire to its final location. An advantage to this catheter is that the balloon is silicone, allowing simple balloon preparation. The balloon is inflated ahead of time, and during the initial stages of the procedure, the air in the balloon diffuses through the silicone and vanishes.

A 45-cm neuro sheath (see Chapter 1) allows more direct deployment of the balloon catheter in the aorta, without the tendency for the catheter to "snake" as much in the iliac artery and lower aorta. Exchange of catheters is also facilitated.

Some of the worst disasters in interventional neuroradiology have been secondary to poor choice of exchange wires. The angled-tip hydrophilic exchange wires are the most troublesome. No matter how still the external portion of this wire is held, the intravascular distal tip wanders back and forth as the catheters are being exchanged, with the wire alternately assuming a straight course in the aorta and then a tortuous course. When this occurs, the angled tip can reach a curve in the vessel that is too abrupt forcing the tip to dig subintimally. This can then produce an intimal dissection with a resultant wind sock effect and subsequent vessel occlusion. Soft, straight, regular wires (Bentson wires) also can cause dissection. The Rosen exchange wire is far safer, although it can cause spasm of the vessel. The new Connors neuroexchange wire, from Cook, Inc., is ideal (see Chapter 1).

TECHNIQUE

The technique of temporary occlusion depends on the type of occlusion catheter used. The patient is well hydrated before the procedure. A standard four-vessel cerebral angiogram is first performed. If there is no evidence of collateral supply to the vessel to be tested (e.g., no anterior or posterior communicating artery), no temporary occlusion of the internal carotid artery should be performed, or, if done, it should be performed with trepidation and alertness to early failure. Occasionally, it appears that there is no collateral supply to the ipsilateral carotid artery, but with a cross-compression carotid angiogram (occlusion of one common carotid artery during injection of the opposite side), some cross flow (through the anterior communicating artery) may be evident.

For certain practitioners, good examination of intracranial hemodynamics and collateral hemispheric supply is adequate for evaluation of the feasibility of permanent occlusion; however, this is a nonquantifiable procedure. For most practitioners, a true occlusion test, with neurologic and other testing, is performed.

Preocclusion neurologic testing is performed either by the attending neurologist or by the interventional neuroradiologist. The baseline neurologic examination is noted. Clinical sedation is not a part of this procedure; the patient should be fully awake. In addition electroencephalogram (EEG) monitoring can be performed during the occlusion procedure, and a technetium-99m (^{99m}Tc) hexamethylpropyleneamine oxime (HMPAO) single-photon emission computed tomography (SPECT) scan can be performed as part of the evaluation. A xenon-133 (^{133}Xe) computed tomography (CT) scan can also be performed.

A bolus of 10,000 units of heparin (personal preference) should be administered after the sheath is in place or just after the balloon occlusion catheter has been introduced into the vascular tree (the temporary occlusion being the intended eventual result of this maneuver). A repeat neurologic test can be performed while allowing time for adequate distribution of this drug and adequate placement of the balloon catheter. This should consist of at least motor and sensory evaluation of the upper and lower extremities as well as cognitive ability, speech, and cranial nerve function. We carry on a conversation with the patient during this entire procedure.

The carotid artery is selected by a routine diagnostic catheter, and then, after the diagnostic baseline angiogram, a safe exchange wire (see Chapter 1) is used to place the temporary occlusion balloon. Again, some of the worst disasters in interventional neuroradiologic procedures have occurred during simple catheter exchanges, almost all secondary to the type of *exchange wire*. Extreme care should be taken during this portion of the procedure, and a safe exchange wire should be used. If the proper wire is used, this is a safe procedure.

Whenever a balloon will be placed in the head or neck region, it should be prepared beforehand to remove any air and to check for leaks (see Chapter 3). It is easier to prepare a silicone balloon, in which the air simply diffuses through the balloon. We use a microtube to connect the inflation syringe to the balloon port of the catheter. This allows the balloon catheter to be manipulated with finesse and the balloon to be inflated while contrast is being injected through the other port of the catheter (through the guidewire lumen).

The Medi-Tech latex balloon may not deflate because the balloon may inflate eccentrically on the side *opposite* the side port, keeping this orifice covered with the noninflating latex. Slight advancement and retraction of the catheter with a wire in place may help free the port. During preparation, these balloons can also be "trained" to inflate over the side port by manipulating the balloon as it is inflated and deflated.

Care must be taken to place the temporary balloon occlusion catheter carefully in the internal carotid artery so that the blunt end of the catheter does not damage the vessel while the balloon is inflated. (The catheter tip moves up and down with respiration and heart beat [Fig. 34–1], with the vessel flexing at this point.) The tip can cause an intimal tear, particularly in a patient with intrinsic vascular pathology. This is of more concern with the older models of temporary occlusion balloons; the newer models and the Swan-Ganz types have extremely short, soft tips. The correct location should be chosen from the previously performed biplane angiogram of the cervical internal carotid artery.

The balloon should not be placed in the bulb of the internal carotid artery because of the possible hemodynamic effects caused by compression of the carotid body during inflation of the balloon (and thus subsequent vasoactive response).

Note that the balloon is not yet inflated.

After the temporary occlusion balloon catheter has been placed in the correct position, a contrast injection is made to confirm its position in a comfortable segment of the internal carotid artery. A three-way stopcock is placed on the hub of the temporary occlusion balloon catheter. A pressure bag terminating in an air filter (see Chapter 1), which has been adequately purged, is hooked to one limb. The other limb is used for purging air out of the system and for injecting contrast material. After the system has been set up, the balloon occlusion catheter is ready for use.

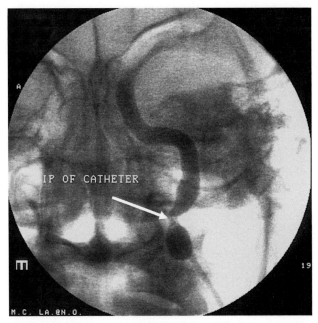

Figure 34-1 Case 1. An example of the difficulty encountered with temporary occlusion balloons. This catheter will move up and down several centimeters during cardiac and respiratory cycles, thus causing buckling of the catheter within the vessel while it is fixed in position by the inflated balloon. A temporary occlusion balloon with a very soft shaft would be ideal to buckle benignly along with the vessel itself. In addition, a soft benign tip is mandatory.

The balloon is then gradually inflated. Distortion of its shape reveals that the balloon is filling the vessel, but any significant distortion may indicate overinflation (Case 2, Fig. 34–2). Overinflation should be avoided because intimal damage can be caused by even a soft silicone or latex balloon, or the balloon may rupture. Aneurysmal dilation has been reported (verbally) after test occlusion, as have intimal dissections.[3] Occlusion is therefore checked by injection of contrast to reveal stagnation of flow, rather than by watching for distortion of the balloon.

After occlusion has been achieved, confirmation is made by contrast injection through the side port of the three-way stopcock (the guidewire lumen) and by observation of a standing column within the distal occluded vessel. A documentary film is obtained.

This contrast is then aspirated and the flush turned on to a *very* slow rate. In prior years, it was observed that some patients suffered eye pain during a test occlusion. This symptom was most disconcerting to the interventionist and unexplained, but now has been determined to be a result of the heparinized flush solution filling the occluded internal carotid artery and being the only supply to the ophthalmic artery, thus causing ischemic symptoms.[4, 5] Therefore, the infusion is kept to a very slow rate after the vessel has been cleared of stagnant blood. Occlusion is maintained for 30 minutes or until any neurologic change is noted.

At the termination of the test procedure, the column of stagnant fluid is thoroughly aspirated into the catheter. Contrast injection is then performed to confirm that continued total occlusion has been present; if the vessel was only occluded for the first minute or so of the test, the patient may later fail a permanent occlusion. After the confirmatory test injection, the balloon is deflated, and a repeat control angiogram is performed over the entire intracranial distribution of this vessel to evaluate for the possibility of distal embolization. Thorough evaluation of this examination is made, and the catheter is then withdrawn into the common carotid artery. A repeat injection is then made to evaluate the condition of the internal carotid artery at the point of occlusion (i.e., where the balloon was).

Consideration must be given to the ultimate mechanism of occlusion. If the vessel will be sacrificed under ideal circumstances (i.e., by an interventional neuroradiologist, and then managed by the same), blood pressure management and optimal conditions can be maintained.

If the vessel may be sacrificed after neck surgery, however, the patient may have undergone a long procedure, lost some blood, and be physically exhausted. In addition, the external carotid, as well as the internal carotid artery, may have been sacrificed. This greatly changes the intracranial hemodynamics. An unsuspected borderline pass during a test occlusion can result in a full-blown failure after sacrifice under these circumstances, even though this patient may have tolerated a permanent detachable balloon occlusion. For this reason, testing should include a prolonged hypotensive period if sacrifice during a major procedure is anticipated or if the external supply might be eliminated.

VARIATIONS

Because there are failures of prediction of the safety of permanent occlusion of the internal carotid artery, additional procedures for evaluation of intracranial flow during a temporary occlusion test have been employed.[6] These fall into several broad categories:

- SPECT scan (injection of a radionuclide [^{99m}Tc HMPAO] during occlusion and later performance of a scan to evaluate intracerebral distribution[7–10])
- ^{133}Xe perfusion CT scanning[11]
- Transcranial Doppler flow measurement
- Measurement of internal carotid artery stump pressure during temporary occlusion[11]
- Oxygen-15 (^{15}O) H$_2$O positron emission tomography (PET) scan to measure cerebral blood flow directly during occlusion[12]
- Hypotensive challenge during test occlusion[3]

All these are used in an effort to predict more fully who will pass or fail a permanent occlusion. EEG monitoring is usually performed only if the patient is incapable of being tested neurologically (an infant, for instance), and it appears to be the least sensitive method of evaluation under these circumstances. Unfortunately, none of these tests are foolproof.

There is no real consensus of opinion on what really works best or on what the findings mean. *Firm*

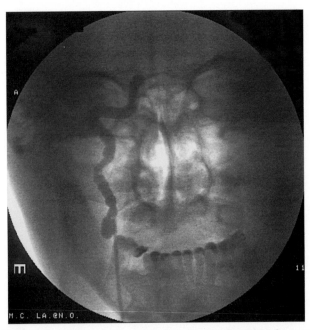

Figure 34-2 Case 2. Note how this latex balloon has become totally asymmetric when inflated. The vessel has obviously become very disturbed. In addition, the balloon is slightly resistant to inflating, and then suddenly overinflates. Contrast has been injected in the stagnant column to confirm total occlusion. Note how the column travels to the first side branch (the ophthalmic artery), at which point it washes into this side branch and appears to stop its ascent.

minimum standards must be met. Fundamental to this is an occlusion lasting at least 20 minutes, unless a sensitive auxiliary cerebral blood flow evaluation is added to the procedure.

This lack of consensus is because of the occasional, but rare, idiosyncratic failure of testing or occlusion. For instance, what does it mean if a patient can tolerate having the carotid artery occluded for 30 minutes with no change seen in neurologic testing, but with some vague change seen on the radionuclide imaging? In multiple cases, a carotid artery has been sacrificed under these circumstances and the patient has done fine. Worse, cases have been reported in which the patient failed both the clinical examination and the cerebral blood flow analysis and yet tolerated permanent occlusion.

Carotid arteries have been occluded that tested negative, and the patient then developed a hemineural deficit (usually temporary, but sometimes not). Delayed deficits have occurred after permanent occlusion, even when the patient passes a temporary test occlusion, and there is some evidence that these delayed failures either were predicted or could have been predicted by SPECT or PET.[7, 12–14] For this reason, failure of SPECT or PET even after the patient has passed a prolonged test occlusion should alert the clinician to a possible increased risk of failure of permanent occlusion.

Most temporary occlusions, however, are done with clinical neurologic (symptomatic) testing alone and with occlusion times ranging from at least 20 minutes to about 30 minutes. Because of the availability of modern technology, it is best to use other means to evaluate cerebral perfusion in addition to the simple functional testing. This permits more accurate identification of and planning for the borderline cases.

Xenon Computed Tomography Perfusion Scan During Test Occlusion

Xenon CT perfusion imaging appears to be an ideal means to evaluate residual supply to the brain. Normal cerebral blood flow is about 50 to 55 ml/100 g brain tissue/min, plus or minus about 12 ml/100 g/min. As people get older, their overall intracranial flow diminishes. No concrete "magic" numbers for ml/100 g brain tissue are known below which the patient is at risk for stroke following permanent vessel occlusion. We have observed some patients who have been able to survive without deficit when the amount of flow to their brain was almost impossible to observe (such as the patient with spontaneous bilateral middle cerebral artery occlusions shown in Figs. 59–99 to 59–108). A "safe" level of perfusion of 30 ml/100 g/min has been reported[15] as a level below which permanent occlusion may be associated with an increased risk of stroke. This appears to be a reasonable amount considering the fact that 20 ml/100 g/min is considered the level below which electrical dysfunction begins; 30 ml/100 g/min is a 50% margin of safety.

Asymmetric blood flow is indicative of a greater risk of deficit following permanent occlusion. The degree of risk is unknown and depends on the degree of asymmetry. Generally, there is a consensus that if the flow is asymmetric to the order of two standard deviations, there is a potential problem; from a practical standpoint, this means a blood flow of less than 30 ml/100 g/min on the side of occlusion. This method does not appear to be foolproof, however.

Mathis et al.[15] reported on 500 internal carotid artery balloon occlusion tests utilizing ^{133}Xe CT blood flow and found rates of 1.2% transient and 0.4% permanent neurologic deficits after subsequent permanent occlusion. These are extremely good results. According to their technique, the test is performed first in the angiography suite with clinical testing. The balloon is then deflated and the patient moved to the CT scanner with the occlusion balloon catheter still in place in the internal carotid artery and the patient still fully heparinized. The balloon is then reinflated to a preset volume. A small amount of very dilute (1/10) contrast is then instilled into the central lumen and a scout image obtained. This reveals the location of the balloon and catheter as well as confirms occlusion for the ^{133}Xe test.

Single-Photon Emission Computed Tomography Scan During Test Occlusion

If a radionuclide examination (SPECT scan) is to be performed, injection of ^{99m}Tc HMPAO should be done after a delay of about 5 minutes to allow the intracranial hemodynamics to stabilize.[7] If the patient's blood pressure is elevated during the test (e.g., due to pain, fear), the results may be invalid. Some series have reported patients passing SPECT scans and then suffering strokes after permanent occlusion (three of four patients),[16] while in other series there has been a high rate of correlation between a satisfactory SPECT scan and the ability to tolerate occlusion.[17] In this latter report by Ryu et al.,[17] of 19 patients that clinically passed a temporary occlusion, all had perfusion that remained between 95% and 101% of the contralateral perfusion after temporary test occlusion, as measured by SPECT scan. On the other hand, the five patients who failed the clinical test had perfusion that dropped to 77% to 85% of the contralateral level.

The difference between this study and most others is that, in addition to the tomographic images, quantitative analysis was performed. For many scanners, software is available that allows this analysis (although many institutions are not currently capable of quantitative analysis). This is illustrated in Figure 34–3. Generally, each hemisphere is divided into several sections (e.g., anterior frontal, posterior frontal, temporal, perisylvian). The number of counts detected in each section over a specified period of time is recorded. Several analyses can then be performed. The number of counts in the two corresponding sections (left and right) can be added and the number of counts on each side expressed as a percentage of the total. The average number of counts per section

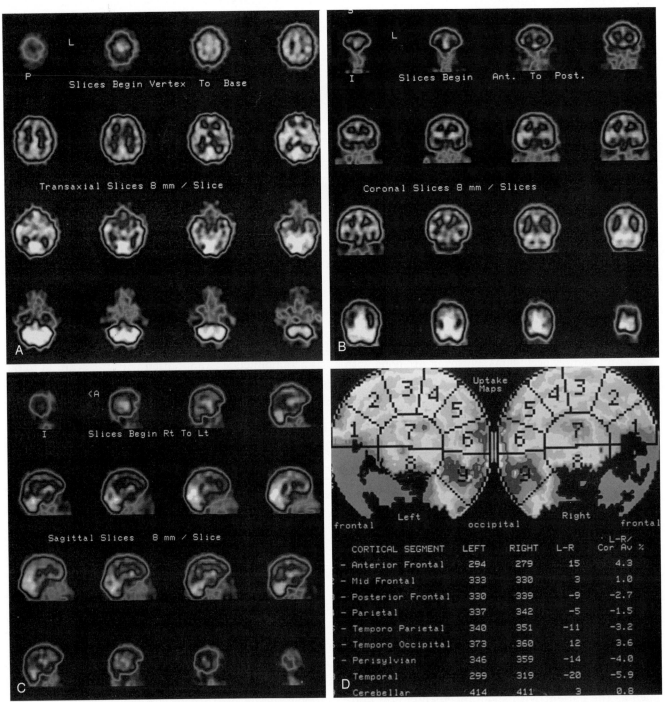

Figure 34-3 Case 3. Single-photon emission computed tomography (SPECT) scan with quantitative analysis. *A–C,* The tomographic images do not demonstrate any appreciable focal abnormality in this patient with a history of multiple transient ischemic attacks and a magnetic resonance imaging (MRI) scan showing white matter ischemic changes bilaterally. *D,* The quantitative analysis demonstrates relative decrease in perfusion in the right anterior frontal (anterior cerebral) and temporo-occipital (posterior cerebral) regions and the left posterior frontal, parietal, temporoparietal, perisylvian, and temporal regions (most of the distribution of the middle cerebral artery).

can be determined for each hemisphere and the number of counts in each section expressed as a percentage of this. The average number of counts for each set of two corresponding sections can be obtained and the difference between the counts in the two sections expressed as a percentage of this. The average number of counts per section for the entire brain can be calculated and the difference between the counts in each corresponding pair of sections expressed as a percentage of this. An analysis performed in this manner can reveal subtle abnormalities that may not be readily apparent upon visual inspection of the tomographic images.

Hypotensive Challenge Test

Perhaps the most accurate means to evaluate the possible sacrifice of an internal carotid artery is to occlude this artery and then slowly lower the blood pressure—a true "stress" test.[3, 13] This should reveal any hemodynamically tenuous situation, the kind that could manifest later. Intellectually, this makes sense. Some reports, however, indicate that this, too, can yield false-negative results. No good data exist concerning what a failed test is. In other words, how low does one lower the blood pressure, and at what point does a change become meaningful? Conceivably, if a patient's carotid artery is occluded and the blood pressure is lowered far enough, at some point *anyone* would fail this test—so what does this mean? Additionally, what symptom is considered a failure? Too rapid a drop in systemic pressure can result in vertigo, nausea, and other posterior fossa symptoms unrelated to the occlusion of the anterior circulation and should not be interpreted as a failure of occlusion.

An interesting report of the work performed at the State University of New York in Buffalo concerning hypotensive challenge during temporary occlusion of the carotid artery appears to offer a rational and practical approach to the problem of predicting which internal carotid arteries can be safely sacrificed and which cannot.[3] This technique is similar to that described previously (see the article for specific variations), but after the patient has passed a 20-minute occlusion test, a nitroprusside drip (or, alternatively, labetalol) is used to lower the main arterial pressure to two thirds the baseline pressure. This pressure is then maintained for an additional 20 minutes. If the patient passes this test, the interventionist should at least be reassured.

Sodium nitroprusside, 2.5 to 7.5 μg/kg body weight, or labetalol, 5 to 20 mg, should be administered by an anesthesiologist (personal preference). If the pressure drops too far and the patient develops symptoms, the temporary occlusion balloon can be immediately deflated. This should reverse any unilateral hypoperfusion problem, independent of the systemic pressure.

The work performed at Yale is discouraging, however. At that institution, after the patients had passed a clinical test occlusion, their mean systolic pressure was decreased by at least 30% (the duration of this hypotension is uncertain). No acute neurologic deficits occurred, but after permanent occlusion, 1 of 12 patients suffered a major permanent deficit (stroke). The technique of permanent occlusion is unknown. This indicates that no method of predicting failure is foolproof.

Hemodynamic Analysis

An additional method of testing for the safety of permanent occlusion has been advocated by Niimi and colleagues.[18] Angiography of the intracranial vasculature is performed to evaluate all supply to the intracranial structures and the circle of Willis. Patients with poor collateral circulation are excluded from further evaluation.

The patients are then tested as just described with occlusion by a double-lumen balloon catheter. While the vessel is occluded, contrast material is injected distal to the occlusion site through the inner lumen of the balloon catheter. The washout of this contrast and its origin is carefully observed. Proximal washout indicates good supply from the ipsilateral posterior communicating artery, whereas the anterior communicating artery will be seen to wash out the contrast at the carotid apex. Although these investigators test the stump pressure, there are no set criteria for failure.

Both clinical neurologic testing and hemodynamic analysis are carried out in addition to the stump pressure measurement. However, the success of their permanent occlusions in part may be a result of their careful postocclusion care. Patients are kept well hydrated and recumbent and are allowed to sit up only over a period of days. Postural hypotension is stringently avoided for several days. In this fashion, they are able to achieve good success, with only 6% temporary deficits developing and no permanent deficits in their last 46 patients.

This method appears to be effective in these circumstances, but the definition of adequate or "good" collateral supply renders this somewhat more a practice of the "art" rather than of the "science" of interventional neuroradiology.

A similar approach is to occlude the internal carotid artery while simultaneously injecting the vertebral and contralateral carotid arteries. This will also provide information concerning collateral supply to the occluded territory and may provide this information in a clearer "visual" manner that interventional neuroradiologists are familiar with. A delay of more than 1 second in the capillary phase is said to be a warning of potential failure of permanent occlusion (see Chapter 36).

WHAT IS A TEMPORARY TEST OCCLUSION FAILURE?

Clinical Neurologic Testing

The most common sign of failure of a test occlusion using simple neurologic testing is arm weakness, usually within the first 5 minutes. The patient may or may not be aware of this. The patient may claim to be squeezing just as hard as before, so careful attention must be paid to the force. In addition, it is a good idea to have the same person perform this portion of the test the entire time; any subtle change must be identified.

If the patient has good pial collaterals between the posterior cerebral artery and the middle cerebral branches, an adequate posterior communicating artery, and a small or nonexistent anterior communicating artery, the watershed zone can shift so that it becomes the *territory of the anterior cerebral artery that is most ischemic*, thus perhaps yielding *failure in the leg more quickly than in the arm*. This must be diligently looked for as well.

Speech disturbance may be one of the more subtle but significant findings during a test occlusion. Again, if there is a shift in watershed zones, Broca's area may be the first affected. This can occur during a test of the left internal carotid artery, with a poor posterior communicating artery, a decent anterior communicating artery, and good pial collaterals between the posterior cerebral branches and the middle cerebral branches.

Finally, headache is an underappreciated sign of cerebral infarction and may be a symptom during test occlusion. Its meaning is unclear, and no large series has proved its significance, but ignoring this finding is unwise.

Single-Photon Emission Computed Tomography Scan Failure

The pattern desired for this imaging modality is one of absolute uniformity. Several abnormal patterns exist, the most abnormal of which is a hole in the image, usually caused by prior infarct or embolus. Tumor (or a space-occupying lesion) is another cause. If any of these are preexisting, accurate analysis of the test occlusion findings can be difficult, even with preocclusion and postocclusion comparison.

Depending on where the watershed has been shifted, a subtle decrease in activity in a region is the most usual finding in a failed SPECT scan. The absolute degree of failure cannot be given with this technique unless quantitative analysis can be performed (this option is not available in many locations, as discussed previously); xenon perfusion imaging is more specific for this. This decreased activity may be particularly difficult to determine in the region of the deep structures of the brain, but these are not the usual watershed zones.

Quantitative analysis may help identify more subtle changes in activity and may be helpful when there is preexisting asymmetry due to a prior insult. If available, it should be utilized.

Some practitioners obtain a pretest baseline SPECT scan, whereas others obtain this only after a failed test or a questionable result, as was the case in Figures 34–4 to 34–7 (Case 4). This case illustrates the subtle nature of a test failure and its results.

Hypotensive Challenge Failure

The goal of a hypotensive challenge is to lower the mean systemic pressure by about 30%. This is a purely arbitrary number; there has been no large series of patients comparing 20% to 40% decreases, but 30% appears to be an adequate degree of challenge. The finding sought is asymmetric neurologic change.

Regulation of the nitroprusside drip while trying to achieve a mean arterial pressure that is actually 30% lower than baseline can be difficult. The operator should be prepared to see a decrease ranging from 20% to 40%. Hypotension should be continued long enough to allow time for subtle change. If the patient passed a routine occlusion, a hypotensive challenge may not produce findings that are evident immediately. The operator should be patient and look for subtle changes. The operator should keep talking to the patient, perform frequent checks, and ask the patient to indicate any changes in sensation as well as motor dysfunction.

If the pressure drops too far too quickly, the patient may experience generalized cerebral hypoperfusion. This manifests as dizziness or lightheadedness, like that experienced with postural hypotension caused by standing too rapidly. As with other forms of decreased cerebral perfusion, posterior fossa symptoms may predominate (e.g., dizziness associated with nausea, vomiting, dimming of vision). The patient may feel hot or cold, as with a vasovagal reaction or a toxic vasoactive response to an intestinal virus. This should not be interpreted as a test occlusion failure when caused by a pressure drop of 50%, for instance. Again, be patient. Testing during this episode demonstrates a nonfocal pattern, and raising the pressure back to 20% below baseline restores normalcy.

Stump Pressure Failure

Measurement of stump pressure is another means to improve the efficacy of testing. This is one of the older methods of testing, but it appears to have fallen by the wayside in favor of more exotic methods. A recent report by Kurata et al.[19] indicates that this is still in use, however. They report no failure to tolerate permanent occlusion in any patient whose postocclusion stump pressure remained above 60% of the preocclusion level.

Transcranial Doppler Flow Failure

Transcranial Doppler is not a widely practiced means of testing for residual perfusion, but it may offer an additional method for determining safety. In a report by Schneweis et al.,[20] if the decrease in flow did not exceed 30%, it was safe to occlude the internal carotid artery.

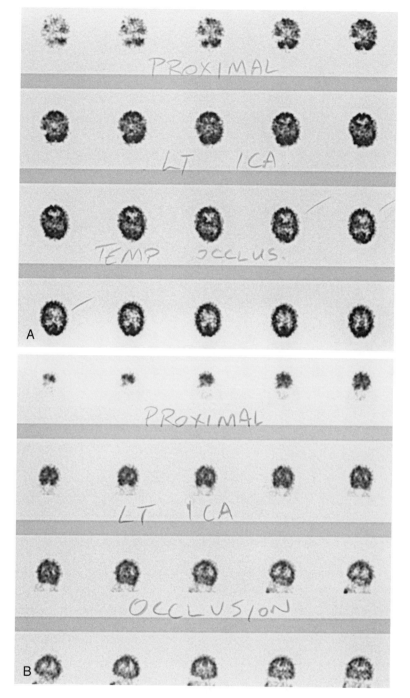

Figure 34-4 Case 4. *A* and *B,* This 63-year-old woman passed a clinical test occlusion of the internal carotid artery (ICA) but failed a permanent ICA occlusion test. These are axial and coronal images of a SPECT scan performed after temporary proximal occlusion of the ICA in this woman with a carotid-cavernous fistula. The occlusion was performed with the balloon proximal to the fistula, in the standard test occlusion location (cervical carotid artery). She was able *clinically* to tolerate the occlusion for a period of 30 minutes with no change in her neurologic status. The radionuclide was injected 10 minutes after occlusion to allow the intracranial hemodynamics to stabilize. *Note the slight decrease in activity over the left cerebral hemisphere and in the basal ganglia region (tick marks on the film). Note also that she passed this clinical test with her steal still present.*

Case 4 continues

TECHNICAL PROBLEMS, COMPLICATIONS, AND SOLUTIONS

Commonly, even though a soft latex (or silicone) balloon has been used, the vessel looks as if it has undergone angioplasty (i.e., it is wider at that point). There is usually no intimal tear, however. This appearance is simply related to the balloon inflation and the expansion of the vessel to its maximal normal size, probably without damage to the wall of the vessel.

A potentially more serious problem occurs when the tip of the catheter has caused intimal damage.

In this case, the patient should remain on heparin for the next 24 hours. In addition, aspirin should be administered orally immediately and continued for 1 month. If the damage appears significant, continued angiographic observation is maintained for at least 30 minutes to ensure that the intimal tear is not extending downstream and that a thrombus is not growing. Although no prospective studies have been performed, a bolus injection of abciximab should be considered.

If there is evidence of intraluminal thrombus formation, preparations for emergency urokinase infusion may be necessary, and the attending neurosur-

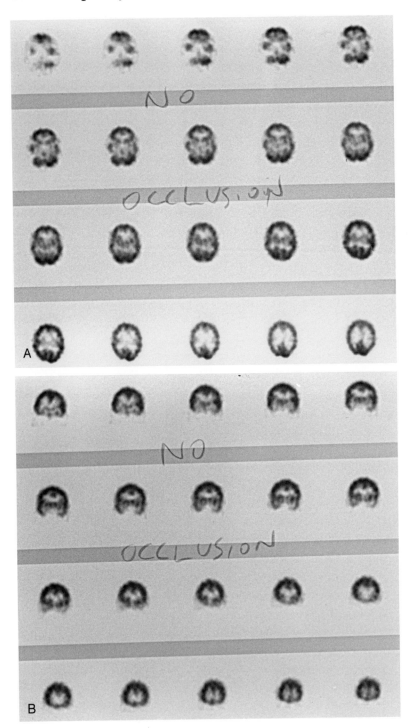

Figure 34-5 *A* and *B,* Because of the vague SPECT scan failure, it was decided to repeat the scan for a normal baseline evaluation to make sure there was no preexisting component of asymmetry. This repeat SPECT scan without occlusion was completely normal.

Case 4 continues

geon should be contacted. If adequate and gentle technique has been employed, these actions are rarely necessary. Aneurysmal distention of the internal carotid artery has been reported secondary to use of temporary occlusion balloons.

An intimal tear in the internal carotid artery can be disastrous and is a result of the choice of exchange wire far more commonly than it is of the choice of the catheter tip. This is discussed in detail in Chapter 1.

A true wind sock effect resulting from the intimal tear can complete the task of occlusion of the vessel, but the patient may not tolerate this. Even if the

tear does not progress to occlusion, this site can act as a nidus for thrombus formation, with subsequent embolization to the intracranial circulation. Heparinization is recommended to allow healing of any intimal damage.

Angioplasty has been advocated to attempt to tack down an intimal tear. Recrossing torn intima is asking for trouble, however, and it is easy for the guidewire tip to seek the subintimal lumen, potentially worsening the situation. Alternatively, if the guidewire has retained position distal to the tear, stenting of the segment is advocated to prevent worsening of

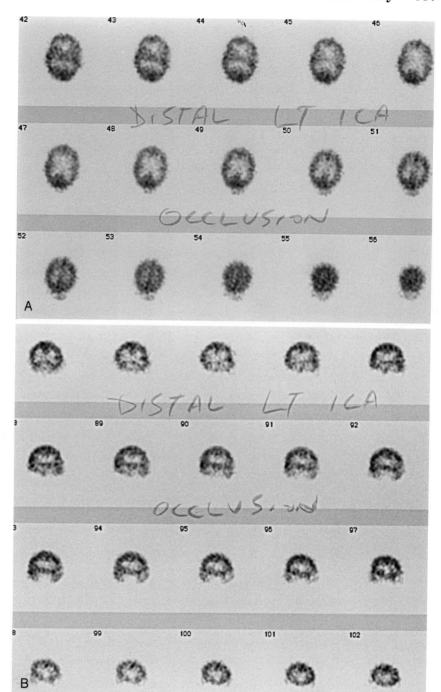

Figure 34-6 *A* and *B,* Because the first test occlusion was performed *with the carotid-cavernous fistula still intact (and with resultant intracranial steal),* it was determined that a repeat occlusion representing a hemodynamic reproduction of the final result of permanent occlusion would be appropriate. Utilizing an Endeavor balloon occlusion catheter (Target Therapeutics), occlusion was performed with the balloon now distal to the fistula in the supraclinoid ICA. The SPECT scan now has an unremarkable appearance. She again tolerated the procedure without difficulty and passed a 30-minute clinical test. We were lulled into complacency by the fact that the patient passed a 30-minute test occlusion with the steal still present and by the apparent passing of the test on the basis of the SPECT, and the vessel was then permanently occluded.

Case 4 continues

the tear. Although this is a routine procedure in the periphery, it raises some concerns in the internal carotid artery, particularly depending on the location of the tear (i.e., whether the tear is in a freely moving segment of the vessel).

Simple heparinization is the usual method of therapy for an intimal tear in the brachiocephalic vessels, and these tears typically are self-healing.

FALSE-NEGATIVE AND FALSE-POSITIVE TEST RESULTS

Various estimates of the rate of clinical failure of temporary carotid occlusion have been made, ranging from 5% to more than 10%. The addition of cerebral blood flow studies tends to bring this overall number of test occlusion failures close to 10%, if not slightly higher. Anyone who passes the clinical test, particularly with hypotensive challenge and a SPECT scan or another form of cerebral blood flow study, is considered to be at low risk of permanent occlusion. At least some of the late failures of permanent occlusion could be secondary to declining ability of the collateral circulation to maintain global perfusion (e.g., progression of atherosclerosis) and thus are totally unpredictable.

Occasional reports have been made of patients passing a test occlusion and failing a permanent oc-

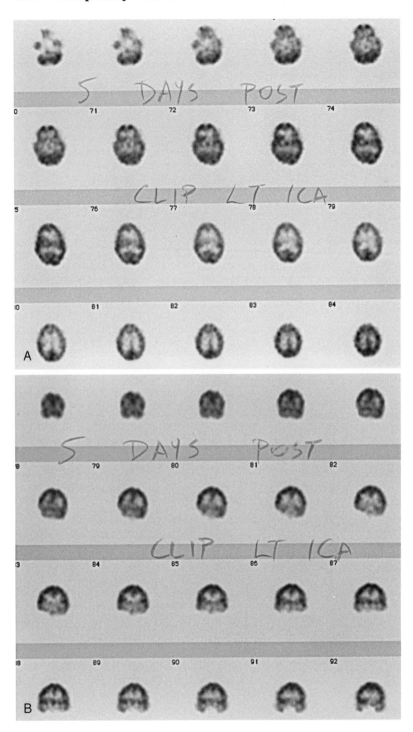

Figure 34-7 *A* and *B*, It was not possible to occlude the ICA distal to the fistula without the balloon slipping farther distally and occluding the orifice of the posterior communicating artery, a vital vessel for intracranial collateral perfusion. Therefore it was necessary *surgically* to trap the ICA by clipping it distal to the transected vessel but proximal to the posterior communicating artery. This was the resultant appearance 5 days after this procedure. Note the vague decrease in activity on the left.

The patient was neurologically symmetric but very lethargic and sleepy. She was not nearly as "bright" and energetic as she had been preoperatively. Her personality has completely changed, her energy level is decreased, and she does not spontaneously chat as she once did. In addition, there is now *bilateral* scattered increased signal in her deep white matter on MRI. She is no longer able to take care of herself in independent living. *Although she has not suffered a focal stroke, the outcome is still disastrous.*

clusion. This is rare and usually temporary or partial. After a permanent occlusion, the patient should be monitored in an intensive care unit for at least 24 hours (and perhaps for as long as 48 hours) to ensure that the systemic mean arterial pressure does not drop; if any symptoms develop, prompt elevation of blood pressure and volume expansion should be undertaken (see Chapter 52). With adequate management, intracranial circulation and collaterals usually adapt, and the patient's condition improves.

The exception is the patient that passes a temporary occlusion test, passes a permanent balloon occlusion test, but then later has a major stroke at surgery. When failure of permanent balloon occlusion that is followed by surgery occurs, it is an indication that current testing methods may be in need of more refinement. In a report of nine patients with permanent balloon occlusion followed by surgery, there were four failures (44%).[14] The mechanism of this outcome may be one of the following three scenarios.

First, the occluded internal carotid artery stump may have provided an embolus to the M1 segment. This could be due to manipulation of the carotid artery with subsequent squeezing of the thrombus downstream. This is the toothpaste theory. Any hyperextension or manipulation of the neck or extracranial carotid artery during surgery should thus be avoided. Second, during surgery, a hypotensive episode may have decreased the perfusion of the hemisphere below the allowable limit of 15 to 20 ml/100 g tissue/min. Third, some collateral supply previously present may have been eliminated for unknown reasons. The actual technique of test occlusion in the series reported is not known, nor the actual technique of permanent occlusion, unfortunately.

What does one do if a patient *does* fail the temporary occlusion test? To a certain extent, it depends on the degree of failure. If there was instant failure on initial occlusion at normosystemic pressure, this is a bad sign. This vessel should probably not be sacrificed, even with a preoperative extracranial-intracranial bypass (unless a good high-flow type of bypass can be achieved).

If the failure occurred under the challenge test conditions only, however, an extracranial-intracranial bypass can be performed preoperatively, and the sacrifice should be tolerated. The argument can be made that the challenge test was too rigorous; even if it was, the risk of any significant permanent harm from the bypass when performed by a skilled surgeon is low (3% to 5%). This added margin of safety is probably warranted in these questionable situations. Several types of bypass grafts are available, depending on the flow rate necessary to be achieved. Superficial temporal artery–to–middle cerebral artery grafts have the lowest initial flow rate of the standard grafts (<50 ml/min) but the highest patency rate. Long vein grafts (external carotid–to–middle cerebral artery branch) have the next highest flow rate, and short vein grafts from the petrous internal carotid artery to the middle cerebral artery have the highest flow rate (80 to 150 ml/min). These short grafts are by far the most technically challenging of the various grafts and require prolonged occlusion of the middle cerebral artery territory during surgery.

The concepts of "barely failing" and "partially failing under hypotensive challenge" are extremely relevant to the concept of global hypoperfusion secondary to atherosclerotic (or other) stenoses involving the internal carotid artery, middle cerebral trunk, and other vessels. Some of the patients described as such, after occlusion of their internal carotid arteries and after seemingly passing a temporary test, experienced a dramatic major delayed failure (a stroke). This implies that *simple global hypoperfusion* can cause true territorial infarcts (not watershed infarcts), probably unrelated to emboli. The appreciation of intracranial hemodynamics may be crucial to the eventual comprehension of and planning for the correct therapy for certain intrinsic vascular diseases involving the head and neck.

REFERENCES

1. Nishioka H. Report on the Cooperative Study of Intracranial Aneurysms and Subarachnoid Hemorrhage, IX. Part I: Results of the treatment of intracranial aneurysms by occlusion of the carotid artery in the neck. *J Neurosurg* 1966;3:660–682.
2. Winn HR, Richardson AE, Jane JA. Late morbidity and mortality of common carotid ligation for posterior communicating aneurysms: a comparison to conservative treatment. *J Neurosurg* 1977;47:727–736.
3. Standard SC, Ahuja A, Guterman LR, et al. Balloon test occlusion of the internal carotid artery with hypotensive challenge. *AJNR* 1995;16:1453–1458.
4. Hurst RW, Goldberg HI. Transient monocular blindness in carotid occlusion testing. *AJNR* 1994;15:255–257.
5. Russell EJ, Goldberg K, Oskin J, et al. Ocular ischemic syndrome during carotid balloon occlusion testing. *AJNR* 1994;15:258–262.
6. Eckard DA, Purdy PD, Bonte FJ. Temporary balloon occlusion of the carotid artery combined with brain blood flow imaging as a test to predict tolerance prior to permanent carotid sacrifice. *AJNR* 1992;13:1565–1569.
7. Mathews D, Walker BS, Purdy PD, et al. Brain blood flow SPECT in temporary balloon occlusion of the carotid artery and intracerebral arteries. *J Nucl Med* 1993;34:1239–1243.
8. Monsein LH, Jeffery PJ, van Heerden BB, et al. Assessing adequacy of collateral circulation during balloon test occlusion of the internal carotid artery with 99mTc-HMPAO SPECT. *AJNR* 1991;12:1045–1051.
9. Moody EB, Dawson RC III, Sandler MP. 99mTc-HMPAO SPECT imaging in interventional neuroradiology: validation of balloon test occlusion. *AJNR* 1991;12:1043–1044.
10. Peterman SB, Taylor A Jr, Hoffman JC Jr. Improved detection of cerebral hypoperfusion with internal carotid balloon test occlusion and 99mTc-HMPAO cerebral perfusion SPECT imaging. *AJNR* 1991;12:1035–1041.
11. Barker DW, Jungreis CA, Horton JA, et al. Balloon test occlusion of the internal carotid artery: Change in stump pressure over 15 minutes and its correlation with xenon CT cerebral blood flow. *AJNR* 1993;14:587–590.
12. Brunberg JA, Frey KA, Horton JA, et al. [15O]H2O positron emission tomography determination of cerebral blood flow during test occlusion of the internal carotid artery. *AJNR* 1994;15:725–732.
13. McIvor NP, Willinsky RA, TerBrugge KG, et al. Validity of test occlusion studies prior to internal carotid artery sacrifice. *Head Neck* 1994;16:11–16.
14. Sekhar LN, Patel SJ. Permanent occlusion of the internal carotid artery during skull base and vascular surgery: is it really safe? [Editorial]. *Am J Otol* 1993;14:421–422.
15. Mathis JM, Barr JD, Jungreis CA, et al. Temporary balloon test occlusion of the internal carotid artery: Experience in 500 cases. *AJNR* 1995;16:749–754.
16. Lorberboyn M, Pandit N, Machac J, et al. Brain perfusion imaging during preoperative temporary balloon occlusion of the internal carotid artery. *J Nucl Med* 1996;37:415–419.
17. Ryu YH, Chung TS, Lee JD, et al. HMPAO SPECT to assess neurological deficits during balloon test occlusion. *J Nucl Med* 1996;37:551–554.
18. Niimi Y, Berenstein A, Setton A, Kupersmith MJ. Occlusion of the internal carotid artery based on a simple tolerance test. *Interventional Neuroradiol* 1996;2:289–296.
19. Kurata A, Miyasaka Y, Tanaka C, et al. Stump pressure as a guide to the safety of permanent occlusion of the internal carotid artery. *Acta Neurochir (Wien)* 1996;138:549–554.
20. Schneweis S, Urbach H, Solymosi L, et al. Pre-operative risk assessment for carotid occlusion by transcranial Doppler ultrasound. *J Neurol Neurosurg Psychiatry* 1997;62:485–489.

ADDITIONAL READINGS

Bailes JE, Deeb ZL, Wilson JA, et al. Intraoperative angiography and temporary balloon occlusion of the basilar artery as an adjunct to surgical clipping: technical note. *Neurosurgery* 1992;30:949–953.

Brunberg JA, Frey KA, Horton JA, Kuhl DE. Crossed cerebellar diaschisis: occurrence and resolution demonstrated with PET during carotid temporary balloon occlusion. *AJNR* 1992;13:58–61.

Eckard DA, Purdy PD, Bonte FJ. Crossed cerebellar diaschisis and loss of consciousness during temporary balloon occlusion of the internal carotid artery. *AJNR* 1992;13:55–57.

Erba SM, Horton JA, Latchaw RE, et al. Balloon test occlusion of the internal carotid artery with stable xenon/CT cerebral blood flow imaging. *AJNR* 1988;9:533–538.

Forsting M, Resch KM, von Kummer R, Sartor K. Balloon occlusion of a giant lower basilar aneurysm: death due to thrombosis of the aneurysm. *AJNR* 1991;12:1063–1066.

Giller CA, Mathews D, Walker B, et al. Prediction of tolerance to carotid artery occlusion using transcranial Doppler ultrasound. *J Neurosurg* 1994;81:15–19.

Gonzales CF, Moret J. Balloon occlusion of the carotid artery prior to surgery for neck tumors. *AJNR* 1990;11:649–652.

Linskey ME, Jungreis CA, Yonas H, et al. Stroke risk after abrupt internal carotid artery sacrifice: accuracy of preoperative assessment with balloon test occlusion and stable xenon-enhanced CT. *AJNR* 1994;15:829–843.

Linskey ME, Sekhar LN, Hecht ST. Emergency embolectomy for embolic occlusion of the middle cerebral artery after internal carotid artery balloon test occlusion: case report. *J Neurosurg* 1992;77:134–138.

Mathis JM, Barr JD, Jungreis CA, Horton JA. Physical characteristics of balloon catheter systems used in temporary cerebral artery occlusion. *AJNR* 1994;15:1831–1836.

Palestro CJ, Sen C, Muzinic M, et al. Assessing collateral cerebral perfusion with technetium-99m-HMPAO SPECT during temporary internal carotid artery occlusion. *J Nucl Med* 1993;34:1235–1238.

Vazquez Añon V, Aymard A, Gobin YP, et al. Balloon occlusion of the internal carotid artery in 40 cases of giant intracavernous aneurysm: technical aspects, cerebral monitoring, and results. *Neuroradiology* 1992;34:245–251.

Wells BA, Keats AS, Cooley DA. Increased tolerance to cerebral ischemia produced by general anesthesia during temporary carotid occlusion. *Surgery* 1963;54:216–223.

Yonas H, Linskey M, Johnson DW, et al. Internal carotid balloon test occlusion does require quantitative CBF [Letter] *AJNR* 1992;13:1147–1152.

CHAPTER 35

Permanent Occlusion of the Internal Carotid Artery

J.J. Connors III

RATIONALE FOR PROCEDURE

Several circumstances may lead to the necessity of occluding the internal carotid artery, including (1) traumatic perforation of the internal carotid artery not amenable to surgical repair, (2) carotid-cavernous aneurysm or fistula, (3) preoperative occlusion before head and neck surgery for tumor, (4) in unusual situations, prophylaxis to prevent thromboembolic insult to the brain (i.e., occlusion of a diseased internal carotid artery may be preferable to the surgical risk of repair in some patients), and (5) other unusual complex vascular problems requiring internal carotid artery sacrifice.

Each indication should be analyzed for its specific need. Experience with this procedure over a span of more than 20 years has resulted in the knowledge that, if performed properly on the correct patient population, this therapeutic modality can yield excellent results with very low morbidity and mortality.

Several methods have been used over the years for occlusion of the internal carotid artery. Originally, surgical ligation was the only means available. For occasions when occlusion was absolutely necessary, but the ability to tolerate occlusion was either questionable or unknown, the Selverstone clamp was developed. This is a screw-type clamp that is placed surgically around the artery but not immediately tightened. The thumbscrew is externally operated, and over a period of days, it is turned slowly until full occlusion is achieved. This technique was intended to decrease flow through the internal carotid artery slowly in order to allow development of collateral supply to vulnerable intracranial territory (usually the middle cerebral artery). Obviously, this was a cumbersome method, revealing the lack of certainty regarding the status of the intracranial hemodynamics and the need for a more elegant solution for carotid occlusion.

In the early 1970s, Serbinenko[1] first introduced the concept of endovascular parent vessel occlusion. He devised a latex detachable balloon by melting rubber bands in a small bowl over a hot plate and then dipping a needle into this latex mass. The resultant latex sock was then placed on the tip of a catheter, and the neck of the sock was hand-tied using a thin latex string.

Since those pioneering days, a multitude of techniques have been explored, resulting in the current effective method that has relatively low morbidity and mortality. Unfortunately, there is still no way to predict with absolute certainty *which patients will tolerate a permanent occlusion* with impunity. (See Chapter 34 for further details concerning patient selection.)

TECHNICAL THEORY

The patient must first be determined to be suitable for permanent occlusion of the internal carotid artery (see Chapter 34). If there is concern about the feasibility of permanent occlusion, a preliminary extracranial-intracranial bypass can be performed to supplement the total flow to the hemisphere. Various bypass options are described in Chapter 49.

The material for permanent occlusion of the internal carotid artery should be permanent and easy to use, resulting in low morbidity and mortality. This has traditionally been achieved by the use of detachable balloons. Unfortunately, none of these is currently approved for manufacture by the U.S. Food and Drug Administration (FDA), and the availability for use under an Investigational Device Exemption no longer exists. Fibered coils are readily available but even these new platinum coils are not approved for carotid sacrifice. Despite the lack of FDA approval, detachable balloons remain the treatment of choice for parent vessel occlusion, either carotid artery or vertebral artery.

Originally, occlusion was performed simply by "tying off" the internal carotid artery above the bifurcation. This was thought to be direct and to the point but led to later problems (i.e., strokes, either immediate or delayed). These strokes were caused either by an inadequate ability of the intracranial circulation to support itself with the carotid artery occluded or by subsequent embolic episodes. The exact cause of these *embolic* strokes is difficult to prove and has been hypothesized to be either via external carotid collaterals to the internal carotid artery developing distal to the occlusion and then blowing off pieces of clot that had formed in the stagnant vessel or via mechanical motion of the neck, squeezing a mass of thrombus downstream into the middle cerebral artery (the "toothpaste" analogy), or both. Direct evidence of the concept of distal migration of thrombotic mass from mechanical cause has been clinically demonstrated.[2–6] We have directly observed a recently occluded internal carotid artery embolizing a mass of thrombus to the middle cerebral artery after mechanical external compression.

Although the use of detachable balloons permits the carotid artery to be occluded on first intent, the addition of a flow-control (occlusive) guide catheter is recommended when using detachable balloons and is *absolutely* required when coils are used[7, 8] (see Chapter 1). This flow arrest is useful for detachable balloons to facilitate their accurate placement and to ensure their stability after they are detached. The downstream force exerted by the systolic pulse is neither radiographically apparent nor measurable, but after the balloon is detached, migration can be disastrous. The proximal occlusion by the flow-control guide catheter maintains stability until further balloons or embolic material can be placed.

The situation with coil use is far different. The mechanism of vascular occlusion with fibered coils is that of accumulation of thrombotic mass (platelet and fibrin plug). For this to occur in the rapidly flowing stream of the internal carotid artery without any dislodgment of particulate matter is highly improbable. As coils are piled on top of other coils, some embolization is virtually guaranteed.[9] This may or may not be of a clinically devastating nature. In addition, coils alone, no matter how firmly packed, can never occlude flow without thrombus. The vessel can be occluded by the flow-control guide catheter, however, which renders the possibility of distal embolization essentially nil. If flow arrest is achieved using a flow-control guide catheter, occlusion of the vessel is possible by dense packing of coils (see below).

Also important is the choice of location for occlusion. Theoretically, occlusion at only the carotid bulb would be fine; indeed, this probably happens in a physiologic manner countless times every day. As seen repeatedly in clinical practice, however, a thrombotic mass can develop distal to a critical stenosis or occlusion, with potentially dire consequences. The previously described rationale concerning mechanical dislodgment of thrombus within the cervical carotid artery or the development of extracranial-intracranial collaterals pushing clot downstream suggests that the proper location of initial occlusion is the cavernous segment of the internal carotid artery. This location provides some degree of stability for the embolic material. Alternatively, some neurosurgeons prefer to clip the internal carotid artery in an intracranial location *in addition to* occluding it in an extracranial location to provide this same degree of safety.

SPECIFIC TECHNIQUE

Temporary test occlusion is performed to confirm the feasibility of permanent occlusion (see Chapter 34). A roadmap of the cervical internal carotid artery is made to allow proper positioning of the guide catheter with its nondetachable balloon. The internal carotid artery is first selected using a standard diagnostic angiography catheter. Once in place, this catheter is exchanged for the flow-control guide catheter (Zeppelin, Medtronic/MIS) by using a safe exchange wire (a Rosen exchange wire is suitable). The 9.4-Fr. Zeppelin is suitable for most detachable balloons and can be placed over its matched dilator or a 7-Fr. Berenstein catheter (Cook, Inc.). This allows placement directly through the skin over the exchange wire. The smooth silicone balloon on the Zeppelin is far better at sliding through the skin puncture site than the floppy latex types, which tend to bunch at the skin (see Chapter 3).

Heparin, 5000 to 10,000 units, is administered intravenously (personal preference). A previous 0.5-mg intramuscular injection of atropine is recommended, or this amount can be administered intravenously at this point; this is to prevent a vasovagal response during inflation of the flow-control balloon or of the final detachable balloon.

After the flow-control guide catheter is in place

and flushed and an adequate control angiogram is performed to confirm its satisfactory position in the internal carotid artery (i.e., without causing spasm or intimal damage), the placement of permanent embolic material can be undertaken.

Silicone Versus Latex Balloons

Although silicone balloons are elegant, easier to prepare, and possibly less traumatic, their use is also fraught with danger. They are semipermeable and thus capable of deflation. Worse, however, is their slippery coat, which allows them to move easily even if not deflated. This threat should not be ignored, and if they are used, abundant care should be taken to reinforce their position. This can be most easily performed with auxiliary coils, as described below.

Where to Occlude

The cavernous segment of the internal carotid artery offers a stable location for deployment of the first balloon. There is no worry of its drifting distally because of the proximal flow arrest produced by the flow-control guide catheter.

When placing the first balloon, and thereafter, no flush should be running through the occluding guide catheter; it will have nowhere to go. The distal internal carotid artery will be a closed system, and any flush would tend to blow the distal (detachable) balloon downstream. Therefore, after the guide catheter has been put into place and flushed, and after the patient has received the heparin bolus, no further fluid should be administered through its inner lumen.

It had been our practice to place a second balloon in the proximal petrous segment of the internal carotid artery and a final balloon just distal to the bulb. Formerly, some practitioners placed a single balloon and stopped (unwise!). Others placed several balloons in a row in the petrous segment. This latter technique resulted in at least one case of inadvertent embolization of the entire mass distally when the cervical carotid artery was later manipulated.

For this reason, our current practice is to place the first balloon as stated previously. This is followed by placement of a long wad of Gianturco coils (0.038″) in the petrous segment of the internal carotid artery. Stainless steel Gianturco coils are the most thrombogenic coils and are less expensive than platinum coils, but either is acceptable (personal preference). These quickly (within weeks if not days or hours) cause a substantial reaction with the vessel wall and are stable. After coil placement, a balloon is placed just below the level of the petrous portion (in the upper cervical ICA), and a final balloon just above the carotid bulb. Alternatively, additional coils can be placed in the cervical carotid artery.

This final placement of the most proximal detachable balloon must be made after the guide catheter has been withdrawn slightly. The detachable balloon is first advanced into the internal carotid artery until it is close to the most proximal balloon just at the skull base. The guide catheter balloon can then be deflated safely and withdrawn slightly into the common carotid artery. The (unsteerable) microcatheter with the balloon will still be in the internal carotid artery and can then be withdrawn to its correct location just above the carotid bulb.

Some interventional neuroradiologists prefer to place the last balloon in the carotid bulb; we think this is unwise. The bulb certainly looks like an inviting location for a balloon and will result in a gorgeous appearance on the postocclusion angiogram, but the hemodynamic effects (from constant pressure on the carotid bulb) are not worth the risk. I who originally described placement of the final balloon in the carotid bulb had to rupture percutaneously more than one balloon because of the life-threatening hemodynamic effects caused by pressure on the carotid body (such as extreme intransigent hypotension and cardiac standstill).[10, 11] The rationale for this particular placement is that there can be an inadvertent thrombotic embolization from the dead-end pouch of the carotid bulb into the external carotid artery, which may traverse a circuitous route through some collateral network into the intracranial circulation. Admittedly, this is possible. Internal carotid arteries, however, have "self-closed" in many cases without causing this particular problem, and a large number of balloon-occluded carotid arteries have had a residual stump, without a great number of problems. Embolic events in the territory of the occluded internal carotid artery have been reported, but the question remains of whether these are from the *current vascular supply* (e.g., the contralateral internal carotid artery) or the ophthalmic artery collaterals and other anastomoses. In any event, the number of emboli through collaterals does not appear to warrant the risk of the hemodynamic dysequilibrium caused by the expansion of a balloon within the carotid bulb and subsequent stimulation of the baroreceptors.

Postocclusion Nursing Care

Perhaps the most important aspect of permanent occlusion of the internal carotid artery, with or without preprocedure testing, is the management of the patient after the procedure to prevent any episode of hypotension. This apparently simple maneuver frequently is overlooked.

Even if a patient passes a test occlusion and the first hours after a permanent occlusion, there is still the possibility that the patient will fail in the first days after this procedure. Typically, patients who fail a test occlusion are not at risk. It is the patients who *pass* a temporary test occlusion (and then the first hours of a permanent occlusion) that yield the few failures that occur with this procedure.

These failures can be mostly eliminated if the postprocedure care optimizes the patient's ability to adapt to the permanent hemodynamic change (i.e., loss of a primary supply to the cerebral circulation). In other words, any period of systemic hypotension or even postural hypotension should be avoided. Circulatory optimization should be maintained, at least for a time. The patient should be well hydrated. Oral intake of food and abundant fluids should be encouraged.

The patient should be kept flat in bed for 24 hours after occlusion. On the night of the day after the procedure, the head of the bed can be raised. The patient is allowed to ambulate only after 48 hours.

A hypercoagulable state can be seen with certain tumors; such tumors are often the reason that the test and procedure were ordered. In these cases, it may be wise not to reverse heparinization with protamine (or even to keep the patient heparinized for 24 to 48 hours) if permanent occlusion is performed in this setting. Indeed, some practitioners routinely leave patients anticoagulated overnight for all permanent occlusions.

SINGLE-PHOTON EMISSION COMPUTED TOMOGRAPHY FOLLOWING BALLOON OCCLUSION

Single-photon emission computed tomographic (SPECT) scans can be used not only for prediction of failure of permanent occlusion of the internal carotid artery, but also to benefit postocclusion clinical management. Hacein-Bey and associates reported that postocclusion SPECT imaging revealed hemodynamic adaptation to occlusion, with an increase in hemispheric perfusion on the occluded side of 5.5%, associated with aggressive hypervolemic hemodilution and hypertension.[12] (Practically speaking, hemodilution is not directly performed.) Although no true control group demonstrates a worse outcome without aggressive therapy, the adaptation shown on SPECT scan (to a hemispheric perfusion at least 90% of that on the contralateral, nonoccluded side) correlated with a good clinical outcome.

ALTERNATIVE TECHNIQUE—FIBERED COILS

Detachable balloon occlusion is an elegant method of achieving the goal of permanent occlusion of a great vessel. Unfortunately, since detachable balloons are not FDA-approved for manufacture in the United States, they are not widely available. An alternative method of occlusion is with fibered coils.

Fibered coils should *never* be placed primarily in a flowing vessel supplying the brain, however. Small emboli can form on the coils and break off before total stasis of flow is achieved, with potentially devastating results.

Fibered coils can still be used, however, if proximal flow arrest is achieved utilizing a flow-control guide catheter (the 5.4-Fr. Zeppelin, Medtronic/MIS, or Berenstein, Medi-Tech/Boston Scientific). After heparinization (10,000 units by intravenous bolus), the flow-control guide catheter is placed in the internal carotid artery and inflated. This proximal location is chosen to allow coil packing as far proximally as possible, because once the balloon is inflated it cannot be deflated and moved. A microcatheter is placed through this flow-control guide catheter into the optimal position for occlusion, as described previously. The coils are then packed in this location.

Additional coils can be placed in the petrous internal carotid artery, or a pack of larger 0.038″ fibered coils can be placed in the cervical internal carotid artery where the flow-control catheter is located. This last large coil pack in the cervical internal carotid artery is recommended for two reasons: (1) as an assurance of proximal occlusion in addition to distal occlusion to prevent distal coil migration, and (2) as a means to achieve *inexpensive* permanent thrombosis (stainless steel Gianturco coils, Cook, Inc.).

After final coil packing has been performed, partial reversal of heparinization is performed (25 mg of protamine administered intravenously). The mass of coils is then allowed to remain undisturbed for 1 hour. The worst possible scenario is to deflate the occlusion balloon before the mass has thrombosed, allowing flow through fibers and clot and potentially dislodging material downstream.

TECHNICAL PROBLEMS, COMPLICATIONS, AND SOLUTIONS

After occlusion, it is necessary to observe the patient closely for at least the first 24 hours to prevent dehydration or episodes of hypotension. If any neurologic symptoms manifest, immediate hydration combined with efforts to increase cerebral perfusion should be undertaken. Initially, simple elevation of the legs can help, followed by alternating peripheral tourniquets until the mean blood pressure is increased. Colloids can be administered, followed by pharmaceuticals, if necessary. Any neurologic change should be temporary, but late infarcts have been known to occur, primarily when inadequate preocclusion testing has been performed.

Higashida and colleagues[13] reported on 68 patients treated with permanent occlusion of the internal carotid artery. A 30-minute simple clinical test occlusion was performed without any additional means of evaluating adequacy of intracranial hemodynamic sufficiency. In this series, 7 patients (10.3%) suffered transient ischemic periods, and 3 (4.4%) had a completed stroke. At the University of Pittsburgh, a series of 54 patients were reported in 1994 by Mathis and associates.[14] Preocclusion testing that included 15 minutes of clinical evaluation followed by cerebral blood flow analysis (using xenon-133 computed tomography) was performed. There were no subsequent transient ischemic episodes, but two patients had permanent strokes (4.8%).

In all significant series, detachable balloons were utilized for occlusion, and the overall permanent complication rate was less than 5%. This figure indicates the relative safety of this procedure, but it also shows the inadequacy of current methods of temporary occlusion testing to predict absolute success; further refinement of this procedure continues.

See "Technical Problems, Complications, and Solutions" in Chapter 34 for management techniques aimed at avoiding these complications.

REFERENCES

1. Serbinenko FA. Balloon catheterization and occlusion of major cerebral vessels. *J Neurosurg* 1974;41:125–145.
2. Nishioka H. Report on the Cooperative Study of Intracranial Aneurysms and Subarachnoid Hemorrhage, IX. Part I: Results of the treatment of intracranial aneurysms by occlusion of the carotid artery in the neck. *J Neurosurg* 1966;3:660–682.
3. Barnett HJM, Peerless SJ, Kaufman JC. "Stump" of internal carotid: a source for further embolic ischemia. *Stroke* 1978;9:448–456.
4. Heros RC. Thromboembolic complications after combined internal carotid ligation and extra-to-intracranial bypass. *Surg Neurol* 1984;21:175–179.
5. Landolt AM, Milliken CH. Pathogenesis of cerebral infarction secondary to mechanical carotid artery occlusion. *Stroke* 1970;1:52–62.
6. Miller JD, Jawad K, Jennett B. Safety of carotid ligation and its role in the management of intracranial aneurysms. *J Neurol Neurosurg Psychiatry* 1977;40:64–72.
7. Roski RA, Spetzler RF, Nulsen FE. Late complications of carotid ligation in the treatment of intracranial aneurysms. *J Neurosurg* 1981;54:583–587.
8. Hughes SR, Graves VB, Kesava PP, Rappe AH. The effect of flow arrest on distal embolic events during arterial occlusion with detachable coils: a canine study. *AJNR* 1996;17:685–691.
9. Hughes SR, Graves VB, Kesava PP, Rappe AH. The effect of flow arrest on distal embolic events during arterial occlusion with detachable coils: a canine study. *AJNR* 1996;17:685–691.
10. Debrun G, Fox A, Drake C, et al. Giant unclippable aneurysms: treatment with detachable balloons. *AJNR* 1981;2:167–173.
11. Fox AJ, Vinuela F, Pelz DM, et al. Use of detachable balloons for proximal artery occlusion in the treatment of unclippable cerebral aneurysms. *J Neurosurg* 1987;66:40–46.
12. Hacein-Bey L, Duong H, Vang MC, et al. Sequential evaluation of cortical perfusion following carotid perfusion: The usefulness of SPECT. Paper presented at the American Society of Interventional and Therapeutic Neuroradiology/World Federation of Interventional and Therapeutic Neuroradiology Scientific Conference. New York, Sept 1997.
13. Higashida RT, Halbach VV, Dowd C, et al. Endovascular detachable balloon embolization therapy of cavernous carotid artery aneurysms: results in 87 cases. *J Neurosurg* 1990;72:857–863.
14. Mathis JM, Barr JD, Jungreis CA, et al. Temporary balloon test occlusion of the internal carotid artery: experience in 500 cases. *AJNR* 1995;16:749–754.

ADDITIONAL READINGS

Braun IF, Battey PM, Fulenwider JT, Per-Lee JH. Transcatheter carotid occlusion: an alternative to the surgical treatment of cervical carotid aneurysms. *J Vasc Surg* 1986;4:299–302.
Countee R, Vijayanathan T, Hubschmann O, Chavis P. Carotid ligation for recurrent ischemia due to inaccessible carotid obstruction. *J Neurosurg* 1980;53:491–499.
Hieshima G, Mehringer C, Grinnell V, et al. Emergency occlusive techniques. *Surg Neurol* 1978;9:293–302.

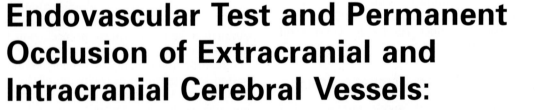

CHAPTER 36

Endovascular Test and Permanent Occlusion of Extracranial and Intracranial Cerebral Vessels:
Indications, Techniques, and Management

J.N. Vallee / A. Aymard / A.E. Casasco / H.S. Jhaveri / E. Houdart / J.-J. Merland

The objective of test occlusion of a vessel is to evaluate the clinical tolerance to occlusion and the effectiveness of the alternative blood supply. This usually is performed when permanent sacrifice of the vessel is contemplated. If the test is well tolerated, the goal of permanent occlusion of a vessel is to stop flow within the vessel, thereby reducing or altering the direction of flow to a lesion at or distal to the site of occlusion.

GENERAL CONSIDERATIONS

Successful and safe test and permanent occlusion requires multidisciplinary collaboration among neurosurgeons, interventional neuroradiologists, and anesthetists. An angiographic room, preferably with digital equipment, is needed. Neuroleptic analgesia is used to enable clinical assessment of the patient during the test occlusion. Strict aseptic technique is essential. Before test (and permanent) occlusion, all patients are evaluated with contrast-enhanced computed tomography (CT), magnetic resonance imaging (MRI), or both, depending on the pathology.

INTERNAL CAROTID ARTERY

Indications

Indications for test and permanent occlusion of an internal carotid artery (ICA) include fusiform aneurysms, giant aneurysms, and wide neck aneurysms (especially of the cavernous segment of the ICA), which cannot be treated selectively by either endovascular technique or surgical technique; post-traumatic lesions of the ICA; and certain carotid-cavernous fistulae (Figs. 36–1 and 36–2). In addition, test occlusion may be performed preoperatively for skull base tumors when intraoperative occlusion of the ICA may become necessary.

Materials for Test and Permanent Occlusion

The standard materials needed for test and permanent occlusion include 5- and 6-Fr. introducers (Terumo, Japan), a 0.035″ hydrophilic-coated guidewire (Terumo, Japan), a 5-Fr. vertebral curve catheter (Terumo, Japan), a 6-Fr. guide catheter (Nycomed, Balt Extrusion, Boston Scientific [Platform], or other), and nonionic contrast media (Omnipaque 300, Nycomed).

A microcatheter with a nondetachable balloon can be used (a B1 balloon preglued on a standard Magic 1.8-Fr. microcatheter [Balt Extrusion]). Alternatively, a microcatheter with a detachable balloon tied with latex ligature at its tip can be used, especially if permanent occlusion of the vessel with detachable balloons is being considered. Catheters used include a coaxial Teflon 2- to 3-Fr. ("red and black") microcatheter (Nycomed, France), a coaxial Teflon 0.5- to 0.7-mm microcatheter (Technofluor, France) with a

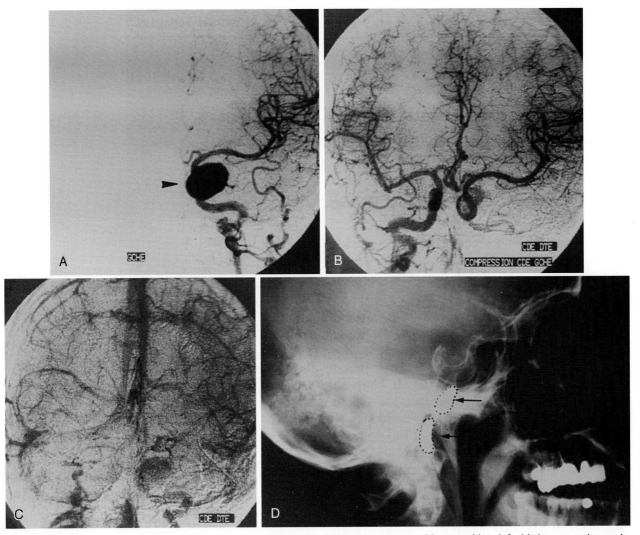

Figure 36–1 Case 1. Test occlusion of the internal carotid artery (ICA) in a 43-year-old man with a left third-nerve palsy and a giant aneurysm. *A,* Left carotid artery injection reveals the giant aneurysm *(arrowhead). B,* Right carotid artery injection (anteroposterior [AP] view, arterial phase) shows perfect, simultaneous filling of both hemispheres by a patent anterior communicating artery. *C,* The venous phase demonstrates adequate filling without delay. *D,* Latex balloons filled with contrast media *(arrows)* were detached at the foramen lacerum and in the high cervical region (for security).

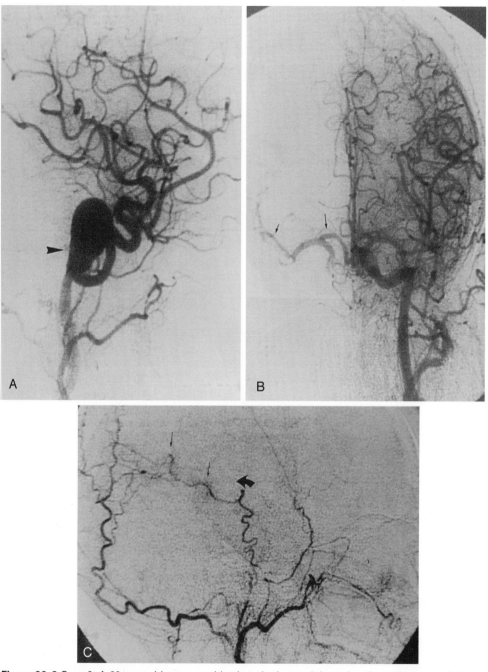

Figure 36–2 Case 2. A 60-year-old woman with trigeminal neuralgia and a giant aneurysm. *A,* Right carotid arteriogram (lateral view) demonstrates a giant aneurysm *(arrowhead),* with the neck arising from the foramen lacerum segment of the ICA. *B,* Left carotid arteriogram (AP view) during occlusion test of the right ICA demonstrates marked asymmetry in the late arterial phase *(arrows).* The patient did not have symptoms, but because of this appearance, bypass was performed. *C,* Right external carotid artery angiogram after an extracranial–intracranial (EC-IC) bypass *(curved arrow)* demonstrates filling of the parietal area *(small arrows).*

universal valve placed through a thermoformable 3.6-Fr. catheter (Balt Extrusion), or a Minitorquer microcatheter (Nycomed). The balloon used varies; commonly used balloons include BAL 1 (9.0-mm length, 6.0-mm diameter) (Balt Extrusion), No. 19 Nycomed (10.5-mm length, 6.0-mm diameter), No. 16 Nycomed (18.9-mm length, 7.0-mm diameter), and L2 Nycomed (16.0-mm length, 7.1-mm diameter). Balloons are secured with a latex ligature (Nycomed).

Procedure of Test Occlusion

Under local anesthesia and using Seldinger's technique, one femoral artery is cannulated with the 5-Fr. Terumo introducer, used as arterial access for performance of angiography during the procedure to evaluate the effectiveness of clamping and of alternative blood flow. The other femoral artery or the common carotid artery on the side to be tested is accessed

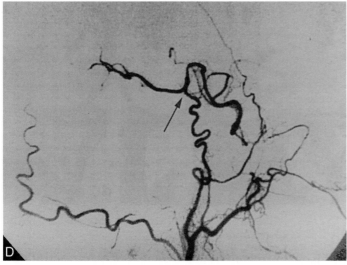

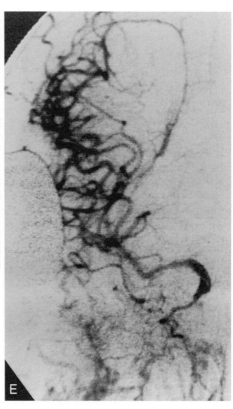

Figure 36–2 *Continued. D,* Right common carotid arteriogram during occlusion test of the right ICA shows extensive filling of the right hemisphere by the enlarged EC-IC bypass (*arrow* at anastomosis). *E,* Right carotid arteriogram (AP view) performed after permanent occlusion shows supply of the middle cerebral artery territory by well-developed anastomoses.

with the 6-Fr. Terumo introducer to perform the test occlusion.

Four-vessel cerebral arteriography is performed with the 5-Fr. vertebral curve Terumo catheter and 0.035″ guidewire to evaluate the complete intracranial hemodynamics and supply.

Preparation of the microcatheter depends on the strategy employed. If a microcatheter is used with a nondetachable balloon, the mandrel is removed from the microcatheter while constantly injecting a mixture of two-thirds nonionic contrast media and one-third normal saline through a 1.0-cc tuberculin syringe at the hub of the catheter to avoid entry of air. The microcatheter and the balloon are then flushed with this mixture to eliminate air, to enable visualization of the balloon under fluoroscopy, and to enable deflation of the balloon promptly. The mandrel is then reintroduced to help push the microcatheter into the guide catheter. Silicon (3M) is sprayed on the tip of the microcatheter and balloon to allow easy, smooth passage of the microcatheter through the guide catheter.

If a microcatheter with a detachable balloon is used, the balloon is attached securely to the tip of the microcatheter with a latex ligature with three knots and three turns after the same preparation is performed as with a nondetachable balloon.

To prevent thromboembolic complications, 25 U/kg of heparin is injected as an intravenous bolus, then 20 U/kg/hr is constantly infused intravenously by electric syringe pump. The ICA is catheterized selectively with the 6-Fr. guide catheter. The entire assembly of the microcatheter and balloon is then ad-

vanced through a Y-type hemostatic valve into the guide catheter. A three-way stopcock is placed on the other arm of the hemostatic valve.

When two thirds of the microcatheter assembly has been advanced into the guide catheter, the mandrel is removed slowly from the microcatheter while the mixture of contrast media and saline in a 1-cc tuberculin syringe is constantly injected at the hub of the microcatheter to avoid re-entry of air into the microcatheter. After the balloon-tipped microcatheter has passed through the guide catheter, the blood flow carries it to the desired location.

All the catheters are flushed continuously with normal saline using a pressure bag to prevent thromboembolic phenomena related to the catheters.

Intraprocedure Care

The test is performed with continuous electrocardiogram (ECG), arterial blood pressure, pulse, and oxygen saturation monitoring (SaO_2) during the entire test occlusion.

Management of Test Occlusion

Level of Occlusion

For tumors and post-traumatic lesions, the balloon is positioned just proximal to the lesion, or in the petrosal segment of the ICA. For aneurysms, the level of occlusion depends on the location of the aneurysm and the final therapeutic strategy (which depends on the presence or absence of reperfusion of the aneurysm by collateral flow during test occlusion). In the case of an aneurysm below the ophthalmic artery, there is no possibility of revascularization of the aneurysm, and the balloon is positioned just proximal to the neck of the aneurysm.

In the case of a carotid-ophthalmic aneurysm, there is some possibility of reperfusion of the aneurysm by the ophthalmic artery. The balloon is positioned either over the neck of the aneurysm, between the aneurysm and the ophthalmic artery if there is more than a 5-mm segment of ICA in which to position the balloon, in front of the ostium of the ophthalmic artery if there is a functional anastomosis from the external carotid artery to the ICA by the ophthalmic artery, or below the ophthalmic artery if there is nonreperfusion of the aneurysm by collateral circulation.

In the case of a supraophthalmic aneurysm, revascularization of the aneurysm depends on the morphology and the hemodynamics of the posterior communicating artery. The balloon is positioned at the level of or proximal to the aneurysm, taking care to respect the posterior communicating artery.

The occlusion test can now be performed, and the balloon is inflated using the prepared mixture until there is occlusion of the artery. This test should not exceed 30 minutes' duration, even under full heparinization.

Evaluation of Tolerance

During the entire duration of the test occlusion, several parameters are evaluated. Clinical tolerance is tested through higher function, sensory and motor function, and cranial nerves. In the case of clinical findings of any minor deficit, the balloon immediately is deflated completely after having aspirated and washed the carotid artery proximal to the balloon with a large volume of normal saline, then having flushed the residual blood into the external carotid circulation.

The integrity of the circle of Willis is verified by injecting the contralateral ICA during occlusion to evaluate the anterior communicating artery and its contribution to the circulation. This is evaluated by the rapidity of emptying of the middle cerebral artery flow and its venous phase on the side of the test occlusion in comparison with the opposite side. The dominant vertebral artery is then injected to evaluate the contribution of the posterior communicating artery on the side of the test occlusion using the same criteria. Finally, the common carotid artery on the side of test occlusion is injected to verify any anastomosis between meningeal branches of internal maxillary artery and cavernous carotid branches as well as retrograde flow in the ophthalmic artery through anastomoses between branches of external carotid artery and ophthalmic artery. This is evaluated better by positioning a 5.0-Fr. pigtail catheter in the ascending aorta and injecting nonionic contrast media using an injector to see the *global* intracranial blood flow as well as the rate of emptying of both sides simultaneously.

Induced Arterial Hypotension Test During Test Occlusion

Objective

A sudden drop of more than 20 mm Hg in systolic pressure is performed after 15 minutes of well-tolerated test occlusion (first confirmed by clinical and arteriographic evaluation). The purpose is to uncover autoregulation irregularities during arterial hypotension that may cause insufficient cerebral perfusion. Neurologic problems have been observed in patients several hours after permanent occlusion of the artery; the cause was modifications in flow rate and volume that were unpredictable on the basis of a clinical and angiographic occlusion test without hypotension.

Technique

Hypotension is induced by infusion of a calcium channel blocker, such as nicardipine (Loxen). After dilution in 5% glucose, 1.0 mg/min of nicardipine is injected as an intravenous bolus, until a drop of more than 20 mm Hg in systolic pressure is achieved for 10 minutes. New clinical neurologic and angiographic evaluations are performed. When nicardipine is stopped, the hypotension reverses rapidly in most cases, with the help of rapid intravenous normal saline infusion. In occasional cases, intravenous colloid infusion may be needed as a supplement for 1 to 2 hours.

Criteria for Tolerance

A patient is said to have tolerated the test occlusion if the following criteria are met:

- Clinically perfect tolerance for 30 minutes
- Cerebral perfusion time and venous phase appearance delayed no more than 1 second on the side of occlusion compared with the opposite side
- No change in clinical status or perfusion when hypotension is induced

If any one of the above three criteria is not met, the patient is considered to have failed the occlusion test. The balloon is rapidly deflated after repeated aspiration and washing of the carotid artery proximal to the balloon with normal saline, then flushing of the residual blood into the external carotid circulation to prevent thromboembolic phenomena.

If the test occlusion is not successful, superficial temporal artery to ipsilateral middle cerebral artery bypass can be considered. Test occlusion is repeated 2 to 4 weeks later. This procedure is especially indicated for giant aneurysm of the carotid artery siphon or of the middle cerebral artery (see Fig. 36–2). As an alternative, test occlusion of common carotid artery can be considered (see below).

At the end of the test occlusion, the balloon is deflated using the same precautions described previously to prevent thromboembolic phenomena. The activated clotting time is verified before removing the introducer. If necessary, protamine can be used to reverse the effect of heparin.

Procedure of Permanent Occlusion

Permanent occlusion of the ICA can be performed immediately after conclusion of the test occlusion if the criteria for tolerance have been satisfied. The balloon is reinflated with the prepared mixture of two-thirds nonionic contrast media and one-third normal saline until occlusion of the vessel occurs and is released by simple traction. A second safety balloon is rapidly released 1 or 2 cm below the first one.

When occlusion distal to the ophthalmic artery or distal to the posterior communicating artery is performed for treatment of an aneurysm, only one balloon is released. Detachable coils can be used and delivered either within the aneurysm, with the tail of the coil extending into the parent vessel lumen to occlude the vessel in conjunction with a safety balloon occlusion, or within the aneurysm to perform a partial selective embolization in association with permanent occlusion of the parent vessel with a balloon overlying the neck of the aneurysm to induce more aneurysmal thrombosis. If coils are used in this manner, they must be positioned before the second balloon placement and detachment. Coils can be used in conjunction with detachable balloons in a similar fashion to treat carotid–ophthalmic aneurysms.

For distal supraophthalmic aneurysms, occlusion preferably is performed at the level of the aneurysm, taking care to preserve the posterior communicating artery. If this is not possible, occlusion can be performed proximal to the posterior communicating artery, reducing the blood flow in the aneurysm, in association with partial embolization of the aneurysm with detachable coils to induce more thrombosis. These aneurysms are the most difficult to exclude and the most susceptible to reperfusion.

Results of Test and Permanent Occlusion

In a series of 40 patients with aneurysms, 32 patients successfully tolerated the test occlusion and were treated by permanent occlusion of the ICA; 4 patients underwent extracranial–intracranial surgical bypass before successful occlusion of the ICA; 4 patients had neurologic deficits (3 patients fully recovered from their transient deficits, whereas 1 patient developed a hemiparesis during test occlusion and did not undergo permanent occlusion; the hemiparesis has not resolved to date); and 39 patients had permanent occlusion of the ICA and at long-term follow-up were found to have complete exclusion of the aneurysm.

COMMON CAROTID ARTERY

Indications

The indications include those for test and permanent occlusion of the ICA with failure of that test, aneurysms of the common carotid artery that cannot be

treated selectively, and post-traumatic lesions of the common carotid artery.

Technique of Test Occlusion

The technique essentially is the same as for test occlusion of the ICA (described above), using the same occlusion microcatheter system. Other balloons also can be used, including the BAL 3 (12.0-mm length, 9.0-mm diameter; 7-Fr. introducer; Balt Extrusion), BAL 4 (11.0-mm length, 10.0-mm diameter; 8-Fr.-introducer; Balt Extrusion), or No. 17 Nycomed (14.7-mm length, 7.8-mm diameter; 7-Fr. introducer), all of which are tied with a latex ligature. Alternatively, a balloon with a valve can be used, such as the gold-valve balloon (GVB) 17 (11.5-mm length, 8.5-mm diameter; 8-Fr. introducer; Nycomed).

Management of Test Occlusion

The evaluation of tolerance is the same as for test occlusion of the ICA (described above) but requires more evaluation of the anastomoses between the ipsilateral external carotid artery, muscular branches of the vertebral artery, and muscular branches of the subclavian artery on the side of test occlusion as well as anastomoses from the opposite external carotid artery that participate in vascularization on the side of occlusion. These anastomoses sometimes can be sufficient to produce tolerance of the test occlusion, even though the circle of Willis is not sufficiently functional. The criteria of tolerance are the same as for test occlusion of the ICA.

Permanent Occlusion

After a properly performed, well-tolerated test occlusion, permanent occlusion by surgical ligature just below the bifurcation of the common carotid artery is much more precise than the detachable balloon technique and avoids potential thromboembolic complications produced by stasis of the blood column between the bifurcation of the carotid artery and the balloon.

Editor's Note: This standing column of stagnant blood (thrombus) has been implicated in embolic complications secondary to proximal permanent occlusion of the ICA. For this reason, permanent occlusion of the common carotid artery should be performed as just described, with a surgical ligature. In addition, permanent occlusion of the ICA should be performed with the occlusion beginning at least as far distal as the petrocavernous junction of the ICA to prevent formation of a free column of thrombus within the cervical carotid artery distal to the occlusion, which can be mashed downstream by simple neck motion.

VERTEBRAL ARTERY

Indications

Indications for test and permanent occlusion of a vertebral artery include vertebrobasilar aneurysms that cannot be treated selectively either by surgery or by selective endovascular technique (Figs. 36–3

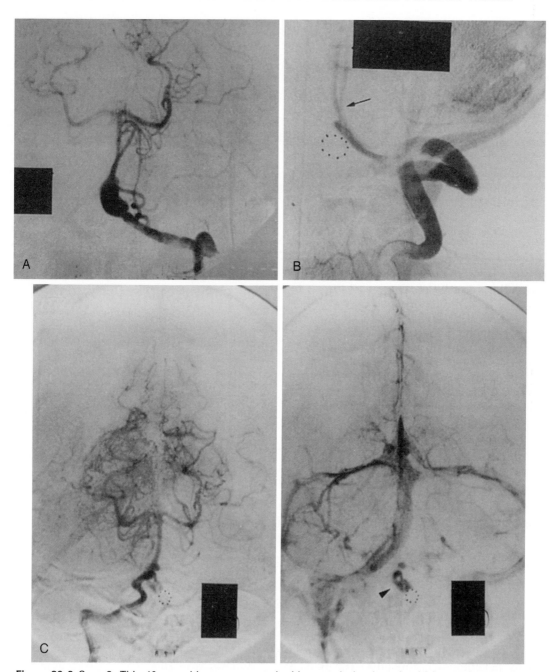

Figure 36–3 Case 3. This 40-year-old man presented with a grade I subarachnoid hemorrhage and was treated 2 weeks later. *A,* AP left vertebral artery (VA) angiogram shows a fusiform aneurysm of the left intracranial VA distal to the posterior inferior cerebellar artery (PICA). *B,* Repeat left VA angiogram during balloon occlusion of the left intracranial VA *distal to the PICA* demonstrates antegrade filling of the ipsilateral PICA *(arrow). C,* Right VA angiogram (midarterial *[left]* and venous *[right]* phases) obtained during treatment shows stagnation of contrast material within the left distal VA aneurysm *(arrowhead).*

and 36–4), tumors of the cervical spine or perispinal region, tumors of the foramen magnum (preoperative), traumatic lesions of the vertebral artery, and certain vertebral arteriovenous fistulae. The goal is to reduce or change the direction of blood flow after permanent occlusion of the dominant vertebral artery, resulting in aneurysmal thrombosis in the case of aneurysms of the posterior fossa, or to occlude the parent vessel in the case of a traumatic lesion of the vertebral artery. In addition, occlusion of the

vertebral artery can be performed in certain cases of aneurysms of the intracranial segment of the vertebral artery and in certain cases of vertebral arteriovenous fistulae that cannot be treated selectively or by venous approach.

Materials for Test and Permanent Occlusion

As noted earlier, a microcatheter with a nondetachable balloon can be used. This can be either the same

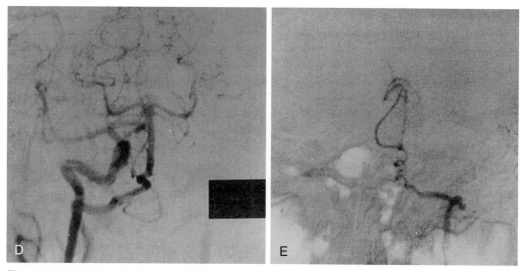

Figure 36–3 *Continued. D,* Right brachial artery retrograde study 12 months after treatment demonstrates complete disappearance of the aneurysm. *E,* Left brachial artery retrograde injection obtained at the same time reveals persistent antegrade filling of the left VA and its PICA.

system used for test occlusion of the ICA (see above) or a standard Magic STD 1.8-Fr. microcatheter (Balt Extrusion) with a balloon tied with ligature or glued by a drop of *N*-butyl-2-cyanoacrylate (NBCA; Histoacryl) to its tip.

Alternatively, a detachable balloon mounted on a microcatheter can be used, particularly if permanent occlusion of the artery is planned if the test occlusion is well tolerated. The same microcatheters are used as for the ICA (see above). Commonly used balloons include the BAL 0 (7.0-mm length, 5.5-mm diameter;

Balt Extrusion) as well as the previously described BAL 1 (Balt Extrusion) and No. 19 Nycomed. As described previously, these balloons are secured to the tip of the catheter by a latex ligature.

Detachable coils can also be used for test and permanent occlusion of the vertebral artery. Either of two systems can be used:

1. TRACKER-18 GDC with Guglielmi detachable coils (GDCs), such as 4 mm × 10 cm GDC-10, 5 mm × 15 cm GDC-18, or 6 mm × 20 cm GDC-18 (all Target Therapeutics)

Figure 36–4 Case 4. This 38-year-old woman presented 1 year before treatment with an aneurysm of PICA that caused a grade IV (Hunt and Hess) subarachnoid hemorrhage. *A,* Right vertebral artery angiogram reveals a 5-mm-diameter saccular aneurysm arising from the PICA. Note the upper cervical anterior spinal artery. Occlusion of the right vertebral artery was performed at the C1–C2 level. *B,* Right brachial angiography was obtained 3 months later. The intracranial right vertebral artery is supplied by cervical anastomoses, the PICA is normal, and the aneurysm has disappeared.

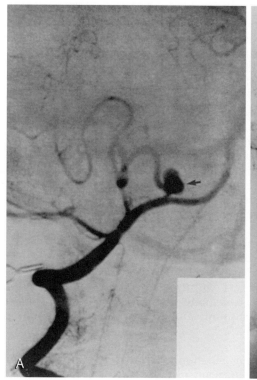
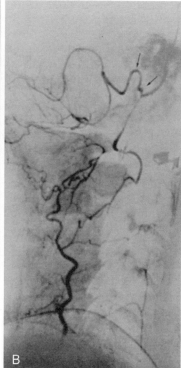

2. MAG 3-Fr./2 Fr. through MDS-N (McCornic Detach System) catheter with SPI-N coils, such as SPID 4* 125N spirale or SPID 5* 150N spirale (all Balt Extrusion)

Technique of Test Occlusion

The technique is similar to that described for the ICA (above), with a minor procedural difference. As in the case of the ICA, two sheaths are placed, with the 5-Fr. sheath in one femoral artery allowing the operator to study the effectiveness of occlusion and of the collateral blood flow. The 6-Fr. sheath is placed in the other femoral artery or in the axillary artery ipsilateral to the vertebral artery to be occluded. This sheath is used to introduce the test occlusion system.

Management of Test Occlusion

Level of Occlusion

For tumoral pathology and post-traumatic lesions of the vertebral artery, test occlusion is performed proximal to the level of the lesion. For vertebral arteriovenous fistulae, test occlusion is performed over the site of the fistula or just proximal to it.

In the case of an aneurysm, the level of occlusion depends on the location of the aneurysm and on whether the therapeutic goal is to reduce or change the direction of flow, inducing thrombosis in the aneurysm, or to occlude the parent vessel. Test occlusion can be performed at two levels:

1. Distal to the origin of the posterior inferior cerebellar artery (PICA) if more than 5 mm of length between the origin of the PICA and the aneurysm is available for placement of either coils or a balloon while preserving the PICA. This occlusion test is performed in the context of parent vessel occlusion as therapeutic strategy in cases in which the aneurysm involves the intracranial segment of the vertebral artery, or in the dominant vertebral artery with the strategy of reducing the inflow or changing the direction of flow in the case of an aneurysm of the basilar artery.

2. At the level of C1, with the goal of reducing the flow, knowing that after permanent occlusion at this level, retrograde flow from the muscular anastomoses with the occipital artery can develop and yield antegrade flow in the vertebrobasilar system. In most cases, unilateral occlusion of the dominant vertebral artery is sufficient to induce thrombosis in the aneurysm. If this is not sufficient, opposite-side vertebral artery occlusion can be performed after 3 or 4 weeks, following a new test occlusion of this vertebral artery to verify adequate retrograde flow from the posterior communicating arteries.

Evaluation of Tolerance

Test occlusion is performed for 30 minutes under systemic heparinization. The neurologic examination is monitored during the entire procedure. The effectiveness of the collateral blood flow and the nonrevascularization of the lesion are assessed by periodic angiographic evaluation of the vertebral artery, which confirms that clamping is effective, that the anterior spinal artery is preserved (if visible), and that the vertebrobasilar system is supplied adequately by the contralateral vertebral artery and by both ICAs through the posterior communicating arteries. The ipsilateral external carotid artery also must be evaluated angiographically to verify the possible reperfusion of the ipsilateral vertebral artery at the C1 level by muscular anastomoses. The criteria for tolerance are the same as those for test occlusion of the ICA.

Technique of Permanent Occlusion

If the criteria for tolerance of test occlusion are satisfied, permanent occlusion is performed. If detachable coils are used, they can be positioned within an aneurysm, with the tail of the coil extending into the vessel lumen, or proximal to an aneurysm or lesion. If detachable balloons are used, the balloon is inflated with the prepared mixture of two-thirds nonionic contrast media and one-third normal saline until occlusion of the vessel occurs; the inflated balloon is detached by simple traction in a position overlying or proximal to the aneurysm or the lesion. A second safety balloon is rapidly released 1 or 2 cm below the first one, taking care to preserve the spinal arteries (if seen). In the case of occlusion distal to the PICA, only one balloon is released.

As noted previously, in most cases, unilateral occlusion of the dominant vertebral artery is sufficient to induce thrombosis in an aneurysm. If this is not sufficient, occlusion of the contralateral vertebral artery can be performed after 3 or 4 weeks, following a new, well-tolerated test occlusion of this vertebral artery.

Editor's Note: Occlusion of large brachiocephalic vessels also can be performed with fibered coils as long as proximal flow arrest is achieved with a flow control guide catheter. See Chapter 35 for further discussion of this technique.

Results of Test and Permanent Occlusion

In one series, 25 patients with posterior fossa aneurysms were treated by this endovascular therapeutic method; most presented with posterior fossa lesions and mass effect. The results were as follows: 15 patients had excellent results, with complete angiographic exclusion of the aneurysm and clinically significant improvement; 8 patients had partial clinical improvement, with about 70% of the aneurysm thrombosed on angiographic follow-up; 2 patients had nonsignificant thrombosis of the aneurysm (one of these patients, who was on systemic anticoagulant therapy for medical reasons, died of fatal hemorrhage; both these cases were aneurysms located at the bifurcation of the basilar artery).

Occlusion of the vertebral artery either distal to

the PICA or at the C1 level is efficient for the aneurysms of the intracranial vertebral artery and is more effective for aneurysms of the middle segment of the basilar artery than for aneurysms of the bifurcation of the basilar artery.

INTRADURAL VESSELS

Indications

Indications for test and permanent occlusion of intradural vessels include carotid-cavernous fistulae, fusiform aneurysms, giant aneurysms, or wide neck aneurysms not suitable for selective treatment (aneurysms of branches of the circle of Willis, such as the middle cerebral artery, anterior cerebral artery, posterior cerebral artery, basilar artery, or intracranial vertebral artery). Endovascular therapy by parent vessel occlusion is the only available method if selective therapy or surgery is not possible.

Materials for Test and Permanent Occlusion

As described above for test occlusion of the ICA and vertebral artery, a microcatheter with either a nondetachable or detachable balloon can be used. In this setting, if a nondetachable balloon is chosen, a Magic STD 1.8-Fr. microcatheter (Balt Extrusion) can be used with a balloon tied with a latex ligature or glued by a drop of NBCA to the tip of the catheter. If a detachable balloon is used, it is mounted on a coaxial Teflon 0.5–0.7-mm microcatheter (Technofluor) advanced through a 3.6-Fr. thermoformable catheter (Balt Extrusion). Commonly used balloons include the previously described BAL 0 and the BAL COLIBRI (5.0-mm length 4.0-mm diameter; both from Balt Extrusion). These balloons are secured to the end of the catheter with latex ligatures, as described previously.

As in the case of the vertebral artery, detachable coils also can be used to occlude intradural vessels *temporarily.* This is especially useful when smaller vessels are to be tested (e.g., M segment). A TRACKER-18 GDC microcatheter generally is used. Commonly used coils include 2 mm × 6 cm GDC-10 Soft and 2 mm × 8 cm GDC-10 (all Target Therapeutics).

Technique of Test Occlusion

The technique of test occlusion is similar to that described previously for the ICA. One femoral artery access (5-Fr. introducer) is used to study the adequacy of occlusion and the collateral blood flow. The other access (6-Fr. introducer) may be the axillary artery (vertebrobasilar system), common carotid artery (anterior circulation), or femoral (either) and is used to introduce the occlusion system. Selective catheterization of the parent vessel is performed with the microcatheter carrying the prepared balloon or with the TRACKER-18 advanced through the guide catheter, which is already positioned either in the ICA or the vertebral artery (according to the localization of the vessel to be occluded). Test occlusion generally is performed for 30 minutes under systemic heparinization. The balloon is inflated with the prepared mixture of two-thirds nonionic contrast media and one-third normal saline, or the chosen coil is advanced into the parent artery until there is occlusion of the vessel.

Management of Test Occlusion of Intracranial Vessels

Middle Cerebral Artery

Test occlusion is performed at the origin of the middle cerebral artery at the M1 segment, *proximal to the origin of the lenticulostriate arteries,* when an aneurysm is located at the trifurcation of the middle cerebral artery. If the aneurysm is located more distally, however, the test occlusion is performed proximal to the aneurysm in the appropriate branch of the middle cerebral artery.

Monitoring of the patient's neurologic status is continued during the 30 minutes of test occlusion. Dominant vertebral and ipsilateral ICA arteriograms are obtained to verify the presence of leptomeningeal anastomotic branches that take over the perfusion of the involved territory.

Criteria for tolerance are clinical tolerance and, above all, angiographic visualization of the leptomeningeal collateral vessels and observation of the rate of opacification and emptying of cerebral vessels in the affected territory. These leptomeningeal vessels arise from the anterior cerebral artery, the posterior cerebral artery, or both.

Anterior Cerebral Artery and Anterior Communicating Artery

Test occlusion is performed at the level of the junction of A1, A2, and the anterior communicating artery for aneurysms of this region (Fig. 36–5). For aneurysms of the pericallosal artery and callosomarginal artery junction, the test is performed in the A2 segment proximal to the level of the aneurysm.

Neurologic evaluation is continued during the 30 minutes of the test, and dominant vertebral artery and ipsilateral ICA arteriograms are obtained to verify the presence of leptomeningeal anastomotic branches that take over the perfusion of the territory distal to the level of occlusion. Injection of the contralateral ICA also is performed to verify nonrevascularization by the anterior communicating artery.

The criteria for determining tolerance are clinical tolerance and angiographic evidence of leptomeningeal anastomoses from the middle cerebral artery and posterior cerebral artery that take over perfusion of the territory of anterior cerebral artery distal to the occlusion.

Posterior Cerebral Artery

For aneurysms of the P1 (precommunicating) segment of the posterior cerebral artery, the test occlu-

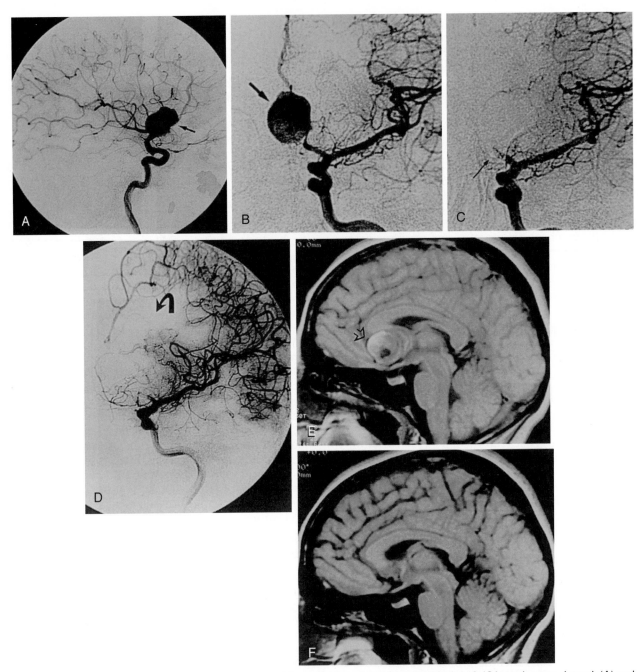

Figure 36–5 Case 5. A case of giant aneurysm treated by occlusion of the parent vessel. Left ICA angiogram, lateral *(A)* and AP *(B)* views, shows a giant aneurysm located at the A1-to-A2 junction of the left anterior cerebral artery *(arrows)*. *C,* During the test occlusion, the balloon is inflated within the A1 segment of the left anterior cerebral artery *(arrow)*. *D,* Left ICA angiogram during the test occlusion demonstrates the effectiveness of the collateral blood flow by leptomeningeal anastomoses from the middle cerebral artery *(curved arrow)*, which provides retrograde perfusion of the territory of the anterior cerebral artery distal to the occlusion. The clinical tolerance of the test was excellent. *E,* Initial MRI scan obtained before the occlusion of the parent vessel reveals the aneurysm *(open arrow)*. *F,* MRI scan obtained 1 year after the occlusion of the left anterior cerebral artery shows that the aneurysm has disappeared.

sion is performed at the origin of posterior cerebral artery. In the case of an aneurysm of the P2 segment, the test occlusion is performed just proximal to the aneurysm (Fig. 36–6). To determine the exact location of the junction of the posterior communicating artery and the posterior cerebral artery, a vertebral arteriogram is performed in the anteroposterior projection during compression of the ipsilateral common carotid artery.

Neurologic monitoring is performed during the 30 minutes of occlusion. It is essential to test visual function. An arteriogram of the ipsilateral carotid artery is performed to assess the leptomeningeal anastomoses that supply the territory distal to the level of occlusion.

As noted previously, the criteria for determining tolerance include clinical tolerance and angiographic demonstration of the leptomeningeal collateral ves-

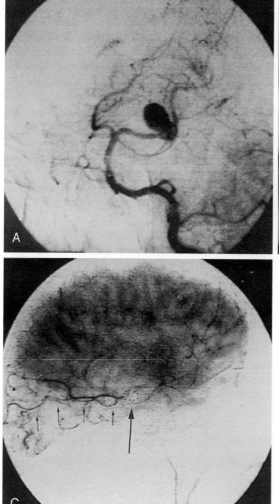
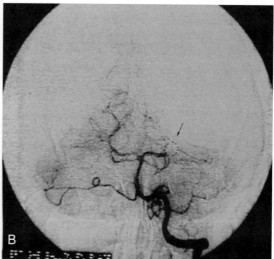

Figure 36–6 Case 6. A 40-year-old woman with severe headache. *A,* Left vertebral artery angiogram reveals a giant aneurysm with a large neck arising from the P2 segment of the posterior cerebral artery. *B,* Left vertebral artery angiogram after permanent occlusion; the balloon is inflated in front of the neck of the aneurysm *(arrow). C,* Left carotid arteriogram performed during test occlusion shows the effectiveness of the collateral blood flow, by leptomeningeal anastomoses, which yields retrograde perfusion of the territory of the posterior cerebral artery *(small arrows)* distal to the occlusion *(large arrow).*

sels from the ipsilateral middle cerebral artery and anterior cerebral artery.

Intracranial Vertebral Artery

Occlusion of the intracranial vertebral artery was described in more detail earlier in the sections on test and permanent occlusion of the vertebral artery. Test occlusion is performed distal to the origin of the PICA if a 5-mm segment of vessel is available proximal to the aneurysm to deliver either coils or a balloon while preserving the PICA (see Fig. 36–4).

Neurologic evaluation is continued for 30 minutes, and angiographic images verify that the vertebrobasilar system is well supplied by the contralateral vertebral artery and by the ICAs through the posterior communicating arteries.

Basilar Trunk

Test occlusion of the basilar trunk is performed over the aneurysm neck. Supply to the basilar trunk above the occlusion by both posterior communicating arteries is studied by injection of each carotid artery. Even so, some of the many small perforating vessels

of the basilar trunk could be occluded by the balloon or the coil, and there is no adequate evaluation for the perforating vessels.

Posterior Inferior Cerebellar Artery

Test occlusion is performed either at the origin of the PICA or within the vertebral artery over the ostium of the PICA. Neurologic monitoring is continued during the 30 minutes of the test occlusion. Angiographic evaluation of both vertebral arteries is performed to verify the effectiveness of the cerebellar and bulbar collateral blood flow that takes over the perfusion of the territory distal to the level of occlusion.

The criteria for determining tolerance are clinical tolerance and angiographic visualization of the degree of cerebellar leptomeningeal anastomoses from the ipsilateral superior and anterior inferior cerebellar arteries as well as the rate of opacification and emptying of the affected region. The uncertainty concerns the evaluation of the bulbar perforating vessels of this region. If the PICA arises proximally on the V4 segment of the vertebral artery (extracranial), the bulbar-perforating branches arise from the intracranial vertebral artery, and test occlusion can be performed with safety. If the PICA arises distally on the V4 segment of the vertebral artery (intracranial), the bulbar-perforating branches arise from the proximal PICA, and the presence of adequate collateral supply to their territory cannot be evaluated safely and adequately.

Technique of Permanent Occlusion of Intracranial Vessels

Permanent occlusion is performed after documenting that the criteria for tolerance (clinical and angiographic) have been met. If coils are used, the coil is delivered either within the aneurysm, with the tail of the coil extending into the vessel lumen, or within the parent vessel proximal to the aneurysm. If detachable balloons are used, the balloon is reinflated with the prepared mixture of two-thirds nonionic contrast media and one-third normal saline until occlusion of the vessel occurs; the balloon is released by simple traction in a position overlying or proximal to the neck of the aneurysm.

Middle Cerebral Artery

For aneurysms of the middle cerebral artery at the trifurcation, the occlusion is performed at the origin of the middle cerebral artery at the M1 segment proximal to the origin of the lenticulostriate arteries. For aneurysms distal to the trifurcation, occlusion is performed in the parent subsegmental branch at the level of or proximal to the aneurysm.

Anterior Cerebral Artery and Anterior Communicating Artery

For the aneurysms of the A1–A2–anterior communicating artery junction, the occlusion is performed precisely at the junction to occlude the anterior cerebral artery at this level. For aneurysms at the percallosal–callosomarginal junction, the A2 segment of the ipsilateral anterior cerebral artery is occluded at the level of or proximal to the aneurysm.

Posterior Cerebral Artery

For lesions of the P1 segment of the posterior cerebral artery, the occlusion is performed at the origin of posterior cerebral artery or at the level of the aneurysm. For aneurysms of the P2 segment of the posterior cerebral artery, occlusion is performed at the level of or proximal to the aneurysm.

Intracranial Vertebral Artery

The occlusion is performed between the PICA and the aneurysm or at the level of the aneurysm if there is more than a 5-mm segment of vertebral artery available, taking care to preserve the PICA.

Basilar Trunk

Occlusion of the basilar artery predisposes to major complications because of the potential occlusion of

perforators, so it is preferable to occlude the dominant vertebral artery. The treatment of giant fusiform basilar artery aneurysms is difficult because occlusion of the basilar artery at the level of vertebrobasilar junction predisposes to occlusion of the brainstem perforators. Occlusion of dominant or bilateral vertebral arteries at level of C1 helps in reducing mass effect.

Posterior Inferior Cerebellar Artery

The occlusion is performed either at the level of the aneurysm, at the origin of the PICA, or within the vertebral artery over the orifice of the PICA.

Results of Test and Permanent Occlusion of Intracranial Vessels

In a series of 18 patients, 14 patients had excellent results with angiographic exclusion of the aneurysm and excellent clinical improvement; 1 patient who had subarachnoid hemorrhage due to rupture of a giant aneurysm of the middle cerebral artery 3 days earlier did not tolerate test occlusion of the M1 segment; and 2 patients died after successful test occlusion of the basilar trunk (in one case at the middle segment, in the other case at the origin) due to acute brainstem infarction.

According to the recent literature, endovascular occlusion has a better outcome than surgical occlusion.

In the case of an unsuccessful occlusion test, extracranial–intracranial surgical bypass could be proposed and the test occlusion repeated 3 or 4 weeks after the surgical bypass; if this is successful, permanent occlusion could then be performed.

COMPLICATIONS

The immediate complications of permanent occlusion are mainly of three types: (1) thromboembolic phenomena; (2) difficulties with detachment of the balloon, with the risk of migration; and (3) premature deflation of the balloon in situations in which only one balloon is released. The use of coils is safer, but they are more expensive. Long-term complications are most often related to reperfusion of the aneurysm.

FOLLOW-UP

After permanent occlusion, the patients in the previously described series were transferred to the neurosurgical intensive care unit for 48 hours of complete bedrest in a horizontal position with the systolic arterial pressure maintained at a level 20 mm Hg higher than normal to maintain adequate distal cerebral perfusion and to prevent hemodynamic hypoperfusion.

Patients were followed up clinically and with serial

skull films to confirm balloon inflation. CT, MRI, and angiography were repeated 1 week after the procedure, at 6 months, and then at yearly intervals thereafter to document disappearance of the aneurysm (or other lesion).

CONCLUSION

Endovascular test occlusion of extracranial and intracranial cerebral vessels, with induced arterial hypotension testing to uncover abnormalities of autoregulation that can cause insufficient perfusion, performed for 30 minutes while taking care to observe whether the criteria for tolerance are met (both clinical tolerance and angiographic demonstration of adequate collateral blood flow through the communicating arteries, leptomeningeal anastomoses, or both) and to verify the nonreperfusion of the lesion through collateral vessels, allows prediction of whether treatment by permanent occlusion can be performed safely. In the case of test occlusion of the basilar artery, there is not enough information to develop criteria for tolerance. These criteria may include stable neurologic status during 30 minutes of occlusion and systemic hypotension, and stable electrophysiologic evaluation of brainstem function. Angiographic evaluation is not adequate to show collaterals to perforating vessels of the brainstem.

ADDITIONAL READINGS

Aymard A, Gobin YP, Hodes JE, et al. Endovascular occlusion of vertebral arteries in the treatment of unclippable vertebrobasilar aneurysms. *J Neurosurg* 1991;74:393–398.

Aymard A, Merland JJ, Rufenacht D, et al. Endovascular treatment of aneurysms of the terminal vertebral artery. *J Neuroradiol* 1987;14:1–9.

Beck DW, Boarini DJ, Kassel NF. Surgical treatment of giant aneurysm of the vertebrobasilar junction. *Surg Neurol* 1979;12:283–285.

Berenstein A, Ransohoff J, Kupersmith M, et al. Transvascular treatment of giant aneurysms of the cavernous carotid and vertebral arteries: functional investigations and embolization. *Surg Neurol* 1984;21:3–12.

Debrun G, Fox A. Interventional neuroradiology in the treatment of cerebral aneurysms. In: Hopkins LN, Long DM (eds). *Clinical Management of Intracranial Aneurysms*. New York: Raven Press, 1982, pp. 273–285.

Debrun G, Fox A, Drake CG, et al. Giant unclippable aneurysms: treatment with detachable balloons. *AJNR* 1981;2:167–173.

Debrun G, Lacour P, Caron JP, et al. Detachable balloon and calibrated leak balloon techniques in the treatment of cerebral vascular lesions. *J Neurosurg* 1978;49:635–649.

Diaz FG, Ausman JI, Pearce JG. Ischemic complications after internal carotid artery occlusion and extracranial intracranial anastomosis. *Neurosurgery* 1982;10:563–570.

Diaz FG, Ohaegbulam S, Dujovny M, Ausman JI. Surgical management of aneurysms in the cavernous sinus. *Acta Neurochir* (Wien) 1988;91:25–28.

Drake CG. Giant intracranial aneurysms: experience with surgical treatment in 176 patients. *Clin Neurosurg* 1979;26:12–95.

Drake CG. Ligation of the vertebral (unilateral and bilateral) or basilar artery in the treatment of large intracranial aneurysms. *J Neurosurg* 1975;43:255–274.

Fox AJ, Vinuela F, Pelz DM, et al. Use of detachable balloons for proximal artery occlusion in the treatment of unclippable cerebral aneurysms. *J Neurosurg* 1987;66:40–46.

Fox JL. Intracranial Aneurysm. Berlin: Springer-Verlag, 1983.

George B, Aymard A, Gobin YP, et al. Traitement endovasculaire des aneurysmes intracraniens: interet et perspectives d'apres une serie de 92 cas. *Neurochirurgie* 1990;36:273–278.

Goto K, Halbach VV, Hardin CW. Permanent inflation of detachable balloons with a low-viscosity hydrophilic polymerizing system. *Radiology* 1998;169:787–790.

Higashida RT, Halbach VV, Cahan LD, et al. Detachable balloon embolization therapy of posterior circulation intracranial aneurysms. *J Neurosurg* 1989;71:512–519.

Higashida RT, Halbach VV, Dowd CF, et al. Intracranial aneurysms: interventional neurovascular treatment with detachable balloons. Results in 215 cases. *Radiology* 1991;178:663–670.

Higashida RT, Halbach VV, Dowd C, et al. Endovascular detachable balloon embolization therapy of cavernous carotid artery aneurysms: results in 87 cases. *J Neurosurg* 1990;72:857–863.

Higashida RT, Hieshima GB, Halbach VV, et al. Intravascular detachable balloon embolization therapy of posterior circulation intracranial aneurysms. *J Neurosurg* 1989;71:512–519.

Higashida RT, Hieshima GB, Halbach VV, et al. Intravascular detachable balloon embolization of intracranial aneurysms: indications and techniques. *Acta Radiol* 1986;369:594–596.

Hodes JE, Fletcher WA, Goodmann DF, Hoyt WF. Rupture of cavernous carotid artery aneurysm causing subdural hematoma and death: case report. *J Neurosurg* 1988;69:617–619.

Kak VK, Taylor AR, Gordon DS. Proximal carotid ligation for internal carotid aneurysms: a long term follow-up study. *J Neurosurg* 1973;39:503–513.

Kempe LG. Aneurysms of the vertebral artery. In: Pia HW, Langmaid C, Zierski J (eds). Cerebral Aneurysms: Advances in Diagnosis and Therapy. Berlin: Springer-Verlag, 1979, pp. 119–120.

Linskey ME, Sekhar LN, Hirsch W, et al. Aneurysms of the intracavernous carotid artery: clinical presentation, radiographic features, and pathogenesis. *Neurosurgery* 1990;26:71–79.

Linskey ME, Sekhar LN, Hirsch W, et al. Aneurysms of the intracavernous carotid artery: natural history and indications for treatment. *Neurosurgery* 1990;26:933–938.

McMurty JG III, Housepian EM, Bowman FO Jr, et al. Surgical treatment of basilar artery aneurysms: elective circulatory arrest with thoracotomy in 12 cases. *J Neurosurg* 1974;40:486–494.

Merland JJ, Rufenacht D. A detachable latex balloon with valve-mechanism for the permanent occlusion of large brain AV fistulas or cerebral arteries. In: Valk J (ed). Neuroradiology 1985/1986. Amsterdam: Elsevier, 1986, pp. 291–293.

Peerless SJ, Drake CG. Management of aneurysms of posterior circulation. In: Youmans JR (ed). Neurological Surgery, 2nd ed. Philadelphia: WB Saunders, 1982, pp. 1715–1763.

Pelz DM, Vinuela F, Fox AJ. Vertebrobasilar occlusion therapy of giant aneurysms: significance of angiographic morphology of the posterior communicating arteries. *J Neurosurg* 1984;60:560–565.

Picard L, Lepoire J, Montaut H. Endarterial occlusion of carotid cavernous fistulas using a balloon tipped catheter. *Neuroradiology* 1974;8:5–10.

Romodanov AP, Cheglov V. Intravascular occlusion of saccular aneurysms of the cerebral arteries by means of a detachable balloon catheter. *Adv Tech Stand Neurosurg* 1982;9:25–48.

Rufenacht D, Merland JJ. A polyethylene microcatheter with a latex balloon as an implant for permanent vascular occlusions: a way for the treatment of distal intracranial or intraspinal large AV fistulas or aneurysms. In: Valk J (ed). *Neuroradiology* 28. Amsterdam: Elsevier, 1986, pp. 291–293.

Scott B, Skwarok E. The treatment of cerebral aneurysms by ligation of the common carotid artery. *Surg Gynecol Obstet* 1961;113:54–61.

Serbinenko FA. Balloon catheterization and occlusion of major cerebral vessels. *J Neurosurg* 1974;41:125–145.

Serbinenko FA, Filatov JM, Spallone A, et al. Management of giant intracranial ICA aneurysms with combined extracranial intracranial anastomosis and endovascular occlusion. *J Neurosurg* 1990;37:57–63.

Spetzler RF, Schuster H, Roski RA. Elective extracranial intracranial arterial bypass in the treatment of inoperable giant aneurysms of the internal carotid artery. *J Neurosurg* 1980;53:22–27.

Sundt TM, Piepgras DG. Surgical approach to giant intracranial aneurysms: operative experience with 80 cases. *J Neurosurg* 1979;51:731–742.

Sundt TM Jr, Piepgras DG, Houser OW, et al. Interposition saphenous vein grafts for advanced occlusive disease and large aneurysms in the posterior circulation. *J Neurosurg* 1982;56:205–215.

Swearingen B, Heros RC. Common carotid occlusion for unclippable carotid aneurysms: an old but still effective operation. *Neurosurgery* 1987;21:288–294.

Vazquez Anon V, Aymard A, et al. Balloon occlusion of the internal carotid artery in 40 cases of giant intracavernous aneurysms: technical aspects, cerebral monitoring and results. *Neuroradiology* 1992;34:245–251.

CHAPTER 37

Endovascular Treatment of Traumatic Lesions in Supra-Aortic Vessels with Stent-grafts

J.C. Parodi / C.J. Schönholz

HISTORY

The vast increase in civilian arterial trauma in recent years has taught that false aneurysms and arteriovenous fistulae in some locations are dangerous to approach and difficult to repair. In supra-aortic vessels, access to the traumatized area can be cumbersome and entails some risks of injury of the adjacent structures.

In 1976, we started to develop a system for endo-

luminally treating aneurysms, traumatic lesions, and dissections of large arteries with a new stent-graft device. In 1990, the first clinical case of an aortic aneurysm repair was performed and reported by us. Between 1992 and July 1996, 25 patients with traumatic arterial lesions were encountered and treated with the stent-graft technique. Sixteen were located in supra-aortic vessels (Table 37–1). Fourteen of the patients were men and two were women. Their ages ranged from 22 to 67 years. The lesions encountered

T A B L E 3 7 - 1   Vascular Trauma in Supra-Aortic Vessels Treated with Stent-grafts

Patient No.	Age/Sex	Arterial Injury	Injury Type	Days	Device	Cause
1	50/M	Axillary	AVF	1	Palmaz/Dacron	Gunshot
2	23/M	Common carotid	FA	2	Palmaz/Vein	Gunshot
3	45/M	Subclavian	AVF	2	Palmaz/PTFE	Gunshot
4	37/M	Internal carotid	FA	4	Palmaz/Vein	Blunt trauma
5	24/M	Subclavian	AVF	3	Palmaz/Dacron	Gunshot
6	56/M	Subclavian	AVF	3	Palmaz/Dacron	Iatrogenic
7	22/M	Subclavian	AVF	2	Palmaz/PTFE	Gunshot
8	56/F	Common carotid	FA	1	CEG	Iatrogenic
9	31/M	Axillary	FA	1	CEG	Gunshot
10	28/M	Subclavian	AVF	2	CEG	Gunshot
11	67/M	Subclavian	AVF	8	CEG + Palmaz/PTFE	Iatrogenic
12	22/M	Common carotid	AVF	2	CEG	Stab wound injury
13	61/M	Subclavian	FA	2	Palmaz/Dacron	Iatrogenic
14	52/F	Subclavian	FA	1	CEG	Iatrogenic
15	65/M	Subclavian	AVF	2	CEG	Iatrogenic
16	32/M	Axillary	FA	1	CEG	Iatrogenic

AVF, arteriovenous fistula; FA, false aneurysm; CEG, Corvita endovascular graft.

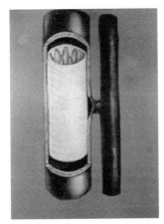

Figure 37-1 Stent-graft device concept for the treatment of an arteriovenous fistula.

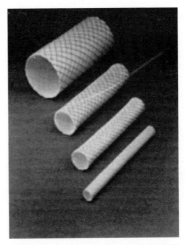

Figure 37-2 Corvita endovascular graft in different sizes.

were nine post-traumatic arteriovenous fistulae and seven false aneurysms. These were located in the subclavian artery (nine), axillary artery (three), common carotid artery (three), and internal carotid artery (one). The cause of the arterial lesion was penetrating trauma in all but one case. The penetrating trauma was gunshot, stab injury, or iatrogenic. The iatrogenic injuries arose from inadvertent arterial puncture during introduction of a central venous catheter.

GENERAL APPROACH

The guiding principle of repair was occlusion of the arterial injury from within the arterial lumen. This was accomplished by implanting a tubular metallic mesh stent covered by Dacron fabric, polytetrafluoroethylene (PTFE), or vein (Fig. 37-1). Occluding the arterial injury from within the lumen then corrected the false aneurysm or arteriovenous communication. In this regard, all the procedures were similar to one another.

The clinical diagnosis in each case was supported by objective imaging, including color duplex ultrasound and arteriography. These methods were employed in every patient.

All procedures were conducted with the patient under local anesthesia, and the stent-graft was introduced from a remote site into the arterial tree, percutaneously or through a small incision designed to expose the entry site. Arteries utilized for access included the common femoral, common carotid, and axillary.

The stent employed was a Palmaz (Johnson & Johnson Interventional Systems) mounted on an angioplasty balloon catheter whose diameter matched that of the artery to be treated. The stent was designed to have a final diameter 10% to 15% in excess of the diameter of the artery in order to obtain secure fixation. The material used for stent coverage included Dacron, PTFE, polycarbonate urethane polymer (Oravein, Corvita Corp.) (Fig. 37–2), and autologous vein (Fig. 37–3). The stent coverings were attached to the stent with four 6-0 polypropylene sutures placed two at either end of the graft at 180 degrees to one another. The Corvita endovascular stent was produced by covering a self-expanding metallic stent with biocompatible elastomeric polycarbonate urethane (Corethane). This is manufactured in a variety of sizes to adapt to the injured vessel.

The entire device of balloon and stent-graft was compressed into an introducer sheath. The smallest sheath possible was used to facilitate introduction and progression into the artery. Guide catheters (9- to 10-Fr.) were used for deployment of the stent.

Choice of Covering

In one patient presenting with acquired immunodeficiency syndrome, autologous vein was used to cover the stent. The vein and not the stent synthetic graft (foreign body) was placed adjacent to the lesion. It was believed that the vein would be more resistant to infection than the synthetic material.

An additional patient with a post-traumatic internal carotid dissection received a vein-covered stent

Figure 37-3 Preparation of a vein-covered Palmaz stent.

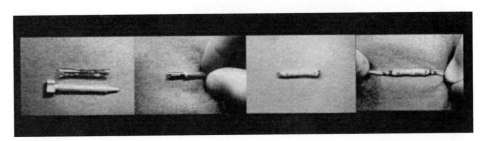

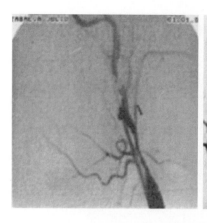
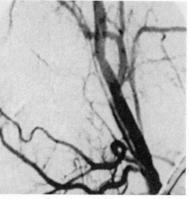

Figure 37-4 Case 1. Internal carotid artery false aneurysm treated with a stent-vein.

placed at the base of the skull. The objective in this case was to create a less thrombogenic surface with which to cover the false aneurysm. The false aneurysm had been the source of thrombus that caused five separate cerebral infarctions. The procedure was successful in preventing further cerebral embolization (Fig. 37–4).

Polycarbonate urethane was used in one case of subclavian artery injury to cover a Palmaz stent.

RESULTS

The false aneurysm or arteriovenous fistulae were closed completely by one or more stent-graft devices in 15 of 16 patients. In the single case of partial failure of the main stent-graft, an additional procedure was necessitated because of an additional arteriovenous fistula in a branch of the subclavian artery. This was closed by a detachable balloon placed in the scapular branch of the thyrocervical trunk (Fig. 37–5). Interestingly, all patients with long-standing arteriovenous fistulae had a significant stenosis of the artery at the site of injury. The stenosis necessitated treatment by inflation with a shorter and stronger balloon. In many of the arteriovenous fistulae, a false aneurysm was present in addition to the direct artery-to-vein connection. This finding did not

change the fundamental strategy employed—the arterial tear was covered with a stent-graft in all cases.

The Corvita endovascular graft is porous. High-flow arteriovenous fistulae therefore remained open up to 24 hours generally after graft introduction and after heparin reversal. In one patient, such a fistula remained open for 7 days and necessitated introduction of a Palmaz stent covered with PTFE. This achieved complete sealing.

COMPLICATIONS

One patient developed a hematoma in the inguinal region that required surgical drainage. No other short- or long-term complications were encountered.

FOLLOW-UP

The follow-up protocol called for color duplex ultrasound evaluation 6 months after arterial repair and yearly after the first year. Fourteen of 16 patients continued to demonstrate stent-graft patency and remained asymptomatic.

One patient with an internal carotid artery false aneurysm became asymptomatic after stent-graft treatment. The Doppler follow-up examination showed flow alteration after 13 months of implantation, and digital arteriography revealed a 90% stenosis due to stent compression. The patient refused further treatment and remained asymptomatic on warfarin (Coumadin) therapy. Spontaneous revascularization through the circle of Willis was seen.

One patient with an iatrogenic common carotid artery false aneurysm was successfully treated (Fig. 37–6). Subsequent neurosurgery to correct an anterior cerebral artery aneurysm led to death from left cerebral infarction.

CONCLUSIONS

The feasibility of endoluminal repair of false aneurysms and arteriovenous fistulae has been demonstrated by this group of cases and the case reports of others. The procedure is new and time is needed to define the future role of this innovative approach. The technique is certainly less invasive, produces

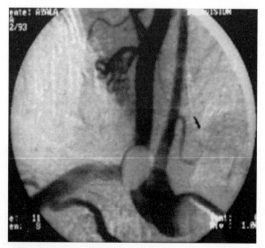

Figure 37-5 Case 2. Subclavian arteriovenous fistula treated with a stent-graft and detachable balloon.

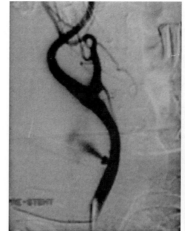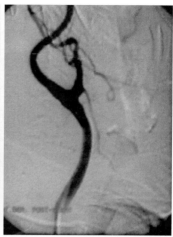

Figure 37-6 Case 3. Common carotid artery false aneurysm treated with a Corvita endovascular graft.

less post-procedural pain and disability, and costs less than conventional surgical repair, largely owing to a markedly shortened recovery time. Thus, the endovascular procedure compares favorably with the approaches used in the past. In the future, stent-grafts may be included in the armamentaria of trauma centers and may be used for civilian and military arterial injuries. The potential of temporary or permanent control of massive bleeding is an attractive one.

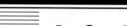

CHAPTER 38

Inferior Petrosal Sinus Sampling

J.J. Connors III / J.C. Wojak

RATIONALE FOR PROCEDURE

Local venous sampling has been performed elsewhere in the body for numerous reasons (e.g., renal vein renin sampling). The primary reason to perform venous sampling in the head and neck region is for evaluation of the secretory nature of a possible pituitary microadenoma. Most commonly, this is to evaluate for a possible tumor-secreting adrenocorticotropic hormone (ACTH) (Cushing's *disease*), as opposed to other causes of the Cushing's *syndrome* (principally ectopic adrenocorticotropin secretion from an occult tumor). The endocrinologist can then use this information to guide therapy. This test has been shown to reliably determine whether or not there is a pituitary tumor, a peripheral ectopic source of ACTH, or primary adrenal disease. In a review of 281 patients with Cushing's syndrome, 215 were surgically proved to have Cushing's disease, 20 had ectopic secretion, and 11 had primary adrenal dysfunction, for a success rate of 100%.[1]

A ratio of peak inferior petrosal sinus (IPS) level compared with peripheral serum level (P), or IPS/P ratio, of >2.0 in the basal metabolic state identified 205 out of 215 patients with Cushing's disease (sensitivity 95%) with no false-positive results (specificity 100%). After administration of corticotropin-releas-

ing hormone (CRH), all 203 patients with Cushing's disease were correctly identified (sensitivity 100%), with no false-positive results (100% specificity). The threshold IPS/P ratio for diagnosis had to be increased to >3.0 for the results to be this impressive.

Of note is the fact that if the results from only one inferior petrosal sinus were used for evaluation, the sensitivity was much lower. In patients with true Cushing's disease (a microadenoma in the pituitary

---

T A B L E   3 8 - 1   Response of Inferior Petrosal Sinus and Peripheral ACTH Levels to CRH in a Patient with Cushing's Disease

Time (Min)	Left IPS Level (pg/ml)	Right IPS Level	Peripheral Level
−5	804	933	48
0 (CRH given)	598	1,382	37
+2	24,170	1,470	46
+5	38,500	1,431	216
+10	13,572	1,451	442

This patient had a surgically proven microadenoma on the left side of the pituitary gland.

CRH, Corticotropin-releasing hormone.

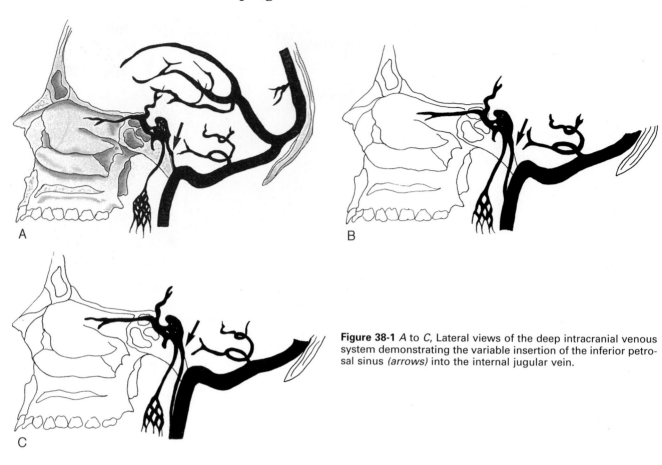

A

B

C

Figure 38-1 *A* to *C,* Lateral views of the deep intracranial venous system demonstrating the variable insertion of the inferior petrosal sinus *(arrows)* into the internal jugular vein.

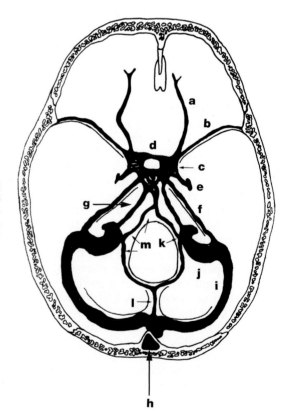

Figure 38-2 Axial view of the venous structures at the skull base, including the superior ophthalmic vein (a), sphenoparietal sinus (b), cavernous sinus (c), intercavernous sinus (d), emissary vein (e), superior petrosal sinus (f), inferior petrosal sinus (g), superior sagittal sinus (h), transverse sinus (i), sigmoid sinus (j), jugular bulb (k), occipital sinus (l), and basivertebral plexus (m).

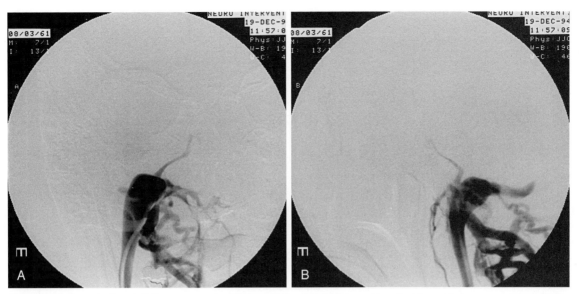

Figure 38-3 Case 1. *A* and *B,* Posteroanterior (PA) and lateral right internal jugular/sigmoid sinus venogram. Reflux into the inferior petrosal sinus was obtained, but the exact origin is still difficult to identify.

gland), a ratio of >1.4 in the detected adrenocorticotropin concentration from one sinus to the other correctly predicted the presence of the adenoma location in 68% in patients during basal sampling and in 71% of 105 patients after stimulation with CRH. An example of results that can be expected from a procedure such as this are presented in Table 38–1. Note the laterality of results in this particular case.

If a primary adenoma is determined to be present in the pituitary gland, the surgeon can use this information to decide which half of the pituitary gland contains the offending secretory tumor, and thus which half to remove, rather than removing the entire gland and potentially causing panhypopituitar-

ism. Usually, however, the presence of a tumor can be detected at surgery. Other indications for venous sampling exist, but the procedure is the same.

TECHNIQUE OF SAMPLING

The venous drainage of the pituitary gland is into the cavernous sinus. The cavernous sinus has a variable drainage pathway but usually drains into the bilateral inferior petrosal sinuses, superior petrosal sinuses, and basilar venous plexus (Figs. 38–1 and 38–2). These all have a variable drainage course into the internal jugular system and paraspinal venous plexus.

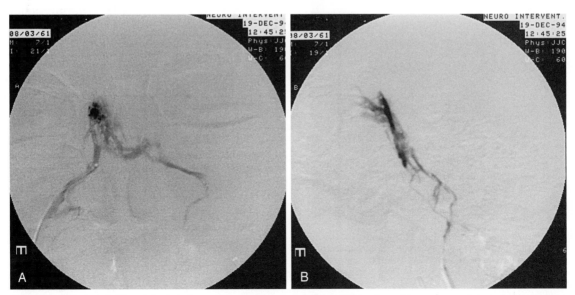

Figure 38-4 A and *B,* The right inferior petrosal sinus was successfully selected by means of the microguidewire followed by the microcatheter. Contrast injection through the microcatheter reveals the anatomy of the ipsilateral inferior petrosal sinus as well as the contralateral side. The selection of the opposite inferior petrosal sinus is now aided by this visualization.

Case 1 continues

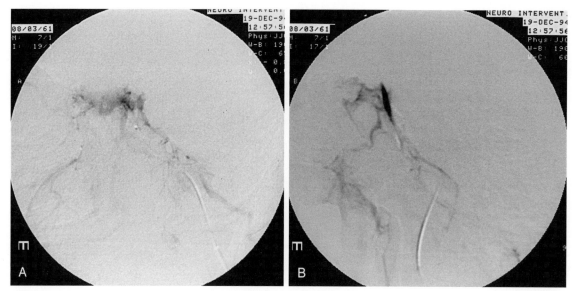

Figure 38-5 A and B, Cannulation of the left inferior petrosal sinus results in the microcatheter being nearly occlusive. Note the course of this left catheter; it is actually in the major drainage path of the pituitary as demonstrated on the previous injection from the opposite side (as desired), but the current venous drainage appears to be via another vessel (owing to the near occlusion by the catheter). (Also note the venous drainage through the retropharyngeal collaterals.) The catheter on the left is in the correct location, but venous sampling needs to be very slow to allow normal flow to the catheter and prevent drawing from other territories (either contralateral contamination of the sample or just ipsilateral dilutional effects).

For evaluation of the side of a possible microadenoma, accurate sampling is required for testing. This is achieved by obtaining simultaneous multiple venous specimens, one from each side of drainage of

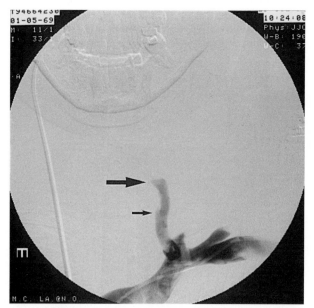

Figure 38-6 Case 2. Once access has been made to the left subclavian vein, a forceful injection can be made to evaluate the anatomy. This reveals the large inferior thyroidal vein (small arrow), the stub of the internal jugular vein (large arrow), and a suprascapular vein as well as the subclavian vein continuing toward the axillary vein. The stub of the jugular vein reveals the location of the proximal large valve, which has to be traversed. It is at this point that repeated probing during various stages of respiration will catch the valve at a point when it is open (see text).

the pituitary (the IPS) along with a concurrent peripheral nonselective sample. Superselective sampling of the cavernous sinus is not necessary and may be self-defeating. Although the catheter may be in the cavernous sinus, the pituitary gland may drain 3 mm anterior to that particular point; a position somewhat downstream (i.e., in the IPS) may catch all the cavernous sinus drainage. Multiple aspirates are necessary because of the possible episodic secretory nature of the tumor and because these sensitive microassays may produce variable individual test results. Several examples of IPS cannulation are given in Figures 38–3 to 38–11.

Anticoagulation

Systemic anticoagulation is maintained during the procedure with a bolus of 5000 units of heparin followed by 2000 U/hr given intravenously after vascular access has been successfully completed from each side. In addition, aspirin (325 mg) is administered before beginning the case. The catheters will be in place for at least 30 minutes, and depending on the ease of catheterization, one side may be indwelling for 1 to 2 hours. Venous thrombosis of the IPS or cavernous sinus is an undesired event.

Venous Access and Jugular Vein Catheterization

Bilateral venous access is necessary, typically by a standard transfemoral approach. On one side, a 6-Fr. sheath is placed for the simultaneous peripheral venous samplings. The ideal catheters are custom steam-shaped Vinuela catheters (Cook, Inc.), but

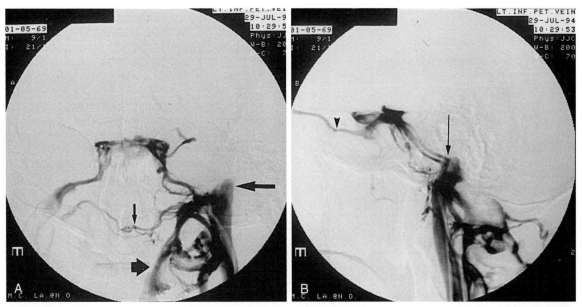

Figure 38-7 A and B, Once the catheter has been maneuvered up the jugular vein, the sudden turn marks the beginning of the sigmoid sinus. An injection at this point reveals the characteristic hook of the inferior petrosal sinus (IPS) *(thin arrow)* as it enters the tissues of the neck near the apex of the jugular vein. Note, however, that the IPS does not appear to drain directly into the internal jugular vein *(large arrow)* but has a short segment separate from this destination. Also note the extensive collateral anastomoses with the paravertebral and occipital venous plexus *(fat arrow)*.

There is not only filling of the entire left IPS but filling of the left cavernous sinus, the clival anastomotic channels to the opposite cavernous sinus, and the right IPS. In addition, there is filling across the retropharyngeal prevertebral venous network anterior to C1 *(arrow)*. Note the superior ophthalmic vein also filling on this injection *(arrowhead)*. The apex of the contrast within the internal jugular vein is superior, posterior, and lateral to the point at which the IPS joins the jugular vein. Once the exploratory catheter or wire reaches this apex without selecting the IPS, it has gone too far.

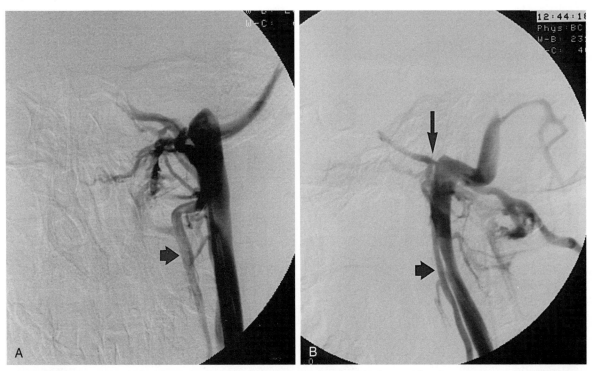

Figure 38-8 Case 3. A and B, Injection of the most cephalad portion of the internal jugular vein, just where it starts to become the sigmoid sinus, reveals an interesting finding. Even though the IPS is opacified, it appears that the communication to the jugular system is very small *(arrow)*. Indeed, the IPS appears to drain primarily via a large sinusoidal vein paralleling the internal jugular vein *(fat arrow)*. While it may be possible to reach the IPS through this tiny channel, it may be necessary to utilize the larger vein, which will probably join the jugular system in the low neck region.

Case 3 continues

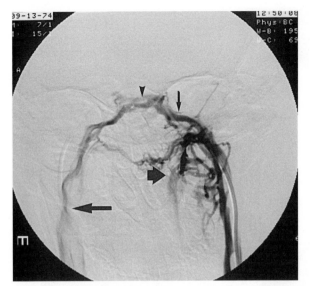

Figure 38-9 The catheter has been steered to the small junction with the IPS seen above. The tip is probably wedged into position. Injection reveals abundant filling of the ipsilateral IPS *(small arrow)*, the cavernous and retroclival sinuses *(arrowhead)*, and the retropharyngeal (prevertebral) venous anastomotic plexus *(fat arrow)*. Note that the internal jugular vein itself is not opacified (probably because of the catheter filling the anastomotic channel seen above).

The long descending vein from the IPS is well seen, as is the IPS on the other side. In addition, the opposite IPS is seen to flow for a few centimeters inferior to the level of the apex of the internal jugular vein before washing into a larger venous structure *(large arrow)*.

other shapes can be used (e.g., JB-1 curve, Berenstein curve, H-1 curve). Both catheters should have a gradual hockey-stick–type curve placed, one with a 70-degree curve and a 1 to 2 cm distal, straight portion, and the other with a 45-degree curve. The radius of the curve should be about that of a quarter. The 70-degree angle catheter is used to cross the midline selectively from the superior vena cava through the innominate vein and then to advance up the proximal left subclavian–left jugular system.[2]

After access has been made on each side, the 70-degree curve catheter is used to access the left subclavian vein region. This catheter should be the one inserted in the left leg because when sampling is being performed, it is easier to keep track of which catheter goes where if the sampling catheters match the side they are sampling.

The innominate vein and its junction with the superior vena cava are relatively large; therefore, the catheter should have a large curve and tip. Once aimed in the right direction, a good hydrophilic-coated guidewire allows easy passage from the right-sided superior vena cava to the left subclavian vein. A forceful injection into the subclavian vein in the region of the sternoclavicular joint on the left shows the anatomy of the inflow veins in the region. Usually only "stubs" are seen because of their valve systems (Fig. 38–6). Other stubs are seen but are smaller, and most are more distal (lateral) than the large jugular inflow tract (except, perhaps, for thyroidal veins).

Catheterization of the internal jugular vein is sometimes tricky; a valve is usually located at the region of the thoracic inlet, and getting the wire past this can sometimes be a matter of luck. Repetitive prodding during various phases of respiration with a J-curved hydrophilic-coated guidewire or an angle-tip wire usually succeeds in getting past this obstruction. This problem is frequently worse on the left.

Accessing the right jugular vein is usually straightforward, but occasionally, the internal jugular vein

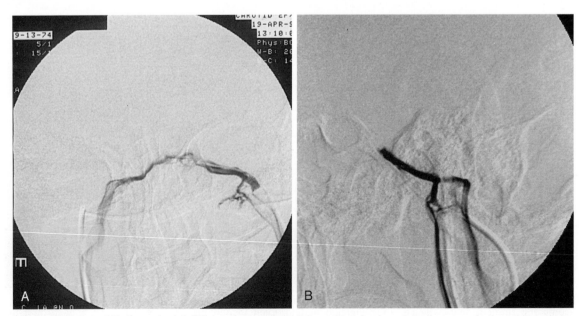

Figure 38-10 A and B, Once the left IPS has been successfully catheterized, an injection reveals the microcatheter tip to be in an ideal location. However, the catheter within the right internal jugular vein is *above* the level at which the IPS appears to drain into the jugular venous system.

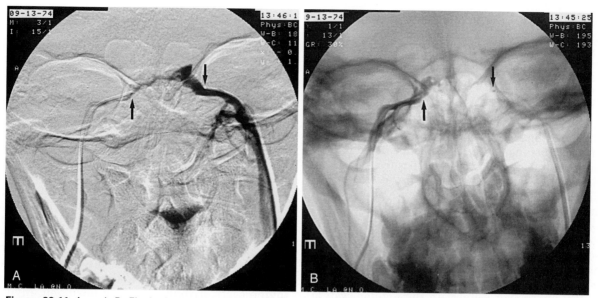

Figure 38-11 A and *B,* Final placement of the two sampling catheters *(arrows).* Injection is made through each microcatheter. Both catheters could be slightly withdrawn (1 cm) and the location would still suffice.

enters the subclavian system slightly lateral to the superior vena cava. The valve can also be a problem on this side but usually is not.

Accessing the Inferior Petrosal Sinus

Once both catheters are in the jugular veins, finding the IPS is the real challenge. The anatomy of the venous drainage in the region of the skull base is inconstant, and the exact entry of the IPS into the jugular system can be difficult to find. In addition, the jugular and sigmoid sinus channels are large, and the entry of the IPS often is very small.[3]

Usually, the IPS enters the internal jugular vein right where the vein turns posteriorly at the skull base and starts its course to the sigmoid sinus. The IPS entrance is typically at the apex of this curve (*beyond* where it looks like it should be) on the medial superior surface. It enters the jugular vein going posteriorly and laterally and thus is at a relatively acute angle to the jugular vein when approached from below (Fig. 38–7). Careful probing with the Vinuela catheter and repeated squirts of contrast eventually are rewarded with visualization of the small passages leading toward the cavernous sinus region. The catheter should never be advanced into the inferior petrosal sinus.

The orifice of the IPS actually may be found slightly around the curve, past where the Vinuela catheter can select its orifice effectively. In this case, selection can be made with the microwire; a custom shape is necessary to provide a large enough curve for selection in a vessel the size of the jugular vein. A typical Seeker Standard type wire works well.

If difficulty is still encountered in locating the origin of the IPS (which is, admittedly, the toughest part of this procedure), then a forceful injection can be made with the Vinuela catheter at the turn in the

jugular vein, with manual compression of the neck over the jugular vein just at the sternal notch. This tends to improve reflux into the true origin of the IPS. Multiplanar viewing is helpful to find the actual entry point.

If this does not work, a more proximal injection (i.e., the catheter lower in the neck) with the same compression technique can be used to evaluate for a possible lower entry of the sinus into the jugular system (Figs. 38–7 to 38–9). Anomalous venous anatomy can frustrate even the most skilled practitioner; if difficulty is encountered, suspect a duplicated jugular vein or anomalous drainage of the IPS.

Evaluation of Venous Anatomy by Arterial Injection

Occasionally it is necessary to catheterize the arterial side, select the internal carotid artery, and perform a standard angiogram to locate the cavernous sinus and visualize its drainage. It can be more rewarding to try to find the IPS from analysis of the venous phase of a good arterial injection. This requires a large volume contrast injection (10 ml) and good digital subtraction equipment and technique.

After the IPS has been found on one side, it is usually a simple matter to advance a microcatheter carefully up to the region just below the cavernous sinus. Frequently the IPS is not actually a well-developed vein but rather a true sinus (a plexus of small channels, hence the name). Careful advancement of the microcatheter is then indicated because of the lack of a true large channel, and care should be taken with the initial aspiration and injection to ensure that the catheter is not wedged and that an overinjection is not made. A contrast injection in this location confirms the correct position for venous sampling. In addition, a forceful injection almost invariably fills across the midline, clearly demonstrating the contralateral IPS. It is then possible to locate the exact entry point of the IPS into the opposite sigmoid sinus.

Anatomic Variants

On one occasion, we almost found it necessary to cross the midline with the microcatheter (through the cavernous sinus and basilar plexus anastomoses) and perform the sampling of the opposite side in this manner because of the difficulty in accessing the opposite IPS. Eventually, the junction of the IPS with the jugular vein was found *at the base of the neck;* the two veins (the jugular and the IPS) coursed parallel to each other for about 12 cm before anastomosing, separated by only a thin web the entire distance. Anatomic variants such as this are not infrequent and can frustrate the process of catheterization.

The IPS may never connect to the jugular system but may drain by means of a plexus into the deep cervical plexus (paravertebral plexus), either anterior or posterior to the brainstem. This can present a real challenge. Arterial injection should be used to define this anatomy.

The microcatheter should be in a final location in which adequate flow goes past the microcatheter to maintain a good secretory rate for sampling; that is, if there is any flow restriction, some of the drainage may go to the opposite side, contaminating the samples. The catheter tips should be slightly below the level of the sella to sample the total output on that side accurately.

Never attempt to advance the 5-Fr. catheter into the IPS, because this can cause venous damage or perforation. In addition, sampling from the 5-Fr. catheter at the base of the IPS can yield false results (venous inflow from the jugular vein may contaminate the sample). Care should be maintained when dealing with the IPS; venous drainage from the pons and brainstem can be directly or indirectly into the inferior petrosal sinus and basilar venous plexus, and occlusion or damage to these venules can be devastating. If the orifice of the inferior petrosal sinus is occluded, the venous samples may be inaccurate. If the microcatheter is in correct position, a slight withdrawal of the macrocatheter while keeping the microcatheter in position may allow better, more hemodynamically normal flow.

Sampling Procedure

After the catheters are in position bilaterally, samples are obtained from each microcatheter and the peripheral sheath simultaneously and labeled as such, with times and locations given. Five samples are obtained from each location, spaced at 5-minute intervals. The microcatheters each require about 2 minutes to aspirate a 3-ml sample. For ACTH, these samples are placed in the tubes used for complete blood counts (usually "lavender-top") and kept on ice. Prolactin and growth hormone samples are placed

in serum-chemistry or "red-top" tubes (not serum-separator types). Prior contact should be made with the appropriate laboratory for confirmation of these instructions and for coordination in handling to ensure that the samples get to the right location. It is extremely frustrating for the patient, the clinicians, and the interventional neuroradiologist to have a laboratory error necessitate repeating the whole procedure.

Challenge or stimulation testing can be performed. For these testing purposes, prestimulation sampling can be performed, as described earlier, followed by hormonal stimulation and subsequent sampling. Alternatively, prestimulation followed by sampling can be performed. This procedure has not been uniformly adopted, but reports have suggested the possibility of an increased positive test rate.

For ACTH testing, corticotropin-releasing hormone (Corticobiss, Bissendorf, Wedemark FRG) or Acthrel (ovine corticotropin-releasing hormone, investigational under FDA evaluation in the United States) can be administered in a 100-µg intravenous bolus just before sampling (or 1 µg/kg). ACTH levels respond rapidly, within 5 to 30 minutes, whereas cortisol levels rise in 30 to 120 minutes. In addition 200 µg of Thyroliberin (Merck, Darmstadt, FRG) can be administered; this has more influence on prolactin secretion.[3] Multiple samples can be obtained as described earlier. This technique may increase the sensitivity to detection of adenomas (for which there is about a 10% false-negative sampling rate). There is some concern regarding these pituitary extracts, owing to the recent increase in incidence of spongiform encephalopathies among cows and sheep and the possible association with Jakob-Creutzfeldt disease in humans.

After the samples have been obtained, the heparin is reversed with protamine, and the catheters and sheath are withdrawn.

Sampling Errors Due to Anatomic Variation

Although the anatomy of most patients is conducive to venous sampling, variants may render these samples inaccurate, as when there is asymmetric drainage of the pituitary gland with more drainage going naturally to one side or the other. This variant may cause the hormone level to be high on one side or the other whether the tumor is located right or left. Presampling visualization of the anatomy may give an indication of this possibility.

TECHNICAL PROBLEMS, COMPLICATIONS, AND SOLUTIONS

Inferior petrosal sinus sampling is a safe and reliable procedure. In the past, the primary complications were related to direct damage to the sinus from forceful catheterization or from thrombosis of the sinus. Both of these conditions are preventable.

Never catheterize the sinus with a 5-Fr. catheter. Always use the 5-Fr. catheter simply to select the distal jugular vein and do roadmapping. Use a microwire to select the sinus and a microcatheter to catheterize the sinus and do the sampling.

Always anticoagulate the patient during the procedure. If care is maintained during catheterization, bleeding should not be a problem. We always use a micropuncture set to catheterize the femoral veins bilaterally, so there is no inadvertent puncture of the artery. This can be an outpatient procedure if there are no untoward events.

REFERENCES

1. Oldfield EH, Doppman JL, Nieman LK, et al. Petrosal sinus sampling with and without corticotropin-releasing hormone for the differential diagnosis of Cushing's syndrome. *N Engl J Med* 1991;325:897–905.

2. Miller DL, Doppman JL. Petrosal sinus sampling: technique and rationale. *Radiology* 1991;178:37–47.
3. Miller DL, Doppman JL, Chang R. Anatomy of the junction of the inferior petrosal sinus and the internal jugular vein. *AJNR* 1993;14:1075–1083.
4. Strack TR, Schild HH, Bohl J, et al. Selective bilateral blood sampling from the inferior petrosal sinus in Cushing's disease: effects of corticotropin-releasing factor and thyrotropin-releasing hormone on pituitary secretion. *Cardiovasc Intervent Radiol* 1993;16:287–292.

ADDITIONAL READINGS

Merola B, Colao A, Rossi E, et al. Hormonal gradients between inferior petrosal sinuses in various pituitary diseases. *Acta Endocrinol* 1992;126:419–424.
Miller DL. Neurologic complications of petrosal sinus sampling [Letter]. *Radiology* 1992;185:878.
Miller DL, Doppman JL, Peterman SB, et al. Neurologic complications of petrosal sinus sampling. *Radiology* 1992;185:143–147.

CHAPTER 39

Nerve Blocks and Discectomy

J.C. Wojak / J.J. Connors III

NERVE BLOCKS

Nerve blocks should be performed by interventional neuroradiologists. They are commonly employed by oncologists or pain management specialists for certain types of chronic pain or cancer. They can also be used as a diagnostic tool in the evaluation of chronic pain. Nerve blocks have been performed in certain locations by personnel with no real training in percutaneous fluoroscopic work, with resultant questionable results.

Nerve blocks not only block pain impulses but also can interrupt motor and sympathetic reflexes. The clinical pain relief, analgesia, and reflex interruption have been noted to outlast the duration of effect of the agent used; this is the rationale for treatment of chronic pain with repeated blocks.[1]

Agents

The agents used in nerve blocks fall into the general categories of local anesthetics, corticosteroids, and neurolytic agents. Commonly used local anesthetic agents include lidocaine, procaine, and bupivacaine. Lidocaine has the fastest onset of action but is intermediate in duration between procaine and bupivacaine. Lidocaine is used in concentrations of 1% to 1.5%, up to 7 mg/kg. Procaine is used in concentrations of 1% to 2%, up to 15 mg/kg. Bupivacaine is used in 0.25% to 0.5% concentrations, up to 2.5 mg/kg.

Corticosteroids can be used alone or in conjunction with local anesthetics. The mechanism of action is presumed to be reduction of edema in the irritated nerve and surrounding tissue.

Neurolytic agents are used to achieve a prolonged or permanent block. The most commonly used agents are ethanol (50% to 100%) and phenol (5% aqueous solution). These agents are most often used in sympathetic ganglion blocks.[1]

General Technical Aspects

Nerve blocks generally are performed without major sedation. It is important to have a thorough understanding of the anatomy in question as well as a knowledge of the maximal amount of agent that can be used. Frequent aspiration to verify that a vessel has not been entered is necessary, especially immediately before injection of the blocking agent. Contrast injection can also be used to confirm an extravascular location.

Most complications are due to toxic reactions to high blood levels of the agent. When caused by local anesthetic agents, these manifest as central nervous system excitement followed by depression, hypotension, decreased cardiac output, and bradycardia. Treatment is supportive. Allergic reactions are rare.

Paravertebral Somatic Nerve Block

Paravertebral somatic nerve blocks are used to block conduction in a selected spinal nerve at the point of its exit from the intervertebral foramen. This produces anesthesia confined to a single dermatome, which can be useful in localizing somatic pain and in identifying the affected root or roots.

For blocks in the thoracic and lumbar regions, the patient is positioned prone. Spinal needles (22-gauge, 7.5 to 10 cm long) are usually employed. After the spinous processes are identified and marked, a point 3 to 4 cm lateral to the superior edge of the appropriate process (on the side to be blocked) is identified and anesthetized. The spinal needle is inserted perpendicular to the skin until it touches the transverse process. Note is made of the depth of the needle. The needle is then withdrawn slightly and angled caudally until it passes below the transverse process. It is then advanced until the final depth is equal to the depth to the transverse process plus 2 cm (thoracic) or 3 cm (lumbar). The position is verified radiographically with fluoroscopy or spot film. Sacral nerves are approached by the sacral foramina under fluoroscopic guidance. Again, the needle should be advanced until it touches the surrounding sacrum. The depth of the needle tip is noted. The needle is then manipulated to advance it into the foramen about 2 cm beyond the distance to the sacrum.

Once the needle is situated properly, gentle aspiration is performed to make sure that a vessel has not been inadvertently entered. If blood is obtained, the needle must be repositioned. Once a negative aspiration is obtained, about 3 ml of the chosen agent is injected.

For a cervical block, the patient is positioned supine, with the head turned away from the side to be blocked. The anterior tubercle of C6 is identified fluoroscopically and by palpation, along with the transverse processes of C2 to C5, which usually lie about 5 mm below a line from the tip of the mastoid process to the anterior tubercle of C6. These transverse processes should be marked. A 22-gauge needle (4 to 5 cm in length) is carefully advanced, under local anesthesia and fluoroscopic guidance, in a slightly caudal direction until it rests on the appropriate transverse process. A nerve stimulator can be used to adjust the needle position so that maximal response is obtained from the nerve. Care must be taken to avoid the vertebral artery; it is important to aspirate before injection of the agent. Injection of 2 to 3 ml of the chosen agent should be sufficient.

Sympathetic Ganglion Block

Sympathetic ganglion blocks are used to interrupt the sympathetic pathways where they are separated from somatic nerves. They are most commonly performed at the stellate ganglion, the celiac plexus, and the lumbar ganglia. Blocks in these locations affect the upper body quadrant, abdomen, and lower body quadrant. Stellate and lumbar ganglion blocks are used for the diagnosis and treatment of reflex sympathetic dystrophy and vasospastic disorders. In the case of reflex sympathetic dystrophy, repeated blocks may be curative in mild cases, especially when the relief outlasts the duration of effect of the anesthetic agent used. Celiac block can be used to differentiate between abdominal wall pain (somatic) and visceral pain. Celiac block with neurolytic agents is used as a palliative treatment for intractable visceral abdominal pain (such as that caused by pancreatic cancer).

Stellate Ganglion Block

The stellate ganglion is approached at the C6 level by a paratracheal approach. The patient is positioned supine with the head tilted back. The anterior tubercle of C6 is identified at the anterior margin of the sternocleidomastoid muscle. The muscle and carotid sheath are gently retracted laterally by a finger placed on the tubercle. The carotid artery should be felt pulsating lateral to the finger. A 22-gauge needle (4 to 5 cm) is attached to a syringe (10-cc) containing the anesthetic agent of choice and inserted under local anesthesia to the tubercle. Careful aspiration is performed; bony contact should be maintained. A small test dose is injected, followed by injection of 10 ml of agent. This spreads along the sympathetic chain from the middle cervical ganglion to the upper thoracic ganglia. Slight elevation of the patient's head after injection helps the agent to spread. A successful block results in Horner's syndrome and in increased temperature and absence of sweating of the affected hand. Transient hoarseness due to recurrent laryngeal nerve block is not uncommon. Other complications are rare; they include total brachial plexus block and phrenic nerve block.[2]

Celiac Ganglion Block

The patient is positioned prone for a celiac ganglion block. The 12th ribs and L1 spinous processes are marked. A horizontal line is drawn through the caudal edge of the L1 spinous process, extending about 7 cm laterally in either direction. Lines are drawn from the lateral limits of this line to the cranial edge of the L1 spinous process. This is the projection of the pathway of the needles. Local anesthesia is administered at the lateral point on one side. A 20-gauge spinal needle is inserted at this point, directed medially at a 45-degree angle. It is advanced slightly cranially along the line previously drawn (a second 22-gauge needle can be placed along this line to serve as a marker for fluoroscopy) until it touches L1. It is then withdrawn slightly and readvanced at a steeper medial angle (about 60 degrees) until it passes anterior to the vertebral body. The procedure is repeated from the other side. Both needles are carefully aspirated. For a temporary block, 20 ml of diluted anesthetic solution (e.g., 0.5% lidocaine) is then injected through each needle. For neurolysis, an equal amount of 50% ethanol can be used. If ethanol is used, the needle should be cleared with saline before withdrawal to avoid tracking the alcohol along the path, with possible damage to other structures. A proper anesthetic block produces short-lived burning. Alcohol blocks take several days to reach full effect. Side effects include transient (2 to 3 days) back pain and orthostatic hypotension, which are treated symptomatically.[2]

Lumbar Ganglion Block

The patient is positioned prone for lumbar ganglion block (the lateral decubitus position can be used if lateral fluoroscopy is available). Long (10 to 15 cm) spinal needles are used (20- or 22-gauge). The L2 spinous process is marked. Local anesthesia is used 4.5 to 5 cm lateral to this. A spinal needle is inserted at this point and directed slightly cephalad until the transverse process is reached. The depth is noted, and the needle is withdrawn partially and directed slightly more caudally and medially to clear the transverse process. The final depth is equal to the depth to the transverse process plus 3.5 to 4 cm. If the vertebral body is struck before this depth, less medial angulation should be used. The needle tip should be just lateral to the anterior aspect of the vertebral body on lateral and posteroanterior images. As usual, careful aspiration is then performed, followed by injection of 10 ml of the chosen anesthetic agent.

Facet Block

Many patients presenting with low back pain and leg pain do not have disc herniation, compression of a radicular nerve from other causes, or a neurologic deficit; these patients are said to have a *pseudoradiculopathy*. The posterior primary ramus of the radicular nerve, which innervates the apophyseal joints, paraspinal muscles, and interspinous ligament, is thought to be the primary mediator of pain in these patients. Immediately after the dorsal and ventral root join to form a radicular nerve, the nerve splits into a larger anterior ramus and a smaller posterior primary ramus. The posterior primary ramus passes through the intertransverse ligament dorsally, then follows the groove at the junction of the transverse process and inferior pedicle. The articular nerve then separates and branches over the inferolateral aspect of the facet joint to enter the joint capsule;

the remainder of the ramus continues dorsally to innervate other structures.

Patients experiencing pain related to the articular nerve or primary ramus typically complain of low back pain and vague hip or thigh pain. The pain is relieved by slumping and rest and is exacerbated by motion. Once other causes of radicular pain have been excluded, facet block can be considered. Patients with lateral spinal fusions are generally not candidates for this procedure because of distorted anatomy.

Several methods of block can be used. In one technique, a 20-gauge spinal needle is advanced under fluoroscopic guidance and local anesthesia, with the patient prone, to lie along the lateral aspect of the facet joint. Alternatively, the tube or the patient can be obliquely turned with the side of interest toward the image intensifier, so that the central ray is pointing down the plane between the articulating facets. The needle is then advanced under local anesthesia to enter or nearly enter the facet joint. In either case, 1 to 2 ml of the chosen anesthetic agent is instilled after aspiration (we prefer to use celestone, 2 ml, along with 1 ml of bupivacaine). Blocks are usually performed at the L3-4, L4-5, and L5-S1 levels bilaterally.

A third approach is to block the posterior primary ramus before the origin of the articular nerve. With the patient prone, the junction of the inferior pedicle of the selected facet joint and its transverse process is identified. Under local anesthesia, the spinal needle is inserted sightly lateral to this point. The needle is advanced until it reaches the transverse process, then walked medially until it lies at the lateral, cephalad margin of the pedicle. After aspiration, 2 ml of the chosen agent is instilled.

When properly performed, this procedure is safe and relatively complication free. If patients are chosen appropriately, a significant number achieve at least some relief from pain.

DISCECTOMY

The initial foray of neuroradiologists into the realm of treatment of lumbar disc disease was the percutaneous injection of chymopapain into the disc space to dissolve the nucleus pulposus (chemonucleolysis).[3] This procedure fell into disfavor because of a combination of technical and anaphylactic complications.

Several techniques have since been developed for the performance of percutaneous lumbar discectomy. Two of these involve mechanical manipulation of the disc.[4] The nucleus pulposus can be selectively removed from the site of herniation using a variety of automated and manual instruments under endoscopic visualization. This is a procedure best left to surgeons. Alternatively, the nucleus pulposus can be removed from the center of the disc space (intradiscal decompression) by means of a single automated instrument (nucleotome). This instrument combines a suction and irrigation device with an oscillating knife. Although direct decompression of the nerve

is not achieved, the intradiscal pressure is lowered, supposedly allowing a decompressive shift of the remaining (herniated) portion of the nucleus. This instrument is inserted under fluoroscopic control, and this procedure can be performed by interventional neuroradiologists (see Chapter 40).

Selective percutaneous discectomy performed under endoscopic control can yield results comparable to open microdiscectomy, but only in a carefully selected patient population.[4] No organized trial has been performed to compare automated percutaneous lumbar discectomy with surgical microdiscectomy, chemonucleolysis, or selective percutaneous discectomy with endoscopic control. Early results suggest that rigorous patient selection is necessary for this procedure to result in an acceptable rate of success. A systematic percutaneous approach to the treatment of disc disease with encouraging results is presented in Chapter 40.

An exciting new technique is percutaneous laser discectomy.[5] Adjustable fibers (quartz) placed under endoscopic or fluoroscopic control are used to apply the laser energy. The type of laser best suited to this procedure, how best to perform the procedure, and the appropriate patient population are still being investigated, but the early results are promising and indicate that this is potentially a safe and useful method of treatment. To the extent that it can be performed under fluoroscopic guidance, percutaneous laser discectomy could fall into the realm of the interventional neuroradiologist.

REFERENCES

1. Bonica JJ. Clinical Applications of Diagnostic and Therapeutic Nerve Blocks. Springfield, IL: Charles C Thomas, 1959.
2. Moore DC. Regional Block: A Handbook for Use in the Clinical Practice of Medicine and Surgery, 4th ed. Springfield, IL: Charles C Thomas, 1965.
3. Smith L. Chemonucleolysis: personal history, trials and tribulations. *Clin Orthop* 1993;287:117–124.
4. Mayer HM. Spine update: percutaneous lumbar disc surgery. *Spine* 1994;19:2719–2723.
5. Liebler WA. Percutaneous laser disc nucleotomy. *Clin Orthop* 1995;310:58–66.

ADDITIONAL READINGS

Buy J-N, Moss AA, Singler. CT guided celiac plexus and splanchnic nerve neurolysis. *J Comput Assist Tomog* 1982;6: 315–319.

Haaga JR, Kori SH, Eastwood DW, Borkowski GP. Improved technique for CT-guided celiac ganglia block. *AJR* 1984;142:1201–1204.

Hegedus V. Relief of pancreatic pain by radiography-guided block. *AJR* 1979;133:1101–1103.

Lee MJ, Mueller PR, vanSonnenberg E, et al. CT-guided celiac ganglion block with alcohol. *AJR* 1993;161:633–636.

Lieberman RP, Lieberman SL, Cuka DJ, Lund GB. Celiac plexus and splanchnic nerve block: a review. *Semin Intervent Radiol* 1988;5:213–222.

Moore DC, Bush WH, Burnett LL. Celiac plexus block: a roentgenographic, anatomic study of technique and spread of solution in patients and corpses. *Anesth Analg* 1981;60:369–379.

Whiteman MS, Rosenberg H, Haskin PH, Teplick SK. Celiac plexus block for interventional radiology. *Radiology* 1986; 161:836–838.

Percutaneous Treatment of Cervical and Lumbar Disc Herniations

J.G. Theron

Most of the disc herniations responsible for lumbar or cervical radicular pain resistant to medical treatment can be treated using percutaneous interventional techniques without open surgery. It is beneficial for the patient in the long term to preserve the function of the intervertebral discs as fully as possible.

The main goal of percutaneous intradiscal techniques is to reduce the increased pressure developed in the whole disc and consequently in the herniated portion compressing the nerve root and the posterior longitudinal ligament. Based on experience with 3500 cases since 1980, I routinely use two techniques: chemonucleolysis[1, 2] and percutaneous automated discectomy.[3]

TREATMENT OPTIONS

Chemonucleolysis is an efficient technique that consists of the injection of an enzyme (chymopapain) that chemically lowers the intradiscal pressure. An efficacy of close to 80% in lumbar herniations has been confirmed by numerous authors, taking into consideration both short-term and long-term results.[4–8] In cervical herniations, the efficacy is even better, close to 85%.[9]

Percutaneous automated discectomy is a technique that also lowers the intradiscal pressure by the mechanical process of retrieving a small amount of disc material from within the disc, ordinarily without trying to reach the herniation; this technique also has been used to treat cervical herniations.[10]

The approach to patient treatment is based on these two intradiscal techniques used alone, successively, or conjointly. A recent addition to these tools is the simultaneous injection of the facet joints with local steroids, based on the belief that in most cases, there is regional inflammation and not only a disc problem to be solved (Case 1, Fig. 40–1).

INDICATIONS

The general philosophy concerning the therapeutic indications is based on three points: (1) totally asymptomatic herniations are frequently observed on computed tomography (CT) scans performed for an indication other than a spine problem,[11] and consequently, any images should be correlated with the clinical presentation; (2) the natural history and non-operative treatments of lumbar disc herniations lead to recovery in most cases[12]; and (3) progressively

aggressive therapeutic techniques should be selected and used as indicated in specific cases.

In contrast to the statements of others, I have routinely used chemonucleolysis in voluminous disc herniations (Case 2, Fig. 40–2), in herniations with extrusion of disc material (Case 3, Fig. 40–3), and in patients with an epidural leak demonstrated on the discogram (see Fig. 40–7B). A discogram is always performed at the start of the procedure. A minor motor weakness is common and is not a contraindication to percutaneous techniques. Recent studies have confirmed most of these nonclassical indications.[13]

Medical treatment remains indicated and should be attempted for 4 weeks. This is successful in most cases of discal radiculalgia, but it should be stopped rapidly if the patient develops hyperalgia and sleeplessness because percutaneous techniques usually are able to relieve these symptoms rapidly.

Recurrent disc herniation after surgery at the same level or a herniation occurring in a pregnant woman is not treated percutaneously. Neurologic deficit consistent with a cauda equina syndrome and a history of anaphylactic reactions are other contraindications.

CHOICE OF PROCEDURE

Percutaneous discectomy is used as the primary technique for treatment of lumbar herniations with moderate volume and without canal stenosis or associated degenerative changes. Chemonucleolysis can yield a higher degree of decompression than percutaneous discectomy but is a more aggressive procedure. This technique has advantages: it is extremely well tolerated and almost totally innocuous, and it has an efficacy of nearly 75% for lumbar herniations[14, 15] and of 80% for cervical herniations,[10] including, in this location, extruded herniations (Case 4, Fig. 40–4 and Case 5, Fig. 40–5).

Percutaneous discectomy usually is my primary technique for cervical herniations, unless there are several levels to treat associated with narrow vertebral interspaces. The patient is informed that the goal is to treat and cure the herniation by use of progressively more aggressive techniques and that a complementary decompressive technique might be necessary; the long-term goal is preservation of disc integrity. This way of explaining the possible necessity of a second procedure usually is well understood by the patient. The patient usually accepts an attempt at percutaneous discectomy because of its excellent immediate tolerance and reasonable chance of success. In my experience with lumbar hernia-

Figure 40-1 Case 1. Standard percutaneous treatment of a lumbar disc herniation. *A,* Right posterolateral L5–S1 disc herniation. The patient has a right S1 radiculalgia. The nerve root is in the lateral recess between the herniation and the ligamentum flavum. *B,* An L5–S1 discogram was performed, using a high posterolateral approach with a curved needle. The contrast fills the herniated material. *C,* Injection of local anesthetic and steroids was performed into the L4–L5 and L5–S1 facet joints after chemonucleolysis at L5–S1. An oblique projection is shown. The L5–S1 disc is still opacified *(single open arrowhead).* Note the site of puncture in the inferior recesses of the joints, approached by using curved needles. The joint space is opacified *(black arrowheads).* The medial portion of the joint cavity, limited by the ligamentum flavum, is filled *(double open arrowheads). D,* A lateral projection demonstrates the close relation of the treated disc to the joint (filled with contrast) *(arrowhead).*

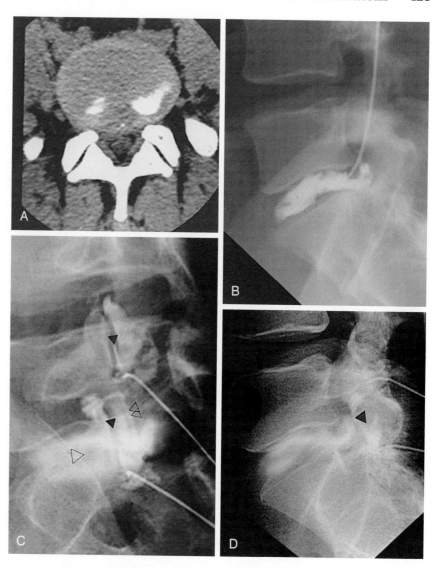

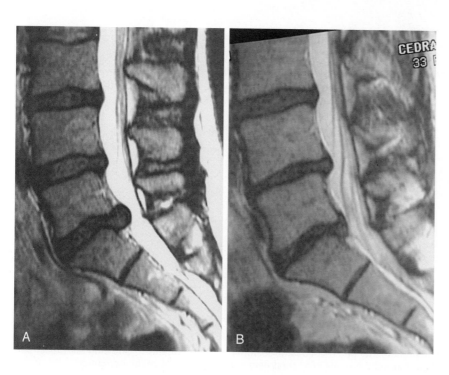

Figure 40-2 Case 2. Treatment of two disc herniations by chemonucleolysis. *A,* Pretreatment magnetic resonance imaging (MRI) demonstrates a moderate disc bulge at L4–L5 and a voluminous herniation at L5–S1. *B,* MRI performed 3 months after treatment, with a good clinical result. Note the marked decrease in the L5–S1 herniation.

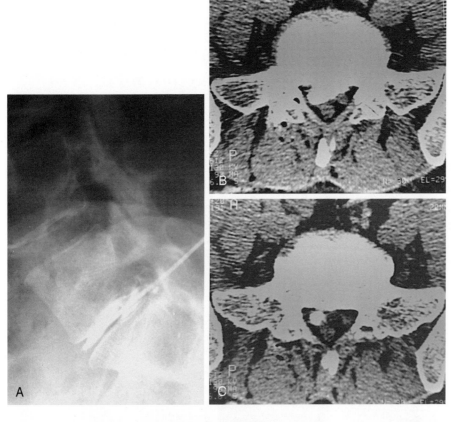

Figure 40-3 Case 3. Patient with an extruded herniation successfully treated by chemonucleolysis. *A,* An L5–S1 discogram was performed via a direct posterolateral approach with a straight needle (compare with Fig. 40–1*B*). *B,* Computed tomography (CT) performed after the discogram and treatment reveals extruded material opacified with contrast. *C,* On a slightly lower slice, the inferior part of the extruded material is opacified and consequently will be reached and treated by the chymopapain.

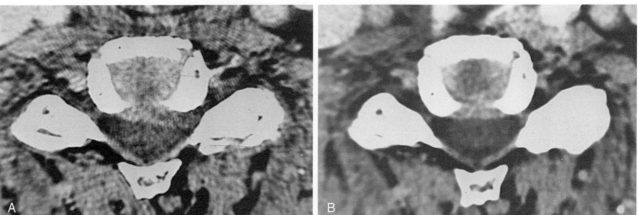

Figure 40-4 Case 4. Case of cervical disc herniation treated by percutaneous discectomy. *A,* Pretreatment CT demonstrates a left posterolateral disc herniation. *B,* CT performed 3 months after treatment shows an excellent result.

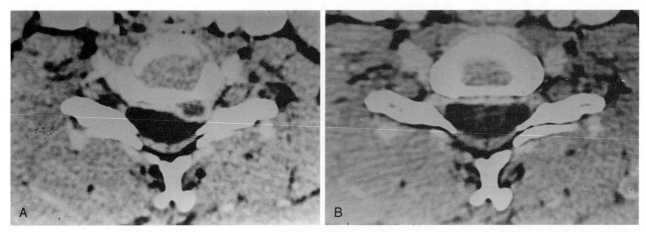

Figure 40-5 Case 5. Extruded cervical disc herniation treated by percutaneous discectomy. *A,* Pretreatment CT showing left posterolateral herniation with an extruded fragment. *B,* CT performed 2 months after treatment shows resolution of the herniation.

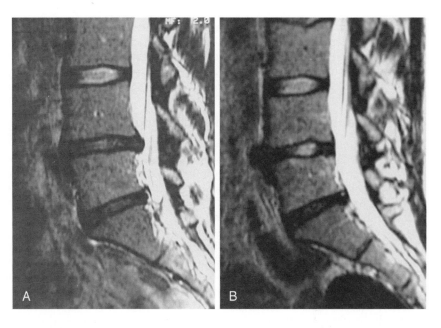

Figure 40-6 Case 6. An L4–L5 disc herniation treated by percutaneous discectomy with incomplete resolution of symptoms. Chemonucleolysis was performed 6 weeks later. *A,* Pretreatment MRI demonstrates the L4–L5 herniation. *B,* MRI performed 3 months after chemonucleolysis. Note the significant reduction in size of the herniation and that the signal of the treated disc has partially normalized. The patient had an excellent clinical result.

tions, 85% of patients who have been treated with complementary chemonucleolysis after a suboptimal result from percutaneous discectomy have had good results (Case 6, Fig. 40–6). Only 1% have required open surgery. In cervical herniations, complementary chemonucleolysis[10] often is even more rapidly successful (Case 7, Fig. 40–7), presumably because of the smaller volume of the disc.

Disc Herniation and Facet Joints

There is an associated involvement of the ligamentum flavum at the same or adjacent level when there is a disc herniation. Thus, the nerve root compression was in part due to the disc bulge but also was in part due to an inflammatory process of the ligamentum flavum and the adjacent facet joint. Consequently, supplementation of all types of intradiscal treatment with an injection of a mixture of a local anesthetic agent and long-lasting steroids is appropriate (see Fig. 40–1). This technique results in much better tolerance of the chemonucleolysis and decreased pain immediately after the procedure as well as during the following days. This especially helps with the common 10th-day painful crisis rarely mentioned in the literature, the mechanism of which is not well understood.

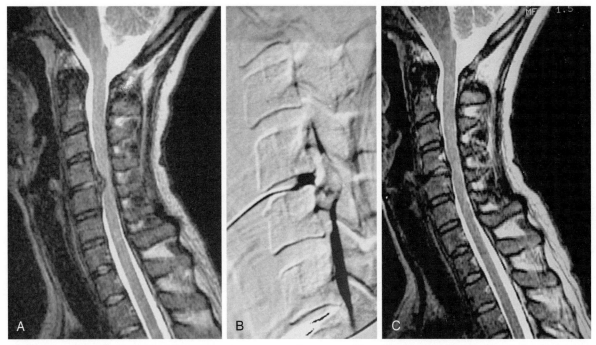

Figure 40-7 Case 7. A C4–C5 herniation treated by percutaneous discectomy. The patient had incomplete resolution of symptoms and underwent chemonucleolysis 6 weeks later. *A,* Pretreatment MRI demonstrates a large herniation in a canal of borderline diameter at this level. *B,* A C4–C5 discogram was performed. Note the epidural leakage of contrast. Chemonucleolysis was performed despite this. *C,* MRI performed 2 months later reveals a dramatic reduction in size of the herniation. An excellent clinical result was achieved.

To be effective, the injection of anesthetic and steroids should reach the inner part of the facet joint, which is medially closed by the ligamentum flavum. This is best achieved by puncturing the joint in the inferior recess (see Fig. 40–1).

Full Percutaneous Decompressive Technique

Disc herniations occurring in narrow canals are more difficult to treat using percutaneous techniques, and the results are not as good. A more efficient decompressive technique involves associating at the same level and in the same procedure a chemonucleolysis followed by a nucleoaspiration, and then injecting the two corresponding facet joints with local steroids. This full decompressive technique has been used on more than 30 patients and has been effective and particularly rewarding when used on elderly patients with associated canal stenosis, degenerative changes, disc herniation, and bilaterally hypertrophied ligamentum flavum at one level (commonly L3–L4), whose associated general medical conditions preclude any kind of surgery (Case 8, Fig. 40–8). This full percutaneous decompressive technique also can be used in patients presenting with a sleepless hyperalgic radiculalgia. The technique is particularly rewarding in this situation because the pain relief is rapid.

A significant palsy is an emergency that also

should be treated by this technique. It appears reasonable, however, to treat the patient rapidly by open surgery if a marked improvement has not been obtained in the following hours. The success of surgery, is however, just as uncertain in this type of presentation.

PRETHERAPEUTIC CONSULTATION

In the pretherapeutic consultation, indications for percutaneous treatments are discussed with the patient and referring physician. It is important to examine the patient as carefully as other specialists who usually deal with spine diseases. This is the only way for the radiologist to manage this type of treatment; otherwise, the radiologist's role will be that of a technician, without real clinical responsibilities and consequently without control over the treatment decision making and patient follow-up.

TECHNIQUE

For the past 5 years, I have performed percutaneous treatments only on an outpatient basis. All of the procedures are performed under local anesthesia, which should be particularly patient and complete. The anesthesiologist is not present in the room but is easily reachable.

Lumbar Chemonucleolysis

The patient is placed in the right lateral position (this avoids the risk of a colon puncture), and a posterolateral approach is used. A 22-gauge needle (BD 3½″) is used for local anesthesia. An 18-gauge needle (BD) is used for disc puncture. For several years, I curved this needle with a clamp to reach the L5–S1 disc more easily (see Fig. 40–1*B*), but I now use a straight direct approach (see Fig. 40–3*A*). Bupivacaine (Marcaine) 0.5%, 1 ml, is injected into the disc before chymopapain injection to reduce the occurrence of low back pain. Chymopapain (Chymodiactin), 2000 U in 1 ml, is then injected into the disc. Rifampicin (Cassenne) 5%, 0.5 ml diluted by 10 in sterile water, is injected after all types of percutaneous intradiscal procedures.

Cervical Chemonucleolysis

The patient is positioned supine, and a right anterolateral approach is used. The right-sided approach facilitates the procedure for a right-handed operator and limits the risk of injuring the esophagus (Fig. 40–9). The same procedure is followed as for a lumbar injection, but the disc puncture is performed with the 22-gauge needle, slightly curved with a clamp to facilitate steering.

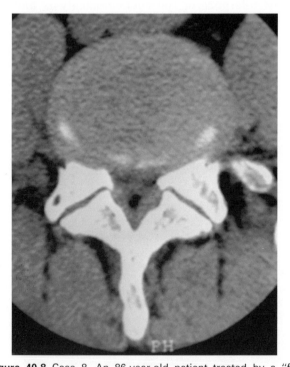

Figure 40-8 Case 8. An 86-year-old patient treated by a "full decompressive percutaneous technique." The patient was totally disabled by severe back pain radiating to both legs, which corresponded to the broad-based L3–L4 herniation superimposed on a narrow canal, as shown. There were cardiac contraindications to surgery. Chemonucleolysis followed by percutaneous discectomy was performed in one procedure, along with injection of the facet joints. The hypertrophied ligamentum flavum contributed to the stenosis. A rapid and lasting relief of symptoms was achieved.

Lumbar Percutaneous Discectomy

The patient is positioned in the right or left lateral position (depending on the side of the herniation),

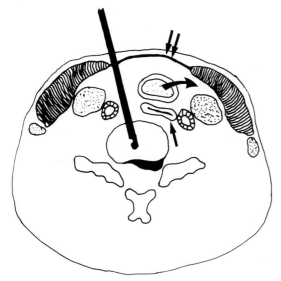

Figure 40-9 An axial diagram of the neck (in standard CT orientation) shows the relationship of the nucleotome to the surrounding anatomic structures. A right anterolateral approach has been used. The trachea is manually displaced *(curved arrow)*. Note the slightly left position of the esophagus *(single straight arrow)* and the thickness of the cervical subcutaneous tissues *(double arrows)*.

and a posterolateral approach is used. A 2.5-mm automated percutaneous lumbar discectomy set (Surgical Dynamics) is used. A sharp needle is used to dilate the soft tissues and facilitate the introduction of the system (Fig. 40–10 demonstrates this at the cervical level). Rifampicin is injected at the end of the procedure using a Chiba needle (22-gauge Nycomed).

Cervical Percutaneous Discectomy

The patient is placed in the supine position, and a right anterolateral (paramidline) approach is used (see Figs. 40–9 and 40–10). This facilitates the proce-

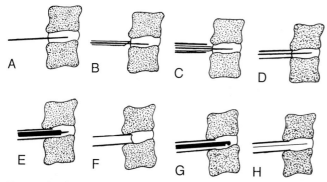

Figure 40-10 Various steps involved in percutaneous cervical discectomy. *A,* Trocar placement. *B,* Placement of a dilating sharp needle. *C,* Advancement of the cannula with a tapered dilator. *D,* The dilator is removed and the cannula is advanced against the margin of the disc. *E,* The trephine is placed over the trocar and the annulus is incised. The cannula is advanced into the disc when possible. *F,* The trephine is removed, leaving the cannula in place. *G,* The nucleotome is placed. *H,* The nucleotome is retrieved and a Chiba needle is advanced to inject antibiotics.

dure and avoids trauma to the esophagus. A 2-mm automated percutaneous lumbar discectomy set (Surgical Dynamics) is used. The same other tools are used as for lumbar discectomy.

Steroid Injections in the Facet Joints

A 20-gauge lumbar puncture needle (yellow BD, 3½″) is used with the mandrel of the 22-gauge lumbar puncture needle (black BD, 3½″). This allows curving of the needle with a clamp to facilitate puncture of the inferior recess of the joint (see Fig. 40–1). Triamcinolone acetonide (Kenacort retard 80), 0.5 ml, is injected in the joint, along with 0.5 ml of bupivacaine, after the correct position of the needle has been verified by contrast injection.

TECHNICAL PROBLEMS, COMPLICATIONS, AND SOLUTIONS

Among the complications of percutaneous techniques, most can be avoided by use of adequate technique. The posterolateral approach at the lumbar level and anterolateral approach at the cervical level (see Fig. 40–9) should be performed as gently as possible. Otherwise, damage may be inflicted on the surrounding structures. This risk usually is reduced significantly by correct training.

Infectious complications leading to discitis were a major concern of mine for several years. I now systematically inject antibiotics in the disc after any intradiscal diagnostic or therapeutic procedure, which has solved this problem.

Considering all the potential complications of chemonucleolysis, a recent review of the literature of the past 30 years has concluded that this technique is 3 to 20 times safer than surgery in the management of disc herniations.[16]

Allergic Reaction

Anaphylactic reactions are not considered as common now as believed in the past. I have experienced one significant allergic reaction per 700 cases, all controlled successfully with medication. Although the risk of allergic reaction is lower than was previously believed, it is essential to be ready to react rapidly to an allergic reaction in the patient undergoing chemonucleolysis. The patient should be given intravenous atropine and hydrocortisone immediately and should be observed overnight in the intensive care unit. The patient usually can be discharged the following day.

CONCLUSION

Disc herniation is the result of several factors, including a predisposing postural alignment, an asymmetry of the facet joints, and a weakness of the corresponding parasagittal muscles, all focusing the postural stresses on one disc level. It is not in the scope of this chapter to develop this theory. An understanding of the causes of a disc herniation is now at hand, and this should soon allow the prevention of recurrence after percutaneous techniques as well as prophylactic treatment before clinical signs occur.

Medical treatment of disc herniation often is effective and should be attempted. When this treatment fails, various percutaneous techniques used alone, successively, or simultaneously in most cases allow cure of the patient with preservation of full disc function.

REFERENCES

1. Smith L. Enzyme dissolution of the nucleus pulposus in humans. *JAMA* 1964;187:137–140.
2. Smith L. Chemonucleolysis: personal history, trials, and tribulations [Review]. *Clin Orthop* 1993;287:117–124.
3. Onik G, Helms C, Ginsburg L, et al. Percutaneous lumbar diskectomy using a new aspiration probe. *AJNR* 1985;6:290–293.
4. Theron J, Blais M, Casaseo A, et al. La radiologie therapeutique du rachis lombaire: chemonucléolyse discale, infiltrations et coagulation des articulaires posterieures. *J Neuroradiol* 1983;10:209–230.
5. Theron J. Percutaneous lysis of the vertebral disk. In Dondelinger R (ed): Interventional Radiology. Thieme, 1990.
6. Gogan WJ, Fraser RD. Chymopapain: a 10-year, double blind study. *Spine* 1992;17:388–394.
7. Nordby EJ, Wright PH. Efficacy of chymopapain: a review. *Spine* 1994;19:2578–2583.
8. Nordby EJ, Wright PH, Schofield SR. Safety of chemonucleolysis: adverse effects reported in the United States, 1982–1991 [Review]. *Clin Orthop* 1993;13:122–134.
9. Krause D, Drape JL. Cervical nucleolysis: indications, technique, results 190 patients. *J Neuroradiol* 1993;20:42–59.
10. Theron J, Huet H, Coskun O. Cervical automated diskectomy: report of 150 cases and evolution in the management of failure cases. *Intervent Neuroradiol* 1996;2:35–44.
11. Wiesel SW, Tsourmas N, Feffer HL, et al. A study of computer assisted tomography. *Spine* 1984;9:549–551.
12. Saal J. Natural history and nonoperative treatment of lumbar disc herniations. *Spine* 1996;21(suppl.):2S–9S.
13. Wapner KL, Vaccaro AR, Albert TJ, et al. The result of chemonucleolysis as a function of three dimensional volumetric analysis of disc herniation. *J Spinal Disord* 1993;6:324–332.
14. Gobin P, Theron J, Courtheoux F, et al. Percutaneous automated lumbar diskectomy. *J Neuroradiol* 1989;16:203–213.
15. Leonardi M, Fabris G, Lavaroni A. Percutaneous treatment of lumbar disk herniation. *Ann Chir Gynaecolo* 1993;82:141–148.
16. Brown MD. Update on chemonucleolysis. *Spine* 1996;21 (suppl.).

PART IV

BRACHIOCEPHALIC ANGIOPLASTY AND STENTING

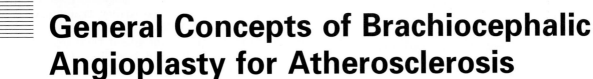

CHAPTER 41

General Concepts of Brachiocephalic Angioplasty for Atherosclerosis

J.J. Connors III

Brachiocephalic angioplasty is now applied routinely to patients with atherosclerotic disease. It has also been used successfully, however, in patients with fibromuscular dysplasia,[1] Takayasu's arteritis,[2, 3] vasculitis (either postsubarachnoid bleed or radiation-induced disease; see Figs. 58–15 to 58–54 in Chapter 58), and stenoses associated with neurofibromatosis.[4] Angioplasty is considered an excellent means of treatment of most atherosclerotic lesions, with varying degrees of success and permanency depending on the location of the lesion, underlying vascular pathology, and operator skill and experience. Angioplasty almost invariably can be accomplished without any permanent worsening of the situation; the brain, however, is far less forgiving than other structures, including the heart.

All cerebrovascular structures, as far distal as the secondary branches of the anterior, middle, and posterior cerebral arteries, can be reached with an angioplasty balloon. The areas of specific concern to interventional neuroradiologists are the origins of the great vessels from the aorta, the carotid bifurcation, the vertebral artery origin, the vertebrobasilar junction, the mid-basilar artery, the carotid siphon, and the main trunk of the middle cerebral artery. Each of these has its own set of indications, contraindications, techniques, pitfalls, complications, and alteratives.

The specific techniques for intracranial and extracranial angioplasty are still not perfected, and only skilled and specifically trained operators should perform this procedure. Intracranial vessels do not appear to react to angioplasty for atherosclerotic disease in the same manner as peripheral or coronary vessels; thus, a technique that may suffice in the periphery or heart may not be appropriate for brachiocephalic angioplasty. Coronary angiography and angioplasty are technically simple but are not performed by untrained practitioners (radiologists) because of lack of knowledge of and training for rescue procedures as well as interpretive acumen, not because of lack of catheter skills. Anyone performing brachiocephalic angioplasty should be proficient at endovascular rescue of all types and particularly with the intracranial use of microcatheters and fibrinolytics. In addition, the varying idiosyncratic reactions of specific vessels in this region should be well understood before these procedures are attempted. Performance of head and neck angioplasty and stenting by a practitioner who does not understand the concept of reversal of flow in the circle of Willis, compensatory hemodynamics, the low-resistance and high-flow nature of intracranial hemodynamics, the potential tolerance for safe permanent occlusion of a great brachiocephalic vessel, and the nature of the end organ, is reckless and unacceptable. Technical prowess does not automatically confer competence to perform certain procedures, and competence to perform a procedure does not confer correct decision-making ability.

Detection of embolic complications is not as straightforward and obvious a task in the head as it is in the periphery or heart. Even trained neuroradiologists have difficulty identifying an intracranial embolus. As stated elsewhere (see Chapter 57), an intracranial embolus is only rarely evidenced by an intraluminal filling defect, or even by a vessel stub. Extensive training in intracranial hemodynamics is necessary for accurate identification of a vascular occlusion. A common trick question posed to residents and fellows is to show an image from a carotid angiogram and ask the student to point to the intracranial occlusion. The correct response is that, without the entire arterial, capillary, and venous phases (i.e., the entire "run"), the question cannot be answered accurately. Slow flow in a branch vessel (i.e., persistence of this artery while the other vessels are in the capillary phase) is the most frequent and reliable clue to the presence of an occlusive lesion.

For these reasons, the interventionist pioneers have had extensive experience in endovascular therapy and brachiocephalic work and are associated with multispecialty teams.

IMPORTANCE AND IMPLICATIONS OF DEGREE OF STENOSIS

With critical hair-like stenoses, it is unknown whether watchful waiting while the patient is anticoagulated is wise; the failure of anticoagulation may be abrupt and total (see Fig. 48–21). Therefore, the simple presence of such a lesion may be an indication for intervention.

Webster et al. have determined that a critical hemodynamically significant stenosis with evidence of only marginal intracranial hemodynamic reserve results in a major infarct in about one fourth of patients within about 19 months.[5] These authors point out the "surprisingly modest attention" that has been paid to the effect of carotid artery occlusive disease on "intracranial hemodynamics in individual patients and on the correlation of those hemodynamic consequences with the risk of irreversible cerebral ischemia." Another interesting result of this study concerns total occlusion of an internal carotid artery. Of patients without a completed stroke in that territory, not only did 26% of those who had poor hemodynamic reserve demonstrated by an acetazolamide (Diamox) challenge test (see Chapter 3) suffer a stroke in the study period, but 0% (zero) with *adequate* hemodynamic reserve suffered one. Because of the protected nature of the territory secondary to the occluded internal carotid artery, the most probable cause for these strokes is hemodynamic insufficiency, not emboli.

The implications of these data are that at least some patients with symptomatic stenoses, either intracranial or extracranial, would benefit from correction of this problem. In addition, these data offer a rationale for performing angioplasty in patients with intracranial lesions rather taking than a wait-and-see attitude. Hemodynamic insufficiency can cause not only strokes but also vague, nonfocal symptoms such as chronic headaches.

ONGOING CLINICAL TRIALS

North American Cerebral Percutaneous Transluminal Angioplasty Register

In an attempt to define further the risks and benefits of angioplasty in this area, at least one ongoing patient registry is gathering data concerning the best techniques and patient population for this procedure. The North American Cerebral Percutaneous Transluminal Angioplasty Register (NACPTAR), organized by Ferguson, Ferguson, and Lee at the Baptist Memorial Hospital in Memphis, has been accumulating data for more than 5 years and has yielded some surprising preliminary results. Specifically, posterior

fossa (basilar artery) angioplasty is extremely dangerous.

The complete results are not known yet because of a lack of statistically significant numbers, but data are being acquired by the registry and analyzed in a rigid scientific manner. Only in this way can the facts concerning these procedures be ascertained. (Even though they are superficially similar, the specific techniques used and their results are vastly different in different anatomic locations and circumstances.)

Carotid and Vertebral Artery Transluminal Angioplasty Study

The Carotid and Vertebral Artery Transluminal Angioplasty Study (CAVATAS) is an ongoing international multicenter randomized trial aimed at determining the risks and benefits of carotid and vertebral artery angioplasty and at comparing these to the risks and benefits associated with carotid endarterectomy or medical management.[6, 7] Patients with symptomatic stenoses of more than 35% are randomly assigned to surgery, angioplasty, or optimal medical management. As of the most recent report, 179 patients have been enrolled (93 angioplasty, 70 surgery, 16 medical therapy). Most of these patients have carotid disease (163 of 179), and most have more than 70% stenosis (owing to enrollment of patients with 30% to 69% stenoses in the ongoing North American Symptomatic Carotid Endarterectomy Trial (NASCET) and other trials).

The primary endpoint is the safety at 30 days (incidence of complications, morbidity, and mortality). The patients are followed clinically and by duplex ultrasonography. The secondary goals of the study include evaluation of techniques, role of stents, and choice of equipment, such as guidewires, test occlusion balloons, and catheters.

All patients considered for enrollment should have a history of symptoms relative to the target vessel within the previous 6 months. All patients undergo a preprocedure cerebral computed tomographic or magnetic resonance imaging scan, duplex ultrasonography of the carotid and vertebral arteries, and angiography. During performance of the procedure, the interventional neuroradiologist is limited to three balloon inflations, each with a maximal duration of 30 seconds. Neurologic examination, systemic blood pressure, electrocardiogram, and transcranial Doppler findings are tabulated before, during, and after the procedure. Intravenous heparin is continued for up to 48 hours. Follow-up duplex ultrasonography and neurologic examinations are performed after 1 and 6 months and then yearly.

The preliminary analysis of the data on the first 100 patients reveals no difference in safety between carotid endarterectomy and angioplasty. Insufficient numbers of patients are available at this time to evaluate vertebral artery disease.

Integra Carotid Stent Trial

A trial of the Boston Scientific, Inc., Integra stent, designed specifically for carotid angioplasty and stenting, is in progress. The stent is a self-expanding, multisegmented nitinol stent that is deployed in a fashion similar to the Wallstent (Schneider, Inc.). It is available in four different sizes. The 6-mm diameter stent is available in 20- and 31-mm lengths; the 7-mm diameter stent is available in 20- and 31-mm lengths. It is premounted in an over-the-wire delivery system (see "Current Commercial and Investigative Stents" in Chapter 1).

The study is designed to include 150 patients at a maximum of eight centers. They will be followed for 1 year after treatment. The stent itself shows promise. Of interest is that this trial requires the participation of an interventional neuroradiologist at each center, but only as a back-up (other specialists, such as cardiologists, may perform the procedure).

Wallstent Carotid Stent Trial

A trial evaluating the use of the Wallstent (Schneider, Inc.) in the carotid artery is in progress. This stent is already widely used for carotid stenting and the results of its use have been promising. The stent currently used for this purpose is the tracheobronchial model, which is more flexible and of a more appropriate size for use in the carotid artery than the stiffer biliary type.

CREST Trial

A carotid stent trial is being organized to evaluate the procedure itself, rather than the specific stent. This is a large multicenter trial involving neurologists, interventional neuroradiologists, vascular surgeons, neurosurgeons, and cardiologists. The choice of stent is optional.

LOCATIONS OF ATHEROSCLEROTIC BRACHIOCEPHALIC DISEASE

About one third of all stenoses in the head and neck that require therapy are at the carotid bifurcation. Table 48–1 lists the most common sites of atherosclerotic disease.[8] Note the presence of a wide range of locations that potentially require therapy. In this study, extracranial stenosis or occlusion was seen in 41.2% of 3788 patients undergoing four-vessel angiography for evaluation of cerebrovascular disease. Fully one third of patients had extracranial lesions combined with *surgically inaccessible* intracranial or extracranial lesions, whereas 6.1% had *only* surgically inaccessible lesions.

Before this study and others of the same era, it often was stated that the pathogenesis of carotid occlusion as demonstrated angiographically frequently could not be determined. Thromboangiitis obliterans was considered the primary factor and arteriosclerosis a secondary factor.[9] The diagnosis of thromboangiitis obliterans now should only be made when strict criteria are met.[10] These include the following:

- Presence of inflammatory reaction in the cerebral arteries, presence of giant cells and epithelioid cells in the thrombus and intima, and sparing of the media
- Obliteration of long vascular segments in the absence of arteriosclerosis or syphilis and presence of cerebral cortical necrosis
- Associated typical thromboangiitis obliterans in the extremities

Thromboangiitis obliterans, in the head as well as in the extremities, is a disease of small arteries (such as branches of the anterior or middle cerebral arteries).

GENERAL THEORY OF ANGIOPLASTY AND PATHOPHYSIOLOGIC RESPONSE

Mechanism of Angioplasty

The original theory of the mechanism of angioplasty, proposed by Dotter et al.,[11, 12] was that angioplasty produced compression and remodeling of the atherosclerotic plaque, with extrusion of any liquid component. Stretching of the media and increase in the outer diameter of the vessel were also thought to occur.

As percutaneous transluminal angioplasty was more frequently employed, this theory was challenged. If the plaque was truly being compressed and remodeled, it should elongate, even if there was some loss of volume due to expression of fluid. This was almost never observed to occur (but an example of this is presented in Chapter 46). In addition, calcified and fibrotic lesions were seen to respond to angioplasty, yet these should be resistant to remodeling. Linear clefts and filling defects were also observed after successful angioplasty. This led to further research into the true mechanism of angioplasty. Dissections, intimal tearing, and medial stretching were observed, but it was not known whether these represented complications or were part of the process itself.[13, 14]

A series of experiments was then undertaken that was aimed at assessing morphologic and metabolic changes in vessel walls after angioplasty and at determining how various types of balloons and inflation pressures affect results.[15–21]

The first part of the study looked at histologic and radiologic changes associated with angioplasty in human cadaver arteries containing plaque and stenoses (dilated within 24 hours of death).[15, 16] This study demonstrated that all successfully dilated vessels contained rupture or tears of plaques. Intimal dehiscence or tearing (oriented longitudinally) was also noted; this corresponded to the linear defects seen on angiography. No compression or remodeling was seen. A minimal increase in outside diameter of the vessels was noted. Limited lamina widening was demonstrated when circumferential plaque was present, but vessels with asymmetric plaque demonstrated marked stretching and localized medial rupture, often with aneurysmal dilation of the opposite adventitia. No dilation was possible in heavily calcified arteries unless there was plaque rupture.

A series of animal experiments aimed at assessing the effects of balloon size and compliance, inflation pressure, and duration of inflation was then undertaken.[15–18] The initial study looked at the effects of dilating normal vessels. Balloons oversized 25% to 100% were inflated in the aorta, iliac arteries, femoral arteries, and carotid arteries of dogs, using pressures of 4 to 5 atmospheres. At 25% oversizing, histologic changes were seen in the intima and endothelium; there was no measurable widening of the lumen. These lesions healed with intimal hyperplasia. At 60% to 80% oversizing, there was widespread change in the intima and media without injury to the adventitia. This resulted in medial fibrosis and intimal hyperplasia. Further dilation (100% overdilation) resulted in complete medial disruption; adventitial stretching occurred, and aneurysm formation was seen. Again, healing occurred by medial fibrosis and intimal hyperplasia.

The intimal hyperplasia appears to be driven by platelet aggregation and is not proportional to the degree of injury (it may be exuberant compared with the degree of the initial injury), whereas medial fibrosis is proportional. Both intimal hyperplasia and medial fibrosis are long-lasting. These findings suggest that inadequate initial dilation may result in rapid restenosis owing to extensive intimal hyperplasia and that adequate dilation requires damage to the intima, the media, and to a lesser degree, the adventitia.

The next phase of this study evaluated the use of higher inflation pressures and the effect of varying balloon compliance.[19, 20] Polyethylene and polyvinyl alcohol balloons sized equal to the vessel lumen, oversized 30%, and oversized 80% to 100% were used; inflation pressures of 4.5, 6, 10, and 12.5 atmospheres were employed. Again, the carotid and femoral arteries of dogs were the chosen sites. The study demonstrated progressive histologic changes in the arterial wall associated with increasing balloon diameter as well as with increasing inflation pressure. Balloons oversized by 30% or more routinely did not reach their specified diameter unless inflated beyond the manufacturers' recommended working pressures. *It was also found that an oversized balloon with low compliance has greater dilating capacity but may cause vessel rupture.* A balloon of the same size but higher compliance may cause less damage, but the damage is spread out over a longer segment because of deformation of the balloon. With balloons close to the size of the vessel, more damage was caused by higher-compliance balloons because of their ability to overinflate and expand at high pressures. Oversized balloons (80% to 100%) produced extensive medial stretching and frank medial rupture; this was associated with local thrombosis. Medial rupture with adventitial stretching resulted in aneurysm formation. Frank vessel rupture was also seen with these balloons at high pressures.

The final phase of this study entailed a comparison of the effects of dilation with 25% and 50% oversized balloons, with inflation times of 15 to 60 seconds in the aortas of normal and atherosclerotic rabbits.[21] In normal rabbits, there was the expected progressive increase in wall changes with time and balloon diameter. In atherosclerotic rabbits, both circumferential and focal plaques were seen; these were mainly fibrous. The degree of histologic change correlated with thickness and location of plaque rather than with balloon size or inflation time. In particular, the extent of plaque fracture and medial dissection correlated not with balloon size or inflation time but rather with the number of plaques and their size. Vessel segments with minor plaque formation demonstrated stretching similar to that seen in normal vessels. Stretching and medial dissection also occurred at sites of plaque rupture and dehiscence (along the edge of the plaque). Damage penetrating into the media occurred with small balloons and short inflation times in vessels with significant plaque. Dissections were longitudinally oriented. Thrombus formation was again seen but remained localized to regions of extensive medial injury.

The overall conclusions of the study were that the mechanism of angioplasty is a combination of rupture and dissection of plaque and stretching of nondiseased vessel segments; atherosclerotic vessels are much more vulnerable than healthy vessels to damage resulting from angioplasty because there is less stretching (where histologic change increases with inflation time and balloon size and is thus controllable) and more rupture and dissection (where extensive damage can occur with short inflation times and small balloons).

Additionally, the practice of inflating balloons to extremely high pressures is meaningless. *It is the size of the balloon, not its internal pressure,* that determines vessel damage or stretching. *A 5-mm noncompliant balloon at 1 million atmospheres of pressure causes less damage and stretching (and less stent "imbedding") than a 6-mm balloon at 4 atmospheres.* Once the balloon is fully inflated, no further change occurs regardless of the interior balloon pressure.

Stent Injury

The injury caused by insertion of an intravascular stent differs from that of a simple angioplasty in at least four ways:

- The struts of the stent cause deep vascular damage different from the damage of a simple angioplasty.
- Instead of temporary strain caused by angioplasty, a stent will cause permanent strain and lasting change in vessel geometry.
- A foreign body is imbedded in tissue. This is particularly problematic in a moving or flexible vessel where chronic stimulation may induce restenosis at a much higher rate than simple angioplasty would.
- The early thrombus formation induced by stent implantation may act as a nidus for further intimal hyperplasia.

The rationale for the use of a stent as opposed to angioplasty alone is complex. Both the rate and duration of proliferation of cells and the response of mononuclear cells after stenting are higher than after simple angioplasty. *Interestingly, primary stent implantation without predilation by simple angioplasty reduces the amount of neointimal hyperplasia.* Stenting of a vessel *absolutely* stimulates an increased endothelial response, but the stent's ability to decrease vascular *remodeling* may make up for this deficiency. Further discussion of the rationale for stent use is given in Chapter 50, and a discussion of stent use in brachiocephalic intervention is presented in Chapter 43.

Pathophysiologic Rationale for Angioplasty Technique

Stretch, but don't tear.

If a mechanism were to be invented to intentionally cause vascular damage and intimal dissection utilizing catheter techniques, *rapidly inflating a large, noncompliant balloon inside an atherosclerotic lesion* would be an ideal method to achieve this goal.

Slow, gradual inflation of the balloon during angioplasty results in far fewer large intimal tears, flaps, and dissections than does the more commonly employed method of "blowing it up, then letting it down." This is particularly the case with intracranial vessels. Techniques that are acceptable in the heart or periphery may have devastating results in the head that can be difficult, if not impossible, to overcome. The large vessels of the neck and periphery are much more forgiving of intimal damage and retain an adequate lumen even when considerably damaged. This may not be the case, however, with the smaller intracranial vessels that usually are less than 3 mm (or even 2 mm) in size. Extensive intimal damage should be avoided when possible.

The rationale for extremely slow balloon inflation is based on the observation that less intimal tearing has occurred with this technique. In addition, allowing the vessel to stretch slowly (as opposed to tearing the vessel wall purposefully, as with the rapid inflation technique) makes sense. A coronary angioplasty trial using a similar technique showed that inflating the balloon slowly can decrease the incidence of major dissection to one third of that associated with the standard technique (3% vs. 9%).[22] In an intracranial location, this can be extremely important. A major dissection can spell disaster, if not death. A surgical rescue is not possible, nor can the lesion be repaired by the use of a stent. These tears should be avoided at all costs, even to the extent of accepting a less visually appealing result.

The reasons an angioplasty may fail acutely include elastic recoil, platelet aggregation, and thrombus formation. Acute vessel occlusion caused by thrombosis or vasospasm of the damaged artery has been reported to complicate femoropopliteal angioplasty in up to 40% of cases.[23] Chronic or delayed closure is thought to be related to intimal (or cellular)

proliferation. Late restenosis occurs in about 30% of coronary artery angioplasty sites. The mechanisms for these complications are well understood and require different means of prevention.

Undamaged vascular endothelium has an anionic surface charge that, along with a constant release of endothelium-derived relaxing factor (a powerful antiplatelet agent), yields an antithrombotic environment. Any damage to this endovascular covering decreases the antithrombotic nature of this surface and exposes the subendothelial matrix to the circulating blood. This matrix is thrombogenic, and its exposure begins the thrombotic cascade. Experimental angioplasty models have shown that platelets are deposited rapidly at sites of angioplasty injury and that this deposition is nearly complete after 10 minutes.[24, 25] The extent of aggregation is determined by local hemodynamic forces that are directly related to flow velocity and indirectly related to the third power of the arterial diameter,[26] as well as to the severity of the vessel wall injury.[25, 27] These experimental data confirm the observations that platelet accumulation and acute occlusion occur much more frequently in small vessels with slow flow. Intracranial vessels are small and have relatively slow flow. Thus, these lesions must be *observed for a period of time after the angioplasty* to watch for this malignant platelet cascade, as noted in Chapter 48.

Vasospasm related to angioplasty injury is most pronounced *distal* to the dilated segment and is directly related to the amount of platelet deposition[27] because this response is mediated by the release of vasoactive agents such as thromboxane A_2, serotonin, and platelet-derived growth factor, which flow downstream.[28, 29]

Late restenosis secondary to angioplasty is related to intimal hyperplasia and vascular remodeling. This results from the interaction between components in blood and the vessel wall.[30] Damaged endothelium, activated platelets, and neutrophils at the angioplasty site generate reactive intermediary agents. These oxidative metabolites induce chain reactions that result in endothelial dysfunction and oxidation of low-density lipoproteins. Macrophages activated by the oxidized LDL and the dysfunctional endothelium then release several growth factors that promote tissue proliferation. The interaction results in medial proliferation and the migration of vascular smooth muscle cells into the arterial intima.

Probucol (Lorelco, Hoechst Marion Roussel) is a powerful antioxidant agent used for the treatment of high serum cholesterol. *It has been shown to inhibit this restenosis significantly and is the only pharmacologic agent proved to be effective at treating restenosis.* This is discussed later.

ANGIOPLASTY AND FIBRINOLYSIS

Just as in the periphery, angioplasty and fibrinolytic therapy overlap. Therapeutic intervention in many cases of stroke or transient ischemic attack may start with fibrinolytics and later require angioplasty, and therapy for many cases of atherosclerosis may begin with angioplasty and subsequently require fibrinolytic therapy. Indeed, the quandary of whether to begin therapy with angioplasty or fibrinolytic infusion is frequently the first major decision made by the interventional neuroradiologist. If faced with an acute vascular occlusion in a situation in which the use of a fibrinolytic agent is not contraindicated, fibrinolytic infusion usually is our first therapy of choice. Strategic quandaries always exist, however (see Chapter 48).

RESTENOSIS

Restenosis is the bane of endovascular therapists. In various studies, it has been shown to occur in 20% to 40% of postangioplasty and stenting cases, and in periods ranging from 3 months to 4 years. It appears to be more of a problem in small vessel procedures.

This failure rate is unacceptable for brachiocephalic angioplasty in almost any location. A failure leading to ischemia of cerebral structures is much worse than recurrence of claudication symptoms. Efforts to prevent restenosis are ongoing. The process is recognized as a proliferative disorder, and therapies similar to those used for malignancies may be applicable.

Probucol

Probucol has been shown to be effective at preventing restenosis after coronary angioplasty. This is the only pharmaceutic agent shown to do this. Probucol is a lipophilic, serum lipid–lowering drug (it lowers total serum cholesterol and has relatively little effect on serum triglycerides). It also has powerful antioxidant properties. In the study by Tardif et al.,[31] it was compared with antioxidant multivitamins and with a combination of probucol and multivitamins. In a prospective study, 317 patients were randomly assigned 1 month before angioplasty to one of four groups; treatment with placebo, probucol (500 mg), multivitamins (30,000 IU of β-carotene, 500 mg of vitamin C, and 700 IU of vitamin E), or both probucol and multivitamins. All medications were administered twice daily. Patients were treated for the entire month before the procedure and for 6 months afterward. All patients received an extra dose of 2000 IU of vitamin E, 1000 mg of probucol, both vitamin E and probucol, or placebo 12 hours before angioplasty, according to the randomized group to which they were assigned. The restenosis rate for patients receiving probucol was 20.7%, for the combined group 28.9%, for the multivitamin alone group 40.3%, and for the placebo group 38.9% ($p = .003$ for probucol versus no probucol). The rate of repeat angioplasty necessary was 11.2% for the probucol group, 16.2% for the combined group, 24.4% for the multivitamin group, and 26.6% for the placebo group ($p = .009$ for probucol versus no probucol). The lack of benefit of antioxidant multivitamins in prevention of restenosis indicates that there may be a separate mechanism of action of probucol. Its positive effect may be a result of prevention of endothelial dysfunction and LDL oxidation or modified neointimal formation. The weak cholesterol-lowering effect of probucol is not thought to be responsible for this behavior, because lovastatin (a more powerful cholesterol-lowering agent) has been shown to be of no benefit in the prevention of restenosis.

For this reason, we consider the addition of probucol to the regimen to be indicated for any patient at high risk for restenosis (see Chapter 4). Probucol is administered at a dose of 500 mg bid, taken with meals. Restenosis is primarily a phenomenon of the first 6 months after angioplasty; this would therefore be a reasonable period of administration.

The manufacturer of probucol, Hoechst Marion Roussel, stopped producing this drug in 1996 owing to its declining use as a lipid-lowering agent. However, because of the results of this study and the potential new indication for the drug, they are planning more research and resumed production.

Brachytherapy (Radiation)

Intimal proliferation is thought to be the primary cause of postangioplasty and stenting restenosis. Radiation is an attractive means to prevent cellular reproduction; it appears to exert a positive influence on vessel remodeling after angioplasty also. It selectively kills dividing cells. Animal research and pilot clinical studies focused on intraluminal delivery of radiation owing to its site-specific activity and the ability to deliver high doses to a limited area. It seems reasonable that external beam radiation would be much less effective.[32]

Delivery of radiation to the angioplasty site from an intraluminal location can be performed in one of three ways: via the angioplasty balloon itself (inflation utilizing a radioactive fluid),[33] via placement of a radioactive source into an indwelling catheter after the angioplasty procedure,[34, 35] or by implanting an intrinsically radioactive source (the stent).

Filling the angioplasty balloon with a radioactive fluid results in extremely uniform distribution of activity, but only for a limited time. Amols et al. utilized yttrium-90 (^{90}Y) chloride solution.[33] The dose rate at the surface of the balloon was about 0.14 cGy/sec per mCi/ml (3.78×10^{-11} Gy/sec per Bq/ml), with the dose decreasing to 53% at 0.5 mm and less than 5% at 3.5 mm. This enabled the delivery of 20 Gy in less than 5 minutes (but required a 5-minute inflation).

The radioactive dose can be delivered by placement of a solid source within an indwelling catheter; this is feasible.[33, 36] A pure metallic ^{90}Y source (β-emitter) was placed within the introducing system, and the dose (18 Gy) was delivered within a reasonable time (about 6 minutes). The restenosis rate was not significantly different from the expected rate, however (six of 15 patients had more than 50% diameter stenosis at the previously treated site). Therefore, this dose rate did not appear to be effective when delivered using this technique.

The characteristics of β-emissions are ideal for superficial radiation delivery through a stent. There is very rapid distance-related drop-off and minimal leaching of material from the stent. This may therefore be the ideal method of radiation delivery for prevention of restenosis.[37, 38] This method delivers 95% of the dose within 4 mm of the stent edge, and the dose drops off to less than 1/1000 at 5 months after implantation. In the trial by Fischell et al.,[38] a zone of growth inhibition around the radioactive stent wires (phosphorus-32 [^{32}P] was observed that averaged about 6 mm. This was achieved at an activity of 0.0006 μCi/cm of wire. ^{32}P has a short half-life (14.3 days) and a limited range of tissue penetration (about 3 to 4 mm).

In the study by Carter and Laird,[37] an initial activity of 0.14 μCi reduced neointimal formation by 37% at 4 weeks after implantation in a porcine model. Additional studies involving radioactive Co and Fe demonstrated almost complete inhibition of neointimal proliferation in a rabbit model. In both instances, this reduction in neointimal hyperplasia was produced without a concomitant increase in thrombosis.

REFERENCES

1. Hasso AN, Bird CR, Zinke DE, Thompson JR. Fibromuscular dysplasia of the internal carotid artery: percutaneous transluminal angioplasty. *AJNR* 1981;2:175–180.
2. Hodgins GW, Dutton JW. Subclavian and carotid angioplasties for Takayasu's arteritis. *J Can Assoc Radiol* 1982;33:205–207.
3. Martin EC, Diamond NG, Casarella WJ. Percutaneous transluminal angioplasty in non-atherosclerotic disease. *Radiology* 1980;135:27–32.
4. Smith TP, Halbach VV, Fraser KW, et al. Percutaneous transluminal angioplasty of subclavian stenosis from neurofibromatosis. *AJNR* 1995;16:872–874.
5. Webster WW, Makaroun MS, Steed DL, et al. Compromised cerebral blood flow reactivity is a predictor of stroke in patients with symptomatic carotid artery occlusive disease. *J Vasc Surg* 1995;21:338–345.
6. Gaines P. The European carotid angioplasty trial [Abstract]. *J Endovasc Surg* 1996;3:107–108.
7. Sivaguru A, Venables GS, Beard JD, Gaines PA. European carotid angioplasty trial. *J Endovasc Surg* 1996;3:16–20.
8. Hass WK, Fields WS, North RR, et al. Joint study of extracranial arterial occlusion. Part II. Arteriography, techniques, sites and complications. *JAMA* 1968;203:961–968.
9. Krayenbühl H, Weber G. Die Thrombose der A. carotis interna und ihre Beziehung zur Endangitis obliterans. *Helv Med Acta* 1944;11:289–333.
10. Blackwood W. Thrombo-angiitis obliterans (Winiwarter-Buerger's disease). In Blackwood W, et al. (eds.): Greenfields Neuropathology. Baltimore: Williams & Wilkins, 1963, pp. 112–114.
11. Dotter CT, Rosch J, Judkins MP. Transluminal dilatation of atherosclerotic stenosis. *Surg Gynecol Obstet* 1968;127:794–804.
12. Dotter CT. Transluminal angioplasty: pathologic basis. In Zeitler E, Grüntzig A, Schoop W (eds.): Percutaneous Vascular Recanalization. Berlin: Springer-Verlag, 1978, p. 3.
13. Baughman KL, Pasternack RC, Fallon JT, Block PC. Coronary transluminal angioplasty in autopsied human hearts [Abstract]. *Circulation* 1978;57/58 (suppl 2):II–80.
14. Jester HG, Sinapius D, Alexander K, Leitz KH. Morphologische Veranderungen nach transluminaler Rekanalisation chronischer arterieller Verschlusse. In Zeitler E (ed.): Hypertonie-Risikofaktor in der Angiologie. Baden-Baden: Witzstrock, 1976.
15. Castañeda-Zúñiga WR, Formanek A, Tadavarthy M, et al. The mechanism of balloon angioplasty. *Radiology* 1980;135:565–571.
16. Castañeda-Zúñiga WR, Amplatz K, Laerum F, et al. Mechanics of angioplasty: an experimental approach. *Radiographics* 1981;1:1.
17. Zollikofer CL, Castañeda-Zúñiga WR, Amplatz K. Results of animal experiments with balloon dilatation. In Dotter CT, Grüntzig A, Schoop W, Zeitler E (eds.): Percutaneous Transluminal Angioplasty. Berlin: Springer-Verlag, 1983, p. 60.
18. Zollikofer CL, Salomonowitz E, Sibley R, et al. Transluminal angioplasty evaluated by electron microscopy. *Radiology* 1984;153:369–374.
19. Zollikofer CL. Experimentelle Grundlagen der perkutanen transluminalen Angioplastie. *Habilitationsschrift* 1985.
20. Zollikofer CL, Salomonowitz E, Brühllmann WF, et al. Dehnungs-, Verformungs- und Berstungs-Charakteristika haufig verwendeter Balloon-Dilitations-katheter: in vivo Untersuchungen an Hundegefassen (Teil 2). *Röfo* 1986;144:189.
21. Zollikofer CL, Chain J, Salomonowitz E, et al. Percutaneous transluminal angioplasty of the aorta. *Radiology* 1984;151:355–363.
22. Ohman EM, Marquis JF, Ricci DR, et al., for the Perfusion Balloon Catheter Study Group. A randomized comparison of the effects of gradual prolonged inflation versus standard primary balloon inflation on early and late outcome. *Circulation* 1994;89:1118–1125.
23. Jorgensen B, Meisner S, Holstein P, Tonnesn KH. Early restenosis in femoropopliteal occlusions treated with percutaneous transluminal angioplasty. *Eur J Vasc Surg* 1990;4:149–152.
24. Groves HM, Kinlough-Rathbone RL, Richardson M, et al. Platelet interaction with damaged rabbit aorta. *Lab Invest* 1979;40:194–200.
25. Wilenz JR, Sanborn TA, Haudenschild CC, et al. Platelet accumulation in experimental angioplasty: time course and relation to vascular injury. *Circulation* 1987;75:636–642.
26. Heras M, Chesebro JH, Penny WJ, et al. Importance of adequate heparin dosage in arterial angioplasty in a porcine model. *Circulation* 1988;78:654–660.
27. Lam JY, Chesebro JH, Steele PM, et al. Is vasospasm related to platelet deposition? Relationship in a porcine preparation of arterial injury in vivo. *Circulation* 1987;75:243–248.
28. Lam JY, Chesebro JH, Badimon L, Fuster V. The vasoconstrictive response following arterial angioplasty in pigs: evidence for vasoconstriction resulting from, rather than causing, platelet deposition [Abstract]. *J Am Coll Cardiol* 1986;7:12A.
29. Berk BC, Alexander RW, Brock TA, et al. Vasoconstriction: a new activity for platelet-derived growth factor. *Science* 1986;232:87–90.
30. Block PC. Restenosis after percutaneous transluminal coronary angioplasty. Anatomic and pathophysiological mechanisms: strategies for prevention. *Circulation* 1990;81:Suppl IV2–4.
31. Tardif JC, Côté G, Lespérance J, et al. Probucol and multivitamins in the prevention of restenosis after coronary angioplasty. *N Engl J Med* 1997;337:365–372.
32. Koh WJ, Mayberg MR, Chambers J, et al. The potential role of external beam radiation in preventing restenosis after coronary angioplasty. *Int J Radiat Oncol Biol Phys* 1996;36:829–834.
33. Amols HI, Reinstein LE, Weinberger J. Dosimetry of a radioactive coronary balloon dilatation catheter for treatment of neointimal hyperplasia. *Med Phys* 1996;23:1783–1788.
34. Waksman R. Local catheter-based intracoronary radiation therapy for restenosis. *Am J Cardiol* 1996;78:23–28.
35. Popowski Y, Verin V, Urban P. Endovascular beta-irradiation after percutaneous transluminal coronary balloon angioplasty. *Int J Radiat Oncol Biol Phys* 1996;36:841–845.
36. Verin V, Urban P, Popowski Y, et al. Feasibility of intracoronary beta-irradiation to reduce restenosis after balloon angioplasty; a clinical pilot study. *Circulation* 1997;95:1138–1144.
37. Carter AJ, Laird JR. Experimental results with endovascular irradiation via a radioactive stent. *Int J Radiat Oncol Biol Phys* 1996;36:797–803.
38. Fischell TA, Carter AJ, Laird JR. The beta-particle-emitting radioisotope stent (isostent): animal studies and planned clinical trials. *Am J Cardiol* 1996;78:45–50.

CHAPTER 42

General Technique of Extracranial Angioplasty and Stenting

J.J. Connors III

TOOLS FOR EXTRACRANIAL ANGIOPLASTY AND STENTING

In addition to the routine catheter tray, the materials needed are listed in Table 42–1.

PRELIMINARY EVALUATION

A thorough patient history and neurologic examination are mandatory; some lesions may not require therapy when the symptoms are found to be inconsistent with the pathology. A preliminary magnetic resonance imaging (MRI) scan is performed to establish a baseline intracranial evaluation and to rule out a recent infarct (perhaps silent). A transient occlusion during angioplasty may cause a recurrence of the symptoms of a prior healing infarct or transient ischemic attack.

After an acute neurologic event, time should be allowed before an elective procedure is performed (about 6 weeks; 4 weeks in the recently established Carotid Stent Supported Angioplasty registry). This delay is needed in case it becomes necessary to use urokinase to treat unwanted thrombus during or after the procedure. Unwanted thrombus is more of a problem with *intracranial* angioplasty than with *extracranial* angioplasty.

Routine blood work includes a complete blood count, prothrombin time, partial thromboplastin time, blood urea nitrogen, creatinine, electrolytes, glucose, and cholesterol levels. Depending on the circumstances and lesion location, evaluation for hypercoagulability may be appropriate. Chapter 54 discusses this topic further.

All patients who undergo brachiocephalic or intracranial angioplasty should first undergo a thorough evaluation of their intracranial hemodynamics, not just a good "picture" of the stenosis, extracranial or otherwise. The site selected for angioplasty should be neurologically compatible with the patient's symptoms, and angioplasty should be undertaken only when it is deemed the most appropriate means of therapy for the symptoms by the attending neurologic and vascular specialists. It may be found that the patient's symptoms are caused by a vertebral artery origin stenosis, for instance, rather than by a previously identified carotid siphon stenosis. *Angioplasty of a lesion because it "looks bad" is unacceptable.*

The operator should be familiar with the shifting watershed zones, normal arteriovenous transit times,

and secondary signs of distal embolization. As noted elsewhere, rarely is an intracranial embolus actually seen as an abrupt vessel cutoff. A thorough understanding of intracranial hemodynamics is necessary before undertaking brachiocephalic angioplasty, not only for proper evaluation of the indications for the procedure but also for understanding the results and possibly performing a rescue.

INDICATIONS

The ideal patients for brachiocephalic angioplasty are those with symptoms of ischemia (particularly posterior fossa) or embolic phenomena. Patients who have failed adequate medical therapy, those who have other conditions precluding surgery, and those who have lesions that are impossible or dangerous to treat surgically are candidates for angioplasty and stenting.

The work by Webster et al. indicates that there may be a future role for the therapy of patients without overt symptoms but with hemodynamically significant lesions.[1] Typically, however, brachiocephalic angioplasty should be performed for clinically symptomatic lesions. In a proper clinical trial, angioplasty with or without stenting can be performed as a substitute for endarterectomy or brachiocephalic bypass (see Chapters 43 and 47).

CONTRAINDICATIONS

Contraindications to angioplasty include lesions with associated thrombus, Ehlers-Danlos syndrome, and any other contraindications for angiography. Elective

---

TABLE 42-1 Tools for Extracranial Angioplasty and Stenting

A quarter (for accurate vessel measuring)
Selected angioplasty catheter
Selected stent (if used)
Appropriate guide catheter
Appropriate selecting and exchange guidewires
Microcatheter, microwire, and micro exchange wire (if needed for vessel selection)
Inflator with 6-foot extension microtubing
Rotating hemostatic valves (large bore for guide catheter, standard for angioplasty catheter)
Heparinized flush (pressurized) for the guide catheter, angioplasty catheter, and sheath (if used)

angioplasty should be avoided (when possible) in a patient with a recent history of stroke unless undertaken as part of the acute neurovascular rescue, because either before or after the angioplasty of a vital vessel, infusion of a fibrinolytic agent is frequently necessary. The ability to use fibrinolytics for rescue of the procedure without worry is a luxury.

PREPROCEDURE PREPARATION

Depending on the location of the lesion and its appearance, some operators prefer to maintain the patient on anticoagulant therapy for a period of time before the procedure to aid in "cleaning up" the lesion before therapy. We have found this to be useful on occasion (see Figs. 48–39 to 48–48).

All patients are started on aspirin and ticlopidine. After 6 weeks the ticlopidine is stopped; aspirin is continued for the rest of the patients' lives, if possible. In addition, the combination of aspirin and dipyridamole has been shown to be more effective than aspirin alone. These patients have already demonstrated a propensity for vascular disease, which is a good enough reason to maintain them on aspirin for life.

Nimodipine is given as a cerebral protectant for prophylaxis against ischemia in the case of cerebral embolus. The use of steroids for preoperative cerebral protection is controversial in this instance.

Although low-molecular-weight dextran may be given as a volume expander before the procedure, its primary role is in the control of platelet aggregation, and it is used after therapy by many interventional neuroradiologists for this purpose.

Tobacco products should be absolutely forbidden. This cannot be emphasized enough. Achieving and maintaining patient compliance on this issue is often the most difficult aspect of long-term management and has been observed to be directly related to recurrence of the primary pathology, in both extracranial and intracranial locations. Not only does nicotine cause progression of vasculopathy, it also causes hypercoagulability.

When angioplasty of the carotid bifurcation is performed, atropine should be administered prophylactically to prevent a vasovagal reaction due to carotid body compression. The use of atropine may be unnecessary or contraindicated, however, depending on the patient's cardiac status. Work is being performed in some institutions involving the use of temporary external pacemakers to deal with any significant hemodynamic problem, but this necessity appears rare. A temporary pacemaker should be available for use when needed, however (see Chapter 1).

PROCEDURAL TECHNIQUE FOR EXTRACRANIAL ANGIOPLASTY

This section provides a general description of the techniques and equipment employed for extracranial brachiocephalic angioplasty. Many of the same principles and techniques are employed for both intra-

cranial and extracranial angioplasty. Most of these are presented here. The section on technique in Chapter 48 contains details specific to distal small vessel work.

Guide Catheter

For all lesions above the aorta, a guide catheter is used. The guide catheter has multiple purposes, but primarily it allows accurate placement of the angioplasty balloon by means of test injections. The guide catheter should have enough shaft stiffness to give support to the angioplasty catheter beyond just the support from the guidewire and to avoid recoil of the guidewire, balloon catheter, and guide catheter into the aorta during the manipulations needed to cross some lesions and position the balloon. The guide catheter also allows postangioplasty evaluation of results without making catheter or wire exchanges or losing catheter or wire position.

In addition, if necessary after angioplasty, the guide catheter allows placement of a Palmaz stent (Johnson & Johnson Interventional Systems) mounted on a 5- or 6-Fr. angioplasty balloon without replacing any catheters. We do not use a sheath to introduce the guide catheter in these patients because we want to create as small a puncture site as possible and because we can insert a guide catheter of adequate size without using a sheath (by using a dilator inside the guide catheter to introduce this device through the skin; see Chapter 3). Therefore, a 9-Fr. guide catheter is used in almost all cases.

For lesions directly off the aorta, at the origin of one of the great vessels, a guide catheter with an accentuated S curve (similar to a JB-2 or JB-3) is useful. This allows the guide catheter to be aimed at the lesion without exerting too much force on the vessel origin from the guidewire or balloon catheter tip.

Anticoagulation

There is no firm agreement on the use of anticoagulants during brachiocephalic angioplasty. Some angioplasty and stenting procedures are now performed on an outpatient basis, whereas others are done with a 3-day hospital stay. Many practitioners prefer preprocedure aspirin and intraprocedural heparin of varying amounts. Aspirin therapy is considered the minimum that is necessary and should be continued for the rest of the patient's life. Ticlopidine is used for the first 6 weeks after the procedure.

Abciximab (ReoPro) (see Chapter 4) is gaining more widespread acceptance. This is a powerful intravenous inhibitor of platelet aggregation. It was initially evaluated for use in conjunction with coronary angioplasty, specifically in patients considered at high risk of postprocedure myocardial infarction due to sudden arterial occlusion after angioplasty. It is given as a bolus immediately before the angioplasty, followed by a 12-hour infusion. The same protocol is used by many practitioners during brachiocephalic angioplasty. Abciximab is used for all intracranial angioplasties and for selected extracranial angioplasties.

The possibility of thrombus associated with stenosis is always present, but it appears that this threat is less common than originally feared. It is, however, lesion specific in the extracranial vasculature. Thrombus is a greater threat with a recently symptomatic intracranial stenosis; frequently, these patients receive intravenous heparin before therapy.

Lesions at the vertebral origin are usually smoothly stenotic, but innominate or subclavian artery stenoses can be irregular; fragmentation of plaque is the primary concern associated with these lesions, but superimposed thrombus has been identified. Stenoses off the aorta at the common carotid origin can be either smooth or irregular (see Chapter 47).

Once the guide catheter is in place, 10,000 units of heparin is administered. Cardiovascular surgeons routinely employ boluses of 50,000 units of heparin, so why not give 10,000 units if adequate anticoagulation is the goal? Additional quantities of heparin are not associated with increased complications in brief procedures such as angioplasty. The practitioner should give an adequate bolus.

Oxygen

Intraprocedural supplemental oxygen is administered to all patients.

Measurement of the Lesion and Choice of Balloon Size

The most important object to measure is the normal vessel nearest the stenosis, both proximal and distal to the lesion, *not the stenosis itself*. This is what determines the size of the balloon and stent to be used; the smallest normal vessel size is the maximal size for the angioplasty balloon. We do not overdilate lesions. Accurate measurement of the stenosis and the normal lumen already should have been performed (see Chapter 3); if not, it is performed at this time.

For extracranial angioplasty, a balloon of the same size as the vessel is chosen. For intracranial angioplasty, on the other hand, a balloon smaller than the normal vessel size is chosen (see Chapter 48). For some cases, we wish the smallest available size of these balloons were 1.5 mm instead of 2 mm.

Initial Crossing of the Stenosis

Initial crossing of the lesion is a critical part of this procedure. If the lesion looks at all irregular, crossing should be done with a soft platinum-tipped microwire. This is by far the safest method of gaining distal access. For most lesions, a Platinum Plus guidewire (Medi-Tech, Inc./Boston Scientific) is used in conjunction with the hydrophilic-coated Sub-4 an-

gioplasty balloon (Medi-Tech, Inc./Boston Scientific) or 5-Fr. Diamond angioplasty balloon (Medi-Tech, Inc./Boston Scientific). Alternatively, a microwire can be placed through the stenosis followed by a microcatheter and then by a 5-Fr. diagnostic catheter, all placed coaxially through the guide catheter. This safely places the large-lumen standard catheter past the stenosis. The microwire and microcatheter can then be removed and replaced by a stiffer interventional exchange wire; we prefer the Rosen guidewire for this reasonably atraumatic tip and relatively stiff shaft, although a better guidewire for brachiocephalic intervention is becoming available from Cook, Inc.

This technique of safe distal acquisition is presented in detail in Chapter 3.

Angioplasty Procedure

The angioplasty balloon hub is attached to a long (6-foot), flexible microextension tube (see Chapter 1) to allow easy manipulation of the catheter without having to drag the inflator around. The tubing is then attached to a mechanical screw inflator to allow extremely slow, controlled inflation. This tubing also reduces the concern regarding any bubbles in the line associated with the inflator or pressure meter. The tubing holds several milliliters of fluid and, owing to its small lumen, fills cleanly without bubbles when flushed before use.

The best angioplasty results have been achieved by *gradual inflations* over 1 to 3 minutes, allowing the vessel to stretch slowly rather than to tear. When using a stent, this inflation can be done more quickly. This slow inflation method is an attempt to lessen the degree of intimal injury, not to tack down intimal tears. Stretching the vessel, rather than abruptly tearing it, is the goal.

Balloon pressure is gradually increased from 1 to 1.5 to 2 atmospheres in several stages, allowing a pause of 15 seconds at each stage. The inflator plunger is turned about one fourth to one third of a turn and then stopped. Further pressure increases also are made gradually in stages, allowing the vessel to comply slowly, until optimal balloon expansion has been achieved. Optimal balloon inflation is dependent on rate of expansion, not simply rate of pressure increase. As each new pressure is reached, time should be allowed for additional expansion that can occur slowly without further pressure increase.

For extracranial lesions, the pressure required for balloon inflation can sometimes be high. Intracranial lesions almost routinely require much lower pressures. This slow inflation has resulted in far fewer extreme intimal dissections than occurred with earlier angioplasty procedures.[2]

Extracranial angioplasty rarely results in true cerebral ischemia of any significance in the few minutes of occlusion with this technique (neurosurgeons routinely temporarily occlude intracranial vessels for 10 minutes or more).[3] Very rarely, however, hypoperfusion may occur rapidly during angioplasty of the vertebral artery origin. This vessel may supply a truly isolated territory; occlusion can result in flow arrest in the entire posterior fossa. It may be for this reason that Higashida et al. recommend dilation for less than 10 to 15 seconds, although we consider this degree of rapidity extreme.[4]

After satisfactory dilation has been achieved, balloon inflation is maintained for about 15 to 60 seconds to allow for remodeling and for the intima to adhere in its new location (depending on the location of the lesion; extracranial lesions can be held for periods of minutes). The balloon is then deflated over 5 to 10 seconds. If a stent is used, deflation can be more rapid.

A less than perfect visual appearance (i.e., <100% dilation) is acceptable and compatible with a satisfactory result, particularly in small intracranial vessels. Conversely, for large vessels, the rate of recurrent stenosis increases with the amount of residual stenosis; the subsequent turbulent flow is thought to contribute to this recurrence. The goal of therapy for these large (and safer) extracranial vessels should be to restore them to a nearly normal lumen size.

Stent Use

A thorough discussion of the different products on the market or approaching the market is presented in Chapter 1. The rationale for stent use is also discussed in Chapters 43 and 50.

In certain situations, stents are very important. The dismal results for stent use in small vessels cannot be ignored, however, particularly when considering their use in the intracranial circulation (in the coronary circulation, failure/restenosis is typically on the order of 25% to 40% within 6 months). It is one thing to have an abrupt closure in the coronary vasculature that requires bypass with no ill results; it is another completely to have a failure in the brachiocephalic circulation that leads to a stroke.

In the great vessels off the aorta, however, stents are of great help. These locations are ideal for stent use. These are large vessels with high flow in a noncompressible location. They are frequently associated with irregular plaque that ideally should be tacked down. More specific discussion of these locations is provided in Chapter 47. We routinely use Palmaz stents for lesions in these locations because of the ability to accurately place them and their long-term results. The shortest size available is chosen; the 10-mm length invariably has been long enough and does not risk overlapping the origin of a distal branch.

Occasionally it may be necessary to overlap stents because of a small intimal dissection at one end of a previously placed stent or inaccurate placement of the original stent. Overlapping stents are of no concern except under one circumstance: placement of a balloon-expandable stent (typically a Palmaz stent) inside a self-expanding nitinol stent (typically a Wallstent [Schneider Inc.]) The self-expanding nitinol stent may continue to expand after the procedure, leaving the balloon-expandable stent floating inside the outer stent—a bad situation that may lead to a dead space between two stents. A fixed-size balloon-expandable stent should not be placed inside a self-expanding stent; it is permissible to place a self-expanding stent inside a balloon-expandable stent.

Postdilation Observation

The procedure does not end at the completion of the angioplasty. In a normal vessel with intact endothelium, in a nonhypercoagulable state, static blood should not clot for a long time (i.e., minutes or longer). Uninjured vascular endothelium is antithrombotic, resists platelet adherence, and provides a hostile environment for activation of clotting factors. When vascular injury does occur (e.g., secondary to guidewire manipulation or angioplasty), the rate of coagulation reactions can increase to 300,000 times baseline.[5] Plaque and intimal disruption cause local platelet deposition by the release of thromboxane A_2 and platelet-derived growth factor. Once the endothelium has been scraped by a guidewire or catheter, thrombus formation is unpredictable; therefore, heparin is indicated during the inflation and for a period of time afterward.

Particularly in intracranial small vessel stenoses, the act of angioplasty can stimulate a malignant coagulation cascade. For prolonged angioplasty inflations in the periphery, however (e.g., the superficial femoral artery), heparin is unnecessary, probably because of the vessel size and flow rate.[6] It is the angioplasty site (after deflation of the balloon), not the distal lumen, that is at primary risk of thrombus formation after the procedure. We routinely heparinize patients during brachiocephalic angioplasty procedures.

Continued surveillance of the site for a period is therefore indicated; the more distal and small the vessel, the longer the observation. If progressive thrombus formation is noted, local infusion of urokinase via a microcatheter positioned just proximal to the angioplasty site is indicated. The site should be observed until it appears stable. Thrombotic occlusion is more common with the use of stents, but even then it is rare in large vessels. We observe large-vessel angioplasties and stents for 10 to 15 minutes (while performing serial postprocedure angiography). For intracranial angioplasties, we observe the site for at least 30 minutes. Delayed thrombosis can be evaluated with nuclear scintigraphy (^{111}In platelet scintigraphy; see Chapter 46).

POSTPROCEDURE CARE

For large-vessel angioplasty with good results and high flow, the heparin is reversed and the guide catheter removed in the angiography suite. Pressure is held for 20 to 30 minutes, and a small pressure dressing is applied, followed by a sandbag. Routine postprocedure orders are described in Chapter 7. Ticlopidine (250 mg bid) is continued for 6 weeks; aspirin (325 mg) is continued for life.

Probucol

Probucol, a lipid-lowering agent that has been on the market since the mid-1970s, has been shown to be effective in preventing restenosis following coronary angioplasty; it is the only pharmacologic agent shown to do this. As discussed in Chapter 41, production of this drug was halted, but its reintroduction is being considered by the manufacturer. If probucol becomes available, we consider its addition to the regimen to be indicated for any patient at high risk of restenosis.

Follow-Up

For large-vessel angioplasty, noninvasive follow-up is recommended after 6 months, with a follow-up angiogram in 1 year. The North American Cerebral Percutaneous Transluminal Angioplasty Register (NACPTAR) protocol calls for ultrasound (Doppler), single-photon emission computed tomography, and computed tomography or MRI evaluation at 1 month, ultrasound evaluation at 6 months, angiogram at 1 year, and ultrasound at 2 years. This protocol differs

from that for intracranial angioplasty, in which short-term angiographic follow-up is obtained at 3 months.

REFERENCES

1. Webster WW, Makaroun MS, Steed DL, et al. Compromised cerebral blood flow reactivity is a predictor of stroke in patients with symptomatic carotid artery occlusive disease. *J Vasc Surg* 1995;21:338–345.
2. Ohman EM, Marquis JF, Ricci DR, et al, for the Perfusion Balloon Catheter Study Group. A randomized comparison of the effects of gradual prolonged inflation versus standard primary balloon inflation on early and late outcome. *Circulation* 1994;89:1118–1125.
3. Heros RC. Management of unclippable aneurysms. In Schmidek HH, Sweet WH (eds): Operative Neurosurgical Techniques: Indications, Methods, and Results, 2nd ed. Orlando: Grune & Stratton, 1988, pp 1023–1034.
4. Higashida RT, Tsai FY, Halbach VV, et al. Interventional neurovascular techniques in the treatment of stroke: state-of-the-art therapy. *J Intern Med* 1995;237:105–115.
5. Brott T. Thrombolytic therapy. Cerebral ischemia: treatment and prevention. *Neurol Clin* 1992;10:219–232.
6. Heras M, Chesebro JH, Penny WJ, et al. Importance of adequate heparin dosage in arterial angioplasty in a porcine model. *Circulation* 1988;78:654–660.

CHAPTER 43

General Considerations for Endovascular Therapy of the Extracranial Internal Carotid Artery at the Bifurcation

J.J. Connors III

Because of the extremely important nature of carotid bifurcation disease and the tremendous potential for endovascular therapy that exists, any dogmatic statements are necessarily premature. It has not been determined whether stents will be necessary; for this reason, studies by the current world authorities are presented in this and subsequent chapters.

NATURAL HISTORY OF THE DISEASE

Many recent studies and ongoing work have centered around carotid bifurcation disease, and a considerable amount of information has begun to accumulate on this subject. These data provide a clear picture of the scope of the problem and its manifestations and provide useful guidelines for therapy.

Most patients who have internal carotid atherosclerotic disease do not have warning signs.[1, 2] Pa-

tients who have 75% or greater stenoses have a 2% to 5% risk of stroke during the first year. Ulceration increases the risk of subsequent stroke to about 7.5% per year.[3]

Asymptomatic Carotid Artery Disease

The Veterans Affairs Cooperative Study Group followed 444 men with asymptomatic carotid stenoses of greater than 50% for 4 years.[4] The patients received surgery or aspirin therapy. During the 4 years of the study, there was an incidence of ipsilateral stroke of 9.4% in the group receiving medical therapy—a yearly risk of 2.3%. The total rate of ipsilateral neurologic events in the medically treated patients was 20.6%, a rate of 5.1% per year (mostly transient ischemic attacks, or TIAs).

An additional study by Mackey et al.[5] followed

asymptomatic patients, with stenoses detected by carotid bruit, by carotid duplex ultrasound. Stenosis evaluation therefore did not follow North American Symptomatic Carotid Endarterectomy Trial (NASCET) criteria but more closely simulated real-world medical practice. The annual rate of all vascular events was 11.0% in patients with stenoses of greater than 50%. The annual rate of stroke or vascular-related death was 5.5% in this group. The yearly rate of stroke was 4.2% in subjects with greater than 80% stenosis and 1.4% in those with less than 80% stenosis, but the stroke or TIA was ipsilateral to the measured stenosis in only 66% of these patients.

The Asymptomatic Carotid Atherosclerosis Study (ACAS) trial evaluated 1662 patients with stenoses of greater than 60%.[6] The 5-year relative risk for ipsilateral stroke and any perioperative stroke or death was reduced by 53%, a significant amount. However, major stipulations pertain to these results. First, patients had to have a reasonable life expectancy, and second, angiography and surgery had to be performed with less than 2.3% risk of stroke or death. These are extremely low rates of stroke or death from combined surgery and angiography!

Several points of major importance concerning these relative risk rates are routinely ignored or overlooked when the results of the ACAS trial are discussed. The annual event rate for patients treated medically was only 2.2% (surgery reduced this rate to 1%). This is a very low rate. Additionally, even though the relative risk reduction provided by surgery was 66% for men, it was only 17% for women—an insignificant reduction. Endarterectomy was not shown to benefit women with asymptomatic stenoses, a widely overlooked fact, and there was no significant reduction in the rate of major strokes. In addition, there was no relationship between benefit and the degree of carotid artery stenosis.

Perhaps of greatest significance, however, was the fact that these relative risk reductions were not compared with optimal medical therapy. Patients in the ACAS medical control group were treated only with 325 mg aspirin per day. Subsequent data suggest that this is probably a suboptimal therapy; even high-dose aspirin may work better.[7, 8] Ticlopidine reduces stroke risk more than aspirin.[9] The combination of aspirin and warfarin may be better than aspirin alone at stroke prevention.[10–12] The comparison with suboptimal medical therapy suggests that the conclusions concerning relative reduction in stroke reduction may be erroneous.

The European Carotid Surgery Trialists Collaborative Group evaluated 2295 asymptomatic patients with carotid stenosis with a mean follow-up of 4.5 years.[13] The stroke risk in 127 patients with 70% to 99% stenosis was 5.7% (1.2% per year). Stenosis was measured by the European Carotid Surgery Trial (ECST) method: the percentage of stenosis was determined by the maximum percentage reduction in the diameter of the relevant carotid artery; the correct prestenosis vessel size was estimated.

Symptomatic Carotid Artery Disease

Symptomatic carotid artery disease has a far different prognosis. More than 2500 patients were enrolled in the ECST over a 10-year period; a mean 3-year follow-up for 2200 was obtained and reported on.[13] Of the patients followed, 778 had a severe stenosis (70% to 99% as measured by the ECST method). During the 3-year follow-up, 16.8% of medically treated patients suffered an ipsilateral ischemic stroke; 11.0% of these were disabling or fatal. This yields a risk rate of any ipsilateral ischemic stroke of 5.6% per year. In patients who have had TIAs, the risk of subsequent stroke increases to about 13% within the first year after the onset of symptoms. About one third of these patients have a stroke within the first 5 years.[14] In patients who already have had strokes, the risk of having another stroke is about 5% to 9% per year, with a 5-year risk of 25% to 45%.[15, 16] The type of plaque has been shown to influence the outcome significantly.

In the North American Symptomatic Carotid Endarterectomy Trial (NASCET), there was a stroke risk of 26.0% in 2 years (13% per year) for patients with symptomatic stenoses from 70% to 99%, as compared with a surgical risk of only 9.0% during this 2-year period (4.5% per year).[17] An interesting subgroup analysis of the patients from NASCET was performed. Patients with stenoses of 70% or greater (659 patients) were divided into groups by severity of stenosis: 70% to 79%, 80% to 89%, 90% to 94%, and near-occlusion. The 106 patients with near-occlusion were then divided into those with a stringlike lumen and those without. The risk of stroke increased with the degree of stenosis; the greatest risk was in those with 90% to 94% stenoses (35.1% ± 10.7% per year, a wide range of error). This decreased to only 11.1% for patients with near-occlusion with a string sign, similar to the rate for 70% to 79% (12.8%). For patients with 80% to 89% stenoses, there was an 18.5% risk of stroke. Only 1 out of 58 (1.7%) patients with near-occlusion of the carotid artery who were treated medically had a stroke in the first month, indicating that these lesions do not necessarily represent an emergent situation.

These dire outcome predictions for patients with carotid artery disease are contrasted with the results of the ECST.[13] Patients with 70% to 99% stenoses treated medically had a 21.9% risk of ipsilateral ischemic stroke or any other stroke over a 3-year period, a yearly rate of 7.3%. Surgery reduced this to 12.3%. However, the previously noted rate of ipsilateral ischemic stroke alone, 16.8% over three years (5.6% per year), was considerably different from the NASCET results.

A risk analysis based on clinical symptoms was performed.[18] Data from published studies were reviewed, and stroke rate predictions were made. For asymptomatic carotid artery disease, the rate of subsequent stroke was 1.3% per year (95% confidence interval [CI], 1.0 to 1.6). For patients presenting with transient ischemic attack, the rate of subsequent stroke was 3.7% per year (95% CI, 3.1 to 4.3); for transient monocular blindness, the rate was 2.2% per year (95% CI, 1.3 to 3.0); for minor stroke, the rate was 6.1% per year (95% CI, 5.7 to 6.6); and for major stroke, the rate was 9.0% (95% CI, 8.0 to 9.9).

CAROTID ENDARTERECTOMY

An excellent discussion of the rationale for carotid endarterectomy is presented by Frey.[19] The inadequacy of correct and specific information concerning the natural history of carotid artery disease is a major concern.

Even after successful carotid endarterectomy, the risk of TIA or stroke does not disappear. Patients who had previous TIAs still have a 1% to 2% chance of stroke. Patients who had previous strokes still have a 2% to 3% chance per year of having another stroke even after successful endarterectomy. In these cases, the *underlying cause was not corrected,* or the healing process at the endarterectomy site was not completely successful.[20, 21]

The guidelines for carotid endarterectomy have been well disseminated[22] (Table 43–1). These guidelines are based on the interim NASCET results. The study was begun in 1986; one arm of the study was halted in 1991 because of the marked benefit of carotid endarterectomy for patients with stenoses of greater than 70%. The final results of the trial indicate that there is clear benefit of surgery over medical management for carotid stenoses greater than 50% in men, even in the higher risk categories. For women, the benefits of surgery for stenoses between 50% and 70% do not uniformly outweigh the risks (presentation by Barnett at the 23rd International Joint Conference on Stroke and Cerebral Circulation, Orlando, Florida, February, 1998).

The actual indications, however, are totally dependent on the safety and efficacy of the procedure, not just on the pathology. This is frequently overlooked, and when discussing the need for treatment, the morbidity and mortality of the procedure frequently are erroneously underestimated, even in papers discussing the risk-to-benefit ratio as compared with endovascular procedures. This form of comparison and discussion is inaccurate.

The blanket statements concerning indications for endarterectomy are based on the NASCET trial, and even then are broken down by risk category. Simply quoting the lowest risk or complication category is not accurate. The NASCET study was highly controlled and the procedure was performed by only the best operators and on only carefully selected patients.

A system of grading patients according to the degree of risk associated with carotid endarterectomy was proposed by Sundt et al. in 1975.[23] Patients were divided into four groups: group 1 had no medical or angiographic risk factors and were neurologically stable; group 2 had angiographic risk factors but no medical risk factors and were neurologically stable; group 3 had significant medical risk factors with or without angiographic risk factors and were neurologically stable; and group 4 were neurologically unstable. Angiographic risk factors included occlusion of the opposite internal carotid artery (ICA); ICA stenosis in the region of the siphon; extensive disease with plaque extending more than 3 cm distal to the bifurcation or more than 5 cm proximal to the bifurcation; location of the bifurcation unusually high in the neck (C2); and soft thrombus associated with an ulcerated lesion. Medical risk factors included angina pectoris, myocardial infarction in the preceding 6 months, congestive heart failure, severe hypertension (180/110 mm Hg or greater), chronic obstructive pulmonary disease, severe obesity, and age greater than 70 years. Neurologic instability was defined as progressing neurologic deficit, deficit of less than 24 hours' duration, frequent TIAs, or neurologic deficits secondary to multiple infarctions. As shown in Table 43–2, the total morbidity and mortality increased slightly in group 2 and more dramatically in groups 3 and 4. All perioperative myocardial infarctions occurred in group 3 patients with known medical risk factors, and seven of eight strokes occurred in neurologically unstable patients. Out of 331 total procedures, there were two deaths, both from myocardial infarction (a mortality rate of 0.61%). The overall perioperative stroke rate was 3.0%, and the combined morbidity and mortality rate was 4.8%.

Analysis of the morbidity and mortality associated with carotid endarterectomy in the Cincinnati area was done by Brott and Thalinger in 1984.[24] This analysis indicated a far higher "real-world" risk associated with carotid endarterectomy than the risk in a high-volume, well-trained institution. The results indicated a combined morbidity and mortality rate of 9.5%, with a perioperative stroke rate of 8.6% and death rate of 2.8%. An additional analysis of 51 studies of endarterectomy done since 1980 was performed by Rothwell et al.[25] This review found a risk of death of 1.62%; the risk of stroke, death, or both was 5.64%. There was significant variation in results, however. The risks were highest in studies in which postoperative assessment was performed by a neurologist (7.7% chance of stroke) and lowest for single investigators affiliated with a department of surgery (2.3%). No temporal trend indicated improvement or worsening of these results. In the ECST, surgery performed on 776 patients with severe (70% to 99%) stenosis resulted in stroke or death within 30 days in 7.5% of cases.[13]

Any generalization pertaining to indications for endarterectomy based solely on the surgical category of lowest risk is misspoken and inaccurate. This is certainly true if expanded to apply to every location and practitioner (i.e., "it is established beyond any doubt [grade A recommendation] that carotid endarterectomy is the treatment of choice for symptomatic [recent TIA or nondisabling stroke] stenosis of 70% to 99%.")[26] These statements are based on statistics which most likely do not apply to the real world.

Some practitioners consistently surpass the quality

T A B L E   4 3 - 1   American Heart Association Indications for Carotid Endarterectomy

Asymptomatic Patients With Coronary Artery Disease

For Patients With a Surgical Risk of Less Than 3%

1. Proven indications: none
2. Acceptable but unproven indications: ipsilateral carotid endarterectomy for stenosis ≥75% with or without ulceration, irrespective of contralateral artery status, ranging from no disease to total occlusion
3. Uncertain indications:
   - Stenosis <50% with a B (10–40 mm²) or C (>40 mm²) ulcer, irrespective of contralateral internal carotid artery status
   - Unilateral carotid endarterectomy with coronary artery bypass graft (CABG); CABG required with bilateral asymptomatic stenosis >70%
   - Unilateral carotid stenosis >70%, CABG required; unilateral carotid endarterectomy with CABG
4. Proven inappropriate indications: none defined

For Patients With a Surgical Risk of 3% to 5%

1. Proven indications: none
2. Acceptable but unproven indications: ipsilateral carotid endarterectomy for stenosis ≥75% with or without ulceration but in the presence of contralateral internal carotid artery stenosis ranging from 75% to total occlusion
3. Uncertain indications:
   - Ipsilateral carotid endarterectomy for stenosis ≥75% with or without ulceration irrespective of contralateral artery status, ranging from no stenosis to occlusion
   - CABG required, with bilateral asymptomatic stenosis >70%; unilateral carotid endarterectomy with CABG
   - Unilateral carotid stenosis >70%, CABG required; ipsilateral carotid endarterectomy with CABG
4. Proven inappropriate indications: none defined

For Patients With a Surgical Risk of 5% of 10%

1. Proven indications: none
2. Acceptable but unproven indications: none
3. Uncertain indications:
   - CABG required with bilateral asymptomatic stenosis >70%; unilateral carotid endarterectomy with CABG
   - Unilateral carotid stenosis >70%, CABG required; ipsilateral carotid endarterectomy with CABG
4. Proven inappropriate indications:
   - Ipsilateral carotid endarterectomy for stenosis ≥75% with or without ulceration irrespective of contralateral internal carotid artery status
   - Stenosis ≤50% with or without ulceration irrespective of contralateral carotid artery status

Symptomatic Patients With Coronary Artery Disease

For Patients With a Surgical Risk of Less Than 6%

1. Proven indications:
   - Single or multiple transient ischemic attacks (TIAs) within a 6-month interval or crescendo TIAs in the presence of a stenosis ≥70%, with or without ulceration, with or without antiplatelet therapy
   - Mild stroke within a 6-month interval, in the presence of a stenosis ≥70%, with or without ulceration, with or without antiplatelet therapy
2. Acceptable but unproven indications:
   - TIA (single, multiple, or recurrent) within a 6-month interval, in the presence of a stenosis ≥50%, with or without ulceration, with or without antiplatelet therapy
   - Crescendo TIAs in the presence of a stenosis >50%, with or without ulceration, with or without antiplatelet therapy
   - Progressive stroke in the presence of a stenosis ≥70% with or without ulceration, with or without antiplatelet therapy
   - Mild stroke in the presence of a stenosis ≥50%, with or without ulceration, with or without antiplatelet therapy
   - Moderate stroke in the presence of a stenosis ≥50%, with or without ulceration, with or without antiplatelet therapy
   - Ipsilateral carotid endarterectomy combined with CABG in a patient experiencing TIAs, in the presence of unilateral or bilateral stenoses ≥70%, CABG needed
3. Uncertain indications:
   - TIA (single, multiple, or recurrent) with stenosis <50%, with or without ulceration, with or without antiplatelet therapy
   - Crescendo TIAs, with or without ulceration, with stenosis <50%

- TIAs in a patient who requires CABG and has a stenosis <70%
- Mild stroke with carotid stenosis <50%, with or without ulceration, with or without antiplatelet therapy
- Moderate stroke with carotid stenosis <70%, with or without ulceration, with or without antiplatelet therapy
- Evolving stroke with carotid stenosis <70%, with or without ulceration, with or without antiplatelet therapy
- Global ischemic symptoms with ipsilateral carotid stenosis >75%, but contralateral stenosis <75%, with or without ulceration, with or without antiplatelet therapy
- Acute dissection of the internal carotid artery with persistent symptoms while on heparin
- Acute carotid occlusion, diagnosed within 6 hr, producing transient ischemic events
- Acute carotid occlusion, diagnosed within 6 hr, producing a mild stroke
4. Proven inappropriate indications:
   - Moderate stroke with stenosis <50%; not on aspirin
   - Evolving stroke with stenosis <50%; not on aspirin
   - Acute internal carotid artery dissection, asymptomatic on heparin

For Patients With a Surgical Risk of 6% to 10%

1. Proven indications: none
2. Acceptable but unproven indications:
   - Single or multiple TIAs within a 6-mo interval, in the presence of a carotid stenosis ≥70%, with or without ulceration, with or without antiplatelet therapy
   - Recurrent TIAs, while on antiplatelet drugs, for a carotid stenosis ≥50% in the presence of ulceration, or ≥70% with or without ulceration
   - Crescendo TIAs with a stenosis ≥50%, with or without ulceration, with or without antiplatelet therapy
   - Mild stroke in the presence of a stenosis >70%, with or without ulceration, with or without antiplatelet therapy
   - Moderate stroke with a stenosis >70%, with or without ulceration, with or without antiplatelet therapy
   - Evolving stroke in the presence of a >70% stenosis with large ulceration
3. Uncertain indications:
   - Single TIA with stenosis <70%, with or without ulceration, with or without antiplatelet therapy
   - Multiple TIAs within 6 mo with stenosis <70%, with or without ulceration; not on antiplatelet drugs
   - Recurrent TIAs while on antiplatelet drugs with stenosis <70%, with or without ulceration
   - Crescendo TIAs for stenosis <70%, with or without ulceration, with or without antiplatelet therapy
   - Acute carotid occlusion with transient cerebral ischemia
   - Acute occlusion with mild stroke
   - Acute carotid artery dissection with continued symptoms while on heparin
   - Patient with transient cerebral ischemia secondary to a stenosis ≥70%, in need of CABG, with or without contralateral stenosis; use of combined operation
   - Mild stroke with stenosis <70%, with or without ulceration, with or without antiplatelet therapy
   - Moderate stroke with stenosis <70%, with or without ulceration, with or without antiplatelet therapy
   - Evolving stroke with stenosis <70%, with or without ulceration, with or without antiplatelet therapy
   - Global ischemic symptoms with an ipsilateral stenosis >75%, with or without symptoms, irrespective of contralateral artery status, with lesions up to and including contralateral occlusion
4. Proven inappropriate indications:
   - Single TIA, <50% stenosis, with or without ulceration, not on aspirin
   - Multiple TIAs within 6 mo, stenosis <50%; not on aspirin
   - Mild stroke, stenosis <50%; not on aspirin
   - Moderate stroke, stenosis <50%, with or without ulceration; not on aspirin
   - Evolving stroke, stenosis <50%, with or without ulceration; not on aspirin
   - Global ischemic symptoms with stenosis <50%, with or without ulceration
   - Acute dissection of the internal carotid artery; no symptoms while on heparin
   - Asymptomatic unilateral carotid stenosis ≥70% in patient undergoing CABG

TABLE 43-2 Morbidity and Mortality in Patients Undergoing Carotid Endarterectomy

Group	Procedures (no.)	Mortality (Myocardial Infarctions) (no.)	Morbidity (no.)		Total Morbidity and Mortality (%)
			Myocardial Infarction	Stroke	
1	129	0	0	1	1
2	56	0	0	1	2
3	76	2	3	(1)*	7
4	70	0	0	7	10

*This patient, with a cerebral infarct, also had a postoperative myocardial infarction.

From Sundt TM Jr, Sandok BA, Whisnant JP. Carotid endarterectomy: Complications and preoperative assessment of risk. *Mayo Clin Proc* 1975; 50:301–306. Reprinted by permission.

of treatment referred to in the recommendations concerning endarterectomy, and interventionists should view these outstanding results with the proper respect. Endarterectomy in the proper hands and proper location is still the gold standard for therapy of carotid bifurcation disease.

The cost-effectiveness of surgery for asymptomatic carotid artery disease is not proven. In the ACAS, it was shown that about 50 strokes were prevented by 800 endarterectomies. The cost of these procedures is a combination of angiography, carotid duplex ultrasonography, hospital costs, and surgical costs. The cost of stroke has been shown to be about $15,000 per patient in the first 90 days, so the cost of the 50 strokes would be about $750,000. To be cost-effective, therefore, the cost of the surgical therapy would have to be less than $1000 per patient, a patently impossible figure.

The North American Cerebral Percutaneous Transluminal Angioplasty Register (NACPTAR) group reports a stroke rate of 6% in 147 patients undergoing angioplasty, but this includes poor surgical risk patients and intracranial angioplasty procedures, both acknowledged increased risk categories.[27] The study by Diethrich et al. reported seven strokes in 110 patients, two major and five reversible, and an additional five TIAs.[28] Theron's complication rate of 1% is certainly comparable to any surgical statistics.[29]

Further data are necessary concerning this disease. Information on plaque morphology, systemic risk factors, stenosis progression, and other items is being obtained in the European Trial on Asymptomatic Carotid Stenosis.[30]

All the above information indicates that a correct and reliable method for predicting stroke risk associated with asymptomatic carotid artery stenosis does not exist. Dogmatic statements concerning the efficacy of surgery to treat this condition are therefore inaccurate and incorrect.

For these reasons, general guidelines for angioplasty or stenting of the internal carotid artery at the bifurcation are not fixed. A consensus exists for endovascular therapy in an individual suffering TIAs with more than 70% stenosis *who is not a surgical candidate,* but the definition of what constitutes a surgical candidate varies among locations. At some locations, any patient is a surgical candidate. The consensus concerning indications is based on inadequate information concerning risks and long-term benefits.

In opposition to this viewpoint, others consider the indications for endovascular treatment (angioplasty with or without stenting) to be the same as those presented by the American Heart Association for surgical endarterectomy. As stated earlier, however, this presupposes procedural morbidity and mortality rates equal to those of surgery, which has not been proved, and a *benefit* from endovascular treatment equal to that of surgery (also not proved). Indeed, the proven restenosis rate of stents used elsewhere in the body is far greater than that for endarterectomy. Also, as Diethrich states, "It appears inevitable that manipulation of the carotid artery will unleash a certain amount of microemboli; this situation probably cannot be prevented without some type of protective device or a more efficacious antiplatelet regimen."[28] (This is absolutely correct. See "Cerebral Protection During Internal Carotid Angioplasty" below.) Perhaps a much more rigorous indication for carotid stenting would be for failed angioplasty or arterial dissection.

ADVANTAGES OF CAROTID ANGIOPLASTY

The review by Becquemin et al. gives a good summary of the advantages and disadvantages of carotid angioplasty.[31] The advantages of angioplasty of carotid bifurcation region lesions include the following:

1. There is no cervical incision. Cranial nerve palsy induced by manipulation of the carotid bifurcation region occurs in 2% to 12.5% of cases.[32] Postoperative neck incision problems (infection or hematoma) are absent with the femoral approach.
2. Cerebral ischemia due to clamp occlusion of the carotid artery should not be a problem with angioplasty (although, with protective proximal occlusion during angioplasty, there is the probability that some people may fail this temporary occlusion quickly). Interestingly, 7% of Becquemin's patients required shunting during carotid endarterectomy, a figure consistent with those

obtained during carotid test occlusions with balloons.[31]

3. Lesions that are surgically inaccessible (or difficult to approach, increasing the risk of surgery) can be treated with angioplasty.

4. With angioplasty, there is no need for general anesthesia, and the patient's clinical status during the procedure can be monitored. Treatment can be rendered immediately for any untoward event.

5. Postoperative recuperation is shorter and less intensive than for endarterectomy. This may translate into significant cost savings when compared with endarterectomy as well as increased patient comfort.

DISADVANTAGES AND RISKS OF CAROTID ANGIOPLASTY

The disadvantages and risks of angioplasty in the region of the carotid bifurcation include the following:

1. Although cerebral embolism has not proved to be as great a danger as originally feared, it is still a devastating problem. Prevention may be possible with refinement in technique. Delayed embolism may be prevented with the development of new stents or antiplatelet and anticoagulant regimens. The use of the proximal occlusion guide catheter technique can further lessen this risk (see "Cerebral Protection During Internal Carotid Angioplasty" below).

2. Access site complications may occur. Direct carotid puncture for the purpose of angioplasty or, more particularly, stent placement, is contraindicated. The incidence of severe hematoma requiring emergency repair is far too high.[28] In addition, the simple act of achieving postprocedure hemostasis can slow flow in the newly stented artery, allowing unseen thrombus to form. This pressure could dent the stent as well.

3. It may be impossible to dilate the lesion adequately.

4. The risk of vasospasm may be decreased with the use of a soft guidewire tip, such as that on the new guidewire being developed by Cook Inc. Alternatively, a Platinum Plus or a TAD guidewire can be used. Preoperative application of a 2″ to 4″ strip of nitroglycerin paste may aid in prevention; treatment can be rendered by the intra-arterial injection of nitroglycerin or papaverine.

5. A dissection can be devastating and life-threatening. Careful manipulation and extremely slow inflation may lower the incidence of dissection, and the primary stenting of the artery can further prevent most of these complications.

6. Dissection can cause acute occlusion of the internal carotid artery as well as subintimal

hemorrhage. Acute occlusion can be the result of malignant platelet or thrombus aggregation and can occur over as short a time as 30 minutes, but we have not observed this in the carotid bifurcation region.

7. Delayed thrombosis can also occur by platelet or thrombus aggregation. It can be treated with anticoagulation and antiplatelet therapy and perhaps prevented by the development of newer and better stent materials.

8. Although now uncommon, loss of the external carotid artery probably will occur more frequently with the use of stents than with simple angioplasty. It also occurs with endarterectomy. This complication usually is of no consequence, but the future results cannot be predicted. This vessel may be of critical importance at some later time.

9. The hemodynamic effects of carotid body manipulation can be extreme during angioplasty. Although this is a manageable complication, there are reports of permanent occlusion of the internal carotid artery using detachable balloons placed in the carotid bulb that has resulted in constant severe hemodynamic disturbance requiring puncture of the balloon to reduce the pressure on the carotid body. Deflation of a stent is difficult. With the use of stents, these hemodynamic events have been known to include severe bradycardia and even asystole, which has caused death.[33]

10. Second only to embolic complications, the recurrence of stenosis after stenting may be the greatest inhibitor of its eventual widespread application. In the coronary arteries, there is a high failure rate at 6 months (20% to 40%). There is a commensurately high restenosis rate in stents placed in the common and superficial femoral arteries. Both of these situations are sobering comparisons. Endarterectomy has a high success rate, with good long-term patency and lack of restenosis. Even in this circumstance, however, the restenosis rate is not absolutely defined, nor as low as would be desired; it ranges from 6.7% to 23.9% of patients after "successful" carotid endarterectomy, with symptomatic restenosis in 0.6% to 3.6% of patients.[34] A potential major breakthrough in the treatment of restenosis is probucol. The role of this drug is discussed in detail in Chapter 41.

RATIONALE FOR STENT USE

Stent use has exploded in the last few years for several reasons, not least of which is the initial outstanding radiographic appearance. For certain locations in the periphery, stents have proved worthwhile, if not invaluable. Early results indicate this in some brachiocephalic locations as well. In most locations, however, there is a relatively high failure rate in a comparatively short period of time for stents. These failures are usually secondary to intimal hyperplasia or abrupt thrombotic occlusion.

For coronary stents in coronary applications, the primary failure rate (acute or subacute closure) is 2% to 17% (the higher number is associated with stenting of failed angioplasties). Predictors of acute closure are more complex preprocedure morphology, persistent uncovered dissection after stenting, and greater residual stenosis.[35] In one study, recurrent stenosis (> 50% stenosis at 6 months) occurred in 32% of elective stents and in 50% of stents that were placed because of failed angioplasty.[35] Multiple stents and multivessel disease are independent predictors of restenosis.

Amazingly, this is an accepted failure rate with stent use. When dealing with lower extremity endovascular stent repairs, a 50% failure rate in 2 to 4 years is entirely acceptable. A report on Strecker stents (Medi-Tech, Inc.) stated, "Thirty-four percent of the stented segments progressed from <20% stenosis at 3 months to >50% stenosis at 12 months."[36] This was described as satisfactory! In addition, the "acute thrombosis rate of 10%, only slightly higher than that reported by Strecker et al., is decidedly lower than incidences reported for Wallstents" (Schneider, Inc.) "in the femoropopliteal position."[36]

Another report on long-term patency of Palmaz stents in the femoropopliteal region stated that "at 24 months, cumulative primary patency was 77% and secondary patency 89%."[37]

If only 77% of all carotid arteries were patent at 2 years with any form of treatment, this would be called a disaster!

Although the analogy to the femoropopliteal region may not be entirely accurate, it is not entirely inaccurate, either. After all, these flexible and moving vessels are more similar to the carotid artery in this regard than the iliac artery, for instance. The exact comparison to the carotid artery may fall somewhere in between.

The most commonly used stent (the Palmaz type) can give excellent results in certain locations but is easily compressible by external forces. Abrupt occlusion of superficial femoral artery stents has resulted from patients simply squatting. A carotid stent therefore could be the cause of abrupt accidental occlusion long after a successful angioplasty and stent procedure, and this has been observed. Some practitioners have their patients wear medical alert collars to warn against inadvertent compression of the neck in times of emergency. In addition, the stiffness may provoke reaction at its two ends, where it is flexing with the vessel.

Intimal Hyperplasia

Intimal hyperplasia associated with stents is a major concern, particularly in a moving and flexible vessel. Preliminary results from other vascular locations superficially similar to the carotid artery in this regard appear to imply early failure of carotid stenting, but this concern has not been clinically confirmed.

Stent use increases the tendency of the vessel to react aggressively to the dilation process, based purely on the mechanical nature of the stent, independent of the stent material.[38] It has been repeatedly and clearly shown that balloon angioplasty alone does not provoke the degree of intimal hyperplasia that stents cause.[39–41]

Angioplasty alone causes between three and five times less endothelial vascular injury than stents. The degree of vascular injury directly affects the degree of responsive intimal hyperplasia.[38] The covering of a stent or its wall composition has a direct effect on the thrombogenicity of the stent, but not on its stimulation of intimal hyperplasia. The configuration of the stent, however, helps to determine the degree of vascular injury to a greater degree than either arterial enlargement or stent surface material. As Rogers and Edelman state, "leaving a stent behind within the artery may cause more severe and prolonged vascular injury and provide a chronic stimulus for smooth muscle cell proliferation and neointimal hyperplasia."[38] *The conclusion of their study was that stents increase arterial lumen size at the expense of early thrombosis and prolonged neointimal hyperplasia.*

Several different stents using new materials have been developed in both the United States and in Europe (see Chapter 1). Ongoing trials of these stents in various vascular locations are occurring at numerous sites worldwide. Progress in this area is vital to development of a viable endovascular treatment for head and neck pathology. The technique of stent deployment is yet to be perfected, and the variety of techniques used around the world highlights this situation. The patent for balloon-expandable stents may place a "lock" on the market for the Palmaz stent in the United States at least for the immediate future. This is not necessarily detrimental, however, because many improvements in design and deployment still can be made.

The largest series with long-term results concerning the longevity of stents is available from the University of Alabama at Birmingham.[42] Of 198 patients with stents placed in the internal carotid artery, only 5 had greater than 50% restenosis after 6 months. These results are discussed further in Chapter 44.

The "Tunnel Vision" Concept Concerning Complications

It has been more than 20 years since open heart cardiopulmonary bypass surgery was first widely practiced. Almost immediately after this procedure came into widespread use, cases began to appear of patients complaining of subtle alterations in their mental or neurologic functioning. These complications were unrecognized or ignored by these patients' physicians and were primarily seen by psychiatrists.

It is only now widely accepted that up to 30% of patients who undergo surgery requiring systemic cardiopulmonary bypass suffer some degree of this complication (cerebral emboli or hypoperfusion damage). A recent report indicates that at least 6% of these patients suffer some degree of severe *permanent* brain damage. It is unfortunate that these results were ignored for such a long period of time. A cavalier attitude toward this possibility or any other potential risk from carotid angioplasty or stenting is unacceptable. The true incidence of complications from endarterectomy is not truly known. The widely quoted values of complication rates for this procedure are from one large highly controlled study of only low-risk patients, without critical evaluation of the intracranial structures using modern imaging techniques (e.g., magnetic resonance imaging).

Preliminary results are available from early angioplasty and stent trials. Diethrich et al. reported on a study of 110 patients who had either symptomatic stenoses of 70% or greater, with or without ulceration, or asymptomatic stenoses of 75% or greater.[28] Lesions were in the proximal common, middle common, distal common, internal, and external carotid arteries. Of 110 patients with 117 lesions, 109 (116 lesions) were successfully treated There were seven strokes (two major, five reversible) and five TIAs. After 30 days, the clinical success rate was 89.1% (two stents occluded, three patients underwent endarterectomy, one patient died). The mean follow-up was 7.6 months. During this time, no new neurologic symptoms were reported. One additional stent occluded, and one case of flow-limiting intimal hyperplasia developed.

Roubin et al. reported on the results of 146 procedures in 74 patients, during which 210 stents were placed in 152 vessels.[42] There was only one technical failure. One in-hospital death and two major strokes were reported; there were seven minor strokes (five reversible, two permanent "minor weakness"). At 6 months, 69 patients underwent angiography or ultrasound evaluation; there were eight cases of stent deformation, but the restenosis rate was less than 5%. One patient reported a TIA during the follow-up period; there were no additional strokes or deaths.

Theron et al. reported on their experience with carotid angioplasty using a form of cerebral protection[29] (see next section). Some cerebral protection would appear to be mandatory for this procedure but has not been widely used, for unknown reasons. These investigators reported on a large series of patients, 38 of whom underwent angioplasty without cerebral protection, with a complication rate of 8%. In the 136 patients in whom cerebral protection was used, however, no embolic complications occurred during angioplasty. With Theron's technique, cerebral protection was not possible during the actual stent placement, and two embolic complications occurred during this phase of the procedure, for a complication rate of 1%.

We agree with Theron that "cerebral protection is mandatory to eliminate embolic complications" during angioplasty and stenting in the carotid bifurcation and should be used in some form by everyone performing this procedure.

Restenosis

Although early results of stenting of the carotid artery demonstrate a restenosis rate lower than expected, any restenosis at all is too much. Efforts are being made on several fronts to try to prevent restenosis; one drug and radiation show the most promise.

Probucol

Probucol has been shown to be effective in preventing restenosis in small vessel (coronary) angioplasty. It should be effective in preventing restenosis related to stents as well. As noted earlier, a thorough description of this agent is given in Chapter 41.

Brachytherapy (Radiation)

Brachytherapy shows great promise for the future, particularly the use of radioactive stents. Studies are being performed to evaluate the correct isotope, method of manufacture, and dose. The early results are promising. See the discussion in Chapter 41.

CEREBRAL PROTECTION DURING INTERNAL CAROTID ANGIOPLASTY

Protection during angioplasty can be achieved by two mechanisms: mechanical or pharmacologic. Mechanical means are intended to prevent emboli from arising at the site of the angioplasty or rerouting their course to either the outside of the patient or to a safer vascular destination (i.e., the external carotid circulation). Consideration of the pharmacologic means is presented first.

Pharmacologic Protection

During a carotid revascularization procedure, there is always the risk of ischemic injury, either from vascular compromise during the procedure or from embolic or occlusive events secondary to the procedure. For this reason, because of the availability of neuroprotectant agents, we believe that their use is warranted when cerebral ischemia is a potential problem. These agents are described in Chapters 4 and 54. Of the currently available agents, nimodipine (Nimotop) may be the most useful (60 mg orally before the procedure).

Mechanical Protection

Primary stenting of large vessel angioplasty sites (such as the carotid artery) may reduce the risk of embolic events because it may trap some material beneath the stent; this practice thus can be considered a means of mechanical cerebral protection. Stents, however, have their own associated problems (discussed earlier). Experimental data, however, indicate that stents increase arterial lumen size at the expense of early thrombosis and prolonged neointimal hyperplasia.[38] A discussion of the advantages and disadvantages of stent use is presented next.

Temporary Vessel Occlusion (Flow Control)

Occlusion of flow in the carotid artery is a means of cerebral protection, at least while the temporary occlusion balloon is inflated. This technique can be performed only in patients who can tolerate temporary occlusion of the carotid artery; but this includes nearly all patients. In a large carotid endarterectomy series, 7% of patients required bypass during the procedure secondary to failure during clamping.[43] The occlusion time necessary for this technique of flow control during angioplasty can last from 5 to 30 minutes, depending on the exact technique and operator expediency. Flow control during angioplasty, therefore, would be possible in nearly all patients.

Stopping flow in the carotid artery using an occlusion balloon can be performed by two different methods. First, the balloon can be placed distal to the lesion in the internal carotid artery, downstream from the angioplasty site, to occlude distal runoff. This is an obvious maneuver but is technically complex and invites disaster (i.e., the occlusion balloon, which is relatively large, has to be advanced past the lesion before anything else is done, potentially dislodging embolic material). Also, occlusion just distal to the lesion produces a stagnant column of blood of varying length both distal to the temporary occlusion balloon and proximal to the balloon, over the angioplasty site. Debris may lodge at the balloon, may be difficult to remove, or may stimulate further thrombosis. It may then be washed downstream after deflation of the balloon. However, this form of protection was used by Theron et al., with excellent results.[29]

Theron et al. described a triaxial system of cerebral protection.[44] The system comprises a 9-Fr. guide catheter containing a 5-Fr. angioplasty catheter. Through the lumen of the angioplasty catheter is placed a 3-Fr. microcatheter. Before endovascular placement, the device is prepared. After the tip of the microcatheter has exited the distal end of the angioplasty catheter, an Ingenor latex balloon is mounted on the end (hand-tied with latex string). The entire apparatus is positioned, and the occlusion balloon is advanced through the lesion and inflated. The angioplasty balloon catheter is then advanced over the microcatheter to its intended location.

In agreement with our prior statements concerning temporary occlusion, Theron states: "Because the occlusion time is usually very short (rarely more than ten minutes), only a simple check of the patient's level of consciousness and motor function was necessary."[29] This technique effectively renders downstream flushing (past the occlusion balloon) during the procedure impossible, but it does not appear to be necessary. This same technique is used by many practitioners for temporary occlusion testing of the internal carotid artery.

The results of Theron's study are evidence enough of the validity of the concept of cerebral protection during carotid angioplasty. For an additional slight amount of technical trouble, an increase in safety is

possible. Theron was able to perform 136 carotid angioplasties with cerebral protection, with no embolic complications. In the 38 procedures performed without cerebral protection, there were three embolic complications (8%).

Flow Control Guide Catheters for Internal Carotid Artery Angioplasty

A proximal flow control guide catheter, such as the previously described Zeppelin (Medtronic/MIS; see Chapter 1), is another means to achieve cerebral protection during angioplasty.[45, 46] Kachel describes a similar system in Chapter 46. This technique is closer to what we consider the optimal technique, although not identical (see "Ideal Cerebral Protection Technique" below).

The rationale for use of a catheter such as this is as follows: when an occlusion balloon is placed in the common carotid artery and inflated, the flow in the common carotid artery is stopped. The intraluminal pressure of the distal internal carotid artery is usually nearly systemic, owing to the circle of Willis. The intraluminal pressure in the external carotid artery usually is low, owing to the sump of its capillary bed. This typically results in reversal of flow in the internal carotid artery. Two potential exceptions to this are (1) cases in which a large arterial collateral is present from the posterior (vertebral) circulation to the anterior (occipital artery and external carotid artery) circulation, and (2) cases in which there is no functionally significant circle of Willis. In the latter situation, a temporary occlusion is failed relatively quickly, and mechanical cerebral protection of any kind also would be failed (i.e., internal carotid balloon occlusion). A large collateral from the posterior circulation to the anterior circulation is usually present only if there is a chronic stenosis or occlusion of the *common carotid artery* (fostering development of such a collateral vessel) or of the vertebral artery origin (causing the arterial supply to flow from the anterior circulation to the posterior circulation). Both of these situations can be identified easily at the beginning of the procedure by an adequate brachio-cephalic and cerebral angiogram.

Use of a flow control guide catheter therefore can yield cerebral protection during angioplasty. Usually, with occlusion of the common carotid artery, flow in the internal carotid artery at least is stopped, if not reversed. Any material dislodged during angioplasty flows retrograde down the internal carotid and out the external carotid artery branches or is aspirated out through the occlusion balloon catheter.

This flow control guide catheter (with a 7-Fr. lumen) can be placed in the common carotid artery and the angioplasty balloon introduced through it. Either a 5-Fr. system or a smaller Sub-4 type (Medi-Tech, Inc.) can be used through these guide catheters. These guide catheters allow roadmapping as well as preangioplasty and postangioplasty evaluation without having to move (or remove) the angioplasty catheter. A thorough description and diagrams concerning the use of a flow control guide catheter as part of an ideal cerebral protection technique for carotid angioplasty are given next.

Ideal Cerebral Protection Technique

A technique has been developed that can solve most of the problems associated with internal carotid artery angioplasty and the fear of emboli (Fig. 43–1). The equipment available for use is suboptimal, but improvements are being made. The slight amount of additional trouble involved with the use of available equipment for reduction of embolic consequences is worth the reduction in morbidity (see previous discussion). Avoidance of the complications associated with this procedure is worth some extra effort. We believe that improvements in equipment will render this technique not only the standard of care but also a simple task.

The patient is premedicated with a cerebral protestant; nimodipine, 60 mg given orally, is the available agent. The internal carotid artery is selected using the selective diagnostic dilator supplied with the "ideal" flow control neuro-guide catheter. The flow control guide catheter is then advanced over this dilator into the common carotid artery, and 10,000 units of heparin is administered. The procedure then is performed as illustrated and explained in Figure 43–1.

Certain other custom devices, including guide catheters, are being designed to optimize these specific maneuvers. This technique can eliminate most threats from embolic debris secondary to the technique. The stent then becomes the weak link in this procedure (i.e., its longevity is relative to intimal hyperplasia).

DISTAL PERFUSION DURING ANGIOPLASTY

Attempts have been made to perfuse the distal territory during angioplasty of large brachiocephalic vessels by several means. A custom-designed, triple-lumen "perfusing" angioplasty catheter has been tested in vitro. This catheter has a soft latex occlusion balloon distal to an angioplasty balloon, with a central lumen that also is used as a vascular flow conduit. The distal occlusion balloon, as described previously, prevents embolic material from washing downstream after the angioplasty; the central lumen permits perfusion during and after the angioplasty. It can, however, carry only limited amounts of blood. Also, this triple-lumen catheter is bulky and cumbersome. This is particularly true in relation to smaller vessels and catheters.

Another distal perfusion technique involves power injection of the guidewire lumen of the standard angioplasty catheter with fresh arterial blood or heparinized saline during the occlusive period of the inflation. This maneuver is also cumbersome and may add more risk than benefit. Even if a *very* slow inflation (and subsequent occlusion) is executed, the brief cessation of flow in the target vessel should not cause any significant problem. After all, nearly all patients

(about 90%) can pass a temporary carotid occlusion test for 20 minutes, much less 1 to 5 minutes during an angioplasty. In most of these patients the original problem was not lack of flow in the carotid artery but rather the fact that the lesions function as an embolic source. A temporary cessation (i.e., less than 5 to 10 minutes) of flow, even in a critical flow situation, and even if rapidly symptomatic, should not lead to permanent neurologic deficit, as stated earlier.[47]

We believe that this maneuver (perfusing the distal carotid artery during angioplasty) is not necessary.

In the case of a failed angioplasty of the carotid bifurcation with subsequent intracranial vascular insufficiency due to vascular collapse (e.g., subplaque hemorrhage with vessel occlusion), temporary stenting by means of a "stenting catheter" can allow time for open surgical rescue or stent placement (see Chapter 1 for a description of this custom product supplied by Cook Inc.). This catheter has a large lumen and multiple proximal and distal side holes as well as a large end hole capable of carrying an adequate amount of blood downstream through the angioplasty site (see Figs. 1–22 and 1–23). Usually, a large volume of flow is not needed to keep cerebral tissue alive for a short time. Using this device can "buy time" while other rescue measures are being prepared (e.g., surgery, permanent metallic stenting). *Alternatively, any other catheter can be placed across the stenosis over a wire, and fresh arterial blood or even heparinized saline can be infused through its central lumen.*

Either of these techniques can allow time to prepare for surgical intervention or to prepare a stent that might be suitable for rescue.

ASYSTOLE AFTER CAROTID STENTING

Asystole can occur after stent placement or after angioplasty in the region of the carotid bulb. If it occurs after stent placement, it may be more dramatic and may be accompanied by prolonged and severe hypotension. Atropine is the first line of defense. The transesophageal pacemaker from Bard, Inc. captures very effectively and can be used as an alternative to transvenous pacing. Both hypotension and asystole can be aided greatly by administration of an intravenous bolus of metaraminol bitartrate (0.5 to 5.0 mg) followed by an infusion (50 mg in 500 ml normal saline, at a rate titrated to keep the blood pressure at an appropriate level). The hypotensive effect after carotid stenting at the bifurcation usually is self-limiting, but it may take days to completely resolve.

THE FUTURE OF ENDOVASCULAR CAROTID ARTERY THERAPY

Endovascular treatment eventually will be the preferred means of therapy for carotid bifurcation pathology, but current devices and technique may be suboptimal.

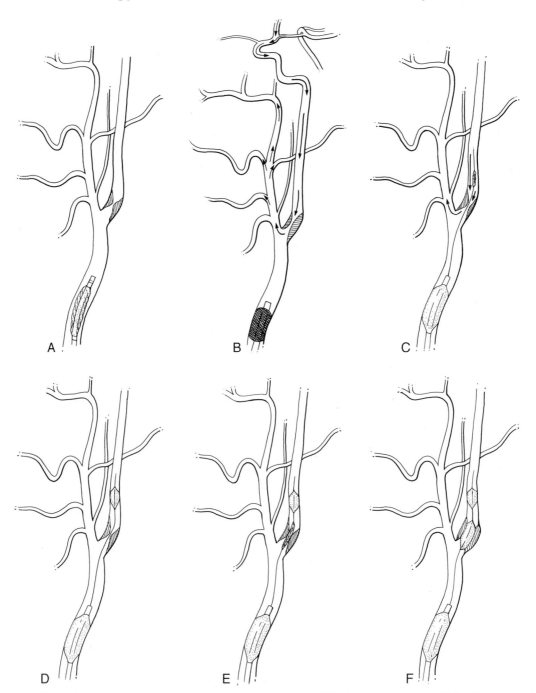

Figure 43-1. A potentially ideal method of cerebral protection for internal carotid artery angioplasty, utilizing flow control for cerebral protection.

A, Initial placement of the flow control guide catheter has been made, but the soft occlusion balloon has not been inflated. Antegrade flow is still present in the common carotid artery and internal and external carotid arteries.

B, Inflation of the guide catheter balloon stops flow in the common carotid artery and reverses or at least stops flow in the internal carotid artery. The high pressure intracranial vascular system (the circle of Willis supplying the pressure and flow) will supply the low-pressure sump of the external carotid artery. Evaluation of the hemodynamics of this carotid system can be made with a gentle contrast injection through the guide catheter. This will reveal the presence or absence of flow reversal in the internal and/or external carotid artery by observing the *washout* of contrast in the vessels. Significant collaterals from the vertebral artery to the external carotid artery would not usually be present in situations of internal carotid artery stenosis but rather with *common carotid artery stenosis* or *occlusion;* this can be evaluated with the gentle injection described above.

C, While flow reversal (or no flow) is occurring in the internal carotid artery (with or without aspiration/drainage from the guide catheter), a soft-tipped balloon on a catheter or wire is advanced safely through the lesion. Any material displaced during passage will flow in a retrograde course out into the external carotid artery or be aspirated into the guide catheter. The flow arrest in the common carotid artery thus protects this initial (potentially dangerous) crossing of the stenosis.

D, The distal occlusion balloon is inflated, stopping all flow in the internal carotid artery.

E, The angioplasty catheter is delivered safely to its intended location.

F, The angioplasty is performed while flow is arrested in the common carotid and internal carotid arteries. The angioplasty can be performed with or without primary stent deployment if necessary.

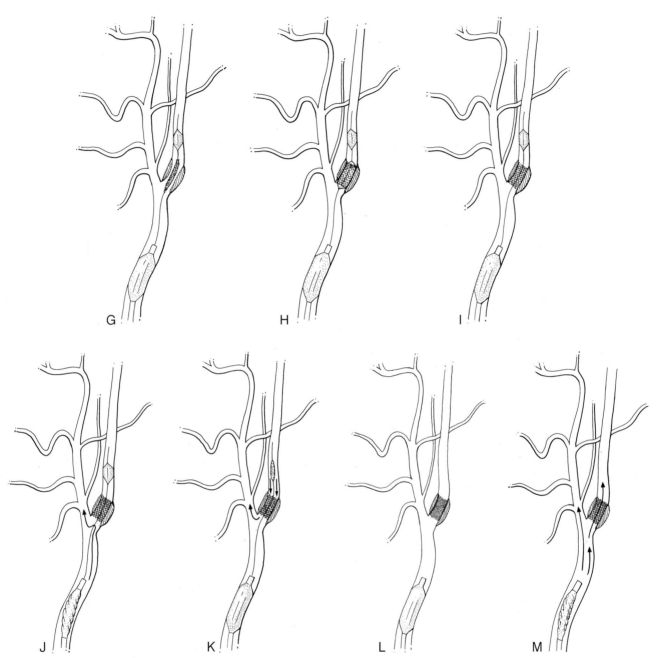

Figure 43-1 *Continued. G,* After initial angioplasty, a stent is delivered into the closed system, again with both the distal and proximal flow occluded, and thus with protection for intracranial structures.

H, The stent is safely deployed under flow arrest.

I, The angioplasty catheter is withdrawn, leaving the stent in place with flow arrested in the carotid arteries.

J, The proximal occlusion balloon (on the guide catheter) is deflated. This allows high-pressure/flow rate antegrade flow into the external carotid artery and permits contrast injection through the inner lumen of the guide catheter for evaluation of the result of the angioplasty/stenting. Any retained debris/plaque/clot material is now forcefully washed out of the system into the external carotid artery territory.

K, The proximal guide catheter occlusion balloon is reinflated and the distal guide wire/microcatheter balloon is deflated, again allowing reversal of flow in the internal carotid artery. Aspiration through the guide catheter (or simply opening the lumen to air) can augment this flow reversal in the internal carotid artery, as determined necessary on the preliminary hemodynamic evaluation.

L, While flow is still occluded in the common carotid artery, the deflated distal wire/balloon is safely withdrawn, again with no chance of dislodging any material into the intracranial flow.

M, Once the inner wire/balloon has been withdrawn, the guide catheter balloon is deflated, allowing final contrast injection through the guide catheter lumen to evaluate the angioplasty results and the intracranial vasculature.

Initial endovascular therapeutic results likely will be as good as or better than open surgical endarterectomy for *selected* patients and when using good technique, but the medium-term or long-term results may not be, using *currently practiced* techniques and *currently available* stents and catheters. Certainly, the issue of possible intimal hyperplasia has to be addressed. What will these vessels be like in 10 years? In the future, the development of improved stenting devices, procedures, and pharmacologic agents to help prevent intimal hyperplasia and to avoid externally induced stent collapse will open doors of opportunity and improve this procedure.

These concerns call for a properly managed, controlled clinical trial of carotid angioplasty and stenting. The enthusiasm of certain interventional neuroradiologists and other practitioners, however, may outweigh technical skills and currently available materials. Any trial should be done with the cooperation, approval, and participation of the appropriate neurologic, neurosurgical, and vascular specialists. Any trial must involve endovascular therapists capable not only of performing the procedure in this location but also of clinically and radiologically evaluating the pretherapeutic and posttherapeutic cerebrovascular territory and the neurologic condition of the patient; they also must be capable of treating any potential complication. The ability to use a microcatheter does not confer expertise in the therapy of a cerebrovascular thromboembolic sequela, as has been demonstrated repeatedly. Preprocedure and postprocedure magnetic resonance imaging scans should be obtained (at a minimum) to evaluate the possibility of subtle sequelae. A neurologic examination alone is inadequate for a rigorous trial because embolic sequelae may yield more subtle neuropsychiatric findings, as has been clearly demonstrated in the past (see previous discussion).

A multicenter trial of carotid angioplasty and stenting with Food and Drug Administration and National Institutes of Health approval is being organized to answer these questions. Carotid angioplasty and stenting, however, also are being performed by physicians with no specific training in brachiocephalic catheterization, no knowledge of intracranial vasculature and hemodynamics, poor understanding of microcatheter rescue techniques, no comprehension of therapy for cerebral ischemia, and no participation in an investigatory protocol.

Any information gained from the conscientiously managed investigatory trials should be of great benefit to patients. This information, along with continuing advances in equipment and technique, eventually should determine the optimal therapy for this common but potentially devastating disease.

REFERENCES

1. Norris JW, Zhu CZ, Bornstein NM, et al. Stroke risks of asymptomatic carotid stenosis. *Stroke* 1991;22:1485–1490.
2. O'Holleran LW, Kennelly MM, McClurken M, et al. Natural history of asymptomatic carotid plaque: five year follow-up study. *Am J Surg* 1987;154:659–662.
3. Autret A, Pourcelot L, Saudeau D, et al. Stroke risk in patients with carotid stenosis. *Lancet* 1987;1:888–890.
4. Hobson RW, Weiss DG, Fields WS, et al. Efficacy of carotid endarterectomy for asymptomatic carotid stenosis. *NEJM* 1993;328:221–227.
5. Mackey AE, Abramowicz M, Laglois Y, et al. Outcome of asymptomatic patients with carotid disease. *Neurology* 1997;48:896–903.
6. Asymptomatic Carotid Atherosclerosis Study Executive Committee. Endarterectomy for asymptomatic carotid artery stenosis. *JAMA* 1995;273:1421–1428.
7. Bornstein NM, Karepov VG, Aronovich BD, et al. Failure of aspirin treatment after stroke. *Stroke* 1994;25:275–277.
8. Helgason CM, Tortorice KL, Winkler SR, et al. Aspirin response and failure in cerebral infarction. *Stroke* 1993;24:345–350.
9. Hass WK, Easton JD, Adams HP, et al. A randomized trial comparing ticlopidine hydrochloride with aspirin for the prevention of stroke in high-risk patients. Ticlopidine Aspirin Stroke Study Group. *NEJM* 1989;321:501–507.
10. Turpie AG, Gent M, Lauacis A, et al. A comparison of aspirin with placebo in patients treated with warfarin after heart valve replacement. *NEJM* 1993;329:524–529.
11. Miller A, Lees RS. Simultaneous therapy with antiplatelet and anticoagulant drugs in symptomatic cardiovascular disease. *Stroke* 1985;16:668–675.
12. Tilley BC. Atrial fibrillation, aspirin, and anticoagulant therapy. (AFASAK 2). *Stroke* 1995;26:352.
13. European Carotid Trialists Collaborative Group. MRC European Carotid Surgery Trial: Interim results for symptomatic patients with severe (70% to 99%) or with mild (0 to 29%) carotid stenosis. *Lancet* 1991;337:1235–1243.
14. Dennis M, Bamford J, Sandercock P, et al. Prognosis of transient ischemic attacks in the Oxfordshire Community Stroke Project. *Stroke* 1990;21:848–853.
15. Meissner I, Whisnant JP, Garraway WM. Hypertension management and stroke recurrence in a community (Rochester, Minnesota, 1950–1979). *Stroke* 1988;19:459–463.
16. Sacco RL, Wolf PA, Kannel WB, et al. Survival and recurrence following stroke: the Framingham study. *Stroke* 1982;13:290–295.
17. North American Symptomatic Carotid Endarterectomy Trial Collaborators. Beneficial effect of carotid endarterectomy in symptomatic patients with high-grade carotid stenosis. *NEJM* 1991;325:445–453.
18. Wilterdink JL, Easton JD. Vascular event rates in patients with atherosclerotic cerebrovascular disease. *Arch Neurol* 1992;49:857–863.
19. Frey JL. Asymptomatic carotid stenosis: Surgery's the answer, but that's not the question. *Ann Neurol* 1996;39:405–406.
20. McCullough JL, Mentzer RM, Harman PK, et al. Carotid endarterectomy after a completed stroke: reduction in long term neurologic deterioration. *J Vasc Surg* 1985;2:7–14.
21. Hertzer NR, Arison R. Cumulative stroke and survival ten years after carotid endarterectomy. *J Vasc Surg* 1985;2:661–668.
22. Moore WS, Barnett HJM, Beebe HG, et al. Guidelines for carotid endarterectomy: a multidisciplinary consensus statement from the Ad Hoc Committee, American Heart Association. *Stroke* 1995;26:188–201.
23. Sundt TM Jr, Sandok BA, Whisnant JP. Carotid endarterectomy: Complications and preoperative assessment of risk. *Mayo Clin Proc* 1975;50:301–306.
24. Brott T, Thalinger K. The practice of carotid endarterectomy in a large metropolitan area. *Stroke* 1984;15:950–955.
25. Rothwell PM, Slattery J, Warlow CP. A systematic review of the risks of stroke and death due to endarterectomy for symptomatic carotid stenosis. *Stroke* 1996;27:260–265.
26. Becker GJ. Should metallic vascular stents be used to treat cerebrovascular occlusive disease? *Radiology* 1994;191:309–312.
27. NACPTAR. Update of the immediate angiographic results and in-hospital CNS complications of cerebral percutaneous transluminal angioplasty. *Circulation* 1995;92:383.
28. Diethrich EB, Ndiaye M, Reid DB, et al. Stenting in the

carotid artery: initial experience in 110 patients. *J Endovasc Surg* 1996;3:42–62.

29. Theron JG, Payelle GG, Coskun O, et al. Carotid artery stenosis: treatment with protected balloon angioplasty and stent placement. *Radiology* 1996;201:627–636.

30. Thomas DJ. The European Trial on Asymptomatic Carotid Stenosis. Platform presentation at the 20th Joint International Conference on Stroke and Cerebral Circulation, Charleston, SC, February, 1995.

31. Becquemin JP, Qvarfordt P, Castier Y, Mellière D. Carotid angioplasty: is it safe? *J Endovasc Surg* 1995;3:35–41.

32. Rosenberg N. Handbook of Carotid Surgery Facts and Figures. Boca Raton: CRC Press, 1989, pp. 171–187.

33. Gaines PA. Carotid angioplasty and sinus arrhythmias [Letter]. *Clin Radiol* 1993;48:431.

34. Bernstein EF, Torem S, Dilley RB. Does carotid restenosis predict an increased risk of late symptoms, stroke, or death? *Ann Surg* 1990;212:629–636.

35. Foley JB, Brown RIG, Penn IM. Thrombosis and restenosis after stenting in failed angioplasty: comparison with elective stenting. *Am Heart J* 1994;128:12–20.

36. Bray AE, Liu WG, Lewis WA, et al. Strecker stents in the femoropopliteal arteries: value of duplex ultrasonography in restenosis assessment. *J Endovasc Surg* 1995;2:150–160.

37. Bergeron P, Pinot JJ, Poyen V, et al. Long term results with the Palmaz stent in the superficial femoral artery. *J Endovasc Surg* 1995;2:161–167.

38. Rogers C, Edelman ER. Endovascular stent design dictates experimental restenosis and thrombosis. *Circulation* 1995;91:2995–3001.

39. Karas SP, Gravanis MB, Santoian EC, et al. Coronary intimal proliferation after balloon injury and stenting in swine: an animal model of restenosis. *J Am Coll Cardiol* 1992;20:467–474.

40. Hanke H, Hassenstein S, Kamenz J, et al. Prolonged proliferative response of smooth muscle cells after experimental intravascular stenting: a stent wire related phenomenon [Abstract]. *Circulation* 1992;86 (suppl I):I–186.

41. Rogers C, Karnovsky MJ, Edelman ER. Inhibition of experimental neointimal hyperplasia and thrombosis depends on the type of vascular injury and the site of drug administration. *Circulation* 1993;88:1215–1221.

42. Roubin GS, Yadav S, Iyer SS, Vitek J. Carotid stent-supported angioplasty: a neurovascular intervention to prevent stroke. *Am J Cardiol* 1996;78:8–12.

43. Becquemin JP, Paris E, Valverde A, et al. Carotid surgery: is regional anesthesia always appropriate? *J Cardiovasc Surg* 1991;32:592–598.

44. Theron J, Courtheoux P, Alachkar F, et al. New triple coaxial catheter system for carotid angioplasty with cerebral protection. *AJNR* 1990;11:869–874.

45. Ferguson RDG, Lee LI, Connors JJ, Ferguson JG. Angioplasty in the extracranial and intracranial vasculature. *Semin Intervent Radiol* 1994;2:64–82.

46. Kachel R. Results of balloon angioplasty in the carotid arteries. *J Endovasc Surg* 1996;3:22–30.

47. Heros RC. Management of unclippable aneurysms. In Schmidek HH, Sweet WH (eds): Operative Neurosurgical Techniques, 2nd ed. Orlando: Grune & Stratton, 1988, pp. 1023–1034.

ADDITIONAL READINGS

Carotid Endarterectomy

Bergeron P. Special series on cerebrovascular disease therapy: part I. *J Endovasc Surg* 1996;3:1–2.

Brott T, Tomsick T, Feinberg W, et al. Baseline silent cerebral infarction in the asymptomatic carotid atherosclerosis study. *Stroke* 1994;25:1122–1129.

Brott T, Toole JF. Medical compared with surgical treatment of asymptomatic carotid artery stenosis. *Ann Intern Med* 1995;123:720–722.

DeBakey ME. Carotid endarterectomy revisited. *J Endovasc Surg* 1996;3:4.

de los Reyes RA, Bederson JB, Germano IM. Direct endarterectomy of the middle cerebral artery for treatment of symptomatic stenosis: case report. *Neurosurgery* 1993;32:464–467.

Diethrich EB. Cerebrovascular disease therapy: the past, the present and the future. *J Endovasc Surg* 1996;3:7–9.

Eastcott HHG. Late thoughts and reflections on carotid reconstruction for the prevention of ischemic stroke. *J Endovasc Surg* 1996;3:3–5.

Gagne PJ, Riles TS, Jacobowitz GR, et al. Long-term follow-up of patients undergoing reoperation for recurrent carotid artery disease. *J Vasc Surg* 1993;18:991–1001.

Harbaugh KS, Pikus HJ, Shumaker GH, et al. Increasing the value of carotid endarterectomy. *J Neurovasc Dis* 1996;1:40–47.

Katz D, Snyder SO, Gandhi RH, et al. Long-term follow-up for recurrent stenosis: a prospective randomized study of expanded polytetrafluoroethylene patch angioplasty versus primary closure after carotid endarterectomy. *J Vasc Surg* 1994;19:198–205.

Katz MM, Jones T, Degenhardt J, et al. The use of patch angioplasty to alter the incidence of carotid restenosis following thromboendarterectomy. *J Cardiovasc Surg* 1987;28:2–8.

Kelly JJ, Callow AD, O'Donnell TF, et al. Failure of carotid stump pressures: its incidence as a predictor for a temporary shunt during carotid endarterectomy. *Arch Surg* 1979;114:1361–1366.

McCormick PW, Spetzler RF, Bailes JE, et al. Thromboendarterectomy of the symptomatic occluded internal carotid artery. *J Neurosurg* 1992;76:752–758.

Meyer FB, Piepgras DG, Fode NC. Surgical treatment of recurrent carotid artery stenosis. *J Neurosurg* 1994;80:781–787.

Motarjeme A, Keifer JW. Carotid-cavernous sinus fistula as a complication of carotid endarterectomy. *Radiology* 1973;108:83–84.

Raithel D. Recurrent carotid disease: optimum technique for redo surgery. *J Endovasc Surg* 1996;3:39–75.

Ranaboldo CJ, Barros D'Sa AAB, Bell PRF, et al. Randomized controlled trial of patch angioplasty for carotid endarterectomy. *Br J Surg* 1993;80:1528–1530.

Rothwell PM, Slattery J, Warlow CP. A systematic comparison of the risks of stroke and death due to carotid endarterectomy for symptomatic and asymptomatic stenosis. *Stroke* 1996;27:266–269.

Schwartz RB, Jones KM, Leclercq GT, et al. The value of cerebral angiography in predicting cerebral ischemia during carotid endarterectomy. *AJR* 1992;159:1057–1061.

Shumway SJ, Edwards WH, Jenkins JM, et al. Recurrent carotid stenosis. *Am Surg* 1987;53:61–65.

Toole, JF. ACAS recommendations for carotid endarterectomy. *Lancet* 1996;347:121.

Treiman GS, Jenkins JM, Edwards WH, et al. The evolving surgical management of recurrent carotid stenosis. *J Vasc Surg* 1992;16:354–363.

Zarins CK. Carotid endarterectomy: the gold standard. *J Endovasc Surg* 1996;3:10–15.

Imaging of Carotid Stenosis

Bluth EI, Stavos AT, Marich KW, et al. Carotid duplex sonography: A multicenter recommendation for standardized imaging and Doppler criteria. *RadioGraphics* 1988;8:487–506.

Castillo M. Diagnosis of disease of the common carotid artery bifurcation: CT angiography vs. catheter angiography. *AJR* 1993;161:395–398.

Castillo M, Wilson JD. CT angiography of the common carotid artery bifurcation: Comparison between two techniques and conventional angiography. *Neuroradiology* 1994;36:602–604.

Cumming MJ, Morrow IM. Carotid artery stenosis: A prospective comparison of CT angiography and conventional angiography. *AJR* 1994;163:517–523.

Dillon EH, van Leeuwen MS, Fernandez MA, et al. CT angiography: Application to the evaluation of carotid artery stenosis. *Radiology* 1993;189:211–219.

Edelman RR. MR angiography: Present and future. *AJR* 1993;161:1–11.

Espeland MA, Craven TE, Riley WA, et al. Reliability of longitudinal ultrasonographic measurements of carotid intimal-medial thickness. *Stroke* 1966;27:480–485.

Faught WE, Mattos MA, van Bemmelen PS, et al. Color-flow duplex scanning of carotid arteries: New velocity criteria based on receiver operator characteristic analysis for threshold stenoses used in the symptomatic and asymptomatic carotid trials. *J Vasc Surg* 1994;19:818–828.

Feussner JR, Matchar DB. When and how to study the carotid arteries. *Ann Intern Med* 1988;109:805–818.

Griewing B, Morgenstern C, Driesner F, et al. Cerebrovascular disease assessed by color-flow and power Doppler ultrasonography. *Stroke* 1996;27:95–100.

Levine RL, Turski PA, Holmes KA, Grist TM. Comparison of magnetic resonance volume flow rates, angiography, and carotid Dopplers: Preliminary results. *Stroke* 1994;25:413–417.

Marks MP, Napel S, Jordan JE, Enzmann DR. Diagnosis of carotid artery disease: Preliminary experience with maximum-intensity-projection spiral CT angiography. *AJR* 1993;160:1267–1271.

Mattos MA, Hodgson KJ, Faught WE, et al. Carotid endarterectomy without angiography: Is color-flow duplex scanning sufficient? *Surgery* 1994;116:776–783.

Moneta GL, Edwards JM, Chitwood RW, et al. Correlation of North American Symptomatic Carotid Endarterectomy Trial (NASCET) angiographic definition of 70% to 99% internal carotid artery stenosis with duplex scanning. *J Vasc Surg* 1993;17:152–159.

O'Leary DH, Polak JF, Kronmal RA, et al. Thickening of the carotid wall: A marker for atherosclerosis in the elderly? *Stroke* 1996;27:224–231.

Pan XM, Saloner D, Reilly LM, et al. Assessment of carotid artery stenosis by ultrasonography, conventional angiography, and magnetic resonance angiography: Correlation with ex vivo measurement of plaque stenosis. *J Vasc Surg* 1995;21:82–88.

Polak JF, Bajakian RL, O'Leary DH, et al. Detection of internal carotid artery stenosis: Comparison of MR angiography, color Doppler sonography, and arteriography. *Radiology* 1992;182:35–40.

Schwartz LB, Bridgman AH, Kieffer RW, et al. Asymptomatic carotid artery stenosis and stroke in patients undergoing cardiopulmonary bypass. *J Vasc Surg* 1995;21:146–153.

Schwartz RB. Helical (spiral) CT in neuroradiologic diagnosis. *Radiol Clin* 1995;33:981–995.

Stehling MK, Lawerence JA, Weintraub JL, Raptopoulos V. CT angiography: Expanded clinical applications. *AJR* 1994;163:947–955.

Steinke W, Meairs S, Ries S, Hennerici M. Sonographic assessment of carotid artery stenosis: Comparison of power Doppler imaging and color Doppler flow imaging. *Stroke* 1996;27:91–94.

Stoney RJ, String ST. Recurrent carotid stenosis. *Surgery* 1976;8:705–710.

Young GR, Humphrey PRD, Nixon TE, Smith ETS. Variability in measurement of extracranial internal carotid artery stenosis as displayed by both digital subtraction and magnetic resonance angiography: An assessment of three caliper techniques and visual impression of stenosis. *Stroke* 1996;27:467–473.

Zwiebel WJ. Duplex sonography of the cerebral arteries: Efficacy limitations, and indications. *AJR* 1992;158:29–36.

Stents

Bergeron P, Chambran P, Benichou H, Alessandri C. Recurrent carotid disease: Will stents be an alternative to surgery? *J Endovasc Surg* 1996;3:76–79.

Iyer SS, Roubin GS, Yadav S, et al. Elective carotid stenting (Abstract). *J Endovasc Surg* 1996;3:105–106.

Jungreis C. The use of stents in endovascular intervention. *AJNR* 1995;16:1974–1976.

Kharrazi MR. Anesthesia for carotid stent procedures. *J Endovasc Surg* 1996;3:211–216.

Parodi JC, Ferreira M, Estol CJ. Treatment of carotid artery disease with an endoluminal stent-venous graft. *J Neurovasc Dis* 1996;1:27–32.

Plat S, Hilaire I, Vuillemin E, Lafaye M. Patient preparation and monitoring for carotid stenting: The operating room nurse's perspective. *J Endovasc Surg* 1966;3:224–227.

Wilson EP, White RA, Vorwerk GE. Utility of intravascular ultrasound in carotid stenting. *J Endovasc Surg* 1996;3:63–68.

CHAPTER 44

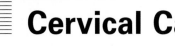

Cervical Carotid Angioplasty and Stent Placement for Atherosclerosis

V. Wadlington / J. Yadav / J. Vitek / M. Parks / S. Iyer / G. Roubin

This chapter provides an overview of the procedure and technique of carotid angioplasty and stenting as practiced at the University of Alabama at Birmingham. The standard treatment for prevention of stroke from cervical carotid stenosis is carotid endarterectomy.[1] Several people have performed angioplasty without stenting to treat this disease and have achieved good results.[2–8] The rationale is to increase the luminal size to allow for more blood flow to the brain. However, a nonstenotic irregular lesion may be a source of emboli causing stroke without hemodynamic compromise. Although this is not always the case, angioplasty can reduce the irregularity of these lesions while increasing the luminal size.

Some of the risks of carotid angioplasty include symptomatic dissection and cerebral embolization. These are thought to be caused by the disruption of plaque by the angioplasty balloon. However, plaque disruption is a necessary event for dilating atherosclerotic lesions, and this can occasionally cause problems.

Deploying a stent may give some security against embolization by preventing fragments from becoming free in the lumen. The stent can smooth the contour of the wall and may reduce embolic events. Its radial force helps prevent restenosis from recoil of the vessel wall. The stent is not intended to be removed and may provide a nidus for more tissue proliferation and restenosis. It may also limit further evaluation with magnetic resonance angiography because of the paramagnetic properties of certain metals used in the stents.

At this time, no stents or balloons are approved for use in the carotid arteries by the Food and Drug Administration. Angioplasty and stenting are being performed at the authors' institution under Institutional Review Board (IRB) approval in cooperation with neurology, radiology, cardiology, neurosurgery, and vascular surgery. It is recommended that this procedure be performed under well-conducted IRB-approved protocols.

PATIENT SELECTION

Since this is a new procedure, the selection criteria for cervical carotid angioplasty have not been definitely established. Techniques have improved significantly (Fig. 44–1) and angioplasty should be used at least in selected cases. Angioplasty is particularly helpful in certain types of stenoses such as fibromuscular dysplasia, stenoses after endarterectomy, postradiation stenoses, or high cervical carotid stenoses or in patients at high risk for myocardial infarction or hypotension during general anesthesia. Its role in initial treatment of atherosclerotic carotid stenoses is not completely established. However, initial analysis of our results reveals comparatively low complication rates in patients with contralateral carotid occlusion, recent unstable neurologic events, and bilateral disease. These groups of patients have traditionally had higher complication rates associated with carotid endarterectomy.

Just as some patients are at high risk for complications related to endarterectomy, some people are at high risk for angioplasty-related problems. The angioplasty procedure can be quite prolonged if the

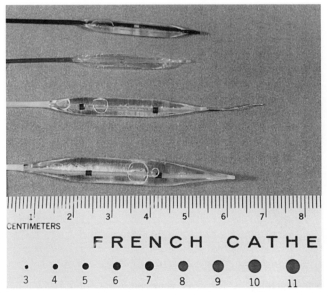

Figure 44-1 Balloon catheters *(top to bottom)*: SciMed Swift, 4 × 20 mm; Cordis Corp., 4 × 20 mm deflated showing balloon wings; Schneider, Inc. Total Cross, 5 × 20 mm inflated with Cook, Inc. Roadrunner 0.018″ guidewire; Total Cross, 7 × 20 mm inflated.

patient has difficult vascular access via the femoral arteries. A tortuous aorta, brachiocephalic artery, and/or common carotid artery can increase the risk associated with manipulating wires and catheters across them. Some of these patients may be best suited for endarterectomy.

For most cases, angioplasty is safe enough for physicians to let patients make their own choice between surgery and angioplasty. However, patients need to understand that surgery is the more established procedure for carotid stenosis.

ANGIOPLASTY RISKS

The main risks of angioplasty are of stroke and inguinal hematoma formation. Strokes can occur from dissection, emboli, or bradycardia with hypotension. The stroke risks should be reduced when these factors are controlled.

Dissection

Dissection is usually necessary during dilation of an atherosclerotic artery. The lumen cannot be enlarged without breaking the plaque. This can cause emboli from plaque fragments that may float distally. It may also cause a low-flow state due to a decreased luminal size. This can occur if the plaque fragment partially occludes the lumen. Mural hematoma formation can also narrow the lumen.

The adverse events of a dissection may be more likely to occur if the balloon is too large. The complexity of the plaque may precipitate these problems even if the balloon is the appropriate size (Fig. 44–2). Angiographically visible dissection has been correlated with transient cervical, ear, scapula, or dental arch pain. The probability of this event has been reported to correlate with increased dilating pressure.[5] It may be related to the resistance that the plaque exerts against the balloon as opposed to the pressure generated inside the balloon. The inflation device may read 20 atmospheres while the plaque is providing no resistance to dilation. Although the dissection may be visible, it may not be symptomatic. Undersizing the balloon may decrease the incidence of problematic dissections, but the lesion may not be adequately dilated this way.

A dissection may be controlled by deploying a stent (Case 1, Fig. 44–2). This has been done many times with excellent results. Long-term evaluation of these patients is awaited.

Emboli Without Dissection

Embolization can originate from plaque or a thrombus on the vessel wall or particles from the catheter system. Occasionally, transcranial Doppler high-intensity transients are detected during contrast or saline injections, immediately after balloon inflation or deflation, or during wire and catheter manipulation.[9] These are almost always asymptomatic. This also occurs during endarterectomy.

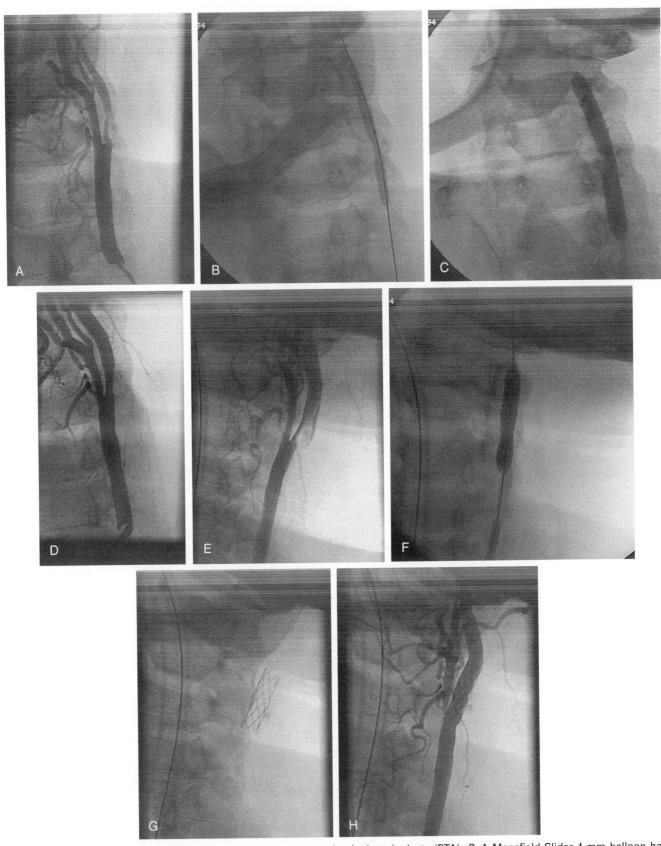

Figure 44-2 Case 1. *A,* Initial appearance pre–percutaneous transluminal angioplasty (PTA). *B,* A Mansfield Slider 4-mm balloon has been advanced. *C,* A Medi-Tech 6-mm PEMT balloon is now in position. *D,* The immediate postangioplasty appearance. *E,* The dissection is clearly seen. The patient became comatose in the recovery room and was returned to the catheterization laboratory. *F,* A 6-mm balloon has been placed. *G,* A Palmaz stent was then placed. *H,* The final post–stent placement appearance.

One study reported a 7.4% incidence of cerebrovascular accidents (4 of 54 cases) during percutaneous transluminal angioplasty (PTA) without stenting. Two of these occurred within 36 hours after the procedure, presumably from emboli.[5] Unilateral amaurosis fugax has occurred in carotid PTA without stenting,[5] but did not occur in our study[10] with stenting.

Bradycardia with Hypotension

Bradycardia arises from stretching of the carotid sinus by the balloon. There is often bradycardia, occasionally severe coughing, and rarely asystole during balloon inflation in the carotid bulb. Bradycardia occasionally causes hypotension, which can be determined immediately by monitoring the pressure in the base catheter. If cuff pressures are being utilized during the procedure, this may not be detected. This is rarely symptomatic because of its short duration, and it almost always resolves after balloon deflation.[8] Bradycardia has been reported in 39% of cases, with hypotension in 2%.[5] Bradycardia may be prevented with intravenous atropine before balloon inflation, but this is not always effective. A transvenous cardiac pacemaker may be required if the bradycardia is refractory.

Hematoma

Another risk of angioplasty is of inguinal or retroperitoneal hematoma formation, the latter being more difficult to detect without a pelvic computed tomographic scan. The catheters used to perform angioplasty can be 6 to 9-Fr. Larger ones are used to facilitate contrast injection around the balloon catheter and to deploy stents. The sheath is removed later. Since heparin is given during the procedure, the risks of inguinal bleeding and hematoma formation are increased. We have not been using protamine to reverse the heparin effects.

Spasm

Spasm may occur anytime a wire or catheter is in a vessel. It seems to be more of a problem in the cerebral circulation because of the risk of low cerebral perfusion pressure and stroke. When wires and catheters are exchanged in the internal carotid artery (ICA) during carotid angioplasty, there may be mild spasm causing no difficulties or severe spasm that may occlude the vessel temporarily. This is usually self-limited. Even if the carotid is occluded, there may be no symptoms. If there are problems, good results have been achieved with intra-arterial nitroglycerin, 100 to 300 μg. No problems have been encountered with nausea or confusion secondary to the nitroglycerin infusion. This agent can be administered much faster than papaverine, which is slightly acidic and needs to be infused slowly.

SURGICAL RISKS

The perioperative stroke rate (surgery to 30 days) associated with endarterectomy is approximately 5.5% (18 of 328); 2 years after carotid endarterectomy, it is approximately 12.6%.[1] Other possible surgical complications include nerve dysfunction (7.6%), wound hematoma, and infection, but most of these are of no lasting consequence.[1] These may be due to difficulties with surgical dissection and carotid artery exposure. If the patient has undergone a previous endarterectomy, the dissection around and within the carotid artery is more difficult. If the stenosis is too far superior, mandibular retraction becomes more difficult. Short, wide necks cause problems of access.

Endarterectomy is often performed with the patient under general endotracheal anesthesia. This involves risks of stroke from hypotension, myocardial infarction, and aspiration. Currently, many surgeons use local anesthesia with intravenous sedation for this procedure if the stenosis is not too high behind the mandibular angle. General anesthesia may be needed if the surgeon decides that the amount of mandibular retraction will be too great for local anesthesia. Some patients may prefer angioplasty if the endarterectomy will require general anesthesia. In any case, patients should understand that angioplasty has not gained the acceptance that endarterectomy has for carotid stenosis treatment.

PREPARATION

A cerebral angiogram is important to demonstrate the status of both carotid and vertebral arteries and the intracranial circulation. This will be helpful if a neurologic deficit occurs during the angioplasty procedure. Detection of abnormalities on the angiogram after the event may be facilitated by comparison with a preangioplasty angiogram.

The carotid ultrasound examination may be accurate but may not correlate with the angiographic findings used to determine whether or not a patient should be treated. For this reason, we perform a carotid angiogram to confirm ultrasound findings. Some surgeons have relied solely on duplex results to perform endarterectomy.[11]

It is not necessary to stop aspirin or ticlopidine before the angioplasty. In our study[10] of carotid stenting, ticlopidine (250 mg bid) and aspirin (325 mg bid) were begun 2 days before the angioplasty to help prevent thrombus formation in the catheter system or in the carotid artery during wire and catheter manipulations.

ANGIOPLASTY AND STENT PROCEDURE
Access and Carotid Artery Catheterization

Most 70-year-old aortic arches are probably too tortuous to deliver a Wallstent (Schneider, Inc.) simply over a 0.038″ wire using a 10- to 20-cm 8-Fr. sheath. This may also cause too much back-and-forth motion of the 0.038″ wire in the ICA. A 0.038″ wire will also have more surface area for small clots to form than a 0.018″ wire. Therefore, a base or guide catheter is used. The following technique is employed for catheterization of the carotid artery.

A 5-Fr. diagnostic catheter (we usually use a Cook, Inc. or Medi-Tech, Inc. HN-2 catheter) is placed in the common carotid artery (CCA) with a Medi-Tech, Inc. 0.038″ angled Glidewire. This catheter is used to view the stenosis. Heparin (5000 U) is then given through the catheter. A 0.038″ exchange wire (a Cook, Inc. or Medi-Tech, Inc. Amplatz Extra Stiff 260-cm 0.038″ wire with a 6-cm floppy end) is then placed in the external carotid artery (ECA) (Fig. 44–3), which is believed to be the safest location in patients with tortuous, diseased vessels.

Base (Guide) Catheter Placement

Once the exchange wire is seated, the diagnostic catheter is removed while the wire tip is kept in the external carotid artery. A 9-Fr. guide catheter or 7-Fr. sheath is needed to deliver a Wallstent. We have been using a 100-cm 9-Fr. Cordis Corp. Brite-Tip (multipurpose tip), which has an inner diameter (ID) of 0.098″, through a 9-Fr. sheath (10.5-Fr. outer diameter [OD]). To reduce the size of the femoral puncture, we have used an Arrow International or Cook, Inc. 90-cm 7-Fr. sheath (9-Fr. OD) with a rotating hemostatic valve. The present Wallstents (7-Fr., 0.091″ OD) do not fit through the 9-Fr. USCI King Multipurpose tip (0.092″ ID); 0.001″ is not enough to account for the friction from curves and length of the catheter. The medium Palmaz (Johnson & Johnson Interventional Systems) stents on a low-profile balloon catheter (e.g., Medi-Tech Symmetry) will pass through this catheter. The medium Palmaz stents can also be mounted on a 3-Fr. catheter with hand crimping and placed through a 7-Fr. guide catheter.

When the 9-Fr. guide catheters are used, a 5-Fr. (0.065″ OD) 120 cm catheter is placed inside the 9-Fr. (0.098″ ID) catheter to smooth the transition between the 0.038″ exchange wire and the tip of the 9-Fr. catheter. This technique, or the use of long

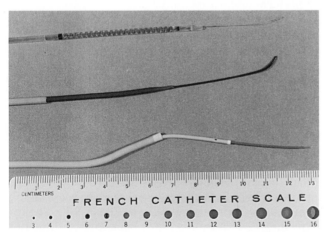

Figure 44-3 *Top,* Schneider, Inc. 7-Fr. 8 × 20 mm Wallstent delivery system with Cook, Inc. Roadrunner 0.018″ wire. *Middle,* Cook, Inc. 80-cm 7-Fr. sheath with dilator and 0.038″ Glidewire (Medi-Tech, Inc.) in it. *Bottom,* Cordis Brite-Tip 9-Fr. (0.098″ inner diameter [ID], multipurpose tip) with Cordis 5-Fr. 0.038″ ID 125-cm catheter and Cook, Inc. Amplatz 0.038″ 260-cm wire.

dilator-sheath combinations, theoretically helps avoid plaque dislodgment while advancing the base catheter. The catheters or sheath and dilator are advanced over the exchange wire into the distal CCA.

If a stent is not going to be deployed, a 6- or 7-Fr. catheter may suffice. After the angioplasty balloon has been inflated, the balloon material may not be as compact as it was in the package. Thus, a larger base (guide) catheter is needed to remove the balloon catheter (if a base catheter is not used and the angioplasty catheter is delivered over a wire, this is only a problem with the femoral sheath).

The activated clotting time is kept between 200 and 250 seconds with intermittent heparin doses through the base catheter. The guide catheter is used to monitor pressure in the CCA and occasionally rinse heparinized saline through it with a 20-cc syringe or via a flush system.

Balloon Catheter Selection and Use

The size of the normal internal carotid and common carotid arteries is measured using the base catheter as a reference measurement. This diameter is typically the final balloon size for each vessel. The ICA is usually 5 to 6 mm and the CCA usually 8 to 10 mm.

We usually begin with an approximately 3-Fr. shaft balloon catheter that accepts a 0.018″ wire. The catheter may be a Mansfield Mighty (2.9-Fr., 0.018″ wire) 4 × 20 mm rated at 15 atmospheres, a SciMed Cobra (3.0-Fr., 0.018″ wire) 4 × 20 mm rated at 15 atmospheres, or another catheter. Balloons 40 mm in length are probably preferable since they are less likely to "melon seed" out of the lesion. Occasionally, a smaller double-lumen balloon catheter is used that may accept only a 0.014″ wire.

The initial balloon catheter is placed across the stenosis with a USCI Standard or Hyperflex 0.014″ or 0.016″ 160- or 175-cm wire, which is easier to steer than a 300-cm wire. This wire is replaced with an exchange length wire, usually a Cook, Inc. Roadrunner (0.018″, 300 cm). The lesion is then dilated. Additional balloon catheters can be placed over the 0.018″ wire if needed.

If the patient is hypertensive, the blood pressure may be controlled with an intravenous nitroglycerin drip before balloon inflation to help prevent reperfusion injury. This should be done judiciously, since there may be a substantial drop in blood pressure after balloon dilation of the carotid bulb. Atropine, 0.5 mg intravenously, and metaraminol bitartrate (Aramine), 1.0 mg intravenously, can be used to increase the heart rate and blood pressure.

A safety balloon catheter can be used in the CCA or ICA, but with current technology this complicates the procedure.[12–14] It provides a second location where the vessel wall can be damaged by a balloon. It also increases the time that the ICA is occluded. Results of this technique do suggest that embolic complications are reduced.[12–14] More refined embolus removal or filter techniques are now in development.

Stent Selection

An ideal stent is not available yet. This would be low-profile, flexible, self-expanding, easy to deploy accurately at both ends, nonthrombogenic, and capable of preventing tissue growth on the inner and outer surfaces. Other stents (Palmaz or Wallstent) are being used in many institutions. The Palmaz is a balloon-expandable stent (not self-expanding) and has plastic properties with a high radial strength. When the medium Palmaz (biliary) stents are inflated to 6 mm diameter, they are 9.4 mm (P104), 14.0 mm (P154), 18.6 mm (P204), or 27.8 mm (P294) long. The Wallstent is self-expanding, but the shortest now available is 20 mm when fully expanded with a 6-mm balloon (H620). If the H820 (8 × 20 mm Wallstent) is expanded maximally with a 6-mm balloon throughout the stent length, the stent is about 40 mm long. However, when the proximal part is in the CCA (approximately 8 mm in diameter), the stent length is 30 to 35 mm.

If a stent is to be deployed, a Wallstent 7-Fr., 0.038″ ID, 160-cm (total length) delivery catheter can be advanced over the 0.018″ wire through the 9-Fr. base catheter. We choose the stent size by the diameter of the CCA, since most lesions cross the CCA bifurcation. A stent is chosen that is 1 to 2 mm larger in diameter than the largest segment to be stented. We usually use an 8 × 20 mm or 10 × 20 mm stent (occasionally 8 × 40 mm or 10 × 42 mm) and deploy it across the CCA bifurcation. The Wallstent diameter is the inner diameter of the fully expanded stent. Since an 8- or 10-mm stent is not fully expanded in the 4- to 6-mm diameter cervical ICA, the total length is approximately 30 mm.

The outer sheath of the Wallstent system is flushed with heparinized saline and the stopcock closed; no additional flush is used. Blood is allowed to reflux around the 0.018″ wire while the stent is advanced; a Y-adapter is not used to provide saline flush around the wire. It takes only a minute or so to deploy the Wallstent.

The stent is positioned distal to the lesion because of the shortening that occurs when the outer sheath is retracted (Figs. 44–4 and 44–5). The stenosis is usually dilated with a 5 × 20 mm or 6 × 20 mm balloon. The authors commonly use the Total Cross

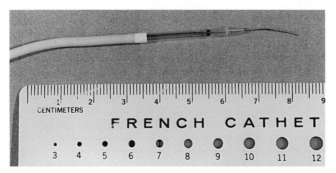

Figure 44-4 A 9-Fr. Brite-Tip (multipurpose tip) with 7-Fr. Wallstent and Roadrunner 0.018″ guidewire.

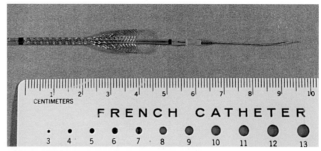

Figure 44-5 Wallstent 8 × 20 mm half deployed with Roadrunner 0.018″ guidewire.

(4.3-Fr., 0.021″ wire) 5 × 20 mm or 6 × 20 mm balloon catheter. The proximal portion of the stent can be seated against the CCA with a larger 8 × 20 mm diameter balloon if necessary. When the CCA is normal, the self-expanding feature of the stent is adequate to seat it against the artery wall. A balloon may be needed to dilate a CCA stenosis. If no significant residual narrowing is seen after stent placement and the stent has been appropriately oversized, no additional balloon inflations are needed. Final views of the head and neck can be obtained at this point.

If the ECA is stenosed or occluded, it can be dilated, usually with a 0.016″ wire and 2.9-Fr. shaft balloon catheter through the Wallstent (Case 2, Fig. 44–6).

POSTANGIOPLASTY AND STENTING RESULTS

Immediately after the procedure, 0% to 10% residual diameter stenosis can be achieved with stent placement (Case 3, Fig. 44–7; Case 4, Fig. 44–8; Case 5, Fig. 44–9). In a study of angioplasty alone, 0% stenosis was reported in 54% (24 of 44 cases) and less than 20% stenosis in 31% (17 of 44 cases) immediately after angioplasty without stenting.[5]

Occasionally the stent traverses a crevice or ulcer, and contrast flows outside the stent into the crevice with washout in a delayed fashion. The rate of washout is probably increased with denser contrast. The crevices are usually posterior, which is the dependent portion of the vessel with the patient supine. Residual (external to the stent) ulceration is of no clinical significance in terms of late results, and most of these lesions fill in with fibrous tissue in the following weeks.

POSTANGIOPLASTY MANAGEMENT

Heparin treatment (continuous infusion or intermittent subcutaneous injections) after angioplasty has not been proved to be beneficial or detrimental. Some practitioners give heparin only during the procedure and begin aspirin treatment immediately. We have used ticlopidine, 250 mg orally bid, 2 days before and for 3 weeks afterward. Routinely, the patient is kept overnight on a regular ward and discharged the next morning. If a case is complicated, the patient is observed in the intensive care unit.

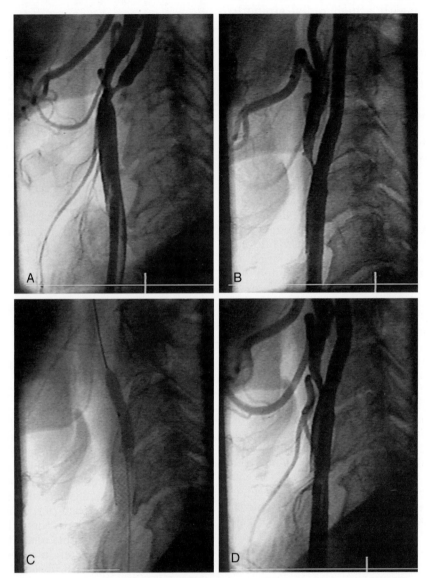

Figure 44-6 Case 2. *A*, Initial pre-PTA image with 9-Fr. catheter in place. *B*, After angioplasty and placement of an 8 × 20 mm Wallstent, the internal carotid artery (ICA) stenosis is relieved, but the external carotid artery (ECA) has become stenotic. *C*, A 4 × 20 mm balloon has been advanced through the Wallstent into the ECA. *D*, The ECA stenosis was relieved after angioplasty.

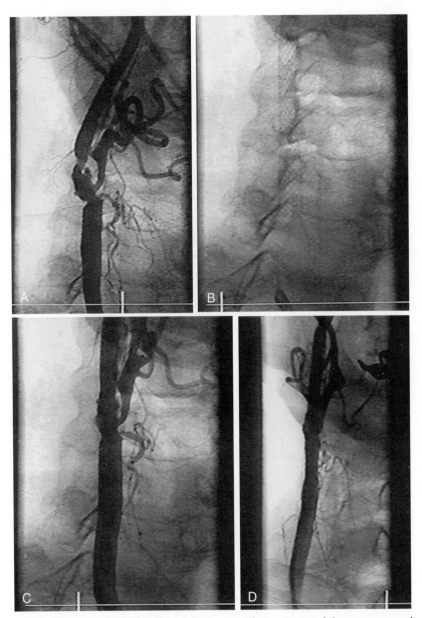

Figure 44-7 Case 3. *A*, The initial angiogram demonstrates right common and internal carotid artery stenoses. *B*, An 8 × 40 mm Wallstent is seen (no contrast was injected). *C*, The post-PTA appearance of the vessel and Wallstent. *D*, At 6-month follow-up, there is less than 50% restenosis.

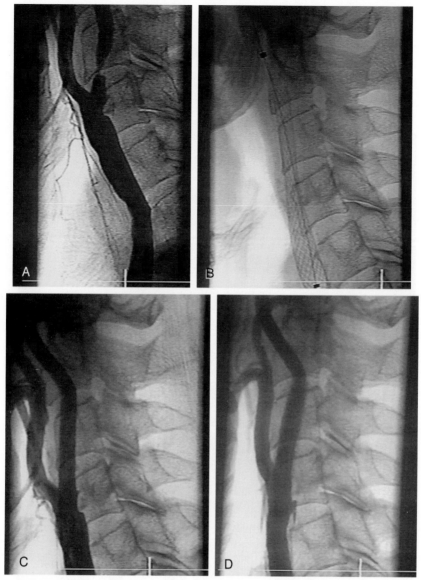

Figure 44-8 Case 4. *A*, The initial view demonstrates 90% stenosis of the right ICA. *B*, A 10 × 42 mm Wallstent was chosen for use. *C*, After PTA, there is no residual stenosis. *D*, At 6-month follow-up, there is less than 50% restenosis.

FOLLOW-UP

Over a 33-month period, 281 patients received 102 Palmaz stents and 222 Wallstents. The periprocedural minor stroke rate was 7% for the Palmaz stent group and 6.3% for the Wallstent group. There were two major strokes in the Palmaz group and one in the Wallstent group, a total of three in 281 (1.06%). The single Wallstent event was due to hypotension and cardiac arrest during coronary angioplasty 4 days after carotid stenting. The other strokes were from a contralateral middle cerebral artery embolus and a stent thrombosis that recanalized. There were four periprocedural deaths (4 of 281 or 1.4%). These were due to pulmonary embolism, retroperitoneal hemorrhage, carotid rupture, and aneurysm rupture after recanalization of a "string sign." One should remember that approximately 80% of the 281 pa-

tients would not qualify for either North American Symptomatic Endarterectomy Trial or Asymptomatic Carotid Atherosclerosis Study because of comorbidity.

Six-month follow-up angiograms were obtained in 75 of 102 patients (74%) in the Palmaz group and 117 of 141 patients (83%) in the Wallstent group. This yielded follow-up on 192 out of 243 eligible vessels. In the Palmaz group, there was a seven of 75 (7%) rate of restenosis (>50% diameter stenosis). In the Wallstent group, the rate was 5% (six of 117). Deformity was seen in 13% (10 of 75) of Palmaz stents; no Wallstents were deformed. One patient with a deformed stent experienced transient ischemic attacks (TIAs); the others were asymptomatic. Five other patients reported TIAs at follow-up (a total of six of 192 or 3.1%). Of these, one had restenosis at the stent, another had a new stenosis distal to the

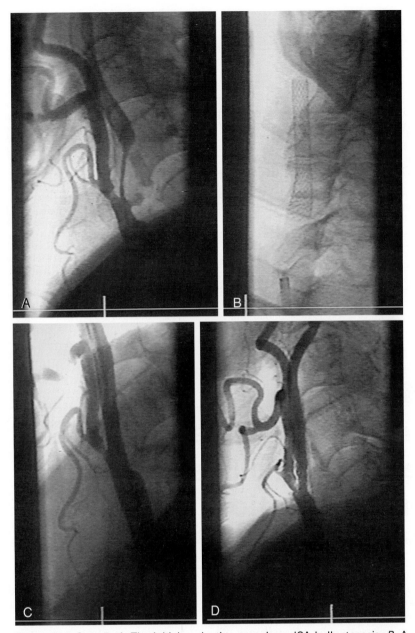

Figure 44-9 Case 5. *A*, The initial evaluation reveals an ICA bulb stenosis. *B*, A 10 × 20 mm Wallstent was used. *C*, The postprocedure image reveals no residual stenosis. *D*, The 6-month follow-up reveals less than 50% stenosis.

stent, and the other three had widely patent vessels. Overall, there were three minor strokes during the follow-up period (3 of 192 or 1.6%) and no major strokes. Seventeen deaths occurred during the follow-up period. Of these, seven were cardiac and four were due to pneumonia or sepsis, two to renal failure, one to a motor vehicle accident, one to a cerebral hemorrhage, one to a pulmonary embolism, and one to an unknown cause.

CONCLUSIONS

Angioplasty with stent deployment provides another treatment modality for carotid stenosis, the same as for other parts of the body. A major difference is that the end organ for the carotid artery is more sensitive to emboli and pressure changes than the end organs in other parts of the body. Problems with plaque fragmentation and restenosis can be reduced with stent placement.

Restenosis (>50%) after angioplasty is due to a combination of elastic recoil and neointimal proliferation at the angioplasty or stent site. This is evident on later ultrasound or angiographic examination. Stenting helps eliminate the elastic recoil. Some animal studies have shown regeneration of smooth muscle after angioplasty.[15]

The results so far look promising and we are awaiting longer follow-up evaluation. In the meantime, work is being done to develop better, smaller-caliber, flexible delivery devices and stents to be placed transfemorally.

REFERENCES

1. North American Symptomatic Carotid Endarterectomy Trial Collaborators. Beneficial effect of carotid endarterectomy in symptomatic patients with high-grade stenosis. *N Engl J Med* 1991;325:445–453 and comments following.
2. Bergeron P, Rudondy P, Benichou H, et al. Transluminal angioplasty for recurrent stenosis after carotid endarterectomy. Prognostic factors and indications. *Int Angiol* 1993;12:256–259.
3. Kachel R, Basche S, Kassel I, Grossmann K. Long-term results of PTA of degenerative supra-aortic arterial changes. *Vasa* 1991;33(Suppl):183–185.
4. Kachel R. Percutaneous transluminal angioplasty of the carotid artery. *Wien Klin Wochenschr* 1993;105:187–193.
5. Munari LM, Belloni G, Perretti A, et al. Carotid percutaneous angioplasty. *Neurol Res* 1992;14:156–158.
6. Kachel R. PTA of carotid, vertebral, and subclavian artery stenoses. an alternative to vascular surgery? *Int Angiol* 1994;13:48–51.
7. Motarjeme A, Gordon GI. Percutaneous transluminal angioplasty of the brachiocephalic vessels: guidelines for therapy. *Int Angiol* 1993;12:260–269.
8. Yamamura A, Oyama H, Matsuno F, et al. Percutaneous transluminal angioplasty for cervical carotid artery stenosis. *No Shinkei Geka* 1995;23:117–123.
9. Markus HS, Clifton A, Buckenham T, Brown MM. Carotid angioplasty. Detection of embolic signals during and after the procedure. *Stroke* 1994;25:2403–2406.
10. Yadav J, Roubin GS, Iyer S, et al. Elective surgery of the extracranial carotid arteries. *Circulation* 1997;95:376–381.
11. Mattos MA, Hodgson KJ, Faught WE, et al. Carotid endarterectomy without angiography: is color-flow duplex scanning sufficient? *Surgery* 1994;116:776–783.
12. Terada T, Yokote H, Nakamura Y, et al. Newly developed blocking balloon catheter for PTA of internal carotid artery. *No Shinkei Geka* 1993;21:891–895.
13. Kinoshita A, Itoh M, Takemoto O. Percutaneous transluminal angioplasty of internal carotid artery: a preliminary report of seesaw balloon technique. *Neurol Res* 1993;15:356–358.
14. Lorenzi G, Domanin M, Constantini A, et al. Intraoperative transluminal angioplasty of recurrent carotid stenosis. *J Cardiovasc Surg* 1993;34:163–165.
15. Okamoto E, Imataka K, Fujii J, et al. Heterogeneity in smooth muscle cell population accumulating in the neointimas and the media of poststenotic dilatation of the rabbit carotid artery. *Biochem Biophys Res Commun* 1992;185:459–464.

CHAPTER 45

Protected Angioplasty and Stenting of Atherosclerotic Stenosis at the Carotid Artery Bifurcation

J.G. Theron

The cervical carotid artery has been considered untouchable from an endovascular approach. Several arguments have been put forth to defend this position, including (1) the observation by any witness of carotid bifurcation surgery that in this location the atherosclerotic plaque is often fragile, ulcerated, and hemorrhagic;[1] and (2) the North American Symptomatic Carotid Endarterectomy Trial (NASCET) demonstration that endarterectomy was superior to medical treatment for symptomatic carotid stenoses (>70% stenosis).[2] Subsequently, the Asymptomatic Carotid Atherosclerosis Study (ACAS) showed a statistically significant reduction in stroke incidence after carotid endarterectomy in patients with asymptomatic carotid stenosis greater than 60%.[3]

The proposition of a therapeutic endovascular alternative certainly disturbs those who practice carotid surgery, since the benefits in specific situations have only just been recognized after the procedure has existed for more than 40 years. The potential application of endovascular techniques of cerebral revascularization is enormous when the aging of the population is considered.

It is considered that the endovascular approach should be applied to carotid pathology only if the following conditions are met:

1. On the technical level, there must be a maximum of technical precautions so that the incidence of complications is greatly lower than that of surgery, the stroke and death risk of which has been precisely evaluated at 5.6% for symptomatic patients.[4] Each technical improvement has to be achieved with maximal concern for safety.
2. With regard to the indications, the endovascular approach must encourage a deeper diagnostic reflection on the cause of cerebral ischemia, and consequently on the possibilities of adapting the revascularization to the exact ischemic state of each patient.

EVOLUTION OF THE TECHNIQUES OF PROTECTED ANGIOPLASTY AND PROTECTED STENTING

The potential cerebral complications of carotid angioplasty have two major isolated or associated anatomic bases: (1) intracerebral embolism of fragments of plaque or clot and (2) dissection leading to carotid occlusion and secondary intracerebral embolic or hemodynamic infarction, most often in the junction region. The clinical expression can be more or less severe. Complications may be asymptomatic or may be expressed as a transient or permanent deficit due to more or less extensive cerebral infarction, which in the extreme may be accompanied by vasogenic edema that eventually leads to death.

Prevention of Intracerebral Embolism by Temporary Distal Occlusion

Experience with cerebral protection by means of temporary occlusion of the carotid artery during therapeutic embolization has led to the adaptation of a cerebral protection technique of angioplasty for atherosclerotic stenosis at the carotid bifurcation.[5] The technique originally used for cerebral protection necessitated a bilateral femoral approach.[6] The technique was simplified by designing a triple coaxial catheter that enabled, from a single femoral approach, angioplasty with temporary carotid occlusion, aspiration of debris, and flushing of the working site (Fig. 45–1).[7] This technique has essentially eliminated the risk of embolic complications during the angioplasty procedure itself (dropping from 8% to 0% in a controlled series), but it did not initially eliminate the embolic risk during the stent placement (which was originally performed using Strecker stents without protection, after protected angioplasty, as discussed further below).[8]

So far, the widespread dissemination of the protection technique has remained limited by the necessity of preparing the 300-cm occlusion balloon catheter before the procedure (attaching the protective microballoon and eliminating the dead space). It is hoped that a ready-made product that addresses these issues may be available in the near future.

Another cerebral protection technique, using proximal occlusion of the common carotid artery (CCA) by a guide catheter with an occlusion balloon, has been proposed.[9] It employs a technique that may not offer sufficient security against the risk of embolism. The carotid bifurcation can be revascularized by retrograde flow in the external carotid artery (ECA), supplied by anastomoses with muscular branches of the vertebral artery. Although proximal flow control is conceivable in the internal carotid artery (ICA), proximal occlusion in the CCA is not recommended.

Stents: Advantages and Early Disadvantages

The risk of dissection[8] has been found to be 5% in a group without protection before the introduction of stenting at the carotid level.[10] The use of stents has eliminated the risk of dissection and allowed treatment of dissections that do occur during angioplasty (Case 1, Fig. 45–2). The risk of embolization initially reappeared (2%) after the introduction of stents, because the Strecker stent[11] was originally used. The

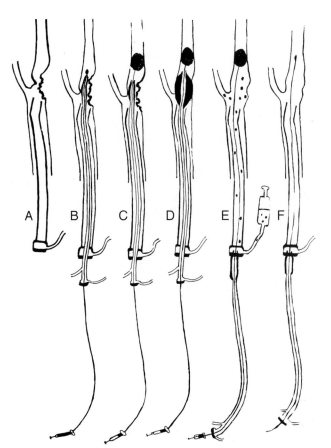

Figure 45-1 Schematic representation of the basic protected angioplasty technique. The femoral introducer is not represented. *A,* The guide catheter (Cordis Corp., vertebral curve) is positioned in the common carotid artery. An 8- or 9-Fr. catheter is used, depending on the potential stent (see Figs. 45-3 and 45-5). *B,* The angioplasty (Cordis Corp. or Medi-Tech 5-Fr., 5- to 7-mm balloon diameter, 2 cm long) and occlusive balloons (Nycomed No. 17 mounted on a 2.6-Fr. 300-cm catheter, Cordis RE658) are gently positioned. It is much more effective to keep the occlusion balloon against the tip of the angioplasty catheter, as there is less dead space to be aspirated and flushed. *C,* The occlusive balloon is inflated after administration of 6000 to 12,000 U heparin. Atropine (1 mg) is injected before inflation of the angioplasty balloon. *D,* Angioplasty is then performed. *E,* The angioplasty balloon is deflated and withdrawn down to the proximal valve of the guide catheter. Potential thrombi or atherosclerotic particles are aspirated through the guide catheter and flushed toward the external carotid artery (ECA). *F,* The occlusion balloon is then deflated. Repeat angiography demonstrates the result of angioplasty. Nimodipine is injected into the internal carotid artery (ICA) via the guide catheter when spasm is observed at the site of the occlusion balloon.

diameter of the stent did not allow its introduction through a guide catheter of a reasonable diameter, and the stents were deployed without cerebral protection, under the assumption that the site had been sufficiently cleared of debris and clots during protected angioplasty. Embolic material that did occur (2%) was obviously fresh because it was possible to clear all such emboli by intra-arterial thrombolysis.[12]

Prevention of Embolization During Stenting

Improvements in the technique of carotid angioplasty and stenting are currently moving in three directions:

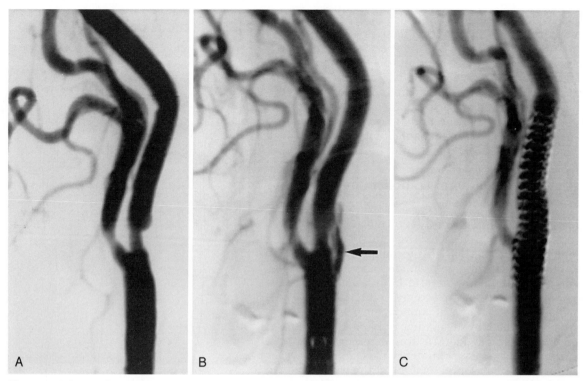

Figure 45-2 Case 1. Stent placement after protected angioplasty. *A,* A short-segment stenosis of the proximal ICA. *B,* After angioplasty with cerebral protection, there is improvement in the diameter of the vessel, but an intimal flap is seen *(arrow). C,* A Strecker stent was subsequently placed, with further improvement in the diameter of the ICA and flattening of the intimal flap. The ECA continues to fill through the interstices of the stent.

1. Prophylactic injection of small doses of fibrinolytic (urokinase, 300,000 IU or t-PA, 20 mg) at the site after angioplasty under temporary carotid occlusion, to clean the freshly dilated artery (angioplasty may cause an aggregation of platelets) (Fig. 45–3 and Case 2, Fig. 45–4). This may allow safer deployment of a Strecker stent (or Wallstent) without cerebral protection.

(*Editors' note*: abciximab (ReoPro) may have a role at this point; see Chapter 42.)

2. Use of a Wallstent *with* cerebral protection by the same system used for angioplasty; this requires a guide catheter of larger diameter (9-Fr.) (Fig. 45–5; Case 3, Fig. 45–6; and Case 4, Fig. 45–7).

3. Development of a simplified system of protection that will allow performance of all the neces-

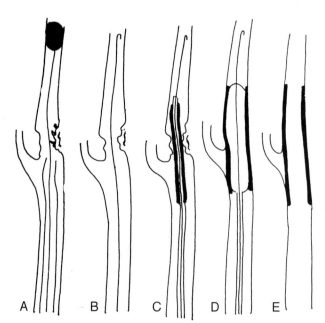

Figure 45-3 These images demonstrate Strecker stent placement without cerebral protection; preparation of the deployment site by local thrombolysis after protected angioplasty is utilized. *A,* After protected angioplasty, the occlusion balloon is reinflated. A thrombolytic agent (urokinase, 300,000 IU or tissue-type plasminogen activator [t-PA], 20 mg) is injected through the guide catheter, left in contact with the potential platelet aggregates for 5 minutes, and then aspirated. *B,* After the occlusion balloon has been deflated, an exchange wire is gently passed. The guide catheter is removed. *C,* The Strecker stent is advanced to the deployment site. *D,* The stent is deployed, in most cases covering the origin of the ECA. *E,* The deployment balloon is deflated and removed. Repeat angiography is performed. The ECA is supplied through the stent.

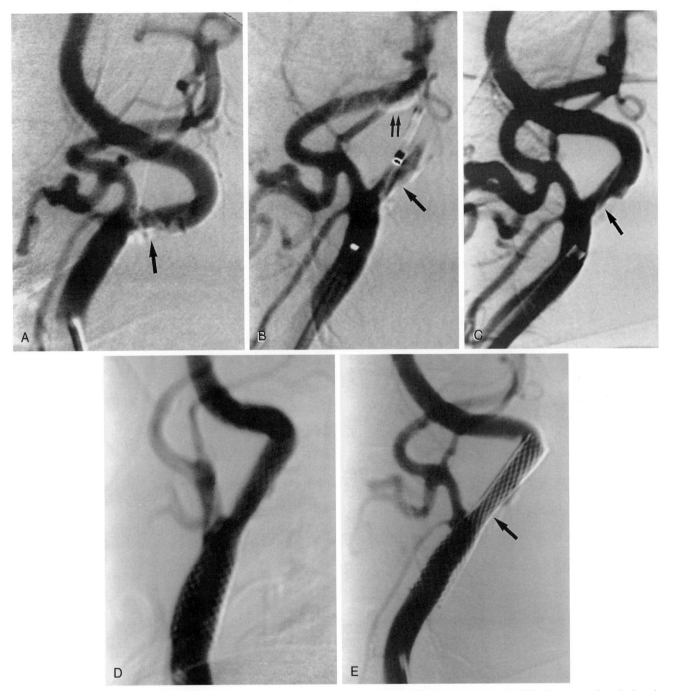

Figure 45-4 Case 2. Protected angioplasty and stenting of an ulcerated and calcified stenosis responsible for a transient ischemic episode in an 86-year-old woman. *A,* The preangioplasty angiogram reveals the irregular and calcified pattern of the stenosis *(arrow).* Protected angioplasty was performed. *B,* An image obtained during balloon occlusion is shown *(double arrows).* The flow is stopped at the angioplasty site *(arrow). C,* An image obtained after cleaning of the angioplasty site with a thrombolytic agent shows the stenosis to be partially opened *(arrow). D,* A Wallstent was then deployed. No preliminary or additional angioplasty was performed. *E,* A follow-up angiogram was obtained 6 months after treatment. The patient remained asymptomatic. Note the slight autoexpansion *(arrow)* of the stent as compared with *D.*

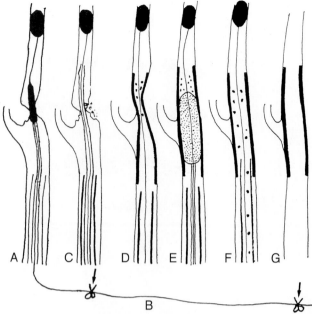

Figure 45-5 Protected Wallstent placement: complete protected procedure in a case of narrow stenosis that necessitates predilation before stent placement. *A,* The protected predilation is performed with a 4- or 5-mm angioplasty balloon catheter. *B,* Without deflating the occlusion balloon, the angioplasty catheter is withdrawn by clamping the microcatheter at two sites *(arrows)* before and after passage of the angioplasty catheter, allowing the hub and stopcock of the microcatheter to be removed without deflation of the occlusion balloon. The same maneuver is repeated at each subsequent step of the procedure. *C,* The Wallstent (mounted on its deployment catheter) is gently passed and positioned. Direct passage of the stent can frequently be performed without predilation. Because of the decrease of caliber between the common and internal carotid arteries, no movement of the stent at deployment is expected. *D,* The Wallstent is then deployed. The hardness of the plaque at this level frequently does not permit immediate full expansion of the stent (as shown in the drawing). Detached fragments of plaque and thrombus remain trapped at the site of deployment. *E,* Complementary protected angioplasty can be performed with a 6- or 7-mm balloon catheter. More fragments can be detached during this maneuver. *F,* Once satisfactory deployment of the stent has been obtained, the guide catheter is gently advanced into the stent. The blood and potential embolic fragments are then aspirated. Further cleaning of the site is obtained by hand or machine injection of saline to flush potential residual fragments into the ECA (as long as the preangioplasty angiogram did not demonstrate open anastomoses between the external carotid and vertebral systems). *G,* Repeat angiography is performed after deflation of the occlusion balloon.

sary steps of the procedure during a single occlusion of the carotid artery, with only one aspiration and flush of the working site. Results of direct stenting without cerebral protection have confirmed that stenting eliminates dissection, but the embolic risk remains between 5% and 10%.[13]

Role of Angioplasty Without Cerebral Protection

Angioplasty of carotid stenoses is performed without cerebral protection in the following cases:

1. Atherosclerotic stenosis of the common carotid artery origin.
2. Atherosclerotic stenosis of the internal carotid artery siphon.
3. Nonatherosclerotic stenosis. However, if there is a substantial risk of an associated atherosclerotic lesion, the use of cerebral protection is recommended. It is also recommended that the balloon be stabilized with a guide catheter in postendarterectomy stenosis or postradiotherapy stenosis to eliminate sliding of the balloon.

The availability of a ready-to-use cerebral protection system could encourage the use of this technique in all types of stenoses.

ROLE OF DIGITIZED PARENCHYMOGRAPHY IN PATIENT EVALUATION

As discussed, studies have shown that carotid endarterectomy is beneficial to symptomatic patients with a stenosis greater than 70%[2] or an asymptomatic stenosis greater than 60%.[3] This information has a statistical value but does not indicate, on an individual basis, what the actual effect of a carotid stenosis is on the intracranial circulation. It also does not take into account patients with multiple stenoses of the brachiocephalic vessels.

The approach to the evaluation of a patient with stenosis of a brachiocephalic vessel starts from the brain and not from the vessel supplying it. Digital parenchymography is employed,[14] which consists of the positioning of a 5-Fr. catheter in the ascending aorta and injection of contrast while anteroposterior images centered on the skull are acquired. Analysis of the images is performed with alteration of the digital angiography windows (low and narrow) to allow demonstration of the perfusion of the parenchyma (Case 5, Fig. 45–8). It is a physiologic technique, as the contrast is injected against the flow in the ascending aorta and then flows where it will. It can be routinely applied during any angiography of the great vessels. This technique yields information that may be summarized by a few concepts:

1. Patients presenting with a carotid stenosis and a normal parenchymogram have only a small risk of a cerebral ischemic event of hemodynamic origin if they are asymptomatic. If the patient presents with a transient ischemic accident, its mechanism is embolic and not hemodynamic.
2. A stenosis can have either insignificant or important hemodynamic cerebral repercussions on the side of the stenosis that are associated with (1) a delay in opacification of the intracranial internal carotid artery, (2) distal parenchymal hypovascularization (see Fig. 45–8), and (3) a prolongation of the cerebral transit time with unilateral stasis in the venous phase. This information is particularly important in the management of asymptomatic patients and encourages the pursuit of revascularization to prevent

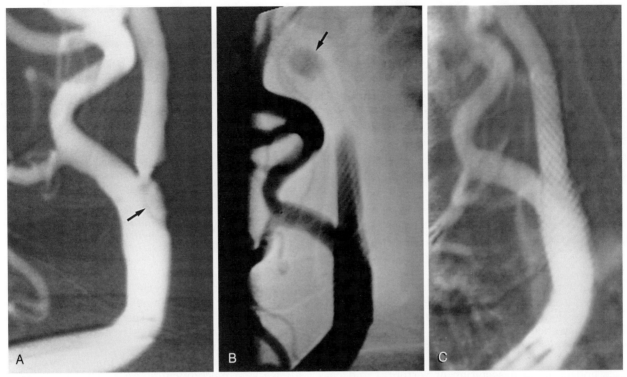

Figure 45-6 Case 3. Protected angioplasty and placement of a Wallstent. *A,* The preangioplasty image demonstrates a tight focal stenosis at the origin of the ICA with an apparent dissection within the carotid bifurcation *(arrow)*. *B,* Angioplasty and stent placement utilizing cerebral protection was then performed. Note the distal occlusion balloon *(arrow)*, with stasis of flow in the ICA. After aspiration and flushing, the occlusion balloon was deflated and withdrawn. *C,* Repeat angiography demonstrates an excellent result.

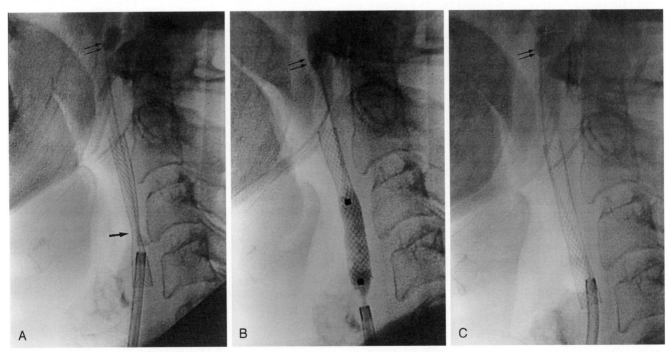

Figure 45-7 Case 4. Three steps of the protected Wallstent technique described in Figure 45-5. *A,* After initial placement, the stent is incompletely deployed because of the hardness of the plaque *(arrow)*. The occlusion balloon is seen at the top of the image *(double arrows)*. *B,* Complementary balloon angioplasty with protection *(double arrows)* is then performed, followed by aspiration and flushing of the angioplasty site *(C)*.

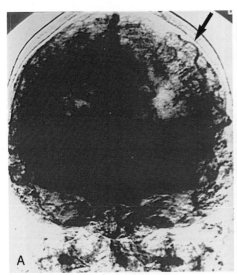
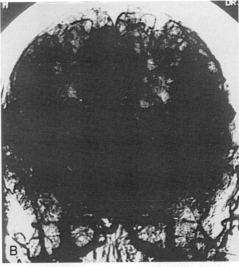

Figure 45-8 Case 5. Digitized parenchymography before and after endovascular treatment of an asymptomatic stenosis. Contrast was injected in the ascending aorta and anteroposterior images were obtained. Display windows (low and narrow windows) have been modified to enhance visualization of the parenchymal supply. *A,* On an intermediate-phase image of the preangioplasty injection, the hypovascularity of the left hemisphere parenchyma is seen *(arrow)*. *B,* Immediately after angioplasty, the same phase (same windows) demonstrates marked improvement of the vascularization on the left side.

hemodynamic complications. Restoration of normal parenchymal supply after the procedure can be demonstrated using the same technique.

3. The parenchymogram allows qualitative comparison with the unaffected side in unilateral stenosis. In patients with a bilateral carotid stenosis or an association of vertebral and carotid stenosis, the parenchymogram is useful only if coupled with an acetazolamide (Diamox) test showing whether a cerebral vascular reserve exists.[15] In "asymptomatic" patients with chronic cerebral ischemia (as demonstrated by a normal unstressed parenchymogram, but little or no reserve on acetazolamide testing), endovascular techniques for treatment of carotid and vertebral stenosis can significantly improve the efficiency of cerebral vascularization. This can be proved by the restoration of cerebral vascular reserve, as demonstrated by parenchymography and acetazolamide testing, and by neuropsychological testing.

CURRENT PERIPROCEDURAL MEDICATION PROTOCOL

The patient is prepared with aspirin, 100 mg twice a day, for 1 week before the procedure. On the day of the procedure, the patient is given 100 mg aspirin before the procedure, 500 mg ticlopidine on the angiography table after the femoral puncture, 1.5 mg/kg heparin at the beginning of the catheterization, 1 mg atropine before the inflation of the angioplasty balloon, and 100 mg aspirin and 250 mg ticlopidine after the procedure (at night). For the first month, the patient is given 100 mg aspirin and 250 mg ticlopidine twice a day. During the next 3 months, this is reduced to 100 mg aspirin twice a day.

COMPLICATIONS AND SOLUTIONS
Hemorrhagic Complications

Complications related to postprocedure bleeding represent a major problem when angioplasty is per-

formed via a direct carotid puncture. When a standard femoral approach is used, there are rarely complications as long as the introducer is removed in a timely fashion. Currently, the introducer is removed the same day by means of a Femstop II system (Radi Medical Systems, Uppsala, Sweden) that allows safe mechanical compression in a patient on heparin.

Restenosis

Before the use of stents, a 16% rate of restenosis after angioplasty was observed. This always occurred at the bifurcation when the immediate postangioplasty result was not satisfactory. These recurrent stenoses were dilated again with satisfactory results in about 60% of cases. Since the introduction of stents, the rate of restenosis appears to have dropped dramatically (to 6%) with the Strecker stent; experience with the Wallstents seems to be even more encouraging.

Editors' note: Over a period of years, Dr. Theron and his team have developed and utilized a technique that has yielded remarkable results. An attention to detail and a willingness to be fastidious and patient are rewarded with an excellently low complication rate.

In the 38 patients who underwent carotid angioplasty without cerebral protection, a dissection occurred in two patients (5%) and embolic complications were seen in three (8%). When cerebral protection was used during angioplasty alone in 136 patients, no embolic complications occurred at all (0%); however, during stent placement without cerebral protection, two embolic complications occurred (1.5%). Although the follow-up periods are variable and possibly inadequate, the restenosis rate after angioplasty without stenting was 16% and after stent placement was only 4%.

The quality of these results is what the rest of the world should aim for in the practice of this procedure.

REFERENCES

1. Imparato AM, Riles TS, Gorstein F. The carotid bifurcation plaque: pathologic findings associated with cerebral ischemia. *Stroke* 1979;10:238–245.

2. North American Symptomatic Carotid Endarterectomy Trial Collaborators. Beneficial effect of carotid endarterectomy in symptomatic patients with high-grade carotid stenosis. *N Engl J Med* 1991;10:445–453.
3. Executive Committee for the Asymptomatic Carotid Atherosclerosis Study. Endarterectomy for asymptomatic carotid artery stenosis. *JAMA* 1995;273:1421–1428.
4. Rothwell PM, Slattery J, Warlow FR. A systematic review of the risks of stroke and death due to endarterectomy for symptomatic carotid stenosis. *Stroke* 1996;27:260–265.
5. Theron J, Cosgrove R, Melanson D, et al. Embolization with temporary occlusion of the internal carotid or vertebral arteries. *Neuroradiology* 1986;28:246–253.
6. Theron J, Raymond J, Casasco A, Courtheoux P. Percutaneous angioplasty of atherosclerotic and post surgical stenosis of carotid arteries. *AJNR* 1987;8:495–500.
7. Theron J, Courtheoux, Alachkar F, Maiza D. New triple coaxial catheter system for carotid angioplasty with cerebral protection. *AJNR* 1990;11:869–874.
8. Theron JG, Paynelle GG, Coskun O, et al. Carotid artery

9. stenosis: treatment with protected balloon angioplasty and stent placement. *Radiology* 1996;201:627–636.
9. Kachel R. Results of balloon angioplasty in the carotid arteries. *J Endovasc Surg* 1996;3:22–30.
10. Theron J. Angioplasty of brachiocephalic vessels. In Vinuela F, Halbach VV, Dion JE (eds): Interventional Neuroradiology: Endovascular Therapy of the Central Nervous System. New York: Raven Press, 1992, pp 167–180.
11. Strecker EP, Hagen B, Lierman D, et al. Current status of the Strecker stent. *Cardiol Clin* 1994;12:673–687.
12. Theron J, Coskun O, Huet H, et al. Local intraarterial thrombolysis in the carotid territory. *Intervent Neuroradiol* 1996;2:111–126.
13. Yadav J, Roubin G, Iyer S, et al. Elective stenting of extracranial carotid arteries. *Circulation* 1997;95:376–381.
14. Theron J, Nelson M, Alachkar F, et al. Dynamic digitized cerebral parenchymography. *Neuroradiology* 1992;34:361–366.
15. Rogg J, Rutigliano M, Yonas H, et al. The acetazolamide challenge: imaging technique designed to evaluate cerebral blood flow reserve. *AJNR* 1989;10:803–810.

CHAPTER 46

Current Status and Future Possibilities of Balloon Angioplasty in the Carotid Artery

R. Kachel

BALLOON ANGIOPLASTY AS A CONTROLLED INJURY

Although Mullan et al performed the first percutaneous transluminal angioplasty (PTA) of a carotid artery as early as 1980,[1] PTA has established itself only in more recent years as a common tool in the treatment of obliterations of the carotid artery.[2–6] One of the reasons was the fear of cerebral embolization resulting in severe neurologic complications (stroke). It is assumed that PTA is a "controlled trauma" of the vascular wall. The rupturing of calcified arteriosclerotic plaques during angioplasty represents the main mechanism of PTA. This mechanism, which is primarily observed in heavily calcified, stenosing arterial disorders, is now generally accepted and is primarily seen in postangioplasty examination of coronary and pelvifemoral arteries.

However, approximately one in four stenosing, arteriosclerotic plaques located in the supra-aortic arteries does not contain major calcifications. As some scholars have correctly assumed, these so-called "soft plaques" are spread along the subintima, compressed and pressed through the adjacent wall segments by the pressure of the inflated balloon segment. This is most frequently seen in short, circular, well-defined, and nonulcerating arteriosclerotic stenoses. It is believed that both theoretically possible mechanisms

play a part in the carotid artery (Fig. 46–1; Case 1, Fig. 46–2; Case 2, Fig. 46–3). Severely calcified stenoses affecting long segments of cerebral arteries should not be dilated unless brain protection and carotid stenting are employed; the act of rupturing the plaque will almost certainly produce debris that will then embolize distally.

INDICATIONS FOR CAROTID ANGIOPLASTY WITHOUT STENTING (CONVENTIONAL)

The indications for PTA are the same as for endarterectomy. To ensure an optimal therapeutic result, each case should be discussed by a team of neurologists, angiologists, vascular surgeons, and interventional neuroradiologists. An accurate case history and clinical and neurologic examinations are indispensable; they help distinguish reliably between patients with and without neurologic symptoms. PTA without stenting or brain protection is indicated only in symptomatic patients, that is, in patients showing neurologic symptoms that are most likely caused by stenosing arterial degeneration, provided that the following morphologic criteria are met:

- Circular, short (<1 cm) stenosis
- Well-defined wall, ulceration not demonstrable
- No circular or rough calcifications of the wall
- No thrombus depositions

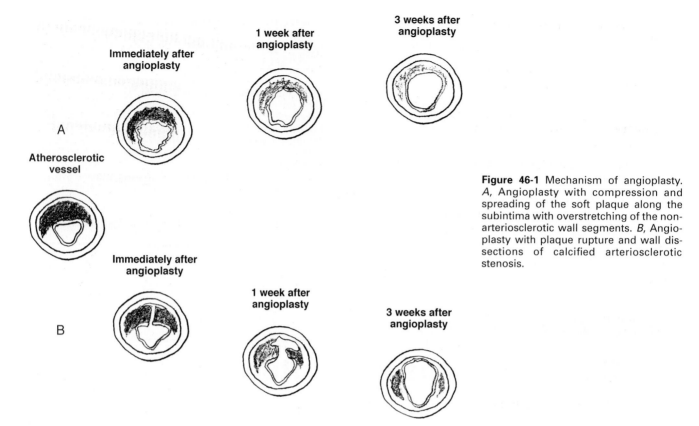

Figure 46-1 Mechanism of angioplasty. *A*, Angioplasty with compression and spreading of the soft plaque along the subintima with overstretching of the non-arteriosclerotic wall segments. *B*, Angioplasty with plaque rupture and wall dissections of calcified arteriosclerotic stenosis.

- No strictures caused by external compression (e.g., tumor, cicatrization)
- No vascular elongation with kinking

The view that only symptomatic and hemodynamically significant stenoses of cerebral vessels should be dilated or corrected surgically has been corroborated by randomized, prospective multicenter studies.[7, 8] I believe that the extension of PTA to stenoses in neurologically asymptomatic patients is not indicated at the present time, because the results of the frequently quoted Asymptomatic Carotid Atherosclerosis Study (ACAS)[9] demonstrated a benefit only for male patients with hemodynamically significant carotid artery stenoses when endarterectomy was compared with medicinal therapy. This study did not show that female patients would benefit from endarterectomy when the postoperative course was compared with the spontaneous progress of the condition.

Whether brain protective measures, including carotid stenting, will result in an improvement of the outcome of PTA will be shown by the findings of the above-mentioned multicenter studies. As far as stenting is concerned, its use may be limited because of the substantial risk of restenosis of the stented vessel. This is discussed further below.

A total of 223 patients (124 men, 99 women) aged 33 to 79 years, average age 54 years, with a total of 252 occlusive lesions in the supra-aortic arteries were candidates for balloon angioplasty. Among these were 76 stenoses in the carotid arteries: proximal common (n = 6), distal common (n = 1), internal (n = 66),

and external (n = 3). All patients but one had symptoms (grades II to IV) of cerebrovascular and/or vertebrobasilar insufficiency:

Grade I. No neurologic symptoms
Grade II. Transient neurologic symptoms
Grade III. Progressive neurologic deficits
Grade IV. Permanent neurologic deficits

The only patient without neurologic symptoms (grade I) had bilateral internal carotid artery (ICA) occlusions and a high-grade stenosis of the right external carotid artery (ECA), which perfused the ipsilateral brain hemisphere.

Combined Surgical and Radiologic Treatment of Brachiocephalic Vascular Obliterations

In multiple brachiocephalic vascular obliterations, PTA can be combined favorably with vascular surgical corrections, with the two techniques applied simultaneously or consecutively. The increased surgical risk for patients with multiple obliterations can be considerably reduced by PTA, provided that the stenosed segments of the carotid, subclavian, or vertebral arteries are dilated before vascular surgical corrections.

Indications for Combined Treatment

Postvascular Surgical Correction

- PTA of a hemodynamically significant stenosis at the origin of the common carotid artery (CCA) or

the brachiocephalic trunk after transposition of the subclavian artery into the CCA or creating a carotidosubclavian bypass (Case 3, Figs. 46–4 and 46–5)
- PTA of a postoperative stenosis after bypass surgery (e.g., carotidosubclavian bypass)
- PTA of a hemodynamically significant subclavian stenosis after creation of an internal mammary coronary artery bypass (presenting with recurrent anginal pain)

Simultaneous Application of PTA and Vascular Surgical Correction

- PTA of a stenosis at the origin of the CCA or the brachiocephalic trunk during endarterectomy of a high-grade ipsilateral ICA stenosis that is impervious to a catheter (lumen narrowed to less than 1 mm, and Z-shaped residual lumen)

Prevascular Surgical Correction

- PTA of a subclavian stenosis before surgical correction of a kinking stenosis of the vertebral artery
- PTA of a stenosis at the origin of the CCA or brachiocephalic trunk before implantation of the ipsilateral subclavian or vertebral artery into the CCA (Case 4, Figs. 46–6 and 46–7)
- PTA of a subclavian artery stenosis before creation of a subclavian-carotid bypass to treat the occlusion of the ipsilateral CCA
- PTA of an ECA stenosis before proposed extra-intracranial bypass surgery (Case 5, Figs. 46–8 and 46–9)

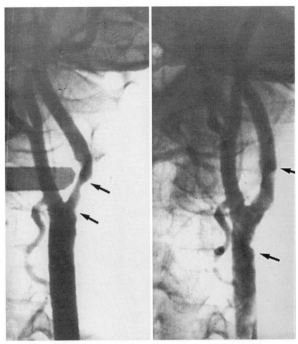

Figure 46-3 Case 2. High-grade ICA stenosis before and immediately after PTA with plaque compression and longitudinal spread along the subintima (*arrows* indicate plaque borders).

PRETHERAPEUTIC DIAGNOSTIC METHODS

The following pretherapeutic diagnostic techniques need to be applied:

- Clinical and neurologic examination
- Duplex or Doppler sonography (ultrasonic tomography)
- Cerebral computed tomography (CT) or magnetic resonance imaging (MRI)
- Hexamethylpropyleneamine-oxime (HMPAO)–single photon emission computed tomography (SPECT) of the brain
- [111]In (indium-111) platelet scintigraphy of the stenosed vascular segment
- Intra-arterial digital subtraction angiography (DSA) in at least two projections

Duplex or Doppler sonography is a noninvasive method that facilitates localization of the carotid stenosis and assessment of its severity. The condition of the vascular wall (e.g., calcification, ulceration, thrombus depositions) is assessed by means of ultrasonic tomography. Thin-layer CT may be indicated in individual cases to study the wall structure more closely in regard to calcifications. Whether CT angiography will become a major diagnostic tool remains to be seen, whereas three-dimensional sonography is already a powerful tool for assessing both the severity of the stenosis and the wall structure.

The purpose of cerebral CT and MRI is to reveal any morphologic parenchymal injuries before treatment is instituted. The purpose of HMPAO-SPECT is to facilitate assessment of the hemodynamic effect of the stenosis in the brain and the compensatory

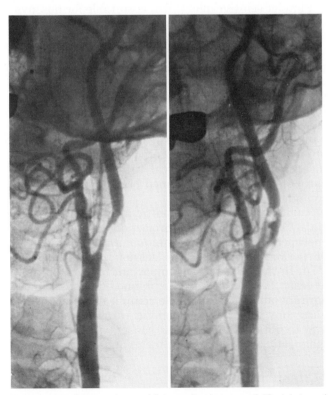

Figure 46-2 Case 1. Long, high-grade, heavy calcified internal carotid artery (ICA) stenosis before and immediately after percutaneous transluminal angioplasty (PTA) with plaque rupture and wall dissection.

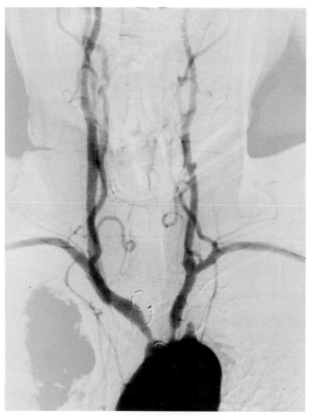

Figure 46-4 Case 3. Patient with stenosis at the origin of the left common carotid artery (CCA) after transposition of the subclavian artery into the CCA.

Case 3 continues

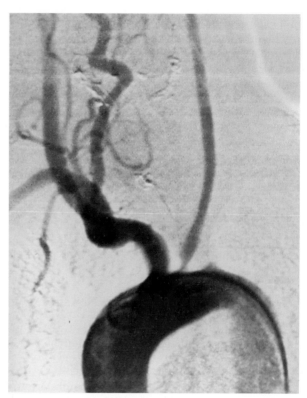

Figure 46-6 Case 4. Patient with severe stenosis at the origin of the left CCA, occlusion of the left subclavian artery, and subclavian steal syndrome.

Case 4 continues

effect of the cerebral arterial circulation. It is believed that angioplasty is especially indicated in cases of insufficient blood supply due to insufficient collateral cerebral arterial circulation.

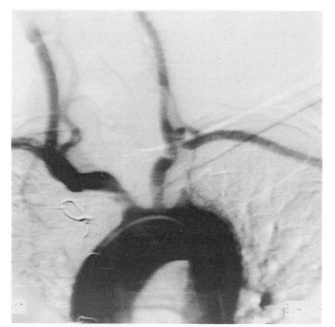

Figure 46-5 Same patient after successful angioplasty at the origin of the left CCA.

Platelet scintigraphy (^{111}In) is suitable for noninvasive detection of thrombus depositions in stenosed arterial walls. As sonographic diagnostic tools for visualizing thrombus depositions advanced, the importance of ^{111}In platelet scintigraphy as a basis of therapeutic decisions (PTA vs. endarterectomy) declined. However, this technique seems to be suitable for diagnosing thrombus depositions and early occlusions after stent applications even before clinical and neurologic symptoms appear. If thrombus deposition or early occlusion in the stented area is identified by means of a scintiscan, local intra-arterial therapy can be successfully performed before any neurologic complications occur.

Angiographic examination by means of intra-arterial DSA in at least two projections is the last pretherapeutic diagnostic technique, and thus it should be performed in the same session as the intended PTA. In this context, it is important to warn patients at least 24 hours before the planned diagnostic angiography about both possible complications of the angiography and the forthcoming carotid angioplasty, and to obtain their written consent to the invasive diagnostic and therapeutic techniques.

PATIENT PREPARATION

Patients must first be informed about their illness, the currently available therapeutic procedures, the results of treatment, and possible complications. They must fast on the day of the operation. Before

PTA is begun, the clotting parameters and blood group must be determined, conserved blood made ready, and venous access ensured for the infusion of electrolyte solution. Sedatives are given only to very anxious patients. Atropine (intravenous) premedication is not foregone, even though—unlike other authors—I have not observed clinically significant bradycardia or asystole in any of my patients during or after PTA in the area of the carotid bulb. Patients undergoing carotid angioplasty are monitored by electroencephalography and electrocardiography.

MATERIALS

The following materials are required for PTA of stenosis of the carotid artery:

- Seldinger initial puncture needle
- Teflon-coated straight guidewire, 0.024″ to 0.035″
- 6-Fr. introducer sheath set (Teflon sheath, vessel dilator, Tuohy-Borst adapter) (7- to 8-Fr. when brain protection is utilized)
- Diagnostic catheter (5-Fr.) (Simmons, Headhunter, Judkins right coronary, multipurpose, cerebral catheter with a tapered tip, Berenstein)
- Terumo guidewire (Medi-Tech), 0.035″
- Long Teflon-coated guidewire (length 250 cm)
- Balloon dilation catheter (2.5-Fr. percutaneous transluminal coronary angioplasty catheter and 5-Fr. dilation catheter; working length, 120 cm; catheter tip, 5 mm; balloon length, 15 to 20 mm; balloon

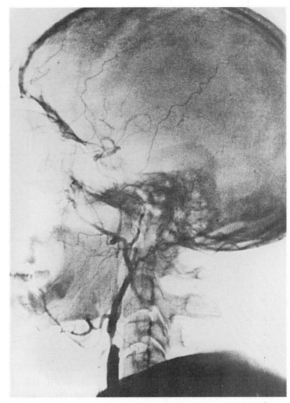

Figure 46-8 Case 5. Patient with occlusion of the ICA and a severe stenosis at the origin of the external carotid artery (ECA); the patient previously underwent extra-intracranial bypass surgery.

Case 5 continues

diameter, 4 to 17 mm; pressure capacity, >8 atmospheres) (see below for further discussion)
- Inflation syringe with pressure manometer
- 10- and 20-cc injection syringes
- Intravascular ultrasound (IVUS) catheter for intravascular sonography

Balloon Catheter Selection

The quality of catheters is of great importance. To ensure minimal traumatization of the arterial wall, the external diameter of diagnostic and dilation catheters should be as small as possible (4- to 5-Fr.). The dilation balloon must withstand high pressure (>8 atmospheres). Furthermore, it must not change its cylindrical form if it is exposed to high dilation pressure, in order to avoid overdilation. The length and diameter of the balloon and the length of the tip are other important factors to be taken into consideration when selecting a dilation catheter. The tip should not exceed 5 mm and should be of conical shape, so that it can pass even high-grade stenoses without giving rise to great tangential shearing forces. A balloon length of 15 mm to not more than 20 mm should be selected for short circular stenoses to avoid unnecessary traumatization of the adjacent healthy arterial wall segments.

The most important aspect is the selection of the diameter of the balloon used for PTA. It must not be greater than the lumen of the normal vessel (this

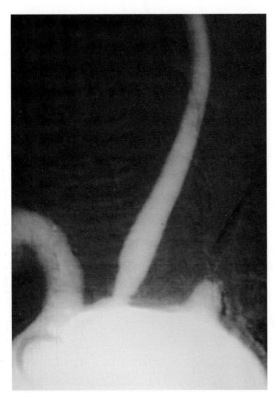

Figure 46-7 Same patient after successful angioplasty of the left CCA at the origin, performed before implantation of the subclavian artery into the CCA.

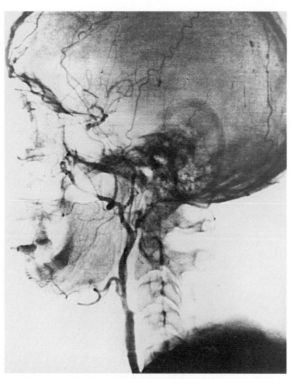

Figure 46-9 Same patient after successful dilation of the severe ECA stenosis. Note the filling of middle cerebral artery branches.

giography is then performed in at least two projections simultaneously (right and left anterior oblique) with a 5-Fr. diagnostic catheter, using DSA technique if feasible, to confirm the suspected diagnosis, precisely locate the stenosis, and rule out recent events such as ulceration, thrombus deposition, and occlusion. Selective angiography of the stenosed vascular region is then performed in at least two projections.

In general, the so-called "guidewire" method is preferred in patients with short, circular, nonulcerated carotid stenosis without heavy calcifications. Heparin, 100 units/kg of body weight, is given intra-arterially. Under fluoroscopic control, a long (200- to 250-cm), straight guidewire is introduced and passed into the distal carotid artery beyond the stenosis. The diagnostic catheter is replaced by a Grüntzig balloon catheter over the guidewire. The diameter of the balloon is usually 4 to 6 mm, depending on the width of the vessel. It is advisable to use a diameter that corresponds to that of the healthy vessel as measured in a distal, undiseased segment of the artery.

After the balloon has been positioned across the stenosis, it is inflated manually by means of a 10-cc injection syringe and a pressure manometer, using a

applies also to the carotid bulb). If this very important criterion is met, no (or only minimal) wall damage and dissection will result.

Assessment of the severity of the stenosis and selection of the diameter of the dilatation balloon are based on North American Symptomatic Carotid Endarterectomy Trial (NASCET) criteria.[7] According to this study, the diameter of the distal healthy segment of the ICA is regarded as the normal vascular lumen (Fig. 46–10).

It is advisable to select a slightly smaller balloon diameter in order to minimize traumatic vascular lesions. In high-grade (greater than 90%) stenoses of the ICA, successive dilation is sometimes necessary. In the first step, a 2.5-Fr. catheter is used for dilation up to 3 mm, and then a 5-Fr. balloon catheter is used to achieve a lumen of 6 mm. It has been found that successive dilation in two sessions performed at an interval of 6 to 8 weeks yields more favorable long-term results than successive dilation to the normal vascular lumen in one session.

The risk of embolic or thromboembolic neurologic complications during PTA increases substantially in high-grade, severely calcified, or substantially ulcerated so-called "toxic" stenoses. For this reason, the performance of PTA without brain protection or carotid stenting is inadvisable. This is discussed further below.

METHOD

Under local anesthesia, an inguinal catheter introducer sheath is inserted. General brachiocephalic an-

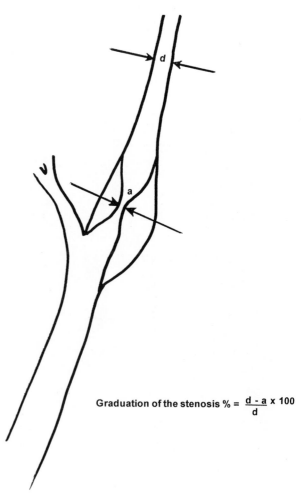

$$\text{Graduation of the stenosis } \% = \frac{d - a}{d} \times 100$$

Figure 46-10 NASCET style measurement of stenosis. The diameter of the distal ICA is indicated by d and the diameter of the stenosis by a.

1:1 contrast medium-to-water mixture. Pressures of more than 800 kPa (>8 atmospheres) are used, depending on the type of balloon catheter. In general, one or two dilations, each lasting 10 to 20 seconds, are required to expand the stenosis. After successful angioplasty, the dilation balloon is deflated with a 20-cc syringe, the catheter is placed in the proximal part of the CCA, and the angioplasty result is documented by angiography in two or more views.

Sometimes, passage with a 5-Fr. dilation catheter is not possible in patients with high-grade carotid stenoses. In these patients, successive dilations are necessary, first using a 2.5-Fr. coronary dilation catheter with a 3- to 4-mm balloon diameter and then a 5-Fr. catheter with a balloon diameter of 5 to 6 mm.

The use of IVUS scanning is also recommended to assess the postdilation structure of the vessel wall for signs of suboptimal angioplasty (e.g., residual stenosis, intimal flaps, plaque fractures, dissections, intramural hematomas) (Case 6, Figs. 46–11 to 46–13). If dissections or flaps are detected, a stent should be applied as a secondary measure to avoid embolic or thrombotic complications.

Angiography and IVUS imaging having been completed, the dilation catheter is removed, but the Teflon sheath with the Tuohy-Borst adaptor is left in place for another 24 hours to facilitate selective angiography and local thrombolysis or redilation in the event of early occlusion or embolization.

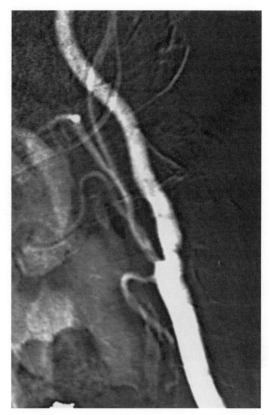

Figure 46-12 Same patient after successful angioplasty.

Case 6 continues

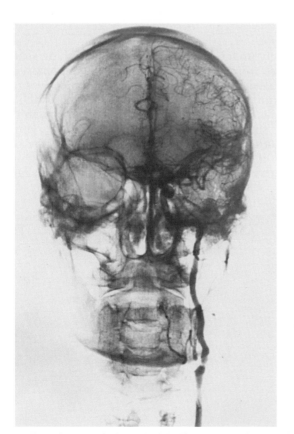

Figure 46-11 Case 6. High-grade left ICA stenosis in a patient with occlusion of the right ICA.

Case 6 continues

On the basis of experience with angioplasty of the subclavian artery, it is believed that good results can be achieved even without carotid stenting, if dilation periods can be increased from 30 to 60 seconds. After the dilation period in high-grade stenoses of the subclavian artery had been increased from 60 to 120 seconds, posttherapeutic angiograms showed relatively smooth walls even in heavily calcified stenoses. This indicates that plaque material is permanently flattened against the artery wall (Case 7, Figs. 46–14 and 46–15).

POSTPROCEDURE MANAGEMENT

Indium-111 platelet scintigraphy is useful to detect thrombus depositions or an early thrombotic occlusion of the stent before neurologic symptoms are diagnosed. In these cases, intra-arterial local thrombolysis is essential to treat the thrombotic stent occlusion.

Posttreatment medication generally includes platelet inhibitors (aspirin). Recommendations are for heparinization for 2 to 3 days with 20,000 to 25,000 units of heparin per 24 hours, overlapping with oral anticoagulants (phenprocoumon [Marcumar] or warfarin [Coumadin]) after the second day. The anticoagulant therapy should be continued for at least 6 months with appropriate monitoring. Aspirin is prescribed if the transaxillary approach was used or if oral anticoagulants are contraindicated, and is now recommended in all patients.

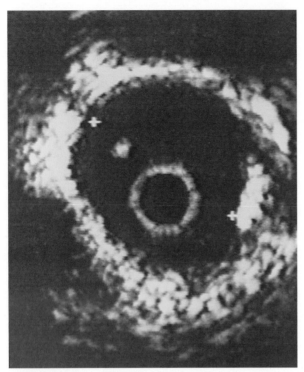

Figure 46-13 Intravascular ultrasound image of the patient in Figure 46-11 immediately after successful angioplasty, without plaque rupture or wall dissection.

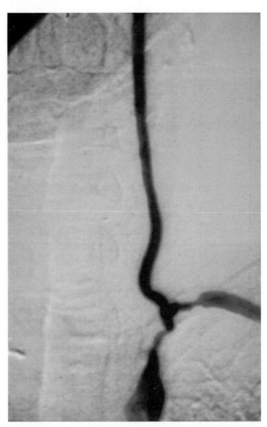

Figure 46-14 Case 7. Long-segment stenosis of the left subclavian artery at the vertebral artery origin.

Case 7 continues

The results of PTA should be followed at intervals of 6 to 12 months by physical examination and duplex or Doppler ultrasound studies. If symptoms recur or if the noninvasive assessment provides objective signs of restenosis, the patient should be informed that a repeat PTA may be necessary during angiography. Repeat angioplasty can then be performed in the same session if hemodynamically significant restenosis is seen.

RESULTS

Angioplasty was successful in 242 of the 252 stenoses of brachiocephalic arteries seen in 223 patients. In these patients, 71 of 76 stenoses of the carotid arteries were successfully dilated: proximal common (n = 5), distal common (n = 1), internal (n = 62), and external (n = 3) carotid arteries. In five high-grade internal stenoses, passage of a 2.5-Fr. PTA catheter was not possible.

Contrary to expectations, the complication rate of PTA is relatively low: 3% to 6% according to the literature.[10, 11] Two deaths have been reported so far.

In the 252 attempted angioplasties in brachiocephalic arteries, there was only one major complication: a hemiparesis after angioplasty of a severely calcified, long, high-grade ICA stenosis (see Fig. 46–2). Mortality was zero.

Minor complications were observed in four patients. There was after bleeding of the puncture site with extensive hematoma formation in two patients (one axillary and one inguinal), which healed com-

pletely under conservative therapy with no sequelae. There were two episodes of transient impaired consciousness during ICA angioplasty, each lasting approximately 5 seconds, during blockage of the blood supply to the brain secondary to balloon inflation. One small thrombus without neurologic symptoms was diagnosed by ^{111}In platelet scintigraphy on the wall of an ICA proximal to the site of a high-grade internal stenosis that resisted the passage of

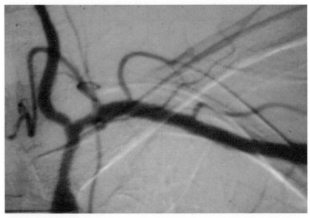

Figure 46-15 Same patient after angioplasty with a 120-second dilation period. Note the smooth wall without dissections or plaque rupture.

T A B L E   4 6 - 1   International Balloon Angioplasty Results in Supra-aortic Arteries

Artery	Procedures		Mortality	Morbidity	Minor Complications
	Attempted	*Successful*			
Carotid	719	693 (96.4%)	1 (0.1%)	1.8%	5.2%
	338*	327 (96.7%)*	1 (0.3%)*	1.4%*	7.5%*
Vertebral	268	255 (95.1%)	0	0.7%	3.3%
Innominate	44	43 (97.7%)	0	0	0
Subclavian	1136	1064 (93.7%)	0	0.4%	3.6%
Totals	2167	2055 (94.8%)	1 (0.05%)	0.9%	4.0%
	2505*	2382 (95.8%)*	2 (0.08%)*	1.0%*	4.6%*

*Angioplasty and carotid stenting.

the dilation catheter. The subsequent carotid endarterectomy was performed successfully without neurologic symptoms.

Table 46–1 combines my results in supra-aortic angioplasty with those reported in the literature. In carotid angioplasty, mortality was zero, morbidity 2.1%, and the minor (transient) complication rate approximately 6%. All transient physical disorders (neurologic and other) without permanent physical disability were regarded as minor complications, whereas all neurologic and other complications resulting in permanent disability were considered to be major complications.

These results correlate well with the endarterectomy results, for which a mortality rate varying between 0.6% and 3.8% and a morbidity rate between 1.0% and 14.5% is reported. If the endarterectomy results of the NASCET and European Carotid Surgery Trial (ECST) studies (which report a combined morbidity and mortality rate of 5.5% and 7.5% after carotid endarterectomy) are used as a basis, the results of PTA compare favorably with surgery.[7, 8] The prospective, randomized Carotid and Vertebral Artery Transluminal Angioplasty (multicenter) Study (CAVATAS) initiated by Brown et al was based on the available results of PTA.[9] So far, the results of endarterectomy and PTA have been compared in more than 600 patients with carotid or vertebral artery stenoses without being able to demonstrate significant advantages or disadvantages of one therapeutic method over the other.

Tables 46–1 and 46–2 also summarize the results of primary and secondary carotid stenting in over 200 patients.[12–14] These indicate that, in the absence of brain protection, secondary stenting is accompanied by an increase in mainly temporary neurologic complications (e.g., minor stroke, transient pareses, transient ischemic attacks). Major complications were largely prevented by primary carotid stenting and could be reduced to 1.8% after secondary carotid stenting as well. This is most likely due to the incomplete, less traumatic dilation by so-called "conventional" angioplasty that preceded the stent application. Complete dilation to the normal lumen was achieved by application of a self-expanding secondary stent that was additionally dilated. This additional dilation is necessary because in severely calcified stenoses the radial forces of the self-expanding stent are insufficient for deployment (Case 8, Figs. 46–16 to 46–18). Self-expanding stents are required because catheter-expanded stents (Palmaz) may be deformed or even occluded by the application of external pressure in the cervical region, resulting in severe neurologic complications.

T A B L E   4 6 - 2   Complications of Carotid Stenting

Author	Procedures		Stent Application	Mortality	Morbidity	Minor Complication
	Attempted	*Successful*				
Mathias[12]	42	42 (100.0%)	Primary stenting: 42 Wallstent	0	0	4.8%
Diethrich et al[13]	117	109 (93.2%)	Secondary stenting: 128 Palmaz-Stent, 1 Wallstent	0	1.8%	11.7% (2.7% CE)
Iyer et al[14]	110	107 (97.3%)	Secondary stenting: 121 Palmaz-Stent, 26 Gianturco-Roubin, 10 Wallstent	1 (0.9%)	2.7%	8.2%
Theron et al[9]	93	69	Secondary stenting: 60 Strecker stents	0	0	2.9%
Totals	362	327 (95.1%)	397 Stents	1 (0.3%)	1.4%	7.5%

CE, carotid endarterectomy.

CEREBRAL PROTECTION

Thromboembolic complications may be prevented by primary stenting (i.e., application of carotid stents without predilation with a Grüntzig balloon catheter). The difficulty in primary stenting is that the dilation catheters currently available for stent application have a minimal size of 2.5-Fr. As a consequence, passage in high-grade ICA stenoses with a diameter of 1 mm or less is not possible without giving rise to great tangential shearing forces entailing the risk of cerebral embolization and vessel wall damage.

Cerebral embolization of plaque material can be prevented by the use of a guide catheter with a proximal occlusion balloon (proximal balloon occlusion) in combination with primary stenting. In light of the continuous upgrading of dilation materials, the routine combined use of vascular occlusion for cerebral protection and primary stenting seems likely in the future.

Cerebral protection with proximal vascular occlusion may facilitate secondary stenting also. After so-called "conventional" angioplasty, this technique provides for substitution of a carotid stent system for the Grüntzig dilation catheter over a guidewire. During the substitution and the secondary stenting, cerebral blood supply via the carotid artery can be

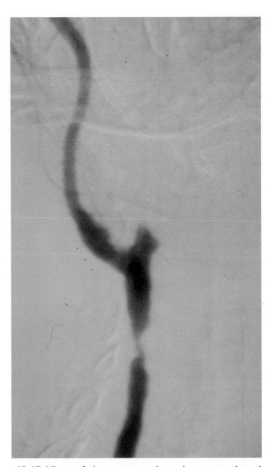

Figure 46-17 View of the same patient demonstrating the CCA stenosis and occlusion of the ECA.

Case 8 continues

blocked to avoid embolization of plaque material into the brain. After successful stent application and removal of the delivery catheter, aspiration of blood from the dilated carotid artery allows detached plaque fragments to be removed with the blood. Future studies will show whether an extended balloon blockage of 1 to 2 minutes' duration has a negative impact on the angioplasty complication rate. In light of experience with carotid artery clamping during implantation of the shunt in carotid endarterectomy, this blockage should not result in an appreciable increase in complications, particularly since the clamping periods during carotid endarterectomy are longer than the occlusion period during catheter therapy.

For treatment of ICA lesions, a new coaxial balloon angioplasty system that affords cerebral protection against microemboli is recommended. The system consists of an 8-Fr. guide catheter with an occlusion balloon on the tip and a 3-Fr. dilation catheter. In patients with stenoses of the middle or distal CCA or ICA, the guide catheter with its occlusion balloon deflated is introduced into the CCA and placed with the balloon segment in the proximal or distal CCA. The dilation catheter is then passed under fluoroscopic control into the stenosed segment, where it is inflated by hand, using the inflation device and dilute

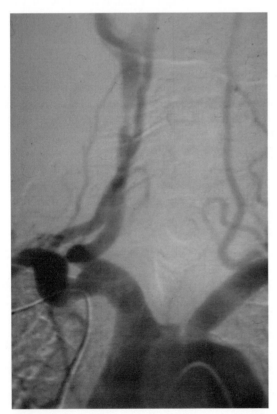

Figure 46-16 Case 8. Arch aortogram after an unsuccessful attempt at vascular surgical treatment of a patient with occlusion at the origin of the left CCA, occlusion of the right ECA, and a long high-grade stenosis of the CCA caused by radiation for hypopharynx carcinoma 25 years previously.

Case 8 continues

contrast medium for about 10 to 20 seconds at 8 to 12 atmospheres of pressure (Fig. 46–19A). In patients with dangerous collaterals (vertebral artery–ECA collaterals) and retrograde blood flow via the ECA during occlusion of the CCA, the orifice of the ECA has to be occluded. In patients with stenoses of the middle or distal ICA, this is accomplished by positioning the occlusion balloon segment of the guide catheter at the level of the origin of the ECA, so that inflation of the balloon results in occlusion of the distal CCA and ECA (Fig. 46–19B). In patients with dangerous anastomoses and more proximal stenoses, the ECA origin is occluded separately with a small (5- to 8-mm) occlusion balloon on a wire, which is positioned before the guide catheter is introduced into the CCA. The guide catheter is positioned with its balloon just proximal to the origin of the ECA (Fig. 46–19C). Before the dilation balloon is deflated, the occlusion balloons on the guide catheter and in the ECA have to be inflated in order to stop the antegrade blood flow to the brain. The dilation balloon is deflated and the dilation catheter removed. Blood is aspirated from the ICA to remove detached plaque material. When aspiration is completed, the occlusion balloons are deflated. After successful dilation, the result must be documented by angiography.

TO STENT OR NOT TO STENT

The currently available stenting materials, which are not compressible by the application of external force

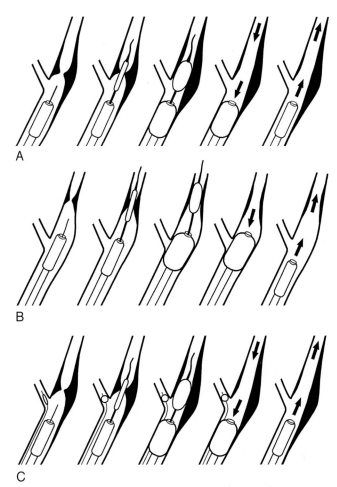

Figure 46-19 Angioplasty with brain protection by a coaxial dilation catheter system. Arrows indicate the direction of blood flow in the internal carotid artery. *A,* Single balloon occlusion of the CCA for patients without dangerous collaterals via the ECA. *B,* Single balloon occlusion of the common and external carotid arteries for patients with dangerous collaterals (for middle and distal ICA lesions). *C,* Proximal ICA angioplasty with brain protection by proximal balloon occlusion of the common and external carotid arteries (separate balloons) for patients with more proximal ICA stenoses and dangerous collaterals via the ECA.

(self-expanding stents), give rise to a relatively high stent restenosing rate in renal, coronary, and peripheral femoral arteries. In light of the restenosis rate after stenting of the renal artery, a restenosis rate of 20% to 40% after carotid stenting cannot be ruled out. This assumption appears realistic, since the hemodynamic conditions and the vascular diameter of the renal artery and ICA are comparable.

The implantation of non–self-expanding Palmaz stents may give rise to stent deformation if external pressure is applied. Such deformations after coronary artery stenting are normally seen only as a result of severe trauma.

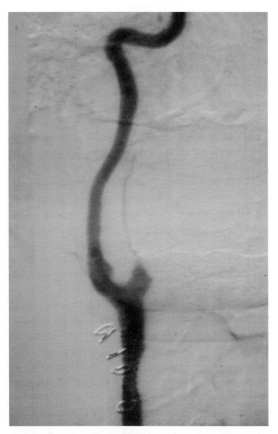

Figure 46-18 Same patient after secondary carotid stenting with a self-expanding Wallstent with a small residual stenosis.

REFERENCES

1. Mullan S, Duda EE, Patronas NJ. Some examples of balloon technology in neurosurgery. *J Neurosurg* 1980;52:321–329.
2. Vitek JJ, Keller FS. Angioplasty in neuroradiology. In Valk J

(ed): Neuroradiology. Amsterdam: Elsevier, 1986, pp 1008–1016.

3. Mathias K. Percutaneous transluminal angioplasty of the supraaortic arteries. In Dondelinger PF, Rossi P, Kurdziel S. (eds): Interventional Radiology. New York: Georg-Thieme-Verlag, 1990, pp 564–583.

4. Theron JG, Courtheoux P, Alachkar F, et al. Techniques endovasculaires de revascularisation cerebrale. *J Mal Vasc* 1990;15:245–256.

5. Munari LM, Belloni G, Perretti A. Carotid percutaneous angioplasty. *Neurol Res* 1992;14:260–269.

6. Higashida RT, Tsai FY, Halbach W, et al. Cerebral percutaneous transluminal angioplasty. *J Heart Dis Stroke* 1993;2:497–502.

7. North American Symptomatic Carotid Endarterectomy Trial Collaborators. Beneficial effect of carotid endarterectomy in symptomatic patients with high-grade-carotid-stenosis. *N Engl J Med* 1991;15:445–453.

8. European Carotid Surgery Trial Collaborative Group. MRC European Carotid Surgery Trial: interim results for symptomatic patients with severe (70–99%) or mild (0–29%) carotid stenosis. *Lancet* 1991;337:1235–1243.

9. Theron J, Payelle G, Coskun O, et al. Carotid artery stenosis: treatment with protected balloon angioplasty and stent placement. *Radiology* 1996;201:627–636.

10. Brown NM, Butler P, Gibbs J. Feasibility of percutaneous transluminal angioplasty for carotid artery stenosis. *J Neurol Neurosurg Psychiatry* 1990;53:238–243.

11. Kachel R. Results of balloon angioplasty in the carotid arteries. *J Endovasc Surg* 1996;3:22–30.

12. Mathias K. Einsatz von Stents in der Therapie von Erkrankungen der supraaortalen Gefässe. In Kollath J, Liermann D (eds): Stents III. Entwicklung, Indikation und Zukunft. Konstanz: Schnetzler-Verlag GmbH, 1995, pp 125–133.

13. Diethrich EB, Ndiaye M, Reid DB. Stenting in the carotid artery: initial experience in 110 patients. *J Endovasc Surg* 1996;3:42–62.

14. Iyer SS, Roubin GS, Yadav S, et al. Elective carotid stenting (abstr). *J Endovasc Surg* 1996;3:105–106.

15. Asymptomatic Carotid Atherosclerosis Study Executive Committee. Endarterectomy for asymptomatic carotid artery stenosis. *JAMA* 1995;273:1421–1428.

CHAPTER 47

Other Extracranial Locations Amenable to Angioplasty and Stenting

J.J. Connors III

The technical details of brachiocephalic angioplasty and stenting are presented in Chapter 42. This chapter presents the approach to specific locations other than the carotid bifurcation.

ORIGIN OF THE LEFT COMMON CAROTID ARTERY FROM THE AORTA

Stenosis at the origin of the left common carotid artery is difficult to reach surgically but usually is easy to reach endovascularly. These stenoses typically occur just at the origin, although they may not be completely ostial. Ulceration is not as prevalent in this location as at the internal carotid artery (ICA) bifurcation. These stenoses can manifest by simple flow restriction before any other signs are apparent. In addition to atherosclerosis, Takayasu's arteritis is a common cause for stenoses at the origin of this vessel.[1]

Treatment of these lesions is straightforward, although the lack of flow control may render these not as easy to treat safely as ICA origin stenoses (Case 1, Figs. 47–1 to 47–6). A retrograde approach from the cervical common carotid artery for an angioplasty has been reported (1) using flow control from this direction. These lesions, however, usually do not appear to be as friable as bifurcation lesions, and the need for flow control is probably infrequent.

From a practical standpoint, there are only two difficulties with this procedure, similar to those for the innominate artery: (1) the stenosis may be difficult and hazardous to cross, and (2) a large balloon may be necessary. Almost uniformly, however, the left common carotid artery is not larger than 9 mm, whereas the innominate artery can be up to 15 to 18 mm in size.

The usual cause for presentation is unexplained carotid artery symptoms (transient ischemic attacks [TIAs]). Often, the patient has already had an endarterectomy, but the symptoms are unchanged. Angiographic evaluation finally reveals the true cause of the problem. Because the symptoms are not infrequently due to hypoperfusion, total occlusion of this vessel can have a dramatic presentation.

Surgical bypass has been performed from one common carotid artery to the other in the anterior neck. This can be a safe and successful procedure but is not elegant and can be difficult. In addition, it requires clamping of the primary residual supply to the brain during the surgery, a maneuver that is not well tolerated in most patients. An alternate procedure is bypass from the subclavian artery to the carotid artery. This procedure circumvents the problem of clamping the primary residual supply to the brain (the residual carotid artery) and is often successful.

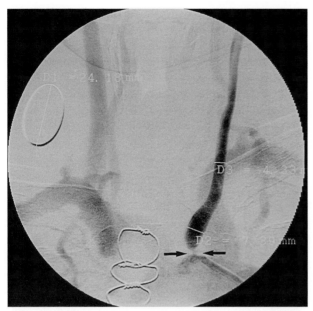

Figure 47-1 Case 1. This man experienced recurrent transient ischemic attacks (TIAs) after previous endarterectomy of the left internal carotid artery (surgery was performed on the basis of carotid Doppler evaluation). The first cerebral angiogram performed now reveals very tight stenosis at the origin of the left common carotid artery *(arrows)*. Note the quarter in the supraclavicular fossa and the corrected measurements of the common carotid artery at two locations. It was thought that the true size of the origin of the common carotid origin was somewhere in between the two measurements; i.e., the 7.39 mm measurement probably represented a degree of poststenotic dilation. It was decided that 7 mm should be the goal for dilation of the origin.

Case 1 continues

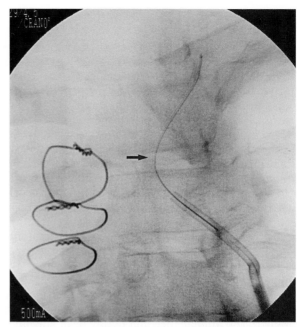

Figure 47-2 A preshaped 9-Fr. guide catheter was chosen and introduced directly through the skin using a 7-Fr. Berenstein catheter (as described in Chapter 3). Through the guide catheter, a very soft microwire (0.014″ Seeker Standard, Target Therapeutics) was used to cross the lesion *(arrow)*, followed by a microcatheter. This microwire was used because of its ability to be preformed so that it can be used for selection in the aorta, and its very soft platinum coil tip, which is safe to cross a stenosis that may be an embolic source.

Case 1 continues

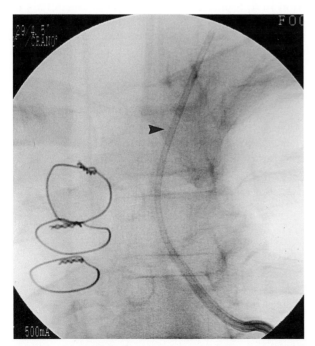

Figure 47-3 Once the microwire and microcatheter were safely downstream, they were followed by a Vinuela catheter (Cook, Inc.), which tapers from a 5.5-Fr. shaft to a 4.5-Fr. tip *(arrowhead)*. This catheter had been advanced into the guide catheter coaxially with the microcatheter and microwire. The microwire and microcatheter were withdrawn.

Case 1 continues

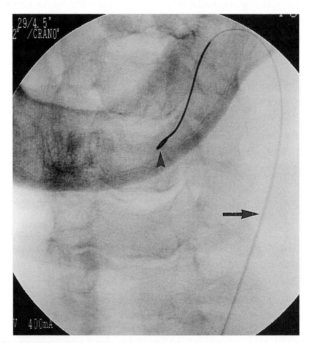

Figure 47-4 A custom-made neuro-exchange wire was then placed through the Vinuela catheter *(arrow)*. The tip of this wire is hydrophilic-coated and has a very tight J curve *(arrowhead)*; the platinum tip tapers to an 0.021″ shaft. This blunt soft tip is capable of extremely safe downstream use owing to its J shape and soft tapered core. It has entered the lingual artery in this case. This safe tip is absolutely mandatory during a case of this nature since no matter how carefully the external portion of the wire is held absolutely still, the movement of the catheter within the aorta combined with respiratory motion will guarantee movement of the tip.

Case 1 continues

INNOMINATE ARTERY

Stenosis in the innominate artery may present an ideal situation for extracranial angioplasty. These lesions are difficult to reach surgically and have a relatively high complication rate for primary repair; bypass procedures are more efficacious.

Surgical bypass has become a more accepted mode of therapy for these lesions than direct repair. Mellière et al. reported on a series of 22 patients with innominate artery stenosis who were treated by direct endarterectomy, direct substernal bypass, or carotid-to-carotid bypass.[2] In agreement with other authors, axillary-to-axillary bypass was not recommended, but carotid-to-carotid bypass with interposed graft yielded good results. As recommended by Owens et al., surgery should be limited to the subclavian artery and supraclavicular fossa and not involve the axillary arteries.[3]

Embolic events may be common with these lesions, which often appear irregular on angiography. This is similar to the appearance and behavior of subclavian lesions but different than the appearance and presentation of vertebral artery origin stenoses, which are typically smooth and tight.

Indications for therapy in this location appear to be related both to embolic events and hypoperfusion, which can be intracranial as well as involve the upper extremity. The series from the University of North Carolina at Chapel Hill indicates that innominate artery stenosis was associated with TIAs in two thirds of patients and with right arm claudication in

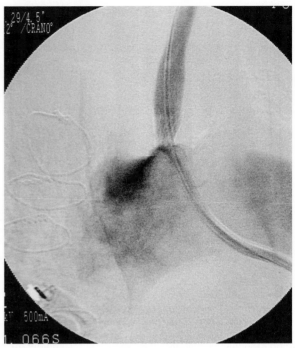

Figure 47-6 After angioplasty and stent placement, and final flaring with an 8-mm balloon inflated to 3 atmospheres, the stent is in ideal location, with a modest residual narrowing at the origin of the common carotid artery; the lumen now measures 6 mm. The struts of the stent are flared proximal to the stenosis for approximately 1 mm.

one third of patients.[3] Mellière found the presenting symptoms to be related to the arm in 11 cases, the vertebrobasilar territory in 7, and the anterior circulation in 4; 5 patients were symptom free.[2] This is in agreement with our small number of cases.

For these reasons, symptomatic, angiographically demonstrable lesions would be considered appro-

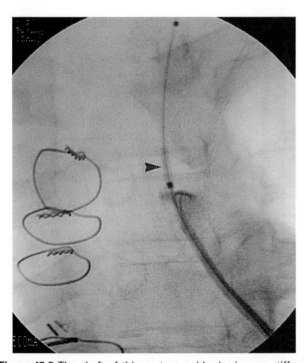

Figure 47-5 The shaft of this custom guidewire is very stiff and therefore carries a stent and balloon with ease and stability. The short 10-mm Palmaz stent (Johnson & Johnson Interventional Systems) *(arrowhead)* is mounted at the proximal marker of a 7-mm balloon catheter. The guide catheter is used for contrast injections to ensure absolutely precise stent placement.

Case 1 continues

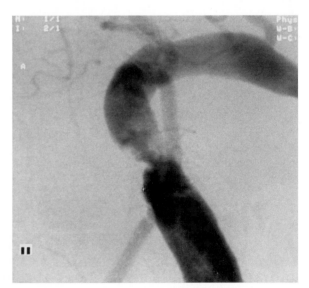

Figure 47-7 Case 2. This patient presented with recurrent posterior fossa TIAs and severe stenosis of the left subclavian artery. The angiogram reveals a very irregular appearance suggesting the possibility of thrombus superimposed on plaque.

Case 2 continues

priate for treatment (i.e., global ischemic symptoms, TIAs, right arm ischemia, or a right subclavian steal phenomenon).

The only real difficulty from the standpoint of endovascular therapy is that of a large vessel with a tight stenosis and an acute origin from the aorta. Although the lesion may be reached easily from the axillary approach, the required size of the catheter and balloon, not to mention the possible need for a stent, may make the axillary approach less than ideal. In our experience, the diameter of the innominate artery can be large, necessitating a huge balloon (and stent).

Achieving an adequate result may or may not require the use of a stent. Angioplasty without a stent is far easier in this location; accurate placement of the stent can be difficult, and the interstices of the stent should adhere closely to the vessel wall, requiring overdilation of the proximal and distal end, which is difficult if the lumen is huge.

SUBCLAVIAN ARTERY

Subclavian angioplasty has been performed for almost two decades and has been shown to be safe and efficacious. The series from the University of North Carolina at Chapel Hill, which included 27 patients,

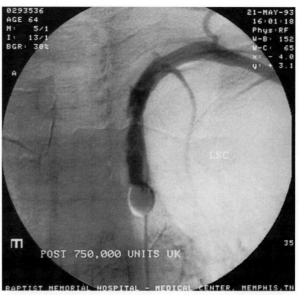

Figure 47-9 After infusion of 750,000 units of urokinase, there appeared to be some slight further clearing and the vessel was now ready for angioplasty. Note the absence of flow in the vertebral artery on this slightly slower injection.

Case 2 continues

indicated that subclavian artery stenosis was associated with simple arm claudication (55%) far more frequently than with vertebrobasilar insufficiency (15%), both of which were present in 30% of patients.[3]

Indications for Treatment of Subclavian Artery Stenosis

The subclavian steal phenomenon is a common indication for therapy of this lesion (Case 2, Figs. 47–7

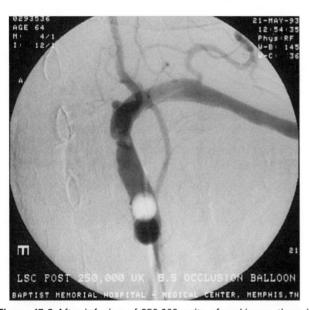

Figure 47-8 After infusion of 250,000 units of urokinase, there is considerable clearing of the lesion. A temporary occlusion balloon has been placed in the origin of the left subclavian artery for flow control. The balloon was inflated enough to achieve *near*-total occlusion, but not complete (note the movement of the balloon during the injection). The near-occlusion creates a subclavian steal with induced retrograde flow in the left vertebral artery, but during the injection the flow through the catheter reestablishes some antegrade flow. For confirmation of the retrograde flow in the vertebral artery, a very slow trickle of contrast can be infused, and absence of filling of the vertebral artery will be seen. Conversely, injection into the opposite vertebral artery would clearly demonstrate this. Urokinase can now be safely infused into the proximal subclavian artery with no risk of embolization to the brain (any emboli from the stenosis will go out the axillary artery).

Case 2 continues

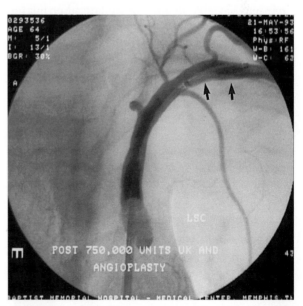

Figure 47-10 Postangioplasty appearance after a gradual inflation over a 5-minute period and a pause with the balloon inflated for 1 minute. The angioplastied vessel appears pristine. Note the angioplasty balloon *(arrows)* past the vertebral artery with the proximal flow control temporary occlusion guide catheter in place in the proximal subclavian artery. Again, note the lack of antegrade flow in the vertebral artery due to the induced steal, effectively protecting the brain during the previous angioplasty.

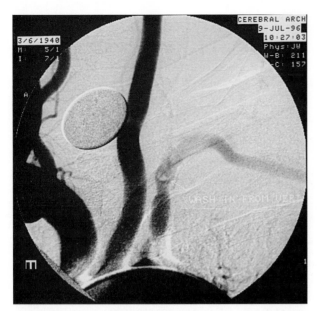

Figure 47-11 Case 3. This 56-year-old woman presented with severe subclavian steal syndrome. An aortogram was performed with a quarter overlying the clavicle for measurement purposes. The stenosis is in the subclavian artery, but just at the origin from the aorta. Note the subtle unopacified wash-in from the vertebral artery in this patient with a true subclavian steal. Note also the poor opacification of the distal subclavian artery itself, secondary to the stenosis.

Case 3 continues

to 47–10; Case 3, Figs. 47–11 to 47–14; and Case 4, Figs. 47–15 to 47–18). The subsequent reversal of flow in the vertebral artery protects the intracranial structures from embolic events during angioplasty. Typical symptoms are episodic dizziness, diplopia, dysarthria, perioral numbness, visual disturbances, and nausea. Variable degrees of unilateral or bilateral

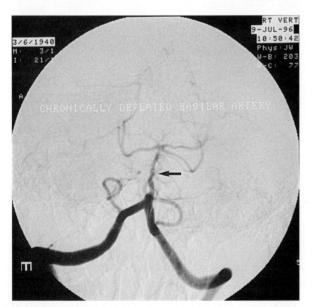

Figure 47-12 A right vertebral artery injection clearly demonstrates the chronic effects of this pathology. The left vertebral artery is the actual continuation of the right vertebral artery, and the basilar artery is chronically deflated *(arrow)*. There is poor filling of the posterior cerebral artery territories bilaterally.

Case 3 continues

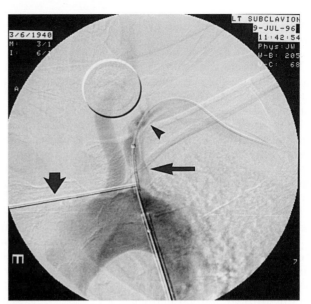

Figure 47-13 A 9-Fr. Brite-Tip catheter (Cordis Corp.) has been placed, and a Palmaz stent *(thin arrow)* is being positioned.

Access to this location had been made utilizing a standard diagnostic catheter (a JB-2 made by Cook, Inc.), with an angled Glidewire (Medi-Tech, Inc.) gaining access to the distal axillary artery. This has to be performed with caution owing to the ability of this guidewire to dissect easily. The diagnostic catheter was then advanced over the wire, and this wire was exchanged for an exchange-length straight Amplatz Superstiff (Cook, Inc.) guidewire.

Before use, the straight Amplatz Superstiff guidewire should have its tip curved into several S turns. This induces the wire to buckle or coil when it encounters resistance, rather than puncturing or dissecting. The Amplatz Superstiff will render interventional procedures much easier and less stressful because of its robust support and extreme resistance to buckling or recoiling.

Note the advantages of the guide catheter also. As usual, this catheter was used instead of a sheath and was placed directly percutaneously as previously described. The large guide catheter permits easy passage of the stent around corners without the worry of the stent becoming dislodged, as well as the ability to inject large volumes of contrast to visualize accurate placement. We use a long guide catheter such as this for every stent case. The rounded lumen distal to the stenosis is not a balloon, but rather a section of normal vessel *(arrowhead)*. The straight object entering the field from the right *(fat arrow)* is a long needle (the outer portion of the Seldinger arterial puncture needle), placed to mark the optimal position for the proximal portion of the stent.

While the inflated size of the Palmaz stent is variable, the shortest length is usually sufficient to cover any stenosis encountered in the subclavian artery.

Case 3 continues

weakness may be present. Classically, these symptoms are worsened or brought on by exercise of the affected arm; however, *this usually is not the case*.[4] Interestingly, symptoms may appear to move around, as opposed to the symptoms of anterior circulation disease, which are more consistently reproducible.

There is no relationship between the degree of stenosis and symptoms.[4] There is a significant association between the presence or absence of subclavian steal and symptomatology, but *steal does not always manifest with symptoms*. Although most patients in the study of Thomassen and Aarli had signs of subclavian steal (42 of 58), only 20 of the 42 (<50%) had symptoms attributable to vertebrobasilar ischemia.[4] Vertebrobasilar symptoms occurred as frequently in

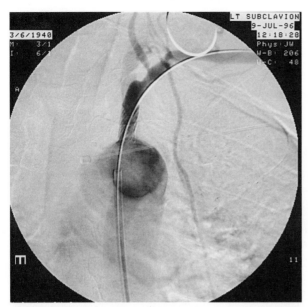

Figure 47-14 Angiogram performed immediately after angioplasty. Note the antegrade flow in the left vertebral artery at this time. While the angioplasty site looks ideal, there is a residual stenosis at the level of the vertebral artery itself, not hemodynamically significant.

patients without steal as in patients with steal. Also, vertebrobasilar symptoms occurred in only 15 of 26 patients with severe steal. *Only 1 of 4 patients with actual reversal of flow in the basilar artery demonstrated symptoms.* Thus, there is no significant association between symptoms and severity of steal or presence or absence of reversal of flow in the basilar artery.

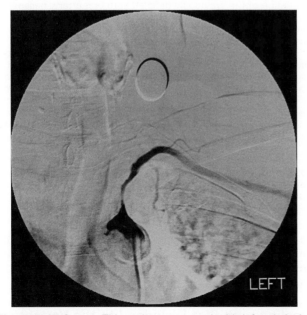

Figure 47-15 Case 4. This patient presented with left subclavian artery stenosis and steal. The baseline angiogram reveals a long segment irregular stenosis with no evidence of the vertebral artery. Again, a quarter is placed in the supraclavicular fossa to give an accurate measurement of vessel size and lesion length.
Case 4 continues

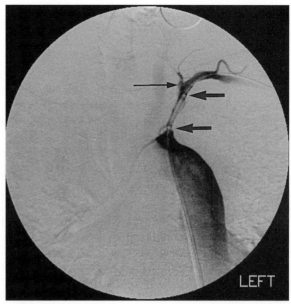

Figure 47-16 A hand-mounted Palmaz stent on a 5-Fr. angioplasty balloon (2 cm in length) has been placed through a 9-Fr. Brite-Tip guide catheter. The Brite-Tip catheter was introduced directly percutaneously in the manner previously described, using a Rosen exchange wire with its safe, tight distal curl. This allows injection of contrast through the guide catheter around the angioplasty catheter to visualize exact placement within the vessel.

Note the two markers on the angioplasty balloon, 2 cm apart *(fat arrows)*. The proximal marker is just distal to the funnel of the stenosis. Note also the visualization of the proximal stub of the vertebral artery overlying another thyrocervical vessel *(thin arrow)*, with the distal balloon marker proximal to this. Note this location on later images.
Case 4 continues

Vertigo, alone or in combination with other focal brainstem symptoms, was the most common symptom in all degrees of steal severity. None of the patients with symptoms, however, had recurrence of symptoms produced by arm exercise or during repeated brachial artery compression–decompression tests. This test entails compression of the brachial artery (generally by means of a blood pressure cuff inflated above systolic pressure) for several minutes to produce hypoxia within the arm. The cuff is then released. As a result of the hypoxia, autoregulation produces vasodilation and hyperemia, worsening the steal. Most patients with subclavian steal appeared to have an adequate supply from the opposite vertebral artery.

These subclavian stenoses commonly are irregular and can have thrombus associated with the stenosis. They commonly occur just distal to the origin from the aorta or at the ostium, similar to the presentation in the innominate artery. Thus, the initial passage of the wire and catheter past this pathology should be performed carefully to avoid plaque disruption.

Restoration of adequate flow by surgical correction or angioplasty does not always relieve symptoms.[5, 6]

Vertebral Artery Protection During Subclavian Angioplasty and Stenting

A transient vertebral artery and subclavian steal can be created during subclavian angioplasty and stenting by creating a hyperemic arm. This can be done in one of two ways: (1) A blood pressure cuff can be inflated above systolic pressure for a few minutes and then released; or (2) a vasodilator, such as nitroglycerin, can be injected intra-arterially into the arm. This can protect the brain during the procedure.

Alternatively, an occlusion balloon guide catheter (Zeppelin, Medtronic/MIS) can be placed at the subclavian origin during the angioplasty or stenting to produce reversal of flow in the vertebral artery, inducing a subclavian steal.

If the lesion is at or near the origin of the subclavian artery, an occlusion balloon can be placed *from the arm* and inflated *over* the vertebral artery origin. It is more effective to infuse saline through the occlusion balloon than to try and aspirate any debris out of the dead end proximal subclavian artery.

Although pretreating a subclavian lesion with urokinase before instrumentation is a subject of debate, it has been unequivocally shown on more than one occasion to improve the appearance of the lesion (with some stenoses reducing to less than 50%). This fact, combined with the observed complications of emboli to the vertebral artery (and brain) after angioplasty and stenting, suggests a need for pretreatment of an irregular lesion with urokinase as well as protection techniques during the procedure. If pretreatment with urokinase is to be performed, it would be wise to protect the vertebral artery from embolization by any fragments of dissolving thrombus that might break free. This can be accomplished by occluding the subclavian artery directly over the vertebral artery as described previously; alternatively, a

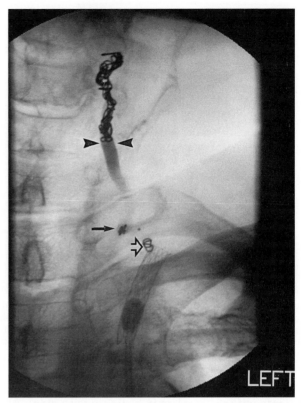

Figure 47-18 A Zeppelin flow control guide catheter (Medtronic/MIS) has been placed into the stent in the subclavian artery and inflated. This again creates a subclavian steal, preventing any distal embolization either from the stent or from the maneuver to permanently occlude the vertebral artery to prevent a possible later embolic event. A TRACKER-18 microcatheter (Target Therapeutics) has been placed through the struts on the stent, and a position in the midportion of the artery was chosen as the location for the occlusion.

Note the coil just within the stent *(open arrow)*. This was the first coil placed and was slightly undersized, owing to the gradual distention of the previously deflated vertebral artery. Because of the reversal of flow in the vertebral artery, the coil migrated in a *proximal* direction rather than a cephalad direction, and its progress was stopped by the stent.

This image was obtained after a mass of coils had been placed in the vertebral artery and the last coil had become jammed in the catheter; its final position is just at the tight curve, where it had become stuck in the catheter *(black arrow)*. After the delivery of a number of coils, the inner surface of microcatheters can become scratched, greatly increasing the friction for delivery of coils. When a microcatheter makes a tight curve, its lumen will become oval, thus potentially causing the coil to jam, as it had in this case. It was therefore deposited in this location, and a final, very gentle injection was made through the microcatheter to confirm occlusion. Note the contrast pooling at the coils *(arrowheads)*, not what the contrast would do if there was any continuing steal!

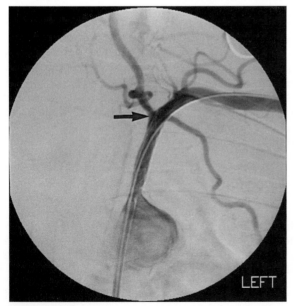

Figure 47-17 After dilation, the angioplasty and stent result is excellent, but a portion of the stent overlies the origin of the vertebral artery *(arrow)*. This is probably unacceptable, but not truly known. This occurred because the only available stent had been 30 mm in length; it was mounted inadvertently on a 20-mm balloon.

Case 4 continues

large-bore guide catheter can be used; a separate micro-occlusion balloon can be placed in the vertebral artery; and infusion can be performed through the guide catheter.

Dealing with Clot Dislodged to the Vertebral Artery Origin

Although it is often said that deploying a stent primarily (without predilation) traps the plaque and thrombus, emboli do occur during stent placement in the subclavian artery. If an embolus or thrombus is present at the vertebral artery origin, a steal should be created by temporary balloon occlusion of the subclavian artery origin, thus reversing flow in the vertebral artery. This will provide protection during the removal of the clot. It may even flush the thrombus down the arm.

This balloon occlusion can be achieved with a 6.4-Fr. or 7.4-Fr. Zeppelin, through which can be placed a Solstice balloon catheter (Medtronic/MIS). (If the subclavian artery is extremely large, a Medi-Tech temporary occlusion balloon should be used.) The low-profile Solstice balloon can then be advanced up the vertebral artery past the clot *while the flow is reversed*, inflated (up to 3.5 mm), and withdrawn. This may extract the clot out of the vertebral artery.

Another means to remove thrombus in the vertebral artery *under the state of flow reversal* described previously is to place a microcatheter past the clot (without dislodging it) and infuse urokinase, which will then flow back past the thrombus.

Alternatively, if there has been no embolus to the brain, it may be possible to occlude the vertebral artery with coils distal to the embolus, thus protecting the brain. If the thrombus is far enough beyond the origin of the vertebral artery, the artery can be occluded proximal to the thrombus.

ORIGIN OF THE RIGHT COMMON CAROTID ARTERY OR RIGHT SUBCLAVIAN ARTERY FROM THE INNOMINATE ARTERY

These locations are similar in appearance and approach. They can be smooth concentric lesions (Case

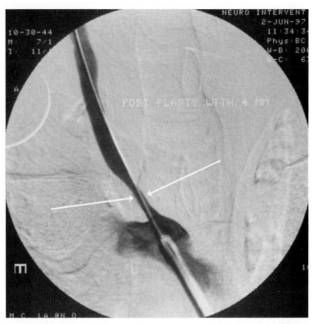

Figure 47-20 Rather than simply try to force a stent through this stenosis, a predilation angioplasty was performed with an undersized balloon (4 mm). Undersizing the balloon helps ensure that there is minimal, if any, intimal damage before placement of the stent. (After the stent is in place, full dilation can be performed to yield the ultimate result.) The result of the angioplasty is good enough to allow the stent to be placed in the proper location without difficulty.

Case 5 continues

5, Figs. 47–19 to 47–22) or extremely irregular and eccentric lesions (Case 6, Figs. 47–23 to 47–26). The vessels can be huge.

Indications for therapy are similar to those given previously and are related either to embolic events or to hypoperfusion. A subclavian lesion can be the cause of subclavian steal, as in the case of left subclavian artery stenosis. Of note is the fact that subclavian steal causes more ischemic symptoms in the arm than in the brain.

A short Palmaz stent is appropriate for use in this location. There is minimal movement of the vessel in this location, the vessel is large, and there is high flow—the ideal situation for stenting.

CERVICAL CAROTID ARTERY OTHER THAN AT THE BIFURCATION

Locations of pathology in the carotid artery other than at the bifurcation obviously exist. These are typically above the bifurcation. Occasionally, lesions may be below the bifurcation, in the common carotid artery, but these are rare in locations other than at the bifurcation. The space between the origin of the common carotid artery and the bifurcation is usually clean if not involved in a generalized vascular pathologic process or traumatic injury.

The cervical internal carotid artery can have focal stenoses, however (Case 7, Figs. 47–27 to 47–29). This usually occurs a short distance from the bifurcation but can occur at any location. These lesions

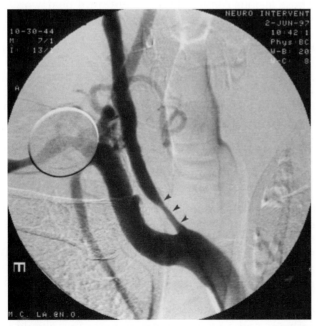

Figure 47-19 Case 5. This patient presented with a stenosis of the origin of the right common carotid artery, just at the innominate artery *(arrowheads)*. This vessel measured about 1 mm at the stenosis and has the typical appearance of a stenosis at this location (i.e., a smooth concentric narrowing). Note the quarter above the clavicle, again used for accurate measurement *(arrow)*.

Case 5 continues

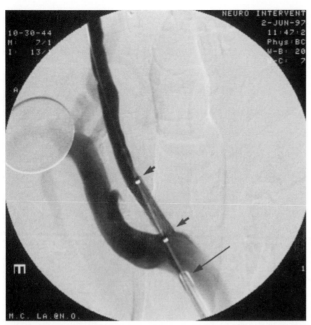

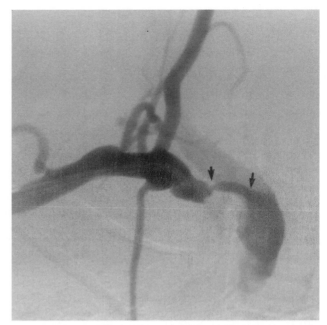

Figure 47-21 The guide catheter (an angled Brite-Tip, *long arrow*) allows injection while precise placement of the stent is made (note the proximal and distal stent location, *short arrows*). This placement is revealed on the angiogram obtained after the Palmaz stent has been deployed, with the balloon catheter still in place.

Case 5 continues

Figure 47-23 Case 6. A very tight irregular appearance of the subclavian artery *(arrows)* is shown in this view from a retrograde axillary injection. The plaque is huge. Even with this irregular appearance, the patient presented with arm ischemia rather than embolic events.

Case 6 continues

usually are not as ulcerated as the carotid bifurcation lesions and respond easily to angioplasty. They do not necessarily need a stent to trap friable plaque material. In a higher location in the internal carotid artery than the bifurcation, however, there is not as much motion, and a stent would probably be safer than at the bifurcation. The lesions in this location are also not as eccentric or as irregular as bifurcation

lesions unless located at a position of extreme ectasia or kinking. There is no series of patients indicating the need for stents in this location.

Indications for Therapy

These lesions commonly are silent until nearly occlusive. They can be the cause of chronic hemodynamic insufficiency and can progress to the point at which they are the source of embolic phenomena; this can occur in the presence or absence of anticoagulation. Stenoses with symptoms (TIAs) in the internal carotid artery (in any location) should be treated because they are associated with recurrent TIAs or stroke at a rate of up to 10% per year.

Remember, TIAs are a warning to the lucky that a stroke is imminent. This sign should not be ignored!

Technique of Therapy

Because of the possible distal location of this pathology, a distal flow control catheter may be impossible to use. A proximal flow control guide catheter can still be used, but the optimal unit is not commercially available. In addition, these lesions are not usually as irregular, friable, or ulcerated as the lesions at the bifurcation, and therefore the fear of emboli is lessened. For this reason, placement of a stable guide catheter and angioplasty without stenting should be adequate (see Figs. 47–27 to 47–29). Avoidance of intimal dissection by use of extremely slow balloon inflation is recommended.

Again, the choice of guidewire over which the angioplasty is to be performed is extremely important. A

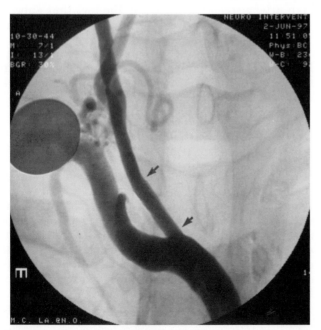

Figure 47-22 The final angiogram reveals ideal placement of the stent with excellent antegrade flow.

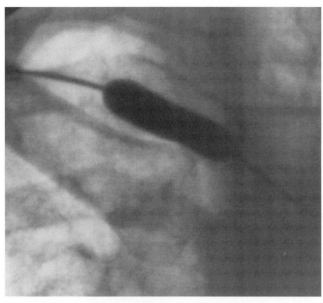

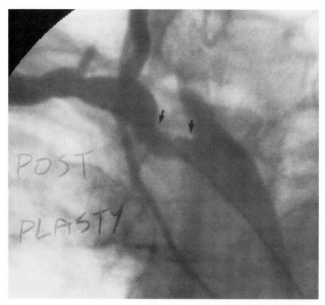

Figures 47-24 and 47-25 Initially, a simple angioplasty was performed, with a poor result. The eccentric nature of the plaque renders simple angioplasty unrewarding.

Case 6 continues

safe tip is mandatory; a Platinum Plus (Medi-Tech, Inc.) or similar wire with a tight curl on the end (similar to a Rosen guidewire) is the safest choice. The prototype Roadrunner "neuro" guidewire made by Cook Inc. has a soft, tapered, tight curl and is ideal.

VERTEBRAL ARTERY ORIGIN

The particular location of this pathology makes a considerable difference to the treatment options as well as to the prognosis. Options for treatment of vertebral origin disease range from angioplasty (with or without stenting), to transplantation of the verte-

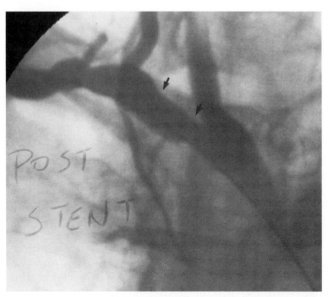

Figure 47-26 It was then necessary to place a Palmaz stent in the vessel. Note that the stent is probably 1 to 2 mm too distal (observe the slight narrowing at the *proximal arrow*). The result was considered to be acceptable, however.

bral artery onto the carotid artery, to placing a jump graft from the subclavian artery to the vertebral artery. All of these options are potentially viable choices with varying degrees of success and failure in individual hands. Most impressive is the large number of cases produced by the St. Thomas Hospital group in Nashville, in which the morbidity and mortality rates for vertebral dislocation with grafting are nearly 0%.

Indications for Therapy

Indications for therapy typically include symptoms of vertebrobasilar insufficiency and are more often related to simple stenosis (and hypoperfusion) than embolic phenomena. There is often minimal communication from the anterior circulation to the posterior circulation through the posterior communicating arteries, thus yielding an isolated posterior fossa and subsequent symptoms. The variation from patient to patient in the severity of lesions causing symptomatology is confounding; in some patients, there is almost no flow and minimal symptoms, whereas in others, there appears to be adequate flow but profound symptoms.

Positional or functional features may also be present; the patient may experience symptoms related to head or neck position in addition to the more classic symptoms related to blood pressure and orthostatic factors.

Embolic events can occur secondary to vertebral origin stenosis. These are typically the result of a critical stenosis at the origin slowing the blood flow enough to allow sludging and thus clot formation, but embolic events can occur even with a moderate stenosis when the flow in the opposite vertebral artery is abundant enough to allow slowing in the artery with the stenosis. In Case 8, Figures 47–30 and

47–31, note the embolism to the posterior cerebral arteries and the only moderate stenosis that was the origin of these emboli. This situation is different from the typical ulcerated carotid lesion, which can cause clot formation (and embolization) in ulcer pits in high flow blood. A carotid stenosis would normally produce symptoms due to ischemia long before it finally reaches a degree of severity sufficient to cause enough slowing to permit thrombus formation. In vertebral artery origin disease, however, the inflow from the opposite vertebral artery generally prevents ischemia caused by hypoperfusion. Therefore, in this particular setting, the stenosis can worsen silently over a period of time until it reaches the point that thrombus may form and migrate downstream, thus causing embolic symptoms without a prior history of ischemic symptoms, even in a smooth stenosis.

Strategic Considerations for Therapeutic Options

From an endovascular standpoint, lesions of the origin of the vertebral artery are easier to treat, are

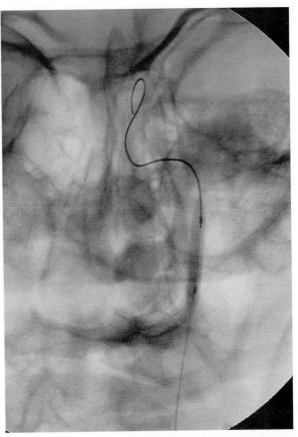

Figure 47-28 After placement of a guide catheter, a custom hydrophilic-coated guidewire with a soft tapered, very tight P-curved tip was used to advance the 5-mm angioplasty catheter to its intended location. Note the ability of the wire to easily advance to the cavernous sinus region with a tip that is entirely safe. This is important, because it is impossible to control the guidewire tip accurately while advancing the catheter to this location. A simple angle-tipped hydrophilic guidewire is unacceptable.

After 10,000 units of heparin had been administered, the angioplasty balloon was gradually inflated over a period of 90 seconds and kept inflated for 60 seconds.

Case 7 continues

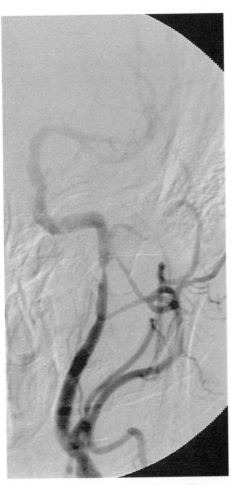

Figure 47-27 Case 7. A 66-year-old woman with a previous left carotid endarterectomy. One year after the endarterectomy, she experienced an episode of dysarthria and arm weakness. The obligatory carotid ultrasound scan was negative, but the patient's persistent neurosurgeon obtained an angiogram, which revealed this stenosis in the upper cervical internal carotid artery. Note the absence of filling of the anterior cerebral artery. It is flowing retrograde to partially fill the middle cerebral artery.

Case 7 continues

safer, and produce more predictable results than more downstream lesions. Distal vertebral artery lesions are much more difficult to access as well as more dangerous; they can dissect. Lesions proximal to the vertebrobasilar junction are treatable, whereas those at the vertebrobasilar junction are the most prone to dissection, occlusion, or perforation.

The anatomy of the proximal 1 to 5 cm of the vertebral artery has a significant influence not only on the safety of the procedure and technique chosen for repair but also on the results. This is the first strategic dilemma to be faced. An inappropriate choice of approach can turn all the vectors of force against the successful completion of the case.

Common iliac artery or superficial femoral artery lesions have minimal variation in anatomy, and the basic approach is hardly variable. This is not the case with the origin of the vertebral artery from the subclavian artery. The choice of access to this location is completely different, depending on which side is approached and on the particular point along

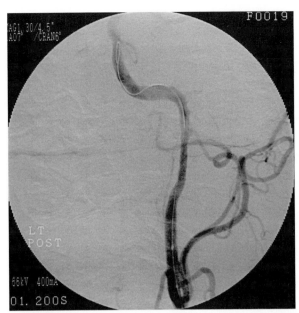

Figure 47-29 After the angioplasty, the wire was kept in place while a repeat angiogram was performed using the guide catheter: a prime reason to use a guide catheter. Note the lack of intimal damage.

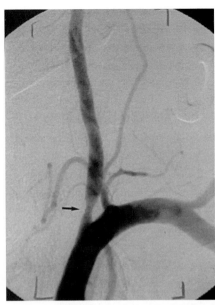

Figure 47-31 The cause of these emboli is seen to be this moderate stenosis *(arrows)*, significant only because the opposite vertebral artery supplied all the flow necessary to the posterior fossa structures. This allowed sludging in this vessel.

the course of the subclavian artery at which the vertebral artery originates. For right-sided lesions, the choice of an axillary approach (or brachial, as cardiologists would employ) is more readily made. There can be extreme tortuosity in the approach to the vertebral artery origin through the innominate artery. In addition, the shape of the vertebral artery has tremendous impact on correct technique.

In addition to changing the choice of approach, anatomy can change the choice of therapy (i.e., whether to place a stent). In certain situations, angioplasty alone should be the rational choice. Although the picture may not be ideal, the clinical

results generally remain adequate (Case 9, Fig. 47–32 to 47–35). In other cases, use of a stent is possible and produces a satisfactory result (Case 10, Figs. 47–36 to 47–38).

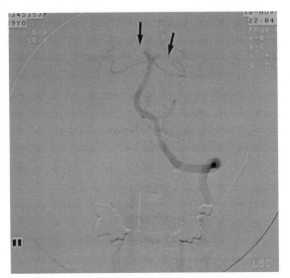

Figure 47-30 Case 8. This young man, with no previous neurologic symptoms of any kind, experienced the sudden onset of complete blindness. Angiography reveals complete occlusion of both posterior cerebral arteries *(arrows)*.

Case 8 continues

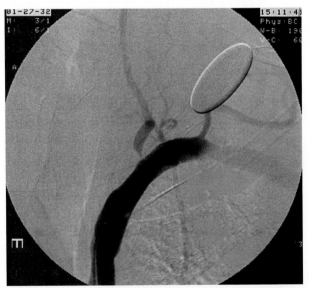

Figure 47-32 Case 9. This 62-year-old woman presented to the emergency room complaining of dizziness, episodic nausea, and periodic generalized weakness. An arteriogram was obtained as part of the work-up. It reveals that posterior fossa insufficiency is likely; the basilar artery is supplied by an isolated left vertebral artery with a high-grade stenosis. The measurement of true vessel size will be made beyond the initial few centimeters of the vessel, above the level of possible poststenotic dilation. Mental allowance must be made, however, for the possibility that the upper vertebral artery (the main trunk seen higher in the image) could be somewhat deflated owing to decreased mean arterial pressure; the vessel could actually be slightly larger once the stenosis is eliminated.

Case 9 continues

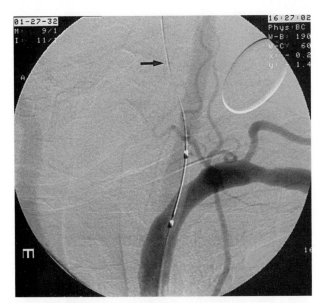

Figure 47-33 Catheterization of the subclavian artery was performed utilizing a Rosen-type tight J-curve wire and a guide catheter placed in the origin of the subclavian artery. The stenotic vertebral artery was selected first with a Seeker Standard guidewire, followed by a microcatheter. The wire was then exchanged for a Platinum Plus exchange wire (*arrow*, in place in the vertebral artery), over which a Sub-4 angioplasty catheter (Medi-Tech, Inc.) was placed. Note the inflated balloon yielding a filling defect in the opacified subclavian artery, verifying accurate positioning for the balloon inflation.

Case 9 continues

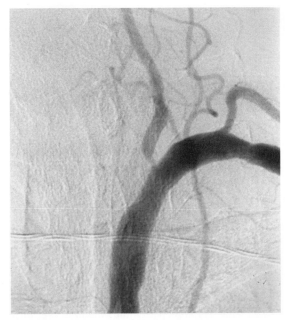

Figure 47-35 Postangioplasty appearance. Rebound of the stenosis is readily apparent—the rationale for primary stenting in many cases. Note the now significantly enlarged downstream vertebral artery lumen, however. While the angiographic appearance may be far less than 100% dilation, the intima is not disrupted and the patient is now asymptomatic. These lesions have a tendency not only to rebound after angioplasty, but also to restenose after stent placement, and should be followed carefully. A stent may eventually be necessary, or a repeat angioplasty.

Safe downstream access to the distal vertebral artery for placement of a control guidewire for angioplasty is mandatory but can sometimes be difficult (and potentially the most dangerous part of this procedure). The origin often is tortuous or at an odd

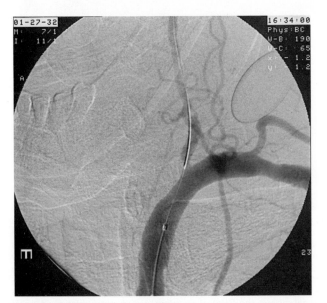

Figure 47-34 After inflation and deflation, the wire is left in place, but the balloon is withdrawn for a follow-up evaluation. Note the elastic recoil of the stenosis, typical for this location. Notice also the increased lumen size of the downstream vertebral artery. The stiff wire can artificially hold open the stenosis, causing a less than ideal appearance once it is withdrawn.

Case 9 continues

angle to the subclavian artery (see Chapter 3). As previously stated, this sometimes necessitates an approach from the arm.

Only the axillary artery is large enough to accept a standard-sized sheath (much less a very large one, which is necessary for a stent). The brachial and radial arteries are too prone to spasm, can be permanently damaged more easily than the larger axillary artery, and are too small to be the site of entry for a case such as this. Even if the radial or brachial artery can be used for most cases, the potential for permanent damage to the artery is too high to risk use of these approaches when a perfectly good site, such as the axillary artery, is available for the competent interventionist.

The technical success rate for angioplasty of the vertebral artery origin is about 80% to 90% (84% in the North American Cerebral Percutaneous Transluminal Angioplasty Register [NACPTAR], personal communication from Robert Ferguson based on early results). This low degree of primary success is related to the fact that the vertebral artery origin, in a manner similar to the renal artery, is subject to severe rebound from elastic properties. In a manner worse than that of the renal arteries, the proximal vertebral arteries are extremely mobile, rendering placement of a stent sometimes difficult.

Symptoms are improved with vertebral artery angioplasty and stenting in only about 75% of cases, and the complication rate is essentially 0%. This situation is much different than for the intracranial distal vertebral artery.

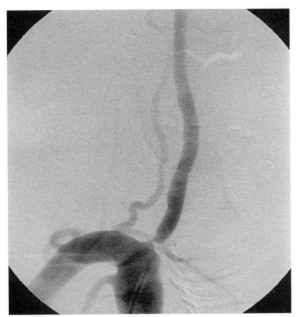

Figure 47-36 Case 10. Initial appearance of right vertebral artery origin stenosis in a patient without a vertebral artery on the other side, and with episodic dizziness consistent with vertebrobasilar insufficiency. The configuration of the takeoff of the vertebral artery would be conducive to an approach from either the arm or the leg. The eccentric nature of the plaque may render simple angioplasty less than ideal.

Case 10 continues

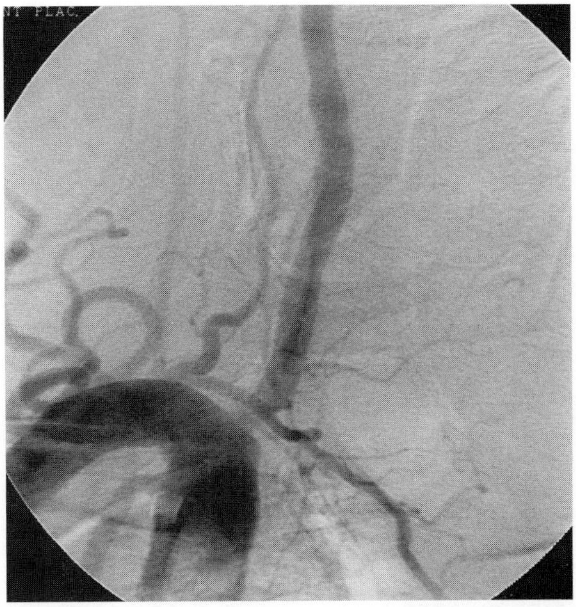

Figure 47-38 Appearance after placement of the Palmaz-Schatz stent. This device is very flexible and comes as a unit with its own delivery sheath (see Chapter 1). Unfortunately, in addition to being nearly invisible radiographically, it is too easily compressed. In this patient, it performed adequately with a good result and no later problem. However, in an anatomically unfavorable situation, a second or even a third stent of this type may be necessary to prevent collapse (much less to even see the stents); if placement of a biliary stent is possible, this is the best choice.

Stent Versus No Stent

With the current popularity of stents, it may come as a surprise that their use has not been proved to

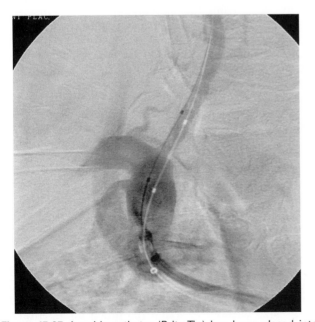

Figure 47-37 A guide catheter (Brite-Tip) has been placed into the innominate artery; angioplasty will take place through this. This allows accurate visualization of the stenosis and the procedure. A Palmaz-Schatz stent (Johnson & Johnson Interventional Systems) has been placed through the stenosis and the stent delivered. Note that the stent is essentially invisible: it is seen poorly with real-time fluoroscopy. This is a potential major drawback to use of this stent, in addition to the fact that it is very weak.

Case 10 continues

be an asset in this location and can even be detrimental. As stated elsewhere in this text, stents provoke a long-term reaction in the vessel wall, with resultant accelerated restenosis. This appears to be true particularly in this location, where it has been shown that severe reaction and restenosis can occur in as few as 3 months.

A stent may not be a viable option in a particular anatomic setting. Even if the result with angioplasty alone is suboptimal, the hemodynamic result may be acceptable and, compared with the potential problems associated with stent use, angioplasty alone may be preferable. In Case 11, presented in Figures 47–39 to 47–41, the option of using a stent should be seriously questioned, particularly in patients with extensive excursion of the subclavian and vertebral artery system during respiration. A fixed kink in a vertebral artery within 1 cm of the subclavian artery is difficult to overcome using a stent.

If a stent is necessary, the small Palmaz-Schatz stent is ideal for access and placement but is easily compressed. It is packaged as a unit that includes a 3-Fr. balloon catheter, a stent expandable to 5 mm, and a sheath cover (to traverse the stenosis), which has a 5-Fr. outer diameter (see Chapter 1). This permits use of a small vascular access, such as the arm. The balloon and stent can be removed from the sheath and placed through a 6-Fr. neuro-guide catheter. If the origin is tortuous or is prone to significant movement with breathing, this stent may not be an ideal choice. The larger Palmaz biliary

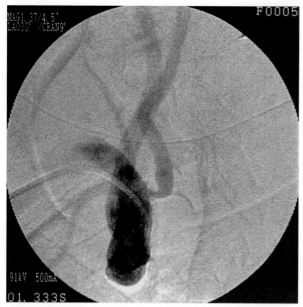

Figure 47-39 Case 11. Right vertebral artery arising from the subclavian artery with a sharp medial kink. This renders catheterization from the femoral approach extremely difficult (impossible in this case) owing to the reversal in vectors. As can be seen, this necessitated an approach from the arm.

Case 11 continues

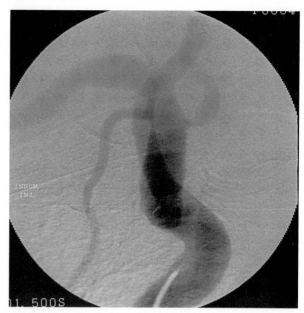

Figure 47-41 After placement of the stent, the lumen was ideal until the patient coughed, causing extreme excursion in the subclavian artery and kinking of the vertebral artery origin, with resultant restenosis. The Palmaz-Schatz stent is too soft to resist this movement and collapsed. Note also the poststenotic dilation.

stents are stronger but difficult to place in certain locations. Their intrinsic length and stiffness are not suitable, and they are intended to be placed using a much larger delivery system.

For these reasons, initial angioplasty should be performed without stent use, and a stent should only be used when absolutely necessary.

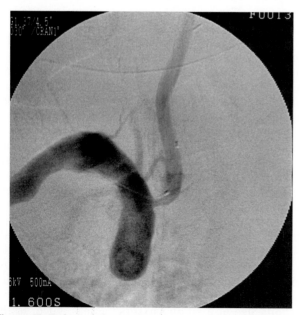

Figure 47-40 Catheterization has been achieved and the angioplasty balloon (with a Palmaz-Schatz stent) is in place. The sheath over the stent is still in place. Note the value of the guide catheter in this situation, rendering visualization of the procedure possible.

Case 11 continues

Poststenotic Dilation

Another problem with vertebral artery angioplasty and stenting occurs when a tight stenosis is followed by a short segment of poststenotic dilation and then by the normal-sized vessel. The vertebral artery origin cannot be overdilated without the risk of rupture or avulsion from the subclavian artery. This is an entirely different situation from rupture or perforation of a superficial femoral artery caused by overly aggressive dilation. A ruptured or avulsed vertebral artery origin can cause not only a fatal hemorrhage but also fatal brainstem ischemia.

Poststenotic dilation can be a relative contraindication to stent placement as well as simple angioplasty. Adequate dilation of the stent against the wall of the artery is mandatory to prevent later distal embolization of thrombus from the dead space around the stent struts. Adequate dilation of the stent in the region of the poststenotic dilation is prevented by the smaller vertebral artery origin as well as by the smaller distal main vertebral artery trunk (the poststenotic dilation may be 1 to 3 mm larger than the main vessel lumen over a distance of only 3 to 10 mm). The risk of rupture secondary to angioplasty, however, is less in the main trunk than the origin. This limitation may be overcome by the use of a compliant balloon that is capable of expanding to a large size without exerting too much force. Alternatively, an angioplasty balloon that is too large for the orifice can be used, but only inflated to low pressure. The force exerted should not be too great for the origin or main shaft of the vertebral artery but should be enough to expand a Palmaz-Schatz stent. Force of dilation, *not* the size of the balloon, is the

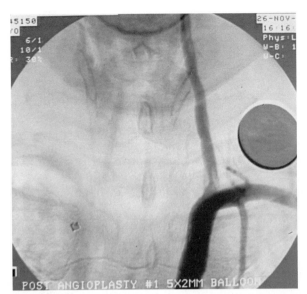

Figure 47-42 Case 12. Choice of a slightly too large angioplasty balloon can result in a dissection at the origin even if there is not true avulsion. Care must be taken not to try to achieve an ideal appearance at the expense of an adequate result.

key to vascular rupture. (A 10-mm balloon with 2 atmospheres of pressure is the same as a 100-mm balloon with 2 atmospheres of pressure.) A Palmaz-Schatz stent can be expanded with minimal force, less than that necessary for rupture of most vertebral origins (which require at least 3 to 4 atmospheres of pressure). A biliary type stent may require more force than this.

Overdilation can result in a severe dissection (Case 12, Fig. 47–42), with or without resultant occlusion. Although the initial angiographic result may not be ideal, the vessel usually heals with a good result. The result illustrated in Figure 47–42, however, is the reason for *not* overdilating this site in an attempt to break the elastic band frequently found at this location. Overdilation can be disastrous and can lead to avulsion.

Technique of Treatment

Angioplasty of the vertebral artery origin is a relatively safe and straightforward procedure as long as excellent technique is employed for initial catheterization of the vertebral artery. Placing a guidewire downstream can be dangerous in the tortuous vertebral artery origin and can result in dissection of the vessel (see Chapter 3).

The angioplasty may result in dissection, but the primary technical difficulty usually is that of an elastic or fibrous band in the origin that is resistant to dilation (see Figs. 47–32 to 47–35). In addition, the eccentric nature of the plaque may render angioplasty suboptimal. Stenting, however, may also be suboptimal, as described previously.

Technical Note

A flow control guide catheter can be placed in the subclavian artery during the angioplasty procedure for the same purpose as that described earlier in the carotid artery. Occlusion of the proximal subclavian artery can create a subclavian steal with reversal of flow in the vertebral artery. During a vertebral artery angioplasty or an angioplasty of the subclavian artery proximal to the vertebral artery origin, any operative debris simply goes down the arm rather than into the vertebral artery and then downstream into the head. Stenoses involving this site typically are smooth, band-like lesions without associated ulceration or thrombus, and the incidence of distal embolization due to angioplasty is low. Conversely, the incidence of elastic stenoses is high, often resulting in suboptimal results.

REFERENCES

1. Hodgins GW, Dutton JW. Subclavian and carotid angioplasties for Takayasu's arteritis. *J Can Assn Radiol* 1982;33:205–207.
2. Mellière D, Becquemin JP, Benyahia NE, et al. Atherosclerotic disease of the innominate artery: current management and results. *J Cardiovasc Surg* 1992;33:319–323.
3. Owens LV, Tinsley EA, Criado E, et al. Extrathoracic reconstruction of arterial occlusive disease involving the supraaortic trunks. *J Vasc Surg* 1995;22:217–222.
4. Thomassen L, Aarli JA. Subclavian steal phenomenon: clinical and hemodynamic aspects. *Acta Neurol Scand* 1994;90:241–244.
5. Ackerman H, Diener HC, Seboldt H, Huth C. Ultrasonographic follow-up of subclavian stenosis and occlusion: natural history and surgical treatment. *Stroke* 1988;19:431–435.
6. Zeumer H. Survey of progress: vascular recanalizing techniques in interventional neuroradiology. *J Neurol* 1985;231:287–294.

CHAPTER 48

Intracranial Angioplasty

J.J. Connors III

GENERAL CONSIDERATIONS

The incidence of atherosclerotic intracranial vascular disease of hemodynamic significance is underappreciated both clinically and diagnostically. Most devastating thromboembolic neurologic events have been "shown" to arise from the carotid bifurcation or the heart, and attention has focused on these areas in recent years. Specifically, however, the apparent ease of correction of carotid bifurcation pathology has distracted the medical community from the active pursuit of treatment of other brachiocephalic vascular causes of stroke.

In a study by Hass et al. in 1968,[1] cerebral angiography was performed in 4748 patients. Intracranial stenoses were found in 22.6% of these patients. This is a considerable amount of pathology. Although the exact nature of these lesions has not been reported, they probably would be treatable by endovascular means. Lesions in the high cervical internal carotid artery (ICA) were present in about 8% of cases, the cavernous ICA in 6%, the siphon in 6%, and the distal ICA and M1 segment in about 6%.

In a large study of transient ischemic attacks (TIAs) and strokes, intracranial stenosis was found in 8% of patients and thought to be the cause of the cerebral ischemia. Intracranial occlusive disease is more common in blacks and females than in whites and males, in whom the lesions tend to be extracranial.[2, 3] Intracranial disease more often presents with an infarct than with TIAs. For this reason, it may be inappropriate to tell a patient to go home and return if he or she has more symptoms (which might, for practical purposes, preclude medical therapy). More likely than not, the next symptom will be a full-blown stroke (see Fig. 48–21, described later), even though it may take 1 to 7 days for symptoms to become maximal (100% of the patients in Caplan's study had infarcts).[3] Data suggest a high rate of subsequent stroke in a relatively short period of time (months) in untreated patients with inadequate cerebral reserve.[4] Unfortunately, the natural history of intracranial stenosis is not clearly known and will be the target of a new multicenter study now getting underway. Previous data from the Extracranial–Intracranial (EC-IC) Bypass Study Group as well as other data indicate that the stroke risk from middle cerebral artery (MCA) stenosis is in the range of 8% per year; this is without the degree of stenosis being accurately known (a residual hairlike lumen may have a far worse prognosis).[5, 6] Early data also indicate a stroke risk of at least 8% per year for intracranial ICA stenosis; this is for lesions with only a moderate degree of stenosis (50% or greater).

With the demise of the feasibility of EC-IC bypass surgery to treat intracranial stenoses, there is a greater need for aggressive therapy. Conversely, in some instances, a combined EC-IC bypass and angioplasty is the correct choice. Again, a thorough understanding of hemodynamics is *fundamental* to the practice of this specialty.

The lack of consideration of intracranial disease by the medical community also has stemmed from two other causes: an underappreciation of chronic ischemic effects and the lack of a realistic way to treat intracranial atherosclerotic disease. When there are tandem lesions, and the worst lesion is intracranial, it often is assumed that improving inflow (i.e., fixing the bifurcation lesion) will correct or improve the situation (this was the only treatment available in the past!). This may not be the case, however, and addressing the intracranial lesion is probably necessary.

Several factors have combined to change the approach to this disease process. These include the emerging appreciation of chronic cerebral ischemic effects; newly developed technologies that can reveal cerebral hypoperfusion (e.g., single-photon emission computed tomography scans and xenon-133 (^{133}Xe) computed tomography (CT) cerebral blood flow studies); the demonstration by acute intracranial thrombolytic therapy that many strokes are caused directly by local, intrinsic intracranial vascular disease; and the growing availability of advanced microendovascular therapeutic capabilities. In addition, many practitioners who treat patients with intracranial stenoses are now finding *nonfocal neurologic symptoms* that are associated with this disease (e.g., chronic headaches, weakness, tiredness, declining vision) and that are cured by angioplasty and revascularization. These soft signs may represent further indications for therapy in selected cases. However, as stated later, the presence of symptoms is not felt to be absolutely necessary before the treatment of certain lesions because the prognosis for intracranial stenoses may be so poor and warnings of impending doom may be lacking.

The diagnosis of intracranial vascular disease also is advancing with the progress in transcranial Doppler ultrasonography and magnetic resonance angiography (MRA). Although these modalities have not been perfected and are not widely available, their increasing use may reveal further the magnitude of this problem. Angiography remains the gold standard for evaluation of intracranial vascular lesions, particularly when symptoms are present.

Previous series do not directly address the underlying incidence of stroke in patients with a hairlike residual lumen of an intracranial vessel; indeed, it is very difficult even to make direct comparisons in studies such as these since measurement of these lesions accurately is very difficult. Statements such as "80% stenosis" have no meaning in a 2.5-mm vessel. This statement would indicate that the residual lumen is 0.5 mm, an extremely difficult size to measure.

LOCATION OF INTRACRANIAL ATHEROSCLEROTIC DISEASE

Typical intracranial atherosclerotic disease presents in primarily five locations: the ICA in the region of the siphon, the main trunk of the MCA, the distal vertebral artery, the vertebrobasilar junction, and the midportion of the basilar artery.

The study by Hass et al.[1] indicates that basilar artery stenoses are more common than any other intracranial stenosis, with an incidence of about 8% of all brachiocephalic lesions, which is surprisingly high. The intracranial vertebral artery accounts for about 4.4% of the lesions. The main branches of the MCA (M2), the main trunk of the anterior cerebral artery (A1), and the proximal portion of the posterior cerebral artery also may be affected. These locations are more rare, however, than those listed previously. An overview of the distribution of these lesions is given in Table 48–1.

Risk factors for development of intracranial stenosis appear to be primarily hypertension and diabetes, but traditional risk factors for atherosclerotic disease are also thought to play a part (e.g., smoking). In white patients, atherosclerotic disease generally affects different arterial trees at different ages: the aorta first, followed by the coronary arteries, peripheral arteries, extracranial carotid and vertebral arteries, and then the intracranial arteries. Blacks, however, have a higher frequency of *intracranial* large vessel occlusive disease than *extracranial* large vessel disease.[7–9] Chinese and Japanese patients are also more likely to develop intracranial vascular stenoses than extracranial stenoses.[10] The influence of lifestyle and diet are not clear at this time, but information suggests that these are significant factors, in addition to genetic influences. African blacks, for instance, do not appear to have the same rate of intracranial stenoses as do blacks who live in the United States. Race is still independently associated with this pattern of vascular pathology.[2, 10] The incidence of strokes among blacks is nearly double that among whites (about 642 per 100,000, compared with 339 per 100,000), and their subsequent death rate is also twice as high. The southeastern United States

T A B L E 4 8 - 1 Incidence of Atherosclerotic Lesions in the Brachiocephalic Vessels and Branches*

Vessel	Location	Side	Stenosis (%)	Occlusion (%)
Subclavian artery	Proximal	Left	12.4	2.5
Innominate artery	Proximal	Right	4.2	0.6
Vertebral artery	Origin	Left	22.3	5.7
		Right	18.4	4.0
	Mid-cervical	Left	5.6	4.4
		Right	5.4	3.2
	Distal	Left	3.8	3.2
		Right	4.9	2.8
Basilar artery			8.0	
Posterior cerebral artery	Origin	Left	2.6	2.6
		Right	1.0	0.7
Common carotid artery	Proximal	Right	3.2	1.0
Internal carotid artery	Origin	Left	34.1	8.5
		Right	33.8	8.5
	Mid-cervical	Left	9.1	8.7
		Right	8.0	8.6
	Petrous	Left	6.6	9.2
		Right	6.7	9.0
	Cavernous	Left	6.0	1.7
		Right	5.5	1.5
	Supraophthalmic	Left	3.3	1.4
		Right	2.8	1.2
Middle cerebral artery	M1	Left	4.1	2.1
		Right	3.5	2.2
Anterior cerebral artery	A1, A2	Left	3.2	1.7
		Right	3.2	1.5
Both extracranial and surgically inaccessible locations			33.3	
Surgically inaccessible			6.1	

*Data are based on a series of 3788 patients with cerebrovascular disease undergoing angiography. The numbers represent the percentage of patients studied with a lesion in the given location.

has a stroke rate that is 10% higher than in the remainder of the nation. Intracranial stenoses also tend to affect younger people far more often than extracranial vascular disease.[8]

Each anatomic location has its own clinical presentation, pathophysiologic development, and underlying implications for therapy. Typically, anterior circulation disease presents with brief, acute episodic unilateral symptoms (*if any*) (e.g., transient numbness, tingling, weakness, clumsiness, usually of the hand, face, or arm) or as a typical acute stroke. Recurrent classic focal TIAs suggest a local vascular cause. Extracranial stenosis causes this pattern more frequently than intracranial stenosis, however; 64% of extracranial lesions have this presentation, whereas only 20% of intracranial anterior circulation stenoses present with this finding, or any symptoms at all.[3] *These statistics indicate that a large number of intracranial lesions may not announce themselves clearly before there is a stroke.*

In a retrospective study of 1770 vessels by Borozan et al., isolated stenosis of the internal carotid artery (>20%) was found in 115 vessels (6.5%).[11] In another study by Keagy et al.,[12] severe stenosis (>80%) was found in 11 of 226 consecutively studied vessels (5%), and moderate stenosis (50% to 79%) was found in an additional 27 (11%). This is further evidence of the prevalence of this disease.

Posterior circulation (vertebral and basilar artery) disease can progress more slowly, with symptoms related to a vague unilateral or generalized clumsiness (such as gait disturbance) or dizziness, diplopia, and nausea (almost pathognomonic of posterior fossa vascular insufficiency when combined with other symptoms) as well as a spectrum of other findings. Drop attacks have been recorded in 10% to 15% of patients with vertebrobasilar insufficiency. Once these symptoms start, they can be relentlessly progressive, either in hours, weeks, or months. No large series has addressed the frequency of TIAs in patients with intracranial vertebral artery or basilar artery stenosis, but it may be as high as 50%.[13]

RATIONALE FOR TREATMENT OF INTRACRANIAL STENOSES

If an incidentally discovered lesion is tight and supplies a vital territory with no collateral support, it may reasonably be judged to require treatment even if it is asymptomatic. Early, nonstatistical data indicate that a tight stenosis (i.e., a hairlike lumen) with evidence of hypoperfusion on cerebral blood flow challenge test (see Chapter 3) is associated with an incidence of major stroke that is markedly above normal.[4] These data are not specific for intracranial vasculature, and extrapolation may not be correct or appropriate. Large-scale studies are necessary for accurate statements to be made concerning the clinical implications of this situation, but it appears that the risk of near-term stroke is high (as many as 25% to 30% may suffer a stroke within 19 months).[4] The outcome of a preocclusive lesion (i.e., a vessel with a hairlike residual lumen) is statistically unknown but precarious, particularly if symptomatic purely from hypoperfusion.

A trial of intracranial angioplasty with evaluation of cerebral perfusion using an acetazolamide challenge test indicated that in patients with an abnormal response to acetazolamide challenge, correction of the stenosis was associated with improvement in symptoms. All patients who showed improvement had failed the challenge test, whereas five of six patients exhibiting no improvement after angioplasty showed normal vasodilatory response to the acetazolamide challenge.[14]

Natural History of Intracranial Stenoses

Degree of Stenosis

Discussion of the natural history of intracranial stenoses is difficult when previous studies with varying patient populations and severity of disease are analyzed. These studies were not performed by scientists with a clear understanding of the disease process, nor, often, with this evaluation being the primary concern of the study.

Part of the difficulty in this situation is technical. When a 2-mm vessel has an atherosclerotic narrowing to a lumen of 0.5 mm, it is only a 75% stenosis; but a 0.5-mm lumen can vanish in an instant. More important, however, is whether it is possible to differentiate a 0.8-mm lumen from a 0.4-mm lumen. Is it truly possible to measure in units of *0.1 mm*, particularly when using digital subtraction equipment with only 512-pixel resolution? Other questions that must be answered include: (1) who is doing the measuring, (2) what projection is to be used, and (3) what magnification is being used. The difference between a 0.4-mm lumen and a 0.8-mm lumen may be crucial, but it is only a difference of *0.4 mm*!

In addition, statements concerning stenoses in comparison with a preexisting large vessel do not take into account finite limits (i.e., a lumen can only get so small before it vanishes). A residual lumen of 0.7 mm in a vessel of 2 mm is not much different from a residual lumen of 0.7 mm in a vessel of 3.5 mm; both situations occur commonly in the intracranial vasculature. However, the degree of stenosis of the first lesion is only 60% whereas the degree of stenosis of the latter is 80%. Is there truly a difference? The 0.7-mm lumen is still teetering on the brink of occlusion and in both cases can carry only a very limited amount of blood. The hemodynamic situation would in all likelihood be identical, but certainly severe and *unpredictable* in both instances. *We therefore believe that statements concerning intracranial stenoses expressed as a degree of stenosis are inaccurate and misleading.*

A tight stenosis with minimal or variable symptoms therefore can present a difficult therapeutic decision. The lesion may have already declared itself (TIAs or reversible ischemic neurologic deficits

[RINDs]) and would seem to require intervention. Cases have been observed that appeared to be similar but, when aggressively followed (with short-interval angiography or clinically), took different courses (i.e., after 3 or 6 months one lesion would be asymptomatic and the other would be abruptly occlusive, resulting in a stroke). Warnings of impending disaster may be absent (only 20% of patients had warnings before a stroke in one study) and the first indication of a problem can be a full-blown stroke.

The dynamic nature of intracranial stenoses was demonstrated in a study by Akins et al,[15a] who reviewed all patients at their institution who underwent more than one cerebral angiogram (at least 6 months apart). After excluding patients with arteriovenous malformations, aneurysms, or vasospasm, they identified 21 patients with 45 intracranial stenoses of at least 50% described in the reports of their initial studies. The mean follow-up interval was 26.7 months. Overall, the average stenosis was 43.9% initially and 51.8% at follow-up ($P = .032$) Internal carotid artery lesions tended to be stable (51.2% initially versus 52.6% at follow-up). Lesions in the anterior, middle, and posterior cerebral arteries progressed from 32.4% to 49.7% ($P = .037$). When lesions demonstrating a minimum of 10% change were analyzed, 20% of internal carotid artery lesions progressed and 14% regressed, while 61% of more distal lesions progressed and 28% regressed. Only four patients experienced TIAs during the follow-up period; of these, only two had progression of their lesion.

It is also appropriate to realize that the stenosis has been slowly growing due to atheromatous process, not thrombus. Anticoagulants would therefore appear to aid only in prevention of an *abrupt final occlusion* caused by thrombus, and not in preventing progression of the disease to an inevitable occlusion. Preventing or delaying this occlusion is not an unworthy form of therapy, however.

Warfarin-Aspirin Symptomatic Intracranial Disease Study

As part of the Warfarin-Aspirin Symptomatic Intracranial Disease (WASID) study,[15] 68 patients with stenoses of 50% or greater were followed. Forty-two were treated with warfarin, whereas 26 received aspirin as therapy (physician's choice); all patients were followed for a mean of 13.8 months. During that time, 15 patients had strokes, of which 10 were in the territory of the target vessel (6 were receiving warfarin and 4 were receiving aspirin, statistically equivalent proportions). The rates of stroke in the same territory were 2/5 (40%) for bilateral vertebral artery stenoses, 2/26 (8%) for unilateral vertebral artery stenosis, 5/28 (18%) for basilar artery stenosis, and 1/9 (11%) for posterior cerebral or posterior inferior cerebellar artery stenosis. Patients with greater than 80% stenosis had only a slightly higher rate of stroke (6/37; 16%) than patients with 50% to 80% (4/31; 13%); this difference is not statistically signifi-

cant. All of these rates are higher than the rate of stroke in most studies examining extracranial carotid artery disease.

Middle Cerebral Artery Stenosis

As stated earlier, data concerning stenoses of the MCA indicate that these lesions carry a risk of stroke of approximately *8% per year*[6]; this is a high-risk lesion. Because many of these lesions occur in younger individuals, there is a very high cumulative stroke risk (e.g., a one in four chance of stroke in only 3 years). This study by Bogousslavsky et al.[6] revealed that 58% of the Asian population enrolled in the EC-IC bypass study were eligible for the MCA atherosclerosis study, whereas only 34% of blacks and only 18% of whites were, again emphasizing the racial differences in this disease. Again, only about one third of patients had a warning TIA prior to stroke. The most common presentation was an immediately completed deficit. During the follow-up period, 11.7% per year of the medically treated (not untreated) patients had additional cerebrovascular events.

Caplan et al.[3] studied patients with MCA occlusive disease. This study demonstrated that occlusion of the MCA is always (100%) associated with stroke (although not necessarily immediately completed), as opposed to occlusion of the ICA, which is associated with stroke only 60% of the time. The incidence of death subsequent to cardiac causes was less in the MCA occlusive group than in the ICA group.

Patients with MCA disease were more often black, female, and younger and had fewer TIAs than the patients with ICA disease (20% versus 64%).[3] About one third had a preceding headache in each group.

About 5% of MCA occlusions are thought on the basis of autopsy data to be caused by intrinsic atherosclerotic lesions of the MCA rather than being embolic in origin.[16]

Internal Carotid Artery Stenosis

The prognosis of intracranial ICA atherosclerotic disease is not clearly known, but several studies have provided a fairly clear idea of the prognosis of this lesion.

In a study of 66 patients, Marzewski et al.[17] found that stenosis was in the intrapetrous segment in 14 patients, intracavernous in 65, and supraclinoid in 6 (some patients had multiple stenoses). Associated conditions were coronary artery disease (57.6%), diabetes (50%), hypertension (more than 150/90 mm Hg, 39.4%), and peripheral vascular disease (15.2%). During the follow-up (average 3.9 years), 18 patients (27.3%) had ischemic events; 8 (12.1%) had one or more TIAs, and 10 (15.2%) had a stroke. The observed rate of stroke for patients 35 years or age or older was 13 times the expected infarction rate for a normal population. This difference was even more dramatic in the subset of patients under 65 years of age, in whom the rate was approximately *300 times normal*.

In this study,[17] 33 patients (50%) died during follow-up (3 times the normal rate); 55% of these deaths were cardiac-related. Intracranial ICA disease is not only dangerous from a direct standpoint but appears to be a marker for heart disease.

In the study by Craig et al.,[18] 58 patients with intracranial ICA stenosis were followed. At the end of the 30-month follow-up period, only 33% were alive and free of subsequent cerebrovascular events. Of the patients studied, 43% died during follow-up; 36% of these deaths were because of stroke and 44% because of cardiac disease. Of the 58 patients, 43% had cerebrovascular events, including 17 strokes (29%), 9 of which were fatal. This resulted in a rate of ipsilateral major stroke of 7.6% per year.

There was no significant difference between patients with symptomatic lesions and those with asymptomatic lesions. Of asymptomatic patients, 36% had cerebrovascular events, whereas 45% of symptomatic patients had events. The mortality rate for asymptomatic patients was 45%, whereas 42% of symptomatic patients died. *The presence of symptoms was therefore not a predictor of increased risk of stroke or death.*

A review by Wechsler et al. in 1986 revealed similar findings.[19]

Basilar Artery Stenosis

The prognosis of basilar artery stenosis is not well known. The outcome of occlusion is more well known; acute occlusion of the basilar artery carries a nearly certain death sentence unless the vessel can be reopened. In the largest series reported (by Hacke et al.[20]), only 3 of 22 patients who received conventional anticoagulant therapy survived; all had a moderate clinical deficit. Of those receiving aggressive fibrinolytic therapy, all patients in whom no recanalization was achieved died (24 of 24). If recanalization was achieved, 14 of 19 patients survived, but only 10 had a favorable outcome.

In another series, the development of the need for intubation was a fatal prognostic sign,[21] but aggressive revascularization efforts were not undertaken. In a series reported by Cross et al. (Washington University, St. Louis, MO) at the Interventional Neuroradiology Morbidity and Mortality meeting (Val d'Isère, France, 1997), there was an overall survival rate (with aggressive intracranial therapy) of only 35%. Distal basilar artery occlusions did not have as grim a prognosis as proximal occlusions: 71% of patients with distal stenoses survived whereas only 15% of patients with proximal occlusions survived. Of these survivors of distal basilar artery occlusion, however, only 27% had a good outcome. Factors that did not predict outcome were age, delay of therapy, and CT scan appearance. However, delay of therapy is difficult to measure in many patients with this disease because of the slow or stuttering progression with resultant delayed presentation and work-up.

In summary, if there are neurologic signs consistent with the diagnosis of basilar artery occlusion, the prognosis is extremely grim. Prevention of occlusion is the goal of therapy in the setting of intracranial stenosis involving the basilar artery.

Extracranial-Intracranial Bypass

Bypassing intracranial stenoses can be devastating. The small residual lumen is open only *because of the antegrade trickle of flow.* If a high flow shunt is placed distally, the arterial pressure gradient that was keeping the flow going and the parent vessel patent is removed. The stenosis then thromboses, and the vessel downstream from the stenosis may then also thrombose all the way to the shunt implant site, thrombosing any tiny perforators along the way. This commonly occurs in the periphery (e.g., loss of collateral flow in the knee region associated with a femoral-popliteal bypass) and is a *predictable* consequence of certain hemodynamic circumstances. It has been demonstrated to occur in the head as well. This is particularly devastating in the posterior fossa where distal bypasses have been performed that resulted in thrombosis of the basilar artery.

In the report by the EC-IC Bypass Study Group, 1377 patients were evaluated, with an average follow-up of 55 months.[5] Of these patients, 714 were assigned to receive optimal medical therapy and 663 to receive the same regimen with the addition of a superficial temporal artery to MCA branch bypass. The postoperative bypass patency rate was 96%.

The 30-day surgical mortality was 0.6%, and the 30-day major stroke rate was 2.5% (an annual rate of 30%). Nonfatal and fatal stroke occurred both more often and earlier in the patients who received the bypasses. A separate analysis of patients with different angiographic lesions did not identify a subgroup that received any benefit from surgery.

Patients with severe MCA stenosis were among those with the worst outcomes. These patients, who were thought to be the most likely to benefit from the bypass procedure, were actually harmed the most. This was later realized to be because the stenosis progressed to occlusion after the bypass was performed; this phenomenon had been described in at least one paper before the EC-IC bypass study.[22] Additional reports indicated further dangers; *in a series of 18 patients with stenotic lesions of the MCA or ICA, 39% (7 patients) had postoperative ischemic complications.*[23] It was postulated that when an alternate means of perfusion of the distal territory of the MCA was offered, there was no longer sufficient flow through the stenotic segment to prevent thrombosis of the proximal main trunk. This resulted in obliteration of the lenticulostriate arteries and thus the basal ganglia and internal capsule, with subsequent devastating neurologic results. This outcome has been shown repeatedly to be the case in subsequent studies.

Diagnosis of Intracranial Large Vessel Atherosclerotic Disease

The gold standard for evaluation of intracranial vascular pathology is cerebral angiography. Performed by a skilled angiographer, the risk of this procedure is less than 1%.

Although MRA is gaining popularity, particularly among neurologists, the fact that this modality misses a large percentage of stenoses renders it inadequate for evaluation of any significant symptomatology. The ability of MRA to detect occlusion is much greater than its ability to detect stenosis. MRA has 97% sensitivity and 99% specificity rates for occlusion but is unable to measure any intracranial stenosis accurately.[24] If there are significant symptoms referable to a single vessel, and no cause is seen on magnetic resonance imaging (MRI) and MRA, this does not constitute a complete evaluation.

The presence or absence of findings on MRI or MRA does not influence whether an angiogram will be obtained if there are symptoms worth investigating. This is particularly true when considering the carotid siphon, a location notorious for artifacts on MRA. If an intracranial reason for the problem is found on MRA, this should be further evaluated with angiography.

MRA has been shown to be unable to detect basilar artery thrombosis in a large percentage of patients with this diagnosis (almost 50%). For this reason, it is mandatory to perform an adequate cerebral angiogram to evaluate any significant symptoms, particularly any that are unexplained by other evaluations (e.g., carotid and vertebral artery duplex ultrasound). Basilar artery occlusion or severe stenosis is a life-threatening disease and should be approached with the appropriate degree of aggressiveness and concern.

Transcranial Doppler ultrasound also can yield useful information if performed by a skilled sonographer. The ability of this modality to detect occlusion is good (but not as good as MRA), but it provides more accurate data concerning hemodynamics than does MRA.[24] This is particularly true of MCA stenosis. Once again, if there is a need to accurately evaluate the intracranial vasculature, an angiogram is mandatory.

Clinical Presentation of Stenoses In Various Vascular Territories

As stated previously, the primary symptoms related to stenoses in various territories are consistent with the symptoms of stroke in these areas but are typically less severe (see Chapter 6). Stenosis of the main trunk of the MCA yields varying degrees (arm worse than leg) of unilateral hemisensory loss, hemiplegia or hemiparesis, dysarthria, neglect (if very severe or if in a completed infarct), and global aphasia (if on the left side). Generally, the symptoms before infarction are not as severe as the typical stroke symptoms and may be confined to a much smaller region of the body (e.g., in the hand alone). Speech difficulties (e.g., word finding problems) are common symptoms as well. These symptoms can be consistent and repetitive from TIA to TIA.

The most common theme in the symptoms of intra-

cranial stenosis without true occlusion is their relationship to blood pressure. When the patient stands, the blood pressure may temporarily drop enough to cause the symptoms to appear; alternatively, the symptoms may be worse in the morning than later in the day. We have had several patients whose symptoms appeared to be brought on by dehydration (e.g., working in the yard in the heat and sun). In addition to degree of hydration, caffeine intake, nicotine serum level, and other factors may also play a role.

Basilar Artery and Intracranial Vertebral Artery Stenosis

Intracranial stenoses in the posterior circulation typically occur in the distal vertebral artery (either at the level of the posterior inferior cerebellar artery [PICA] or just beyond), at the vertebrobasilar junction, or in the trunk of the basilar artery (previously thought to occur most typically at the junction of the proximal and middle third, but now thought to be almost evenly distributed throughout its length).[9] As opposed to anterior circulation occlusive pathologies, the distal vertebral or basilar artery is not typically a destination for embolus (and when it is, the embolus is thought usually to lodge at the basilar apex, not in the midportion of the basilar artery). The basilar artery is a primary occlusive site anywhere along its length.[13]

Clinical Findings

Stenoses in the basilar artery can cause a wide range of clinical findings, depending on whether the stenosis involves the proximal segment, the distal basilar artery, or the basilar tip and the ascending perforators arising from the P1 segments of the posterior cerebral arteries (the usual source of the vascular supply to the reticular-activating system). Usually, these symptoms are vague and often associated with dizziness.

If the basilar artery is only stenotic, the symptoms may be varied and changing. Ataxia, dizziness, and visual disturbance, combined with dysarthria, are classic (similar symptoms can be seen with distal vertebral artery stenosis if the opposite vertebral artery is occluded). All of these symptoms are not necessarily present, however, and dizziness alone can herald the onset of this disease.

If the basilar artery is occluded, there is usually a progressive downhill course, in hours or days. Symptoms can be related to cranial nerve dysfunction or long tract signs to varying degrees. The patient may lapse into coma with varying degrees of bilateral weakness (frequently asymmetric). Dizziness is the most common symptom with or without other brainstem symptoms.[13]

On rare occasions, the basilar artery may gradually occlude and the patient may be asymptomatic. The collaterals have had time to develop sufficiently to keep the territory alive. Trying to open an occlusion, even when absolutely necessary, is fraught with danger, both of dissection and of thrombus formation with perforator occlusion and distal embolization. *If basilar artery occlusion is found incidentally in an asymptomatic individual, it is best to leave this situation alone.*

Thalamic ischemia (resulting from distal basilar artery or posterior communicating artery disease) introduces additional symptoms, including sensory disturbance and alteration in level of consciousness; these symptoms are not usually present without infarct. Amnesia (or memory disturbances) can be caused by the ischemic effects on the thalamus or medial temporal lobe (amygdala-hippocampal complex), and was the presenting complaint in one of our patients. This may be a more common presentation of posterior fossa ischemia than is commonly thought.

The most dreaded outcome of basilar artery occlusion is the locked-in syndrome. This is caused by bilateral infarction of the pons. The patient is awake and paralyzed and can only blink, with or without some vertical eye movement. This can be caused by primary basilar artery occlusion or bilateral vertebral artery occlusion in a patient with an isolated posterior fossa (which is functionally the situation in up to 40% of the population).

Posterior cerebral artery ischemia affects the occipital lobe as well as the medial temporal lobe, resulting in a wide range of symptoms, including hemianopsia, visual agnosia, hemisensory loss (thalamic involvement), and memory disturbance (usually short-term, secondary to the medial temporal lobe involvement). If the top of the basilar artery is occluded with resultant bilateral occipital infarction, cortical blindness occurs. We have had a patient with posterior cerebral artery stenosis and gradual visual decline over a period of years, to the point that he could no longer watch television; after angioplasty of the posterior cerebral artery he is able to read without glasses.

Posterior fossa symptoms associated with vertebral artery stenosis are varied and include vertigo (the most common symptom), drop attacks, ipsilateral ataxia (falling to one side), contralateral weakness (usually affecting the arm and leg equally, as opposed to anterior circulation symptoms, which most frequently involve the arm more than the leg), vertical diplopia, dysarthria, hearing loss, nystagmus, dysphagia, and ipsilateral facial weakness or numbness. Hearing loss (or decline) is caused by occlusion of the internal auditory artery, which arises from the vertebrobasilar system, usually from the anterior inferior cerebellar artery (AICA).[25]

Distal vertebral artery stenosis can also rarely produce generalized weakness that is unilateral or diffusely bilateral (unilateral or bilateral paramedian pontine ischemia), pseudobulbar palsy, various eye movement disorders (unilateral or bilateral), internuclear ophthalmoplegia, and Horner's syndrome. The level of consciousness may be affected if the reticular-activating system is also ischemic; this is a grave sign (as it is in any hypoperfusion state).

In distal vertebral artery stenoses, sensory abnormalities may be absent because the PICA is not affected, and this vessel can supply the posterior pons and cerebellum (and often the entire cerebellum, covering the territory of the superior cerebellar artery through pial collaterals). The sensory tracts may therefore be preserved.

Headache is usually associated with abrupt occlusion of the basilar artery (or a stroke of any kind), and not necessarily with stenosis of the basilar artery. Some patients (with intracranial lesions in any vascular distribution), however, have chronic, unexplained focal headaches, often for a long time, which are cured after angioplasty.

The "top of the basilar" artery syndrome is characterized by emotional or behavioral disturbances, eye movement disorders, and pupillary disorders. Dysar-

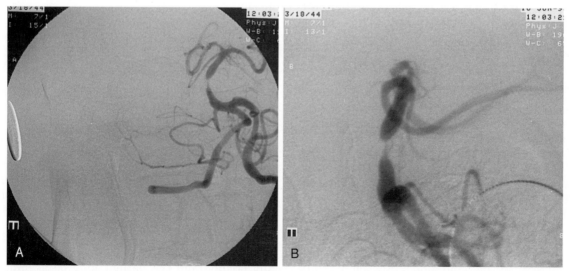

Figure 48-1 Case 1. This 51-year-old diabetic man presented with the acute onset of a right cranial nerve III palsy and dizziness. An angiogram was requested to exclude a posterior communicating artery aneurysm. Instead, severe stenosis of the midportion of the basilar artery was found, as is shown on the posteroanterior (PA) *(A)* and lateral *(B)* views (left vertebral artery injection).

Case 1 continues

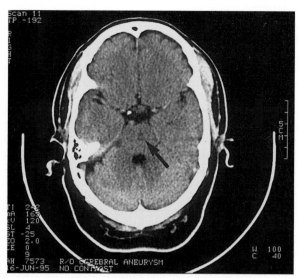

Figure 48-2 Computed tomographic (CT) scan obtained on admission revealed a small pontine infarct *(arrow)*.

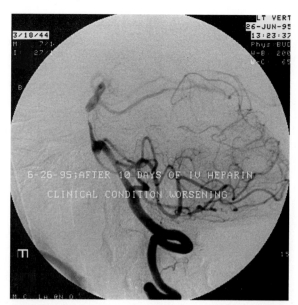

Figure 48-3 After the desperate situation had been revealed by the angiogram, the patient was placed on intravenous heparin as we were out of town. Two days before our return, the patient's clinical condition began to deteriorate; he became more somnolent and developed hiccups, nausea, and vomiting. Repeat angiography revealed near-total occlusion of the basilar artery with only a residual thread of patent lumen. Note that the flow is so slow that the contrast is actually layering in the posterior (dependent) portion of the proximal lumen. Obviously the heparin had not prevented progression of the pathologic process, despite a "therapeutic" activated partial thromboplastin time (aPTT).

thria may be an additional presenting feature. If the posterior communicating artery is deficient or absent, additional deficits occur related to thalamic ischemia and posterior cerebral artery ischemia (which affects the medial temporal lobe as well as the occipital lobe, as noted previously). Short-term memory loss also can occur (because of medial temporal lobe involvement).

All these posterior fossa intracranial lesions are extremely difficult to deal with and are dangerous with or without treatment, and they present either with vague, slowly progressive symptoms or a rapid downhill course (Case 1, Figs. 48–1 to 48–7 and Case 2, Figs. 48–8 and 48–9). The symptoms can be confus-

ing in their vagueness, mostly depending on whether the artery is still patent or recently occluded.

More specific symptoms may appear, depending on which side branch (e.g., the superior cerebellar ar-

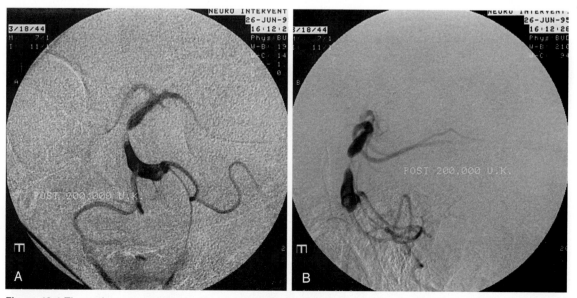

Figure 48-4 The patient was now 2 weeks past the original acute event. Urokinase infusion was begun in the hope of not only returning the basilar artery to the condition it had been in 10 days before, but possibly improving the stenosis to the point where angioplasty might no longer be necessary (basilar artery angioplasty can be a dangerous procedure). After 200,000 units of urokinase had been infused over an hour, PA *(A)* and lateral *(B)* views reveal only minimal improvement. Note the position of the microcatheter tip.

Case 1 continues

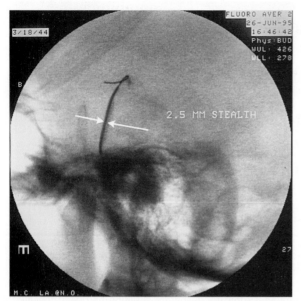

Figure 48-5 A 2.5-mm STEALTH angioplasty balloon (Target Therapeutics) is in place and inflated *(arrows)*. The balloon size was purposely chosen to be undersized; an intimal tear is far worse than an inadequate response, and a 2-mm lumen is entirely adequate for this location. A very gradual inflation was used, with maximal expansion occurring at only 3 atmospheres pressure. Even though the basilar artery was occluded for several minutes, the patient's vital signs were unaffected (his true level of consciousness was not evaluated; he had been sedated intravenously and the anesthesiologist had been warned to watch for any sudden change in clinical or respiratory status).

tery) is most affected. Occlusion of this vessel results in severe ipsilateral cerebellar ataxia (middle or superior cerebellar peduncles, or both), nausea, vomiting, dysarthria, loss of pain and temperature sensation over half the body, and possible partial deafness.

Moderate basilar artery stenosis may be treated with anticoagulants or aspirin. This treatment has been successful in patients with only 50% stenosis,[13] implying a residual lumen of greater than 1 mm. More severe stenosis may lead to occlusion, which is almost invariably fatal, as noted earlier (see Chapter 59).

Another indirect finding associated with posterior fossa stenosis (usually basilar artery stenosis) with secondary ischemia is idiopathic hypertension. We have observed several patients with posterior circulation lesions and hypertension who, after angioplasty to correct the stenosis, have required discontinuing of their antihypertensive medications (to prevent symptomatic *hypotension*) (see Figs. 48–8 and 48–9 and Case 3, Figs. 48–10 to 48–12; both patients experienced this phenomenon).

Typical locations for intracranial vertebral artery stenoses are at the point where the vertebral artery turns cephalad (in the region of the PICA origin) and at the vertebrobasilar junction. When dilating in the region of the PICA origin, care must be taken not to occlude this origin with an intimal dissection. The origin of the PICA is variable and can be immediately proximal, distal, or at the site of a stenosis in this location. Case 4, presented in Figures 48-13 and 48-14 demonstrates an unusual possibility; the PICA arises both before and after the stenosis!

Diagnosis

The primary problems associated with making the correct diagnosis of posterior fossa ischemia are the fact that the onset of symptoms is often vague and that the slow progression of symptoms sometimes results in a nonurgent approach. This may allow time for work-up but may lull one into missing the window of opportunity available when the disease first presents itself. If the patient has been lucky enough to have a warning, the treating physicians are at an advantage and should make the best of it.

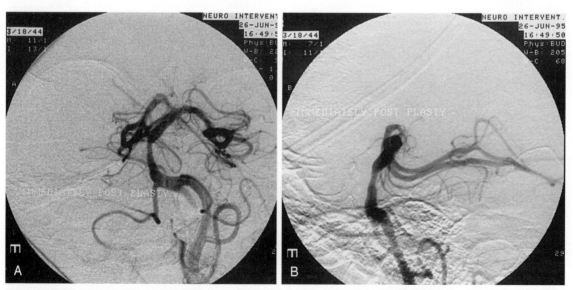

Figure 48-6 PA *(A)* and lateral *(B)* views immediately after angioplasty. The result is excellent; the lumen is clean and adequate for the purpose. No dissection is seen. A clean intima with minimal endothelial damage is less likely to display a hyperactive thrombogenic response. After 1 hour of postangioplasty observation, the angioplasty site was considered to be stable.

Case 1 continues

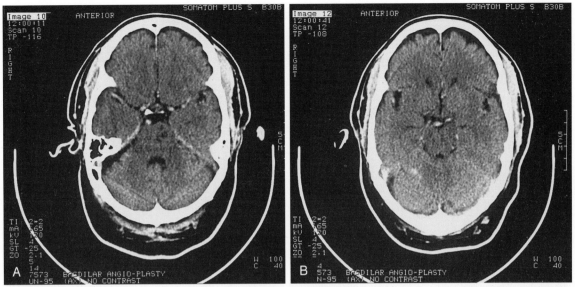

Figure 48-7 CT scan obtained immediately after the angioplasty (the time on the scan is incorrect). Note the preexisting infarcts in the pons *(A)* and the blush in the right cerebellar hemisphere *(B)*. (Is this related to the infusion location of the urokinase?) Although the patient's clinical status was now stabilized, the decision not to treat this lesion by angioplasty immediately (two weeks before) was perhaps unfortunate. This is typical of cases in which a trial of anticoagulation may not be the correct choice. The failure of this "test" may be permanent. This patient went on to make a good neurologic recovery.

Once thrombus has formed or the vessel is occluded, the rescue is far more difficult and dangerous.

MRI combined with MRA, performed specifically to look for this disease, can provide useful information[24] and should be obtained urgently in anyone suspected of having posterior fossa crescendo ischemia. MRI and MRA can demonstrate most vertebral artery etiologies of posterior fossa ischemia. However, in a study performed by Castillo et al., MRI revealed ab-sence of flow in only 6 of 11 basilar arteries that were occluded.[26] This is a very poor record because this lesion is usually fatal and was missed in nearly 50% of cases. The possibility of missing a significant finding, combined with the inability to evaluate the intracranial hemodynamics, renders this form of evaluation (MRI and MRA) inadequate (at least for a

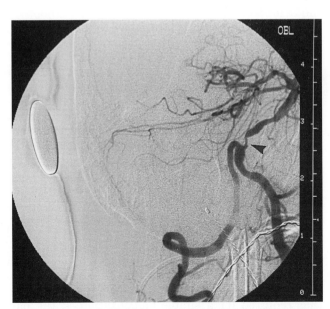

Figure 48-8 Case 2. A 75-year-old woman with posterior fossa symptoms of episodic ataxia, blurry vision, dizziness, and dysarthria, unrelieved by medication. A magnified PA left vertebral artery injection revealed a stenosis *(arrowhead)* just within the basilar artery, beyond the vertebrobasilar junction.

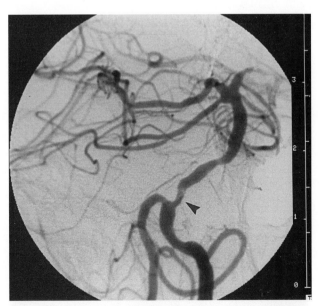

Figure 48-9 Postangioplasty appearance of the vessel. Note that the angioplasty was purposely undersized to prevent intimal damage at this most dangerous location *(arrowhead)*. While the vessel does not look beautiful, the lumen is without dissection. Indeed, the stenosis in the midbasilar artery is now as flow restricting as the proximal lesion. This intentional undersizing is routinely performed in attempt to avoid severe intimal damage.

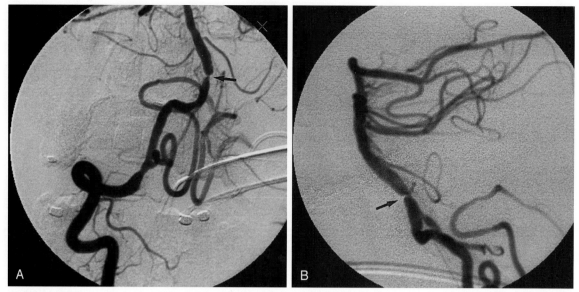

Figure 48-10 Case 3. PA *(A)* and lateral *(B)* right vertebral injection revealing an extremely tight stenosis of the basilar artery *(arrow)* slightly distal to the vertebrobasilar junction. This stenosis was totally inapparent on a previous magnetic resonance imaging (MRI) scan as well as on a previous angiogram. If the angiographic image had been obtained in a straight PA projection, the portions of the artery proximal and distal to the stenosis would overlap, thus obscuring the stenosis.

disease that can be life threatening in a short period of time) unless supplemented by angiography; this has been shown to be the case clinically on several occasions (both our experience and anecdotal reports).

In a patient who has serious posterior fossa symptoms, when there is any confusion whatsoever about the diagnosis (even after MRI), angiography is still the gold standard and should be performed urgently. This is particularly true if there is any possibility that treatment will be rendered from an endovascular standpoint (the only real hope of success for basilar artery thrombosis).[20]

This disease is one of the few diagnostic emergencies for a neurologist and should not be evaluated in a leisurely fashion.

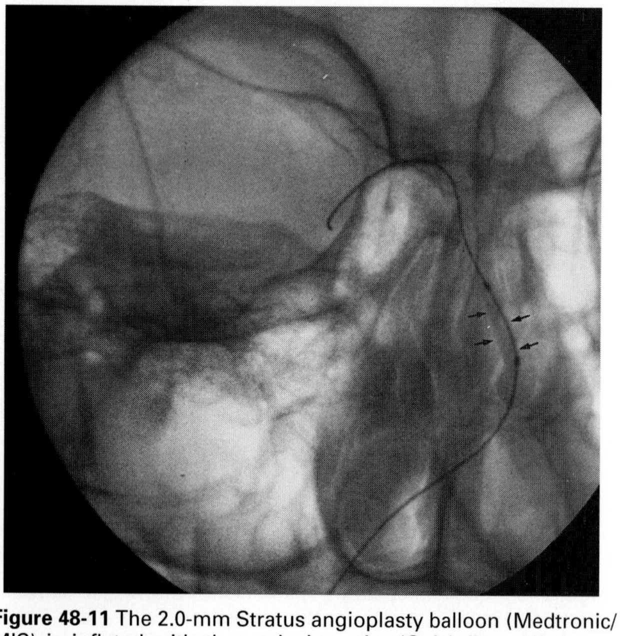

Technical Approach to Posterior Fossa Angioplasty

The overwhelming consideration in the specific technique for treatment of this disease is the pathophysiology of the angioplasty procedure and the vascular response to this process (described in detail in Chapter 41).

The particular vascular approach to each of these posterior fossa stenotic locations is nearly the same and raises issues similar to those raised when planning a vertebral origin angioplasty or stent procedure. Both distal intracranial vertebral artery and basilar artery lesions are approached through the vertebral artery, so safe distal access must be obtained (see Chapter 3).

An adequate guide catheter should be used in all cases, owing to the necessity to deploy a STEALTH (Target Therapeutics) or Stratus (Medtronic/MIS) angioplasty balloon and the need to perform repeated injections of contrast around this (large) microcatheter to evaluate the vascular status. In addition, a stable platform for deployment of the microangioplasty catheter requires a degree of stiffness beyond that required for a simple embolization. If the parent vessel permits, we therefore use a 7-Fr. Lumax Neuroguide catheter (Cook, Inc.). If the parent vessel is too small or tortuous for this catheter, a 6-Fr. FasGUIDE (Target Therapeutics) is used. If the ver-

Figure 48-11 The 2.0-mm Stratus angioplasty balloon (Medtronic/MIS) is inflated with the occlusion wire (Quicksilver-10) downstream in the right posterior cerebral artery. When using this angioplasty catheter, it is possible to leave the wire in a comfortable position and freely move the angioplasty balloon into the correct location.

Case 3 continues

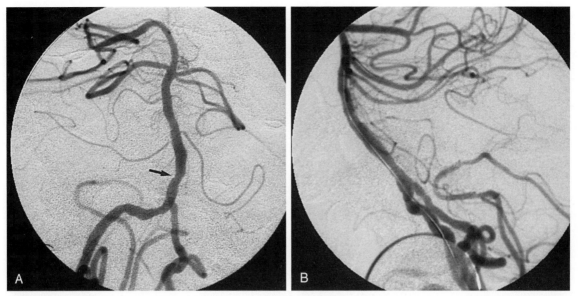

Figure 48-12 Postangioplasty PA *(A)* and lateral *(B)* views of the basilar artery reveal an ideal appearance. The extremely slow dilation did not result in intimal damage, and the risk of this vessel acutely thrombosing after the angioplasty was therefore felt to be low, but delayed observation for 1 hour was still performed to observe for this.

tebral artery is too small for even this catheter, a 5-Fr. Omniguide catheter (Medtronic/MIS) can be used with small angioplasty balloons, or alternatively, a 7-, 8-, or 9-Fr. Brite-Tip catheter (Cordis Corp.) can be placed in the subclavian artery and the angioplasty catheter can be deployed from there. The Brite-Tip is a nontapered guide catheter (in terms of stiffness) that is a very stable platform in this difficult proximal deployment position. If it is necessary to deploy the microangioplasty balloon catheter from this proximal position, a 9-Fr. Brite-Tip is usually used.

The particular vertebral artery to be accessed may be self-evident owing to the lack of choice. The portal of entry into the vascular tree (arm or leg) can make a large difference to the success or failure of the case; more typically, it adds to the ease of the case. Vectors of force are very important in these cases in order to get the angioplasty catheter to its intended target.

Dilation to a less than optimal size is indicated for any posterior fossa location (true for all intracranial angioplasties but particularly for distal vertebral and basilar arteries).[27] As stated previously, the risk of

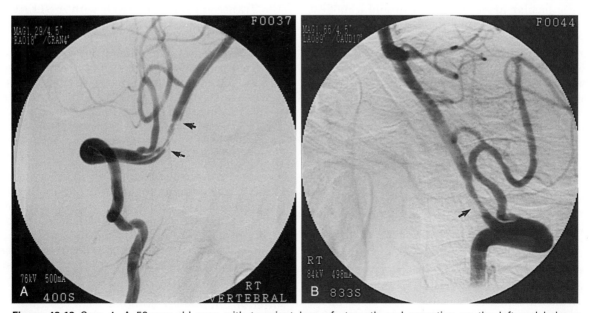

Figure 48-13 Case 4. A 52-year-old man with transient loss of strength and sensation on the left and balance disturbance and dizziness. This persisted for several days and gradually cleared, with only minimal residual dysesthesia. PA *(A)* and lateral *(B)* views of a right vertebral artery angiogram reveal a tight stenosis of the distal vertebral artery at a typical location for atherosclerosis, the acute turn at the skull base *(black arrows)*. The vessel just proximal and distal to the stenosis measured 2.4 and 2.7 mm in diameter, respectively. A 2-mm balloon was used to dilate this lesion (note the wire in place through the lesion, with the balloon marker slightly proximal to the lesion *[A]*).

Case 4 continues

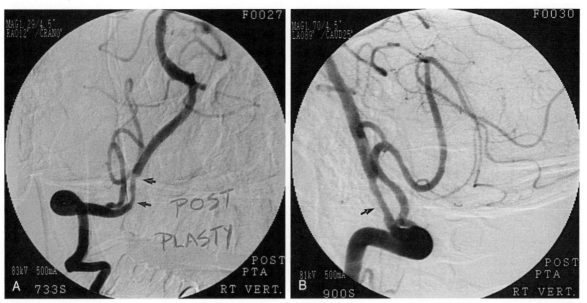

Figure 48-14 PA (A) and lateral (B) views after angioplasty. The stenosis is not much improved. Although it does look smoother on the PA view, it is obviously underdilated. This was achieved without a dissection, however, and the flow was greatly improved. It is against our policy to cross a fresh angioplasty site to retreat a lesion (unless the true lumen can be "saved" with an exchange microwire); the intima is allowed to heal before repeat angioplasty is attempted. This lesion will probably need retreatment with a larger balloon at the 3-month follow-up.

intimal damage is extreme, and a significant increase in flow can be achieved with even a modest increase in size. For this reason, the use of a small angioplasty balloon is required. The basilar artery is usually about 3 mm; as noted earlier, the smallest STEALTH or Stratus angioplasty balloon is 2 mm, which is adequate for good flow. The vessel may not maintain a lumen of 2 mm, however, and an increase in angioplasty balloon size may be required. Starting small is still probably the best choice, because the brittleness of the basilar artery is unknown and a modest increase in the size of the lumen is nearly always adequate to resolve the hypoperfusion.

Even though a less than ideal angioplasty result may be obtained and the chance of restenosis is increased, an undersized result is probably optimal. Purposefully sizing the balloon too small also helps avoid rupture of the basilar artery[28] or a devastating dissection.

Slow dilation of these lesions is required to avoid damaging the vessel (see "Technique of Elective Intracranial Angioplasty"). The presence of small perforators may increase the technical difficulty of angioplasty of the basilar artery. Instead of one prolonged and gradual inflation, it may be necessary to allow several seconds of deflation for reperfusion of any of the small perforators that may be transiently occluded. This has never been proved to be a problem, however. As stated previously, it is extremely important to apply a gradual stretch to the vessel. As we have stated repeatedly, if one were to invent a way to tear up a vessel, putting a balloon inside and blowing it up as fast as possible would be a good choice.

A potential problem with undersizing the balloon is that the lumen may not be large enough to maintain

adequate flow after the angioplasty (see Figs. 59–12 to 59–41). If this occurs, the angioplasty should be repeated with the same balloon, it will get larger. The balloon should also be left inflated for a few minutes. (This is not extremely dangerous; neurosurgeons routinely temporarily clip vessels for *at least* 10 minutes, as discussed later under "Temporary Vessel Occlusion Secondary to Balloon Inflation"). If these maneuvers do not work, the balloon should be exchanged for a larger one over an exchange wire (the Transcend-EX works well with a STEALTH; an 0.010", exchange-length wire is needed for the Stratus).

The angioplasty site should not be recrossed with the guidewire unless it is absolutely necessary. The intima is in all likelihood damaged and it is possible to create a severe dissection with the advancing edge of the guidewire. This has occurred, with fatal results.

Postdilation Observation

As stated later in the general description of the technique of intracranial angioplasty and in Chapter 41, the procedure is not completed when the lesion looks well dilated. A period of watchful waiting is indicated to observe for malignant acute postangioplasty thrombosis (see "Technique of Elective Intracranial Angioplasty," below). This portion of the procedure can be crucial.

Anterior Circulation Stenosis

Intracranial stenoses in the anterior circulation usually occur in the siphon of the ICA (Cases 5 to 7, Figs. 48–15 to 48–20) or in the main trunk of the MCA (M1) (Cases 8 to 12, Figs. 48–21 to 48–35). Addition-

Text continued on page 526

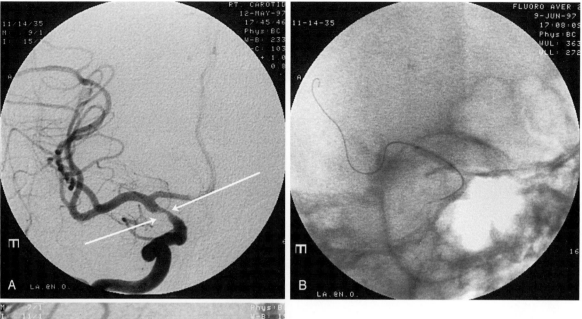

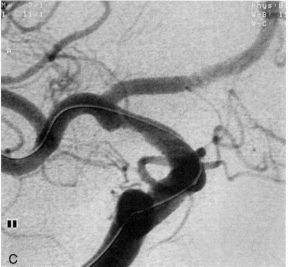

Figure 48-15 Case 5. *A*, PA view of a tight stenosis of the right internal carotid artery (ICA) *(long white arrows)* in a patient with a previous transient episode of left hand weakness associated with speech difficulty. *B*, Stratus angioplasty balloon in place. Note the guidewire with the safe J curve on the tip. *C*, Postangioplasty appearance before the guidewire was removed. Note that this angioplasty catheter allows the balloon to be withdrawn while maintaining the guidewire position across the angioplasty site.

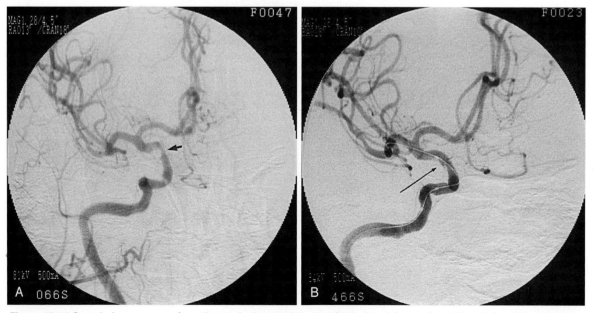

Figure 48-16 Case 6. Appearance of another typical stenosis in the ICA in the siphon before *(A)* and after *(B)* angioplasty. Although the balloon was undersized, there was still an intimal dissection (note the irregularity *[long arrow]*).

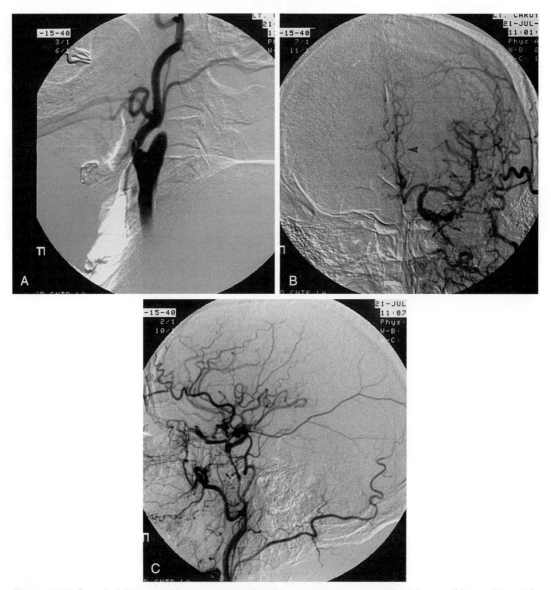

Figure 48-17 Case 7. A 55-year-old man presented to the emergency room with a history of intermittent left-sided weakness but was neurologically intact on presentation. The CT scan was normal. The MRI revealed a vague area of high signal in the frontal lobe–parietal lobe junction area on the left.

A cerebral angiogram was performed. The left common carotid artery injection reveals a totally occluded ICA *(A)*, with an amazing amount of collateral supply provided to the intracranial territory via tremendous collateral flow through the ophthalmic artery as well as cavernous branches of the ICA (*B* and *C*).

What is the immediately noticeable quality of the ICA stub? It looks gorgeous! There is no evidence of typical carotid artery plaque involving the origin of the ICA at the bifurcation. The appearance is characteristic of an occluded vessel stub with a residual pouch kept patent by swirling blood. The occlusion is caused by an intracranial ICA stenosis at the siphon, rather than at the cervical carotid bifurcation.

Note the extensive sphenopalatine branches of the internal maxillary artery *(small arrow, C)*.

The extremely abnormal aspect of this injection, however, is the fact that the extracranial supply to this hemisphere is supplying not only the middle cerebral artery (MCA) on the ipsilateral side, but also the ipsilateral anterior cerebral artery *(arrowhead, B)*. This is extremely unusual. More remarkable than even this, however, is the fact that this collateral supply is also feeding the *opposite* anterior cerebral artery! The implications of this are profound. This vessel is apparently better able to supply the contralateral (right) ICA territory than its own carotid!

Case 7 continues

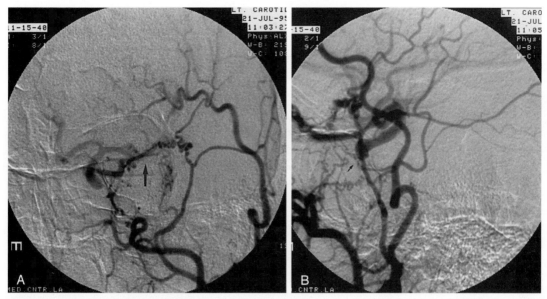

Figure 48-18 Magnification perorbital *(A)* and lateral *(B)* views of the left common carotid artery injection. The ICA is well seen as it "materializes" in its siphon region. Note the excellent example of the middle meningeal artery giving supply to the ophthalmic artery *(arrow)*. Also note the small cavernous collaterals *(small arrow)*. The middle meningeal artery appears to give more supply than the ethmoidal (sphenopalatine) branches of the internal maxillary artery.

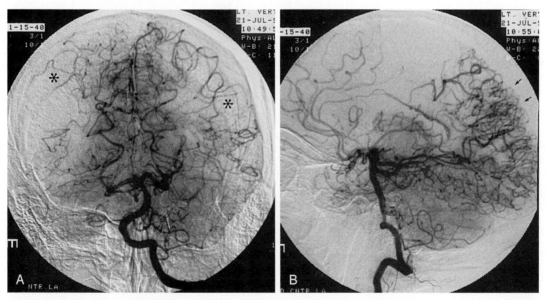

Figure 48-19 The left vertebral artery injection demonstrates the critical nature of this vessel. It is supplying not only its posterior circulation territory, but also an extensive amount of both anterior hemispheres *(asterisks, A)*. The posterior communicating arteries are present bilaterally, but they are not large enough. How is this known? Because the ophthalmic artery is being forced to supply the *opposite* hemisphere, as seen above! (They do not appear to be large on inspection, either.)

Note the extensive microcollateral superficial pial communications *(small arrows, B)*. Also note the anastomotic connection between the anterior pericallosal artery and the supply from the posterior cerebral arteries. The posterior circulation is in the capillary phase while the parietal lobes are still in the arterial phase; this is not normal!

Case 7 continues

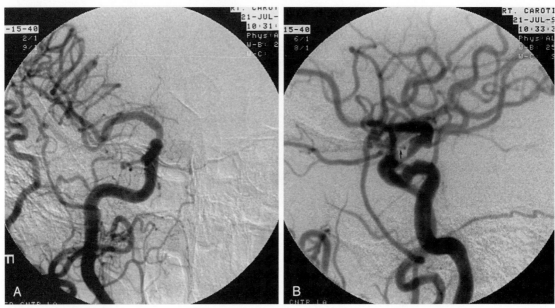

Figure 48-20 Magnification PA *(A)* and lateral *(B)* views of the right ICA. This vessel supplies only its own MCA. The reason for this is the huge plaque in the distal siphon just past the ophthalmic artery. This same type of plaque was probably present on the opposite side (mirror image lesions) and was the cause of the occlusion of the contralateral ICA. The hemodynamics of this situation are ominous.

Note the appearance of this ICA plaque. Is there a thin line separating the plaque from the wall of the vessel *(small arrow, B)*? Various obliquities were used to try to answer this question. If the line were seen to disappear on a different projection, however, this would be essentially meaningless. It would be *expected* to go away unless the view was directly down the channel!

So what is to be done? Work from the University of Pittsburgh reveals the dangerousness of this situation (up to 30% of people with hemodynamically significant stenoses of the internal carotid artery will have an extensive infarct within 18 months).

This man is obviously in trouble. An extracranial-intracranial bypass is an option. This would have to be a high-flow bypass, rather than the standard superficial temporal to middle cerebral artery type. In addition, the presence of the bypass could potentially cause proximal thrombosis at the point where antegrade flow meets retrograde flow. The treatment has to be well planned from a hemodynamic standpoint.

A high-flow bypass to one of the circle of Willis vessels is another possibility. This would require prolonged occlusion of the vessel, with resultant probable hemispheric or global ischemia, possibly with permanent results. Should an angioplasty be performed? This is a difficult location, and, in particular, this lesion is extremely threatening in appearance.

An alternative approach would be to place a bypass and, during the surgery, perform the angioplasty. This would allow potential rescue, if necessary.

Anticoagulants, although necessary, are of no real benefit. The problem is not embolic in origin, but rather purely hemodynamically (flow volume) related. It is our opinion that the natural history of this lesion will be to occlude. When this occurs, the entire hemisphere will be in jeopardy, if not (predictably) infarcted. Relief of some sort should be planned before this time.

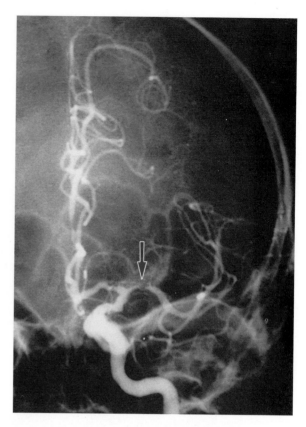

Figure 48-21 Case 8. This 67-year-old woman presented to the emergency room 2 days before this angiogram was performed, with the sudden onset of right arm weakness and aphasia, lasting approximately 30 minutes. A CT scan revealed small left cortical and basal ganglia infarcts. This left common carotid artery injection reveals a tight stenosis of the proximal M1 portion of the left MCA *(arrow)*. The patient was placed on intravenous heparin, and we were consulted. Owing to the recent infarcts, a delay of the proposed angioplasty was thought to be indicated to enable the brain to heal to some degree. (This is our standard practice because of the potential need for urokinase during any intracranial angioplasty. After an acute infarct, a delay of at least 6 weeks is thought to be indicated to decrease the threat of parenchymal bleed if urokinase is used). Unfortunately, *the next day, with the patient's aPTT in the 50- to 70-second range, the vessel occluded and she suffered a devastating MCA stroke.* We have observed stenoses that improve on intravenous heparin, allowing definitive therapy at a later date, and we have seen lesions such as this in which therapy should have been rendered urgently; it is impossible to predict which lesions will occlude.

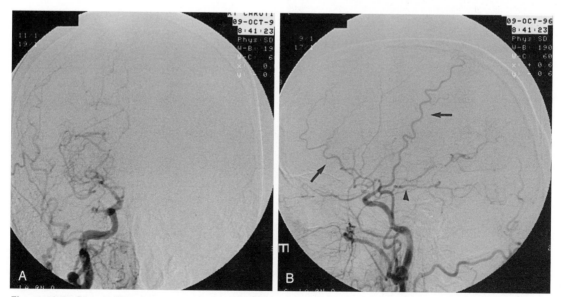

Figure 48-22 Case 9. This 41-year-old man presented with left hemiparesis. The PA *(A)* and lateral *(B)* views of the initial right carotid artery injection reveal total occlusion of the anterior cerebral artery and near-total occlusion of the MCA. Note that the superficial temporal artery branches *(arrows)* fill more rapidly than the ICA branches. More ominously, the posterior cerebral artery is seen to fill from the anterior injection *(arrowhead)*, and even this vessel does not appear to supply much of the hemisphere through pial collaterals.

Case 9 continues

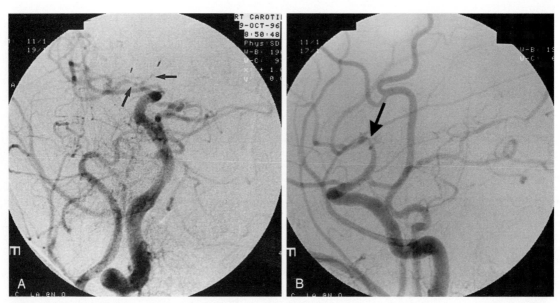

Figure 48-23 Magnification PA *(A)* and lateral *(B)* views of the ICA bifurcation confirm total occlusion of the anterior cerebral artery with a severe stenosis of the MCA (*black marks* and *small arrows, A*). The lateral view is a sharply angled view with acute craniocaudal angulation to look under the MCA trunk. This opens up the proximal MCA to demonstrate the stenosis *(arrow)* and is a useful view during this procedure. The residual lumen in the MCA is far less than 1 mm.

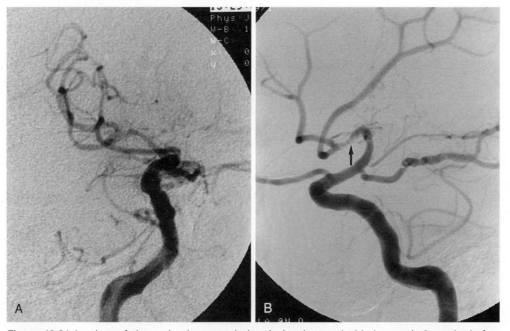

Figure 48-24 In view of the patient's recent ischemic insult, we decided to wait 8 weeks before performing angioplasty, in case the use of thrombolytics was necessary. The patient was kept on warfarin (Coumadin) and made steady neurologic improvement. Uneventful elective angioplasty was performed. PA *(A)* and lateral *(B)* magnification views were obtained after angioplasty following a delay of several minutes. Superficially, the result is acceptable, but actually it is very worrisome. Note the blurry appearance of the arterial lumen and the outline of the vessel *(arrow on lateral view)*. This is due to thrombus within the vessel lumen, which prevents adequate contrast opacification, both in the vessel and along the wall, thus resulting in this appearance. This was aggressively treated with intra-arterial urokinase, which cleared the lumen. The patient was continued on abciximab and heparin after the procedure This is the only patient receiving abciximab that we have had to treat with urokinase.

Case 9 continues

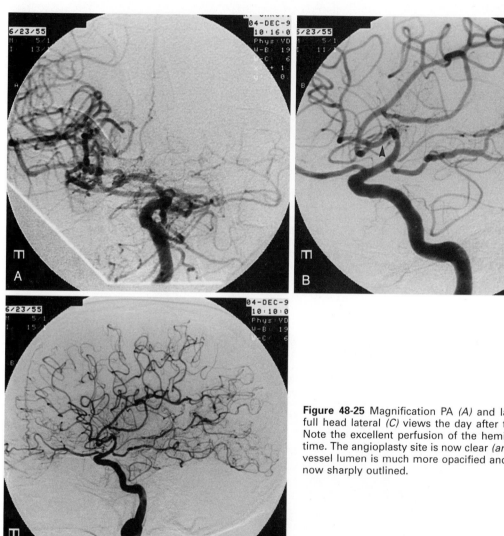

Figure 48-25 Magnification PA *(A)* and lateral *(B)*, and full head lateral *(C)* views the day after the procedure. Note the excellent perfusion of the hemisphere at this time. The angioplasty site is now clear *(arrowhead)*. The vessel lumen is much more opacified and the walls are now sharply outlined.

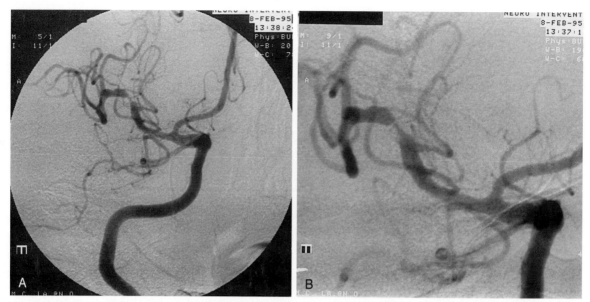

Figure 48-26 Case 10. This 45-year-old woman was experiencing transient ischemic attacks (TIAs) involving the right MCA territory. The initial arteriogram revealed severe stenosis of the right MCA (M1). After the patient had been on intravenous heparin for 10 days, she remained symptomatic. Angiography was repeated at that time, and the angiogram is shown here. Right common carotid artery injection *(A)* with magnification view *(B)* shows an extremely tight stenosis in the distal M1 segment. The incidence of total occlusion within a short time is believed to be high for these lesions, especially when symptomatic on intravenous heparin therapy.

The main trunk of the vessel measures 3 mm in diameter, and the distal portion measures about 2.5 mm. The stenotic segment is hairlike.

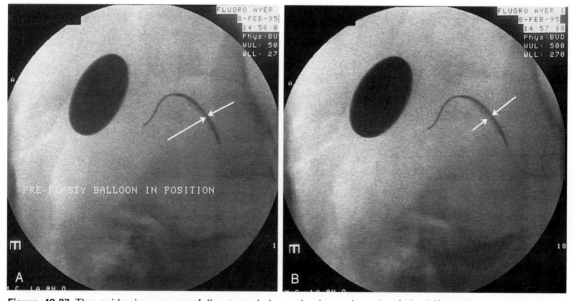

Figure 48-27 The guidewire was carefully steered down the lower branch of the bifurcation and the 2.5-mm FasSTEALTH angioplasty balloon placed across the stenosis. *A,* Note the waist in the balloon at the level of the stenosis *(arrows)*. *B,* Over a period of several minutes, the balloon was gradually inflated to 3 atmospheres, at which point the vessel slowly stretched open *(arrows)*. Gradual increase in pressure up to 6 atmospheres produced no further visible change in the vessel size.

Case 10 continues

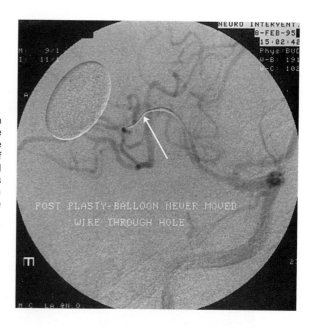

Figure 48-28 The balloon was deflated and the wire slightly withdrawn to back the occlusion bead on the wire out of the distal valve and ensure deflation. Injection of contrast through the guide catheter around the balloon while it was still in place was not revealing as to the success of the angioplasty. The wire was then advanced to re-engage the valve and reinflate the balloon. Note the position of the guidewire *(arrow)*. It has failed to follow the inferior branch, and its exact location is unknown on this injection. Did it enter a very small branch or go directly through the side wall of the bifurcation?

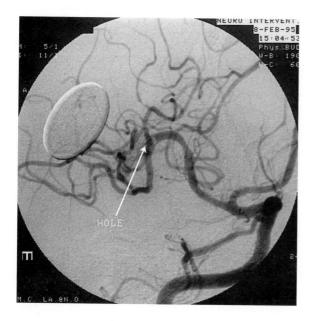

Figure 48-29 After reinflation of the balloon in the same slow fashion, it was deflated and withdrawn. A follow-up angiogram reveals that the angioplasty site looks excellent, but there is now a blush distal to the bifurcation. The *arrow* points to a hole in the wall of the vessel where the wire was.

Case 10 continues

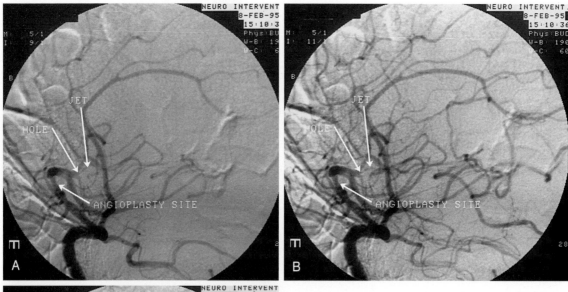

Figure 48-30 *A*, *B*, and *C*. Three lateral images obtained during the same injection of contrast. Note the waving jet effect of the blood and contrast squirting through the hole in the vessel.

Almost every interventional neuroradiologist has experienced a hole such as this; they are almost always self-limiting (the wire is approximately 30 gauge). Anticoagulation (heparin) should be reversed immediately, if present. If there is evidence that the slow bleed is continuing, surgical repair is "extremely simple" (per Issam Awad, Department of Neurosurgery, Yale University School of Medicine). The location of the hole along the course of the vessel is within the subarachnoid space, near the surface in the sylvian fissure. Fibrin glue, Avitene, or Gelfoam placed on the surface of the hole should stop the ooze in most cases. At most, a single microstitch (10–0 suture) could close the hole easily.

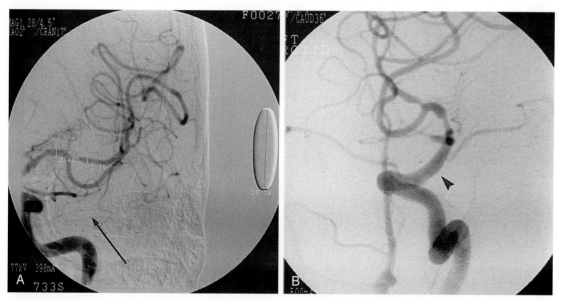

Figure 48-31 Case 11. A man with increasing TIAs. A duplex ultrasound examination revealed a 60% stenosis in the left ICA at the carotid bifurcation, which was repaired. However, 1 month later the man had a small stroke (Wernicke's area), and a review of the previous MRI and magnetic resonance angiogram suggested a lesion in the MCA, the probable cause of his original symptoms. This episode of dysphasia mostly resolved over a period of days. There was a parenchymal change on CT and MRI, and it was decided to wait the standard 6 weeks before undertaking angioplasty. PA *(A)* and magnified oblique lateral *(B)* views from the angiogram performed at the time of the interventional procedure reveal a very tight lesion in the MCA just distal to the first (temporal lobe) branch. There is an additional tight area in the proximal M1 segment just distal to the bifurcation of the ICA.

As usual, a quarter was used to provide a reference for measurement. Remeasurement of the quarter using the outer surface of both the white and black images yielded a measurement of 25.14 mm, only a 4.2% error. The PA projection reveals the main trunk of the MCA to measure 2.44 mm, with the branch vessel measuring 1.75 mm. The stenosis is hairlike.

This renders the choice of angioplasty balloon both difficult and simple. Although we deliberately undersize all balloons for intracranial angioplasty, the smallest balloon available is 2 mm (Target Therapeutics and Medtronic/MIS), larger than we would have preferred to use.

One consoling thought, however, is the fact that the vessel distant to the stenosis could be slightly deflated rather than simply small. Overdilating an intracranial vessel is to be avoided if at all possible, not only because of the risk of rupture, but mostly because of the risk of severe dissection with subsequent possible vessel occlusion.

The lateral view is actually very steeply angled in an oblique manner, with the tube aiming up under the M1 segment (the direction of the *arrow* in *A*). This permits the distal ICA and M1 segments to be projected in profile and usually yields an excellent view, particularly of the distal ICA *(arrowhead)*. The MCA lesion is still slightly "down the barrel."

Case 11 continues

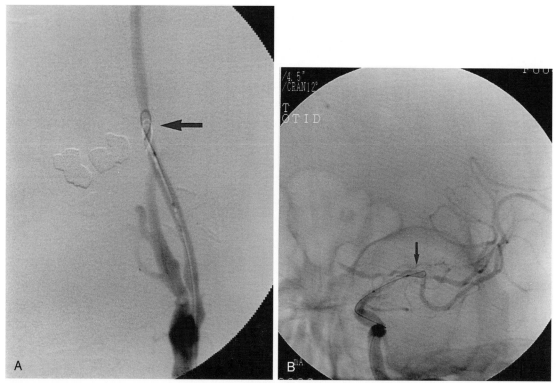

Figure 48-32 It was not possible to advance the guide catheter to its typical distal cervical ICA location owing to the residual tight (postendarterectomy) stenosis at the origin of this vessel. The safest way for a catheter–guidewire combination to advance downstream is by following a tight J curve *(large arrow, A)*. This prevents the wire from selecting any small side branch and allows the catheter to follow the main lumen. It was possible to easily advance the hydrophilic-coated Stratus angioplasty catheter and Quicksilver-10 guidewire into the MCA *(small arrow, B)*.

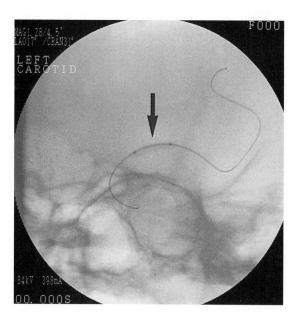

Figure 48-33 The Quicksilver wire was advanced downstream into an M2 branch to ensure that it remained distal to the angioplasty site, and the Stratus was then advanced into position and inflated *(arrow)*. This catheter allows inflation of the balloon with the wire at any position through the end of the catheter. As usual, a very slow and gradual inflation was performed. The patient received a preangioplasty bolus of abciximab followed by the standard 12-hour infusion (see Chapter 4). Both the MCA origin and the more distal lesions were dilated.

Case 11 continues

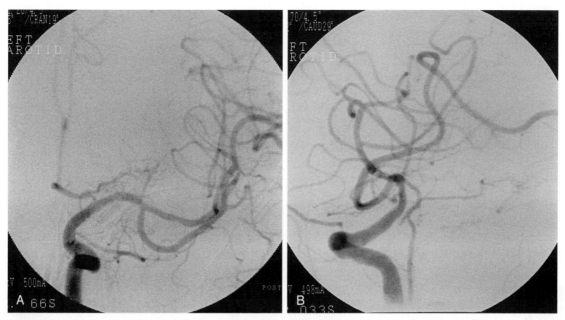

Figure 48-34 After observing the dilated segments for 1 hour after the angioplasty (to watch for any acute hyperthrombotic episode that could necessitate therapy), the final PA *(A)* and lateral *(B)* views reveal an excellent appearance. The patient returned home and reported feeling much more energetic since the angioplasty procedure, a result confirmed by his wife. Increasing energy, unfortunately, has not been the typical response to a standard intracranial angioplasty.

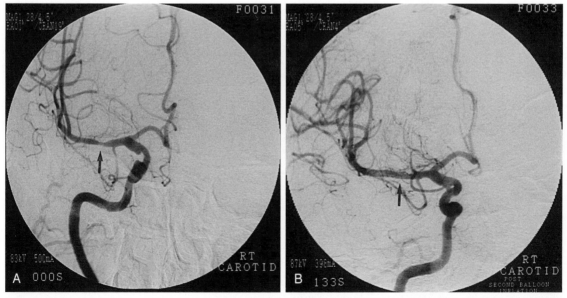

Figure 48-35 Case 12. This patient had recurrent episodes of transient tingling and numbness of the left hand, as well as weakness of grip. *A,* The angiogram reveals a high-grade stenosis in the right MCA *(arrow)*, in the middle of the region in which the lateral lenticulostriate arteries frequently originate. It is imperative not to cause intimal damage during this angioplasty. Measurement of the vessel revealed the normal lumen proximal to the stenosis to be 2.8 mm and the vessel distal to the stenosis to be 2.3 mm. *B,* A 2.0-mm angioplasty balloon was used (the smallest available). *C,* The postangioplasty result is excellent, with the distal vessel now apparently "inflated" and as large as the proximal M1 segment. Distal "inflation" after angioplasty has been observed in numerous locations, including the cervical ICA.

ally, the cavernous portion of the ICA may be involved in the process (Case 13, Fig. 48–36).

If the upper (superior) division of the MCA on the dominant side is stenotic, symptoms may include partial hemiplegia or hemiparesis, hemisensory loss, Broca's aphasia, and/or word finding difficulty. Involvement of the inferior division results in Wernicke's aphasia, hemianopia, or both. Wernicke's aphasia is very difficult to diagnose even when it is secondary to a true infarct, much less when it is only partial and caused by a stenosis with resultant ischemia.

The location of the origin of the primary supply to Wernicke's area determines whether this symptom manifests itself. It may originate from the upper or lower division of the MCA and may even be spared if there are good pial-to-pial collaterals from the posterior cerebral artery. An infarct in Wernicke's area, however, is a devastating insult. On the nondominant side, hemianopia is present, along with confu-

sion and inability to copy or draw accurately (an interesting phenomenon to observe). Speech is only minimally affected. On the dominant side, inability to read, comprehend instructions, describe particular events or feelings, or carry on a coherent conversation render this a serious deficit.

Stenoses of these MCA branches usually are minimally symptomatic until occlusive. Branch stenoses are compensated for to some degree by their neighbors, and therefore the symptoms commonly are vague and sporadic.

Isolated stenoses of the anterior cerebral artery are rare and usually located distal to A1 (see Figs. 48–22 to 48–25). These can cause symptoms ranging from paresis and sensory disturbance of the leg to various disturbances in language or understanding (because of ischemia of the most distal portion of the territory of the anterior cerebral artery). These symptoms are frequently evoked by standing rapidly (postural hypotension).

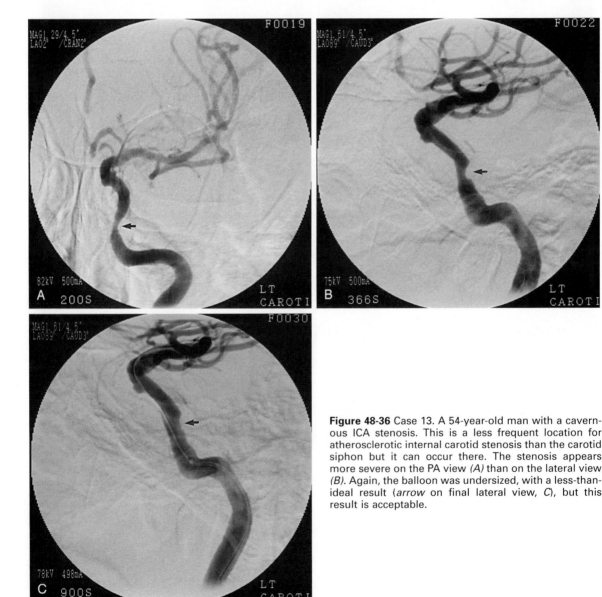

Figure 48-36 Case 13. A 54-year-old man with a cavernous ICA stenosis. This is a less frequent location for atherosclerotic internal carotid stenosis than the carotid siphon but it can occur there. The stenosis appears more severe on the PA view *(A)* than on the lateral view *(B)*. Again, the balloon was undersized, with a less-than-ideal result *(arrow* on final lateral view, *C),* but this result is acceptable.

Strategic Considerations Concerning Anterior
Circulation Angioplasty

Adequate placement of a guide catheter must be achieved before the angioplasty catheter can be placed. The ICA is much larger than most vertebral arteries, and the choice of guide catheters is broadened. The guide catheter, however, must be safely placed in a position where it will cause no harm for the duration of the procedure and still give good support to the distal microcatheter. Stiffer cardiology guide catheters can be used, but these probably should be withheld until they are absolutely needed; a true neuro-guide catheter should be chosen first. Unfortunately, there is no ideal guide catheter available. The Lumax Neuroguide is a hybrid guide catheter and is our choice for this task. While the tip is slightly too stiff, it is relatively safe and provides adequate support. This guide catheter comes with a matching dilator and can be placed directly through the skin over an exchange wire. It comes as a 7- or 8-Fr. size.

Strategic consideration of anatomic approach is limited because of the lack of choice of both destination and access. Approach by the axilla or arm generally is not feasible. A direct puncture of the common carotid artery rarely may be necessary (see Chapter 3). Direct puncture of the carotid artery can improve the vectors of force greatly, but at the risk of worsening the postprocedure problems of hemostasis and possibly of altering the flow in the dilated vessel, with unknown consequences. This technique is not advised for carotid stent placement and carries a tremendously increased incidence of complications (sometimes necessitating emergency vascular repair and evacuation of hematoma owing to threatened airway obstruction).[29]

The carotid siphon is a segment with a tight curve, and attempting to recross this lesion results in the wire tip tracking forcefully along the outside of the turn, seeking any intimal crevice. No matter how skillful the operator is, it will not be possible to avoid having the wire take this outside course, with potentially devastating results. After angioplasty, the position across the stenosis should be saved by leaving the wire downstream and withdrawing the angioplasty catheter; repeating the angioplasty is thus possible with reduced danger. If the true lumen has been lost, it is in this instance that attempting to recross the lesion is the most dangerous. If any postangioplasty narrowing or irregularity manifests, therefore, fibrinolysis should be performed, with or without the addition of papaverine (or nitroglycerin) to treat associated vasospasm. An attempt to recross a suboptimal angioplasty site in the carotid siphon should be avoided if at all possible.

The angioplasty procedure is not completed once the angioplasty has been performed. A period of watchful waiting is necessary to ensure that the vessel does not occlude secondary to the hypercoagulable platelet cascade described previously (see Chapter 41).

Anticoagulant and Antiplatelet Agent Use in Intracranial Atherosclerotic Disease

Although neurologists consider the use of anticoagulants for the treatment of carotid disease with TIAs controversial, this is not necessarily the case for intracranial disease. Analyses have been made comparing medical and surgical therapy for carotid bifurcation disease; even though the infarct rate may be decreased slightly for the anticoagulated group, the rate of intracranial hemorrhage is increased, and surgical therapy for carotid bifurcation disease is relatively safe and effective. The risk-to-benefit ratio tends to support surgical intervention rather than anticoagulation in this setting.

In patients with intracranial disease, even though the risk of intracranial hemorrhage or other bleeding may be increased with anticoagulants, this risk is almost certainly less than the risk of the untreated natural course of the disease. The exact risk of angioplasty is not known, but angioplasty of certain lesions is known to be difficult and dangerous. Operator skill is a tremendous variable; therefore the risk-to-benefit ratio is unknown.

Many in the neuroscience community believe that if an intracranial atherosclerotic vascular stenotic lesion is discovered as an incidental finding (i.e., is asymptomatic), the patient should be placed on antiplatelet or anticoagulant therapy. No large series has been compiled of intracranial lesions that have been followed long enough to prove the need to treat these lesions (by intracranial angioplasty) before they become significantly symptomatic (in contrast to carotid bifurcation disease, which has been shown to require therapy when the pathology has reached a certain degree of severity, regardless of symptomatology). The natural history of these lesions (discussed earlier) would appear to mandate some form of aggressive therapy, but more than that, *effective* aggressive therapy.

Ticlopidine (Ticlid) has been shown to be effective in the medical management of coronary artery disease and posterior fossa atherosclerotic disease; perhaps its use should be considered for any patient with an intracranial lesion who is a candidate for medical therapy. Warfarin is another consideration. Anticoagulants and antiplatelet agents are not without their own risks, however, and their role is uncertain.

Data obtained while examining intracranial stenoses for microemboli with transcranial Doppler indicate that these lesions are *not* sources of emboli.[30] In addition, anticoagulants and antiplatelet agents do not slow the progression of the underlying disease. They may, however, prevent or delay the ultimate occlusive event. For this reason, it would appear that patients with these lesions deserve at least this form of therapy, although it may be of only limited and/or temporary help.

A lesion associated with episodic neurologic manifestations (TIAs or RINDs) may not require direct intervention, but certainly necessitates evaluation and therapy, even if treatment consists of only cessation of smoking and institution of antiplatelet or anticoagulant medication. In some cases, the apparent stenosis simply vanished during the few weeks that it took to obtain the appropriate angioplasty catheters. The implication of this observation is profound; the stenosis was probably just thrombus, and any manipulation could have displaced this mass downstream. Alternatively, a stenosis was seen to vanish in just one day and possibly represented severe spasm of unknown cause (Case 14, Figs. 48–37 and 48–38).

In other cases, lesions that initially appeared severe enough to need therapy improved after an initial course of intravenous heparin (about 1 week), to the point at which it was believed that removal of any hypercoagulable stimuli (e.g., smoking), combined with continued antiplatelet or anticoagulant therapy, would forestall further intervention for at least some time. If correction of a preexisting hypercoagulable state has been and will continue to be achieved, it may be possible to avoid (or delay) a high-risk intracranial procedure.

Conversely, cases have been observed in which the patient presented with a nearly occlusive lesion; when the patient was placed on intravenous heparin, the lesion continued to progress (see Figs. 48–1 to 48–7 and 48–21). At this point, angioplasty in these

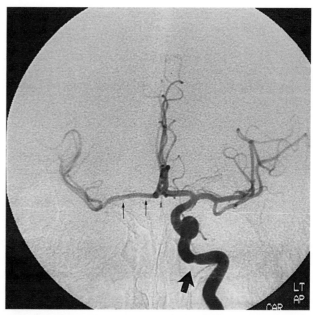

Figure 48-38 The patient was returned to the angiography suite the next day for angioplasty of the ICA stenosis. At this time, the ICA was selectively catheterized for the first time (note the lack of external carotid artery branches on this injection, whereas the previous injection had been a common carotid artery injection). Amazingly, the petrous segment carotid stenosis has nearly vanished. Note the excellent perfusion of the opposite hemisphere.

At no point during either procedure was the catheter or guidewire in the distal ICA. It is unlikely that this was thrombus that disappeared; the lesion in this case is thought to have represented spasm.

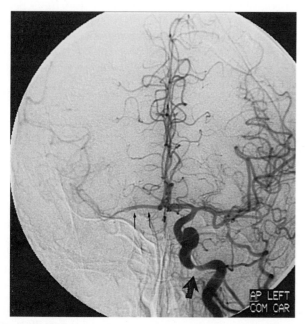

Figure 48-37 Case 14. This man had previously suffered an occlusion of the right ICA and now presented with episodic weakness of the left arm and face with some associated sensory disturbance. He was a long time sufferer of migraine headaches and had been on warfarin for many months. The angiogram reveals a severe stenosis of the petrous portion of the left ICA *(large arrow)*. Although the flow through the lesion is limited, it is obvious that there is a tremendous need for this blood in the contralateral hemisphere. The density and flow rate in the right hemisphere are, however, markedly lower than they should be. The right MCA and A1 segment of the anterior cerebral artery appear somewhat deflated *(small arrows)*.

Case 14 continues

cases became a neurovascular rescue rather than prevention, and even though most vital neurologic function was recovered, some function had been irrecoverably lost before the angioplasty was performed.

As stated previously, intracranial stenosis is not felt to be a primarily embolic problem. Anticoagulation does not stop progression of the disease. Anterior circulation intracranial stenosis leads to about a 1 in 4 chance of stroke in 3 years, or a risk about thirteen times baseline, even with medical therapy. Therefore, while anticoagulant use may be necessary, it is truly a minimum therapy. Intracranial angioplasty can be performed with a reasonable degree of safety and should therefore be considered a primary means of therapy.

Generic Risks of Intracranial Angioplasty

No firm data exist concerning the risk of therapy as related to lesion location. In several series, there was no clear statistical indication of which lesions are more responsive or of which are more dangerous. It appears that the primary risk is operator-dependent, followed closely by the risks related to location and type of lesion.

In our series of 67 intracranial angioplasty cases, the risk has been related more to equipment (catheter) technology and experience than to the location. With the new hydrophilic-coated microangioplasty catheters and better guide catheters, the struggle to advance the catheter is much less and there is much more finesse to the procedure.

In the series of 67 elective cases, there have been four major permanent complications:

- An intimal dissection led to vessel occlusion. The lesion was a very tight stenosis of the ICA in the siphon. The dissection was typical of dissection following angioplasty in this location, but there was still excellent antegrade flow. The dissection was caused by an attempt to recross the already dilated lesion to treat a downstream embolus with direct local urokinase infusion.

  Recrossing a fresh intracranial angioplasty site is attempted only when it is certain that there is no intimal damage and when the vessel segment to be traversed is relatively straight, without a severe narrowing at the stenosis. Almost any downstream thrombus can be cleared by infusion from a proximal location (see Figs. 59–109 to 59–112). This complication was an error in judgment.

- A dissection (with occlusion) at the vertebrobasilar junction occurred as a direct result of angioplasty. At the time, the complication was thought to be secondary to the brittleness of the vessel in this location. Although this is still considered to be a contributing factor, we now believe that the balloon may have been oversized. The vertebrobasilar junction has proved to be a difficult location for other interventional neuroradiologists, and we are particularly careful to undersize balloons in this location.

- The guidewire of the STEALTH catheter punctured the wall of the vessel just distal to the angioplasty site, at an acute curve in the vessel (see Figs. 48–26 to 48–30). The occluding wire of the STEALTH catheter was advanced to a certain point (beyond the site where the balloon needed to be positioned) and inadvertently was forcefully pushed into the curve of the vessel as the balloon was inflating. This was caused by a loss of finesse and "feel" related to the amount of force necessary to advance the catheter and the inability to deflate the balloon without removing the guidewire and then readvancing the wire and catheter as a unit to hold position across the lesion. Depending on how the wire is loaded in the STEALTH catheter, the wire cannot be advanced beyond the angioplasty site and the catheter then withdrawn. We now backload the occlusion wire when using a STEALTH catheter in order to do this. If the wire is backloaded in this fashion, however, it cannot be exchanged for another wire during the case without removing the entire catheter, and it is truly a spear, without the ability to be withdrawn past a certain point. If the wire is loaded from the typical antegrade direction, it is *never* withdrawn back into the catheter to allow deflation; deflation is performed with the guidewire in position using firm aspiration. With the guidewire in position and the valve locked,

however, the STEALTH catheter–guidewire combination can be rigid and may cause a downstream perforation, as occurred in this case. For these reasons, we generally use a Stratus catheter for intracranial angioplasty procedures (see Chapter 1).

- A patient presented with an evolving vertebrobasilar stroke. Both distal vertebral arteries were occluded and the angioplasty was performed as part of a rescue maneuver following successful recanalization using urokinase. The vessel, however, slowly reoccluded over a period of about 15 minutes (elastic rebound). A stent was needed, but a stent suitable for this location was unavailable. An attempt at another angioplasty utilizing a larger balloon resulted in dissection of the vessel during the attempt to recross the occlusion; the vessel was subsequently unable to be reopened. Sometimes there are only poor choices.

Further discussion of the complications of intracranial angioplasty is presented later in "Complications of Intracranial Angioplasty and How to Avoid Them."

Successful Angioplasty as Defined by Cardiology Criteria

The possibility of severe (irrecoverable) damage caused by intracranial angioplasty is the reason that a "suboptimal" result is not only adequate, but also *desirable*. The risk of gross dissection, with subsequent loss of perforators or occlusion, may rise exponentially with the degree of vessel wall distention. The goal is to achieve results adequate to treat the immediate problem without damaging the vessel wall enough to injure the perforators or causing enough vascular damage to prompt occlusion. Unlike cardiology procedures (e.g., coronary angioplasty), there is no emergent surgical rescue available.

In coronary angioplasty, success is defined as a 20% relative improvement with a decrease in stenosis to less than 50%.[31] This definition of success is appropriate for intracranial angioplasty as well, but a less than perfect result is difficult to accept. Interventional neuroradiologists need to understand that less than perfect is good enough.

Risk of Angioplasty Based on Location

Even though an M1 lesion may contain perforators (the lateral lenticulostriate arteries), the loss of a few of these perforators may not be as devastating as the loss of a few pontine perforators arising from the basilar artery (particularly if the M1 perforators supply only the extreme capsule). In addition, the MCA does not appear to be as routinely fragile as the basilar artery or to dissect as easily and therefore appears to respond to angioplasty in a much more favorable manner (see Fig. 48–35). The MCA does not intrinsically tend to calcify as much as the vertebrobasilar system, the access is more direct, and angioplasties are more straightforward. Inflation pressures required in the MCA appear to be less than those required in a calcified basilar artery, and the lesion responds with less cracking. Simple angioplasties of the MCA are therefore felt to be associated with the lowest risk of complication of any intracranial stenosis. Again, the key is undersizing the balloon.

Internal carotid lesions in the siphon fall between the two extremes of the basilar artery and the MCA. Traversing a carotid siphon lesion safely with finesse is difficult in a vessel that takes a 180-degree turn within less than 1 cm. The wire invariably tends to follow the outside of the curve of the siphon. In addition, in this location, the vessel can be very friable. Trying to dilate a vessel in the middle of a curve is potentially dangerous. Blowing up the angioplasty balloon can tear the vessel simply by straightening it out.

Lesions in the petrous ICA are very rare. In the straight (horizontal) petrous portion of the ICA, the vessel is surrounded by bone. The vessel cannot be stretched or cracked as in the typical angioplasty, but lesions in this location have been treated successfully with high pressure.[32] The plaque may be simply smashed flat, or the vessel may be expanded at the expense of the bone. We would be interested to know if there has been a fracture in the very thin bone in the roof of the petrous canal associated with angioplasty in this location.

Lesions in the petrocavernous junction of the ICA are more common. They can be at the curve in the vessel, however, and therefore somewhat more dangerous to treat; they can dissect. There are no dangerous collaterals in this region, however.

Distal vertebral artery lesions, unassociated with the vertebrobasilar junction, have been treated with a reasonable degree of success and safety. There are no dangerous perforators in this area, and the lesions respond to reasonable inflation pressures. The origin of the PICA is a primary concern in this location (as is the proximity of the stenosis to the vertebrobasilar junction). Dissection can occlude this vessel, with devastating results.

The major risk associated with treating lesions of the distal vertebral artery is that these patients often are undergoing therapy for poor posterior fossa perfusion secondary to an absent or occluded vertebral artery on one side and stenosis on the other. Loss of this remaining vessel can be life-threatening. Extension of a tear to the vertebrobasilar junction could also be a problem. In Higashida's series of posterior circulation intracranial angioplasties, two of five patients suffered severe complications (vessel occlusion and death) and a third patient had a TIA related to posterior fossa ischemia during the procedure.[33] Temporary occlusion of the posterior fossa circulation may be similar to generalized systemic flow arrest, in that there may be no collateral supply to this territory. This may result in immediate symptoms and a long-term or permanent deficit after a brief occlusion. Expeditious technique should be employed in this region, making the technique of slow balloon

inflation difficult. In cases in which immediate symptoms develop during occlusion, the technique of slow balloon inflation can still be used, but it should be done in stages with deflations in between the inflations.

Another potential problem associated with angioplasty in the distal vertebral artery is that the vessel makes a cephalic turn at this point. The stenosis may be located at a point where there is an acute angle; even if dilated, the vessel may kink, thus yielding a poor result. The solution for this problem is a flexible stent capable of reaching this location and not promoting restenosis. The success rate for treatment of a distal vertebral stenosis is about 90%, but the complication rate (stroke and death) is about 10% (verbal report from Robert Ferguson, North American Cerebral Percutaneous Transluminal Angioplasty Register). The complication rate associated with dissection and loss of perforators appears to be dramatically worse in the posterior circulation than in the anterior circulation (most particularly in the basilar artery).

Vertebrobasilar junction lesions and basilar artery stenoses appear to be the most dangerous of any intracranial lesions to treat because of their tendency to dissect and occlude vital perforators. In the basilar artery, an excellent angiographic result can be obtained with optimal dilation, but a severe pontine infarct may result.

In the study by Clark et al. of intracranial angioplasty,[34] there were two strokes, one secondary to dissection and subsequent occlusion of the MCA and the other probably caused by occlusion of a perforator off the basilar artery, most likely related to a small dissection of the basilar artery crossing this vessel. Small dissections are almost unpreventable and can be devastating in the basilar artery. Large dissections may be prevented by intentional undersizing of the angioplasty balloon (see "Technique of Elective Intracranial Angioplasty," below).

Patient Counseling

We quote a risk of vessel occlusion of 10% to 20% (10% for anterior circulation lesions and 20% for posterior circulation locations). There is about a 95% chance that the lesion can be accessed and the angioplasty balloon delivered. The reaction of the vessel to the angioplasty is an unknown quantity; this is the source of the less than ideal results. We believe that the overall success rate for intracranial angioplasty should be higher than 80% with the addition of abciximab and continuing improvement in angioplasty balloons (closer to 90% to 95%), but this has not been proved.

The issue of restenosis has not been resolved. We monitor patients with short-term angiographic follow-up (at 3, 6, and 12 months), which is repeated at intervals (the optimal interval has not been determined). In addition, the institution of the use of probucol (discussed later) may lessen the threat of restenosis.

Rationale of Therapy for Stenosis Associated with Acute Infarction

The decision to treat a stenosis can be extremely difficult when it is discovered during the evaluation of an unrelated or directly related acute infarct that presents too late for acute intervention. Most acute infarcts present after the critical first few hours when aggressive intervention (fibrinolytic therapy) may be possible. A stenotic lesion may then be found that needs therapy acutely, but recent damage (infarct) has already occurred (hours or days previously, not weeks), precluding the use of fibrinolytic agents for any reason.

Delayed presentation of a potentially worsening or progressive neurologic deficit with an underlying stenosis or occlusion is fraught with hazard; preangioplasty or postangioplasty fibrinolytic therapy is an important part of our armamentarium that we are loath to forgo. Urokinase has been instrumental in rescuing a certain percentage of intracranial angioplasty procedures. The ability to use urokinase has allowed us to snatch victory from the jaws of defeat. When trying to achieve an ideal angioplasty result (even if less than 100%), modest intimal tears should be planned for and the use of postangioplasty urokinase has succeeded in maintaining vessel patency more than once.

In the neuroscience community, there is some consensus concerning the time interval after an acute infarct beyond which infusion of fibrinolytic agents should not be performed (6 to 9 hours). No consensus has been achieved, however, concerning how long to wait before it is again acceptable to use these agents. In the neurology and interventional neuroradiologic community, there is an extremely wide divergence of opinion on when, after an infarct, the use of intra-arterial fibrinolytics would be acceptable; opinions range from 4 days to 4 months or longer. Obviously, hard facts are lacking in this area.

The guidelines for the ongoing Prolyse for Acute Cerebral Thromboembolism trial for acute stroke therapy specify waiting 6 weeks after an infarct before administration of intra-arterial prourokinase (Prolyse). This appears to be a reasonable time and is the guideline we use for elective therapy of any intracranial stenosis that has possibly been associated with a prior infarct.

What should be the approach when faced with an apparent acute or subacute occlusion or stenosis and possible infarction, but not total downstream tissue death (which, however, may be incipient) (see Case 1, Figs. 48–1 to 48–7 and Case 15, 48–39 to 48–48)? If an underlying stenosis has progressed to the point at which the local microcirculation stimulates thrombus formation on top of the plaque and thus has

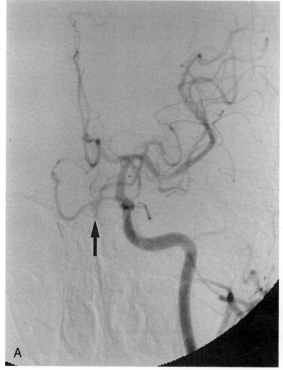
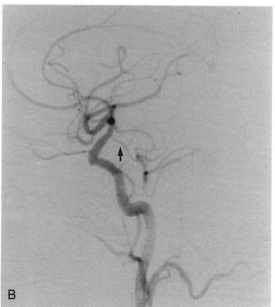

Figure 48-39 Case 15. This 53-year-old man presented to the emergency room with acute discoordination and mild dizziness. An amazing amount of information can be ascertained from analysis of the hemodynamics in this situation. The PA *(A)* and lateral *(B)* views of the left common carotid artery injection demonstrate an abnormal flow to the basilar artery through a very small posterior communicating artery *(small arrow)*, not just to the ipsilateral posterior cerebral artery. Indeed, there is flow into both superior cerebellar arteries as well as inferiorly into the midbasilar artery *(large arrow)*, a most abnormal distribution through such a small communicating artery.

This finding also suggests that there is minimal supply to the infratentorial circulation from the right posterior communicating artery via the right ICA.

Case 15 continues

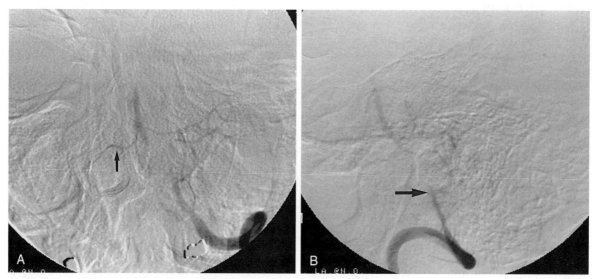

Figure 48-40 PA *(A)* and lateral *(B)* views of the left vertebral artery injection reveal an occlusion of the distal vertebral artery, just past the origin of the posterior inferior cerebellar artery (PICA) *(large arrow)*. There is reconstitution of the basilar artery via the anterior inferior cerebellar artery (AICA), a somewhat unusual communication. There is no supply to the superior cerebellar territory, the more common collateral pathway for the PICA. This is because there is some supply to the superior cerebellar territory via the previously demonstrated retrograde flow down the basilar artery from the left posterior communicating artery. Note the filling of the opposite (right) AICA *(small arrow)*, part of the sump causing the retrograde flow in the left AICA via the PICA.

On the lateral view *(B)*, note that the posterior extent of the flow in the distribution of the PICA does not reach the farthest peripheral portion of the cerebellar hemisphere, as is usually the case (and certainly when the PICA is supplying most of the cerebellum and the superior cerebellar artery territory, which is not infrequently the case [as demonstrated in Figs. 59–12 to 59–41]). Indeed, the flow from the left PICA does not even supply the midportion of its normal territory! Remember this. This is because the left superior cerebellar artery is trying to supply most of the cerebellum (a tough job under the circumstances), while the left PICA supplies the right lower cerebellar hemisphere. There obviously is no right vertebral artery; if there were, there would not be the sump from the left hemicerebellum into the right AICA, nor the filling of the right superior cerebellar artery via retrograde flow in the basilar artery (as described in Figure 48–39). Any supply from a normal PICA on the right would have supplied a good portion of the territory of the superior cerebellar artery and the AICA. Indeed, any normal supply to any part of the right cerebellar hemisphere would have supplied the majority of all right cerebellar territories.

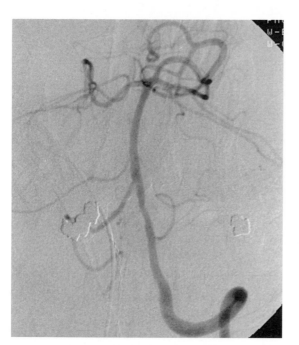

Figure 48-41 Upon repeat angiography after 1 week of intravenous heparin, the vessel had indeed opened up to the point that it was thought that angioplasty was unnecessary. The size of the vessel is amazingly good and the flow is good. Short-term follow-up was planned. We did not want to be surprised by a major infarct at a later time.

Case 15 continues

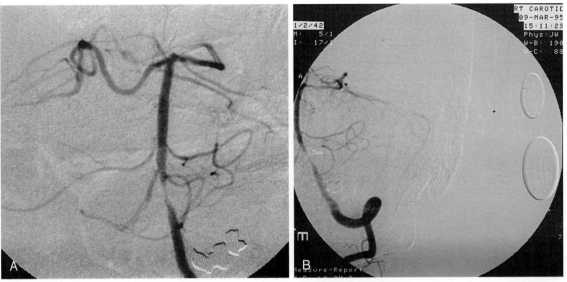

Figure 48-42 The follow-up examination was hastened by recurrent episodic symptoms consisting mostly of ataxia and dysarthria. The repeat PA *(A)* and oblique *(B)* views reveal a very small, but still patent, distal vertebral artery. The oblique PA view *(B)* has been obtained with overlying coins (a quarter and a dime) placed for measuring purposes. As can be seen from the measurement, the residual lumen is about 0.7 mm, not a reassuring size. Angioplasty was now considered necessary. However, unforeseen scheduling circumstances necessitated delaying the procedure for 5 days, during which time the patient was maintained on heparin.

become symptomatic, occlusive, or both, acute therapy is required, at least in the form of aggressive anticoagulation. This may be enough to reopen the occlusion, leaving behind a stenosis that could rethrombose without therapy.

In the study presented by Pessin et al., chronic anticoagulant administration succeeded in stopping recurrent infarcts in most patients, but all these patients had stenoses of less than 50%.[13] For a stenosis resulting in a residual hairlike lumen, the response of this lesion to anticoagulant therapy alone is hard to predict, and treatment (angioplasty) may well be

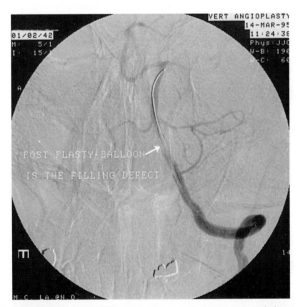

Figure 48-43 The patient was brought back to the angiography suite for angioplasty. On the off-chance that some of the narrowing was due to additional thrombus, an infusion of low-dose urokinase was performed: 100,000 units over approximately 25 minutes (i.e., 250,000 units per hour). This resulted in a clean but very tight lumen, as shown here, and angioplasty was undertaken.

Figure 48-44 A STEALTH angioplasty catheter was used through an Envoy guide catheter (Cordis Corp.). After the angioplasty, an injection of contrast through the guide catheter does not give a clear demonstration of the result. This is commonly the case with small-vessel as opposed to large-vessel angioplasty. In this instance the catheter itself (much less the deflated balloon) is very close to the size of the vessel and thus tends to fill the lumen even after dilation. The image suggests that there is at least residual stenosis if not a major intimal dissection *(arrow)*.

Case 15 continues

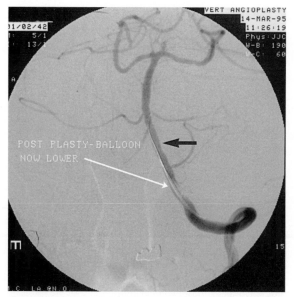

Figure 48-45 Simply repositioning the balloon *(white arrow)* and making another injection clearly changes the appearance of the vessel, now showing a gorgeous result *(black arrow)*.

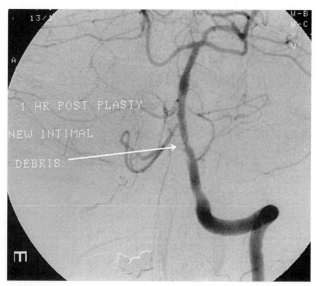

Figure 48–47 One hour after the angioplasty, some early thrombus formation is seen (remember, we always observe for any delayed thrombosis). This does not appear to warrant any intervention, and indeed it could actually be minimal thrombus and a slight tear. In any event, there was no malignant reaction and the procedure was terminated. Again, note the opposite distal vertebral artery filling retrograde to supply its PICA.

urgently necessary (see "Rationale for Treatment of Intracranial Stenosis," above).

If there is superimposed thrombus on top of a stenosis, simple angioplasty would appear to guarantee at least some distal embolization. How much thrombotic bulk is actually present? Would the effect of this distal embolization after angioplasty outweigh the end result of occlusion of the proximal main trunk? This is obviously a decision that has to be based on the particular situation. Additionally, a pe-

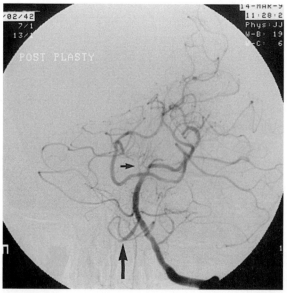

Figure 48-46 Removal of the STEALTH angioplasty balloon confirms the result. Note the asymmetric posterior cerebral arteries. The right P1 segment is hypoplastic *(small arrow)*, part of the reason that, as noted above, there was no effective supply from the right anterior circulation to the infratentorial circulation. Note also the filling of the distal right vertebral artery and right PICA *(large arrow)*.

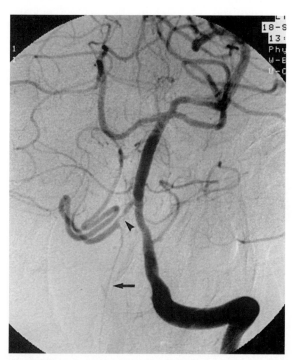

Figure 48-48 Six months after the procedure, the patient returned to the emergency room with recurrent symptoms, including ataxia and some dysarthria. On re-examination it was seen that the real problem was not restenosis at the angioplasty site, but a new stenosis in the opposite vertebral artery *(arrowhead)*. This was decreasing flow not only to the opposite PICA, but also to the anterior spinal artery *(arrow)*, which still needed this supply, and was therefore (amazingly) still present. We could not safely reach a vessel this small and treated this medically, as described in the text. The patient's symptoms waxed and waned but stabilized with no worsening.

riod of heparinization before treatment should allow time for at least a certain amount of thrombus superimposed on the stenosis to clear (see Figs. 48–39 to 48–48).

Heart versus Brain (Myocardial Infarction versus Stroke)

In the cardiology field, acute angioplasty for developing myocardial infarction can be performed instead of fibrinolysis with satisfactory, and even improved, results. Apparently, reestablishing flow is a priority for at least some of these lesions. This is not necessarily the case with the cerebral vasculature, however, but might be applicable under some circumstances.

The heart is a structure that acts primarily as a unit, with a limited number of separate functions. Preserving its bulk function mode is of primary importance; if a small portion of the overall substance is lost, the total strength may be affected, but its mission may be accomplished relatively unchanged. This is decidedly not the case with the brain. Small, strategically placed cerebral insults can be devastating.

It has been shown experimentally (but perhaps not conclusively) that multiple branch occlusions are worse than a single proximal trunk occlusion in the brain.[35] Specifically, multiple embolic microclots result in more brain damage than a single proximal macroclot (although in this trial, the total volume of microclot used was more than the volume of macroclot). Angioplasty of a proximal mass of clot, however, does not necessarily guarantee widespread dissemination of the clot into multiple vital vessels; it may simply move as a unit into the first side branch and thus increase flow to distal territories.

Collateral circulation also is different in the heart than in the brain. Distal branches in the brain can frequently survive for extended periods, whereas small perforators off the main trunk of M1 die rapidly. Angioplasty of clot in the M1 segment, therefore, is not a rational approach to the problem of clot in this location; it could simply mash thrombus into the origins of these lenticulostriate vessels.

For this reason acute angioplasty is not recommended in circumstances involving clot in intracranial vessels. In the setting of proximal large vessel occlusion secondary to thrombus, there is limited time for reperfusion by fibrinolysis. Mechanical reestablishment of flow can be performed by simply poking a hole in the thrombus with the wire and catheter, followed by fibrinolytic therapy (see Chapter 58).

Alternatively, mechanical reperfusion can be obtained by means of snares or other clot-retrieval devices (see Chapter 58).

Strategic Analyses of Specific Cases

The two cases presented here are not typical of the truly elective angioplasty situation, but are presented to demonstrate the strategic dilemma and therapeutic choices that have to be made at the time of therapy. While these cases had rewarding results, every situation is unfortunately different. These two cases are illustrative of the stages of reasoning necessary when formulating a rationale for therapy.

Case Study. This case is illustrated in Figures 48–39 to 48–48. A 53-year-old man presented with sudden onset of dizziness, slurred speech, and balance problems, which worsened over 3 days. He experienced several falls and felt "drunk." Twenty-four hours before presentation to the emergency room, he began to experience "heaviness" and weakness in his right arm and leg. He had a history of smoking the equivalent of one pack of cigarettes per day for 45 years and a family history of hypertension and strokes. On physical examination, he was hypertensive (162/88 mm Hg). He was noted to have slurred speech, a mild right facial droop, 3 out of 5 strength in his right upper and lower extremities, increased right-side muscle tone, right pronator drift, right-sided dysmetria, right-sided sensory disturbance (hyperesthesia and disturbance of vibration sense and proprioception), and a positive right Babinski reflex. On CT and MRI scans, he had a right PICA infarct, lacunar infarcts in the cerebellar hemispheres bilaterally, and bilateral cerebral white matter changes consistent with small vessel ischemia, predominantly in the parietal regions.

After 3 days in the hospital, an angiogram was obtained (see Figs. 48–39 and 48–40) that revealed absence of the right vertebral artery and occlusion of the left vertebral artery just past the origin of the PICA, with reconstitution of the lower basilar artery through PICA to AICA collaterals. There was filling of the right AICA, but not of the right PICA, from the lower basilar artery. The upper basilar artery, both posterior cerebral arteries, and both superior cerebellar arteries were supplied by a small left posterior communicating artery. Because of the delay in presentation to angiography, thrombolysis was not considered.

The patient was placed on heparin. One week later, repeat angiography revealed reopening of the left vertebral artery, with a stenosis between the PICA origin and the vertebrobasilar junction. There was now antegrade flow through the basilar artery and some retrograde flow into the distal right vertebral artery to the opposite PICA origin (see Fig. 48–41). Angioplasty was thought not to be absolutely necessary at the time (because of the hemodynamic improvement) and potentially dangerous in view of his recent infarct. The patient was maintained on warfarin (Coumadin) and aspirin, and he stopped smoking. His clinical condition was stable, and he underwent physical therapy and speech therapy.

He returned in 2 months with worsening symptoms. Repeat angiography at that time revealed that the left vertebral stenosis was now worse (indeed, critical), and he underwent angioplasty with good results (see Figs. 48–42 to 48–47). He again did well and was maintained on aspirin and warfarin. Repeat angiography 3 months later showed the angioplasty site to be stable. The patient, however, had developed an ulcerated plaque at the origin of the left ICA. Two weeks after his angiogram, he experienced a left anterior circulation TIA and underwent an uneventful endarterectomy.

The patient did well for 2 months, then returned with recurrent right cerebellar symptoms (arm and leg stiffness). Angiography revealed a tight stenosis of the residual distal right vertebral artery between the vertebrobasilar junction and the PICA origin (Fig. 48–48). The origin of the anterior spinal artery from the right vertebral artery was identified downstream from the stenosis (flow is retrograde from the vertebrobasilar junction). Flow to both PICA and the anterior spinal artery was thought to be compromised, but the vertebral segment was thought to be too small to access safely for angioplasty. The patient was maintained on aggressive anticoagulation, instructed to avoid caffeine and nicotine, and taught about maintenance of adequate hydration. His symptoms have waxed and waned, with no further permanent worsening, for more than 2 years.

Case Study. Case 16, Figures 48–49 to 48–57 illustrates this case. This 62-year-old man was referred to cardiology with a history of falling off his lawn mower repeatedly because of fainting spells. He was found to have third-degree heart block; his symptoms were thought to be cardiogenic. On closer questioning, it became apparent that his spells were more than just fainting spells that could be accounted for by periods of heart block and poor systemic perfusion. His spells also entailed periods of severe ataxia, falling and stumbling (always to the right), and dizziness to the point that he had to "hold onto a tree" to keep from falling. These episodes lasted for a matter of minutes.

The patient had experienced an increasing number of the staggering episodes in recent weeks and a major episode 4 to 5 weeks previously, at which time he had an MRI. He was informed that this study showed three "white spots" in his brain.

The angiogram at the time of coronary angiography was similar to that shown in Figure 48–49. During this coronary angiogram, the patient once again experienced complete atrioventricular dissociation with idioventricular rhythm, and a pacemaker was inserted. (Incidentally, he had no neurologic symptoms during this period.)

Treatment of the vertebral artery stenosis was requested. Because antiplatelet medication had not stopped the attacks, and because of the severity of the stenosis and the isolated posterior fossa, it was determined that the lesion should be treated with angioplasty. Because of the possibility that the patient had suffered an infarct several weeks before, it was thought prudent to delay therapy until at least 6 weeks had passed since the last cerebrovascular event and he had recovered adequately. (The MRI could not be repeated because of the now present pacemaker.) Angioplasty was then performed (Fig. 48–50), and the results are shown in Figure 48–51.

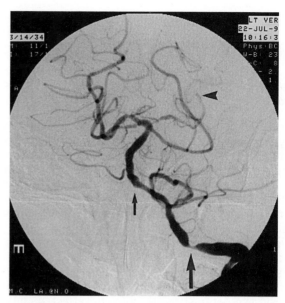

Figure 48-49 Case 16. A 62-year-old man with periodic episodes of dizziness associated with falling to the right. He was diagnosed with third-degree heart block; the neurologic symptoms were ascribed to cardiogenic syncope. In recent years he had developed visual difficulties and been told he had "white spots" in the back of his brain, seen on MRI. Note the threadlike remnant of the left vertebral artery at the atlanto-occipital junction, a typical location for stenosis as well as dissection *(large arrow)*. In addition, note the similar appearance of the origin of the left posterior cerebral artery.

The left vertebral artery injection allows analysis of the hemodynamics of the left posterior cerebral artery and reveals this vessel to be the sole supply to the proximal posterior cerebral artery territory. If the posterior communicating artery had been present, the flow rate in the P2 segment *(arrowhead)* and distal posterior cerebral artery territory would be more rapid, although more dilute. This is not the case. Note that the density of the vessel is essentially unchanged throughout its visualized path and consistent with the limited supply through the stenosis, but no distal perfusion of the territory is seen at this point in the runoff. The flow is slow but not washed out. Note also the lack of inflow from the opposite vertebral artery where it should join the basilar artery *(small arrow)*.

Case 16 continues

The day after the procedure, the patient was able to watch (and see) television for the first time in 3 years because of the increased perfusion of the occipital lobes (Fig. 48–52), although there remained a stenosis of the left posterior cerebral artery P1 segment (see Fig. 48–51).

The decision was made not to treat the P1 lesion at that time, owing to the need to cross the fresh angioplasty site in the vertebral artery to reach the stenosis in the posterior cerebral artery. The patient returned for treatment of this lesion 4 months later. At that time, the previous angioplasty site demonstrated minimal restenosis. The patient underwent an uneventful angioplasty of the P1 lesion, using a 2-mm Stratus balloon (Medtronic/MIS), with further improvement in his vision (Figs. 48–53 to 48–57). He can now read a newspaper without glasses, whereas prior to therapy he could not even watch television.

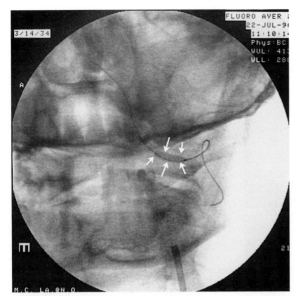

Figure 48-50 A Stratus angioplasty balloon is in place through the stenosis. An Envoy guide catheter has been placed in the vertebral artery by first selecting the vessel with a diagnostic catheter and exchanging for the Envoy over a Rosen-type exchange wire (Cook, Inc.). The Envoy was chosen for this particular case because, while the tip is not as atraumatic at the FasGUIDE, the body of the catheter is stiffer and offers more support for the advancement of the angioplasty balloon catheter. The Stratus has an excellent profile and hydrophilic coating. Even so, it was difficult to advance the balloon microcatheter without forcing the guide catheter to back down the vessel. Newer guide catheters such as the Lumax Neuroguide (Cook, Inc.) or cardiology guide catheters can help with this problem.

TECHNIQUE OF ELECTIVE INTRACRANIAL ANGIOPLASTY

The role of emergent angioplasty is covered in Chapter 58. This procedure should be part of the armamentarium of anyone truly performing direct therapy for acute stroke. As stated previously, an overwhelming consideration in this procedural technique is the pathophysiology of angioplasty and the vascular response to this process (described in detail in Chapter 41).

Preprocedure Preparation

Aspirin

Aspirin (325 mg) is given the morning of the procedure.

Antioxidants (Probucol)

Although the use of antioxidants is controversial, if probucol was readily available, we would place all patients on this drug before and after the intracranial angioplasty procedure to prevent restenosis. It is not known how long before a procedure these patients should be started on probucol. In the initial study of this drug for coronary angioplasty, patients were placed on probucol 1 month before the procedure and maintained on this drug for 6 months afterward.[36] This would appear to be the indicated

regimen for patients undergoing intracranial angioplasty.

Anticoagulants

We always place patients on oral or parenteral anticoagulants for a time before elective intracranial angioplasty, as a test of best medical therapy or lesion stability. If the patient will remain hospitalized, intravenous heparin can be given. This can be converted to oral warfarin before discharge, or the patient can be reevaluated angiographically while still in the hospital, depending on the clinical circumstances. Rarely, a tight stenosis is observed that resolves to the point at which angioplasty does not appear to be necessary; continued anticoagulation is then considered the appropriate therapy. In more than one case, during the time that the proper angioplasty catheters were being acquired (a matter of weeks), the stenosis simply went away. In addition, a case has been reported in which, after a typical carotid endarterectomy, an intracranial internal carotid artery stenosis simply vanished.[36a] We have observed this same phenomenon, as well as a patient with a history of severe migraines and an internal carotid artery stenosis that had caused an infarct, but which probably represented malignant vasospasm rather than atherosclerotic disease. This stenosis was not treated after it improved dramatically in only one day (see Figs. 48–37 and 48–38).

These cases imply that at least a portion of some lesions was simply thrombus, for which angioplasty should not be performed at all. For this reason, we routinely pretreat patients with anticoagulants for a period of time and initiate the angioplasty procedure with a brief infusion of urokinase (1 hour) in selected

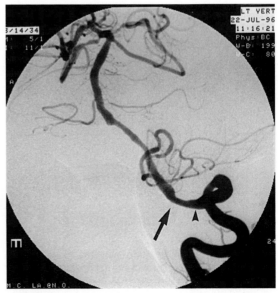

Figure 48-51 This injection reveals the postangioplasty result *(arrow)*. Note that the result is not that of a vessel with a lumen equal to the size of the vessel both immediately before and after the lesion *(arrowhead)*, but a size that is adequate for perfusion of the distal territory, and indeed larger than the somewhat more distal vertebral artery before its junction with the basilar artery.

Case 16 continues

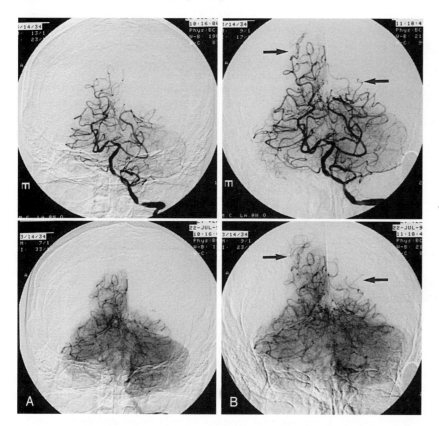

Figure 48-52 A comparison of preangioplasty *(A)* and postangioplasty *(B)* images. Note the significantly increased perfusion of both posterior cerebral territories *(arrows)*. Additional branches are filling on both sides, but most particularly, there is more perfusion of the posterior cerebral territory on the left. This is significant, because this increased perfusion is seen in spite of the fact that *the origin of the posterior cerebral artery still has a critical stenosis with severe flow restriction*. If the supply to this territory from MCA collaterals was adequate, there would not have been this increase in the runoff in these vessels, particularly the left. The patient's ataxia and dizziness resolved.

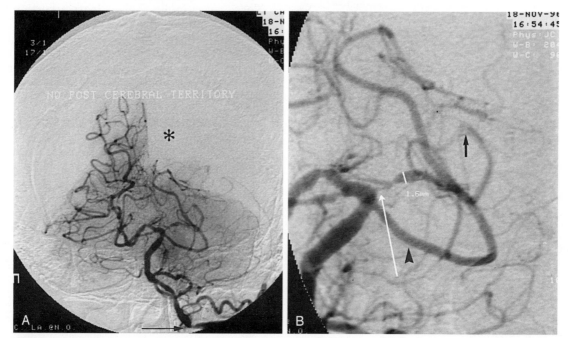

Figure 48-53 PA *(A)* and magnification *(B)* views of the left vertebral artery obtained when the patient returned 4 months later for treatment of the left P1 lesion. Note that the previously treated stenosis in the vertebral artery *(long black arrow, A)* looks slightly worse than on the immediate postangioplasty images. Note also the severe stenosis of the origin of P1 on the left *(white arrow, B)*. There was no posterior communicating artery on this side.

Also note the almost total absence of perfusion of the posterior cerebral artery territory on the left *(asterisk, A)*. The only territory actually filling is below the tentorium from the large superior cerebellar artery *(arrowhead, B)*. On the magnification view, it is noted that the posterior cerebral artery itself is only 1.6 mm and practically ends in the distal P2 segment *(small arrow, B)*. This is smaller than the smallest intracranial angioplasty balloon now available (Medtronic/MIS is in the process of making a 1.5-mm balloon). This renders an angioplasty more dangerous in this location owing to the possibility of severe vessel damage due to overdistention of the normal vessel during the angioplasty procedure.

Case 16 continues

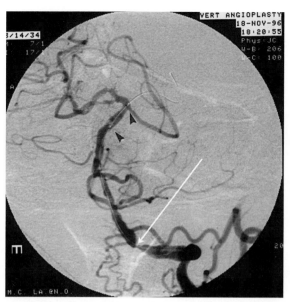

Figure 48-54 A 2-mm Stratus balloon angioplasty catheter is being advanced through the P1 lesion; note the marker bands on the catheter *(arrowheads)*. The contrast injection through the guide catheter still perfuses the posterior fossa (the microcatheter does not occlude the stenotic segment of the vertebral artery). The microwire (0.010″) does occlude the posterior cerebral artery, however. The balloon in the P1 segment was inflated to only 3 atmospheres because of concern about overdilation of the normal vessel.

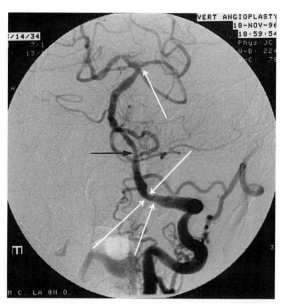

Figure 48-56 The postangioplasty angiogram reveals that the vertebral stenosis is not ideally dilated *(proximal white arrows)* but is the same size as the more distal stenosis *(black arrow)* at the PICA origin. It is no longer a flow-restricting lesion and will carry adequate blood to the posterior fossa. Note the left posterior cerebral artery, now filling normally *(distal white arrow)*.
Case 16 continues

cases. If any change is observed, the infusion is continued until stability is reached and the angioplasty can be performed or the angioplasty is no longer needed (see "Lesion Stability," below).

Even when a patient is maintained on anticoagu-

lants before the procedure, this does not guarantee that the lesion will be free of thrombus. A case presented in Chapter 59 demonstrates this dramatically (see Figs. 59–109 to 59–112). The fact that urokinase infusion succeeded in cleaning up the embolus relatively easily in this case implies that the lesion (and embolus) was not entirely old plaque.

Pharmacologic Cerebral Protection

This topic is discussed in Chapter 43. Nimodipine, 60 mg given orally before any intracranial procedure, appears to be a safe, worthwhile adjunct, and is routinely administered.

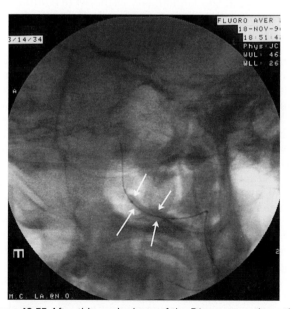

Figure 48-55 After this angioplasty of the P1 segment, the catheter was withdrawn and the vertebral artery stenosis dilated with a 3-mm balloon (purposely undersized to prevent severe intimal tears). It was considered acceptable to withdraw the balloon catheter system completely since the proximal lesion had not been dilated and therefore there was no worry about recrossing a lesion. The 3-mm balloon is now inflated in position *(arrows)*.

Procedural Technique

At the start of any procedure involving intracranial vessels, a control angiogram is performed to ascertain the supply to all parts of the brain and the flow rates, in addition to the baseline status of the vessel in question.

For cases that are not emergencies, the initial goals are to evaluate the lesion thoroughly and to measure both the parent vessel and the lesion accurately. The stenosis is evaluated thoroughly to find the projection that yields the best profile of the lesion; it is then measured with the use of an external marker, typically a quarter (see Chapter 3).

The stenosis is not the object of measurement, but rather the vessel just proximal and distal to the abnormality. It does not matter if the stenosis is 0.4 mm or 0.9 mm. It is the minimum measurement of the *normal vessel* that determines the size of the balloon to be used.

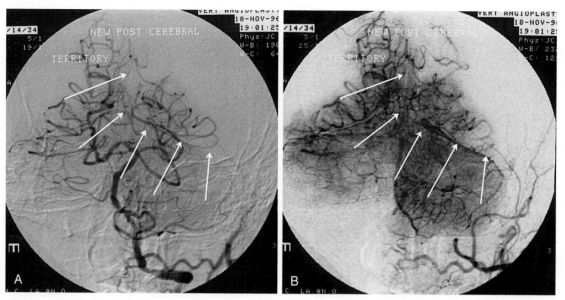

Figure 48-57 The final angiogram reveals newly seen left posterior cerebral artery perfusion *(arrows, A)* with newly seen blush in the occipital lobe *(arrows, B)* (compare with Figure 48–52). After these areas had been observed for 1 hour for any delayed thrombus formation, the patient was returned to his room and was now able to read a newspaper without glasses for the first time in 3 years.

Oxygen

Oxygen is administered during all procedures at a rate of 2 L/min by nasal cannula.

Vascular Access

In any case in which prolonged postprocedural anticoagulation is almost certainly needed, a micropuncture set (Cook, Inc.) is used. This is always true if there is the probability (or possibility) that fibrinolytic agents will be required. Once the vessel is entered, the diagnostic angiogram is performed in a routine fashion. After this has been done, the diagnostic catheter is exchanged for a guide catheter. If a sheath is needed, a long 6-Fr. sheath is used (see Chapter 1). If a guide catheter larger than 6-Fr. is needed, one that can be introduced directly percutaneously over its own dilator (without a sheath) is used to avoid creating a large hole in the artery (see Chapter 3).

Diagnostic Angiogram

Selection of the brachiocephalic vessel is made using a diagnostic catheter. These catheters are designed for this purpose and can accomplish this task effectively and safely. We do not use angled guide catheters for this purpose; these are not intended for vessel selection, and the angled tip of the guide catheter does not sit well in the intended location. Safe downstream access is obtained with the diagnostic catheter (see Chapter 3).

We routinely evaluate the *entire* vascular supply to the brain prior to angioplasty because changes do not occur just in the target vascular distribution. After the intended lesion has been dilated, there may be a shift in the watershed zone. If the watershed zone is not well understood prior to the angioplasty, it may appear after the angioplasty that there is slow flow in a large branch arising from the treated vessel (suggestive of embolus). This may simply represent a distal shift of the watershed in this branch due to the newly increased inflow. For this reason, we routinely examine the supply to all parts of the brain, not just what the target vessel supplies.

Guide Catheter

An adequate guide catheter is mandatory not only to inject around the angioplasty catheter to evaluate its position and the angioplasty results but also to give firm, stable support to the actual delivery and advancement of the angioplasty catheter. It is extremely frustrating to get the microangioplasty catheter almost to where it needs to be and then have a buckle develop proximally in the delivery system (causing everything to recoil into the aorta).

The design criteria for an intracranial angioplasty guide catheter are different than for catheters for the large proximal brachiocephalic stenoses discussed earlier and also for guide catheters suitable for simple intracranial embolization procedures. In large vessel angioplasty procedures, the angioplasty balloon needs to be larger, a stent may be needed, and the parent vessels are larger. This permits the use of a larger guide catheter. Injections to check for results also require large boluses of contrast, and thus a large lumen.

Particularly in the posterior fossa, where the size of the vertebral artery is limited, a smaller guide catheter is almost always mandatory. The vertebral artery is fragile and tortuous, even if it looks relatively straight on the posteroanterior view.

Larger, stiffer guide catheters can damage the endothelium of the vessel during the time they sit there, simply as a result of respiratory motion. Due to scratching from the catheter tip over the course of a case, thrombus can build up around the outside of the guide catheter and be unsuspected until it is noticed that the runoff is not as fast as expected. Even though the distal 1 mm of the guide catheter tip is soft, the catheter can damage the lining of the vessel or even cause an intimal tear. Thus, a softer guide catheter should be used even though support may be sacrificed (the reason that neuro-guide catheters were developed). Support is not as important as not damaging the inside of the vessel.

No ideal guide catheter is available for delivery of an intracranial angioplasty catheter. The Envoy (Cordis Corp.) has a large lumen, but the tip is not as benign as desired. The FasGUIDE has by far the best tip of any guide catheter, but the lumen is slightly too small to inject around the angioplasty balloon (particularly larger balloon sizes) for a follow-up angiogram after angioplasty; worse, the shaft is far from stiff enough. Although the Omniguide has thin wall construction, and thus a larger lumen, and a relatively benign tip, it is even less stiff than the FasGUIDE, and not nearly stiff enough to retain its position. Both the Envoy and Omniguide catheters are available in a 5-Fr. size and are capable of carrying a microangioplasty catheter. These catheters are all discussed in Chapter 1.

The Guidezilla (Schneider, Inc.) and the Lumax have sturdy shafts but are not truly intended for head and neck work (their distal tips are too stiff; they are actually cardiology designs). They may give a stable platform for deployment of an angioplasty balloon if placed with great caution in a section of vessel that accommodates their shape and watched carefully during the case. We prefer the FasGUIDE for any case with questionable vascular status.

The Lumax Neuroguide design is a good compromise. It provides excellent support for advancement of the angioplasty catheter and allows good bolus injection around the indwelling catheter. If the vessel is capable of accommodating a 7-Fr. guide catheter, we use this catheter because of its relative safety as well as the good support and adequate lumen. The distal shaft is still too stiff, however. The lumen of the 7-Fr. guide catheter is adequate for injection when using 2-, 2.5-, or 3-mm balloons, while the 8-Fr. version provides the larger lumen needed when using 3.5- or 4-mm balloons. As mentioned previously, these catheters are packaged with a dilator; they can be advanced directly through the skin without a sheath. The 8-Fr. catheter produces a hole in the artery no larger than that made by a 6-Fr. sheath.

When using microangioplasty balloons in a (relatively) small vertebral artery, it may not be possible to place a large guide catheter within this vessel. In this instance, the guide catheter must be left within the subclavian artery. In this proximal location, there is the need for very strong stable support. The guide catheter must be able to deliver the microcatheter, sit in its place without moving (there is no room for "back-up"), and deliver a large bolus of contrast so that visualization of downstream structures is possi-

ble even though the injection is in the subclavian artery. We choose a 9-Fr. guide catheter without a distal taper, such as the Brite-Tip, introduced without a sheath over a 7-Fr., 110-cm Berenstein catheter (USCI) (see Chapter 3). This allows deployment of the microcatheter from a very stable location in the subclavian artery, as well as good bolus injections for distal opacification, yet it produces a hole in the skin and vessel only as large as that made by a 7-Fr. sheath. It is necessary to predilate the puncture site with a 9-Fr. dilator.

Guide Catheter Placement

Once the guide catheter has been selected, it should be seated as far distally as feasible, depending on which guide catheter has been chosen. The operator should observe for the effects of respiration and make sure that the tip of the guide catheter is in a good position and not in a curve of the vessel where respiration could make it buckle and cause intimal damage, thrombus, or spasm. The sheath (if one is used) and guide catheter should be secured in position with Steri-Strips and connected to flush systems.

Posterior Circulation

Generally, for any posterior circulation intracranial angioplasty, it is desirable to place the guide catheter as far distally in the vertebral artery as possible. The safest guide catheter for this purpose is the FasGUIDE. The flow rate in the vertebral artery is not very high and the relatively small lumen of this catheter does not make a significant difference. A bolus injection around the microangioplasty catheter will opacify the distal territory adequately.

If the 6-Fr. FasGUIDE is too large for the vertebral artery, the 5-Fr. Omniguide may fit. This catheter is small and has a very large lumen, but it offers very little support for the deployment of the angioplasty catheter. Alternatively, the 5-Fr. Envoy can be used. This has a slightly smaller lumen but offers more support.

If even the Omniguide catheter is too large for the vertebral artery, it may be necessary to deploy the microcatheter from the subclavian artery. If this is the case, an extremely stable platform is necessary, as discussed earlier.

Under these circumstances, the notion of a small puncture site becomes secondary to the ability to achieve the goal at hand, and a large, stable guide catheter should be used. As discussed previously, it is possible to advance a 9-Fr. Brite-Tip catheter placed over a 7-Fr. Berenstein catheter directly through the skin to the correct position (using an appropriate exchange wire). The correct shape of Brite-Tip catheter (to fit the deployment direction) is chosen in advance.

Once this guide catheter has been placed, the microangioplasty balloon catheter can be delivered. It may be necessary to use the angioplasty catheter to select the vessel (the vertebral artery), but this is relatively simple with the choice of guidewires available.

Anterior Circulation

Intracranial stenoses involving the anterior circulation present a different technical problem. Catheterizing the parent vessel (the internal carotid artery) is typically not a significant challenge. Placement of a stable guide catheter will render the remainder of the procedure far easier. In this location, the flow rate is more rapid than in the vertebral artery and larger bolus injections are needed. Depending on the size of the angioplasty balloon required, either a 7-Fr. or an 8-Fr. Lumax Neuroguide is chosen. If the vessel containing the stenosis to be dilated is 3 mm or less in diameter, the 7-Fr. size is used; if the vessel requires a balloon larger than 3 mm, an 8-Fr. catheter is placed. This is placed directly over an exchange wire into the distal cervical internal carotid artery, utilizing the dilator that comes with the guide catheter. If necessary, it is possible to perform the angioplasty from the common carotid artery, but firm purchase within the internal carotid artery will make the task much easier.

The real challenge in this situation is the tortuosity of the internal carotid artery just distal to the bifurcation of the common carotid artery (i.e., the proximal cervical internal carotid artery). It may not be possible to place a guide catheter into the distal internal carotid artery without inducing a significant amount of spasm.

Intraprocedural Parent Vessel Vasospasm

Proximal parent vessel vasospasm can be more of a problem for intracranial angioplasty than for the usual case. Aggressive intravascular maneuvers are being performed, thus potentially causing spasm. Any slowing of flow can also precipitate further problems downstream either before the angioplasty (when there may be sluggish flow) or after angioplasty (when the endothelium is disrupted). Careful attention to catheter and guidewire technique is therefore indicated.

It is frequently the exchange wire that is the cause of spasm. We have begun using the neuro-exchange wire from Cook, Inc. for this reason.

We routinely use nitroglycerin paste (2") at the start of the procedure to avoid vasospasm. Other operators routinely use nifedipine for the same purpose (see Chapters 3 and 4).

For treatment of vasospasm during the case, papaverine, nitroglycerin, or amyl nitrate can be used (see Chapter 66). We use nitroglycerin, 50 μg/ml in normal saline, infused slowly (1 to 3 ml over 1 to 3 minutes, repeated if necessary). Papaverine has been shown to be toxic when used in concentrated doses infused with a syringe; therefore we no longer use this technique routinely.

Air Filters

We use air filters (see Chapter 1) on all brachiocephalic flush systems for peace of mind, not to remove debris but to trap an inadvertent air bubble coming down the intravenous tubing. One never knows when an unsuspected air bubble may make its way downstream or when a flush solution bag may be changed and a bubble inadvertently introduced into the system during the procedure.

Lesion Stability

If stability of the lesion has not been demonstrated by repeated angiography over a period of time, the possibility exists that at least a portion of the identified stenosis is actually thrombus. This is not usually a problem (but see Figs. 59–109 to 59–112).

If there is some doubt, and there is no possibility of a recent infarct, infusion of urokinase (125,000 units) is indicated to try to clean up the angioplasty site (see Chapter 60). This is continued for 1 hour, and then the lesion is reassessed. If a change is noted, the infusion is continued until no further progress is made. A determination is then made about the continued necessity for an angioplasty (i.e., if significant reduction in the amount of occlusive material results, the stenosis may not require angioplasty).

Although the infusion of urokinase might clear the stenosis to some degree, it is usually not cleared enough to avoid the necessity of an angioplasty. About half the practicing interventional neuroradiologists perform this preangioplasty urokinase infusion (verbal communications), but this practice may be fading. If the patient has been receiving heparin for a period of time, or if a comparison with a prior angiogram reveals stability of the lesion, this maneuver probably is not necessary.

If no change has occurred during the infusion, the remaining 125,000 units of urokinase is then available for use after the angioplasty (if needed for emergency infusion for a postangioplasty platelet and thrombus cascade). Since the advent of abciximab (ReoPro), we have used urokinase only once on an angioplasty site.

Measurement of the Lesion and Choice of Balloon Size

If a control angiogram with an external marker has not been performed, now is the time to do it (see Chapter 3). Accurate measurement of the vessel is *mandatory*. It is unacceptable to guess; an error of 0.5 mm may be a potential error of 20% or more and will result in selection of a different balloon size. Accidentally oversizing a balloon may result in a potentially fatal vascular rupture or intimal dissection.

Once an accurate size has been obtained, a balloon size is chosen that is at least one size or 0.5 mm smaller than the measurement of the vessel. In other words, if the vessel measures 2.4 mm, a 2.0-mm balloon is used. If the lesion measures 3.3 mm, a 2.5-mm (or, at most, a 3-mm) balloon is used. We try to use a balloon that is at least 0.5 mm smaller than the vessel.

Measurement of the vessel by comparison with the catheter size is difficult; an error of 1 pixel on the screen may easily be a margin of error of 10% to

20%. The Brite-Tip catheter can be used for this purpose. Its tip is easier to see than the vague outline of other catheters, and a 9-Fr. tip is exactly 3 mm. Measuring the shaft of a microcatheter for sizing, however, is asking for trouble. The margin of error is great. We always use an external quarter because of the predictability and accuracy of sizing (see Chapter 3).

The size of angioplasty balloon is chosen to give a result that is intentionally undersized. These patients present not because of embolic events from these lesions, but because of lack of flow through them. Opening the vessel to three to five times the previous size (in cross-sectional area) increases the flow exponentially. Simply doubling the diameter will increase the cross-sectional area four-fold and will increase flow proportional to the fourth power of the radius.

What is to be avoided at all costs is vessel damage to the extent that a severe intimal dissection occurs and the vessel occludes. Therefore, we *always* undersize balloons. Even if the angioplasty result does not look perfect, the result will be adequate and the vessel is not torn up. If needed, the balloon can be reinflated to try to stretch the vessel a little more. Increasing the inflation pressure also increases the dilation size of the balloon slightly. This increase in pressure can substitute for a change to a larger balloon.

If the angioplasty result is suboptimal (as it may be, since the balloon is intentionally undersized), *an attempt to recross the lesion with a larger balloon should only be made in extreme circumstances.* If absolutely necessary, a delay of a week or two will allow the intima to heal and the lesion can be redilated. We have never had to do this, however. Almost any improvement in lumen is adequate, and the lesion can be re-treated at the time of the 3-month follow-up angiogram if necessary.

Procedural Anticoagulation

As noted previously, patients receive 325 mg aspirin prior to the procedure. Heparin is used during all intracranial angioplasties. A bolus of 5000 units is given, followed by an infusion of 1000 U/hour.

We now use abciximab (ReoPro) for all elective intracranial angioplasties. This drug is a powerful antiplatelet agent (see Chapter 4) and has been shown to offer some protection from thrombus formation following angioplasty in the coronary arteries.[37, 38] This agent is currently being used as an adjunct to percutaneous transluminal coronary angioplasty (PTCA) to prevent acute cardiac ischemia in patients at high risk for abrupt closure of the treated vessel, and is used in conjunction with heparin and aspirin. It is administered intravenously as a bolus (0.25 mg/kg) 10 to 60 minutes before PTCA and is followed by a continuous infusion for 12 hours (10 μg/min). Abciximab has been shown to add to the activity of heparin, prolonging the activated clotting time by 30 to 40 seconds. The bolus dose provides activity for at least 2 hours, and residual activity

following administration of the entire dose can last up to 96 hours. There is an increased incidence of hemorrhagic complications associated with its use (as compared with the same procedure performed without abciximab). In addition, there is a risk of development of thrombocytopenia; this risk appears to be greater in thin patients. Although no clinical trials have been completed that have evaluated this agent as an adjunct to brachiocephalic (or peripheral) angioplasty and stenting, it appears to control the tendency to develop local thrombosis following angioplasty that is so troublesome to interventional neuroradiologists.

Prolonged infusion may not be necessary because most hyperacute thrombus formation occurs within the first 15 to 30 minutes. This has not been established, however, and we are so concerned about thrombus formation that we continue the infusion as recommended for coronary angioplasty.

Other agents that inhibit the platelet fibrinogen receptor glycoprotein IIb/IIIa (e.g., Integrelin) are undergoing clinical evaluation.[39] These agents may prove to have a role in the prevention of restenosis as well as acute occlusion following angioplasty.[38]

Intracranial Angioplasty Catheters

The introduction of a monolumen angioplasty catheter incorporating a dedicated guidewire for distal catheter tip occlusion and based on the original TRACKER (Target Therapeutics) technology opened new possibilities for distal access, which have more recently been expanded on. The original STEALTH design is essentially unchanged except for the addition of a hydrophilic coating (FasSTEALTH) and modest improvements in the occlusion guidewire. Additional sizes are also available. Cardiology or other microangioplasty catheters can be potentially forced into fairly distal or tortuous locations, but not with the finesse, ease, steerability, and safety of the STEALTH catheters. Medtronic/MIS has introduced a microangioplasty monolumen design with some improvements; this design is available with a relatively noncompliant balloon for dilatation of atherosclerotic lesions (the Stratus) and a softer, more compliant balloon (Silastic) for angioplasty of vasospasm (the Solstice).

Angioplasty catheters used by cardiologists are inappropriate for intracranial use. The stiffness of their design, while making them easier to push, deters finesse, and a dissection is far easier to produce with these little spears. All "feel" for intracranial maneuvering is lost, and these catheters can jump forward forcefully after going around a corner. Coronary angioplasty balloons are generally at least 2 cm in length, far too long for intracranial use. In addition, it is not possible to completely purge these balloons of air.

Getting the angioplasty catheter into place can be a challenge. The newer intracranial designs, incorporating a hydrophilic coating, make the procedure much easier than the older designs. The numerous, extremely tortuous curves leading to the angioplasty site result in a great deal of friction on the surface of the catheter, and even with the hydrophilic coating, placement can be difficult. There are two strategies that can be used when this is encountered.

When using the STEALTH catheter, we prefer to have the occlusion wire backloaded in the catheter. This permits the tip of the wire to protrude as far past the catheter as necessary to select the correct path and give some support to the trailing catheter. This strategy, however, does not permit the use of a standard microguidewire for downstream selection and then exchange of this wire for the occlusion wire; if this is required, the occlusion wire is loaded from

the typical (antegrade) direction. This usually is not a significant problem if the catheter is already in position at the lesion. The use of the long-tipped occlusion guidewire allows the tip of the guidewire to be well out of the catheter without engaging the valve. Engaging the valve increases the pushability of the unit, but renders the catheter-guidewire combination very stiff.

When using the STEALTH, we no longer have the wire and catheter prefixed as a unit, with the lumen already prepared with diluted contrast and the wire occluding the tip. This is too difficult to maneuver as a unit and defeats the purpose of having the ability

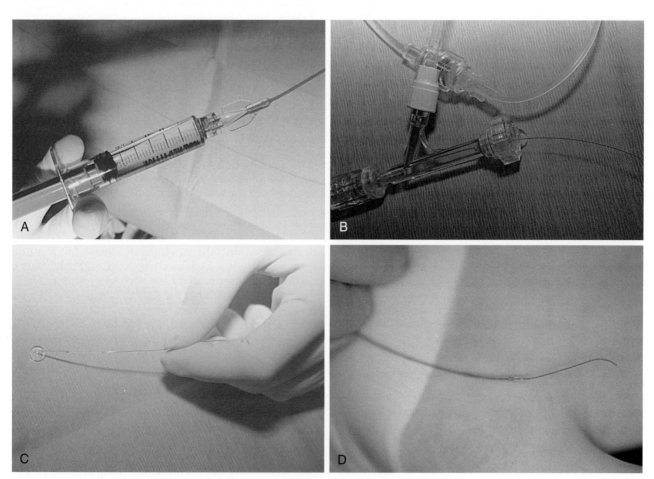

Figure 48-58 The technique of preparation of a Stratus microangioplasty catheter:

A. The Stratus microangioplasty catheter is flushed with a solution of three-quarter strength contrast. This contrast density is necessary for visualization of the balloon when it is inflated (a 2-mm balloon is very difficult to see).

B. A Y-connector is attached to the hub of the microangioplasty catheter. The Quicksilver-10 occlusion guidewire (Medtronic/MIS) has been placed through the Y-connector into the Stratus catheter, but *not all the way out the end of the catheter*. The side port of the Y-connector is connected a 3′ to 6′ microtubing extension set (see Chapter 1) attached to an inflation device. This flexible microtubing is used because it allows free movement of the system once it has been placed into position in the guide catheter without having to move the inflation device unnecessarily. The three-quarter strength contrast is injected into the system through the side port while holding the O-ring end of the Y-connector up to purge any air; contrast is allowed to leak out the valve of the Y-connector.

C. As stated previously, the Quicksilver occlusion guidewire is not advanced out the end of the catheter; the tip is positioned about 5 cm proximal to the end of the catheter. Once the valve is closed on the Y-connector at the hub of the microangioplasty catheter, the tip of the Y-connector is held up and the three-quarter strength contrast (and any remaining bubbles) is forced into the microangioplasty system and allowed to drip out the end of the catheter. The system is now purged.

D. Once the system has been purged, the Quicksilver guidewire is advanced out the end of the angioplasty catheter and shaped. A simple arc shape is sufficient (as shown) for distal selection during the angioplasty procedure; alternatively, a true J can be placed for safety.

to move or remove the wire. It is not possible to steer the wire when loaded in this fashion either.

Both the Stratus and Solstice balloon angioplasty catheters are similar to the STEALTH except for one important detail. They are designed so that the wire can occlude the catheter tip at any location along the distal portion of the wire (over a certain range) by utilizing a watertight slip-ring (O-ring) connection. This allows the wire to lead the catheter. The catheter is advanced as far as necessary to reach the lesion while allowing the wire to remain in position beyond the lesion in a comfortable location. This offers a certain freedom not present with the STEALTH. In addition, after the angioplasty is performed, the guidewire can be left downstream while the catheter is withdrawn, thus permitting evaluation of the angioplasty site without losing access to the true lumen of the vessel.

How to Prepare Microangioplasty Catheters

The instructions supplied with the Stratus and Solstice catheters themselves are much better than most such instructions. The procedure we use to prepare and introduce these balloon catheters is shown in Figure 48–58 and described in the accompanying legend. This procedure allows for meticulous purging of the catheter system prior to insertion but permits the operator to take advantage of the ability of the

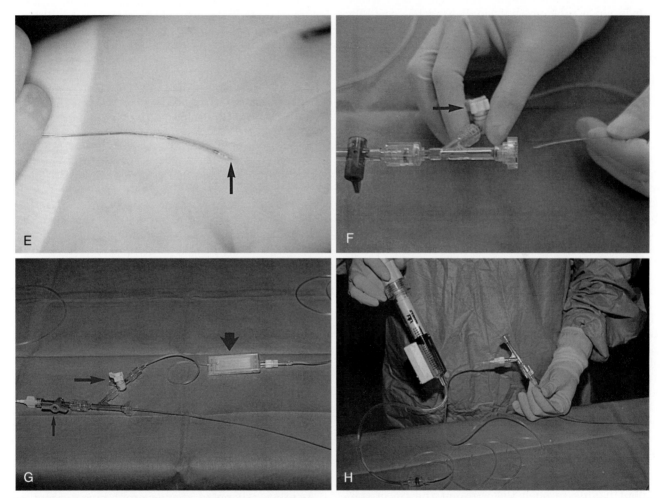

Figure 48–58 *Continued. E.* The shaped Quicksilver guidewire is withdrawn back into the Stratus catheter tip, resulting in a blunt end *(arrow).* This configuration is necessary for advancement of this system into the Y-connector of the guide catheter.

F. The Stratus angioplasty catheter (containing the guidewire just within its tip) is advanced into the Y-connector on the end of the guide catheter. Note the three-way stopcock on this Y-connector *(arrow),* allowing injection of contrast around the microcatheter during and after the dilation procedure. Note also the one-way valve on the guide catheter (on the left, turned off), permitting loading of the angioplasty catheter without significant blood loss.

G. Close-up view of the assembled operating system. Note the air filter (Pall Medical; *large arrow,* always used in flush systems) leading to the side port of the Y-connector of the guide catheter. Note also that the one-way stopcock between the guide catheter and the main Y-connector *(thin arrow)* is now open, since the Stratus is being advanced to its intended site. Once the Stratus has been advanced about halfway into the guide catheter, the Quicksilver occlusion guidewire is advanced several centimeters out the end of the Stratus.

H. The overall view of the operating system reveals the inflation device connected to the long (3′ to 6′) microtubing, which is connected to the side port of the Y-connector on the Stratus microangioplasty catheter. This arrangement allows free movement (and finesse) when using the angioplasty balloon catheter.

occlusion wire to act as a selecting guidewire. It also allows for easy manipulation of the microangioplasty catheter without having to move the bulky inflation device around.

It is also crucial to be sure that contrast material is actually filling the entire catheter and balloon before the angioplasty is performed. We use three-quarter strength contrast to ensure visualization of these tiny balloons, particularly the 2-mm size. All flushing during preparation is performed with this dilute contrast rather than with saline.

How to Use Microangioplasty Catheters

When performing angioplasty for intracranial stenoses, roadmapping capability is not necessary but is helpful in most circumstances. Generally, the anatomy is not extremely complex and finding the correct path is not a problem, but small branches (usually perforators) should be avoided with the guidewire, and accurate localization of the stenosis is necessary before balloon inflation.

The projection that gives the most truly perpendicular view of the stenotic vessel both proximal and distal to the stenosis should be chosen; this is necessary for accurate balloon positioning for the angioplasty. If the vessel makes a curve just at the stenosis, a projection between the two extremes should be used, not one with an ideal view of one portion of the vessel and a "down the barrel" view of the other; this destroys the depth perception necessary for accurate placement of the balloon. A view perpendicular to the *lesion* should be chosen.

There are at least three different techniques for reaching the lesion, placing the angioplasty balloon, and performing the angioplasty. The method used depends on the choice of microangioplasty catheter and the anatomy encountered.

A standard wire may be necessary to advance the STEALTH around tortuous loops to the region of the stenosis. When using the STEALTH catheter, the lesion can be crossed with a standard microguidewire followed by the balloon catheter (the balloon tip is placed all the way through the lesion and left in a relatively straight segment distal to the lesion). The standard guidewire is then replaced with the dedicated occluding wire. Ideally, this wire should be placed just proximal to the tip of the angioplasty catheter and then the catheter pulled back, thus exposing the tip of the wire and ensuring safe deployment of the occluding wire distal to the stenosis without having to push the wire out the tip of the catheter (a potentially dangerous maneuver). When the occlusion wire exits the tip of the STEALTH, subtle feel will be limited. The occlusion wire can also be used as a selecting wire when loaded in an antegrade fashion if a long-tipped occlusion wire is used.

Alternatively, the occlusion wire can be used as the leading guidewire and the STEALTH system placed as a unit. The occlusion wire can be backloaded with the occluding portion of the guidewire (the bead) distal to the tip of the catheter. As noted previously, this is the method we prefer. The tip of the wire should always have a curve placed before use to deter inadvertent impact at a vulnerable turn; this allows the soft distal tip to probe gently. This careful probing as the catheter is advanced is mandatory. The standard "feel" associated with the use of microcatheters and microguidewires is somewhat lost when using the STEALTH, and care should be maintained during its use.

The longer the soft coil tip segment of the wire that is protruding from the catheter, the safer the advancement will be. This is why many practitioners prefer to backload the wire. If a short-tipped occlusion wire is utilized in a standard antegrade manner, there may not be enough soft tip beyond the catheter to allow recoil if the wire hits a dead end. If the wire is partially withdrawn into the catheter in order to soften the shaft strength of the catheter, it will leave only a minimal amount of wire external to the tip. Three lengths of exposed coil tip are available: 0, 2, and 4 cm. The 2-cm coil tip does not provide a long distance for the wire to absorb an impact if it does encounter an obstruction while the valve is engaged, but does not require as extensive a length of usable vessel distal to the lesion as the 4-cm length. The 4-cm tip is better at absorbing impact force if it does hit an obstruction, even if it is partially withdrawn.

As noted above, we prefer the Stratus catheter. The ability to occlude the balloon at any point along the distal wire is a great advantage. It permits the use of the guidewire as a selecting wire, with a variable length of wire protruding from the tip of the catheter. It also allows freer motion of the guidewire, resulting in more precise steering. This allows much more delicate work without the risk of the stiff catheter-guidewire unit acting as a spear. It does not, however, permit the use of a standard (0.014″) microguidewire to aid in the initial advancement of the catheter; the lumen of these catheters is smaller than that of the STEALTH and accepts only 0.010″ wires. This is not a major disadvantage.

Lesion Dilation

Once the angioplasty balloon is in place, *extremely* slow inflation is begun. This is not possible by a hand inflation of the balloon using a standard syringe. A true screw-type inflation device must be used; this allows not only accurate assessment of the pressures generated but also finesse in the control of the rate of inflation and its duration.

As previously noted, if one were to invent a method of tearing up the inside of a vessel, one of the best would be to place a balloon inside the lumen and inflate it as rapidly as possible. When I first started performing angioplasties more than a decade ago, I routinely observed extensive intimal damage and dissections. This is almost never seen now with the technique of extremely slow inflation of the angioplasty balloon. Although a large vessel dissection may be well tolerated, an intracranial dissection is a potential disaster.

We now use an extremely long (2-meter or 6-foot)

microtubing extension set to connect from the inflation device to the rotating hemostatic valve around the occlusion wire for two reasons: (1) to avoid the hassle and fear of bubbles in the line coming from the connections and (2) this long, flexible tubing makes manipulation of the angioplasty catheter much easier and allows nonacrobatic hand positioning during catheter manipulation and balloon inflation.

As noted in Chapter 42, our best results have been achieved by these extremely gradual inflations, over several minutes (3 to 5), allowing the vessel to slowly stretch rather than tear. Balloon pressure is gradually increased from 1 to 1.5 to 2 atmospheres in several stages, allowing a pause of at least 15 seconds at each stage.

Vascular dilation is dependent on the rate of expansion, not on the rate of pressure increase. The vessel can be slowly stretching while the pressure never increases above 2 atmospheres. Therefore, extremely slow instillation of contrast should be performed combined with observation of the balloon, *not just the pressure*. As each new fluid injection is made, time should be allowed for additional slow expansion to occur.

Intracranial lesions are not extremely resistant to dilation (with the possible exception of the vertebrobasilar junction, midbasilar artery, and petrous ICA). The stenosis can begin dilating even before the pressure is much above 1 atmosphere. Usually, once the balloon reaches 2 atmospheres of pressure, visible expansion starts to occur; simply waiting and watching can reveal further dilation without instillation of additional fluid. Further pressure increases are made gradually in stages, allowing the vessel to comply slowly, until optimal balloon expansion has been achieved.

These slow increments of inflation are continued until the balloon reaches a maximum of about 6 atmospheres of pressure (the recommended limit); no further inflation of the balloon is made. Usually, nearly full vascular distention is reached at about 3 atmospheres; continuing increase in pressure gives the last 10% of the distention, if needed. Although extracranial lesions can sometimes require high pressures, intracranial lesions almost routinely require much less pressure.

The balloon is left inflated at the maximal pressure reached for 15 to 30 seconds and then gradually deflated. An angiogram can then be performed to confirm the results by injecting through the guide catheter with the angioplasty balloon still in place. Almost invariably, however, the deflated balloon blocks the flow of contrast enough to result in a poor image of the angioplasty result if it is still in the stenotic segment. Only after the balloon is removed from the angioplasty site is the actual result evident. This can be done by advancing the catheter or withdrawing it, with the guidewire maintained distal to the angioplasty site. This latter maneuver is easily performed with the Stratus balloon. It is not possible with a STEALTH balloon if the wire has been loaded

in an antegrade fashion, but can be used if the wire is backloaded.

Once the angioplasty has been performed, the balloon should be fully deflated. This is achieved not by simply releasing pressure, but by actively withdrawing fluid. This is particularly apparent with the STEALTH angioplasty catheter; simply pulling the occlusion wire back will move the occluding bead away from the tip and release pressure. However, *once the pressure is released, the balloon can remain inflated.* The fluid can stay within the inflated balloon at systemic blood pressure; it will not be pressurized, but will not depart the balloon, either. Therefore, it is imperative that the fluid be actively aspirated and not just allowed to leak out.

Temporary Vessel Occlusion Secondary to Balloon Inflation

Neurosurgeons routinely temporarily occlude intracranial vessels for periods longer than 10 minutes with no ischemic damage, even though periods of occlusion in excess of 10 minutes should be avoided, and, if necessary, periods of unclamping are used.[40] Batjer has noted that temporary occlusions up to 18 minutes are without consequence (verbal report).

Although temporary occlusion of a vessel may be tolerated in almost all cases, there may be circumstances in which this is not possible. The possible exception to the recommendation of slow balloon inflation is in the main trunk of the basilar artery. Temporary neurologic change (fainting) was noted once during an angioplasty in the posterior fossa, and such change should be viewed with the appropriate concern. Specifically, in the posterior circulation, there can be isolated perfusion of the brainstem and cerebellum, supplied by only one stenotic vessel. In this circumstance, rapid neurologic change can be noted with brief occlusion. This situation may be more analogous to general systemic flow arrest, in which permanent cell death can be produced by cessation of flow for as briefly as 10 minutes when there is absolutely no collateral perfusion or drift. In addition, invisible small perforators can be occluded by any prolonged inflation. These small perforators should not be occluded for any longer than 3 minutes. For this reason, the procedure should be broken down into several small stages, allowing reperfusion of any small branches in between. This complicates the procedure considerably. The goal of the procedure is to dilate the vessel adequately without severe intimal disruption, particularly in the region of these perforators.

Postdilation

Once the stenosis has been dilated to the optimal extent with this catheter, no further manipulation is undertaken (but this is not the end of the procedure, as noted below). Almost any improvement is acceptable, but usually the result is good or at least adequate. A less-than-perfect visual appearance (i.e., less than 100% dilation) is acceptable and compatible with a satisfactory result, particularly in the smaller intracranial vessels. As stated previously, a moderate improvement in lumen size for intracranial angioplasty is adequate; if the intima is minimally damaged, the chance of restenosis is lessened, at least over the short term.

The almost universal indication for intracranial angioplasty is arterial insufficiency, not for treatment of a thrombogenic source. Increasing a threadlike lumen to 2 to 3 mm is a vast increase in cross-sectional area and thus flow rate. The vessel does not have to be returned to its adolescent appearance. Remodeling of the surface also is accomplished with this process, which reduces thrombogenic turbulence. It is more important to dilate the vessel without the risk of severe intimal injury and the consequent acute or subacute closure rate. Angioplasty of these intracranial lesions cannot be rescued by stent placement at this time. In addition, stent placement in

and of itself increases the incidence of acute thrombosis and long-term restenosis.[41]

For these reasons, a period of watchful waiting is instituted to observe for any dynamic endothelial thrombotic response. Although spasm can be a problem, thrombosis is the primary concern, as described next.

Dynamic Endothelial Response to Angioplasty: Thrombosis

The procedure does not end at the completion of the angioplasty. In a normal vessel with intact endothelium, in a nonhypercoagulable state, static blood should not clot for a long period of time (minutes, certainly, and usually much longer). Uninjured vascular endothelium is antithrombotic, resists platelet adherence, and provides a hostile environment for activation of clotting factors. When vascular injury

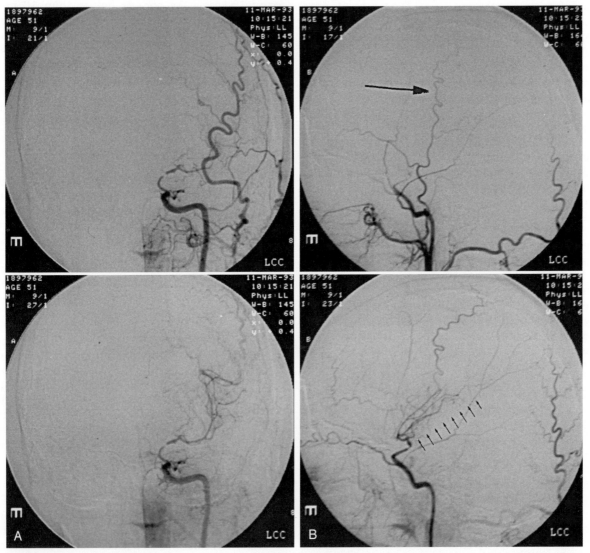

Figure 48-59 Case 17. Postangioplasty malignant thrombosis. PA *(A)* and lateral *(B)* left common carotid angiogram in a 51-year-old man with symptoms typical of stenosis of the distal ICA (i.e., episodic weakness and numbness of the hand with occasional speech difficulty). The angiogram reveals severe hemodynamic abnormality; note that the superficial temporal artery *(arrow)* reaches the crown of the head long before intracranial vessels are even perfusing their own territory *(arrows)*.

Case 17 continues

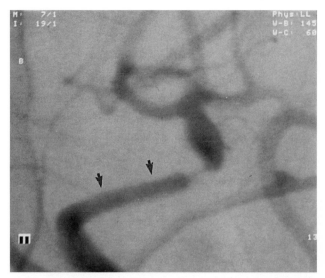

Figure 48-60 A magnified view of the focal stenosis reveals only a residual hair; the entire ICA also appears small *(arrows)*.

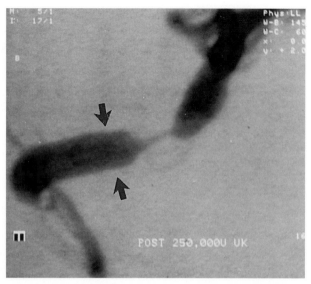

Figure 48-61 As per our standard procedure, 250,000 units of urokinase was infused for 1 hour to assess the possibility of thrombus superimposed on the plaque. Note that the urokinase has had minimal effect on the stenosis, but the urokinase infusion has produced *vasodilation*, a phenomenon we have observed on other occasions.

does occur (e.g., secondary to guidewire manipulation or angioplasty), the rate of coagulation reactions can increase to 300,000 times baseline.[42] Plaque and intimal disruption causes local platelet deposition by the release of thromboxane A_2 as well as platelet-derived growth factor. Once a guidewire or catheter has scraped the endothelium, thrombus formation is unpredictable and therefore heparin is indicated during the inflation and for a period of time afterward. Pharmacologic agents with platelet antiaggregation action (e.g., abciximab) are proving to be of great benefit in controlling this thrombotic cascade.

It is the angioplasty site itself (after deflation of the balloon), and not the distal lumen, that is at primary risk for thrombus formation following angioplasty. For prolonged angioplasty inflations in the periphery (e.g., the superficial femoral artery), our

experience has shown heparin to be uniformly unnecessary, probably due to the vessel size and flow rate. In intracranial small vessel stenoses, however, the process of angioplasty is a dynamic one, not ending simply at deflation of the balloon. The act of angioplasty can stimulate a malignant coagulation cascade. The damaged vessel wall undergoes immediate thrombotic reaction involving platelet aggregation, which can progress to occlusion (Case 17, Figs. 48–59 to 48–65). Even though it has been shown experimentally that the platelet cascade is essentially ended after about 10 minutes,[43, 44] this activity can continue on to occlusion even after that time. This endothelial

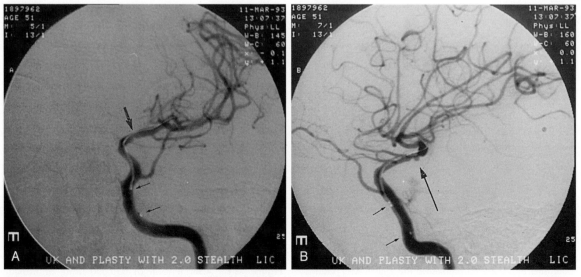

Figure 48-62 Angioplasty with a 2.0-mm STEALTH balloon was performed. After the angioplasty, the occluding wire was left in the vessel across the stenosis while the catheter was withdrawn slightly (note the markers on the balloon, *short arrows*). The angioplasty result appears acceptable *(long arrows)*. The antegrade intracranial flow is excellent.

Case 17 continues

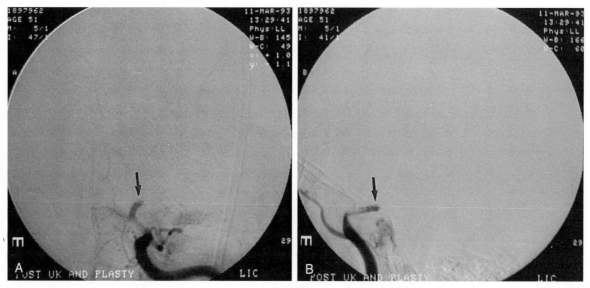

Figure 48-63 The PA *(A)* and lateral *(B)* angiograms 37 minutes later demonstrate that the ICA is completely occluded *(arrows)*. It was only at this time (more than 30 minutes after the angioplasty) that the patient began to experience some neurologic difficulty.

damage can be greatly lessened with the slow stretch described previously. The posterior fossa is the most likely location for this reaction, but it can occur in any location.

This delayed thrombus formation may not be noticed, however, if no delayed imaging is performed after the angioplasty and the initial appearance (which looks great) is the last one seen. This is a common practice among interventional radiologists. The procedure is done, the initial result looks great, and everyone goes home. Standing around waiting for an infrequent complication is difficult; it is boring,

inefficient, and usually unrewarding; when there is a complication, it is unwelcome information and a hassle.

Although some occlusions may be asymptomatic (and are classified as late vascular occlusions on follow-up), some can be dramatically symptomatic, manifesting when the patient is in the holding area or the recovery room. Continued periodic angiographic observation of the angioplasty site is therefore mandatory. We routinely observe all angioplasty sites for 1 hour after the procedure, but most thrombus cascades reveal themselves within the first 15 to 30 minutes (see Figs. 59–1 to 59–11).

Usually, the platelet aggregation cascade stops in

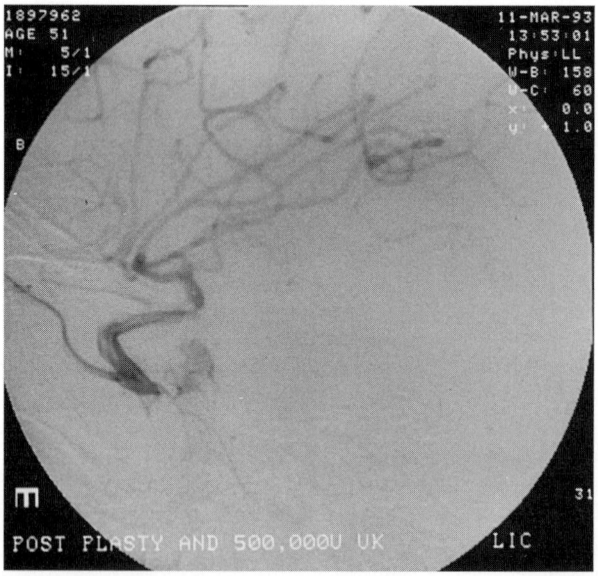

Figure 48-64 Infusion of urokinase was begun immediately, and after 250,000 units had been administered the vessel was patent, with good antegrade flow. Streaming from injection though the microcatheter renders accurate evaluation of residual thrombus difficult (no true guide catheter was used).

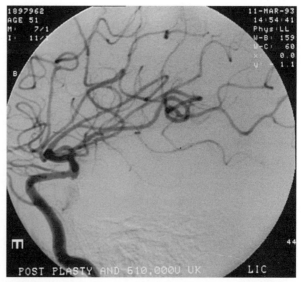

Figure 48-65 After a total of 610,000 units of urokinase was infused, the vessel and angioplasty site appear pristine. Further observation of the site revealed no further evidence of malignant thrombosis.

less than 30 minutes, and during the second half hour the angioplasty site either stabilizes or begins to clear to the appearance it had immediately after the angioplasty. It typically clears spontaneously, without any intervention. As discussed below, if the situation requires treatment, when this cascade has been stopped and cleaned up using urokinase or another agent, the lesion stabilizes without further malignant occlusive tendency.

The site may, however, rapidly begin to appear irregular after the angioplasty, and the tendency may be to interpret this as an intimal flap necessitating redilation, or tacking down. Remanipulation of a damaged vessel and its intima should be avoided. The intracranial vessels are not only small but also tortuous, and it is not possible to skillfully select the true lumen; the wire takes the outside curve and tends to find any extraluminal channel. Any attempt to recross the angioplasty site is therefore fraught with danger.

Fibrinolysis

If thrombus or angioplasty site irregularity has formed, an infusion of fibrinolytics usually clears the fresh angioplasty site easily (see Figs. 48–59 to 48–65). After the initial clotting reaction has subsided and there has been clearance by fibrinolytics, the site usually stabilizes and no further intervention or infusion is necessary.

Angioplasty Site Vasospasm

As noted previously, a less-than-ideal postprocedure appearance may be partially caused by vasospasm, although it is mostly caused by intimal damage. Urokinase appears to have a slight vasodilatory effect, and this may be part of the reason for the apparent good results obtained by infusing urokinase after an angioplasty site begins to look less than ideal.

Papaverine or nitroglycerin may also be of benefit, especially if thrombolytics are being avoided. A safe method of administration of papaverine is to mix 300 mg of papaverine in 100 ml normal saline and infuse slowly over 30 to 60 minutes. The major risks of papaverine infusion are infusion of the ophthalmic artery, which can cause blindness, and infusion of the posterior fossa. It has been reported verbally that bolus infusion in the posterior fossa can lead to death, probably related to its propensity to precipitate when infused in too concentrated a solution.

We use nitroglycerin rather than papaverine for this reason. A solution of 50 μg/ml in normal saline is prepared and 1 to 5 ml is infused over 1 to 2 minutes. This does not have the potential for problems such as the precipitation encountered when using papaverine, and is usually effective.

Postprocedure Care

As noted above, since the advent of abciximab and its proven efficacy in coronary angioplasty and stenting, we use it for all intracranial angioplasty cases. The protocol for administration of abciximab for high-risk coronary angioplasty (which is applicable to all intracranial angioplasty cases) calls for institution of therapy prior to the angioplasty or stenting and continued infusion for 12 hours after the procedure.

This regimen appears to be effective at preventing the malignant thrombotic cascade immediately after angioplasty. We leave a sheath in place and continue the abciximab for 12 hours. The sheath is pulled the morning after the procedure and the patient is discharged that afternoon.

Patients are placed on ticlopidine, 250 mg twice daily, for 1 month after the procedure. Aspirin, 325 mg daily, is continued for the rest of the patient's life.

Probucol

Restenosis is the bane of both vascular surgeons and endovascular surgeons. A solution for this problem would be particularly helpful to cardiologists and interventional neuroradiologists. No pharmacologic agent has previously been shown conclusively to prevent restenosis after coronary or any other type of angioplasty. A potentially exciting addition to the armamentarium for angioplasty of atherosclerotic sites, however, is the use of antioxidants (specifically probucol) to help prevent restenosis.

Antioxidants such as vitamins C and E have shown promise in preventing restenosis. However, probucol (Lorelco, Hoechst Marion Roussel) has been shown to be beneficial in preventing restenosis in a way never before demonstrated.[46–49] This is discussed further in Chapter 41.

We believe that the addition of probucol (if available) to the regimen is indicated for any patient at high risk for restenosis. Restenosis is primarily a phenomenon seen in the first 6 months after angioplasty; this would appear to be a reasonable period of administration, and was used in the coronary angioplasty study.

Follow-Up

The correct time interval for follow-up has not been determined. Small vessel angioplasty, particularly with a suboptimal response, may result in recurrence in a short period of time. In one series reported by Hyodo et al. at the annual meeting of the American Society of Interventional and Therapeutic Radiologists (New York, September 1997), 28 patients who had undergone intracranial angioplasty were followed for more than one year. Of these patients, 5 patients had recurrent stenosis and one lesion had progressed to occlusion (a restenosis rate of 21.4%). Aggressive follow-up should be performed to watch for a malignant vasculopathic response, which should be dealt with before it is too late. Coronary angioplasty has a failure rate of 20% to 40% in a matter of months. For this reason, we prefer 3-month, 6-month, and 1-year follow-up.

With the advancements in MRA, it may be possible

to follow these cases noninvasively in the future, but we evaluate our patients angiographically.

STRATEGY AND TECHNIQUE OF PENETRATING A TOTAL INTRACRANIAL VASCULAR OCCLUSION WITH DOWNSTREAM ISCHEMIA

In most cases of total occlusion, the goal should be to clean the occlusive site as completely as possible with fibrinolytics. After this has been done, mechanical means can be employed to recanalize the vessel.

If a microcatheter can be advanced through a stenosis or occlusion, a lumen of 0.67 mm can be formed (about 2-Fr., the typical size of the tip of a microcatheter). Probing blindly with an angled-tip microguidewire may lead to inadvertent complications (e.g., intimal dissection or vascular perforation, particularly with the gold angle-tip micro Glidewire) as the normal see-and-feel relationship between the operator and this tool is lost in this situation. The guidewire might also advance into any unseen and invisible small arterial branch or perforator, or a curve, with unknown or unpredictable consequences, perhaps puncturing the vessel or causing an intimal tear, both of which have been reported more than once.

In agreement with Berenstein,[50] a complete J curve placed on the tip of the wire allows safer advancement into unknown territory. The curve of the wire presents a larger face to the obstruction, and the leading edge is not absolutely against the wall of the vessel as an angled-tip guidewire would be; it will tend to find its own way. A considerable amount of force may be necessary to traverse the stenotic area, but the tight J tip will potentially seek the correct lumen.

Although probing with a J-curved tip may be the ideal method of penetrating an occlusion, the soft leading edge of a platinum-tipped microwire can be used, but very gently. The tips of monofilament guidewires are the most dangerous.

If it is possible to advance the guidewire through the occlusion, the operator should not then simply withdraw the wire. Microwires are about 0.33 mm in diameter (0.013″) and tend not to leave a passage behind when withdrawn. Therefore, when the wire is through the stenosis, the operator should determine whether it behaves as if it is in an intravascular location by trying to spin the wire and watching the tip and by advancing it gently to see if it looks like it is following the correct arterial branching pattern. This may be difficult to tell, but it is reassuring if it behaves predictably. It is then necessary to advance the catheter to follow the wire through the occlusion. It might still be difficult to advance the catheter through the stenosis, however, and a disturbing degree of force may be necessary (thus, knowledge that the distal wire tip is intraluminal is reassuring). Use of a hydrophilic-coated microcatheter is mandatory.

Frequently, the lumen distal to a stenosis will be free of thrombus. As stated previously, normal endothelium is a hostile environment for thrombus.

When the catheter is past the occlusion, it is imperative that withdrawal of the wire, flushing of the catheter, and contrast injection be done with abnormally slow and meticulous caution. Saline should be dripped into the hub of the catheter while the wire is being very slowly withdrawn. When the wire has exited the catheter, the saline in the hub should be observed for any tendency to back up into the hub. If so, the hub should again be filled with saline and a contrast-filled syringe very carefully attached.

An attempt at flushing the catheter should not be made unless blood return (or at least back-up of the saline) is seen on withdrawal of the guidewire. An attempt to aspirate blood simply invites air or nitrogen gas to enter or form in the catheter lumen. An extremely slow injection of isotonic iso-osmolar nonionic contrast should be performed to evaluate catheter position. There should be minimal, if any, movement of the contrast column (i.e., no antegrade flow) and thus no need to inject rapidly. The abnormally slow injection is performed because the exact location of the tip of the catheter is not known, and if it is in an intravascular location, it is in a theoretically closed system (i.e., there is no inflow and therefore no room for reflux back around the catheter — the distal runoff is into capillaries that may be considerably damaged or occluded). Any injection may therefore rupture these dead-end vessels.

As stated in Chapter 60, a nonionic isotonic iso-osmolar contrast agent should be used in any situation in which perfusion of an injured capillary bed may occur; half-strength contrast is a suitable substitute. (If the contrast is diluted with normal saline, however, the tonicity and osmolarity are not significantly changed, and the contrast opacity suffers considerably. Therefore, sterile water, not saline, should be used for dilution).

Once an intravascular location is confirmed, and if fibrinolysis is not contraindicated and is planned, a concentrated solution of the agent can be infused as the catheter is withdrawn (250,000 units of urokinase mixed in 10 ml normal saline).

A suitable exchange wire should be placed through the microcatheter and the catheter withdrawn, leaving the guidewire behind to hold the intraluminal position and to lead the angioplasty balloon catheter into place (300-cm microwires are available in 0.018″, 0.014″, and 0.010″ sizes). Recrossing the lesion with the guidewire for the angioplasty balloon is one more potentially dangerous step that should be avoided if at all possible. If a hydrophilic-coated microcatheter following a J-curved wire cannot pass through the stenosis, it will be very difficult to advance any microangioplasty balloon catheter through this lesion.

In this situation, the goal of the therapy should be to achieve an adequate lumen to prevent short-term (weeks to months) reocclusion without doing enough intimal damage to stimulate a vigorous thrombogenic cascade that may or may not be treatable with urokinase under the circumstances. Therefore, undersizing of the balloon for angioplasty is in order. An ideal angioplasty result giving years of carefree living is not necessary at this point. Simply allowing the brain to recuperate until definitive therapy can be rendered at some future time should be the goal.

The smallest STEALTH or Stratus angioplasty balloon available is 2 mm in diameter (the catheter itself is 1 mm or 3-Fr.). It would appear that a 2-mm lumen would be adequate for at least a moderate amount of flow. Indeed, if a 2-mm lumen is the result, it would be. After all, a normal M2 branch is hardly this size, and frequently the M1 or A1 segment is as small or smaller (i.e., about 1.5 to 3 mm).

Assuming the decision has been made to abstain from using urokinase, there are several options for rescue if the angioplasty result is less than ideal:

1. High concentrations of heparin can be infused through the guide catheter. The patient, however, should already be adequately systemically heparinized, and heparin does not truly prevent a platelet aggregation cascade even though it inactivates thrombin and thus the coagulation cascade.
2. Oral aspirin can be administered, but this takes at least 30 to 120 minutes to work and should have been administered beforehand.
3. Abciximab can be administered. Again, this should be started before the angioplasty is performed; there are no trials assessing its effectiveness if begun after angioplasty, even in coronary arteries, but it is worth considering. Its antiplatelet effect is almost immediate and it has been anecdotally reported to "dissolve clot before your very eyes." Its effect on the risk of intracranial hemorrhage is also unknown, however!
4. The systemic blood pressure can be raised; this is part of the routine treatment of hypoperfusion, whether caused by atherosclerotic disease or aneurysmal subarachnoid hemorrhage vasospasm. Hypertension has been shown to increase the risk of hemorrhage after stroke therapy and probably will not maintain vessel patency unless the pressure is high.
5. A slow infusion of papaverine or nitroglycerin can be instituted in the hope that at least some of the less-than-ideal result is due to vasospasm. If the balloon was truly undersized, the muscularis should be intact and only minimally disturbed, but vasospasm could still be producing some or all of the suboptimal appearance. We currently prefer to use nitroglycerin. This has proved to be successful in several cases, and should be the first choice under these circumstances. Ideally, neither a large intimal tear or dissection nor a coagulation cascade is present. Treatment of the coagulation cascade precipitated by endothelial damage is best handled by combinations of fibrinolytic agents, heparin, and antiplatelet agents.

COMPLICATIONS OF INTRACRANIAL ANGIOPLASTY AND HOW TO AVOID THEM

Dissection

The best treatment for dissection is to avoid it. As stated previously, the goal of therapy for an intracranial angioplasty is to increase the absolute flow through the vessel by increasing the lumen size to an acceptable cross-sectional area. The vessel does not have to look like it did when the patient was 20 years old. It simply has to be adequate. A successful coronary angioplasty is defined as only *a 20% relative improvement with a decrease in stenosis to less than 50%*.[30] This would appear to be a reasonable goal and has proved to be adequate. The restenosis rate associated with our method of undersizing the balloon for intracranial angioplasty is unknown because of the limited time available for evaluation, but so far the rate has been low (only one patient has needed retreatment).

Thrombus

Adequate heparinization during the procedure is necessary at a minimum. As discussed previously, we use abciximab in all intracranial angioplasty procedures to minimize the possibility of thrombus formation.

Parent Vessel Damage

Parent vessel damage usually is caused by the guide catheter. It is imperative to choose a suitable location to place the tip of this catheter. In addition, the correct guide catheter must be selected. This issue is discussed at length in "Technique of Elective Intracranial Angioplasty."

Emboli

There are two principal causes of downstream emboli. First, thrombus or plaque can be dislodged from the original lesion. This can be prevented by ensuring that the lesion to be dilated is clean to begin with. An initial course of urokinase is administered if the lesion has not been shown to be stable following either prolonged treatment with oral anticoagulants or in-hospital administration of heparin. Second, thrombus can form at the angioplasty site and migrate downstream.

If either of these two events occurs, proximal infusion of urokinase without recrossing the angioplasty site should be sufficient to treat the problem. The embolus should be relatively small and should migrate to a second-order or third-order vessel; the time for rescue can be prolonged in this setting. An evaluation of the efficacy of this strategy can be made by observing the diagnostic angiogram; if contrast reaches the thrombus, urokinase will also. Fresh thrombus is exquisitely sensitive to fibrinolysis.

Delayed Occlusion

As stated previously, there are three components to the effective management of this problem: (1) prevention, (2) detection, and (3) treatment. All three components are important. Prevention is achieved by adequate use of anticoagulants and antiplatelet agents. Detection is accomplished by patiently observing for thrombosis. Delayed occlusion is treated with fibrinolytic agents combined with platelet anti-aggregates.

Rebound Stenosis

Rebound constitutes the major weakness of our technique. Purposely undersizing the balloon will prevent major intimal damage as completely as possible. This process will, however, cause some lesions not to be properly dilated. A certain amount of damage may be necessary to produce optimal dilation, but an inadequate result that must be retreated at a later date is preferable to either a ruptured vessel or a damaged vessel leading to occlusion. Intrinsic elastic recoil does not appear to be as great a problem in intracranial lesions as in extracranial lesions such as the vertebral artery origin. Vessel geometry, however, can be a problem. The bend of a vessel (e.g., the curve of the distal vertebral artery at the skull base) is a poor location for effective angioplasty. An effective stent would solve this problem, and one may be forthcoming.

Lesion Access

Initial crossing of a lesion is typically a minor problem. Most intracranial stenoses are smooth, tapering lesions. The exception to this is in the carotid siphon, where lesions can be shelf-like, and in the mid basilar artery, where lesions can be particularly jagged. The only recommendations in these instances are to consider using a tight J-shaped curve to initially cross the lesion and to be very careful.

Distal Vessel Damage from the Guidewire or Occlusion Wire

This problem has been greatly helped by the advent of the Stratus balloon. It is our practice to keep the wire well downstream from the tip of the balloon and to carefully place the tip in a comfortable, safe location. This wire is very soft and very safe.

Avoid Recrossing an Angioplasty Site

As repeatedly stated throughout this chapter, no matter how adept the operator believes himself or herself to be, it is not possible to skillfully advance the guidewire through the center of the lumen of a newly dilated vessel; trying to accomplish this is an invitation to disaster. If absolutely necessary to recross a fresh angioplasty site, placement of a tight J-shaped curve on the tip of the guidewire will encourage it to remain in the center of the vessel and is a safe method to use when trying to recross this segment.

Even this maneuver can be dangerous in a tight curve such as the carotid siphon. The operator should beware.

REFERENCES

1. Hass WK, Fields WS, North RR, et al. Joint study of extracranial arterial occlusion. II. Arteriography, techniques, sites and complications. *JAMA* 1968;203:961–968.
2. Gorelick PB, Caplan LR, Langenberg P, et al. Clinical and angiographic comparison of asymptomatic occlusive cerebrovascular disease. *Neurology* 1988;38:852–858.
3. Caplan L, Babikian V, Helgason C, et al. Occlusive disease of the middle cerebral artery. *Neurology* 1985;35:975–982.
4. Webster WW, Makaroun MS, Steed DL, et al. Compromised cerebral blood flow reactivity is a predictor of stroke in patients with symptomatic carotid artery occlusive disease. *J Vasc Surg* 1995;21:338–345.
5. EC/IC Bypass Study Group. Failure of extra-intracranial arterial bypass to reduce the risk of ischemic stroke: results of an international randomized trial. *N Engl J Med* 1985;313:1191–1200.
6. Bogousslavsky J, Barnett HJM, Fox AJ, et al. Atherosclerotic diseases of the middle cerebral artery. *Stroke* 1986;17:1112–1120.
7. Gorelick PB, Caplan LR, Hier DB, et al. Racial differences in the distribution of anterior circulation occlusive disease. *Neurology* 1984;34:54–59.
8. Heyden S, Heyman A, Goree JA. Nonembolic occlusion of the middle cerebral and carotid arteries — a comparison of predisposing factors. *Stroke* 1970;1:363–369.
9. Gorelick PB, Caplan LR, Hier DB, et al. Racial differences in the distribution of posterior circulation occlusive disease. *Stroke* 1985;16:785–790.
10. Feldmann E, Daneault N, Kwan E, et al. Chinese-white differences in the distribution of occlusive cerebrovascular disease. *Neurology* 1990;40:1541–1545.
11. Borozan PG, Schuller JJ, LaRosa MP, et al. The natural history of isolated carotid siphon stenosis. *J Vasc Surg* 1984;1:744.
12. Keagy BA, Poole MA, Burnham SJ, Johnson G Jr. Frequency, severity, and physiologic importance of carotid siphon disease. *J Vasc Surg* 1986;3:511.
13. Pessin MS, Gorelick PB, Kwan ES, Caplan LR. Basilar artery stenosis: middle and distal segments. *Neurology* 1987;37:1742–1746.
14. Toucho H. Percutaneous transluminal angioplasty in the treatment of atherosclerotic disease of the anterior cerebral circulation and hemodynamic evaluation. *J Neurosurg* 1995;82:953–960.
15. The Warfarin-Aspirin Symptomatic Intracranial Disease (WASID) Study Group. Prognosis of patients with symptomatic vertebral or basilar artery stenosis [Abstract]. *Stroke* 1995;26:35.
15a. Akins PT, Pilgram TK, Cross DT, Moran CJ. Natural history of stenosis from intracranial atherosclerosis by serial angiography. *Stroke* 1998;29:433.
16. Escourelle R, Poier J. Manual of Basic Neuropathology. Philadelphia: W.B. Saunders, 1978, p. 91.
17. Marzewski DJ, Furlan AJ, St. Louis P, et al. Intracranial internal carotid artery: Longterm prognosis. *Stroke* 1982;13:821–824.
18. Craig DR, Megura K, Watridge C, et al. Intracranial internal carotid artery stenosis. *Stroke* 1982;13:825–828.
19. Wechsler LR, Kistler P, Davis KR, et al. The prognosis of carotid siphon stenosis. *Stroke* 1986;17:718.
20. Hacke W, Zeumer H, Ferbert A, et al. Intra-arterial thrombolytic therapy improves outcome in patients with acute vertebrobasilar occlusive disease. *Stroke* 1988;19:1216–1222.

21. Wijdicks EF, Scott JP. Outcome in patients with acute basilar artery occlusion requiring mechanical ventilation. *Stroke* 1996;27:1301–1303.
22. Chater NL, Weinstein PR. Progression of the middle cerebral artery stenosis to occlusion without symptoms following superficial temporal artery bypass: case report. In Fein JM, Reichman OH (eds). Microvascular Anastomoses for Cerebral Ischemia. New York: Springer Verlag, 1974, pp. 269–271.
23. Gumerlock MK, Ono H, Neuwelt EA. Can a patent extracranial-intracranial bypass provoke the conversion of an intracranial arterial stenosis to a syptomatic occlusion? *Neurosurgery* 1983;12:391–400.
24. Röther J, Wentz K-U, Rautenberg W, et al. Magnetic resonance angiography in vertebrobasilar ischemia. *Stroke* 1993;24:1310–1315.
25. Baloh RW. Vertebrobasilar insufficiency and stroke. *Neck Surg* 1995;112:114–117.
26. Castillo M, Falcone S, Naidich TP, et al. Imaging in acute basilar artery thrombosis. *Neuroradiology* 1994;36;426–429.
27. Ahuja A, Guterman LR, Hopkins LN. Angioplasty for basilar artery atherosclerosis. *J Neurosurg* 1992;77:941–944.
28. Piepgras DG, Sundt TM, Forbes GS, et al. Balloon catheter transluminal angioplasty for vertebrobasilar ischemia. In Berguer R, Bauer RB (eds). Vertebrobasilar Arterial Occlusive Disease: Medical and Surgical Management. New York: Raven Press, 1984, pp. 215–224.
29. Diethrich EB, Ndiaye M, Reid DB, et al. Stenting in the carotid artery: initial experience in 110 patients. *J Endovasc Surg* 1996;3:42–62.
30. Sliwka U, Klotzsch C, Popescu O, et al. Do chronic middle cerebral artery stenoses represent an embolic focus? *Stroke* 1997; 28:1324–1327.
31. Ryan TJ, Bauman WB, Kennedy JW. Revised guidelines for percutaneous transluminal coronary angioplasty: a report of the American College of Cardiology/American Heart Association Task Force on Assessment of Diagnostic and Therapeutic Cardiovascular Procedures (Subcommittee on Percutaneous Transluminal Angioplasty). *Circulation* 1993;88:2987–3007.
32. Rostomily RC, Mayberg MR, Eskridge JM, et al. Resolution of petrous internal carotid stenosis after transluminal angioplasty. *J Neurosurg* 1992;76:520–523.
33. Higashida RT, Tsai FY, Halbach VV, et al. Transluminal angioplasty for atherosclerotic disease of the vertebral and basilar arteries. *J Neurosurg* 1993;78:192–198.
34. Clark WM, Barnwell SL, Nesbit G, et al. Safety and efficacy of percutaneous transluminal angioplasty for intracranial stenosis. *Stroke* 1995;26:1200–1204.
35. Overgaard K. Thrombolytic therapy in experimental embolic stroke. *Cerebrovasc Brain Metab Rev* 1994;6:257–285.
36. Tardif JC, Côté G, Lespérance J, et al. Probucol and multivitamins in the prevention of restenosis after coronary angioplasty. *N Engl J Med* 1997;337:365–372.
36a. Day AL, Rhoton AL, Quisling RG. Resolving siphon stenosis following endarterectomy. *Stroke* 1980;11:278–281.
37. The EPIC Investigators. Use of a monoclonal antibody directed against the platelet glycoprotein IIb/IIIa receptor in high-risk coronary angioplasty. *N Engl J Med* 1994;330:956–961.
38. LeBreton H, Plow EF, Topol EJ. Role of platelets in restenosis after percutaneous coronary revascularization. *J Am Coll Cardiol* 1996;28:1643–1651.
39. Schulman SP, Goldschmidt-Clermont PJ, Topol EJ, et al. Effects of Integrelin, a platelet glycoprotein IIb/IIIa receptor antagonist, in unstable angina. A randomized multicenter trial. *Circulation* 1996;94:2083–2089.
40. Heros RC. Management of unclippable aneurysms. In Schmidek HH, Sweet WH (eds). Operative Neurosurgical Techniques: Indications, Methods, and Results, 2nd ed. Orlando: Grune & Stratton, 1988, pp. 1023–1034.
41. Rogers C, Edelman ER. Endovascular stent design dictates experimental restenosis and thrombosis. *Circulation* 1995; 91:2995–3001.
42. Brott T. Thrombolytic therapy. Cerebral ischemia: treatment and prevention. *Neurol Clin* 1992;10:219–232.
43. Groves HM, Kinlough-Rathbone RL, Richardson M, et al. Platelet interaction with damaged rabbit aorta. *Lab Invest* 1979;40:194–200.
44. Wilenz JR, Sanborn TA, Haudenschild CC, et al. Platelet accumulation in experimental angioplasty: time course and relation to vascular injury. *Circulation* 1987;75:636–642.
46. Regnstrom J, Walldius G, Nilsson S, et al. The effect of probucol on low density liproptein oxidation and femoral atherosclerosis. *Atherosclerosis* 1996;125:217–229.
47. Magil A. Inhibition of progression of chronic puromycin aminonucleoside nephrosis by probucol, an antioxidant. *J Am Soc Nephrol* 1996;7:2340–2347.
48. Olsson AG, Yuan XM. Antioxidants in the prevention of atherosclerosis. *Curr Opin Lipidol* 1996;7:374–380.
49. Sasaki S, Nakagawa M, Nakata T, et al. Efficacy and safety of the 3-hydroxy-3-methylglutaryl coenzyme A reductase inhibitor fluvastatin in hyperlipidemic patients treated with probucol. *Cardiology* 1997;88:160–165.
50. Berenstein A, Lasjaunias P. Surgical Neuroangiography, Vol 4: Endovascular Treatment of Cerebral Lesions. New York: Springer-Verlag, 1992, pp. 252–258.

CHAPTER 49

Surgical Alternatives to Interventional Neuroradiology

J. R. Tompkins / F. Culicchia

In recent years, interventional neuroradiology has achieved great progress in the treatment of cerebrovascular disease. Current endovascular techniques permit treatment of problematic vascular disease when surgery is associated with significant morbidity. Unfortunately, there still remain lesions that are inaccessible or unresponsive to endovascular treatment. In patients with such lesions, surgical intervention may be indicated. The purpose of this chapter is to discuss the indications and available procedures for the surgical management of vascular disease affecting the central nervous system.

HISTORY

Cerebral revascularization was first attempted in 1942 by Kredel,[1] who directly applied a flap of temporalis muscle to the surface of the brain in five stroke patients, with reported improvement. In 1967, Goldsmith et al[2] described a procedure in which omentum was tunneled to the surface of the brain of dogs, where microvascular connections could later be demonstrated. Subsequently, Karasawa et al[3] demonstrated that collateral circulation to the brains of patients with moyamoya disease could be provided using temporalis muscle grafts or free omental grafts that were anastomosed to the superficial temporal artery (STA) and applied directly to the brain. Spetzler et al[4] in 1980 described a technique that involved suturing a mobilized STA segment to the arachnoid. Subsequent angiography revealed excellent collateral circulation to the middle cerebral artery (MCA) territory.

Bypassing occlusions in the cerebral vasculature by establishing direct connections between the extracranial circulation and the intracranial circulation (EC-IC bypass) began in the 1960s. Woringer and Kunlin[5] first described a procedure of this type in 1963 when they used a saphenous vein graft to provide flow from the common carotid artery (CCA) to the intracranial internal carotid artery (ICA) distal to an occlusion. In 1964, Pool and Potts[6] used a plastic tube to shunt blood from the STA to the distal anterior cerebral artery during surgery for an anterior cerebral artery aneurysm. Yasargil et al[7] then reported the first STA-to-MCA bypass procedure. Similar procedures were then used to revascularize the posterior circulation.

By the 1970s, these operations were being used by many surgeons to treat symptomatic patients with occlusive pathology of the ICA and MCA, and later the posterior circulation. EC-IC bypass also found use in supplementing cerebral blood flow before planned occlusion of a cerebral artery for treatment of an unclippable aneurysm.

In 1977, the EC-IC Bypass Study[8] was begun to assess the efficacy of this treatment. In 1985, the group reported that STA-MCA bypass did not prevent stroke in the group studied at a rate higher than that achieved with optimal medical care alone. This conclusion generated considerable controversy; the reliability of the conclusion was brought into question. It is evident that the EC-IC bypass trial did not succeed in establishing generally acceptable guidelines for selection of patients for cerebral revascularization procedures. Since the publication of the EC-IC Bypass Study in 1985, the number of intracranial bypass procedures has fallen dramatically. However, there are still certain specific situations in which bypass grafting may be indicated.

INDICATIONS FOR CEREBRAL REVASCULARIZATION

Surgical cerebral revascularization is indicated in patients with symptomatic cerebral ischemia if the following criteria are established: (1) symptoms are unresponsive to optimal medical/neurointerventional treatment, (2) symptoms are secondary to a vascular lesion that is not amenable to direct surgical attack, and (3) an appropriate region of reduced cerebral perfusion is documented using some measurement of regional cerebral blood flow. The last-named criteria, reduced cerebral perfusion, can be suspected in patients with neurologic deficits that are manifested when blood pressure is lowered as a result of treatment of hypertension, or in whom such deficits appear with postural changes in arterial pressure. Likewise, patients who describe a "graying out" of monocular vision (as opposed to the sudden monocular blindness of embolic amaurosis fugax) are more likely to have a fixed hemodynamic basis for their symptoms. Despite these symptoms, objective measures of hemodynamic insufficiency are invaluable. Angiography provides indirect but important evidence of such insufficiency when it reveals limited collateral flow, slow filling, and slow washout of the arteries distal to the stenosis or occlusion. Quantitative assessment of cerebral blood flow is available utilizing ^{133}Xe-enhanced computed tomography (CT), single-photon emission computed tomography (SPECT), or the more costly positron emission tomography (PET).

Bypass surgery is also indicated when a planned surgical procedure will require occlusion of an artery supplying a region of the brain in which there is evidence of inadequate collateral circulation.[9] Many patients are able to tolerate acute internal carotid occlusion because of preexisting adequate collateral circulation. Test balloon occlusion techniques (discussed in Chapters 34 and 36) reveal those patients who are in need of a revascularization procedure as a component of their treatment.

For the indications discussed above, arterial bypass surgery is preferred to the technique of omental or temporal muscle transposition, except when the donor artery is not of sufficient caliber or there is no recipient vessel of sufficient caliber to accept a bypass graft (as in the case of moyamoya disease).

EXTRACRANIAL-INTRACRANIAL SURGICAL REVASCULARIZATION

Surgical revascularization by EC-IC bypass is most frequently used in occlusive cerebrovascular disease. Other indications include treatment of an occlusion of the ICA by trauma, nontraumatic dissection, and involvement by a neoplasm or an unclippable aneurysm.

Anterior Circulation Revascularization

STA to MCA Branch

The standard surgical method of cerebral revascularization is the STA anastomosis to a cortical branch of the MCA.[7] In this procedure, the frontal branch of the STA is mobilized and redirected intracranially, where it is sutured to a suitable cortical branch of the MCA, typically the angular branch. There are inherent advantages to this procedure: no brain retraction or dissection is required, and the cortical vessel provides blood to a restricted region of the brain normally provided with an adequate collateral circulation from adjacent cortical branches (via pial collaterals), thereby decreasing the risk of a major stroke during surgery or if this branch becomes occluded as a result of surgery. The disadvantages of this procedure are the relatively low flow obtained from the STA and the frequency with which this vessel is involved by atherosclerotic disease. The STA has been demonstrated to dilate and provide a gradual increase in the rate of flow over time. In some situations, there are advantages to anastomosing the STA to the proximal (M2) portion of the MCA. Alternatives to the standard STA-MCA bypass and the indications are described below.

STA to Proximal MCA

This is most commonly performed when the cortical vessels are too small in diameter to be used in the anastomosis.[10] This anastomosis, even if technically accomplished, is likely to result in an ischemic brain owing to the low-flow bypass. There is positive correlation between outcome and the degree of filling of the intracranial vessels after EC-IC bypass. Finding a more suitable recipient in the proximal M2 will ensure a more adequate blood supply to the cerebral tissue at risk.

Anastomosis to the proximal MCA is also considered when there is a proximal stenosis in the MCA. The sylvian fissure must be dissected to identify the stenosed branch of the MCA and to perform the anastomosis close to the distal end of the stenosis.

Saphenous Vein Interposition to Proximal MCA from Various Sources

Superficial Temporal Artery

This procedure is considered when the donor vessel is not of sufficient caliber or length to complete the bypass successfully.[9] In this situation, the disproportionate size of the vein graft and the cortical artery significantly jeopardizes the bypass. Spetzler and Chater[11] studied the relationship between the donor/recipient vessel diameter ratio and the subsequent patency rates, finding that a ratio of 1.6:1 leads to a maximal rate of graft patency. With this information, it is suggested that a saphenous vein graft should be anastomosed to one of the proximal branches of the MCA. The use of a short vein graft from the STA to the MCA may provide a more rapid increase in the rate of flow when this vessel tapers quickly or is involved with atherosclerotic disease.

Occipital Artery

When the STA is not available, the occipital artery may be used.[11] This vessel is usually difficult to dissect owing to its dense connective tissue investment and its tendency to branch extensively early in its course. A short vein graft can be interposed between the occipital artery and the MCA, averting this problem.

Other Sources

High-flow bypasses using a saphenous vein graft can also be constructed between the CCA and the MCA, or between the subclavian artery and the MCA if the more distal vessels are unsatisfactory.[12, 13] These same donor vessels and interposition grafts can be used in the posterior circulation, utilizing the proximal posterior cerebral artery (PCA) as a recipient vessel.

This technique has obvious advantages in that it supplies an immediate large volume of flow into the appropriate vascular territory. Also, because it is a large-vessel anastomosis, there is a higher patency rate. The disadvantages include the need for two anastomoses, the need to harvest the saphenous vein, a larger vascular territory at risk during the operative procedure, and the risk associated with extensive dissection of the sylvian fissure or ambient/interpeduncular cistern. All of these must be taken into consideration in planning the appropriate surgical revascularization procedure.

Posterior Circulation Revascularization

EC-IC bypass techniques can also be used to treat vertebrobasilar disease that is not amenable to direct surgical or endovascular therapy.[14]

Occipital Artery to Posterior Inferior Cerebellar Artery

This procedure is utilized to bypass an occlusion or severe stenosis in the distal vertebral artery, usually when the opposite vertebral artery is occluded.[15] The site of the anastomosis is the perimedullary portion of the posterior inferior cerebellar artery (PICA). As noted above, difficulty can be encountered because the occipital artery is difficult to dissect and often has proximal branches.

Occipital Artery to Anterior Inferior Cerebellar Artery

This anastomosis can be used when there is an occluding or stenotic lesion at the vertebrobasilar junction or distal to the PICA origin.[16] The occipital artery is anastomosed to one of the two major branches of the anterior inferior cerebellar artery (AICA)—the one with the fewest collaterals to the brainstem. In addition to the difficulties associated with using the occipital artery described above, the anastomotic site is near the anterior surface of the foramen of Luschka. This is a longer distance to reach than in the case of the perimedullary PICA and is technically more difficult. The AICA is often a small vessel, adding to the complexity of this procedure.

STA to Posterior Cerebral Artery or Superior Cerebellar Artery

This approach can be used for the treatment of basilar artery disease distal to the AICA origins.[9] The superior cerebellar artery (SCA) has a more extensive collateral network and is therefore a better choice. It is also easier to reach. The risk of producing cortical blindness is another factor making the PCA an inferior choice compared with the SCA.

Saphenous Interposition from Various Sources to PCA or SCA

As mentioned previously, saphenous vein interposition grafts can be used to construct bypasses between the CCA or subclavian artery and the PCA or SCA.[9] The same advantages and disadvantages discussed above regarding saphenous vein grafts to the MCA apply.

Other Approaches to Revascularization

In situ bypass is accomplished when a vessel near the pathologic segment can be anastomosed to the involved vessel, providing continued flow in that vascular territory.[17] This is utilized when a giant aneurysm must be trapped or a diseased segment of artery removed, thereby not allowing a primary reanastomosis.

On occasion, a satisfactory recipient vessel is not identified. This is most commonly seen in moyamoya disease. Implanted muscle, galea, or omentum can be used to supply an arterial network to the brain. Encephalomyosynangiosis (EMS) involves mobilizing the temporal muscle and fascia, performing a craniotomy, opening the dura and placing the muscle in contact with the cortex, and suturing the temporal fascia to the dura. The arachnoid must be carefully removed to achieve direct contact with the cortex. A variation of this procedure is encephaloduroarteriosynangiosis (EDAS), in which the STA is surgically isolated as previously described but allowed to remain intact and in contact with the temporal muscle and fascia. The galea, intact artery, and muscle are sutured to the open dura, keeping a more vascular portion of tissue in contact with the cortex. Omentum has been utilized in similar circumstances. The omentum is harvested by means of laparotomy, with the arteries and veins anastomosed to the scalp vessels to allow vascularization of the omentum.

OPERATIVE PROCEDURES

STA to MCA

The surgical procedure must be planned in detail once the patient has been considered appropriate for surgical revascularization.[10] Careful study of all the intracranial and extracranial cerebral vessels provided by conventional angiography is mandatory. Preoperative identification of the donor vessel and the appropriate intracranial recipient vessel best suited to supplement the vascular territory in question is determined by comparing angiography with cerebral blood flow studies. The possible need for an interposition saphenous vein graft is also determined at this time.

The case is discussed with the anesthesiologist, alerting him or her of the impending temporary closure of a major vascular structure and the need for a stable blood pressure, as well as for the use of brain protective agents such as barbiturates or etomidate. Continuous electroencephalographic (EEG) monitoring is utilized and these agents are titrated to achieve burst suppression of the EEG recording. This EEG pattern corresponds to the maximal brain protection offered by these medications, while still allowing the monitoring of possible ischemic complications.

Patients not receiving an antiplatelet agent are started on one before surgery. Aspirin, 5 grains (325 mg) taken three times daily, is adequate to decrease platelet adhesiveness and reduce the risk of postoperative thrombosis of the bypass graft. Other antiplatelet agents are available for patients allergic to aspirin.

Once an adequate level of anesthetic is obtained, the patient is positioned supine on the operating table with the head secured in tongs. The STA is identified by palpation or Doppler, and the skin overlying the vessel is marked. The frontal or parietal branch may be used, relying on the angiogram for assistance. The operative field is properly prepared, and a skin incision is placed overlying the path of the vessel. Branches of the artery are ligated and cut. If bipolar coagulation is used, it is performed a distance away from the STA to avoid injury. The STA remains intact until the bypass is completely prepared. A margin of 0.5 cm of fascia is dissected with the STA, protecting the adventitia and nutrient vessels. At least 6 cm of vessel is necessary to accomplish the bypass.

With the dissection of the STA complete, the temporalis muscle and fascia are incised and the proposed site of the craniotomy is exposed. An adequate recipient vessel is usually identified approximately 6 cm above the external auditory meatus. A burr hole is placed in this area and a 3- to 5-cm diameter craniotomy accomplished. The dura is tacked up along the edges of the craniotomy site and meticulous hemostasis is maintained. The dura is opened in a cruciate fashion and held in retraction with sutures. The operating microscope is brought into the field along with a chair, providing a resting place for the arms during the intracranial dissection and anastomosis.

Under the microscope, a careful inspection of the cortical vessels reveals which one is most likely to provide the best recipient vessel. The vessel should be over 1 mm in size and have a segment of at least 6 to 8 mm available for microanastomosis preparation. Branches of the recipient vessel can be occluded with temporary microclips during anastomosis, or coagulated and divided if very small. A piece of Silastic is placed under the vessel to protect the underlying brain and provide an improved background for visualization.

Upon completion of the preparation of the recipient vessel, the final preparation of the STA is accomplished. The distal end of the STA is ligated and cut proximal to the ligature. The STA is allowed to bleed, ensuring that it is an adequately functioning artery. A temporary clip is applied to the proximal vessel, and the distal end of the vessel is prepared under the microscope. The distal end of the vessel is stripped of its fascia, exposing a 6- to 8-mm portion. The distal end is cut once again to fashion a fish-mouth appearance for the anastomosis.

The recipient vessel is prepared for anastomosis first by determining the direction of flow so that the bypass will be directed *proximally*. Temporary clips are then applied to the proximal as well as the distal ends of the recipient vessel, and a small arteriotomy is begun in the vessel with a scalpel. This arteriotomy is extended with sharp micro-scissors so that clean edges are obtained. The recipient segment is irrigated free of blood with heparinized saline. Using 10–0 monofilament nylon suture, a stitch is placed first through the heel of the temporal artery and into the portion of the recipient artery to direct the flow proximally. The suture is tied and then the toe stitch is placed and tied. The anastomosis may be completed with running or individually tied 10–0 suture. The toe and heel stitch described above are crucial in that they should evert the edges of the vessel. They should be placed close to the edge of each vessel to allow a widely patent yet secure anastomosis. The STA should be of adequate length so that there is no tension on the anastomosis, which would risk disastrous complications of breakdown and subsequent bleeding.

Upon completion of the anastomosis, the distal recipient vessel clip is removed first, followed by the proximal clip, and lastly the clip from the STA. One should visualize or palpate good pulsation through the anastomosis. A micro-Doppler can document good flow if necessary. Intraoperative angiography is rarely necessary. Once again, meticulous hemostasis is obtained. Leaks at the anastomosis are managed with local hemostatic agents or 10–0 individual sutures if necessary. The dura is closed without disturbing the STA, and Gelfoam is placed over the dural opening. The bone is secured into place after a passage is created for the STA. The temporal muscle and fascia are loosely closed around the STA, and the skin is closed with individual nylon sutures.

Occipital Artery to PICA or AICA

A very similar technique is employed for posterior fossa bypass surgery, using the occipital artery as a donor vessel.[15] As mentioned earlier, the occipital artery in its deep fascial layer is more difficult to dissect but can be utilized in a bypass procedure.

Saphenous Vein Grafts

As described above, when a high-flow bypass is necessary or when the STA is not sufficient, a vein graft may be used to fashion a bypass.[9] The vein graft may be interposed between the proximal STA, carotid artery, subclavian artery, or vertebral artery and an appropriate intracranial vessel. The saphenous vein can be harvested from either lower extremity by a second team of surgeons while the bypass is under preparation. Careful dissection of the vein will increase the probability of a successful bypass. All tributaries should be suture ligated and divided. The vein is marked in situ so that it does not become twisted when tunneled from the donor to the recipient site. This is accomplished with methylene blue or a 10–0 prolene suture along the outer surface of the vessel. Great care is taken to direct the flow in the vein so that the valves do not pose a problem. Once the vein is harvested, it is distended with heparinized saline, and leaks are repaired with 10–0 monofilament nylon.

The proximal anastomosis is addressed first. The same suture technique described for the STA-MCA anastomosis is employed. The vein is tunneled beneath the skin and behind the ear between the two incisions. The vessel is allowed to bleed to ensure that the proximal anastomosis is patent and the vein not twisted. A temporary clip is applied proximally and the vessel is filled with heparinized saline, washing out any potential blood clots.

The distal anastomosis is carried out once an appropriate recipient vessel is identified. Proximal M2 branches, the ICA, the PCA, the anterior cerebral artery, and the vertebral artery can accept this graft. The distal anastomosis to the chosen vessel is carried out with 9–0 monofilament nylon. As this anastomosis involves a major vessel, a protective agent such as a barbiturate is administered before temporary vessel occlusion to obtain an EEG recording of burst-suppression. Upon completion of the bypass, the distal recipient vessel clip is removed, followed by removal of the proximal clip. Any leak at the site of the anastomosis is managed with topical hemostatic agents or individual sutures. The clip on the feeding vessel is now removed to establish bypass circulation. Wound closure is accomplished in the same manner described for the STA-MCA bypass.

RESULTS

Graft patency rates of 90% to 95% should be obtained. The EC-IC Bypass Study reported a graft patency rate of 96% in 663 patients randomized to surgery.[9, 10]

Flow Rates

There are limited data on how much of an increase in blood flow occurs as a result of bypass grafting. The STA is thought to provide approximately 25 ml/min of additional blood flow (range 10 to 100 ml/min), with some increase over time. Compared with the mean cerebral blood flow of approximately 50 ml/100 gm/min, the STA is capable of augmenting flow to marginally perfused brain, but it is not sufficient to replace the contributions of major cerebral vessels. Short vein grafts may provide up to 50 to 150 ml/

min, whereas long vein grafts may supply up to 75 to 200 ml/min, which is almost enough to compensate for the loss of an ICA.[10]

POSTOPERATIVE CARE

Postoperative care is much the same for those undergoing a routine craniotomy. Antiplatelet agents are continued and the patient is observed in the intensive care unit for 24 to 48 hours after surgery. Close observation of blood pressure is mandatory. The optimal blood pressure is decided on an individual basis, taking into consideration the patient's preoperative pressure. Parameters are set for a blood pressure range within 10 to 20 mm Hg of preoperative pressure. Intermittent administration of a β-adrenergic blocker or a calcium-channel blocker is utilized to accomplish these goals. Antiplatelet agents are continued postoperatively and for the indefinite future. Anticoagulation is avoided. Intravenous fluids such as normal saline or lactated Ringer's solution are administered at a maintenance rate. The patency of the graft can be followed by Doppler scan or palpation. Angiography is carried out before discharge to ensure the patency of the bypass. Cerebral blood flow studies are utilized to determine the effect of the bypass on cerebral circulation.

CONCLUSIONS

Surgical alternatives to interventional neuroradiologic procedures do exist and should be kept in mind when dealing with lesions refractory to or not amenable to such treatment. Preoperative evaluation with complete, high-resolution conventional angiography, along with cerebral blood flow measurements, significantly aids surgical planning and the achievement of goals.

Surgical revascularization is fashioned to maximally augment blood flow to the affected area. If adequate donor vessels are not available, vein grafts are used. If adequate recipient vessels are not available, temporalis muscle or omentum is available to improve blood flow to the area in jeopardy. This is a constantly evolving field, with new indications for surgical intervention created by the advancing technology of interventional radiology.

REFERENCES

1. Kredel FE. Collateral cerebral circulation by muscle graft. Technique of operation with report of three cases. *South Surg* 1942;10:235–240.
2. Goldsmith HS, de los Santos R, Beattie EJ Jr. The relief of chronic lymphedema by omental transposition. *Ann Surg* 1967;166:572–585.
3. Karasawa J, Kikuchi H, Furuse S, et al. A surgical treatment of "moyamoya" disease: "encephalomyosynangiosis." *Neurol Med Chir (Tokyo)* 1977;17:29–37.
4. Spetzler RF, Roski RA, Kopanicky DR. Alternative superficial

5. Woringer E, Kunlin J. Anastomose entre la carotide primitive et la carotide intracranienne ou la sylvienne par greffon selonia technique de la suture suspendice. *Neurochirurgie* 1963;9:181–188.
6. Pool JL, Potts DG. Aneurysms and Arteriovenous Anomalies of the Brain. New York: Hoeber, 1964, pp 221–222.
7. Yasargil MG, Krayenbuhl HA, Jacobson JH. Microneurosurgical arterial reconstruction. *Surgery* 1970;67:221–233.
8. EC-IC Bypass Study Group. Failure of extracranial-intracranial arterial bypass to reduce the risk of ischemic stroke. Results of an international randomized trial. *N Engl J Med* 1985;313:1191–1200.
9. Sundt TM Jr, Piepgras DG, Houser W, Campbell JK. Interposition saphenous vein grafts for advanced occlusive disease and large aneurysms in the posterior circulation. *J Neurosurg* 1982;56:205–215.
10. Carter LP, Tenaltas O, Guthkelch A. Cerebral revascularization. In Carter LP, Spetzler RF (eds): Neurovascular Surgery. New York: McGraw-Hill, 1995, pp 441–456.
11. Spetzler RF, Chater N. Occipital artery–middle cerebral artery anastomosis for cerebral artery occlusive disease. *Surg Neurol* 1974;2:235–238.
12. Samson DS, Gerwetz BL, Beyer CW Jr, Hodash RM. Saphenous vein interposition grafts in the microsurgical treatment of cerebral ischemia. *Arch Surg* 1981;116:1578–1582.
13. Hadeishi H, Yasui N, Okamoto Y. Extracranial-intracranial high flow bypass using the radial artery between the vertebral and middle cerebral arteries. *J Neurosurg* 1996;85:976–979.
14. Diaz FG, Zinkle JF. Surgical management of vertebrobasilar ischemic disease: intracranial. In Carter LP, Spetzler RF (eds): Neurovascular Surgery. New York: McGraw-Hill, 1995, pp 405–414.
15. Sundt TM Jr, Piepgras DG. Occipital to posterior inferior cerebellar artery bypass surgery. *J Neurosurg* 1978;48:916–928.
16. Ausman JI, Diaz FG, de los Reyes RA, et al. Extracranial-intracranial anastomoses in the posterior circulation. In Berger R, Bauer BB (eds): Vertebrobasilar Arterial Occlusive Disease. New York: Raven Press, 1984, pp 313–319.
17. Cowell RM, Ogilvy CS, Choi IS, Gress DR. Direct brain revascularization. In Schmidek HH, Sweet WH (eds): Operative Neurosurgical Techniques, 3rd ed. Philadelphia: WB Saunders, 1995, pp 909–928.

ADDITIONAL REFERENCES

Beebe HG, Stark R, Johnson ML, et al. Choices of operation for subclavian-vertebral arterial disease. *Am J Surg* 1980;139:616–623.
de los Reyes RA, Ausman JI, Diaz FG, et al. The surgical management of vertebrobasilar insufficiency. *Acta Neurochir* 1983;68:203–216.
Diethrich EB, Garrett HE, Ameriso J, et al. Occlusive disease of the common carotid and subclavian arteries treated by carotid-subclavian bypass. *Am J Surg* 1967;114:800–808.
Kaul TK, Fields BL, Wyatt DA, et al. Surgical management in patients with coexistent coronary and cerebrovascular disease: long term results. *Chest* 1994;106:1349–1357.
Kinugasa K, Mandai S, Kamata I, et al. Surgical treatment of moyamoya disease: operative technique for encephalo-duro-arterio-myo-synangiosis, its follow-up, clinical results, and angiograms. *Neurosurgery* 1993;32:527–531.
Morrison E. The surgery of extracranial vascular occlusive disease. *J S C Med Assoc* 1994;90:327–329.
Origitano TC, Al-Mefty O, Leonetti JP, et al. Vascular considerations and complications in cranial base surgery. *Neurosurgery* 1944;35:351–363.
Schlosser V. Subclavian steal syndrome. Correction by transthoracic or extra-anatomic repair. *Vasc Surg* 1984;18:289–293.

CHAPTER 50

Clinical Applications of Intravascular Ultrasound

S.P. Jain / S.R. Ramee

Editor's note: With the growth of brachiocephalic angioplasty, and particularly carotid angioplasty and stenting, it has become evident that the tools and experience available to other disciplines should be used to their fullest extent by anyone practicing interventional neuroradiology. This discussion is an excellent overview of this field.

Since its introduction in 1958 by Sones and Shirey[1] selective angiography has been accepted as the clinical gold standard for the assessment of atherosclerosis. Angiography provides only a two-dimensional "silhouette" image of a three-dimensional arterial tree, highlighting areas of significant stenoses. Based on the relative severity of stenosis as assessed by angiography, revascularization procedures, such as percutaneous transluminal angioplasty or bypass surgery, are performed. The inherent limitations of contrast angiography, including accuracy, reproducibility, interobserver and intraobserver variability, and the underestimation of stenosis severity in a diffusely diseased artery, are well known and have been reported extensively in the literature.[2–7] In addition, angiography provides little information about atherosclerotic plaque morphology, its composition, and vessel wall thickness. Although quantitative coronary angiography, including computerized image analysis and automated edge detection techniques, has improved the reproducibility issue, it still suffers from all the limitations of conventional angiographic interpretation.[8–12]

New insights into the pathophysiology of atherosclerosis and plaque composition in the past decade have renewed interest in an imaging modality that can show plaque morphology and its geometry within a vessel wall. Intravascular ultrasound (IVUS) imaging offers a unique advantage over angiography because it allows the operator to visualize the arterial wall and its components from within the lumen. Thus, it provides a cross-sectional tomographic image of the arterial wall and lays out the full-thickness slices of an artery like a histopathologic section. The serial cross-sectional images obtained by the passage of the ultrasound catheter across the arterial lumen allow full circumferential visualization of the vessel wall and enable the quantitative measurement of lumen dimensions, plaque area, and total vessel area. In addition, IVUS can visualize structural details within an atherosclerotic plaque, which has important prognostic implications in the natural course of atherosclerosis and the outcome of interventional procedures. Its capability to provide instantaneous visual monitoring of various mechanical interventions (balloon angioplasty, directional and rotational atherectomy, stenting) of the atherosclerotic plaque and vessel wall is responsible for its rapid growth as a diagnostic and clinical imaging tool.

CURRENTLY AVAILABLE DEVICES

Two different types of transducers are available that generate intravascular ultrasound images: mechanical and phased-array. Each system possesses a unique set of advantages and disadvantages.

Mechanical Catheter System

In the mechanical catheter system, a single piezoelectric transducer (12.5 to 30 MHz) is mounted near the distal end of the catheter encased in a clear plastic housing. An external motor drive is used to rotate the transducer at a speed of 1800 rpm, yielding images at 30 frames/sec. Mechanical catheters are being manufactured by various companies (Cardiovascular Imaging Systems (CVIS)/SciMed, Inc./ Boston Scientific Corporation; Mansfield/Boston Scientific Corporation; and Dumed, Rotterdam, The Netherlands). The quality of ultrasound images generated by these mechanical catheters is generally good in terms of dynamic range (gray-scale level), lateral resolution, and penetration. Tortuous vessels, however, can cause an uneven rotation of the driving cable, leading to nonuniform rotational distortion (NURD) in the ultrasound image. Advances in the drive cable design have minimized this problem. In addition, the catheter needs to be flushed with normal saline at the beginning of the procedure to remove trapped air bubbles surrounding the transducer. Any tiny bubbles near the transducer can lead to a significant degradation of image quality. Available catheters have a low profile (2.9 to 3.2 Fr.; 0.9 to 1.0 mm) and can be used to image smaller distal vessels.

Phased-Array Imaging Catheter

The phased-array imaging catheter (Endosonics Corporation) is composed of a ring of 64 narrow elements arranged radially near the catheter tip. Because of size constraints, each element does not have a dedicated transmission line. The ultrasound image is constructed using an electronic processing known as *synthetic aperture*. There are five integrated circuits at the catheter tip to control the switching of the elements in sequential order to create an ultrasound image. The advantages of this system include the absence of a moving cable or transducer and the ability to adjust the beam electronically, which enables optimal focusing throughout the effective imaging zone. The disadvantages include limited lateral resolution, owing to the effective aperture size. In addition, a "ring-down" artifact seen as a halo around the catheter needs to be subtracted electronically. Available catheters are 3.5 Fr. (1.1 mm) and operate at center frequency of 20 MHz (band-width, 15 to 25 MHz).

NEW DEVICES

Intravascular Ultrasound Guidewire

The IVUS guidewire is actually a modification of the drive cable used in the 2.9-Fr. ultrasound catheter (CVIS/SciMed, Inc.). A 30-MHz piezoelectric crystal is mounted at the distal end of the cable, which is connected to a motor unit and is rotated at a speed of 1800 rpm. Although it has the diameter of a normal angioplasty guidewire, its tip is nonsteerable and cannot be used to cross a lesion. IVUS imaging with this technique involves placing a balloon at the lesion, removing the regular guidewire, and inserting the IVUS guidewire through the balloon catheter. Repeated negative pressure must be applied to the balloon catheter before IVUS imaging can be performed with the balloon inflated at 4 atmospheres. Any amount of air within the balloon can cause significant image distortion. Second, at high-pressure balloon inflation (10 to 20 atmospheres), malrotation artifacts occur as a result of the pinching of the guidewire lumen; rupture of the driving cable also has been noted. The available prototype has been used for guidance in endoluminal stenting.[13]

Combined Balloon and Ultrasound Device

There are two combination devices available, a balloon plus imaging catheter (Oracle Micro Plus, Endosonics Corp.) and an atherectomy plus imaging catheter (ACS/DVI). These devices allow immediate IVUS assessment, which can be used to evaluate the need for further modification of mechanical interventions.[14, 15] There are no data available to support their routine use over stand-alone IVUS catheters.

Three-Dimensional Reconstruction

Three-dimensional reconstruction of IVUS images requires the acquisition and digitization of two-dimensional cross-sectional images, necessitating the use of a continuous pullback at a constant speed or an electrocardiogram-gated, motorized pullback. Images are acquired at a pullback speed of 0.5 to 1 mm/sec over 1 to 2 minutes. The second step involves the segmentation of the digitized images, leading to differentiation between the blood pool and structures of the vessel wall. The vessel then can be displayed in sagittal, cylindrical, and lumen cast format. The sagittal format is similar to the longitudinal profile of an arteriogram and allows the direct assessment of the vessel lumen, dissection length, plaque area, and arterial wall in a 360-degree rotational view. The cylindrical format allows the visualization of the endoluminal surface, whereas the lumen cast format allows the assessment of the luminal area of the diseased compared with the reference segment. The details of this technique, its pitfalls, and its limitations can be found in the articles written by Rosenfield et al.[16] and DiMario et al.[17] Although three-dimensional reconstruction of IVUS images has enhanced the understanding of vascular pathology, its clinical utility remains to be defined.

ULTRASOUND IMAGE INTERPRETATION

Differentiating the layers of the arterial wall can be accomplished using 20- to 40-MHz transducer frequency. The ultrasonic appearance of the arterial wall differs according to the type of artery examined. A number of investigators have compared IVUS images with the corresponding histopathologic specimens and have found different ultrasonic characteristic features in muscular than in elastic arteries. A three-layered appearance is characteristic of muscu-

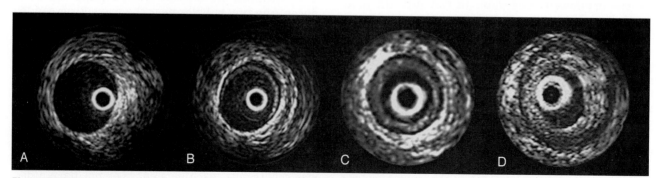

Figure 50-1 Atherosclerotic disease progression as documented by ultrasonography. *A,* Normal coronary artery without the three-layered appearance. *B,* Mild atherosclerotic disease. Note the presence of a typical three-layered appearance due to intimal thickening (9 to 5 o'clock position). *C,* Moderate atherosclerotic disease with the typical three-layered appearance due to circumferential intimal thickening. *D,* Severe atherosclerotic disease.

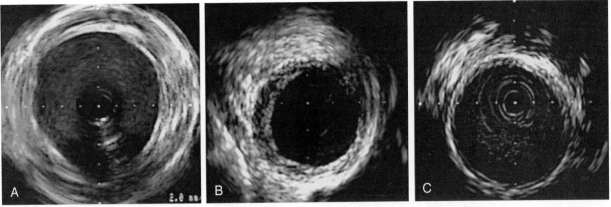

Figure 50-2 Examples of elastic arteries. *A,* Abdominal aorta. *B,* Subclavian artery. Note the absence of a three-layered appearance despite the presence of a circumferential atheromatous plaque. *C,* Common carotid artery.

lar arteries, which include coronary, renal, iliofemoral, and popliteal arteries.[18–21] The bright inner layer is produced predominantly by the internal elastic lamina and, in part, by the intima. The middle layer, which is relatively echolucent, is produced by the media. This echolucency is due to a lower content of collagen and elastin. The outermost echogenic layer represents the external elastic lamina surrounded by the adventitia (Fig. 50–1). Normal coronary arteries with intimal thicknesses of less than 178 microns produce a homogenous circle without layering.[22] In contrast, the wall morphology of elastic arteries, such as the carotid, subclavian, pulmonary, and aorta, do not produce a three-layered appearance (Fig. 50–2). This is because the media in these arteries consist of densely packed elastin and collagen that are highly echogenic. Thus, there is no distinction between the media and adventitia.[21]

Morphometric Assessment

One of the main advantages of IVUS is the ability to provide information about plaque composition, extent, and distribution within the vessel wall. Atherosclerotic disease in coronary, peripheral, and brachiocephalic arteries produces a wide variety of plaques with different tissue compositions. Ultrasound imaging of these plaques reveals distinctive acoustic characteristics corresponding with specific tissue composition.[23–28] For clinical purposes, atherosclerotic plaques can be divided into three subtypes, depending on the relative echodensity of the plaque compared with the adventitia. A plaque containing lipids, thrombus, or loose connective tissue is less echogenic than the surrounding adventitia and is classified as a *soft plaque.* A plaque that produces bright homogenous echoes similar to the adventitia is termed *fibrous plaque.* A plaque with a combination of soft, fibrous, and calcified deposits is classified as a *mixed-type plaque* (Fig. 50–3). Calcified deposits within the plaques produce highly reflective echoes and a drop in signal intensity projecting beyond the lesion, resulting in a characteristic acoustic shadow. Plaque calcification can be classified into four types, depending on the arc of circumference occupied by the calcified segment. An arc of 90 degrees or less is classified as grade I, 91 to 180 degrees is grade II, 181 to 270 degrees is grade III, and more than 270 degrees is grade IV (Fig. 50–4). Dissection after coronary intervention is defined as an echo-free space behind the atherosclerotic plaque extending circumferentially and having a thickness of more than 0.3 mm. The degree of dissection severity can be graded on a scale of 1 to 4, similar to that used for calcified lesions (Fig. 50–5). Intra-arterial thrombus usually produces a finely speckled appearance and can be difficult to differentiate from a soft atheroma.[29, 30] In an animal model, the echodensity of thrombus varied

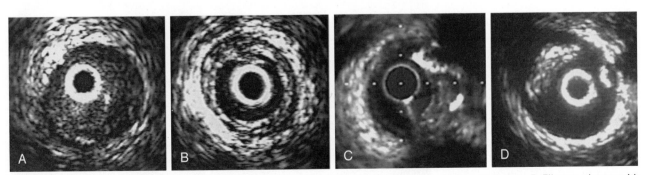

Figure 50-3 Ultrasonic plaque tissue characterization. *A,* Soft plaque with a relatively echolucent plaque. *B,* Fibrous plaque with a relatively echogenicity. *C,* Mixed plaque with segments of soft, fibrous, and calcified areas. *D,* Calcified plaque with characteristic "acoustic shadowing" in areas behind the calcific deposits (between 9 and 1 and at 3 o'clock positions).

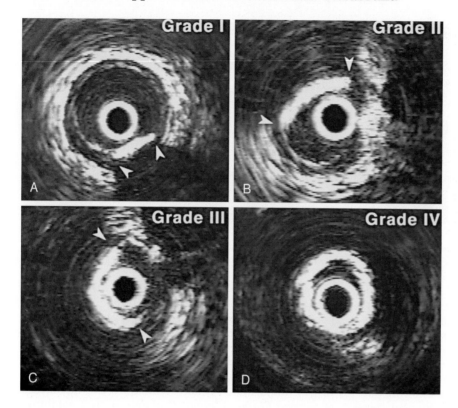

Figure 50-4 *A* to *D,* Four grades of calcification based on degree of circumferential arc subtended by calcified plaque. Note the presence of acoustic shadowing beyond the calcified plaque *(arrowheads).*

Figure 50-5 *A* to *D,* Ultrasonic grading of dissections based on the arc of echolucent space *(arrows)* behind the atherosclerotic plaque.

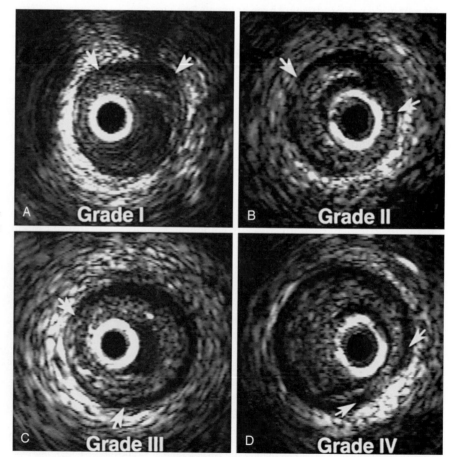

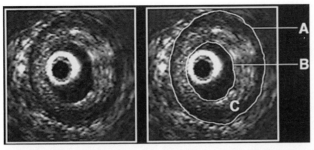

Figure 50-6 Quantitative analysis from an ultrasound image. Total vessel area is defined as the area bounded by the external elastic membrane (A). Luminal area is defined as the interface between atherosclerotic plaque and the lumen (B). Plaque plus media area is calculated by subtracting luminal area from total vessel area (C).

from a predominantly speckled appearance in the early phase (3.8 ± 4.1 hr) to a layered pattern at a later stage (16.8 ± 9.8 hr). A significant correlation was found between the fibrin content of the thrombus and ultrasonic echodensity.[31]

Quantitative Assessment

The various parameters that can be analyzed from IVUS imaging include plaque thickness, eccentricity, minimal luminal diameter, cross-sectional stenosis, luminal area, vessel wall area, and the plaque plus media area, which is derived from the difference between the external elastic lamina area and the lumen area (Fig. 50–6). Residual plaque burden is defined as the ratio of the plaque cross-sectional area to the area bounded by external elastic lamina. Plaque eccentricity is calculated as the ratio of the width of the thinnest plaque divided by the width of the opposite wall plaque. A plaque is considered *eccentric* if the ratio is less than 0.5 and *concentric* if the ratio is 0.5 or greater (Fig. 50–7).

Several studies have demonstrated a close correlation between the lumen cross-sectional area measured from ultrasound images and histopathologic cross-sections.[18, 20, 23, 32] The correlation between ultrasound images and the angiographic measurements of

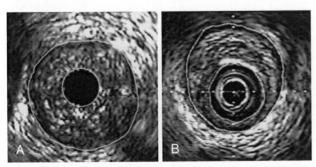

Figure 50-7 Ultrasound plaque distribution. A, Concentric plaque; note the presence of an evenly distributed plaque surrounding the ultrasound catheter. B, Eccentric plaque; note the uneven distribution of the plaque, with the thinnest portion at the bottom half and the thickest portion in the remaining half of the cross-section.

luminal dimensions has been shown to be excellent (r = 0.92 to 0.95) in normal vessels.[33–36] In cases of advanced atherosclerosis, the correlation coefficient decreases significantly (r = 0.46 to 0.63). Similarly, after balloon angioplasty, ultrasound measurements of luminal dimensions correlate poorly with the angiographic measurements (r = 0.12 to 0.28).[26, 33–36] The discrepancies between angiographic and IVUS measurements represent the differences in orientation of these imaging modalities (silhouette versus tomographic). The presence of a complex, irregular lumen with plaque fissuring and dissection hardly can be analyzed accurately by a luminal silhouette technique such as angiography. On the contrary, the tomographic cross-sectional imaging provided by IVUS is a superior method of assessing luminal dimensions after mechanical interventions.

Quantitative measurements obtained from ultrasound images tend to be slightly smaller than angiographic luminal dimensions, particularly after percutaneous intervention.[35, 37, 38] Nakamura et al[39] reported that the presence of a deep injury causing medial dissection (assessed by IVUS) is responsible for the poor correlation between angiography- and ultrasound-derived measurement of minimal luminal diameter and lumen cross-sectional area. A significant correlation between angiography- and IVUS-derived measurement of minimal luminal diameter and lumen cross-sectional area (r = 0.67 and 0.69, respectively) was observed when IVUS imaging demonstrated either no plaque fracture or only a small plaque tear that did not extend into the media.

REPRODUCIBILITY

The issue of reproducibility of IVUS-derived quantitative measurements has been addressed by various groups in the past and has been reported to be excellent.[23, 40] In a study by Hausmann et al.,[41] a close agreement (>87%) was noted for morphometric parameters, which included presence of plaque, calcification, and nondiseased wall. For quantitative measurements (minimal and maximal lumen diameters, luminal area, area within the internal elastic lamina, arc of calcium plaque), the correlation coefficient was high (r > 0.90), and the differences between measurements were low (mean difference, <10%). The ultrasound tissue characterization and measurements are based on the acoustic reflections of the tissue, which in turn depend on the dynamic range of the ultrasound system. Therefore, caution should be exercised in drawing definite conclusions about plaque morphology and quantitative measurements when analyzing images acquired by different systems with different parameter settings.

SAFETY ISSUES

Although invasive in nature, IVUS imaging has been associated with a low incidence of complications. Among 2207 coronary IVUS studies performed at 28 centers, no complications were reported in 2034

(92.2%) patients.[42] Vasospasm was the most common (2.9%) acute event. Other procedure-related events included occlusion, embolism, dissection, and thrombosis (0.4%). The incidence of major complications (myocardial infarction and emergent bypass surgery) was 0.1%. The complication rate was higher in patients with unstable angina (2.1%) than in those with stable angina (0.8%) and in patients without symptoms (0.4%). Even in patients who undergo IVUS imaging as part of an annual surveillance for cardiac allograft vasculopathy, no evidence of accelerated atherosclerosis has been noted in the instrumented arteries.[43]

LIMITATIONS

Although IVUS offers several advantages over contrast angiography, it has certain limitations that need to be mentioned. Plaque morphologic features (soft, fibrous, or calcified) and various quantitative measurements are potentially subjective variables that also are influenced by technical factors, such as the position (coaxial or eccentric), dynamic range, and axial resolution of the transducer.[44–46] Acoustic shadowing due to calcified plaque precludes the definition of underlying tissue structures and thus prevents the measurement of plaque thickness and vessel wall area. A minor degree of dissection can be missed when the intimal flap is compressed against the vessel wall by the ultrasound catheter.

CLINICAL UTILITY OF INTRAVASCULAR ULTRASOUND

Ambiguous Angiographic Lesions

Angiographic assessment of certain lesions, such as ostial stenosis, bifurcation lesions with overlapping branches, or short napkin-ring–type lesions, often remains suboptimal, despite multiple angiographic views.[47] IVUS imaging permits the precise evaluation of luminal dimensions and cross-sectional area stenosis at the suspected site (Case 1, Fig. 50–8). Our initial experience involved a series of seven patients in whom angiographic assessment was inconclusive and, therefore, IVUS imaging was performed.[48] In two patients, angiography significantly overestimated the stenoses severity, and the planned intervention was canceled (Case 2, Fig. 50–9). In the remaining five patients, lesions that appeared nonobstructive by angiography and that were inconsistent with the clinical evidence of significant coronary ischemia revealed significant stenoses when imaged by IVUS. Of the five patients in whom angiography underestimated the stenoses, two were referred for bypass surgery, two underwent balloon angioplasty, and one was treated medically. The ability of IVUS to clarify these ambiguous angiographic stenoses was of critical importance in the management of these patients. Assessment of such ambiguous lesions has become a routine indication for intracoronary ultrasound in many centers.

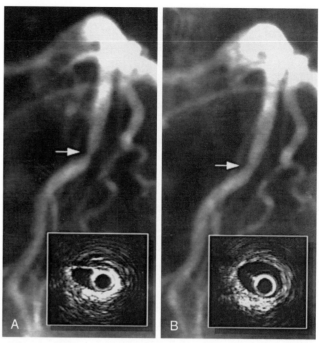

Figure 50-8 Case 1. Ultrasound imaging of a de novo myocardial bridge in a heart transplant recipient. *A,* The angiogram shows an area of mild stenosis in the mid left anterior descending artery *(arrow)* in a left anterior oblique (LAO) projection (systolic frame). *B,* A diastolic cine frame shows minimal stenosis *(arrow).* Corresponding intravascular ultrasound (IVUS) inset images show systolic compression and diastolic relaxation of the artery and the absence of atherosclerotic disease.

Left Main Coronary Artery Disease

The presence of left main coronary artery disease (LMCAD) is a poor prognostic sign for patients with coronary artery disease. The diagnosis of LMCAD is critical because surgical revascularization improves the survival substantially in patients with symptomatic as well as asymptomatic disease.[49, 50] Because of

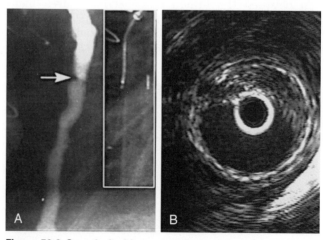

Figure 50-9 Case 2. Ambiguous angiography. *A,* An angiogram of a saphenous vein graft to a right coronary artery shows a greater than 70% lesion in its midportion *(arrow).* Inset shows the fluoroscopic confirmation of the IVUS catheter at the lesion site. *B,* IVUS cross-sectional imaging demonstrates an eccentric plaque with less than 30% diameter stenosis.

the anatomic variations in the origin, length, and course of the artery, angiographic assessment of LMCAD often is unsatisfactory. Frequent foreshortening and the overlapping of the left anterior descending and circumflex arteries often make it impossible to obtain a true orthogonal angiographic view for calculating lesion severity.[51] IVUS has the ability to provide a precise cross-sectional image of the area of interest, thereby allowing more accurate assessment of the severity of the left main lesions. We evaluated 15 patients in whom the diagnosis of LMCAD was in question on angiography.[52] In this study, most of the left main plaques were eccentric and composed of fibrocalcific tissue. Two patients had an angiographic filling defect in the left main coronary artery, indicating the possibility of intracoronary thrombus. Intravascular ultrasound imaging revealed the presence of a severely calcified atheroma while ruling out the presence a thrombus. The comparison between IVUS and angiographically calculated diameter stenosis showed a poor correlation (r = 0.30). In this series, eight patients underwent bypass surgery, six of whom were sent to surgery based on the IVUS findings (Case 3, Fig. 50–10). Angiography overestimated LMCAD in two patients in whom intravascular ultrasound revealed insignificant disease and bypass surgery was deferred. IVUS appears to be a better imaging modality for assessing LMCAD because it provides both morphologic and quantitative information about atherosclerotic narrowing. In the wake of similar findings reported by other investigators,[53, 54] we believe that IVUS should be the new gold standard for the diagnosis of LMCAD. It should be used cautiously or not at all in patients with obvious critical stenosis on angiography. Wedging an IVUS catheter into a stenotic area occasionally can lead to profound ischemia and hemodynamic instability.

Progression of Cardiac Allograft Vasculopathy

Cardiac allograft vasculopathy (CAV) remains a major cause of death in cardiac transplant recipients 1 year after transplantation. Until recently, annual angiographic surveillance has been used to assess the progression of CAV. Because of the diffuse nature of CAV, the extent of disease commonly is underestimated by angiography (Case 4, Fig. 50–11). Several studies from our center and other centers have shown that IVUS is a more sensitive method for detecting development and progression of CAV (Case 5, Fig. 50–12).[55–58] A study by Mehra et al.[59] has shown that the presence of severe intimal hyperplasia is associated with a higher risk of cardiac events, even in the presence of normal angiographic results.

Intravascular Ultrasound During Coronary Interventions

Intravascular ultrasound imaging before percutaneous interventions has shown that the angiographically normal reference segment has significant atherosclerotic disease occupying 51% ± 13% of the luminal cross-sectional area.[60] This confirms the theory of adaptive vascular remodeling in human coronary arteries proposed by Glagov et al. in 1987.[61] Several studies have confirmed the presence of adaptive vascular remodeling in native coronary arteries.[62, 63] Similarly, we also have documented the presence of this vascular remodeling in cardiac allograft vasculopathy.[64] IVUS has proved to be more sensitive in the detection of calcium deposits in the atheromatous plaques than angiography (73% versus 38%).[65] Similarly, most of the plaques (69%) have been noted to be eccentric in nature.[66]

The impact of IVUS imaging during coronary re-

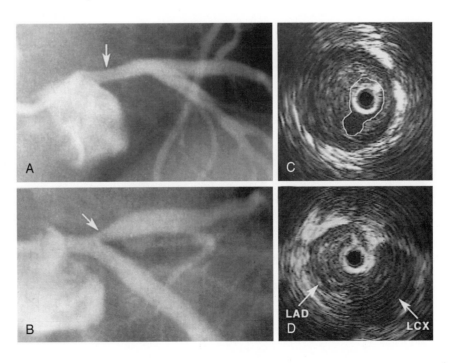

Figure 50-10 Case 3. *A* and *B,* Different angiographic projections in a patient with suspected left main coronary artery stenosis. Note the absence of any significant stenosis in the left main trunk (*arrow* in *A*) and the presence of a mild ostial lesion at the origin of the LAD artery (*arrow* in *B*). *C* and *D,* IVUS images show significant stenosis in the left main trunk extending into the origin of the LAD artery. LCX, left circumflex artery.

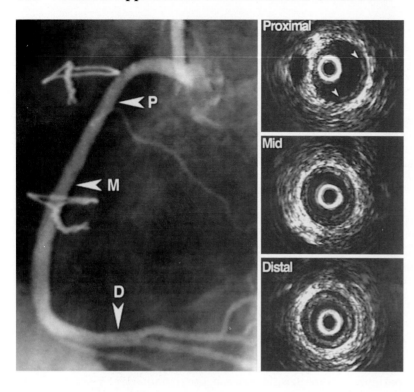

Figure 50-11 Case 4. Cardiac allograft vasculopathy. A "normal" right coronary angiogram taken 2 years after orthotopic heart transplantation. IVUS imaging at proximal (P), mid (M), and distal (D) sites demonstrates diffuse intimal thickening, which is not apparent on the angiogram.

vascularization has been well illustrated by the Guidance by Ultrasound Imaging for Decision Endpoints (GUIDE) study, in which IVUS imaging changed the therapeutic approach in 48% of the total procedures.[67] In the balloon angioplasty group, this resulted in the use of either a perfusion balloon for dissection or a larger balloon for suboptimal results. The detection of superficial calcium in the atheroma led to a decision to abandon directional coronary atherectomy (DCA) in nine cases, whereas significant residual plaque burden led to the upsizing of DCA devices in five cases. Mintz et al.[68] from the Washing-

ton Heart Center reported similar findings in 301 patients in whom the revascularization strategy intended before IVUS imaging was compared with the treatment actually performed.[68] A change in therapy was documented in 40% of the lesions, which included coronary revascularization when none was planned (6%), avoiding planned surgery or intervention (7%), changes in revascularization strategy based on plaque composition (6%), and changes in selection of revascularization strategy (20%).

Assessment After Various Interventional Techniques

Balloon Angioplasty

Before the advent of IVUS, information about the mechanism of balloon angioplasty was limited and was derived either from in vitro studies or from necropsy of patients who died after the procedure.[69, 70] IVUS imaging can provide instantaneous imaging of the arterial lumen after mechanical interventions and has been used successfully to demonstrate the effects of balloon angioplasty in both in vitro and in vivo studies.[26, 71–77] Various IVUS studies have shown that plaque fractures with varying degrees of dissection and stretching of the arterial wall are the predominant mechanisms of successful balloon angioplasty (Case 6, Fig. 50–13). Plaque compression does not appear to be a significant factor in most cases. Based on the IVUS plaque characteristics, Potkin et al.[71] reported that arterial expansion occurred in only 29% of the calcified plaques, as compared with 86% of the noncalcified plaques. In eccentric plaques, the stretching of relatively nondiseased segments without plaque fractures has been noted more

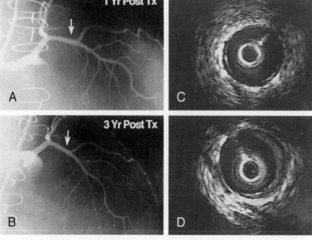

Figure 50-12 Case 5. Progression of cardiac allograft vasculopathy. A and B, Serial angiographic follow-up images of the LAD artery in a heart transplant recipient. Note the absence of significant luminal narrowing (arrows) on the follow-up angiogram at 3 years. C and D, Corresponding IVUS images show significant intimal thickening.

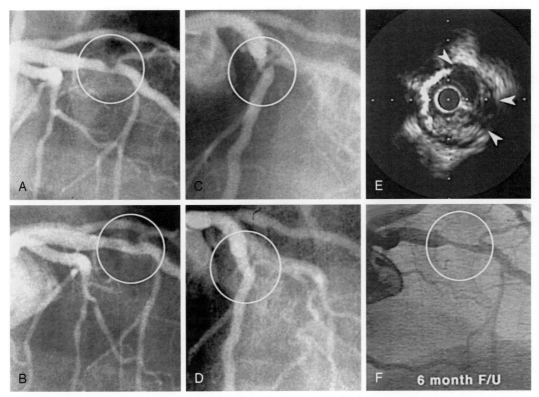

Figure 50-13 Case 6. Effects of balloon angioplasty. *A* to *D,* Angiographic pictures of an LAD artery stenosis before and after balloon angioplasty in right anterior oblique (RAO) and LAO projections. *E,* IVUS imaging after balloon angioplasty demonstrates an irregular lumen with a high residual plaque burden and calcification (9 to 12 o'clock position). Note the presence of plaque fracture at the junction of the calcified and noncalcified portions of the plaque *(arrowhead)*. Also note the plaque fissuring between the 3 and 4 o'clock positions *(arrowheads)*. *F,* Angiographic follow-up at 6 months demonstrates severe restenosis.

commonly.[72, 77] The extent and depth of arterial dissection after balloon dilation can be depicted clearly with high-quality IVUS imaging and has been noted more often by IVUS imaging (83%) than contrast angiography (23%).[71] IVUS imaging before intervention also can predict the site of the tear. The junction between the eccentric plaque and normal wall is the most frequent site of dissection.[71] Another frequent location for tearing is the junction between a localized calcium deposit and relatively soft plaque.[78] Small plaque tears or dissections, however, can be missed by IVUS because of the splinting of the atheroma by the IVUS catheter. Based on the IVUS cross-sectional images obtained after balloon angioplasty, different classifications of luminal morphologies have been proposed;[72, 73] however, none of these classifications has been studied prospectively. Currently, there is a lack of uniform definitions for plaque fissures, superficial versus deep plaque tears, and subintimal versus submedial tears.

Directional and Rotational Atherectomy

Directional coronary atherectomy was introduced with the hope of reducing postangioplasty plaque burden and ultimately leading to a lower restenosis rate. Initial clinical studies comparing balloon angioplasty and DCA did not show clinically significant differences in the restenosis rate.[79] IVUS imaging

after DCA has shown that tissue removal remains the major mechanism of luminal improvement.[80, 81] The "Dottering effect," caused by passage of the device, and stretching of the vessel wall after balloon dilation also contribute significantly to overall luminal improvement (Case 7, Fig. 50–14). The effect of plaque composition, particularly calcific deposits, is a strong determinant of the success of tissue retrieval. Tissue retrieval was reduced by half when a plaque had superficial calcium deposit, compared with plaques containing calcium deep inside the plaque or media.[82] The ability of IVUS to provide a direct assessment of plaque volume and its geometric distribution within the vessel area makes it an excellent device for monitoring the debulking process by DCA. Results from the Optimal Atherectomy Restenosis Study (OARS), a prospective, multicenter trial, have demonstrated the benefits of optimal atherectomy using IVUS guidance for plaque removal.[83] Procedural success was achieved in 97.5% of 199 patients, a mean residual stenosis of 7% was achieved in the 213 lesions, and only 19% of the lesions required target lesion revascularization at a median follow-up of 366 days.

As mentioned previously, plaques with superficial calcium deposits do not respond well to DCA and are better suited for rotational atherectomy (Fig. 50–15). Selective ablation of these calcific plaques has been demonstrated by Mintz et al.[84] and Kovach et al.[85]

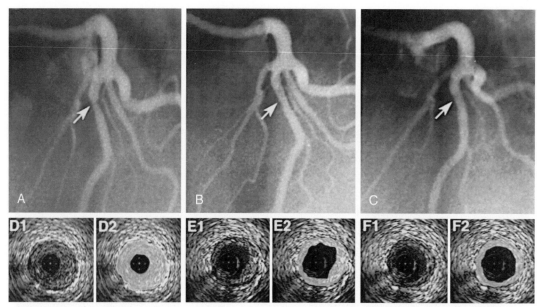

Figure 50-14 Case 7. Mechanisms of directional atherectomy. Angiograms of a proximal LAD artery lesion *(arrows)* in an LAO projection at baseline *(A)*, after directional atherectomy *(B)*, and after adjunctive balloon angioplasty *(C)*. *D1* and *D2*, Corresponding IVUS images demonstrate severe atherosclerosis at baseline. *E1* and *E2*, A large, irregular lumen after tissue excision by atherectomy. *F1* and *F2*, A relatively circular lumen after balloon angioplasty.

The neolumen after rotational atherectomy usually is circular or elliptical, with dissections occurring in 26% of the treated lesions. The resultant lumen tends to be slightly larger (15% to 20%) than the largest burr used, probably because of lateral movement of the burr during the procedure.

Endovascular Stenting

Stent struts are highly echogenic and thus easy to visualize by IVUS. Application of IVUS imaging during stent deployment has revolutionized the entire approach of intracoronary stenting. During initial human studies, intracoronary stenting was shown to be an effective therapy to treat abrupt or threatened closure and reduce the restenosis rate in de novo lesions. Subacute thrombotic occlusions and bleeding complications related to antithrombotic therapy, however, remained a cause of concern that increased both the hospital stay and procedural costs (Case 8, Fig. 50–16). Based on IVUS imaging after stent

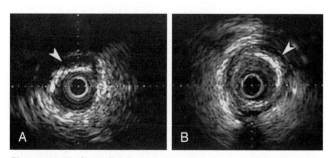

Figure 50-15 Superficial versus deep calcium. *A*, IVUS image shows a superficial rim of calcium near the luminal border *(arrowhead)*. *B*, IVUS image shows a rim of deep calcium at the base of an atherosclerotic plaque near the medial border.

deployment, Colombo et al.[86, 87] were the first to show that most of the Palmaz-Schatz stents were deployed suboptimally and that incomplete apposition of the stent struts to the vessel wall was responsible for an increased rate of subacute thrombosis. These investigators used IVUS to optimize stent expansion either with high-pressure balloon dilations or using larger balloons and discharged patients on antiplatelet therapy only.[88] This strategy not only reduced the rate of subacute stent thrombosis but also reduced the rate of vascular complications, thereby shortening the hospital stay and procedural cost. The experience with the Gianturco-Roubin stent has shown similar results.[89] In a series of 16 patients, significant improvements were observed in minimal luminal diameter and intrastent cross-sectional area measurements after high-pressure balloon dilation compared with the IVUS measurements performed immediately after initial stent deployment. No significant angiographic difference could be detected before and after high-pressure dilations (Case 9, Fig. 50–17). A number of IVUS studies have demonstrated that poststent high-pressure balloon dilations significantly increase the stented lumen diameter, yet angiography fails to reveal any significant improvement.[90, 91] In calcified lesions, however, optimal stent expansion does not occur, even after high-pressure balloon dilations (Case 10, Fig. 50–18). Severe target lesion calcification has been associated with lower procedural success, smaller postprocedural diameter, and poor clinical outcome compared with noncalcified lesions.[92–94]

Whether IVUS guidance should be a routinely used during stenting procedures remains controversial. Goods et al.[95] and Morice et al.[96] have demonstrated that in selected patients, intracoronary stenting can

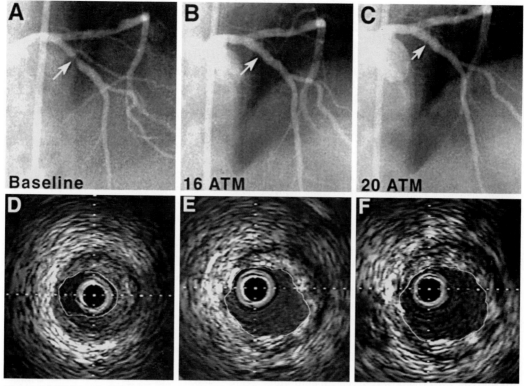

Figure 50-16 Case 8. Ultrasound imaging during intracoronary stenting. Angiograms of an LAD artery in an RAO view. *A,* A baseline image shows a severe narrowing *(arrow). B* and *C,* The next images were obtained after deployment of a 4-mm Palmaz-Schatz stent using a noncompliant balloon at 16 and 20 atmospheres, respectively. Note the absence of any significant improvement in the angiographic luminal dimensions *(arrows). D* to *F,* Corresponding IVUS images reveal inadequate stent expansion at 16 atmospheres and complete expansion after balloon dilation at 20 atmospheres, which is not apparent by angiography.

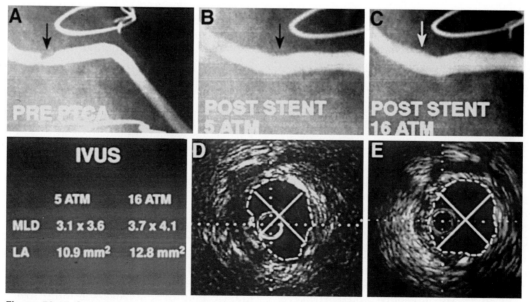

Figure 50-17 Case 9. Ultrasound imaging during intracoronary stenting. *A,* Baseline angiogram of a saphenous vein graft to the obtuse marginal branch with an eccenteric stenosis *(arrow). B* and *C,* Images after deployment of a 4-mm Gianturco-Roubin stent at 5 atmospheres and after dilation with a noncompliant balloon at 16 atmospheres. *D* and *E,* Corresponding IVUS images show significant improvement in the luminal dimensions and areas, not apparent by angiography *(arrows in B and C).* PTCA, percutaneous transluminal coronary angiplasty; MLD, minimal luminal diameter; LA, luminal area.

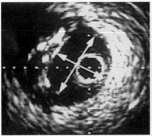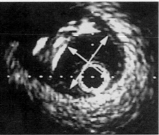

5 ATM   MLD 2.3x2.8 mm   18 ATM   MLD 2.6x3.1 mm

Figure 50-18 Case 10. Effect of a calcified lesion on intracoronary stenting. Left and right panels demonstrate minimal improvement in the intrastent diameters and luminal areas despite high-pressure balloon dilations.

be performed safely without anticoagulation or IVUS guidance. Whether IVUS-guided stenting can further reduce the restenosis rate in stented segments is a subject of ongoing studies[97–100]; so far, these studies have not demonstrated any impact on 30-day clinical event rates. Long-term results of these trials are awaited.

Editor's note: In brachiocephalic stenting, it is sometimes difficult to ascertain whether the stent is fully deployed. This is particularly true with the large curved innominate arteries but also is applicable to other arteries. Because brachiocephalic stenting is in the early period of its development, particularly as performed by most interventional neuroradiologists (who have not had the experience of peripheral vascular interventional training), many potential problems may occur that most interventional neuroradiologists are not aware of and that will be identified when patients return with either recurrent stenoses or embolic events secondary to suboptimal stenting.

Predictors and Mechanism of Restenosis

Earlier data from animal and human necropsy studies showed that excessive neointimal proliferation in response to mechanical trauma was responsible for restenosis.[101–105] Platelet aggregation and thrombus formation, activation of smooth muscle cells, and elastic recoil were proposed as mechanisms to be involved in the restenosis process.[106–110] However, all the clinical trials using pharmacologic agents to reduce intimal proliferation were unsuccessful.[111]

To investigate whether IVUS-defined parameters of plaque morphologic features and luminal dimension can predict the development of restenosis after percutaneous transluminal coronary angioplasty, several IVUS studies were performed to address the restenosis issue. Honye et al.[72] found higher restenosis rates in patients with concentric plaques without fracture or dissection. On the contrary, in a study by Tenaglia et al.,[112] the presence and severity of dissections assessed by IVUS were associated with increased risk of restenosis. The authors also studied 30 patients immediately after angioplasty and compared IVUS-derived parameters in patients who developed restenosis with parameters in those who did not.[113] Plaque fracture frequently (74%) was seen in

patients who did not develop restenosis and infrequently (30%) was seen in those who did develop restenosis. Plaque composition (soft, fibrous, or calcified) and lesion eccentricity did not differ between the two groups, nor was there a difference in the severity of calcification. Of the various quantitative parameters, plaque burden (defined as the ratio of the planimetered cross-sectional area of residual plaque to the planimetered cross-sectional area of the region bounded by external elastic membrane) was the only IVUS predictor of restenosis. Overall, 78% of patients with a plaque burden of more than 0.40 developed restenosis. Follow-up IVUS studies were not performed in patients with restenosis; therefore, the authors could not confirm the relative contribution of intimal proliferation and chronic recoil to the restenosis process. A recent multicenter study (GUIDE II) of 390 patients also found that residual cross-sectional narrowing and minimal luminal diameter were the most powerful predictors of restenosis.[114]

Data from follow-up ultrasound studies have challenged the prevailing theory that neointimal proliferation is mainly responsible for restenosis. Mintz et al.[115] analyzed the results of 360 nonstented lesions for which follow-up quantitative angiography or IVUS data were available. IVUS measurements of external elastic membrane (EEM, a measure of total arterial cross-sectional area), lumen cross-sectional area (CSA), plaque plus media area (P + M = EEM − lumen CSA), and cross-sectional narrowing (CSN = P + M/EEM) were performed before and after intervention and at follow-up. At follow-up, 73% of the late lumen loss was attributed to arterial remodeling (a decrease in external elastic membrane cross-sectional area), and 27% was due to tissue growth (an increase in plaque plus media cross-sectional area). Among the various parameters, IVUS-derived postprocedural CSN (i.e., plaque burden) was the most powerful predictor of restenosis and was related to the change in EEM as a mechanism of restenosis.

Two other studies have found similar results and confirmed these findings. In the OARS, late lumen loss was shown to be almost entirely the result of pathologic remodeling, which accounted for 84% of late lumen loss.[116] Additional data about the role of arterial remodeling came from the Serial Ultrasound Analysis of Restenosis (SURE) trial.[117] In this study, IVUS was performed in native vessel lesions before intervention, immediately after intervention, 24 hours after intervention, after 1 month, and at 6-month follow-up. During the early (first month) follow-up, there was adaptive remodeling (an increase in external elastic membrane cross-sectional area); a late pathologic remodeling (a decrease in external elastic membrane cross-sectional area) was noted from 1 month to 6 months. The changes in lumen cross-sectional area paralleled the changes in external elastic membrane cross-sectional area. Recent data from animal studies also support the findings that arterial remodeling is the predominant cause of late lumen loss and therefore plays a major role in the process of restenosis as compared with neointimal hyperplasia.[118–122] IVUS-guided aggressive reduction of residual plaque burden using multiple devices, however, has resulted in an increased restenosis rate (77%).[123] Severe vessel wall injury due to multiple devices can negate the benefit of reduced plaque burden and may result in increased restenosis owing to both neointimal proliferation and pathologic remodeling.

On the other hand, neointimal hyperplasia appears to be solely responsible for restenosis in stented arteries.[124] Serial follow-up studies of patients with intracoronary stents have shown that stenting prevents acute as well as chronic remodeling.[125, 126] Although the degree of neointimal hyperplasia is greater in stented segments than in nonstented segments, the vessels can accommodate a greater amount of neointimal tissue because the stent eliminates the process of remodeling, a predominant factor in restenosis.

Utility During Peripheral and Brachiocephalic Vascular Interventions

Although IVUS has not been studied as extensively in the peripheral or brachiocephalic vessels as it has been in the coronary arteries, its clinical utility has been demonstrated. IVUS imaging before and after percutaneous transluminal angioplasty (PTA) in peripheral arteries has shown mechanisms of luminal enlargement similar to those reported in the coronary arteries. Using a combined balloon and ultrasound imaging catheter, Isner et al.[127] demonstrated plaque fracture (at 2 atmospheres of balloon inflation pressure) in 60% of the patients undergoing PTA of the iliac arteries. Varying degrees of recoil (35% to 54%) were observed immediately after balloon deflation. Subsequently, this same group demonstrated that plaque fractures and atherosclerotic plaque "compression" were the principal mechanisms of successful PTA in the iliac arteries, whereas arterial wall stretching provided only a minor contribution to the overall increase in luminal dimensions (Case 11, Fig. 50–19).[128] In contrast, The et al.,[129] who studied the effects of balloon angioplasty on the superficial femoral artery with IVUS imaging, reported that luminal enlargements after PTA were primarily the results of an overstretched arterial wall, whereas the lesion volume remained unchanged (Case 12, Fig. 50–20). Most lesions in this study were classified as soft (60%) and eccentric (57%) plaques. Dissections and plaque ruptures were associated more commonly with soft plaques than with hard plaques (56% versus 28%). The differences in plaque morphology and composition may have been responsible for the observed difference in these two studies.

Katzen et al.[130] performed IVUS imaging in 140 patients after peripheral atherectomy (100 patients) and stent placement (40 patients). Residual stenoses were significantly underestimated by digital subtraction angiography in 80% of the patients who underwent atherectomy. In all patients, IVUS demonstrated the presence of more residual plaque, resulting in the decision to pursue further intervention. In eight (20%) patients undergoing stent deployment, IVUS demonstrated incomplete expansion that was not visible by angiography (Case 13, Fig. 50–21). Further dilations with larger balloons were performed in all of these cases to achieve optimal expansion. Similarly, Navarro et al.[131] have shown that

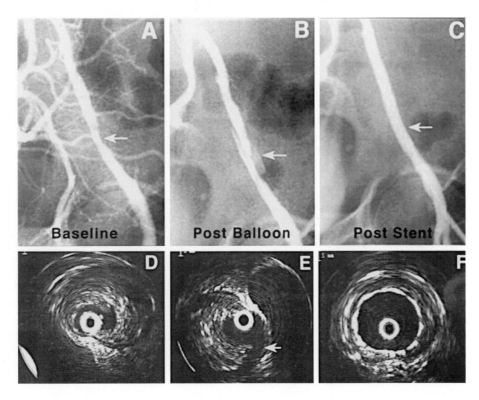

Figure 50-19 Case 11. Ultrasound imaging during iliac artery angioplasty. *A*, Baseline angiogram demonstrates mild stenosis *(arrow)* while the corresponding IVUS image *(D)* demonstrates severe stenosis. *B*, Angiogram showing dissection *(arrow)* following balloon dilation. IVUS image *(E)* also demonstrates the dissection *(arrow)*. *C*, Angiogram following stent placement demonstrates a smooth lumen *(arrow)*, which is confirmed by IVUS imaging *(F)*.

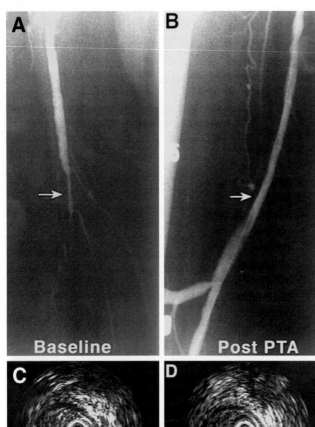

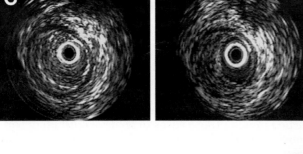

Figure 50-20 Case 12. Peripheral angiograms before *(A)* and after *(B)* balloon angioplasty of a superficial femoral artery lesion *(arrows)*. *C,* IVUS imaging before percutaneous transluminal angioplasty (PTA) demonstrates the presence of severe atherosclerotic narrowing. *D,* Note the presence of a high residual plaque burden despite a successful angiographic result.

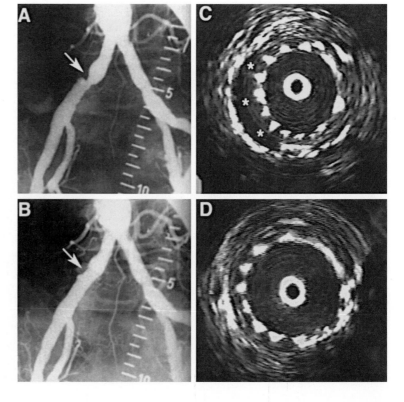

Figure 50-21 Case 13. Ultrasound imaging of an incompletely expanded Palmaz (biliary) stent in a common iliac artery. *A,* Baseline angiogram showing an eccentric stenosis in a right common iliac artery *(arrow)*. *B,* Poststent angiogram showing mild residual stenosis at the lesion site *(arrow)*. *C,* IVUS imaging demonstrates incomplete stent expansion with a gap between the stent struts and the arterial wall *(asterisks)*. *D,* After dilation with a larger-size balloon, IVUS shows full stent expansion with complete stent strut-wall apposition.

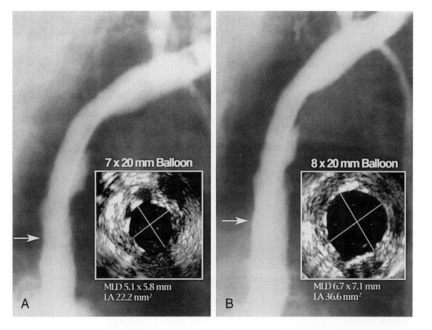

Figure 50-22 Case 14. Example of an ultrasound-guided subclavian artery stenting. *A,* Angiography after Palmaz (biliary) stent deployment in a subclavian artery using a 7 × 20 mm balloon demonstrates suboptimal stent expansion by IVUS *(inset). B,* Angiography and IVUS imaging *(inset)* after dilation with an 8 × 20 mm balloon demonstrate optimal stent expansion and a significant improvement in the intrastent luminal dimensions and the area, which was not apparent on the angiogram *(arrows* in *A* and *B*).

despite a satisfactory angiographic appearance, 25 of 101 (25%) stents deployed in the common or external iliac arteries were either undersized or incompletely deployed, and IVUS imaging was helpful in optimizing the final results. With the technological advances in the field of endovascular therapy for peripheral vascular disease, precise measurements of arterial lumen, lesion length, location, and plaque composition have become important issues (Cases 14, 15, and 16, Figs. 50–22 to 50–24). IVUS provides unique complementary information during endovascular procedures, such as endovascular grafting for the

exclusion of an aneurysm or bypass of long atherosclerotic lesions.[132–135]

CONCLUSIONS

Intravascular ultrasound's usefulness as an adjunct to coronary angiography has spurred its growth as an integral part of many interventional laboratories. Intravascular ultrasound is adept at defining the plaque morphology and intraluminal changes after various therapeutic modalities. It has enhanced the understanding of the mechanisms of various percutaneous interventions and has significantly changed

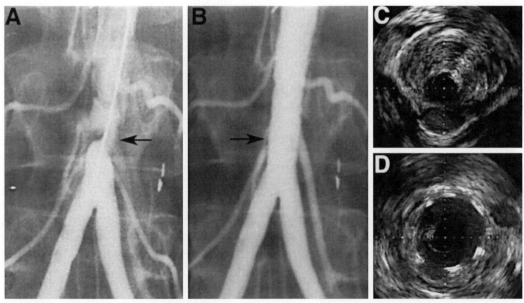

Figure 50-23 Case 15. Distal abdominal aortic stenting. *A,* Baseline angiogram shows a severe, eccentric stenosis *(arrow). B,* After placement of a Palmaz-Schatz stent, a smooth lumen without residual stenosis is seen *(arrows). C* and *D,* Corresponding IVUS images show irregular, severe luminal narrowing at the baseline, while a smooth circular lumen is noted after stenting.

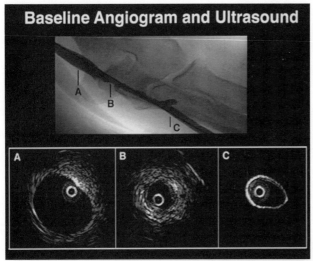

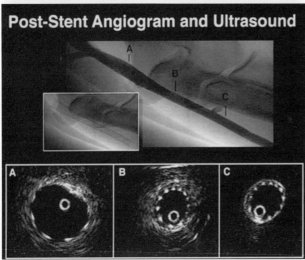

Figure 50-24 Case 16. Angiographic and corresponding ultrasound images before and after deployment of a wall stent in a hemodialysis fistula with recurrent stenosis.

the understanding of the restenosis process. As a diagnostic modality, it is useful in cases with ambiguous angiographic results and in the quantitative assessment of left main coronary stenosis. It is far superior to conventional angiography in detecting the extent and progression of cardiac allograft vasculopathy. Its utility in atherectomy device selection, based on the presence of superficial versus deep calcium, has been helpful in optimizing the final results. It has revolutionized the entire approach of intracoronary stenting and has markedly reduced the procedural-related morbidity as well as the cost. Whether it should be used routinely during all endoluminal stenting will depend on whether ongoing trials demonstrate the clinical benefit of imaging in terms of further reduction in restenosis rate. Finally, in this era of cost-containment, ongoing and future trials should identify a subset of patients or lesion morphologies in which IVUS imaging will be the most cost beneficial.

Editor's note: Brachiocephalic angioplasty and stenting

will be a growth industry in the future. Many aspects of the skill and art of this procedure are yet to be determined, but we, as interventional neuroradiologists, should be at the forefront of their development.

REFERENCES

1. Sones FM, Shirey EK. Cine coronary arteriography. *Mod Concepts Cardiovasc Dis* 1962;31:735–738.
2. Pepine CJ, Feldman RL, Nichols WW, et al. Coronary arteriography: potentially serious sources of error in interpretation. *Cardiovasc Med* 1977;2:747–752.
3. Arnett EN, Isner JM, Redwood CR, et al. Coronary artery narrowing in coronary heart disease: comparison of cineangiographic and necropsy findings. *Ann Intern Med* 1979;91:350–356.
4. Spears JR, Sander T, Baim DS, et al. The minimum error in estimating coronary luminal cross-sectional area from cineangiographic diameter measurements. *Cathet Cardiovasc Diagn* 1983;9:119–128.
5. White CW, Wright CG, Doty DB, et al. Does visual interpretation of the coronary arteriogram predict the physiologic importance of a coronary stenosis? *N Engl J Med* 1984; 310:819–824.
6. Marcus ML, Skorton DJ, Johnson MR, et al. Visual estimates of percent diameter coronary stenosis. "a battered gold standard". *J Am Coll Cardiol* 1988;11:882–885.
7. Katritsis D, Webb-Peploe M. Limitations of coronary angiography: an underestimated problem? *Clin Cardiol* 1991;14:20–24.
8. Spears JR, Sander T, Als AV, et al. Computerized image analysis for quantitative measurements of vessel diameter from cineangiograms. *Circulation* 1983;68:453–461.
9. Reiber JHC: An overview of coronary quantitation techniques as of 1989. In: Reiber JHC, Serruys PW (eds): Quantitative Coronary Angiography 1991. Dordrecht, the Netherlands: Kluwer Academic Publishers, 1991, pp. 55–132.
10. Mancini GBJ, Simon SB, McGillen MJ, et al. Automated quantitative coronary arteriography: morphologic and physiologic validation in vivo of a rapid digital angiographic method. *Circulation* 1987;75:452–460.
11. Whiting JS, Ptaff JM, Eigler NL. Advantages and limitations of video densitometry in quantitative coronary angiography. In: Reiber JHC, Serruys PW (eds): Quantitative Coronary Angiography 1991. Dordrecht, the Netherlands: Kluwer Academic Publishers, 1991, pp. 43–54.
12. Herrold EM, Goldberg HL, Borer JS, et al. Relative insensitivity of densitometric stenosis measurement to lumen edge detection. *J Am Coll Cardiol* 1990;15:1570–1577.
13. Tobis J, Hall P, Maiello L, et al. Clinical feasibility of an 0.018″ intravascular ultrasound imaging device [Abstract]. *Circulation* 1995;92(suppl I):I-400.
14. Hodgson J, Nair R, for the Endosonics Oracle Investigators. Efficacy and usefulness of a combined intracoronary ultrasound-angioplasty balloon catheter: results of the multicenter Oracle™ trial [Abstract]. *Circulation* 1992;86(suppl I):I-321.
15. Yock PG, Fitzgerald PJ, Jang YT, et al. Initial trials of combined ultrasound imaging/mechanical atherectomy catheter [Abstract]. *J Am Coll Cardiol* 1990;15:17A.
16. Rosenfield K, Losordo DW, Ramaswamy K, et al. Three dimensional reconstruction of human coronary and peripheral arteries from images recorded during two dimensional intracoronary ultrasound examinations. *Circulation* 1991; 84:1938–1956.
17. DiMario C, von Birgelen C, Prati F, et al. Three dimensional reconstruction of cross sectional intracoronary ultrasound: clinical or research tool? *Br Heart J* 1995;73(suppl 2):26–32.
18. Gussenhoven EJ, Essed CE, Lancee CT, et al. Arterial wall characteristics determined by intravascular ultrasound imaging: an in vitro study. *J Am Coll Cardiol* 1989;14:947–952.
19. Fitzgerald PJ, Cogburn MA, Law VK, et al. Determination of arterial wall components using intravascular backscatter analysis [Abstract]. *Circulation* 1990;82(suppl III):III-441.

20. Nishimura RA, Edwards WD, Warnes CA, et al. Intravascular ultrasound imaging: in vitro validation and pathologic correlation. *J Am Coll Cardiol* 1990;16:145–154.
21. Lockwood GR, Ryan LK, Gotlieb AI, et al. In vitro high resolution intravascular imaging in muscular and elastic arteries. *J Am Coll Cardiol* 1992;20:153–160.
22. Fitzgerald PJ, St Goar FG, Connolly AJ, et al. Intravascular ultrasound imaging of coronary arteries. Is three layers the norm? *Circulation* 1992;86:154–158.
23. Potkin BH, Bartorelli AL, Gessert JM, et al. Coronary artery imaging with high frequency ultrasound. *Circulation* 1990;81:1575–1585.
24. Bartorelli AL, Potkin BH, Almagor YA, et al. Plaque characterization of atherosclerotic coronary arteries by ultrasound. *Echocardiography* 1990;7:389–395.
25. Siegel RJ, Ariani M, Fishbein MC, et al. Histopathological validation of angioscopy and intravascular ultrasound. *Circulation* 1991;84:109–117.
26. Tobis JN, Mallery J, Mahon D, et al. Intravascular ultrasound imaging of human coronary arteries in vivo: analysis of tissue characterizations with comparison to in vitro histological specimens. *Circulation* 1991;83:913–926.
27. DiMario C, The S, Madretsma S, et al. Detection and characterization of vascular lesions by intravascular ultrasound: an in vitro study correlated with histology. *J Am Soc Echocardiogr* 1992;5:135–146.
28. Peters RJG, Kok WEM, Havenith MG, et al. Histopathologic validation of intracoronary ultrasound imaging. *J Am Soc Echocardiogr* 1994;7:230–241.
29. Pandian HG, Kreis A, Brockway B. Detection of intraarterial thrombus by intravascular high frequency two dimensional ultrasound imaging in vitro and vivo studies. *Am J Cardiol* 1990;15:1280–1283.
30. Jain A, Ramee SR, Mesa J, et al. Intracoronary thrombus: chronic urokinase infusion and evaluation with intravascular ultrasound. *Cathet Cardiovasc Diagn* 1992;26:212–214.
31. Jain A, Jain SP, Paulson DB, et al. Characteristics of in vivo forming intravascular thrombi: intravascular ultrasound imaging evaluation [Abstract]. *Circulation* 1991;86(suppl I):I-576.
32. Tobis JM, Mallery JA, Gessert J, et al. Intravascular ultrasound cross-sectional arterial imaging before and after balloon angioplasty in vitro. *Circulation* 1989;80:873–882.
33. Davidson CJ, Sheikh KH, Harrison JK, et al. Intravascular ultrasonography versus digital subtraction angiography: a human in vivo comparison of vessel size and morphology. *J Am Coll Cardiol* 1990;16:633–636.
34. St Goar FG, Pinto FJ, Alderman E, et al. Intravascular ultrasound imaging of angiographically normal coronary arteries: an in vivo comparison with quantitative angiography. *J Am Coll Cardiol* 1991;18:952–958.
35. Nissen SE, Gurley JC, Grines CL, et al. Intravascular ultrasound assessment of lumen size and wall morphology in normal subjects and patients with coronary artery disease. *Circulation* 1991;84:1087–1099.
36. De Scheerder I, De Man F, Herregods MC, et al. Intravascular ultrasound versus angiography for measurement of luminal diameters in normal and diseased coronary arteries. *Am Heart J* 1994;127:243–251.
37. Davidson CJ, Sheikh KH, Kisslo KB, et al. Intracoronary ultrasound evaluation of interventional technologies. *Am J Cardiol* 1991;68:1305–1309.
38. DeFranco A, Tuzcu EM, Moliterno DJ, et al. Overestimation of lumen size after coronary interventions: implications for randomized trials of new devices [Abstract]. *Circulation* 1994;90(suppl I):I-550.
39. Nakamura S, Mahon DJ, Maheswaren B, et al. An explanation for discrepancy between angiographic and intravascular ultrasound measurements after percutaneous transluminal coronary angioplasty. *J Am Coll Cardiol* 1995;25:633–639.
40. Crowe TD, Kim MH, Ziada KM, et al. Reproducibility and sources of variability in intravascular ultrasound measurements [Abstract]. *Circulation* 1996;94(suppl I):I-654.
41. Hausmann D, Lundkvist A, Friedrich GJ, et al. Intracoronary ultrasound imaging: intraobserver and interobserver variability of morphometric measurements. *Am Heart J* 1994;128:674–680.
42. Hausmann D, Erbel R, Alibelli-Chemarin M, et al. The safety of intracoronary ultrasound: a multicenter survey of 2207 examinations. *Circulation* 1995;91:623–630.
43. Pinto FJ, St Goar FG, Gao SZ, et al. Immediate and one year safety of intracoronary ultrasound imaging: evaluation with serial quantitative angiography. *Circulation* 1993;88(part I):I709–I714.
44. Chae JS, Brisken AF, Maurer G, Seigel RJ. Geometric accuracy of intravascular ultrasound imaging. *J Am Soc Echocardiogr* 1992;5:577–587.
45. Benkeser PJ, Churchwell AL, Lee C, et al. Resolution limitations in intravascular ultrasound imaging. *J Am Soc Echocardiogr* 1993;6:158–165.
46. DiMario C, Madretsma S, Linker D, et al. The angle of incidence of the ultrasonic beam: a critical factor for the image quality in intravascular ultrasonography. *Am Heart J* 1993;125:442–448.
47. Honye J, Mahon DJ, Nakamura S, et al. Enhanced diagnostic ability of intravascular imaging compared with angiography [Abstract]. *Circulation* 1992;86(suppl I):I-324.
48. White CJ, Ramee SR, Collins TJ, et al. Ambiguous coronary angiography: clinical utility of intravascular ultrasound. *Cathet Cardiovasc Diagn* 1992;26:200–203.
49. Mock MB, Killip T. Effect of coronary bypass surgery on survival patterns in subsets of patients with left main coronary artery disease: report of the collaborative study in coronary artery surgery (CASS). *Am J Cardiol* 1981;48:765–777.
50. Taylor HA, Deumite JH, Chaitman BR, et al. Asymptomatic left main coronary artery disease in the coronary artery surgery study (CASS) registry. *Circulation* 1989;79:1171–1179.
51. Isner JM, Kishel J, Kent JM, et al. Accuracy of angiographic determination of left main coronary arterial narrowing: angiographic–histologic correlative analysis in 28 patients. *Circulation* 1981;63:1056–1064.
52. Jain SP, White CJ, Ramee SR, et al. Comparison of coronary angiography and intravascular ultrasound in the diagnosis of left main coronary artery disease (abstr). *Cathet Cardiovasc Diagn* 1993;29:88.
53. Hermiller JB, Buller CE, Tenaglia AN, et al. Unrecognized left main coronary artery disease in patients undergoing interventional procedures. *Am J Cardiol* 1993;71:173–176.
54. Davies SW, Wintertown SJ, Rothman MT. Intravascular ultrasound to assess left main stem coronary artery lesion. *Br Heart J* 1992;68:525–526.
55. Goar FG, Pinto FJ, Alderman EL, et al. Intracoronary ultrasound in cardiac transplant recipients: in vivo evidence of angiographically silent intimal thickening. *Circulation* 1992;85:979–987.
56. Ventura HO, White CJ, Jain SP, et al. Assessment of intracoronary morphology in cardiac transplant recipients by angioscopy and intravascular ultrasound. *Am J Cardiol* 1993;72:805–809.
57. Escobar A, Ventura HO, Stapleton DD, et al. Cardiac allograft vasculopathy assessed by intravascular ultrasound and nonimmunologic risk factors. *Am J Cardiol* 1994;74:1042–1046.
58. Mehra M, Ventura HO, Chambers R, et al. Predictive model to assess risk for cardiac allograft vasculopathy: an intravascular ultrasound study. *J Am Coll Cardiol* 1995;26:1537–1544.
59. Mehra M, Ventura HO, Stapleton DD, et al. Presence of severe intimal thickening by intravascular ultrasound predicts cardiac events in cardiac allograft vasculopathy. *J Heart Lung Transplant* 1995;14:632–639.
60. Mintz GS, Painter JA, Pichard AD, et al. Atherosclerosis in angiographically "normal" coronary artery reference segments: an intravascular ultrasound study with clinical correlation. *J Am Coll Cardiol* 1995;25:1479–1485.
61. Glagov S, Weisenberg E, Zarins CK, et al. Compensatory enlargement of human atherosclerotic coronary arteries. *N Engl J Med* 1987;316:1371–1375.
62. Gerber TC, Erbel R, Gorge G, et al. Extent of atherosclerosis

and remodeling of left main coronary artery determined by intravascular ultrasound. *Am J Cardiol* 1994;73:666–671.

63. Ge J, Erbel R, Zamorano J, et al. Coronary artery remodeling in atherosclerotic disease: an intravascular ultrasound study in vivo. *Coron Artery Dis* 1993;4:981–986.

64. Jain SP, White CJ, Ramee SR, et al Coronary remodeling in cardiac allograft vasculopathy detected by intravascular ultrasound. *Circulation* 1993;88(suppl I):I-550.

65. Mintz GS, Popma JJ, Pichard AD, et al. Patterns of calcification in coronary artery disease: a statistical analysis of intravascular ultrasound and coronary angiography in 1155 lesions. *Circulation* 1995;91:1959–1965.

66. Hausmann D, Lundkvist AJS, Friedrich G, et al. Lumen and plaque shape in atherosclerotic coronary arteries assessed by in vivo intracoronary ultrasound. *Am J Cardiol* 1994;74:857–863.

67. The GUIDE Trial Investigators. Impact of intravascular ultrasound on device selection and endpoint assessment of interventions: phase I of the GUIDE Trial [Abstract]. *J Am Coll Cardiol* 1993;21:134A.

68. Mintz GS, Pichard AD, Kovach JA, et al. Impact of preinterventional intravascular ultrasound imaging on transcatheter treatment strategies in coronary artery disease. *Am J Cardiol* 1994;73:423–430.

69. Block PC, Baughman KL, Pasternak RC, et al. Transluminal angioplasty: correlation of morphologic and angiographic findings in an experimental model. *Circulation* 1980;61:778–785.

70. Waller BF, Garfinkel HJ, Rogers FJ, et al. Early and late morphological changes in major epicardial coronary arteries after percutaneous transluminal coronary angioplasty. *Am J Cardiol* 1984;53(suppl C):42C–47C.

71. Potkin BH, Karen G, Mintz GS, et al. Arterial response to balloon coronary angioplasty: an intravascular ultrasound study. *J Am Coll Cardiol* 1992;20:942–951.

72. Honye J, Mahon DJ, Jain A, et al. Morphological effects of coronary balloon angioplasty in vivo assessed by intravascular ultrasound imaging. *Circulation* 1992;85:1012–1025.

73. Gerber TC, Erbel R, Gorge G, et al. Classification of morphologic effects of percutaneous transluminal coronary angioplasty assessed by intravascular ultrasound. *Am J Cardiol* 1992;70:1546–1554.

74. Jain SP, Roubin GS, Nanda NC, et al. Intravascular ultrasound imaging of saphenous vein graft stenosis. *Am J Cardiol* 1992;69:133–136.

75. Tenaglia AN, Buller CE, Kisslo KB, et al. Mechanism of balloon angioplasty and directional coronary atherectomy as assessed by intracoronary ultrasound. *J Am Coll Cardiol* 1992;20:685–691.

76. Hodgson J, Reddy KG, Suneja R, et al. Intracoronary ultrasound imaging: correlation of plaque morphology with angiography, clinical syndrome and procedural results in patients undergoing coronary angioplasty. *J Am Coll Cardiol* 1993;21:35–44.

77. The GUIDE Trial Investigators. Lumen enlargement following angioplasty is related to plaque characteristics: a report from the GUIDE Trial [Abstract]. *Circulation* 1992;86(suppl I):I-531.

78. Fitzgerald PJ, Ports TA, Yock YG. Contribution of localized calcium deposits to dissection after angioplasty: an observational study using intravascular ultrasound. *Circulation* 1992;86:64–70.

79. Topol EJ, Leya F, Pinkerton CA, et al. for the CAVEAT Study Group. A comparison of directional atherectomy with coronary angioplasty in patients with coronary artery disease. *N Engl J Med* 1993;329:221–227.

80. Matar FA, Mintz GS, Farb A, et al. The contribution of tissue removal to lumen improvement after directional coronary atherectomy. *Am J Cardiol* 1994;74:647–650.

81. Baim DS, Simonton C, Popma JJ, et al. Mechanism of luminal enlargement by optimal atherectomy: IVUS insights from the OARS study [Abstract]. *J Am Coll Cardiol* 1996;27:291A.

82. Fitzgerald PJ, Muhlberger VA, Moes NY, et al. Calcium location within plaque as a predictor of atherectomy tissue retrieval: an intravascular ultrasound study [Abstract]. *Circulation* 1992;82(suppl I):I-516.

83. Popma JJ, Baim DS, Kuntz RE, et al. Early and late quantitative angiographic outcomes in the Optimal Atherectomy Restenosis Study (OARS) [Abstract]. *J Am Coll Cardiol* 1996;27:291A.

84. Mintz GS, Potkin BH, Karen G, et al. Intravascular ultrasound evaluation of the effect of rotational atherectomy in obstructive atherosclerotic coronary artery disease. *Circulation* 1992;86:1383–1393.

85. Kovach JA, Mintz GS, Pichard AD, et al. Sequential intravascular ultrasound imaging characterizes mechanism of lumen enlargement after rotational atherectomy [Abstract]. *Circulation* 1992;86(suppl I):I-532.

86. Nakamura S, Colombo A, Gaglione S, et al. Intravascular ultrasound observations during stent implantation. *Circulation* 1994;89:2026–2034.

87. Goldberg SL, Colombo A, Hakamura S, et al. Benefits of intracoronary ultrasound in the deployment of Palmaz-Schatz stents. *J Am Coll Cardiol* 1994;24:996–1003.

88. Colombo A, Hall P, Hakamura S, et al. Intracoronary stenting without anticoagulation accomplished with intravascular ultrasound guidance. *Circulation* 1995;91:1676–1688.

89. Jain SP, Liu MW, Iyer SS, et al. Do high pressure balloon inflations improve acute gain within flexible metallic coil stents? An intravascular ultrasound assessment [Abstract]. *J Am Coll Cardiol* 1995;25(suppl A):49A.

90. Mudra H, Klauss V, Blasini R, et al. Ultrasound guidance of Palmaz-Schatz intracoronary stenting with a combined intravascular ultrasound balloon catheter. *Circulation* 1994;90:1252–1261.

91. Gorge G, Haude M, Ge J, et al. Intravascular ultrasound after low and high inflation pressure coronary artery stent implantation. *J Am Coll Cardiol* 1995;26:725–730.

92. Fitzgerald PJ for the Strut Registry Investigators. Lesion composition impact size and symmetry of stent expansion: initial report from the STRUT registry [Abstract]. *J Am Coll Cardiol* 1995;25(suppl A):49A.

93. Komiyama N, Stone GW, Alderman E, et al. Relative stent expansion is dependent upon target lesion calcification: an intravascular ultrasound assessment [Abstract]. *Circulation* 1996;94(suppl I):I-262.

94. Yokoi H, Nobuyoshi M, Nosaka H, et al. Palmaz-Schatz stent implantation in calcified lesions: immediate and follow-up results [Abstract]. *Circulation* 1996;94(suppl I):I-453.

95. Goods CM, Al-Shaibi KF, Yadav SS, et al. Utilization of the coronary balloon expandable coil stent without anticoagulation or intravascular ultrasound. *Circulation* 1996;93:1803–1808.

96. Morice MC, Breton C, Bunouf P, et al. Coronary stenting without anticoagulant, intravascular ultrasound: results of the French registry [Abstract]. *Circulation* 1995;92(suppl I):I-796.

97. Russo RJ, Teirstein PS, for the AVID investigators. Angiography versus intravascular ultrasound directed stent placement [Abstract]. *Circulation* 1996;94(suppl I):I-263.

98. Metz JA, Fitzgerald PJ, Oshima A, et al. Impact of intravascular ultrasound guidance on stenting in the CRUISE substudy [Abstract]. *Circulation* 1996;94(suppl I):I-199.

99. Strain JE, Rehman DE, Fischman D, et al. Stress III: preliminary acute results of IVUS vs. non-IVUS stenting [Abstract]. *Circulation* 1996;94(suppl I):I-200.

100. Hodgson J, Frey AW, Mueller C, et al. Comparison of acute procedure cost and equipment utilization with strategies of ICUS guided vs. angiographic guided PTCA and stenting: preliminary results of the Strategy of ICUS-guided PTCA and Stenting (SIPS) Study [Abstract]. *Circulation* 1996;94(suppl I):I-325.

101. Clowes A, Reidy M, Clowes M. Mechanism of stenosis after arterial injury. *Lab Invest* 1983;49:208–215.

102. Schwartz RS, Murphy JG, Edwards WD, et al. Restenosis after balloon angioplasty: a practical proliferative model in porcine coronary arteries. *Circulation* 1990;82:2190–2200.

103. Austin GE, Ratlif NB, Hollman J, et al. Intimal proliferation of smooth muscle cells as an explanation for recurrent coronary artery stenosis after percutaneous transluminal coronary angioplasty. *J Am Coll Cardiol* 1985;6:369–375.

104. Farb A, Virmani R, Atkinson JB, et al. Plaque morphology and pathologic changes in arteries from patients dying after coronary balloon angioplasty. *J Am Coll Cardiol* 1990; 16:1421–1429.

105. Nobuyoshi M, Kimura T, Ohishi H, et al. Restenosis after percutaneous transluminal coronary angioplasty: pathologic observations in 20 patients. *J Am Coll Cardiol* 1991;17:433–439.

106. Ip J, Fuster V, Israel D, et al. The role of platelets, thrombin, and hyperplasia in restenosis after coronary angioplasty. *J Am Coll Cardiol* 1991;17:77B–88B.

107. Chesebro J, Lam J, Badimon L, Fuster V. Restenosis after arterial angioplasty: a hemorrheologic response to injury. *Am J Cardiol* 1987;60:10B–16B.

108. Casscells W. Migration of smooth muscle and endothelial cells: critical events in restenosis. *Circulation* 1992;86:723–729.

109. Nobuyoshi M, Kimura T, Nosaka H. Restenosis after successful percutaneous transluminal angioplasty: serial follow-up of 229 patients. *J Am Coll Cardiol* 1988;12:616–623.

110. Liu MW, Roubin GS, King SB. Restenosis after coronary angioplasty: potential biologic determinants and role of intimal hyperplasia. *Circulation* 1989;79:1374–1387.

111. Franklin S, Faxon D. Pharmacologic prevention of restenosis after coronary angioplasty: review of randomized clinical trials. *Coron Artery Dis* 1993;4:232–242.

112. Tenaglia AM, Buller CE, Kisslo KB, et al. Intracoronary ultrasound predictors of adverse outcome after coronary artery interventions. *J Am Coll Cardiol* 1992;20:1385–1390.

113. Jain SP, Jain A, Collins TJ, et al. Predictors of restenosis: a morphometric and quantitative evaluation by intravascular ultrasound. *Am Heart J* 1994;128:664–673.

114. The GUIDE Trial Investigators. IVUS-determined predictors of restenosis in PTCA and DCA: final report from the GUIDE trial, phase II. *J Am Coll Cardiol* 1996;27:156A.

115. Mintz GS, Popma JJ, Pichard AD, et al. Intravascular ultrasound predictors of restenosis after percutaneous transcatheter revascularization. *J Am Coll Cardiol* 1996;27:1678–1687.

116. Mintz GS, Fitzgerald PJ, Kuntz RE, et al. Lesion site and reference segment remodeling after directional coronary atherectomy: an analysis from the Optimal Atherectomy Restenosis Study (OARS) [Abstract]. *Circulation* 1995;92(Suppl I):I-93.

117. Kimura T, Kaburagi S, Tashima Y, et al. Geometric remodeling and intimal regrowth as a mechanisms of restenosis: observations from Serial Ultrasound Analysis of Restenosis (SURE) Trial [Abstract]. *Circulation* 1995;92(Suppl I):I-76.

118. Luo H, Nishioka T, Eigler H, et al. Chronic vessel constriction is an important mechanism of restenosis after balloon angioplasty: an intravascular ultrasound analysis [Abstract]. *Circulation* 1994;90(Suppl I):I-318.

119. Post MJ, Borst C, Kuntz RE. The relative importance of arterial remodeling compared with intimal hyperplasia in lumen renarrowing after balloon angioplasty: a study in the normal rabbit and the hypercholesterolemic Yucatan micropig. *Circulation* 1994;89:2816–2821.

120. Kakuta T, Currier JW, Haudenschild CC, et al. Differences in compensatory vessel enlargement, not intimal formation, accounts for restenosis after angioplasty in the hypercholesterolemic rabbit model. *Circulation* 1994;89:2809–2815.

121. Shi Y, Pieneik M, Fard A, et al. Adventitial remodeling after coronary arterial injury. *Circulation* 1996;93:340–348.

122. Lafont A, Guzman L, Whitlow P, et al. Restenosis after experimental angioplasty: intimal, medial, and adventitial changes associated with constrictive remodeling *Circ Res* 1995;76:996–1002.

123. Tobis J, Colombo A, Almagor Y, et al. Intravascular guidance of multiple interventions does not reduce restenosis rate [Abstract]. *Circulation* 1995;92(Suppl I):I-148.

124. Painter JA, Mintz GS, Wong SC, et al. Serial intravascular ultrasound studies fail to show evidence of chronic Palmaz-Schatz stent recoil. *Am J Cardiol* 1995;75:398–400.

125. Hoffman R, Mintz GS, Pompa JJ, et al. Chronic arterial responses to stent implantation: a serial intravascular ultrasound analysis of Palmaz-Schatz stents in native coronary arteries. *J Am Coll Cardiol* 1996;28:1134–1139.

126. Mudra H, Regar E, Klauss V, et al. Serial follow-up after optimized ultrasound-guided deployment of Palmaz-Schatz stents: in-stent neointimal proliferation without significant reference segment response. *Circulation* 1997;95:363–370.

127. Isner JM, Rosenfield K, Losordo DW, et al. Combination balloon-ultrasound imaging catheter for percutaneous transluminal angioplasty: validation of imaging, analysis of recoil and identification of plaque fracture. *Circulation* 1991; 84:739–754.

128. Losordo DW, Rosenfield K, Pieczek A, et al. How does angioplasty work? Serial analysis of human iliac arteries using intravascular ultrasound. *Circulation* 1992;86:1845–1858.

129. The SHK, Gussenhoven EJ, Zhong Y, et al. Effect of balloon angioplasty on femoral artery evaluated with intravascular ultrasound imaging. *Circulation* 1992;86:483–493.

130. Katzen BT, Benenati JF, Becker GJ, et al. Role of intravascular ultrasound in peripheral atherectomy and stent deployment [Abstract]. *Circulation* 1991;84(Suppl II):II-542.

131. Navarro F, Sullivan TM, Bacharach JM. The use of intravascular ultrasound to assess peripheral vascular interventions [Abstract]. *Circulation* 1995;92(Suppl I):I-649.

132. White RA, Donayre CE, Scoccianti M, et al. Ultrasound guidance in peripheral interventions. *J Intervent Cardiol* 1994;7:84–85.

133. Parodi JC, Palmaz JC, Barone HD. Transfemoral intraluminal graft implantation for abdominal aortic aneurysms. *Ann Vasc Surg* 1991;5:491–499.

134. Chuter TAM, Green RM, Ouriel K, et al. Transfemoral endovascular aortic graft placement. *J Vasc Surg* 1993;18:185–197.

135. Cragg AH, Dake MD. Percutaneous femoro-popliteal graft placement. *J Vasc Intervent Radiol* 1993;4:455–463.

POSTSUBARACHNOID HEMORRHAGE VASOSPASM

Endovascular Therapy of Postsubarachnoid Hemorrhage Vasospasm

CHAPTER 51

J.J. Connors III / J.C. Wojak

Vasospasm after subarachnoid bleed from an aneurysm is the single most significant complication of this disease process. Of patients reaching a center that treats aneurysms, 5% to 20% subsequently die from the damage caused by vasospasm. This number has declined in recent years, mostly because of the use of nimodipine but also because of improved medical management.

Elsewhere in the body, vasospasm generally refers to either an iatrogenic temporary problem (mechanical stimulation of the vessel), a reactive protective mechanism for bleeding, or a response to local trauma. Intracranially, however, vasospasm can be a devastating complication related to subarachnoid blood arising from an aneurysmal or other rupture (e.g., arteriovenous malformation, cortical vein).

Vasospasm secondary to subarachnoid hemorrhage can be defined as either angiographic or clinical. After a subarachnoid bleed, up to 70% of individuals suffer some degree of intracranial vasospasm. This usually reaches maximum intensity from 4 to 12 days after the acute hemorrhage but still can be present as late as 3 weeks (or longer) after a bleed. Angiographic vasospasm manifests more often than clinical vasospasm. True clinical vasospasm affects only 20% to 30% of patients with subarachnoid hemorrhage. It presents as a decrease in level of consciousness, confusion, delirium, or focal neurologic deficits. Clinical vasospasm can be reversible even when the symptoms are profound.

The grading scale developed by Fisher et al.[1] describes the computed tomography (CT) findings associated with an increased chance of vasospasm. The scale is outlined in Table 51–1.

Numerous techniques have been tried over the years to alleviate the problem of postbleed intracra-

nial vasospasm, including washing away all blood in the subarachnoid space with saline at the time of surgery; applying papaverine, tissue type plasminogen activator, urokinase, or other drugs onto the intracranial vessels at the time of surgery; or using other systemic drugs, such as calcium-channel blockers and antioxidants, postoperatively. This last approach (systemic pharmacologic therapy) has begun to achieve some degree of success.[2–4] In addition, endovascular therapy (angioplasty or infusion of vasodilators) is now available for treatment of intracran-

T A B L E   5 1 - 1   The Fisher Grading System for Computed Tomographic Scan Findings in Aneurysmal Bleed

Grade/ Group	Findings on CT	Predicted Severity of Vasospasm
1	No detectable blood	No severe spasm
2	Diffuse blood not dense enough to represent a large, thick homogeneous clot	No severe spasm
3	Dense collection of blood appearing to represent a clot >1 mm thick in the vertical plane (interhemispheric fissure, insular cistern, ambient cistern) or >5 × 3 mm in longitudinal and transverse dimension in the horizontal plane (stem of the Sylvian fissure, Sylvian cistern, interpeduncular cistern)	Severe spasm
4	Intracerebral or intraventricular clots but with only diffuse blood or no blood in the basal cisterns	No severe spasm

ial vasospasm secondary to subarachnoid bleed or intracranial surgery.

The exact physiologic reason for intracranial vasospasm and the associated microendovascular changes have been studied for years, are still not absolutely clear, and are beyond the scope of this discussion. It is known, however, that subarachnoid blood is a direct stimulant for vasospasm, possibly as a protective mechanism against further intracranial hemorrhage. Reactive vasospasm can protect injured downstream parenchymal structures from full pulse pressure, a potentially appropriate adaptive mechanism for ischemically injured tissues.

An interesting observation was reported by Rosenwasser et al. at the American Society of Therapeutic and Interventional Neuroradiology/World Federation of Therapeutic and Interventional Neuroradiology Scientific Conference (New York, September 1997). They retrospectively studied 35 patients with ruptured aneurysms who were treated using Guglielmi detachable coils (GDC) and compared them with similar patients treated by open surgical procedures. Standard medical management and vasospasm prophylaxis were identical for the two groups. The patients undergoing endovascular therapy also received intravenous heparin for 48 hours and low-molecular-weight dextran for 24 hours.

All patients in the endovascularly treated group who developed neurologic deficits because of vasospasm responded to elevation of blood pressure; none required angioplasty or papaverine infusion. In the surgically treated group, seven out of nine patients who were Hunt-Hess grade III (see Chapter 24) preoperatively developed clinical vasospasm. These patients had significant elevation of the transcranial Doppler velocities and required maximum hemodilution, hypervolemia, and hypertension. Out of this group of seven, two also required active intervention (angioplasty and papaverine infusion).

Although this retrospective analysis is not a statistically powerful proof, these preliminary data suggest that endovascular treatment of aneurysms with GDC may be associated with decreased clinical and transcranial Doppler evidence of vasospasm.

EVALUATION OF INTRACRANIAL VASOSPASM

Transcranial Doppler ultrasonography is the most common means for preliminary evaluation of possible intracranial vasospasm (see Chapter 52). If vasospasm occurs postoperatively, it should first be treated by medical means, including hypertension (volume expansion and, if needed, pharmacologic support), hypervolemia (volume expansion with crystalloid and colloid solutions), and hyperventilation (if the patient is intubated) to lower intracranial pressure and thus increase perfusion. If there is no improvement in 1 to 2 hours, endovascular therapy is warranted. An angiogram is performed at this time to evaluate the status of intracranial blood flow. Any

delay after clinical symptoms have ensued decreases the likelihood of therapeutic success.

The results of vasospasm treatment are not ideal; this may be related at least partially to the delay in therapy. In many clinicians' minds, if symptoms have developed, it may already be too late. Spetzler believes that treatment of vasospasm should be proactive rather than reactive (verbal communication). We agree with this opinion. This fundamental shift in approach may open the door to more positive results but will require a change in attitude among clinicians. In addition, more aggressive therapy (mechanical angioplasty) appears to be indicated.

RADIOGRAPHIC MANIFESTATIONS

Postbleed, postoperative vasospasm manifests angiographically in three broad patterns, mostly affecting the circle of Willis vessels at the skull base, with some degree of overlap: (1) one or a few small focal areas of spasm, (2) long-segment vascular narrowing, or (3) a generalized or patchy pattern that can affect more peripheral second- and third-order branches in addition to the vessels at the skull base. Additionally, a malignant peripheral pattern of hypoperfusion can develop related to an incipient infarct and can be resistant to therapy. These patterns can develop in one or more vascular territories.

In the anterior (carotid) circulation, spasm typically begins just beyond the origin of the ophthalmic artery; in other words, where the internal carotid artery enters the subarachnoid space. There can be a tight segment in the distal internal carotid artery or additional involvement of the main trunk of the middle cerebral artery.

THERAPEUTIC OPTIONS

Two techniques are available for endovascular treatment of vasospasm: mechanical angioplasty and pharmacologic infusion (papaverine or another vasodilator). Each of these options is described with the knowledge that no controlled trials have been performed and that the strategy of therapy is still in evolution.

Clinical response to therapy appears to be related more to the rate of increase in clinical symptoms than to the degree of radiographic vasospasm; some patients with incredible spasm may be essentially intact, whereas others with only moderate vasospasm may display profound symptoms. It is important to understand that the earlier therapy is performed, the better. Rosenwasser et al. presented their experience at the American Society of Therapeutic and Interventional Neuroradiology/World Federation of Therapeutic and Interventional Neuroradiology Scientific Conference (New York, September 1997). They treated 367 patients between 1993 and 1997; 92% of these patients underwent surgery within the first 24 hours after bleeding. All patients were aggressively managed postoperatively with prophylactic hypervolemia and hypertension and were evaluated by transcranial Doppler twice daily. If a patient's neurologic condition worsened and did not respond to medical management within 60 minutes, emergency endovascular therapy was performed.

During this study, 80 patients (22%) underwent emergency treatment. In all cases, angioplasty was performed utilizing a STEALTH or Endeavor system (Target Therapeutics: described below), followed by a papaverine infusion (300 mg over 30 to 45 minutes). Low-molecular-weight dextran was given intravenously.

Analysis of their data indicated a 1- to 2-hour window in which this therapy resulted in reversal of deficit, with a sustained clinical improvement. Forty-nine patients (61%) were treated within this 2-hour period. The rest were treated between 2 and 8 hours after the onset of vasospasm. In patients treated within 2 hours, there was a 90% rate of angiographic improvement and a 70% rate of immediate and sustained clinical improvement. In patients treated between 2 and 8 hours, however, there was an 88% rate of angiographic improvement but only a 40% rate of sustained clinical improvement. In addition, asymptomatic dots of reperfusion microhemorrhage were noted on the post-therapy CT scans of patients undergoing delayed treatment. No patients developed intraparenchymal hematomas that necessitated surgical evacuation or dangerously elevated intracranial pressure. Eight patients required retreatment, all of whom were Fisher grade III or higher and had sustained transcranial Doppler velocities greater than 200 cm/sec. No procedural complications occurred. This study suggests an actual time window for optimal therapy and should act as a stimulus for rapid and aggressive intervention.

The advantages of papaverine infusion are simplicity, safety (no chance of mechanical intracranial vascular rupture), and the ability to reach small distal vessels. The disadvantages are that the treatment results may be temporary, the results are inconsistent and frequently poor (as few as 25% of patients show clinical improvement), and the procedure can be time-consuming. Papaverine has been shown to have risks; infusion has been associated with injury to the brainstem and even death. In addition, if spasm recurs, it may be resistant to further infusion.

The advantages of balloon angioplasty are that it appears to be more consistently successful; it yields rapid, dramatic results; and retreatment of a site is almost never needed (the results are satisfactory and durable).

Relative contraindications to endovascular therapy of vasospasm include a fixed neurologic deficit or the presence of a completed infarct. The definition of *fixed* can be difficult to specify, however, because patients may experience recovery from neurologic deficits of a profound and prolonged nature (hemiparesis of 10 to 48 hours' duration). Also, it may be difficult to differentiate acute edema without infarct from a completed infarct in the particular clinical circumstances. An additional note of caution is warranted with regard to any remaining unclipped aneurysms at the time of treatment; spasm proximal to an unclipped aneurysm may be present for a real reason. Also, caution is advised when angioplasty of a narrowed segment associated with an aneurysm clip is attempted. It is possible to move the clip, with unpredictable consequences.

Mechanical (Balloon) Angioplasty of Vasospasm

Rationale

For focal stenoses in a proximal location along a primary intracranial vessel, direct angioplasty yields excellent results and is a straightforward solution.[5] In addition, downstream vascular dilation may result from the increased pressure head after removal of a proximal stenosis, thus giving a more generalized result. This may be true even if there was a more generalized vasospastic pattern initially and if an attempt at papaverine infusion did not relieve the problem.

Angioplasty is the treatment of choice for experienced interventional neuroradiologists. The angiographic results are more dramatic and immediate, and the clinical results appear to be more significant. The value of angioplasty has been demonstrated by cerebral blood flow measurements as well as by single-photon emission computed tomography. The vasodilation is also permanent.

Angioplasty requires more technical skill than simple infusion. The possibility of vascular rupture or intimal tear makes this procedure more risky than papaverine infusion.

Tools

Two microcatheters are commonly used for intracranial angioplasty of vasospasm, and an additional two atherosclerotic angioplasty balloons can be used if necessary. The general consensus in the interventional neuroradiologic community is that soft silicone balloons are more appropriate for vasospasm angioplasty and that harder, less compliant balloons are more appropriate for atherosclerotic disease. This is not absolute, and soft silicone balloons are capable of generating significant dilation forces. Atherosclerotic lesions require 3 to 6 atmospheres of pressure for dilation, whereas vasospasm requires only 2 to 3 atmospheres. The soft silicone balloons will develop this much force when nearly fully inflated. The blunt Endeavor balloon tends to keep expanding longitudinally at its distal tip, whereas the Solstice cannot expand longitudinally and can develop higher radial pressures (at least 6 atmospheres).

The two soft balloons available for this purpose are the Endeavor (formerly the NDSB) from Target Therapeutics and the Solstice from Medtronic/MIS. Using the closed-ended Endeavor balloon, angioplasty for spasm in the anterior circulation is possible in the internal carotid artery, the main trunk of the middle cerebral artery (M1), and possibly one

M2 branch (Cases 1 and 2, Figs. 51–1 to 51–8). In the posterior circulation, it is possible to advance the balloon all the way up the basilar artery and then usually into one posterior cerebral artery, but not the other (Case 3, Figs. 51–9 and 51–10). Once the soft balloon has expanded one branch, it repeatedly seeks this same course. Using the guidewire-steerable Solstice, it is possible to select the anterior cerebral artery, multiple branches of the middle cerebral artery, and either of the two posterior cerebral arteries (Cases 4 and 5, Figs. 51–11 to 51–26).

Technique

Endeavor Balloon

The technique for using the Endeavor soft microballoon is relatively straightforward. The balloon–catheter system is delivered through a large-lumen guide catheter (at least 0.060″ inner diameter). Target Therapeutics provides a guide catheter for this use, but the Omniguide (Medtronic/MIS) and Envoy (Cordis Corp.) are more sophisticated guide catheters. The Cook, Inc. Lumax Neuroguide is more supportive and is our choice. The use of an 0.014″ guidewire inside the balloon catheter makes advancement of the system easier, with inflation achieved by using a rotating hemostatic valve (see Chapter 3) to seal around the wire.

The balloon first should be prepared to remove any air (see Chapter 3). A 50% to 70% contrast solution is less viscous and aids in rapid inflation and deflation. Introducing the floppy catheter into the backbleeding guide catheter can be difficult or impossible. This is best done by preplacing the balloon–catheter system into a rotating hemostatic valve (one with a large

lumen), with the balloon just at the exit. This unit is then attached to the guide catheter with no fluid flowing in the side part of the valve. The microcatheter is advanced about halfway through the guide catheter before the valve is loosened, bubbles are removed, and the flush system is turned on.

The balloon–catheter system is then advanced to the area of stenosis and *slowly* inflated. The balloon inflates in its proximal portion first and slowly pushes downstream, dilating a length of about 10 mm. It is then deflated, advanced to the end of this dilated segment, and again inflated. This process is repeated. In this stepwise fashion, it is possible to work the catheter downstream slowly, similar to the crawling of a caterpillar.

As can be discerned from this description, steering of this system is not possible. When the catheter comes to the tip of the basilar artery or the bifurcation of the internal carotid artery, it will go where it will go, and once dilation has progressed down one branch, it will seek this path repeatedly.

The Solstice System

Endovascular use of the Solstice balloon is slightly more complicated than use of the Endeavor, but it is possible to treat spasm in multiple vessels because of the ability to steer the catheter. Preparing the balloon is easier than preparing the Endeavor. The preparation of this balloon is similar to the preparation of the Stratus microangioplasty balloon (Medtronic/MIS) except that a mechanical inflator is not used; the balloon is inflated by hand, using a syringe (see Fig. 48–58).

The microcatheter is flushed with a solution of two-

Text continued on page 592

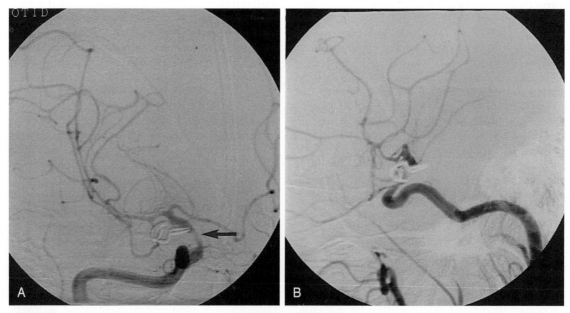

Figure 51-1 Case 1. *A,* Posteroanterior (PA) and *B,* lateral views of a right internal carotid artery (ICA) injection in a patient with typical severe postintracranial bleed, postoperative (aneurysm clipping) vasospasm. Severe narrowing of the supracavernous carotid artery and almost all intracranial vessels is seen. Note the very poor contrast density in the segment proximal to the clip, indicative of circumferential narrowing *(arrow).*

Case 1 continues

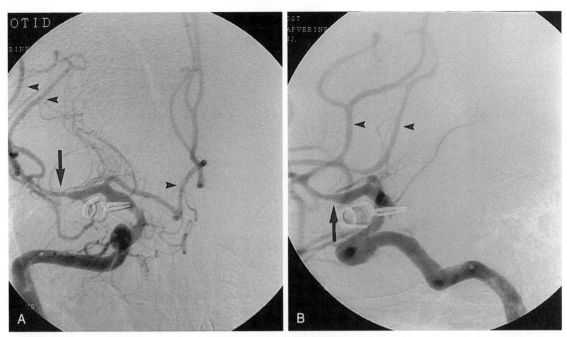

Figure 51-2 *A,* PA and *B,* lateral views after an Endeavor (Target Therapeutics) silicone balloon (4 × 10 mm) was used to dilate the proximal vasospastic segment. The supracavernous carotid and proximal middle cerebral artery (MCA) main trunk are now nearly normal. Note the abrupt transition from the angioplastied section to the vasospastic portion in the M1 segment *(arrows).* Note also that the peripheral branches appear to be larger after the angioplasty *(arrowheads).* This is commonly seen when there is severe vasospasm involving the carotid artery itself, thus decreasing the pressure head to the intracranial vessels; the pressure head is increased after the angioplasty.

There is now also the suggestion of a density at the base of the clip on the lateral view. Did the clip actually move secondary to the balloon distention, exposing some of the aneurysm neck?

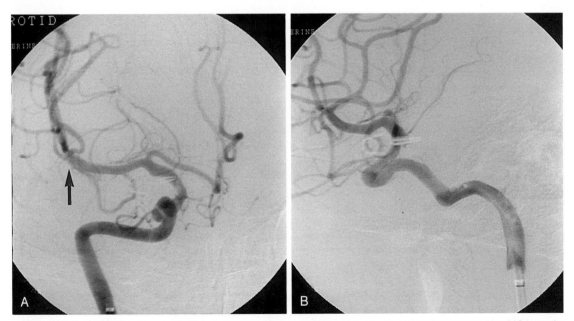

Figure 51-3 *A* and *B,* Final angiographic appearance after the balloon was advanced further into the MCA, to the trifurcation region *(arrow).* In addition, 300 mg papaverine was infused over 30 minutes after this process, with this result. The distal distention of the vascular tree is probably due to the combination of these two factors: chemical relaxation and an increase in the pressure head secondary to dilation of the ICA.

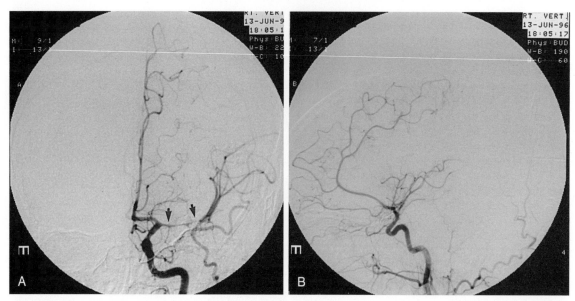

Figure 51-4 Case 2. This woman had experienced subarachnoid hemorrhage, with severe increase in transcranial Doppler velocities after surgery for an MCA aneurysm. During that time, she had no clinical symptoms. Therefore, intravascular therapy was not requested.

Two weeks later, she was admitted with variable dysphasia (mostly word-finding difficulty). PA *(A)* and lateral *(B)* left carotid angiograms reveal *severe* spasm of the main (M1) segment of the MCA and the proximal portion of the M2 divisions *(arrows)*. Note the delayed filling of the distribution of the MCA territory compared with the anterior cerebral artery territory. This is clear evidence of a hemodynamic alteration secondary to the MCA stenosis, even without clinical sequelae (which have finally manifested themselves in this situation).

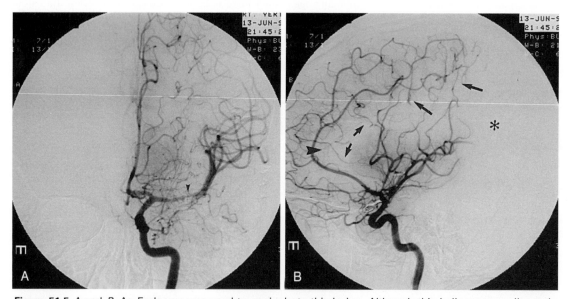

Figure 51-5 *A* and *B*, An Endeavor was used to angioplasty this lesion. Although this balloon generally works very well, this particular stenosis had become fixed owing to its age and was therefore very resistant to simple stretching. The soft silicone balloon was suboptimal for this procedure, and it was very difficult to even advance the balloon into the narrowed origin of the MCA or to dilate particular sections of the vessel. Rather, it would squeeze through focal stenosis and form a "sausage," without distending the stenotic section. The result was an uneven dilation.

The upper division of the MCA *(small arrowhead)* was not dilated because of the presence of the aneurysm clip and a doubt concerning its location and security. The neurosurgeon thought that some of the aneurysm neck could have been left unclipped. This resulted in the angiographic pattern seen here. There is now some increased perfusion of the midportion of the MCA territory. Note that the posterior angular region (Wernicke's area) *(asterisk)* is still not perfusing well from the MCA, nor the lateral midfrontal lobe (Broca's area) *(large arrowhead)* from this ICA injection. Note also the retrograde filling of the superior division territory by branches *(arrows)*. The patient, however, had improved neurologically at this point (while still on the angiogram table), and the procedure was considered to have achieved a maximal benefit versus risk ratio. The patient was returned to her room, the plan being to re-examine her the following day.

Case 2 continues

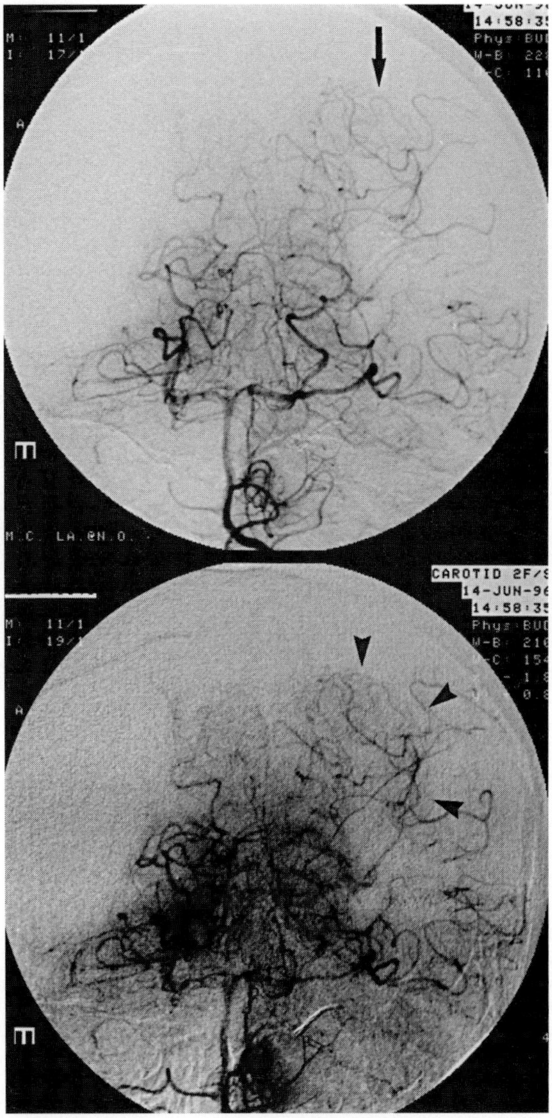

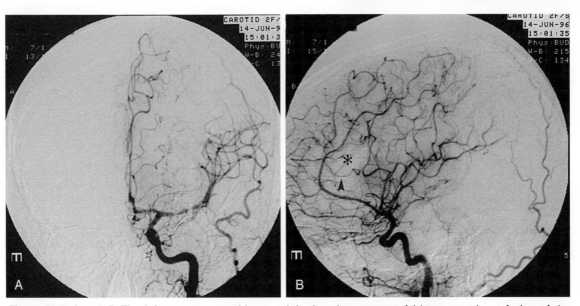

Figure 51-6 The following day, the vertebral artery injection still reveals some perfusion of the MCA territory via pial collaterals *(arrow)*. Note the blush in Wernicke's area on this "blush-o-gram" image *(arrowheads)*. This indicated suboptimal flow through the MCA; this would not otherwise occur. The patient's excellent pial collaterals, however, have prevented her from being more symptomatic all along.

Figure 51-7 *A* and *B*, The left common carotid artery injection demonstrates fairly symmetric perfusion of the hemisphere with the anterior cerebral and middle cerebral arteries flowing at approximately the same speed, although the volume of flow and pressure head in the MCA are probably still diminished. The overall hemisphere is supplied fairly well with the exception of the posterior angular region, as previously described, and Broca's area in the lateral midfrontal lobe *(asterisk)*. Note the retrograde flow in the same anterior MCA branch *(arrowhead)*. The symptoms had again resolved and the patient was clinically intact.

Case 2 continues

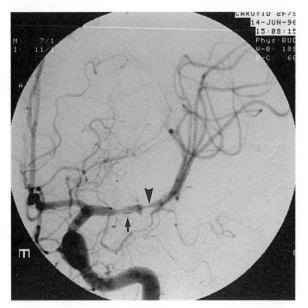

Figure 51-8 Magnified view showing the postprocedure appearance of the MCA. A less than ideal angioplasty result is seen, with a possible residual nub of aneurysm at the bifurcation of the MCA (previously seen but thought to possibly be the origin of the inferior division of the MCA). Note the residual stenosis in the upper division *(arrowhead)*. Note also the intimal tear in the inferior portion of the MCA *(arrow)*, a relatively unusual appearance for vasospasm angioplasty using the very slow and gentle technique previously advocated. This technique was not possible with the silicone balloon catheter being used (the Endeavor), as described earlier.

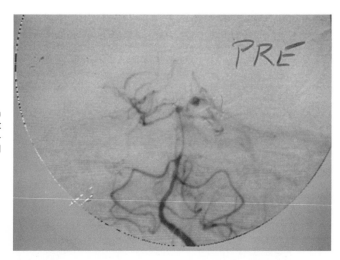

Figure 51-9 Case 3. Initial evaluation of the posterior circulation in a patient after clipping of an aneurysm reveals extremely tight basilar artery and downstream vessel spasm (both superior cerebellar arteries and posterior cerebral arteries). Note the opacified round object in the left posterior cerebral artery territory.

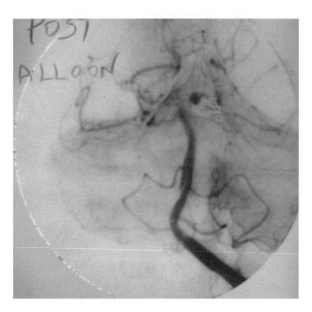

Figure 51-10 Left vertebral angiogram after angioplasty with an Endeavor. The balloon was advanced only up to the basilar tip, but notice the tremendous increase in flow to the posterior fossa. The right posterior cerebral artery also fills better, but the left does not. This is due to (1) the inability of the Endeavor to select individual vessels and (2) the fact that this vessel (the left posterior cerebral artery) was in spasm for a reason, to protect *the residual aneurysm*, which is now seen very well.

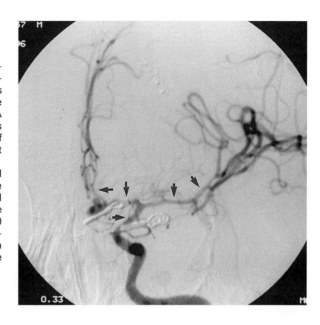

Figure 51-11 Case 4. A 38-year-old man with a ruptured anterior communicating artery aneurysm and an additional posterior communicating artery aneurysm. Both were clipped without difficulty. Six days after the original bleed, he became poorly rousable and plegic on the right side. Angiography reveals moderate vasospasm in the distal ICA with moderately severe spasm of the MCA and proximal branches, as well as the A1 and A2 segments *(arrows)*. There is the suggestion of residual filling of the anterior communicating artery aneurysm, but some of this could be nonspastic normal vessel.

Angioplasty typically has more permanency than papaverine as well as a greater degree of benefit, and should be used as the initial mode of therapy in most cases. In this particular case, it was not initially used because of the degree of vasospasm in peripheral vessels and the involvement of multiple territories. Papaverine was infused locally (300 mg in 100 ml normal saline over 45 minutes) in preparation for angioplasty of the M1 segment. This infusion was somewhat slower than usual owing to the severe cardiac response to the infusion (the pulse rate increased to over 170).

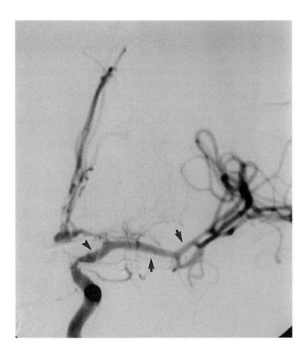

Figure 51-12 After the infusion, the angiogram reveals some improvement in the appearance of all the vessels, but not as impressive as desired. Note the generalized pattern of improvement in caliber of the distal ICA *(arrowhead)* and M1 and M2 segments *(arrows)*. While A1 is still tight, A2 is somewhat improved. Although there is some improvement after the papaverine infusion, angioplasty can still be of additional benefit to a territory of critical significance, such as the MCA.

The Solstice balloon catheter (Medtronic/MIS) can be placed through an Envoy catheter (Cordis Corp.) with relative ease, but this guide catheter is too flexible in its proximal portion to offer enough support for distal positioning of the Solstice without the risk of the guide catheter recoiling downward into the aorta. For this reason, placement of the Solstice through a stiffer guide catheter such as a Brite-Tip (Cordis Corp.) or Lumax Neuroguide (Cook, Inc.) is probably advisable, although the tips of these catheters are far too stiff and traumatic for routine use in the carotid and vertebral arteries.

Figure 51-13 Inflated Solstice balloon catheter in place in the main trunk of the MCA *(arrow)*. This system allows the guidewire to double as the catheter occluder, and is capable of functioning with a variable amount of wire extending out of the catheter. The soft silicone balloon is inflatable to approximately 3.5 to 4.0 mm, similar to that of the Endeavor. The guidewire capability of this catheter renders it steerable, however: a significant benefit. As can be seen in this slightly oblique projection, the guidewire has entered the lower branch of the bifurcation *(arrowhead)*, while the balloon is near the distal end of the M1 segment of the MCA. The distal ICA was also dilated.

Case 4 continues

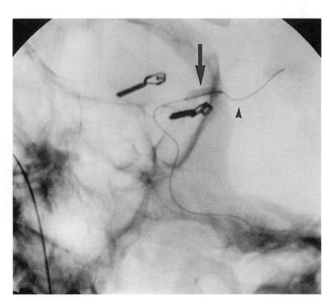

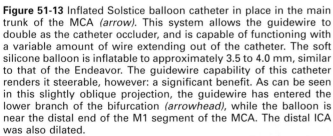

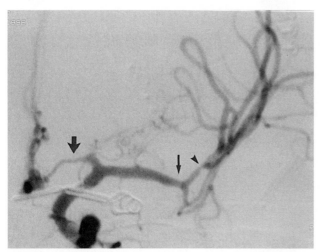

Figure 51-14 The postangioplasty result 3 days later. The angiogram was repeated owing to an abrupt deterioration in the patient's condition; he suddenly became weak on the right side and mute. Note the tapered appearance of the distal M1 segment where the original angioplasty was suboptimal *(thin arrow)*. Note also the severe stenosis in the superior division of the MCA *(arrowhead)*. This was thought to be the origin of the recurrent symptoms.

Note the severe residual or recurrent stenosis of the A1 segment *(fat arrow)*. Not only does this potentially affect the anterior cerebral artery territory, it prevents this vessel from supplying collateral perfusion to the distal territory of the MCA.

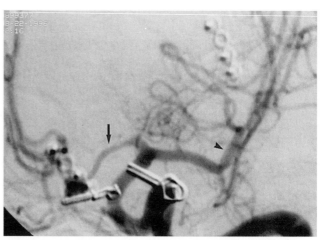

Figure 51-15 Using the ability to steer the Solstice balloon, it was possible to select the superior division of the MCA and angioplasty this branch *(arrowhead)*. Care was taken not to overinflate the balloon while it was in this branch, in view of the intrinsically small size of this vessel. Note the now uniform optimal size of the entire MCA as well as the superior division.

After the repeat angioplasty of the MCA, it was necessary to try to improve the anterior cerebral artery flow, but we were unable to advance the catheter around the bend at the bifurcation of the ICA into the anterior cerebral artery without buckling the Envoy back into the aorta. Therefore, papaverine was reinfused selectively into this vessel with satisfactory results *(arrow)*. The patient again recovered completely, almost immediately, and remained neurologically intact.

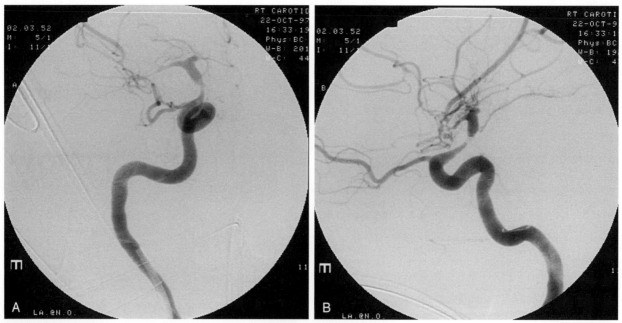

Figure 51-16 Case 5. PA *(A)* and lateral *(B)* right carotid angiograms reveal severe vasospasm of the distal ICA, the anterior cerebral artery, and the MCA. Note the threadlike appearance of the supracavernous ICA. This ICA cannot supply enough blood to the hemisphere to keep it alive.

Case 5 continues

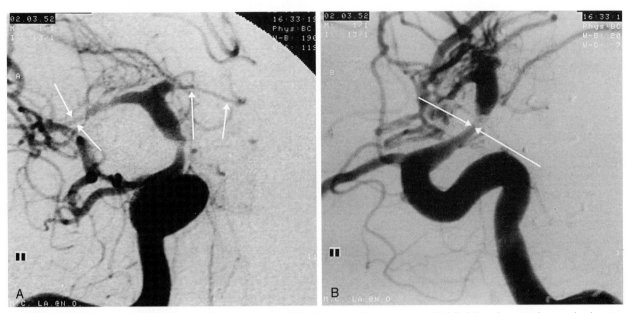

Figure 51-17 PA *(A)* and lateral *(B)* magnification views of the intracranial vasospasm, highlighting the anterior cerebral artery vasospasm and the threadlike ICA *(arrows).*

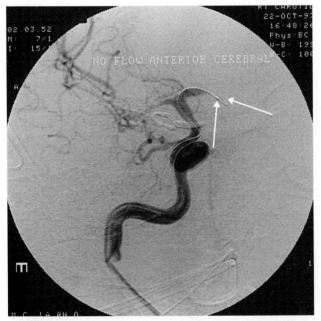

Figure 51-18 Flow is temporarily occluded by the Quicksilver wire and Solstice balloon *(arrows)* during selective dilation of the anterior cerebral artery. This is of no real consequence because this vascular territory has had essentially no flow for a prolonged period before this procedure. However, angioplasty of this vessel is mandatory and possible only with the Solstice system.

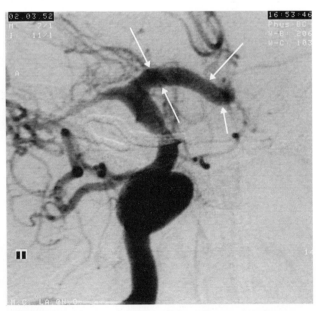

Figure 51-19 After angioplasty of the A1 segment, the appearance of the vessel is excellent *(arrows).*

Case 5 continues

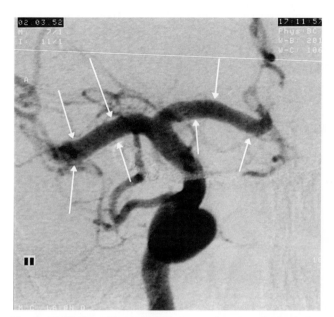

Figure 51-20 The M1 segment has now been angioplastied as well, resulting in a dramatic change in the appearance of and flow in these vessels *(arrows)*.

thirds contrast solution and one-third normal saline (the contrast is seen more readily than if a "half-and-half" solution is used). A Y connector is placed on the hub of the balloon catheter; a 3- or 6-foot microtubing extension set is connected to this; and a 20-cc syringe filled with the two-thirds contrast solution is connected to the tubing. An uncurved Quicksilver-10 wire (Medtronic/MIS) is advanced through the Y connector into the balloon catheter until its tip is about 5 cm from the distal end. The 20-cc syringe is used to flush all bubbles out of the Y connector, and the valve is tightened about the wire. The Y connector is then held *with the catheter end up* (to facilitate exit of bubbles through the catheter) and is "thumped" vigorously while additional contrast mixture (about 5 ml) is instilled and allowed to drip out the end of the catheter.

One or two minutes should be allowed for the fluid to exit the tip of the catheter; it takes time for the intracatheter pressure to equalize. If this delay is not allowed, the balloon will inflate slightly on its own once the wire is advanced out the end of the catheter.

Once pressure equalization has occurred, it is possible to advance the wire out the tip of the catheter and then to place a curve on it. At this point, the 20-cc syringe is exchanged for a 1-cc syringe filled with the two-thirds contrast solution. Because this balloon is *not* pressure-dependent but rather *volume-dependent*, very accurate control of volume during angioplasty is mandatory. *This can be best performed by using a 1-cc syringe.*

The occlusion guidewire should then be withdrawn back inside the microcatheter so that the tip of the wire is just within the tip of the catheter; this allows the catheter to be placed through the Y connector and the entire unit to be loaded into the guide catheter in the standard fashion. The wire is *never* withdrawn back past the O-ring valve of the Solstice (just proximal to the balloon), particularly when the catheter is in the vascular tree (this allows blood to enter the balloon, making it invisible).

Once the catheter assembly is loaded into the guide catheter, the guidewire tip is advanced 3 to 5 cm to allow downstream advancement of the angioplasty

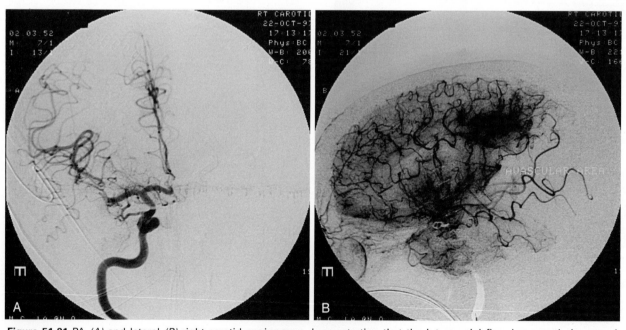

Figure 51-21 PA *(A)* and lateral *(B)* right carotid angiograms demonstrating that the intracranial flow has greatly increased, along with the supply to the opposite anterior cerebral artery distribution (seen on the PA view), but perhaps not enough to supply adequate flow to this vascular distribution if this vessel is the only supply. Note on the lateral view that there is a large avascular area in the territory of the angular branch of the MCA—a typical location for hypoperfusion defects.

Case 5 continues

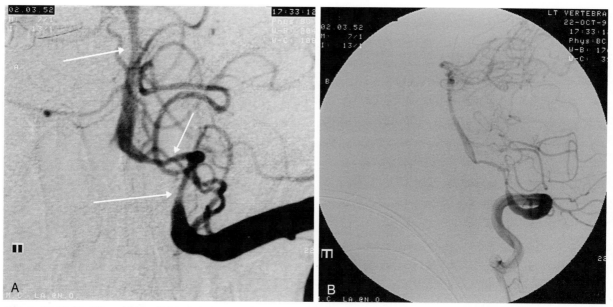

Figure 51-22 PA *(A)* and lateral *(B)* views of a left vertebral artery injection. Note the severe vasospasm of the vertebral and basilar arteries *(arrows)*.

balloon system. This catheter quickly slides into position; the guidewire will allow selection of difficult vessels, such as the anterior cerebral artery, if it is necessary to treat vasospasm in such a location.

Other Options

Use of a FasSTEALTH or Stratus angioplasty balloon catheter also may allow selection of the P1 segment of the posterior cerebral artery, the anterior cerebral artery, or specific M2 branches that the soft Endeavor balloon does not normally select. Care should be used because of the stiffness of these balloons and consequent possible vascular damage, but if care is taken,

these balloons can be used successfully for the treatment of vasospasm. If the vasospasm has persisted for several days, the vessel may be resistant to both papaverine and soft balloons, and the FasSTEALTH or Stratus may be successful when all else fails.

Another new soft (silicone) balloon microcatheter is available: the Grapevine (Medtronic/MIS), a dual-lumen balloon microcatheter that allows wire guidance. It is not as soft as the Solstice but is useful in

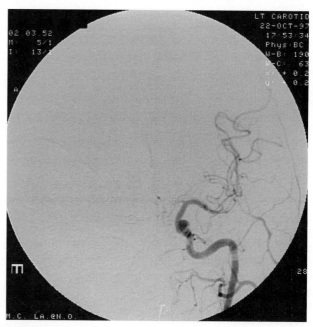

Figure 51-24 PA view of a left carotid artery injection after preliminary angioplasty demonstrates modest improvement in the ICA and MCA compared with the pretreatment images. The perfusion of the MCA territory is still poor, but the anterior cerebral territory is perfused even more poorly. *It is supplied by the previously angioplastied opposite A1 segment* (see Fig. 51-19).

Figure 51-23 After angioplaty with the Solstice balloon, these vessels appear satisfactory. Each posterior cerebral artery can be treated individually, if desired.

Case 5 continues

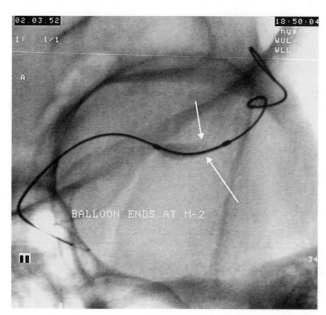

Figure 51-25 Magnified image demonstrating the use of the Solstice balloon. Note that the balloon is filled only to the point at which the vessel *intrinsically* becomes smaller. It is extremely difficult to manually obtain this degree of finesse because the total volume of the balloon is only 0.1 ml and the volume instilled at the time of this image was only about 0.05 ml. If the balloon is overinflated, it may rupture or damage the distal, smaller portion of the vessel.

proximal locations and the double-lumen design is easier to use than the single-lumen design of the Solstice.

Potential Complications, Problems, and Solutions

Care also should be taken when using these balloons in the secondary branches of any of the intracranial vessels because of their intrinsically small size. Rarely do normal M2, A2, or P2 branches exceed 2 mm; they usually do not exceed even 1.5 mm. Most of the soft balloons available expand to 4 mm, with serious potential consequences.

Even with the soft silicone balloons, inflating the balloon too rapidly can produce intimal dissection with resultant possible occlusion, just as with atherosclerotic angioplasty. *Very slow inflation,* allowing the vessel to slowly stretch, is safer.

Inadvertent aspiration of blood into the tip of a guidewire-detectable balloon catheter can result in inability to see the balloon during inflation; this may result in inadvertent overinflation. The lumen of the catheter and balloon should always be filled with contrast. As noted previously, the wire should *never* be drawn back into the microcatheter, as this can allow blood to enter the system. If there is any question, the balloon catheter should be withdrawn and prepared again.

The occlusion wire can be spearlike if not enough length is advanced to allow the wire to be soft when it protrudes past the tip of the balloon. At least 1 cm of wire should be exposed beyond the catheter tip. By far the safest occluding wire is that of the Solstice,

which is very soft and can be advanced far distal to the balloon (up to 9 cm if necessary).

Results

The limited data available indicate that rapid, aggressive treatment of vasospasm with balloon angioplasty can satisfactorily treat this condition. Angioplasty for treatment of intracranial vasospasm is essentially completely effective (angiographically) and permanent (with extremely rare exceptions). Cases 1 to 5, Figures 51–1 to 51–26, illustrate the results that can be achieved.

It is important to remember that it may not be possible to effectively treat all affected arteries by mechanical angioplasty if there is distal spasm. In the hands of a trained operator, it should be possible to treat the proximal portions of the vessels arising from the circle of Willis as well as some more distal branches.

More importantly, as in the case of acute stroke therapy, time is brain. Effective treatment of vasospasm is an emergency procedure; the patient is essentially in the process of suffering a stroke. Not only is delaying treatment (e.g., until the next morning) unacceptable, but delaying accurate and timely diagnosis can render subsequent therapy of any type (medical or interventional) ineffective.

Chemical Angioplasty (Papaverine Infusion)

Papaverine is a member of the benzylisquinline group of alkaloids. It has potent, nonspecific smooth muscle relaxant ability and has been shown to increase regional blood flow in humans, whether given intravenously or intra-arterially.[6] Its half-life is ques-

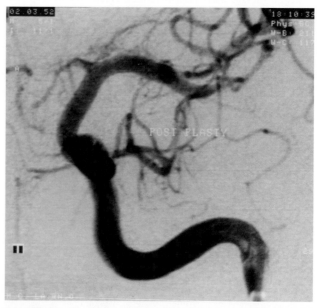

Figure 51-26 After angioplasty of the M1 segment, the vessel is dilated optimally but the distal branches are still very narrow; the use of papaverine may help in this situation. Note that A1 is still extremely narrow. Note also the abrupt transition at the point where balloon angioplasty ended.

tionable and appears to be longer than the stated average blood half-life of 45 to 60 minutes; possibly as long as 24 hours.[7] It is supplied as a 3.0% solution with a pH of 3.3 either with (Eli Lilly and Co.) or without (Frosst, Kiriland, Quebec, Canada) a preservative (chlorobutanol). It is incompatible with ioxaglate meglumine (Hexabrix).

Any of the previously mentioned angiographic patterns of vasospasm can be treated by means of intracranial infusion of papaverine, with variable results (Cases 6 to 8, Figs. 51–27 to 51–32). Although small series of patients have shown benefit,[8–10] there has been no large controlled series that verifies the efficacy of intra-arterial papaverine infusion for treatment of postsubarachnoid hemorrhage vasospasm. (The variability in severity of symptoms, combined with the delays in therapy, is a major cause of the variability of response.)

Rationale of Therapy

The indications for therapy are the same for papaverine as for angioplasty. It is important to treat vasospasm as soon as possible for two reasons: vascular response is better, and permanent ischemic damage is minimized. If there is true downstream parenchymal damage, even if there is good response to infusion, spasm recurs shortly after the infusion has ceased and can be even worse than before treatment, extending on occasion down to the extracranial (cervical) internal carotid artery and even down to the region of the carotid bifurcation. This appears to be a true protective mechanism, rather than a pathologic vascular behavior (i.e., the brain is trying to prevent normal pressure from reaching the damaged territories).

If there is a single, focal, high-grade stenosis in a location reachable by a soft vasospasm angioplasty balloon, this procedure offers a quick and relatively safe solution and should be employed first. If the spasm is more diffuse or more peripheral, infusion of intra-arterial papaverine can be performed before an attempt at angioplasty is made. This is a judgment call. Mechanical angioplasty can increase the pressure head to these areas, with subsequent "inflation" of these branch vessels and is also effective in this situation.

Technique

Use of papaverine requires intracranial catheterization with a microcatheter. Three hundred milligrams of papaverine is mixed with 100 ml of normal saline; this is then infused directly through the microcatheter into the target area over a period of 1 hour. The rate of infusion has been increased to 200 to 300 ml/hr by some operators; although this would amount to 600 to 800 mg of papaverine if infused for 1 hour, the dose is usually kept down, and the infusion is performed faster.[11] Infusion of the ophthalmic artery should be avoided because of the reported incidence of eye or retinal infarction; infusion should be at least supraophthalmic. If infusion is intended for the distal internal carotid artery, steaming a curve on the end of the catheter is beneficial; otherwise, it is difficult to get the catheter tip to sit just past the ophthalmic artery without popping back into the cavernous segment or jumping into the middle cerebral artery or posterior communicating artery. The catheter also tends to pop back directly into the ophthalmic origin, so periodically checking it during the infusion is wise. Care must be taken in certain

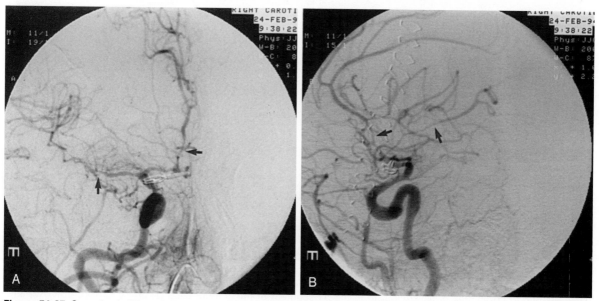

Figure 51-27 Case 6. *A*, PA and *B*, lateral right carotid angiograms obtained after aneurysm clipping, demonstrating severe diffuse vasospasm in both anterior and middle cerebral artery distributions. The pattern is diffuse, peripheral, and in more than one territory *(arrows)*; thus, mechanical angioplasty would probably be less than ideal. Papaverine infusion was performed.

Case 6 continues

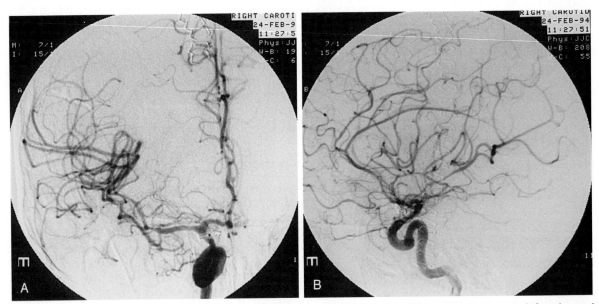

Figure 51-28 *A,* PA and *B,* lateral right carotid angiograms were performed after 300 mg papaverine was infused over 1 hour. Note the greatly increased perfusion of both territories and significant increase in size of even the distal branches. Branches of the MCA that were hardly visible at all are now well perfused. After infusion, continued observation for the next 30 minutes is indicated, since spasm can recur and additional infusion or angioplasty may be indicated (see text).

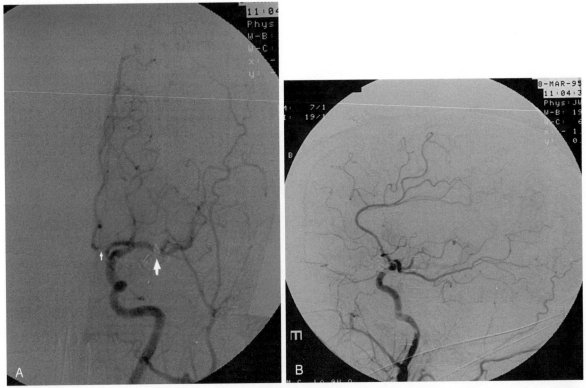

Figure 51-29 Case 7. *A,* PA and *B,* lateral left carotid angiograms performed the day after a patient began doing poorly following clipping of an aneurysm. Note the moderately severe, generalized poor perfusion of the intracranial vessels. This was due to (1) an area of severe spasm in the A1 segment of the anterior cerebral artery *(small arrow)*; (2) an area of narrowing at the level of the clip, poorly seen on these views *(large arrow)*; and (3) no sign of the upper division of the MCA.

Case 7 continues

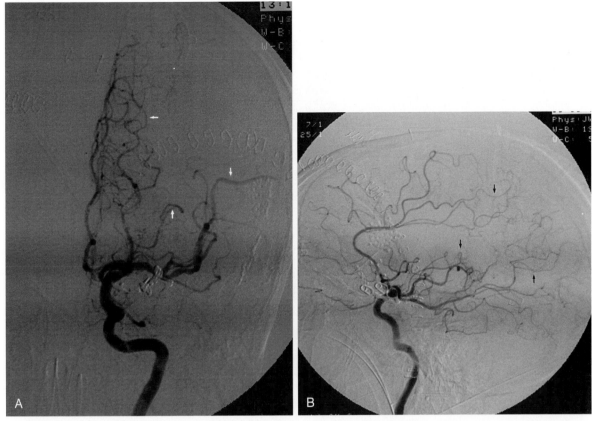

Figure 51-30 *A* and *B*, After infusion of 300 mg papaverine over 1 hour, the results are less than spectacular, but there is slight improvement. Note that the caliber of the distal vessels has improved *(arrows)*.

The patient's clinical response, however, was suboptimal. This was thought to be due to (1) the long delay in institution of therapy (the time is noon on the day after the patient's deterioration started—not infrequently, such deterioration begins in the middle of the night) and (2) the fact that a significant portion of the symptoms are due to the occlusion of a branch of the MCA.

circumstances to avoid allowing all the flow to enter the posterior communicating artery; a slow injection of contrast will reveal any streaming into this vessel.

Strategic Considerations

The choice of infusion location is important. Occasionally, spasm is located in peripheral branches of the anterior and middle cerebral arteries, and it may be necessary to infuse all of the territory supplied by the internal carotid artery, depending on the clinical symptoms. In addition, the dose may need to be divided between territories. For instance, diffuse vasospasm may be present in the territory of one internal carotid artery (or both), but spasm of the A1 segment on the side most affected may divert most of the flow from that internal carotid artery to its middle cerebral distribution. If peripheral spasm of the anterior cerebral artery on this side requires treatment, it is sometimes possible or necessary to infuse the opposite (contralateral) internal carotid artery or anterior cerebral artery because the anterior communicating artery may supply the affected side better than the ipsilateral vasospastic A1 segment. This strategy is similar to that used for treatment with fibrinolytics in the periphery in certain circum-

stances (i.e., hemodynamics can be used to help deliver the drug to the target area in the most efficient manner).

Care should be taken to use this drug wisely. There can be more than one cause of slow flow in an intracranial vessel; one is spasm of arteries or arterioles, but another, potentially important cause is lack of a downstream capillary bed to accept this flow. This can be due to an evolving infarct in the brain parenchyma. The angiographic appearance of an infarct is that of an adequate-sized vessel with flow slower than normal and associated with a poor capillary blush, or with flow slower than that of a nearby companion vessel of similar size (a vessel supplying an area of infarct is relatively large but distinctly slower in flow). With high-quality digital subtraction equipment, the lack of parenchymal blush (in the capillary phase) is evident if the fluoroscopic monitor controls are adjusted to accentuate the contrast (use of a narrow window). A vasospastic vessel supplying viable brain, although small and carrying less blood than is normal or necessary, still flows rapidly. The capillary bed may be normal or even show a stain from the attempts by the distal vasculature to increase its perfusion (a hyperemic response). Although we have not had a patient develop hemorrhagic con-

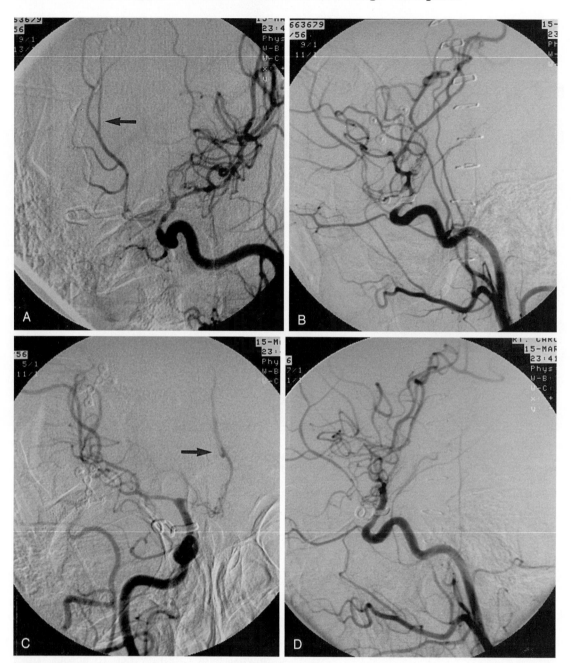

Figure 51-31 Case 8. PA and lateral views of the left (*A* and *B*) and right (*C* and *D*) ICA. These angiograms were obtained when the patient's neurologic status began to deteriorate after subarachnoid hemorrhage and subsequent craniotomy and aneurysm clipping. Severe vasospasm is identified in all territories, but worst in the anterior cerebral arteries. Note the clip in the region of the posterior communicating artery on the right. The ICA spasm is worse on the left; note the classic beginning of this spasm at the entry into the subarachnoid space (just at the ophthalmic artery).

Note also that the MCA branches have filled to a more peripheral point well ahead of either anterior cerebral artery *(arrows)*. Neither of these vessels (the anterior cerebral arteries) can help the other through the anterior communicating artery (if present) because of their own desperate situation.

Note also the very poor filling of the lenticulostriate arteries on both sides.

The strategy for treatment of this situation could be aimed at correction of the ICA on the left by angioplasty, but the anterior cerebral artery would not be easily treated by mechanical means in view of its origin and size.

Case 8 continues

version of ischemic brain after papaverine infusion, this is a concern.

Side Effects of Papaverine

The response to papaverine infusion is variable and unpredictable. Although some patients reportedly have demonstrated improved clinical status on the angiogram table, this has not been our observation. Instead, after maximal therapeutic response has been achieved, continued medical therapy generally leads to slow clinical improvement, if it is to occur at all.

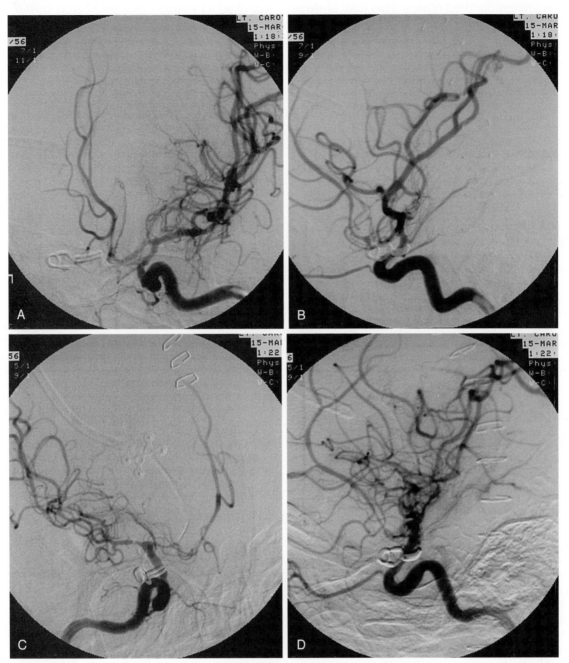

Figure 51-32 *A* to *D*, After infusion of a divided dose of papaverine (150 mg per side), there is significantly improved flow, particularly in the MCA territory bilaterally. The left MCA is now nearly normal.

In addition, note the appearance of vessels that were not even seen before (e.g., the frontopolar branch on the left). The recurrent artery of Heubner, barely visible previously, is now well seen bilaterally. The posterior communicating artery and anterior choroidal arteries are now well seen on the left (the posterior communicating arteries were not seen at all previously).

Note, however, the less than optimal response on the side of surgery, the right. This could be due to true downstream tissue damage with resultant appropriate protection by the cerebral vasculature (spasm), a more intense insult from the bleed to begin with, a more intense insult from the surgery, or an inadequate dose of papaverine. If we were to treat this patient today, we would reinfuse this right side with an additional 300 mg in the hope of obtaining a better response and angioplasty any vessels we could reach.

A reason why this patient responded better than some could be related to the time of treatment: in the middle of the night, soon after symptoms appeared, not the next day when it would possibly have been too late. It would have been very difficult to treat the anterior cerebral arteries on either side in this patient with the standard angioplasty balloons available at the time. The Solstice guidewire-directable balloon is of use in these situations.

In addition, certain territories may respond more promptly or profoundly than others. This may be due to laminar flow distribution of the drug, or, more likely, to a better or worse preexisting condition. In addition, the response may be transient, as described previously. If the spasm is resistant or response is transient, a repeat infusion can be performed with the caveat that papaverine can have profound cardiovascular systemic effects and may not help the intracranial situation. Close physiologic monitoring by the appropriate personnel is indicated at all times during a case such as this. There have been cases in which the infusion appeared to worsen the condition and at least one case occurred in which there appeared to be embolic consequences. Potential damage from the pH of the papaverine has been suggested, as has the precipitation of papaverine out of solution in certain circumstances (discussed later).

When infusion is performed proximal to the ophthalmic artery, mydriasis commonly occurs. This does not imply intracranial herniation. In slow-flow vasculature, such as the ophthalmic artery, papaverine precipitation may also occur (as described later). This may cause microvascular embolization with unknown consequences (thought to be minimal, if any). Damage to the eye has been reported, however. It is for this reason that the catheter tip should be beyond the ophthalmic artery during infusion.

Infusion of the posterior circulation may result in unpredictable results and may be more dangerous, resulting in respiratory arrest or cardiac dysfunction. Transient worsening of the patient's clinical condition may occur. Brainstem infarction has been reported, presumably from crystal deposition (microemboli), but this is not proved.

Pitfalls of Papaverine Pharmacokinetics

Papaverine has been noted to form crystalline precipitates when mixed with human blood at 3.0% or 0.3% concentrations. Additionally, when a 3.0% solution is mixed with a heparinized saline solution, a precipitate can form. As mentioned previously, it is incompatible with Hexabrix. The solution used for intracranial intra-arterial administration of papaverine is a 0.3% solution; it should therefore be administered slowly and with caution.

This instability is related to concentration density. The precipitate formed is spicules of 30 to 100 microns. These could be a significant cause of microemboli during administration. The concentration of papaverine in saline *should not be increased* to more than 300 mg/100 ml (0.3%). This concentration may be too high and, in conditions of stagnant blood flow, perhaps should be decreased. Precipitate forms when the infusion volume equals the quantity of serum (a rarity).[12]

In addition, symptoms similar to those associated with transient ischemic episodes have occurred that may be related to crystal precipitation or the direct action of papaverine or chlorobutanol. These are almost uniformly transient. Permanent neurologic deficit has been reported, however. Whether this was a sequela of the vasospasm or an additional insult secondary to therapy has not been determined.

Papaverine infusion has also been associated with systemic side effects, such as nausea, diaphoresis, hypotension, and tachycardia.

If papaverine appears to work better in some vascular territories than in others, it may be for a reason. When true parenchymal damage is present, these particular vessels may be serving a purpose by remaining vasospastic. In addition, vasospasm has been seen to persist in a particular territory when the incorrect aneurysm has been clipped and the one that actually bled is still present.

Even though it appears that the use of papaverine is not as beneficial as direct angioplasty, this agent remains a useful part of the vasospasm treatment armamentarium, particularly when used in conjunction with angioplasty.

Other Agents

Alprostadil

Early experience with the use of an entirely new agent, alprostadil (prostaglandin E1), has been reported. This drug may be of value in the treatment of vasospasm, but no large series is available to assess its effectiveness. Indeed, no widespread use of this agent has been attempted, but the drug has intriguing qualities and has been used for this purpose. Alprostadil is mentioned here because of its potential usefulness and the fact that papaverine may not be the ideal agent. It is currently used to maintain patency of the ductus arteriosus in newborns. This drug is discussed further in Chapter 4.

Nimodipine

Early reports have been made of the use of intra-arterial nimodipine, mostly in Japan. It is not readily available in the United States in injectable intra-arterial form. Verbal anecdotal reports indicate that this drug does not work as well as papaverine, even though it appears to have a more long-lasting effect.

Nitroglycerin

We have used intra-arterial nitroglycerin with some success. It has not been shown which is more effective, papaverine or nitroglycerin. A solution of 50 µg/ml in normal saline is prepared and then infused as a slow drip; systemic hypotension is an end point, and systemic effects should be observed for. The vasodilatory response to nitroglycerin may be more transient than to papaverine, but it has worked well on occasion.

REFERENCES

1. Fisher CM, Kistler JP, Davis JM. Relation of cerebral vasospasm to subarachnoid hemorrhage visualized by computerized tomographic scanning. *Neurosurgery* 1980;6:1–9.
2. Mee E, Dorrance D, Lowe D, Neil-Dwyer G. Controlled study of nimodipine in aneurysm patients treated early after subarachnoid hemorrhage. *Neurosurgery* 1988;22:484–491.
3. Allen GS, Ahn HS, Prezoisi TJ, et al. Cerebral arterial spasm:

a controlled trial of nimodipine in patients with subarachnoid hemorrhage. *N Engl J Med* 1983; 308:619–624.

4. Zuccarello M, Marsch JT, Schmitt G, et al. Effect of the 21-aminosteroid U-74006F on cerebral vasospasm following subarachnoid hemorrhage. *J Neurosurg* 1989;71:98–104.

5. Eskridge JM, Hartling RP. Angioplasty of vasospasm [Abstract]. *AJNR* 1989;10:877.

6. McHenry LC, Stump DA, Howard G, et al. Comparison of the effects of intravenous papaverine hydrochloride and oral Pavabid HP capsules on regional cerebral blood flow in normal individuals. *J Cereb Blood Flow Metab* 1983;3:442–447.

7. Cook P, James I. Cerebral vasodilators. *N Engl J Med* 1981;305:1508–1513.

8. Kassell NF, Helm G, Simmons N, et al. Treatment of cerebral vasospasm with intra-arterial papaverine. *J Neurosurg* 1992;77:848–852.

9. Kaku Y, Yonekawa Y, Tsukahara T, Kazekawa K. Superselective intra-arterial infusion of papaverine for treatment of cerebral vasospasm after subarachnoid hemorrhage. *J Neurosurg* 1992;77:842–847.

10. Clouston JE, Numaguchi Y, Zoarski GH, et al. Intraarterial papaverine infusion for cerebral vasospasm after subarachnoid hemorrhage. *AJNR* 1995;16:27–36.

11. Dion JE. Intraarterial papaverine hydrochloride therapy with or without angioplasty in the treatment of cerebral vasospasm. Paper presented at the 1995 Course in Interventional Neuroradiology of the American Society of Interventional and Therapeutic Neuroradiology.

12. Mathis JM, DeNardo AJ, Thibault L, et al. In vitro evaluation of papaverine hydrochloride incompatibilities: a stimulation of intraarterial infusion for cerebral vasospasm. *AJNR* 1994;15:1665–1670.

ADDITIONAL READINGS

Alksne JF, Greenhoot JH. Experimental catecholamine-induced chronic cerebral vasospasm: myonecrosis in vessel wall. *J Neurosurg* 1974;41:440–445.

Barr JD, Mathis JM, Horton JA. Transient severe brain stem depression during intraarterial papaverine infusion for cerebral vasospasm. *AJNR* 1994;15:719–723.

Brothers MF, Holgate RC. Intracranial angioplasty for treatment of vasospasm after subarachnoid hemorrhage: technique and modifications to improve branch access. *AJNR* 1990;11:239–247.

Eckard DA, Purdy PD, Girson MS, et al. Intraarterial papaverine for relief of catheter-induced intracranial vasospasm. *AJR* 1992;158:883–884.

Erba M, Jungreis CA, Horton JA. Nitropaste for prevention and relief of vascular spasm. *AJNR* 1989;10:155–156.

Higashida RT, Halbach VV, Cahan LD, et al. Transluminal angioplasty for treatment of intracranial arterial vasospasm. *J Neurosurg* 1989;71:648–653.

Higashida RT, Halbach VV, Dormandy B, et al. New microballoon device for transluminal angioplasty of intracranial arterial vasospasm. *AJNR* 1990;11:233–238.

Higashida RT, Halbach VV, Dowd C, et al. Intravascular balloon dilatation therapy for intracranial arterial vasospasm: patient selection, technique, and clinical results. *Neurosurg Rev* 1992;15:89–95.

Hughes JT, Schianchi PM. Cerebral artery spasm. *J Neurosurg* 1978;48:515–525.

Hurst RW, Schnee C, Raps EC, et al. Role of transcranial Doppler in neuroradiological treatment of intracranial vasospasm. *Stroke* 1993;24:299–303.

Kim C-J, Bassiouny M, Macdonald L, et al. Effect of BQ-123 and tissue plasminogen activator on vasospasm after subarachnoid hemorrhage in monkeys. *Stroke* 1996;27:1629–1633.

Kinoshita A. Intra-arterial papaverine for vasospasm [Letter]. *J Neurosurg* 1993;79:797.

Kobayashi H, Ide H, Aradachi H, et al. Histological studies of intracranial vessels in primates following transluminal angioplasty for vasospasm. *J Neurosurg* 1993;78:481–486.

LeRoux PD, Newell DW, Eskridge J, et al. Severe symptomatic vasospasm: the role of immediate postoperative angioplasty. *J Neurosurg* 1994;80:224–229.

Linskey ME, Horton JA, Rao GR, Yonas H. Fatal rupture of the intracranial carotid artery during transluminal angioplasty for vasospasm induced by subarachnoid hemorrhage. *J Neurosurg* 1991;74:985–990.

Livingston K, Hopkins LN. Intraarterial papaverine as an adjunct to transluminal angioplasty for vasospasm induced by subarachnoid hemorrhage. *AJNR* 1993;14:346–347.

Marks MP, Steinberg GK, Lane B. Intraarterial papaverine for the treatment of vasospasm. *AJNR* 1993;14:822–826.

Mathis JM, DeNardo A, Jensen ME, et al. Transient neurologic events associated with intraarterial papaverine infusion for subarachnoid hemorrhage-induced vasospasm. *AJNR* 1994;15:1671–1674.

Newell DW, Eskridge JM, Mayberg MR, et al. Angioplasty for the treatment of symptomatic vasospasm following subarachnoid hemorrhage. *J Neurosurg* 1989;71:654–660.

Powers WJ, Grubb RL, Baker RP, et al. Regional cerebral blood flow and metabolism in reversible ischemia due to vasospasm. *J Neurosurg* 1985;62:539–546.

Ropper AH, Zervas NT. Outcome 1 year after SAH from cerebral aneurysm. *J Neurosurg* 1984;60:909–915.

Toni D, Frontoni M, Argentino C, et al. Update on calcium antagonists in cerebral vascular diseases. *J Cardiovasc Pharmacol* 1991;18:s10–s14.

Zubkov YN, Nikiforov BM, Shustin VA. Balloon catheter technique for dilatation of constricted cerebral arteries after aneurysmal SAH. *Acta Neurochir* 1984;70:65–79.

Medical Management of Vasospasm and Hemodynamic Alterations in the Neurosurgical ICU

C. Paoletti / C. Dematons / C. Bellec / J.L. Raggueneau / D. Payen de la Garanderie / L. Do / G. Lot / B. George / J. Cophignon / J.-J. Merland

Multidisciplinary management of intracranial aneurysms requires well-equipped units in very specialized centers so as to be able to apply adequate specific treatments.

Postoperative problems in cases of aneurysmal rupture are different from those in incidental cases. This chapter deals mainly with complications occurring after subarachnoid hemorrhage (SAH). Management of these complications requires the patient to be in a neurosurgical intensive care unit (ICU) for monitoring of intracranial pressure, hemodynamic parameters, transcranial Doppler, pulmonary status, and neurologic condition.

POSTEMBOLIZATION CARE AFTER ANEURYSMAL SUBARACHNOID HEMORRHAGE

General Considerations

The choice of procedure depends primarily on the location and anatomic and morphologic features of the aneurysm and also on the patient's clinical grade and age. Other factors such as the time since hemorrhage, intracranial hypertension, ventricular dilation, and vasospasm may also influence the choice of treatment.

There is general agreement on the need for early treatment of ruptured aneurysms in order to prevent rebleeding; the rate is estimated at 4% during the first 24 hours and 1% to 2% per day during the following month.[1]

Early treatment permits application of medical therapy (hemodilution, hypervolemia, and hypertension ["triple H"]) or interventional treatments of vasospasm more safely, as well as ventricular drainage. In fact, after endovascular procedures, the aim of patient management in the ICU is to prevent or reduce all post-SAH complications that may worsen the final outcome. However, overall results are principally related to the initial clinical grade (Table 52–1).

Similar posttherapeutic problems are observed after surgery and endovascular treatment. In high-grade, generally comatose patients, intubation and assisted ventilation must be applied. Ventilation parameters need to be adjusted if pulmonary aspiration

has occurred. The arterial P_{CO_2} has to be maintained between 33 and 38 mm Hg in these patients at high risk for ischemia. There is always intracranial hypertension after rupture, and autoregulation mechanisms are later impaired in the territories involved by vasospasm. Nevertheless, hypocapnia may reduce the flow through these territories by limiting the compensatory distal vasodilation; it should therefore be avoided.

Cardiovascular Problems

In some patients, cardiac rhythm disorders of sympathetic origin are observed. These are generally benign and resolve without treatment. However, severe myocardial lesions, disturbances of electrical conduction, or ventricular dyskinesia may sometimes be seen;[2-4] these are generally transient. However, they must be treated, as they may lead to cellular necrosis. They may also induce a low flow in the carotid

---

T A B L E 5 2 - 1 Clinical Grading Scales for Patients with Acute Aneurysmal Subarachnoid Hemorrhage

Hunt and Hess

Grade	Examination Findings
I	Normal neurologic examination, mild headache, slightly stiff neck
II	Moderate to severe headache and stiff neck; no confusion or neurologic deficit except for cranial nerve palsy
III	Persistent confusion and/or focal neurologic deficit
IV	Persistent stupor; moderate to severe neurologic deficit
V	Coma with moribund appearance

World Federation of Neurological Surgeons

WFNS Grade	Glasgow Coma Scale Score	Motor Deficit
I	15	Absent
II	13–14	Absent
III	13–14	Present
IV	7–12	Present or absent
V	3–6	Present or absent

territory, with consequences for the whole brain in the case of intracranial hypertension, or for particular territories in the presence of vasospasm.

The treatment of systemic hypertension remains controversial. In hypertensive patients, the goal is only to limit a further elevation of systemic pressure, never to "normalize" the numbers. Practically, the aim is to avoid systolic pressures greater than 180 mm Hg, except in the presence of intracranial hypertension related to intracerebral hematoma (Cushing's reflex). In this case, the treatment is emergent and consists of aspiration of the hematoma. After aneurysm obliteration, no antihypertensive drug is given, in order to preserve cerebral blood flow (CBF) as much as possible. Nimodipine, 2 to 3 mg/hr, routinely employed to prevent vasospasm, is generally sufficient to control the arterial pressure. However, in some cases, another antihypertensive drug must be added, or another calcium channel blocker is used, such as nicardipine, which is a more powerful antihypertensive agent and also has some vasoactive effect against vasospasm. The dose recommended is 0.15 mg/kg/hr intravenously.[5]

Fluid and Electrolyte Disorders

The most common fluid and electrolyte disorders are hypovolemia and hyponatremia. These are more likely related to excessive urinary sodium elimination than to inappropriate antidiuretic hormone secretion.[6, 7] Hypovolemia is generally observed in high-grade patients; its development roughly parallels the time course of vasospasm. Hypovolemia must be corrected, since it worsens the effects of vasospasm on brain parenchyma and consequently increases the risk of neurologic deficits.[8] Correction of hypovolemia is best achieved with isotonic solutions, supplemented with sodium chloride to balance urinary loss related to secretion of atrial natriuretic factor (cerebral salt wasting).

Epilepsy

Epileptic seizures after aneurysmal rupture are frequent (25% of cases).[1] Routine treatment is therefore the rule even if seizures are related to the initial intracranial hypertension.[9]

Most studies in the literature were carried out on patients treated surgically. One might consider that endovascular treatment, avoiding manipulations of the cortex, will eventually lead to fewer patients needing to be treated and to treatment for a shorter period. However, it seems safer to continue using this treatment in cases of intracerebral hematoma, cerebral infarction, previous status epilepticus, and incomplete obliteration of the aneurysm (because of the risk of rebleeding).[1]

Hydrocephalus

Obstructive hydrocephalus is observed in 20% to 25% of patients with aneurysmal ruptures, most commonly after severe hemorrhage (high-grade patients). Since hydrocephalus aggravates the intracranial hypertension and later worsens the consequences of vasospasm, it should be treated by ventricular drainage during the acute phase. However, because ventricular drainage increases the risk of rebleeding, aneurysm obliteration has to be performed on an emergent basis by surgery or endovascular technique. Since hydrocephalus is mainly seen in high-grade patients, the endovascular technique appears more suitable.

In addition, ventricular drainage permits monitoring of intracranial pressure, even when ventricular dilation is moderate; it is useful despite risks of infection. Such drainage in comatose patients with low middle cerebral artery (MCA) diastolic velocities frequently improves their neurologic status.

Vasospasm

Vasospasm is the most frequent cause of secondary deterioration, occurring in 33% of cases of aneurysmal rupture, and responsible for 7% of deaths and 7% of permanent deficits. Since the introduction of nimodipine, the rate of infarction observed on computed tomography (CT) has been reduced by 34%.[10] Although some studies reported a 5% rate of permanent deficit when early surgery, nimodipine, and "triple H" therapy were employed, this has not been confirmed by a cooperative study.[11] The incidence of angiographic vasospasm (40% to 50%), and of symptomatic vasospasm (32%) leading to permanent deficit or death (20%) appears stable.[11, 12]

Compared with the data reported before 1980, the present results are largely improved. This may stem from the avoidance of fluid restriction for hyponatremia and hypovolemia associated with hypertensive therapy in the presence of vasospasm.[13]

The clinical signs indicating vasospasm range in severity from headaches and fever to dementia or a comatose state with focal deficit. Unfortunately, these symptoms are not specific, since they can be observed during other complications such as ventricular enlargement, rebleeding, infectious disorders, and fluid and electrolyte disorders. Moreover, subclinical epileptic seizures or thromboembolic complications may induce similar symptoms. A coil protruding into the arterial lumen or the mass effect of a packed aneurysm compressing the parent artery after endovascular treatment may reduce the flow, with consequences similar to those of vasospasm.

The ability to tolerate vasospasm depends on the vessel diameter reduction, blood viscosity, length of vasospasm, state of autoregulation, development of collaterals, and cerebral perfusion pressure. Current therapies for vasospasm modify one or more of these factors.

Transcranial Doppler

Transcranial Doppler (TCD), introduced by Aaslid in 1982, is becoming the "gold standard" for bedside detection of vasospasm and follow-up of the evolution

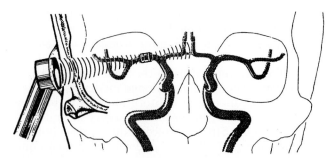

Figure 52–1 Frontal view of the ultrasound probe directed toward the middle cerebral artery (MCA). The cylinder around the MCA indicates the observation region (sampling volume) for Doppler recording. The distance from the middle of the cylinder to the probe corresponds to the depth setting. (From Aaslid R, Markwalder TM, Nornes H. Noninvasive transcranial Doppler ultrasound recording of flow velocity in basal cerebral arteries. *J Neurosurg* 1982;57:769–774.)

of the process. This noninvasive examination can be easily repeated and has a sufficiently high sensitivity and specificity to avoid the need for repeated angiography.[14–16]

The increase in velocity always precedes clinical and angiographic signs of vasospasm.[14, 17, 18] TCD permits one to follow the evolution of vasospasm and the therapeutic effects. The normal values of mean velocities are 62 ± 12 cm/sec, 51 ± 12 cm/sec, 44 ± 11 cm/sec, and 37 ± 6.5 cm/sec for the MCA, the anterior cerebral artery (ACA), the posterior cerebral artery, and the extracranial internal carotid artery (ECICA), respectively. The normal ratio between the mean velocities of MCA and ECICA is 1.7 ± 0.4.[14] The ECICA is recorded at a depth from 50 to 65 mm, and the probe is positioned high in the neck, near the angle of the jaw.

The MCA is most commonly used for TCD studies because of the low interrogation angle, the functional importance of its territory, and a good correlation between vessel narrowing and velocity (Figs. 52–1 and 52–2).

Blood flow in a particular artery depends on the cross-sectional area (Πr^2) of the artery and the mean velocity (V) of the blood flowing through it (F = $\Pi r^2 V$). As reported by Lindegaard et al, a reduction of 25% in the MCA diameter corresponds to a 56% reduction in the surface of the vessel section and induces a velocity increase of 178%.[19]

Other factors must be considered, such as arterial pressure, intracranial pressure, variations of the perfusion territory, and the P_{CO_2} level. TCD and ^{133}Xe blood flow recordings measure different parameters in different territories. However, some studies have shown parallel changes in velocity and MCA-dependent territory blood flow during tests of vascular reactivity.[20, 21] These tests should be performed to evaluate the hemodynamic reserve in the presence of vasospasm and the efficacy of therapy. Mean velocity is decreased in the elderly and in hypertensive patients compared with controls.[22] Conversely, mean velocity increases with cardiac output increase and decreases when hematocrit is low.[15] With TCD, the relative changes of average velocity (V_mMCA) are more useful than the absolute values (time-averaged mean).

Significant correlations between Fisher score on CT scan (no clot, thin clot, thick clot), velocity on TCD, vasospasm on angiography, and clinical symptoms have been described.[17, 18, 20, 23–27] Velocity increases on day 3 or 4, reaching the highest value between days 7 and 15. This high velocity starts to decrease during the end of the third week. However,

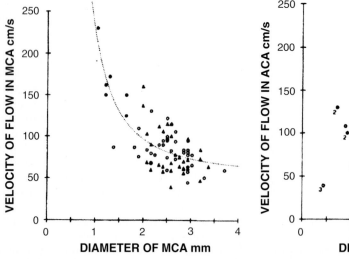

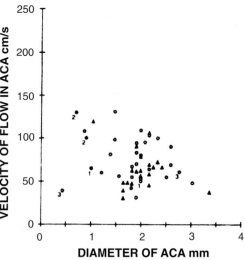

Figure 52–2 *Left,* Flow velocity in the MCAs as a function of the diameter of that section of the lumen as measured on angiography. *Triangles:* Cases without angiographic evidence of aneurysm. *Filled circles:* Cases with aneurysms and clear angiographic evidence of vasospasm. The dotted line, y = 55 + 167/x², was found by nonlinear regression analysis of the entire series. The correlation was r = 0.75. *Right,* Flow velocity in the anterior cerebral artery (ACA) as a function of the diameter of that section of lumen as measured on angiography. Symbols as in *left.* (From Aaslid R, Huber P, Nornes H. Evaluation of cerebrovascular spasm with transcranial Doppler ultrasound. *J Neurosurg* 1984;60:37–41.)

only 20% to 30% of patients experience no velocity increase, which is a lower rate than the absence of vasospasm on angiography. It has been observed that elderly patients have a lower rate of delayed ischemic deficits and also a less frequent increase in velocity.[28]

Along with the improvements in vasospasm treatment, the critical values for velocity have changed. In 1987, Harders et al. suggested that hypertensive therapy (induced arterial hypertension [AHT]) should be applied when the velocity was over 80 cm/sec even in asymptomatic patients (systolic arterial pressure up to 150 to 170 mm Hg).[23] With this strategy, they reported a decrease in the rate of delayed ischemic deficits. Such a concept has been supported by the observation of a velocity over 120 cm/sec in patients developing delayed ischemic deficits. Such a threshold is still widely accepted, although some authors admit a higher threshold (130 or 140 cm/sec) for 100% sensitivity.[29-31]

Harders et al. proposed to add the slope of velocity increase during the first days to this threshold to detect the high-risk patients (Doppler index of delayed ischemic deficit).[23] They observed that patients with delayed ischemic deficit increased their velocity by more than 20 cm/sec per day between days 3 and 7. A similar value was observed by many authors, but patients with high grades on Fisher score were excluded. In this case, the velocity increase is blunted by intracranial hypertension.

The index proposed by Aaslid et al. in 1982, using the ratio between mean velocity in the MCA and mean velocity in the ECICA, has the advantage of being independent of variations in cardiac output induced by vasospasm treatments.[14] Lindegaard et al. considered a value of 3 for this index to be diagnostic of vasospasm. A value greater than 5 is consistent with severe vasospasm.[32] However, this increased index may result from a low internal carotid artery (ICA) velocity, which requires specific treatment, such as correction of hypovolemia and/or induced AHT.

If intracranial hypertension is present, the degree of vasospasm is underestimated, since velocity increase cannot occur. According to Romner et al., this mechanism explains the low velocity values observed in the first 48 hours after aneurysmal rupture.[33] Some authors use Pourcelot's resistance index: systolic velocity minus diastolic velocity divided by systolic velocity ($V_{syst} - V_{diast}/V_{syst}$), which reflects the level of distal arterial resistance (normal value: 0.5–0.6). In Klingerhofer et al.'s study, all patients with permanent deficit had an index greater than 0.6.[34] The pulsatility index of Gosling ($V_{syst} - V_{diast}/V_{mean}$) has similar significance, with normal values ranging between 0.65 and 1.10. Its use is recommended in patients with high Fisher grades and with intracranial hypertension.

TCD studies on the basilar trunk are seldom performed, but it is possible to obtain them by suboccipital access. Normal velocity at this level is 40 ± 8 cm/sec. The sensitivity of vasospasm detection in the basilar trunk is 76.9% for a velocity of 60 cm/sec and 100% for a velocity of 95 cm/sec.[35]

The intracranial ICA velocity is recorded via transorbital access with a 25% sensitivity for a mean velocity of 90 cm/sec.[31]

Limits of Transcranial Doppler After Aneurysmal Rupture

There is no correlation between the degree of vasospasm in the ACA and TCD recordings because of the anatomic variations of the anterior communicating artery (Fig. 52–2). Therefore, the MCA velocity recording may give a false-negative result if vasospasm develops only on the ACAs. The same limitation is present when vasospasm occurs in distal branches or on a segment upstream of the recorded vessel. Finally, 5% to 9% of patients with thick temporal bones cannot be properly evaluated.

These data and false-negative results explain why angiography remains the reference method for detection of vasospasm and should be performed in doubtful cases. TCD is a very useful tool for daily use but cannot replace angiography. TCD patterns are considered more a warning detector than a diagnostic procedure.

Personal Observations

Every patient systematically receives nimodipine, 2 mg/hr, as soon as aneurysmal rupture is confirmed and hypovolemia corrected. The usual fluid and electrolyte intake (40 ml/kg/day) is complemented by colloids (except albumin), 10 to 20 ml/kg/day. Greater intake has proved useless in young patients because of increased diuresis, and hazardous in older patients because of frequent pulmonary edema associated with myocardial dyskinesia.

For each patient, the clinical status is monitored and a noncontrast CT scan is repeated as needed to assess for early ventricular enlargement.

In grades I, II, and III patients (Cases 1 and 2, Figs. 52–3 and 52–4), if arterial pressure is less than 120 mm Hg, dopamine is given and titrated to maintain systolic arterial pressure at greater than 140 mm Hg. If diuresis increases, increased fluid and electrolyte intake is necessary to maintain normovolemia (which is evaluated by fluid balance and protidemia). In grades IV and V patients (Case 3, Figs. 52–5 and 52–6), induced arterial hypertension and volume expansion are routinely used and monitored by central venous pressure. A Swan-Ganz catheter is inserted only when volume expansion seems to be poorly tolerated or when a cardiopulmonary problem occurs. Systemic arterial pressure is raised to maintain cerebral perfusion pressure over 80 mm Hg in the presence of intracranial hypertension. In the absence of severe intracranial hypertension, TCD parameters are used, including mean velocities in the MCA and extracranial ICA, diastolic velocity in the MCA, and pulsatility index. Intracranial hypertension is treated medically and occasionally by external ventricular drainage even if the ventricles are only slightly dilated.

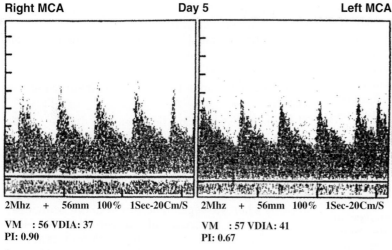

Right MCA   **Day 5**   **Left MCA**

2Mhz   +   56mm   100%   1Sec-20Cm/S   2Mhz   +   56mm   100%   1Sec-20Cm/S

VM   : 56 VDIA: 37   VM   : 57 VDIA: 41
PI: 0.90   PI: 0.67

A

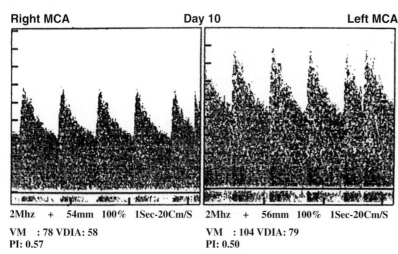

Right MCA   **Day 10**   **Left MCA**

2Mhz   +   54mm   100%   1Sec-20Cm/S   2Mhz   +   56mm   100%   1Sec-20Cm/S

VM   : 78 VDIA: 58   VM   : 104 VDIA: 79
PI: 0.57   PI: 0.50

B

Figure 52–3 Case 1. A 50-year-old man suffered a subarachnoid hemorrhage related to a ruptured left MCA aneurysm, which was clipped the day after (grade II). *A,* After 5 days, velocities were in the normal range. *B,* On day 10, left MCA velocities increased with no clinical deterioration. *C,* On day 12, a right-sided neurologic deficit occurred despite volume expansion and induced arterial hypertension. Mean velocity (V_m) MCA was 125 cm/sec with V_mMCA/V_mICA >3. The pulsatility index (PI) was 0.38 and the diastolic velocity (VDIA) was elevated. We thought that mechanical angioplasty was necessary because of impaired hemodynamic reserve.

Case 1 continues

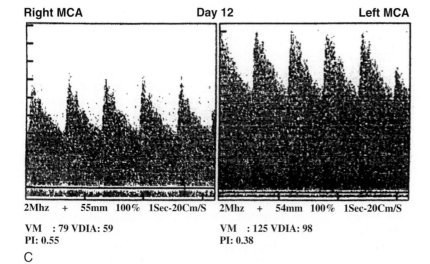

Right MCA   **Day 12**   **Left MCA**

2Mhz   +   55mm   100%   1Sec-20Cm/S   2Mhz   +   54mm   100%   1Sec-20Cm/S

VM   : 79 VDIA: 59   VM   : 125 VDIA: 98
PI: 0.55   PI: 0.38

C

As emphasized by Aaslid et al. in 1986,[36] TCD is very useful to identify the risk of ischemia when the ratio V_mMCA/V_mICA is elevated in relation to low V_mICA values. Such a velocity has to be increased but not normalized, to be adjusted to the CBF and cerebral metabolic rate of oxygen consumption ($CMRO_2$) reduction after aneurysm rupture.[37] During the acute phase, CBF/$CMRO_2$ is unchanged. At the site of vasospasm, the vessels contract under the influence of oxyhemoglobin and activated comple-

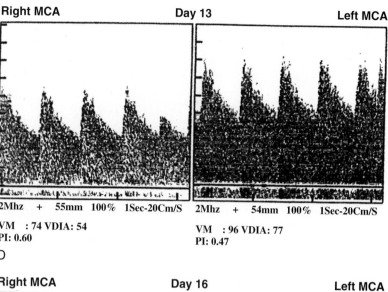

Right MCA   Day 13   Left MCA

2Mhz   +   55mm   100%   1Sec-20Cm/S   2Mhz   +   54mm   100%   1Sec-20Cm/S

VM   : 74 VDIA: 54   VM   : 96 VDIA: 77
PI: 0.60   PI: 0.47

D

Figure 52–3 *Continued. D,* After this treatment, velocities decreased immediately, the right deficit disappeared the day after and velocities remained within the normal range on day 21 *(E and F).* The time course of left MCA vasospasm is shown. The low PI indicates distal vasodilation (0.38, with a normal range of 0.65 to 1.10). After angioplasty on day 12, spectral analysis shows a lower VDIA and higher PI.

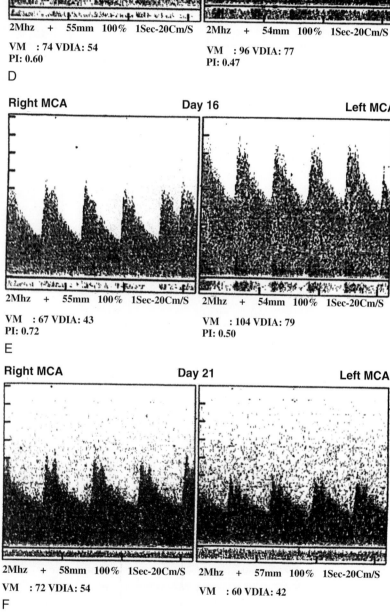

Right MCA   Day 16   Left MCA

2Mhz   +   55mm   100%   1Sec-20Cm/S   2Mhz   +   54mm   100%   1Sec-20Cm/S

VM   : 67 VDIA: 43   VM   : 104 VDIA: 79
PI: 0.72   PI: 0.50

E

Right MCA   Day 21   Left MCA

2Mhz   +   58mm   100%   1Sec-20Cm/S   2Mhz   +   57mm   100%   1Sec-20Cm/S

VM   : 72 VDIA: 54   VM   : 60 VDIA: 42

F

ment. Distal to the vasospasm, vessels conversely dilate to maintain the regional CBF, and oxygen extraction increases. However, these reactions depend on the level of autoregulation. Moreover, if vasospasm is severe and extensive or if perfusion pressure decreases, the dilation of distal vessels may not be sufficient to preserve regional CBF, leading to cellular damage. Therefore, when the ratio V_mMCA/V_mICA reaches 2.5, it is considered indicative of vasospasm, and one should perform adequate fluid loading and increase the arterial pressure to 150 to 160 mm Hg. This may sometimes require a combination

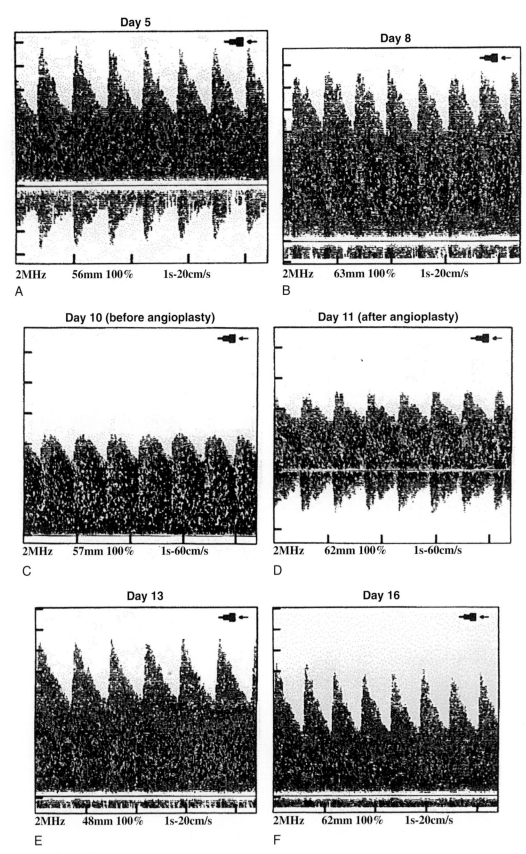

Figure 52–4 Case 2. A 45-year-old woman was admitted 4 days after rupture of a left posterior communicating artery aneurysm (grade III). Endovascular treatment of the aneurysm was performed emergently. *A*, MCA velocity recordings started on day 5 after the subarachnoid hemorrhage. On day 6, the left MCA velocities increased, reaching a maximum on day 10 (174 cm/sec) *(B and C)*. The same day, her clinical condition deteriorated with dysphasia but no motor deficit. The V_mMCA/V_mICA ratio was >5. Maximal distal vasodilation was indicated by high VDIAs and low PI. Mechanical dilation was rapidly performed until the V_mMCA/V_mICA ratio was lower than 3 *(D to F)*. Velocities were so high that their peaks were off the screen, requiring an increase in the scale from 20 to 60 cm/sec.

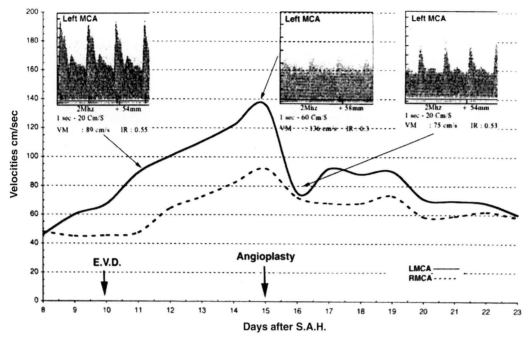

Figure 52–5 Case 3. A 35-year-old woman was admitted after rebleeding from a left posterior communicating artery aneurysm 8 days after first rupture; clinically, she was grade IV. Intracranial hypertension was treated by mannitol, and induced arterial hypertension produced an increase in the low ICA velocities. Two days later, ventricular dilation was discovered on computed tomography. After ventricular drainage, mannitol perfusion was stopped. Increased velocities were then observed, with a V_mMCA of 136 cm/sec and V_mMCA/V_mICA ratio of 4.8 on day 7. Simultaneously, a slight motor deficit of the right upper limb appeared, with no impact on the Glasgow score based on the best motor response. The resistance index was 0.30 (normal range, 0.50 to 0.60). Mechanical angioplasty was successfully performed and the motor deficit disappeared within 2 hours.

of dopamine and dobutamine. When this ratio (V_mMCA/V_mICA) is greater than 3 despite appropriate medical treatment, endovascular therapy (angioplasty) must be considered. High diastolic velocities and a low pulsatility index suggest that distal vasodilation has reached its maximum and indicate a poor hemodynamic reserve. In consequence, medical treatment cannot further improve regional CBF. In fact, the indications for angioplasty rely on the patient's clinical condition. Some severe vasospasm can be well tolerated and does not require such treatment. Conversely, when neurologic deterioration occurs or when the patient is comatose, endovascular treatment is indicated.

The hypervolemic therapies previously described are not to be recommended since they are associated with many general and cerebral complications such as pulmonary edema, infections, cerebral edema, and hemorrhagic cerebral infarction.[38–40] Other pharmalogic treatments are still experimental: bosentan (RO 47–0203), an endothelin receptor antagonist[41, 42]; protein kinase C inhibitors (staurosporin), which facilitate nitric oxide liberation; superoxide dismutase, which produces blockage of nitric oxide oxidation by superoxide anion; and complement inhibitors.[43, 44]

Before these drugs become clinically available, adequate fluid loading, hypertensive therapy, and occasionally endovascular angioplasty are the current

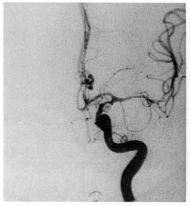
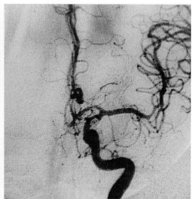

Figure 52–6 Angiographic appearance of the left MCA before and after angioplasty.

modalities available for treating vasospasm. Obviously, angioplasty requires experienced interventional neuroradiologists. In our department, 47 endovascular procedures were performed in 38 patients between January 1993 and December 1996. Mechanical (balloon) angioplasty was applied in 17 patients (21 procedures) who had focal vasospasm limited to the main trunk of the cerebral vessels. Conversely, chemical angioplasty with papaverine (300 mg) or nimodipine (3 mg) was used in 21 patients (26 procedures) with diffuse or distal vasospasm involving the secondary branches that are out of reach for angioplasty balloons. These chemical angioplasties were performed preoperatively in one patient (two procedures); postoperatively in two patients (two procedures); before, during, and after endovascular coiling of the aneurysm in 10 cases (nine patients admitted in vasospasm); and late after endovascular treatment in 12 cases (nine patients). Chemical angioplasty has a short duration of effect (velocity accelerations recur 4 hours later). Therefore, it often has to be repeated at various intervals from a few hours to 48 hours, depending on velocity recordings and the clinical evolution. In one patient presenting with vasospasm involving both carotid systems and the basilar trunk, chemical angioplasty was used three times with a good result.

Mechanical angioplasty has provided an effective and long-lasting result in all cases with a velocity ratio returning below 3. It decreased the diastolic velocity and brought to normal the pulsatility index, indicating that distal vasodilation was no longer necessary. No recurrence of increased velocities was noticed. In four patients, two balloon angioplasty procedures were performed, but in two different territories in each instance. Clinical improvement was observed after various delays, as short as 2 hours in one case. As already mentioned, although the results are better when treatment is early, delayed treatment may also be effective. In one patient, mechanical angioplasty was performed 48 hours after an area of hypodensity in the superficial MCA territory was discovered on CT scan (on day 12 after the aneurysmal rupture). This delay was explained by the very poor condition of this 20-year-old patient, in coma with unilateral decerebration. The V_mMCA/V_mICA ratio was 4.7, with a V_mMCA of 125 cm/sec. Considering the very poor neurologic condition, the angioplasty was performed despite the risk of hemorrhage in the infarcted area. The patient demonstrated flexion response after 24 hours, had purposeful reaction after 3 days, and showed eye opening after 1 week. TCD recordings showed normal velocities around the 26th day. At 6 months, the patient returned to work.

Use of Heparin

In addition to the specific problems observed after an SAH, thromboembolic complications are of importance, especially after a procedure. After an endovascular embolization, with or without SAH, the antithrombotic treatment started during the procedure must sometimes be continued for several days. It is of particular importance when there is encroachment on the parent artery by the mass of the coiled aneurysm or protrusion of a coil into the parent artery.

Another indication for antithrombotic treatment is a high ratio between aneurysm and parent artery diameter. Additionally, the risk of emboli coming from the aneurysmal wall is higher when either the neck is wide or the aneurysm is partially clotted.

When any of these conditions are present, close follow-up in a neurosurgical ICU is necessary. The antithrombotic treatment must be maintained at various doses and for a variable duration. Sometimes, it is necessary to use antiplatelet aggregant agents as a complement therapy for a couple of weeks, especially when there is a high risk of thromboembolic complications.

The typical clinical manifestation of a thromboembolic event is a focal deficit or dysphasia occurring soon after the procedure. It is crucial to diagnose this complication, since the success of fibrinolytic treatment is time dependent.

MONITORING AND CARE AFTER BALLOON OCCLUSION OF THE INTERNAL CAROTID ARTERY

Balloon occlusion is used mostly for giant ICA aneurysms, skull base tumors, carotid cavernous fistulae, and carotid artery injury. A review of the literature of recent years indicates that there is great heterogeneity in the criteria used to define tolerance of ICA occlusion. Some authors describe the use of positron emission tomography (PET) and CBF.[45] Others report a high risk of ischemia when CBF is less than 30 ml/100 gm/min.[46, 47] Other studies report the use of TCD for predicting tolerance to ICA occlusion. Transient ischemic attacks have been reported in patients whose V_mMCA decreased more than 65% during the test.[48]

Tolerance to ICA occlusion implies adequate cerebral vasoreactivity, which is an indicator of the hemodynamic reserve of the cerebral circulation. There is a good correlation between change in regional CBF and V_mMCA.[20, 49–51]

Acetazolamide (ACZ) is used as a vasodilatory stimulus. By increasing the H^+ concentration, ACZ induces acidosis, which provokes vasodilation of small arterioles.[52, 53] This effect is usually obtained 10 to 30 minutes after intravenous administration of 1 gm of ACZ. In normal subjects, ACZ causes a rapid 55% increase in CBF related to a decrease in arteriolar resistance without transmural pressure modification.[54] Diastolic velocity increases by 50% compared with basal values.[21] Reduced cerebral vasoreactivity during balloon test occlusion may therefore be an early indicator of reduced collateral potential, with a subsequently greater risk of ischemic stroke after ICA occlusion.

Since hypotension is supposed to be one of the causes of stroke in ICA occlusion, balloon test occlusion with hypotension is thought to be the best test to predict tolerance of ICA occlusion. Standard et al. performed occlusion for 20 minutes under normotension and induced hypotension by 30% of the initial pressure value during 20 minutes.[55] The other methods reported concern the use of transcranial cerebral oximetry,[56] magnetic resonance imaging and HMPAO scintigraphy,[57] color Doppler guided Matas test, and continuous electroencephalography.

Because of the risks of ischemia and a thromboembolic complication, patients undergoing ICA occlusion must be observed in a neurosurgical ICU. Clinical examination must be repeated regularly and arterial blood pressure monitored, since hemodynamic factors are prominent in ischemic complications.

Generally, all antihypertensive drugs given as a regular treatment are withdrawn. Moreover, the patient should lie down for 2 days, with sitting allowed on the third day. If necessary, hypotension can be treated with cardiovascular agents: dopamine or dobutamine with a starting infusion rate of 5 µg/kg/min. Hypovolemia should be avoided and plasma expanders should be employed.

One must keep in mind that ischemia can result from embolic factors. Embolic stroke is a possibility, originating from the wall of an aneurysm (mostly carotid-ophthalmic aneurysms) treated by carotid occlusion. In this case, intravenous heparin is administered to obtain effective anticoagulation. Balloon migration can also lead to ischemia. Skull x-ray films allow one to check balloon position by comparison with previous x-rays. If migration results from balloon deflation, an injection of ether close to the balloon may be useful.

Headaches occurring in this context are claimed to result from thrombosis and related mass effect, justifying the use of steroids. Decreased visual acuity (in the case of carotid-ophthalmic aneurysms) has been reported after ICA occlusion.[58]

As previously stated, repeated clinical examination remains the basis of monitoring of patients with ICA occlusion in neurosurgical ICUs. TCD represents another way of monitoring, since a noninvasive measurement of blood flow velocities in the basal brain arteries can be obtained. Moreover, it is inexpensive and easy to perform, with direct access to the MCA, which supplies 60% of CBF. For these reasons, TCD is a suitable technique for routine clinical use. Cerebral oximetry (near-infrared spectroscopy) appears useful and convenient for monitoring patients with ICA occlusion, because it provides real-time information regarding the regional brain oxygen saturation, which changes before the occurrence of adverse clinical events.[56, 59] Accordingly, repeated TCD measurements, transcranial oximetry, and appropriate adjustment of therapy in the neurosurgical ICU may prevent ischemic stroke. Rebleeding of an aneurysm treated with ICA occlusion is a possibility. In this setting, CT can help confirm the diagnosis. Nevertheless, it must be remembered that CT performed after angiography shows densities mimicking SAH.

The authors wish to acknowledge the contributions of Martine Randon, Joel Barnavon, and Georges Moret.

REFERENCES

1. Mayberg MA, Batjer HH, Dacey R, et al. Guidelines for the management of aneurysmal subarachnoid hemorrhage. *Circulation* 1994;90:2592–2605.
2. Yasu T, Owa M, Omura N, et al. Transient ST elevation and left ventricular asynergy associated with normal coronary artery in aneurysmal subarachnoid hemorrhage. *Chest* 1993;103:1274–1275.
3. Szabo MD, Crosby G, Hurford WE, Strauss HW. Myocardial perfusion following acute subarachnoid hemorrhage in patients with an abnormal electrocardiogram. *Anesth Analg* 1993;76:253–258.
4. Kono T, Morita H, Kuroiwa T, et al. Left ventricular wall motion abnormalities in patients with subarachnoid hemorrhage: neurogenic stunned myocardium. *J Am Coll Cardiol* 1994;24:636–640.
5. Haley EC, Kassel NF, Torner JC. A randomized controlled trial of high-dose intravenous nicardipine in aneurysmal subarachnoid hemorrhage: a report of the Cooperative Aneurysm Study. *J Neurosurg* 1993;7:537–547.
6. Nelson PB, Seif SM, Maroon JC, Robinson AG. Hyponatremia in intracranial disease: perhaps not the syndrome of inappropriate secretion of antidiuretic hormone (SIADH). *J Neurosurg* 1981;55:938–941.
7. Diringer MN, Wu KC, Verbalis JG, Hanley DF. Hypervolemic therapy prevents volume contraction but not hyponatremia following subarachnoid hemorrhage. *Ann Neurol* 1992;31:543–550.
8. Solomon RA, Post KD, McMurtry JG III. Depression of circulating blood volume in patients after subarachnoid hemorrhage: implications for the management of symptomatic vasospasm. *Neurosurgery* 1984;15:354–361.
9. Hart RG, Byer JA, Slaughter JR, et al. Occurrence and implications of seizures in subarachnoid hemorrhage due to ruptured intracranial aneurysms. *Neurosurgery* 1981;8:417–421.
10. Allen G, Ahn H, Preziosi T, et al. Cerebral arterial spasm: a controlled trial of nimodipine in patients with subarachnoid hemorrhage. *N Engl J Med* 1983;308:619–624.
11. Haley EC, Kassel NF, Torner JC. The international cooperative study on the timing of aneurysm surgery: the North American experience. *Stroke* 1992;23:205–214.
12. Longstreth WT Jr, Nelson LM, Koepsell TD, Van Belle G. Clinical course of spontaneous subarachnoid hemorrhage: a population based study in King County, Washington. *Neurology* 1993;43:712–718.
13. Kassel NF, Peerless SJ, Durward QJ, et al. Treatment of ischemic deficits from vasospasm with intravascular volume expansion and induced arterial hypertension. *Neurosurgery* 1982;11:337–343.
14. Aaslid R, Markwalder TM, Nornes H. Noninvasive transcranial Doppler ultrasound recording of flow velocity in basal cerebral arteries. *J Neurosurg* 1982;57:769–774.
15. Newell D, Aaslid R. Transcranial Doppler: clinical and experimental uses. *Cerebrovasc Brain Metab Rev* 1992;4:122–143.
16. Miller J, Smith R. Transcranial Doppler sonography in aneurysmal subarachnoid hemorrhage. *Cerebrovasc Brain Metab Rev* 1994;6:31–46.
17. Aaslid R, Huber P, Nornes H. Evaluation of cerebrovascular spasm with transcranial Doppler ultrasound. *J Neurosurg* 1984;60:37–41.
18. Seiler RW, Grolimund P, Aaslid R, et al. Cerebral vasospasm evaluated by transcranial ultrasound correlated with clinical grade and CT-visualized subarachnoid hemorrhage. *J Neurosurg* 1986;64:594–600.
19. Lindegaard KF, Bakke SJ, Worteberg W, et al. A noninvasive Doppler ultrasound method for the evaluation of patients with subarachnoid hemorrhage. *Acta Radiol* 1986;369:96–98.
20. Dahl A, Russel D, Nyberg-Hansen R, et al. Cerebral vasoreactivity in unilateral carotid artery disease. A comparison of

blood flow velocity and regional cerebral blood flow measurements. *Stroke* 1994;25:621–626.

21. Mancini M, Dechiara S, Postiglione A, Ferrara LA. Transcranial Doppler evaluation of cerebro-vascular reactivity to acetazolamide in normal subjects. *Artery* 1993;20:234–241.

22. Ekelund A, Saveland H, Romner B, Brandt L. Transcranial Doppler ultrasound in hypertensive versus normotensive patients after aneurysmal subarachnoid hemorrhage. *Stroke* 1995;11:2071–2074.

23. Harders AG, Gilsbach JM. Time course of blood velocity changes related to vasospasm in the circle of Willis measured by transcranial Doppler ultrasound. *J Neurosurg* 1987;66:718–728.

24. Sekhar LN, Wechsler LR, Yonas H, et al. Value of transcranial Doppler examination in the diagnosis of cerebral vasospasm after subarachnoid hemorrhage. *Neurosurgery* 1988;22:813–821.

25. Kaech DL, Despland PA, De Tribolet N. Le Doppler transcrânien dans l'évolution des vasospasmes après hémorragie sous-arachnoïdienne. *Neurochirurgie* 1990;36:279–286.

26. Grosset DG, Straiton J, Dutrevou M, Bullock R. Prediction of symptomatic vasospasm after subarachnoid hemorrhage by rapidly increasing transcranial Doppler velocity and cerebral blood flow changes. *Stroke* 1992;23:674–679.

27. Grosset DG, Straiton J, McDonald I, et al. Use of transcranial Doppler sonography to predict development of a delayed ischemic deficit after subarachnoid hemorrhage. *J Neurosurg* 1993;78:183–187.

28. Boescher-Schwarz HG, Ungersboeck K, Ulrich P, et al. Transcranial Doppler diagnosis of cerebral vasospasm following subarachnoid hemorrhage: correlation and analysis of results in relation to the age of patients. *Acta Neurochir (Wien)* 1994;127:1–2, 32–36.

29. Langlois O, Rabehenoina C, Proust F, et al. Diagnostic du vasospasme: comparaison arteriographie-Doppler transcranien. Une série de 112 examens comparatifs. *Neurochirurgie* 1992;38:138–140.

30. Lennihan L, Petty GW, Finck ME, et al. Transcranial Doppler detection of anterior cerebral artery vasospasm. *J Neurol Neurosurg Psychiatry* 1993;56:906–909.

31. Burch CM, Wozniak MA, Sloan MA, et al. Detection of intracranial internal carotid artery and middle cerebral artery vasospasm following subarachnoid hemorrhage. *J Neuroimaging* 1996;6:8–15.

32. Lindegaard KF, Nornes H, Bakke SJ, et al. Cerebral vasospasm diagnosis by means of angiography and blood velocity measurement. *Acta Neurochir (Wien)* 1989;100:12–24.

33. Romner B, Ljunggren B, Brandt L, Saveland H. Correlation of transcranial Doppler sonography findings with timing of aneurysm surgery. *J Neurosurg* 1990;73:72–76.

34. Klingerhofer J, Dander D, Holzgraefe M, et al. Cerebral vasospasm evaluated by transcranial Doppler ultrasonography at different intracranial pressures. *J Neurosurg* 1991;75:752–758.

35. Sloan MA, Burch CM, Vozniak MA, et al. Transcranial Doppler detection of vertebro-basilar vasospasm following subarachnoid hemorrhage. *Stroke* 1994;25:2187–2197.

36. Aaslid R, Huber P, Nornes H. A transcranial Doppler method in the evaluation of cerebrovascular spasm. *Neuroradiology* 1986;28:11–16.

37. Carpenter DA, Grubb PL, Tempel LW, Powers WJ. Cerebral oxygen metabolism after aneurysmal subarachnoid hemorrhage. *J Cereb Blood Flow Metab* 1991;11:837–844.

38. Levy M, Giannotta S. Cardiac performance indices during hypervolemic therapy for cerebral vasospasm. *J Neurosurg* 1991;75:27–31.

39. Medlock MD, Dulebohn SD, Elwood PW. Prophylactic hypervolemia without calcium channel blockers in early aneurysm surgery. *Neurosurgery* 1992;30:12–16.

40. Shimoda M, Oda S, Tsugane R, Sato O. Intracranial complications of hypervolemic therapy in patients with delayed ischemic deficit attributed to vasospasm. *J Neurosurg* 1993;78:423–429.

41. Shigeno T, Clozel M, Sakai S, et al. The effect of bosentan, a new potent endothelin receptor antagonist, on the pathogenesis of cerebral vasospasm. *Neurosurgery* 1995;37:87–90.

42. Zimmermann M, Seifert V, Loffler BM, et al. Prevention of cerebral vasospasm after experimental subarachnoid hemorrhage by RO 47–0203, a newly developed orally active endothelin receptor antagonist. *Neurosurgery* 1996;38:115–120.

43. Findlay JM, McDonald RL, Weir BKA. Current concepts of pathophysiology and management of cerebral vasospasm following aneurysmal subarachnoid hemorrhage. *Cerebrovasc Brain Metab Rev* 1991;3:336–361.

44. Hans P. Perspectives thérapeutiques nouvelles du vasospasme. *XVIIe Journées de Neuro-Anesthésie Réanimation de Langue Française* 1995:193–214.

45. Brunberg JA, Frey KA, Horton JA, et al. (150)H20 positron emission tomography determination of cerebral blood flow during balloon test occlusion of the internal carotid artery. *AJNR* 1994;15:725–732.

46. Linskey ME, Jungreis CA, Yonas H, et al. Stroke risk after abrupt internal carotid artery sacrifice: accuracy of preoperative assessment with balloon test occlusion and stable xenon-enhanced CT. *AJNR* 1994;15:829–843.

47. Witt JP, Yonas H, Jungreis C. Cerebral blood flow response pattern during balloon test occlusion of the internal carotid artery. *AJNR* 1994;15:847–856.

48. Giller CA, Mathews D, Walker B, et al. Prediction of tolerance to carotid artery occlusion using transcranial Doppler ultrasound. *J Neurosurg* 1994;81:15–19.

49. Kofke WA, Brauer P, Policare R, et al. Middle cerebral artery blood flow velocity and stable xenon-enhanced computed tomographic blood flow during balloon test occlusion of the internal carotid artery. *Stroke* 1995;26:1603–1606.

50. Dahl A, Lindegaard KF, Russel D, et al. A comparison of transcranial Doppler and cerebral blood flow studies to assess cerebral vasoreactivity. *Stroke* 1992;23:15–19.

51. Muller M, Voges M, Piepgras U, Schimrigk K. Assessment of cerebral vasomotor reactivity by transcranial Doppler ultrasound and breath-holding. A comparison with acetazolamide as vasodilatory stimulus. *Stroke* 1995;26:96–100.

52. Dahl A, Russel D, Rootwelt K, et al. Cerebral vasoreactivity assessed with transcranial Doppler and regional cerebral blood flow measurements. Dose, serum concentration and time course of the response to acetazolamide. *Stroke* 1995;26:2302–2306.

53. Okudaira Y, Bandoh K, Arai H, Sato K. Evaluation of the acetazolamide test. Vasoreactivity and cerebral blood volume. *Stroke* 1995;26:1234–1239.

54. Vorstrup S, Brun B, Lassen NA. Evaluation of the cerebral vasodilatory capacity by the acetazolamide test before EC-IC by-pass surgery in patients with occlusion of the internal carotid artery. *Stroke* 1986;17:1291–1298.

55. Standard SC, Ahuja A, Guterman LR, et al. Balloon test occlusion of the internal carotid artery with hypotensive challenge. *AJNR* 1995;16:1453–1458.

56. Samra SK, Dorje P, Zelenock GB, Stanley JC. Cerebral oximetry in patients undergoing carotid endarterectomy under regional anesthesia. *Stroke* 1996;27:49–55.

57. Simonson TM, Ryals TJ, Yuh WT, et al. MR imaging and HMPAO scintigraphy in conjunction with balloon test occlusion: value in predicting sequelae after permanent carotid occlusion. *AJR* 1992;159:1063–1068.

58. Vasquez Anon V, Aymard A, Gobin YP, et al. Balloon occlusion of the internal carotid artery in 40 cases of giant intracavernous aneurysm: technical aspects, cerebral monitoring and results. *Neuroradiology* 1992;34:245–251.

59. Dujovny M, Slavin KV, Luer MS, et al. Transcranial cerebral oximetry and carotid cavernous fistula occlusion. Technical note. *Acta Neurochir* 1995;133:83–86.

EMERGENCY TREATMENT OF ACUTE ISCHEMIC STROKE

CHAPTER 53

General Considerations in Emergency Stroke Therapy

J.J. Connors III / J.C. Wojak

HISTORY

Stroke is the third leading cause of death in the United States and perhaps the greatest cause of morbidity. It ranks as the leading cause of expenditure of health care dollars and affects about 550,000 people per year. To many, the fact that 10% of stroke victims die within 1 month and about one third die after living 6 months with horrible disability catapults this illness even beyond the category of malignant cancer.[1-3] Data specifically concerning angiographically proven occlusion of the main trunk of the middle cerebral artery indicate that the initial mortality rate may approach 25% to 30%.[4-6] Caplan et al.[7] reported a 33% mortality rate in 3 months; if there was a branch occlusion (M3), the 3-month mortality rate was "only" 14.3%.

Consequently, to many people, a rapid death would be preferable to a lingering terminal existence; this reality stimulates even further the aggressive attempts to rescue people suffering this terrible fate. The nearly unanimous choice of patients offered enrollment in the National Institute of Neurological Disorders and Stroke (NINDS) tissue-type plasminogen activator (t-PA) trial and the Abbott Prolyse for Acute Cerebral Thromboembolism (PROACT) trials to undergo treatment confirms this attitude.

Although there is abundant ongoing research in the field of neurovascular pathology, the treatment of acute stroke has been nearly stagnant for several decades. Continuing developments in cytoprotective and fibrinolytic agents, combined with technologic advances, have raised the possibility of acute stroke intervention. The question has become not *whether* to intervene in acute stroke, but *how* best to do this. Although most early interventional investigative studies were done in Europe, particularly by Zeumer and others in Germany,[3] a large number of sites in the United States are performing emergency intracranial revascularization on a regular basis. At present, at least three active studies are evaluating the emergency treatment of stroke by intracranial intra-arterial local fibrinolytic therapy. The oldest is a registry organized by Ferguson at the Baptist Memorial Hospital (Memphis, TN), which continues to accumulate information on the specifics of this therapy. An additional NINDS trial of combination intravenous and intra-arterial administration of t-PA has been halted because of the results of the intravenous arm of the trial (see later). Abbott Laboratories has started a new phase in its investigation of the direct local intra-arterial administration of prourokinase (the core radiology group is at the University of California, San Francisco, headed by Higashida). The first phase showed promising results concerning recanalization and safety, which are encouraging enough to warrant further investigation into this area. These trials are all discussed at length, later.

Associated Costs

Amazing as it sounds, the decision whether to treat patients is largely made by health care management companies and hospital administrators. The up-front costs of therapy can be high, particularly with the more labor-intensive, intra-arterial therapies. Even though the patient's life can be greatly benefited by these techniques, the eventual money-saving aspects of having a functional person rather than a disabled person are not necessarily obvious to health care delivery systems. Therefore, aggressive stroke therapy is being considered as a money-losing proposition in some locations.

Pharmaceutical companies, one of the primary driving forces for research, do not see this as a great marketing area (the volume of patients is too low) and are not supporting this work any further in Europe. As of this writing, Abbott Pharmaceuticals is still supporting the intra-arterial trial of acute stroke therapy with prourokinase in the United States (see later).

Studies have shown that even if the long-term positive benefits to the patient are ignored, *there can be monetary benefit to the hospital by reducing the number of patients and the length of stay in the intensive care unit and inpatient rehabilitation.* The study by Lanzieri et al.[8] demonstrated that emergency treatment of stroke is not only cost-effective but also humanitarian. During a 1-year period, 34 patients with acute strokes caused by thromboembolic occlusion of the middle cerebral artery were seen. Of these, eight were treated aggressively with intracranial intra-arterial fibrinolysis (urokinase). The difference between the initial and the 24-hour follow-up National Institutes of Health Stroke Scale Score,[9] the hospital costs, and the length of stay in the hospital of the 8 treated patients and the 26 control patients were compared. In addition, the risk of nursing home admission and the projected costs of the nursing home were calculated for the two groups.

The results of the analysis indicated that for the untreated group, the stroke score deteriorated by an average of 0.5 points. *In the treated group, the score improved by 5.125, a difference that was both statistically and clinically significant.* The two groups had a similar length of stay. The cost of hospitalization per patient was $13,478 for the untreated group and $15,202 for the treated group, an insignificant difference.

The risk of nursing home admission was reduced by one third in the treated group, representing a savings of $3,435 per patient in the treated group. Nursing home care can result in expenditures of hundreds of thousands of dollars in a short time; this estimate should thus be considered extremely conservative. In certain locations, this estimate of savings would represent only the savings in in-hospital *rehabilitation* costs, before the patient was even sent to a nursing home.

The ongoing efforts by Berger and Callahan in Nashville (see Chapter 63) demonstrate that this service can be delivered with excellent medical and monetary results.

Mechanism of Insult

There are two basic types of stroke: ischemic and hemorrhagic. With regard to ischemic stroke, there are basically two mechanisms of occlusion of intracranial arterial flow: intrinsic thrombus and migratory embolus. There are also primarily two territories affected by thromboembolic occlusion: the anterior (carotid) and the posterior (vertebrobasilar) territories. Each of these has its more common means of occlusion and clinical presentation; the posterior circulation more frequently is caused by intrinsic

thrombus formation than anterior circulation ischemia (percentages unknown), whereas the anterior circulation typically is caused by embolus. Cardiac sources account for 15% to 30% of emboli; the remainder come from cervical and cranial vessels (commonly the carotid bifurcation). Table 48–1 in Chapter 48 gives the distribution of atherosclerotic disease involving the carotid and vertebrobasilar systems. It is the opinion of many of the neurologic specialists participating in the Abbott trials of acute stroke therapy (see later) that a higher percentage of true mainstem middle cerebral artery embolic occlusions than previously thought may arise from the heart as opposed to carotid bifurcation disease. In younger patients in particular, this appears to be the case[10, 11] (see Figs. 59–49 to 59–62 in Chapter 59).

This variability of the mechanism of insult results in variability of the rapidity and severity of ischemic insult and subsequent damage. Combined with the intrinsic danger of the specific location of ischemia, this necessitates at least two broadly different approaches to the treatment of stroke. Additionally, each patient has tremendous variability in his or her ability to withstand certain occlusions related to their intrinsic collateral pathways. At the core of any *targeted* therapy is the identification of thrombus (occlusion) in a clinically appropriate location with symptoms sufficient to warrant therapy. This is the only appropriate target of fibrinolysis.

RATIONALE FOR EMERGENCY CEREBRAL REVASCULARIZATION

The most obvious therapeutic choice for the treatment of an intracerebral arterial occlusion is revascularization. The varying means of occlusion and varying locations, however, necessitate different strategies for treatment. In addition, the variable preexisting collateral supplies to areas of insult give some patients a wider window of opportunity for treatment as well as a better chance for a good response. At present, however, it is impossible to predict accurately which patients these are.

About one third of patients with a transient ischemic attack (TIA) eventually have a stroke, with 20% of these occurring within the first month after the initial event. A TIA is defined as a sudden neurologic disturbance lasting more than 15 minutes but with complete resolution within 24 hours. The mechanism of insult is thought to be inadequate blood supply to a focal brain region, usually small. A reversible ischemic neurologic deficit (RIND) is a deficit that persists for more than 24 hours, but with "complete" recovery within 3 weeks. A completed stroke has a duration greater than 3 weeks. Even a RIND with apparent complete recovery, however, may result in some area of true infarct. *This has significant implications for emergency treatment of acute stroke in a patient who has had sentinel events in the recent past.* If there has been a TIA or RIND within the several days (or weeks) before the acute stroke, there is a much increased chance of an intraparenchymal bleed secondary to any revascularization effort. This may be totally patient dependent and difficult or impossible to predict. Accurate history and astute evaluation of the preprocedure computed tomography scan is mandatory.

The quotation marks above concerning recovery from a RIND infer that the definition of "complete" recovery can be slightly flexible. Many experienced neurologists will admit that when they see a certain kind of stroke presentation, they know whether the outcome will be bad or good. When major symptoms last longer than 1 hour, only 14% of patients show full resolution within 24 hours. Indeed, when severe symptoms persist for longer than 4 hours, the chance of significant recovery is slim.

Interestingly, 6.5% to 8.7% of all first-time strokes occur while a patient is in a hospital, and these patients may be the ideal recipients for emergency revascularization.[12] In addition, in a 1-year review of strokes among 71,874 hospital admissions to a major medical center, 38% of in-hospital strokes were found to be iatrogenic in origin.[13] About 55% of these patients would qualify for a hypothetical protocol using a 3-hour enrollment window.

Furthermore, it is well known that about 20% of all major strokes end in death within 1 month. Indeed, in the NINDS t-PA stroke trial, the placebo group had a 21% incidence of death at 3 months, and the t-PA group had a statistically insignificantly different rate of death of 17%. Commonly quoted figures are that there are 150,000 deaths from stroke per year, and about 550,000 new strokes per year. This yields a resultant death rate of about 25% per year, although not necessarily in the 1-month time frame.

Ischemic Penumbra

In most ischemic insults, there is an area of irrecoverable tissue damage surrounded by a region that may be viable and teetering on the brink of cell death—the *ischemic penumbra*.[14, 15] Even though saving all tissue in jeopardy would be ideal, it is this potentially salvageable ischemic penumbra that results in the clinical improvement in many cases and that is the true target of therapy. It is possible that there will be total cure in only a small number of patients; in most, however, the salvage of a portion of this viable ischemic penumbra is possible, resulting in a significant improvement in clinical condition.

The ischemic penumbra generally is thought to represent a geographic area of tissue surrounding a more profoundly ischemic central core; basically a concentric circle model. This concept was once considered hypothetical but is now an accepted fact. The amount of collateral supply to the insulted territory determines the volume of recoverable tissue. The volume of tissue "teetering on the brink" can range from none to almost all of the insulted territory and is not truly circular. This fact can give hope while rendering predictions of outcome difficult.

Disruption of the normal physiologic activity of cerebral tissue occurs well before the decreased blood flow becomes critical to tissue survival. This means that if the flow is within a certain critical range, neurologic abnormality can occur earlier than infarction and for an almost indefinite period (in the context of the standard time frame for an emergency). (See Figs. 58–15 to 58–54 in Chapter 58, illustrating the case of a patient with a major neurologic deficit of more than *2 days*' duration that was successfully and totally reversed.)

The average regional blood flow is about 55 ml/100 gm/min of cerebral tissue, specifically 65 to 75 ml/100 gm/min in the gray matter and 15 to 20 ml/100 gm/min in the white matter. The ischemic threshold (for electrical dysfunction) is about 15 to 20 ml/100 gm/min (average). Tissue death does not usually ensue until perfusion falls below about 10 to 12 ml/100 gm/min.[16] A rate of flow of 10 to 20 ml/100 gm/min may result in functional failure without cell death.

REFERENCES

1. Kappelle LJ, Adams HP Jr, Heffner ML, et al. Prognosis of young adults with ischemic stroke: a long-term follow-up study assessing recurrent vascular events and functional outcome in the Iowa Registry of Stroke in Young Adults. *Stroke* 1994;25:1360–1365.
2. Vogel J. Five-year follow-up of stroke patients over age 65. *Rehabilitation* 1994;33:155–157.
3. Zeumer H, Freitag H-J, Zanella F, et al. Local intra-arterial fibrinolytic therapy in patients with stroke: urokinase versus recombinant tissue plasminogen activator (r-TPA). *Neuroradiology* 1993;35:159–162.
4. Andreoli A, Limoni P, DeCarolis P, et al. Prognosis of middle cerebral artery occlusion: cooperative study on 178 cases. In Spetzler R, Selman W, Carter LP, Martin MA (eds). Cerebral Revascularization for Stroke. New York: Thieme/Grune & Stratton, 1985, pp. 53–56.
5. Moulin DE, Lo R, Chiang J, Barnett HJM. Prognosis in middle cerebral artery occlusion. *Stroke* 1985;16:282–284.
6. Saito I, Segawa H, Shiokawa Y, et al. Middle cerebral artery occlusion: correlation of computed tomography and angiography with clinical outcome. *Stroke* 1987;18:863–868.
7. Caplan L, Hier D, D'Cruz I. Cerebral embolism in the Michael Reese Stroke Registry. *Stroke* 1983;14:530–536.
8. Lanzieri CF, Tarr RW, Landis D, et al. Cost effectiveness of emergency intra-arterial intracerebral thrombolysis: a pilot study. *AJNR* 1995;16:1987–1993.
9. Brott T, Adams HP, Olinger CP, et al. Measurements of acute cerebral infarction: a clinical examination scale. *Stroke* 1989;20:864–870.
10. Adams HP, Butler MJ, Biller J, Toffol GJ. Nonhemorrhagic cerebral infarction in young adults. *Arch Neurol* 1986;43:793–796.
11. Lisovoski F, Rousseaux P. Cerebral infarction in young people: a study of 148 patients with early cerebral angiography. *J Neurol Neurosurg Psychiatry* 1991;54:576–579.
12. Kelley RE, Kovacs AG. Mechanism of in-hospital cerebral ischemia. *Stroke* 1986;17:430–433.
13. Azzimondi G, Nonino F, Fiorani L, et al. Incidence of stroke among inpatients in a large Italian hospital. *Stroke* 1994;25:1752–1754.
14. Overgaard K. Thrombolytic therapy in experimental embolic stroke. *Cerebrovasc Brain Metab Review* 1994;6:257–286.
15. Heiss WD, Graf R, Weinhard J, et al. Dynamic penumbra demonstrated by sequential multitracer PET after middle cerebral artery occlusion in cats. *J Cereb Blood Flow Metab* 1994;14:892–902.
16. Grosset DG. What have drugs to offer the patient with acute stroke? *Br J Clin Pharmacol* 1992;33:467–472.

CHAPTER 54

Medical Aspects of Cerebral Ischemia

L.A. Weisberg

Stroke is the most common serious life-threatening neurologic disorder. It is the third most frequent cause of death (150,000 deaths per year) and the most frequent cause of disability. There are almost 600,000 new stroke cases per year and 3 million stroke survivors, many of whom have not regained functional or vocational independence. These numbers probably underestimate stroke prevalence. For example, there are other patients who have stroke risk factors (e.g., hypertension, cardiac disease, lipid abnormalities) and are at high stroke risk. They may have no clinical stroke episodes; however, computed tomography (CT) or magnetic resonance imaging (MRI) shows silent (asymptomatic) cerebral infarction or leukoaraiosis (white matter changes that frequently represent vascular ischemic demyelination). Although these patients never suffered clinical stroke, neuropsychological evaluation may show evidence of cognitive or behavioral abnormalities, probably related to silent stroke; recognition of such patients may elude clinical detection.

Stroke is symptomatic manifestation of cerebrovascular disease due to degenerative changes in arterial or arteriolar circulation, less commonly involving venous circulation. These may lead to vascular occlusion due to embolism or thrombosis, or weakness in the arterial wall may lead to aneurysm formation (berry aneurysms cause subarachnoid hemorrhage; Charcot-Bouchard aneurysms rupture to cause hypertensive intracerebral hemorrhage).

Stroke is defined as *sudden* onset of focal neurologic deficit in which maximal dysfunction is reached rapidly (minutes to several hours) and in which delayed (several days later) neurologic deterioration does not usually occur unless there is a complicating medical condition. The deficit stabilizes, and subsequent neurologic improvement occurs; however, 25% of stroke patients rapidly deteriorate and die from cerebral edema, increased intracranial pressure, cerebral herniation, cardiac arrhythmia, myocardial infarction, or pulmonary embolism. Death usually occurs in patients with major cerebral (carotid, basilar, stem of middle cerebral) artery occlusion and is less common with arteriolar occlusion.

RISK FACTORS FOR ISCHEMIC STROKE

Stroke risk factors are listed in Table 54–1.[1] Stroke is *not* a random occurrence, as implied by the term *cerebrovascular accident*. Stroke represents a summation of detrimental effects of multiple identified risk factors. Because about 30% of strokes have no identified cause, there must be many other unidentified risk factors. Hypertension (isolated systolic as well as diastolic) and cardiac dysfunction (atrial fibrillation, congestive heart failure, prior myocardial infarction, electrocardiographic abnormality) are major stroke risk factors. Hypertension may accelerate atherosclerosis and enhance arteriolar wall damage (lipohyalinosis, fibrinoid degeneration). Control of elevated blood pressure is the most important element of a stroke prevention strategy. Although aggressive management of hypertension is warranted, blood pressure lowering should be performed carefully and judiciously in patients after acute stroke. Some patients with a "warning stroke" or transient ischemic attack (TIA) who have high-grade carotid or basilar artery stenosis may have hemodynamic disturbances. Their condition could be worsened or symptoms precipitated by rapid blood pressure reduction.

Cardiac abnormalities may lead to cardiogenic cerebral embolism, especially with left atrial thrombus formation in atrial fibrillation patients or left ventricular thrombus formation after myocardial infarction. Diabetes mellitus is an independent stroke risk factor, but there is no evidence that careful normoglycemic control prevents stroke. Increased blood lipids are a modifiable risk factor for coronary artery disease and accelerate carotid atherosclerosis[2]; this may be reduced by administration of hydroxymethylglutaryl-coenzyme A (HMG-CoA) reductase inhibitors.[3] It appears that elevated blood lipids are related to large vessel atherosclerotic stroke but not to small vessel lacunar stroke. After acute ischemic stroke, lipid levels are temporarily reduced, and a lipid profile should be repeated 1 month later before initiating lipid-lowering strategies.[2]

T A B L E   5 4 - 1   Potential Risk Factors For Cerebrovascular Disease

Modifiable Risk Factors	Nonmodifiable Risk Factors
Hypertension	
Systolic	Gender:
Diastolic	Male
Left ventricular hypertrophy	Race
Cardiac disease	Black
Glucose intolerance	Hispanic
Lipid abnormalities	Asian
Cigarette smoking	Age
Coagulation factors	Family history
Elevated hematocrit	
Elevated fibrinogen	
Obesity	
Alcohol consumption	
Sedentary lifestyle	
Illicit drug use	

Cigarette smoking increases stroke risk. Oral contraceptive pill use is a stroke risk factor correlating with high estrogen content, positive family history of stroke, age older than 35 years, history of hypertension, and positive smoking history. Estrogen influences stroke risk by its effect on endothelial wall morphology, causing an adverse effect on lipid metabolism and enhancing hypercoagulability. Postmenopausal estrogen may lower stroke risk.

Alcohol may increase stroke risk, especially with moderate and high levels of use.[4] At low levels, alcohol has a *protective* effect on the cardiovascular and cerebrovascular system, owing to its beneficial effect on lipid metabolism and blood pressure. With binge drinking, alcohol may trigger cardiac rhythm disturbances to cause cardiogenic cerebral embolism. High alcohol levels may increase ischemic stroke risk by increasing blood viscosity, inducing hypertension, and having a deleterious effect on lipid metabolism.[4]

Elevated fibrinogen levels are most common in heavy smokers and enhance coagulability. Elevated hematocrit and hemoglobin levels act as risk factors by increasing blood viscosity and impairing blood rheology. Coagulation disorders, including protein S or C deficiency, antithrombin III factor deficiency, antiphospholipid antibody syndrome, or hemoglobinopathies (including sickle cell disease), may predispose to stroke, involving arterial or venous circulation. Head or neck trauma may predispose to carotid or vertebral artery dissection.

Certain nonmodifiable stroke risk factors are important. The incidence of stroke is higher in men than in women, although since women live longer than men, the incidence of stroke is increasing in older women. Blacks and Asians have a higher incidence of stroke than whites. Whites have a higher incidence of extracranial arterial disease; blacks and Asians have more intracranial disease. The incidence of stroke increases with age.

NEUROLOGIC RISK FACTORS FOR STROKE

Asymptomatic Carotid Stenosis

Carotid bruit implies that flow is turbulent, not laminar; however, its presence does not necessarily indicate carotid stenosis.[5] Bruits occur in 4% of the population older than 45 years and in 8% older than 75 years. The stroke risk for patients with asymptomatic carotid bruits is 1%; however, for asymptomatic patients with greater than 75% carotid stenosis, the stroke risk is 5%. In patients with carotid stenosis of 75%, 30% have CT evidence of silent (asymptomatic) cerebral infarction.[6] This indicates that carotid stenosis is not good for the brain.

In patients with asymptomatic carotid stenosis (ACS), stroke may occur; however, TIA *usually* precedes stroke, allowing the physician time to intervene.[7] Patients with ACS should have serial vascular imaging procedures to determine progression of disease. Management should be more aggressive with progression of carotid stenosis. Treatment with anti-

platelet or anticoagulant medication does not reduce stroke risk in ACS patients; however, treatment with HMG-CoA reductase inhibitors may cause carotid plaque regression. Based on the results of ACS studies, carotid endarterectomy reduces relative stroke risk if stenosis is greater than 60%.[8]

Transient Episodes of Neurologic Dysfunction of Vascular Origin

In patients experiencing transient episodes of focal neurologic deficit, it is presumed that the mechanism is vascular; however, there are other potential mechanisms (Table 54–2). In focal seizures, there is rapid spread of neurologic symptoms (the jacksonian march). If focal seizures are suspected because of the quality of the symptoms and their rapid spread, an electroencephalogram (EEG) should be performed. If a focal deficit spreads more slowly and symptoms consist of disturbances moving across visual fields, followed by contralateral headaches, migraine should be considered.

In TIAs, symptoms develop suddenly, do not spread, and are not followed by headache. TIAs represent "mini-strokes" and may be harbingers of cerebral infarction.[9] Their occurrence indicates that the arterial circulation is compromised and in jeopardy of being occluded. If brain perfusion is not rapidly returned to normal, cerebral infarction may occur unless adequate collateral circulation develops to restore flow.

Transient ischemic attacks may occur in the carotid or vertebrobasilar distribution. Carotid TIA symptoms include (1) cerebral hemispheric attacks (hemiparesis, hemianesthesia, aphasia, homonymous hemianopia), or (2) retinal attacks with transient monocular blindness (amaurosis fugax). Patients with transient monocular blindness due to vascular ischemic disturbances involving the ophthalmic or central retinal artery describe the illusion that a curtain is being pulled over one eye or the impression of fog, blur, or mist obscuring vision. In cerebral hemispheric TIAs due to vascular disturbance in the anterior or middle cerebral artery, patients may develop monoparesis, hemiparesis, hemianesthesia, or aphasia. In vertebrobasilar TIAs, characteristic symptoms include diplopia, dysarthria, dizziness and vertigo, difficulty swallowing (dysphagia), ataxia or gait incoordination, bilateral visual loss (homonymous hemianopia), weakness (hemiparesis or tetraparesis), and drop attacks (the patient suddenly falls

T A B L E   5 4 - 2   **Differential Diagnosis of Transient Ischemic Attacks**

Migraine	Drug intoxication
Focal seizures	Vertigo
Syncope	Transient global ischemia
Hyperventilation	Psychogenic conversion reaction
Metabolic disorder	

to the ground without losing consciousness). These symptoms are due to brainstem, cerebellar, or occipital lobe ischemia. Isolated symptoms (e.g., dizziness or diplopia) are rarely manifestations of vertebrobasilar TIAs.

The onset of TIAs is sudden. There is no spread of neurologic deficit. Most are brief, usually lasting less than 30 minutes. If a TIA lasts longer than 1 hour, there is likelihood that the neurologic deficit will not resolve within 24 hours. Long-duration (several hours) TIAs are unlikely to resolve completely and are more likely to show lesions on CT or MRI consistent with ischemia or infarction. When patients with TIAs have ischemic lesions on CT or MRI, this is called *cerebral infarction with transient signs* (CITS). The finding of silent or asymptomatic ischemic lesions visualized by CT occurs in 13% to 50% of TIA patients.[10] This abnormality represents an additional risk factor. These patients are at higher risk of subsequently developing a major clinical stroke than are TIA patients with normal CT findings.[11]

Transient ischemic attacks may be single or recurrent. If recurrent, they may increase in frequency and duration (crescendo TIA); these crescendo TIAs are associated with a high risk of carotid stenosis and completed stroke.

Neurologic deficit of vascular origin that persists for longer than 24 hours and resolves within several days is called *reversible ischemic neurologic deficit* (RIND). Other ischemic stroke patients have rapid clearing of most neurologic impairment (minor stroke). These terms—TIA, CITS, RIND, and minor stroke—represent subgroups of ischemic stroke based on temporal profile. They tell the clinician nothing about the underlying vascular disorder.[12] For example, small vessel lacunar disease or large vessel atherosclerotic disease may cause any of these stroke subtypes. Thirty-five percent of patients with transient or minor ischemic stroke subsequently develop major stroke. *The high-risk period for stroke occurrence is the 12 months after the initial TIA.*

The pathogenesis of TIAs can vary.[13] Most commonly, they are due to embolic disturbances. The embolism may originate from the heart (rhythm disturbances such as atrial fibrillation, myocardial infarction, valvular heart disease) or from thrombus forming on ulcerated carotid plaque. This thrombus may dislodge and embolize to the distal intracranial circulation.

In cardiogenic cerebral embolism, there is *red thrombus* formation (clot forming in a stagnant region, such as a dilated left atrium; clot is composed of red blood cells, fibrin, and thrombin). If the source is an ulcerated plaque (artery-to-artery), this is *white thrombus*, composed of platelet–fibrin material. Cardiogenic cerebral embolism (red thrombus) is prevented with anticoagulation; artery-to-artery embolism (white thrombus) is best prevented with antiplatelet medication.[14]

Transient ischemic attacks may result from abnormal hemodynamics with reduced perfusion in the borderzones between the distal portions of two arterial systems (middle and posterior cerebral arteries, middle and anterior cerebral arteries). These distal borderzone territories are most vulnerable to tissue ischemia, especially when cardiac output is reduced.

To determine appropriate treatment strategies for TIA patients, it is necessary to delineate any underlying arterial lesion and to visualize brain morphologic changes by CT or MRI. It would be ideal to assess physiologic or metabolic brain changes using positron-emission tomography (PET), single-photon emission computed tomography (SPECT), or diffusion or perfusion weighted MRI.

DIAGNOSTIC AND TREATMENT STRATEGIES

Neuroimaging and neurovascular studies should be performed in all patients suspected of having acute stroke. These include the following:

1. CT to exclude intracerebral hemorrhage or nonvascular lesion. MRI is more sensitive for detection of early ischemic lesions; however, detection of ischemic lesions is not absolutely necessary if anticoagulant, thrombolytic, or antiplatelet medication is considered.
2. SPECT may detect perfusion defects when CT and MRI are normal. Ideally, PET studies delineate abnormal brain flow and metabolism.
3. Vascular imaging studies are imperative in all TIA patients to delineate any underlying arterial obstructive lesion. Despite the excellent screening capabilities of Doppler (duplex) carotid ultrasound, magnetic resonance angiography, and CT angiography, conventional catheter angiography is necessary. If the patient has a TIA referable to the left cerebral hemisphere, the left carotid artery, and then the right, should be studied; however, it is not necessary to study the vertebral arteries or arch if a causal lesion is identified. After injection of the suspect vessel, the patient should be briefly assessed neurologically for any deficit before injecting the opposite carotid artery.[15] If the TIA patient shows no arterial obstructive lesion, careful cardiac examination and hematologic studies should be performed (Table 54–3).

MANAGEMENT OF THE PATIENT WITH TRANSIENT ISCHEMIC ATTACKS

If a TIA occurs in the carotid artery distribution, duplex ultrasound has a sensitivity of 90% to 95% for detecting angiographically proven stenosis of at least 50%.[16] Based on results of European[17] and North American[18] carotid endarterectomy (CEA) studies, surgery is beneficial for symptomatic (cerebral ischemia) patients with angiographically documented cervical carotid stenosis of at least 70%. With less than 30% carotid stenosis, CEA is not beneficial; for patients with 30% to 69% stenosis, the value of CEA is unknown. The complication rate for CEA has

T A B L E 5 4 - 3   **Laboratory Evaluation of Patients with Transient Ischemic Attacks**

Complete blood count, including platelet count
Erythrocyte sedimentation rate
Activated partial thromboplastin time and prothrombin time
Lipid profile
Lupus anticoagulant and anticardiolipin antibodies
 (antiphospholipid syndrome)
Urine and serum toxicology
Syphilis serology
Plasma fibrinogen
Hemoglobin electrophoresis
Serum glucose
Urinalysis (for hematuria to suggest renal embolism and
 proteinuria to suggest hypertensive vascular disease)
Renal and hepatic function panels
If no atheroembolic or cardioembolic source is demonstrated,
 the patient is young (less than 40 years old), and an
 unusual source of stroke is suspected, these lower-yield
 studies may be considered:
Protein S and C and antithrombin III levels
Urine amino acid screen for homocysteinuria
Immune complex screening studies, including studies for
 systemic lupus erythematosus and rheumatoid arthritis
Serum and whole blood viscosity
Platelet function studies
Human immunodeficiency virus, Lyme disease, and
 cysticercosis screening tests
Pregnancy test
Serum protein electrophoresis
Coagulation factor analysis
Chest radiogram for sarcoidosis

been documented at 5.5%; however, in many centers, the surgical complication rate is less than 3%.

After CEA, there is no evidence that prophylactic treatment with aspirin prevents vascular ischemic events. Despite this, I routinely prescribe 325 mg of aspirin daily to prevent carotid restenosis and to prevent coronary artery occlusion. Aspirin has been shown to reduce intimal hyperplasia after coronary artery bypass surgery because it inhibits platelet aggregation on endothelial surfaces and has similar effects on the carotid artery.[19]

For TIA patients with an established cardiogenic cerebral embolic source, anticoagulation is indicated. In five studies of patients with nonvalvular atrial fibrillation but no clinical TIA or ischemic stroke, oral warfarin (Coumadin) treatment reduced stroke occurrence. In these studies, the average international normalized ratio (INR) for prothrombin time was 2.7. This was associated with an incidence of major hemorrhagic complications of 1.2% per year. The INR should be kept between 2.0 and 3.0 to minimize hemorrhagic complications and maximize stroke prevention. If there are contraindications to warfarin, antiplatelet medication should be used.[20]

If the angiogram shows high-grade stenosis of a large intracranial artery (internal carotid, middle cerebral, or basilar) in a TIA patient, the stroke risk is high. In this circumstance, neurologists frequently initiate intravenous heparin. This should be followed by oral warfarin. Despite this bias toward anticoagu-

lation in these clinical settings, evidence on efficacy is inconclusive.

If surgery and anticoagulation are not indicated in TIA patients, antiplatelet medication should be considered as follows:

1. Dipyridamole (Persantine) has not been clinically proved to be more effective than aspirin alone, although their mechanisms of action are different and theoretically should be synergistic. Recent evidence suggests that their effects are additive.
2. Pentoxifylline (Trental) is not an antiplatelet drug.[21] It reduces blood viscosity, enhances erythrocyte flexibility, and increases tissue oxygen content. It is effective in patients with peripheral vascular disease but has *not* been shown to be effective in TIA patients, although its use in multi-infarct dementia is being investigated.
3. Aspirin is effective in reducing the risk of cardiovascular and cerebrovascular events.[22] There is a relative risk reduction of 30% for stroke, 22% for stroke and death, and 15% for vascular mortality. Studies have demonstrated that doses of 300 to 1300 mg of aspirin are effective in stroke prevention; however, it is uncertain whether low-dose (40 to 325 mg) aspirin is equally effective.

Aspirin inhibits cyclo-oxygenase to prevent thromboxane A_2 formation (proaggregatory and vasoconstrictive effect); at high dose, aspirin inhibits prostacyclin (vasodilation effect and inhibition of platelet aggregation). There is theoretical advantage to low-dose aspirin because prostacyclin inhibition is avoided at low doses; however, this enhanced effectiveness of low-dose aspirin has not been demonstrated in clinical trials. In fact, clinical studies have shown that *high-dose* aspirin is more effective for stroke prevention in TIA patients.

In TIA patients, it has not been established if aspirin reduces stroke severity in patients who suffer cerebral infarction. Because of aspirin's effect on the clotting mechanism, it may increase the risk of brain hemorrhage. In one study, aspirin was used as prophylactic stroke therapy in asymptomatic patients. There was no reduction in ischemic stroke incidence compared with placebo, and hemorrhagic stroke was more frequent in aspirin-treated patients.[23] With improved brain imaging techniques (CT, MRI), it is possible to detect clinically silent strokes. These patients are at increased risk for development of multi-infarct dementia. Clinical trials are being performed to determine if progression of these lesions seen on CT or MRI can be reduced with prophylactic agents. Although aspirin is effective in stroke prevention in men, its beneficial effect in women is unclear. Because risk of stroke after a TIA is lower in female patients than in male patients, it is important to analyze studies with large numbers of female patients to determine the value of different antiplatelet medications in stroke prevention.

4. Ticlopidine (Ticlid) is an antiplatelet drug that interferes with platelet–fibrinogen binding.[22] Ticlopidine is not a cyclo-oxygenase inhibitor and does not reduce stomach prostaglandins; it causes less gastric irritation than aspirin. Ticlopidine acts to reduce platelet–fibrinogen binding within plaques and reduces white (platelet–fibrin) thrombus size. The dose of ticlopidine is 250 mg given twice daily. Most clinical studies have used this dose; however, some studies have used lower doses to minimize cost and side effects. In the Ticlopidine-Aspirin Stroke Study (TASS), patients with TIAs and mild ischemic strokes were treated with ticlopidine or aspirin (1300 mg daily). In the first year, ticlopidine-treated patients showed a 47% risk reduction for stroke and death, and there was a 26% reduction at 2 years. Ticlopidine is more effective than aspirin in blacks, those with angiographic evidence of diffuse atherosclerotic disease, and female patients. In the Canadian-American Ticlopidine Study (CATS), patients who suffered major stroke were treated with ticlopidine. This was a placebo-controlled study because aspirin has not been demonstrated to prevent *recurrent* stroke; however, it is illogical to believe that aspirin is effective in TIA patients and not effective in patients with other types of ischemic stroke when the vascular mechanism is identical. Ticlopidine was associated with a 30% relative risk reduction for stroke, myocardial infarction, and vascular disease. Potential side effects of ticlopidine include diarrhea, skin rash, dyspepsia, hepatic dysfunction, bleeding episodes, and mild elevation of total blood cholesterol levels. A major side effect is reversible neutropenia; in several cases, neutropenia was irreversible. Complete blood count monitoring should be performed biweekly for 3 months because all cases of neutropenia have occurred within this time period. The incidence of serious side effects with ticlopidine is 1%, comparable to that of warfarin and aspirin.

CEREBRAL BLOOD FLOW AND METABOLISM

The brain requires 25% of the total cardiac output to obtain a continuous supply of adequate energy substrates (oxygen, glucose) to maintain cell membrane electrical potentials.[24–26] Cerebral blood flow (CBF) is 55 ml/100 gm/min. The brain maintains the capability to autoregulate CBF such that it remains constant despite moderate or severe levels of hypotension or hypertension. During cerebral ischemia, CBF is reduced. When CBF is reduced to 30 to 35 ml/100 gm/min, extracellular H^+ increases, resulting in brain acidosis. At a CBF of 20 ml/100 gm/min, evoked potentials are no longer obtainable, and the EEG of the ischemic cortex becomes isoelectric. At a CBF of 15 ml/100 gm/min or less, the following changes occur: (1) extracellular potassium concentration increases, (2) intracellular calcium increases, and (3) the cell membrane depolarizes. If the CBF is less than 15 ml/100 gm/min and is not restored rapidly to normal, irreversible cellular brain injury (infarction) occurs. When CBF falls because of an arterial obstructive lesion, and collateral blood flow is not adequate to compensate, treatment strategies to salvage the brain include *reperfusion* (administration of thrombolytic agents, anticoagulation, surgery) and *neuroprotection* (prevention or reversal of ischemic cascade events).

The central ischemic core receives minimal or no blood flow during arterial occlusion. This region is probably incapable of being salvaged unless reperfusion is immediately achieved; however, the surrounding penumbra may be salvaged if the ischemic cascade events are rapidly reversed.

After arterial occlusion, there is depletion of high-energy phosphates, glycogen, glucose, and oxygen. If oxygen is reduced, anaerobic glycolysis results in increased carbon dioxide and lactic acid production with reduced tissue pH. With low tissue pH, mitochondrial function is inhibited, and there is reduced adenosine triphosphate (ATP) production. This results in failure of the sodium–potassium pump system. Intracellular potassium is extruded into extracellular spaces, and sodium concentration is increased intracellularly. There is depolarization in presynaptic terminals, initially seen in the central (core) infarct area and subsequently spreading outward to the periphery (penumbra). Depolarization waves initiate activity in voltage-sensitive calcium and sodium channels to cause glutamate release from presynaptic terminals.[27]

In cerebral ischemia, depletion of oxygen and glucose impairs mitochondrial function, leading to free radical formation. These are highly reactive compounds that have an unpaired electron in their outer orbit and that normally are part of the mitochondrial electron transport system. With mitochondrial dysfunction, free radicals cause oxygen-dependent peroxidation reactions. Compounds such as glutathione and ascorbic acid act as free radical scavengers. After ischemia, there is an increase in brain free fatty acids (palmitic, oleic, stearic, linoleic, and arachidonic acids). When cerebral ischemia occurs, there is reduction of intracellular ATP, phospholipid breakdown, and increased intracellular free fatty acids.[28, 29]

The release of L-glutamate from presynaptic terminals activates postsynaptic receptors, including N-methyl-D-aspartate (NMDA) and D-amino-3-hydroxyl-5-ethyl-4-isoxazole propionate (AMPA) receptors. Free radicals enhance glutamate release from presynaptic terminals. When NMDA receptors are activated, there is influx of calcium into neurons; when AMPA receptors are activated, this opens sodium channels, and intracellular concentration rises. When cellular energy production is normal, glutamate is rapidly removed from extracellular spaces by glial cells and neurons; however, in cerebral ischemia with reduced ATP, calcium and sodium channels remain open owing to glutamate that remains present.[28]

After vascular ischemia, there is increased tissue accumulation of toxic metabolites, including lactate and glutamate. After large vessel occlusion, there are microcirculatory changes resulting in thromboembolism in smaller distal vessels; these microvascular occlusions impair cerebral perfusion. Endothelial cells are damaged because of vascular ischemia. There may be intraluminal thrombus formation, detachment of endothelial wall fragments, platelet aggregation, polymorphonuclear cell adherence to endothelial cells, and vasoconstriction. This worsens the cerebral ischemia.

Edema occurs with vascular ischemia because of impaired cell energy metabolism. Damage to the sodium pump mechanism, which is high-energy dependent, results in increased intracellular sodium. This leads to metabolic or cytotoxic edema. Cytotoxic edema may be triggered by glutamate, which affects AMPA receptors to keep sodium channels open. When the blood–brain barrier is injured, there is extracellular (vasogenic) edema in vascular ischemia. In addition, ischemia causes nitric oxide production in endothelial cells to enhance water diffusion into cells.[29]

If a major artery is occluded, the ischemic region receives collateral blood supply. CBF is pressure dependent because arterioles are maximally dilated owing to the ischemia, with resultant increased lactate. There is loss of autoregulation, and brain parenchyma is sensitive to small reductions in blood pressure; therefore, blood pressure reduction is a greater risk than arterial hypertension. The clinician should make careful decisions regarding blood pressure reduction in acute stroke. If major arterial occlusion is relieved by use of thrombolytic agents or the embolus fragments, restoring flow, the ischemic region is exposed to systemic arterial pressure. This may worsen extracellular edema and enhance red blood cell extravasation through blood vessel walls into the parenchyma, which may be minimized by blood pressure reduction.[30] These divergent effects of blood pressure reduction emphasize the dilemma of blood pressure management in acute ischemic stroke.

MANAGEMENT OF ACUTE CEREBRAL ISCHEMIA

Several treatment strategies have been proposed,[31] including prevention of clot propagation, restoration of cerebral blood flow (reperfusion), and neuroprotection.

Prevention of Clot Propagation

The appropriate use of anticoagulation in patients with acute ischemic stroke remains unsettled. If a patient is in a prothrombotic or hypercoagulable state (e.g., protein S or C deficiency), in which recurrent thromboembolism is likely, anticoagulation is warranted. If the patient has an underlying cardiac disorder (e.g., atrial fibrillation), and stroke recurrence due to cardiogenic cerebral embolism is considered likely, anticoagulation is also warranted. In cardiac-source stroke, the embolic material occluding the artery may fragment, resulting in restoration of blood flow to the infarcted region and hemorrhagic transformation. This risk of hemorrhagic transformation is enhanced with anticoagulation but may occur in its absence (spontaneous). In cardiogenic cerebral embolism, it is prudent to delay anticoagulation for 24 to 48 hours to minimize hemorrhage.[32] In patients with acute partial thrombotic stroke treated with heparin, one study showed a slight but statistically significant reduction in neurologic progression.[33] In patients with suspected impending basilar artery occlusion and risk of brainstem infarction, intravenous heparin frequently is used, although there are no studies to support this approach.

In patients with acute cerebral ischemia, intravenous heparin administration should be considered in the following settings:

- Established cardiogenic source of ischemic stroke
- Severe arterial stenosis or occlusion seen on noninvasive vascular imaging
- History of continued neurologic deterioration (progressing stroke)
- Hemorrhage excluded by CT or MRI
- Evidence of venous sinus thrombosis

Heparin should be used in this manner:

1. Infuse at 800 to 1000 U/hr (0.25 U/kg/min) without initial bolus. The use of a bolus increases the intracranial hemorrhage risk.
2. Maintain the partial thromboplastin time (PTT) at 1.5 to 2 times normal.
3. Obtain daily hematocrit and platelet counts to exclude occult bleeding or heparin-induced thrombocytopenia.

An ongoing study using low-molecular-weight heparinoids to prevent clot propagation or recurrent embolism is not yet completed. These compounds have less antithrombin III activity and more factor X_a activity than heparin. They cause less PTT elevation and reduced bleeding risk and thrombocytopenia occurrence than does heparin.[34]

Restoring Cerebral Blood Flow

The four possible means of restoring CBF are as follows[35]:

1. *Vasodilating medications.* These medications are not effective because the infarcted region is already maximally vasodilated owing to local tissue acidosis, and these drugs have more effect on nonischemic brain. Blood is diverted from the infarcted region and potentially salvageable surrounding penumbra to nonischemic regions. Drugs that have been used include

prostacyclin, which has vasodilatory and platelet antiaggregation effect, and calcium-channel blockers, which may vasodilate, reduce blood pressure, and prevent vasoconstriction (vasospasm). Vasodilating agents are efficacious in preventing ischemic complications in subarachnoid hemorrhage but have not been shown to be effective in acute cerebral ischemia. It is possible, however, that they have not been used early enough after stroke occurrence. If treatment is initiated at an early stage, these drugs might be effective.

2. *Improving perfusion pressure.* In patients with acute stroke, rapid lowering of blood pressure represents a potential hazard unless the blood pressure elevation is high enough to cause end-organ damage (heart, kidney) and unless lowering the pressure is necessary to protect these organs, hypertensive encephalopathy is present (neurological dysfunction is reversed when blood pressure is rapidly lowered in this circumstance), intracerebral hemorrhage has occurred, or the patient is receiving anticoagulant medication. In ischemic stroke, blood pressure may be elevated in the acute stage because of increased intracranial pressure, catecholamine release, or sympathetic hyperactivity. The theoretical benefits of lowering blood pressure in acute stroke include (1) reduction of edema, (2) reduced risk of hemorrhagic transformation, and (3) prevention of endothelial wall damage. The theoretical disadvantage of lowering blood pressure is that reduction in perfusion pressure and extension of damage into the ischemic penumbra may result.

3. *Improving blood rheology.* Blood viscosity is predominantly dependent on red blood cell mass and fibrinogen.[32] Because of arterial obstruction, there is stasis, resulting in thrombosis and clot propagation. Fibrinogen may be reduced with defibrinating agents, such as ancrod (see later).[36] Hematocrit reduction by hemodilution is an efficacious technique for blood viscosity reduction. Lowering blood viscosity by 15% increases CBF. Reduced tissue oxygenation is a potential side effect of lowered hematocrit; therefore, the hematocrit should not be lowered below 33%. Hemodilution techniques include (1) isovolemic technique, using a loading dose of dextran followed by phlebotomy; (2) hypervolemic technique, using synthetic starch (hetastarch) followed by phlebotomy (pulmonary wedge pressure and cardiac output should be monitored); and (3) normovolemic technique, using 20% albumin and crystalloid infusion followed by phlebotomy. Clinical trials of hemodilution have not shown efficacy. In isovolemic hemodilution studies, hematocrit reduction frequently was not reached in 24 hours. In hypervolemic studies, volume expansion was achieved before hemodilution developed, and some patients developed cerebral edema and herniation.

Normovolemic hemodilution appears to help if patients are dehydrated or have increased hematocrits, but not in most cases of ischemic stroke. Use of fluids for hemodilution may increase the risk of pulmonary edema and congestive heart failure. Theoretically, pentoxifylline should improve rheology. It improves red blood cell deformability and reduces viscosity (especially at the capillary level). This drug should enhance microcirculation; however, it has not been effective in clinical studies.

4. *Removal of arterial obstruction (revascularization).* This is covered extensively elsewhere in this chapter.

Neuroprotectant Agents

Neurologic deficit after acute arterial obstruction is due to metabolic brain failure. The central core is probably irreversibly damaged, and this triggers a series of metabolic derangements that involve the penumbra. These penumbra neurons are viable but physiologically impaired and therefore unable to maintain synaptic function.

Agents that interrupt the ischemic cascade have been the subject of intense investigation, particularly in the setting of acute ischemic stroke, head trauma with cerebral edema, and postsubarachnoid hemorrhage vasospasm.

The role of cerebral protective agents in acute stroke is a topic of great interest at present. The use of these agents alone, as well as in conjunction with revascularization, is being addressed. The early administration of a neuroprotectant agent may increase the window of opportunity for revascularization and decrease the incidence of complications, such as hemorrhage.[37]

Calcium-Channel Blockers

Immediately after vascular ischemia, calcium influx into cells begins.[38, 39] Cytotoxic free radicals are produced by calcium-activated phospholipases and proteases. Calcium entry into cells occurs after membrane depolarization; this initiates glutamate release. The calcium-channel blocker nimodipine has been shown to be effective in improving the outcome in patients with vasospasm due to subarachnoid hemorrhage. These patients still develop spasm, but nimodipine enables the brain to withstand the ischemia better. In one study of oral nimodipine in acute stroke (30 mg every 6 hours for 28 days), there was reduced morbidity and mortality when therapy was initiated within 24 hours;[32] however, in other studies, nimodipine was not effective.[39] Further studies of calcium channel blockers in acute ischemic stroke are warranted but treatment probably should be initiated within 12 hours and hypotension should be avoided.

Glutamate-Blocking Agents

Calcium entry into ischemic neurons is inhibited by glutamate receptor blockade.[25, 26] Ischemia induces release of L-glutamate, which is an excitatory neurotransmitter. Agents that prevent glutamate receptor activation include (1) calcium-channel antagonists, (2) sodium-channel antagonists (including derivatives of the anticonvulsants lamotrigine and phenytoin), and (3) lubeluzole, which interferes with nitric oxide activity, prevents buildup of extracellular glutamate, and normalizes neuronal excitability (but is not an NMDA receptor antagonist). Lubeluzole has shown promise in reducing stroke mortality. It does not produce microvacuolization within the brain or behavioral toxicity (psychosis, hallucinations), which occur with NMDA receptor antagonists.[40]

An alternative strategy to reducing the glutamate excitatory effect is activation of inhibitory receptors. Drugs that increase postsynaptic inhibition reduce ischemic injury. Adenosine may block glutamate's effect to reduce vascular ischemia. Pentoxifylline is an adenosine agonist and may reverse glutamate's effect on cell membranes. As calcium and sodium enter cells, they cause membrane depolarization. It is possible to hyperpolarize the membrane using γ-aminobutyric acid agonists, such as clomethiazole, to block the excitatory (depolarizing) effect of glutamate.

Free Radical Scavengers

As calcium enters cells, proteases and phospholipases are activated.[41] Formation of free radicals leads to lipid peroxidation with subsequent damage to the blood–brain barrier. The 21-aminosteroids block lipid peroxidation and appear to reduce cerebral edema. The 21-aminosteroid tirilazad (Freedox) is undergoing phase III testing, with promising early results.[42] Superoxide dismutase is another drug that may inhibit free radical formation and has the potential to be effective in reducing ischemic brain injury. Clinical trials are in progress, but efficacy has not yet been demonstrated.

Gangliosides

Gangliosides are part of the neuron membrane.[43] They may act to prevent membrane inositol hydrolysis. In one study, they did not reduce morbidity or improve outcome.

Glucocorticosteroids

Glucocorticosteroids may reduce vasogenic edema and act as free radical scavengers.[44, 45] There is no evidence that they are effective in acute cerebral infarction.

General Measures

When an acute stroke patient has increased intracranial pressure and shows signs of neurologic deterioration, the following treatment measures should be considered:

- Intubation and hyperventilation to PCO_2 of 25 mm Hg. Lowering PCO_2 below 25 mm Hg should be avoided because this may cause worsened vasoconstriction and ischemia.
- Ventriculostomy and CSF drainage using an indwelling ventricular catheter
- Osmotic therapy with mannitol or glycerol
- High-dose barbiturate (pentobarbital) therapy

Cerebral edema may worsen ischemic brain injury because of intracranial hypertension, lowered cerebral perfusion pressure, and brain herniation. Fluids should be restricted to two thirds of maintenance amount, and hypo-osmolar fluids should be avoided.

Factors That May Worsen Neurologic Deficit in Acute Cerebral Ischemia

Many factors may worsen neurologic deficits associated with acute ischemia and should be avoided. These include hyperthermia, hyperglycemia, hypoxia, hypercarbia, seizures, hyponatremia, infection, reduced cardiac output, arrhythmias, and venous thrombosis (risk of pulmonary embolism). These are all general systemic factors that influence the brain's ability to either withstand the insult or better tolerate the ischemia by intrinsic metabolic factors affecting the cells.

Reperfusion Injury

In focal cerebral ischemia, tissue injury correlates with duration and severity of CBF reduction.[46, 47] The hypothesis that reperfusion of brain tissue leads to further tissue damage seems inconsistent with logic. Perhaps reperfusion can cause tissue damage when flow restoration is not adequate to salvage brain tissue or when tissue has been ischemic for a prolonged time, so that it is not possible to reverse the injury after reperfusion has been accomplished. In most cases, tissue reperfusion causes no injury; however, in rare instances, reperfusion has been identified as a possible cause of tissue injury.

If reperfusion causes tissue injury, what are the possible mechanisms?

1. When perfusion is restored, microcirculatory endothelial vascular walls damaged by ischemia may rupture.
2. Reperfusion pressure may result in edema by leakage through damaged endothelial–capillary junctions.
3. Reperfusion can result in calcium influx into cells.
4. Reperfusion increases free radical formation and activation of lipid peroxidation.
5. Reperfusion attracts leukocytes and platelets to enhance leukocyte adherence and vasoconstriction.
6. Leukocyte adherence and vasoconstriction may increase blood viscosity and impair blood rheology. Blood flow in microvascular channels may decrease despite reperfusion through large arteries. This may result in decreased tissue perfusion despite angiographically patent arteries after reperfusion.

It is important to determine whether reperfusion injures brain or whether tissue was irreversibly injured and could not be resuscitated by reperfusion techniques. As clinicians develop reperfusion techniques, it will be important to assess the function (electrophysiology) of the affected brain to assess the severity of cerebral ischemia and help predict salvageability.

REFERENCES

1. Wolf PA, Kannel WB, Verter J. Current status of risk factors for stroke. *Neurol Clin* 1983;1:317–343.
2. Hachinski V, Graffagnino C, Beaudry M. Lipids and stroke: a paradox resolved. *Arch Neurol* 1996;53:303–308.
3. Furberg CD, for the Asymptomatic Carotid Artery Progression Study (ACAPS). Effect of lovastatin on early carotid atherosclerosis and cardiovascular events. *Circulation* 1994;90:1679–1687.
4. Gorelick PB. The status of alcohol as a risk factor for stroke. *Stroke* 1989;20:1607–1610.
5. Wolf PA, Kannel WB. Asymptomatic carotid artery bruit and risk of stroke. *JAMA* 1981;245:1442–1443.
6. Norris JW, Zhu CZ. Silent stroke and carotid stenosis. *Stroke* 1992;23:483–485.
7. Norris JW, Zhu CZ, Chambers BR. Vascular risks of asymptomatic carotid stenosis. *Stroke* 1991;22:1485–1490.
8. Executive Committee for Asymptomatic Carotid Atherosclerosis Study. *JAMA* 1995;273:1421–1428.
9. Toole JF. TIA: scientific method and new realities. *Stroke* 1991;22:99–104.
10. Bogousslavsky J, Regli FF. Cerebral infarction with transient signs. *Stroke* 1984;15:536–539.
11. Koudstaal PJ. TIA with and without a relevant infarct on CT. *Arch Neurol* 1991;48:916–920.
12. Caplan LR. Terms describing brain ischemia by tempo are no longer useful. *Surg Neurol* 1993;40:91–95.
13. Russell RWR. Pathogenesis of transient ischemic attacks. *Neurol Clin* 1983;1:279–290.
14. Caplan LR. Coagulation factors. In Caplan LR (ed): Brain Ischemia. London: Springer-Verlag, 1992, pp. 121–126.
15. Caplan LR, Wolpert SM. Angiography in patients with occlusive cerebrovascular disease. *AJNR* 1991;12:593–603.
16. Polak JF, Kalina P. Carotid endarterectomy: preoperative evaluation. *Radiology* 1993;186:325–333.
17. European Carotid Surgery Trialist Collaborative Group MRC European Surgical Trial in Carotid Stenosis. *Lancet* 1991;337:1235–1242.
18. North American Symptomatic Carotid Endarterectomy Trial Collaborators. Beneficial effect of carotid endarterectomy in symptomatic patients with high-grade carotid stenosis. *N Engl J Med* 1991;325:445–453.
19. Chesbro JH, Fuster V, Elveback LP. Effect of dipyridamole and aspirin on vein-graft patency after coronary bypass operations. *N Engl J Med* 1984;310:209–214.
20. Laupacis A, Albers G, Dalen J. Antithrombotic therapy in atrial fibrillation. *Chest* 1995;108:352(s)–359(s).
21. Pentoxifylline Study Group. Pentoxifylline in acute ischemic stroke. *Stroke* 1987;18:298–305.
22. Sherman DG, Dyken ML, Gent M. Antithrombotic therapy for cerebrovascular disorders. *Chest* 1995;108:444(s)–456(s).
23. The Steering Committee of Physicians Health Study Research Group. Final report on aspirin component of ongoing physician health study. *N Engl J Med* 1989;321:129–135.
24. Siesjo BK. Pathophysiology and treatment of focal cerebral ischemia. *J Neurosurg* 1992;77:169–184.
25. Zivin JA, Choi DW. Stroke therapy. *Sci Am* 1991;14:56–63.
26. Buchan A. Advances in cerebral ischemia. *Neurol Clin* 1992;40:49–57.
27. Hossmann KA. Viability thresholds and the penumbra of focal ischemia. *Ann Neurol* 1994;36:557–565.
28. Choi DW. Excitotoxicity and stroke. In Caplan L (ed): Brain Ischemia. London: Springer-Verlag, 1992, pp. 29–36.
29. O'Brien MD. Ischemic cerebral edema. In Caplan L (ed): Brain Ischemia. London: Springer-Verlag, 1992, pp. 43–50.
30. Powers W. Acute hypertension after stroke: scientific basis for treatment decisions. *Neurology* 1993;43:461–467.
31. Grotta JC. Pharmacologic modification of acute cerebral ischemia. In Barnett HJM (ed): Stroke. New York: Churchill-Livingstone, 1992, pp. 943–951.
32. Hornig CR, Bauer I, Simon C. Hemorrhagic transformation in cardioembolic stroke. *Stroke* 1993;24:465–468.
33. Duke RJ. IV heparin for prevention of stroke progression in acute partial stable stroke. *Ann Intern Med* 1986;105:825–828.
34. Biller J, Massey ED. A dose escalation study of ORG-10172 in stroke. *Neurology* 1989;39:262–268.
35. Grotta JC. Current medical and surgical therapy for cerebrovascular disease. *N Engl J Med* 1987;317:1505–1516.
36. Sherman D. Ancrod for the treatment of acute ischemic stroke. *Ann Neurol* 1993;34:251–256.
37. Aronowski J, Strong R, Grotta JC. Combined neuroprotection and reperfusion therapy for stroke: effect of lubeluzole and diaspirin cross-linked hemoglobin in experimental focal ischemia. *Stroke* 1996;27:1571–1577.
38. The American Nimodipine Study Group. Clinical trial of nimodipine in acute ischemic stroke. *Stroke* 1992;23:3–8.
39. Gelmers HJ, Gorter K, de Weerdt CJ. Controlled trial of nimodipine in acute ischemic stroke. *N Engl J Med* 1988;318:203–207.
40. Dueber HC, Hacks J, Hennerici M. Lubeluzole in acute ischemic stroke. *Stroke* 1996;27:76–81.
41. Southorn PA, Powis G. Free radicals in medicine. *Mayo Clin Proc* 1988;63:381–389.
42. The RANTTAS Investigators. A randomized trial of tirilazad mesylate in patients with acute stroke (RANTTAS). *Stroke* 1996;27:1453–1458.
43. Argentino G. GM ganglioside therapy in acute ischemic stroke. *Stroke* 1989;20:1143–1148.
44. Ropper AH, Shafran B. Brain edema after stroke. *Arch Neurol* 1984;41:26–29.
45. Caronna JJ, Levy DE. Clinical predictors of outcome in ischemic stroke. *Neurol Clin* 1983;1:103–118.
46. Hallenback JM, Butka AJ. Background review and current concepts of reperfusion injury. *Arch Neurol* 1990;47:1245–1254.
47. Hallenback JM, Frerichs KU. Stroke therapy. *Arch Neurol* 1993;50:768–770.

ADDITIONAL READINGS

Cerebral Protection

Alps BJ. Drugs acting on calcium channels: potential treatment for ischaemic stroke. *Br J Clin Pharmac* 1992;34:199–206.
Barinaga M. Finding new drugs to treat stroke. *Science* 1996;272:664–666.
Clemens JA, Saunders RD, Phebus LA, Panetta JA. The antioxidant LY231617 reduces global ischemic neuronal injury in rats. *Stroke* 1993;24:716–723.
Coimbra C, Drake M, Boris-Moller F, Wieloch T. Long-lasting neuroprotective effect of postischemic hypothermia and treatment with an anti-inflammatory/antipyretic drug. Evidence of chronic encephalopathic processes following ischemia. *Stroke* 1996;27:1578–1585.
Leistra HPJM, Dietrich WD. Effect of the histamine antagonist cimetidine on infarct size in the rat. *J Neurotrauma* 1993;10:83–89.
Umemura K, Gemba T, Mizuno A, Nakashima M. Inhibitory effect of MS-153 on elevated brain glutamate level induced by rat middle cerebral artery occlusion. *Stroke* 1996;27:1624–1628.

General

Adams HP Jr, Brott TG, Crowell RM, et al. Guidelines for the management of patients with acute ischemic stroke: a statement for healthcare professionals from a special writing group of the Stroke Council, American Heart Association. *Circulation* 1994;90:1588–1601.

Alberts MJ, Bertels C, Dawson DV. An analysis of time of presentation after stroke. *JAMA* 1990;263:65–68.

Alberts MJ, Perry A, Dawson DV, Bertels C. Effects of public and professional education on reducing the delay in presentation and referral of stroke patients. *Stroke* 1992;23:352–356.

Astrup J, Siesjö BK, Symon L. Thresholds in cerebral ischemia—the ischemic penumbra [Editorial]. *Stroke* 1981;12:723–725.

Besson G, Bogousslavsky J. Medical treatment of acute ischemic stroke. *J Cardiovasc Pharmacol* 1991;18(Suppl 8):S6–S9.

Biller J. Medical management of acute cerebral ischemia. *Neurol Clin* 1992;10:63–85.

Broderick JP, Phillips SJ, Whisnant JP, et al. Incidence rates of stroke in the eighties: the end of the decline in stroke? *Stroke* 1989;20:577–582.

The Canadian Cooperative Study Group. A randomized trial of sulfinpyrazone in threatened stroke. *N Engl J Med* 1978;299:53–59.

Cerebral Embolism Task Force. Cardiogenic brain embolism. *Arch Neurol* 1989;46:727–743.

Chambers BR, Norris JW, Shurvell BL, Hachinski VC. Prognosis of acute stroke. *Neurol* 1987;37:221–225.

Chew W, Kucharczyk J, Moseley M, et al. Hyperglycemia augments ischemic brain injury: in vivo MR imaging/spectroscopic study with nicardipine in cats with occluded middle cerebral arteries. *AJNR* 1991;12:603–609.

Fieschi C, Argentino C, Leni GL, et al. Clinical and instrumental evaluation of patients with ischemic stroke within the first six hours. *J Neurol Sci* 1989;91:311–322.

Fisher CM. The posterior cerebral artery syndrome. *Can J Neurol Sci* 1986;13:232–239.

Fisher CM, Curry HB. Pure motor hemiplegia of vascular origin. *Arch Neurol* 1965;13:30–44.

Garraway WM, Whisnant JP, Furlan AJ, et al. The declining incidence of stroke. *N Engl J Med* 1979;300:449–452.

Gent M, Blakely JA, Easton JD, et al. The Canadian American Ticlopidine Study (CATS) in thromboembolic stroke: design, organization, and baseline results. *Stroke* 1988;19:1203–1210.

Haley EC, Kassell NF, Torner JC. Failure of heparin to prevent progression in progressing ischemic infarction. *Stroke* 1988;19:10–14.

Horowitz DR, Tuhrim S, Weinberger JM, Rudolph SH. Mechanisms in lacunar infarction. *Stroke* 1992;23:325–327.

Jones TH, Morawetz RB, Crowell RM, et al. Thresholds of focal cerebral ischemia in awake monkeys. *J Neurosurg* 1981;54:773–782.

Jovicic A, Ivanisevic V, Nikolajevic R. Circadian variations of platelet aggregability and fibrinolytic activity in patients with ischemic stroke. *Thromb Res* 1991;64:487–491.

Kay R, Wong KS, Yu YL, et al. Low-molecular-weight heparin for the treatment of acute ischemic stroke. *N Engl J Med* 1995;333:1588–1593.

Li P-A, Kristian T, Shamloo M, Siesjo B. Effects of preischemic hyperglycemia on brain damage incurred by rats subjected to 2.5 or 5 minutes of forebrain ischemia. *Stroke* 1996;27:1592–1602.

Lindgren A, Roijer A, Norrving B, et al. Cerebral lesions on magnetic resonance imaging, heart disease, and vascular risk factors in subjects without stroke: a population-based study. *Stroke* 1994;25:929–934.

Marshall RS, Mohr JP. Current management of ischaemic stroke. *J Neurol Neurosurg Psychiatry* 1993;56:6–16.

Meyer JS, Kawamura J, Terayama Y. White matter lesions in the elderly. *J Neurol Sci* 1992;110:1–7.

Nuwer MR, Jordan SE, Ahn SS. Evaluation of stroke using EEG frequency analysis and topographic mapping. *Neurology* 1987;37:1153–1159.

Olsen T. Regional cerebral blood flow after occlusion of the middle cerebral artery. *Acta Neurol Scand* 1986;73:321–337.

Ono N, Koyama T, Suehiro A, et al. Clinical significance of new coagulation and fibrinolytic markers in ischemic stroke patients. *Stroke* 1991;22:1369–1373.

Pantoni L, Garcia JH, Gutierrez JA. Cerebral white matter is highly vulnerable to ischemia. *Stroke* 1996;27:1641–1647.

Rasmussen D, Køhler O, Worm-Petersen S, et al. Computed tomography in prognostic stroke evaluation. *Stroke* 1992;23:506–510.

Slivka A, Levy D. Natural history of progressive ischemic stroke in a population treated with heparin. *Stroke* 1990;21:1657–1662.

Smucker WD, Disabato JA, Krishen AE. Systematic approach to diagnosis and initial management of stroke. *Am Fam Phys* 1995;52:225–234.

Thomas WS, Mori E, Copeland BR, et al. Tissue factor contributes to microvascular defects after focal cerebral ischemia. *Stroke* 1993;24:847–854.

Timsit S, Sacco S, Mohr J, et al. Brain infarction severity differs according to cardiac or arterial embolic source. *Neurology* 1993;43:728–733.

Tohgi H, Kawashima M, Tamura K, Suzuki H. Coagulation-fibrinolysis abnormalities in acute and chronic phases of cerebral thrombosis and embolism. *Stroke* 1990;21:1663–1667.

Wityk RJ, Stern BJ. Ischemic stroke: today and tomorrow. *Crit Care Med* 1994;8:1278–1293.

Transient Ischemic Attacks

Feinberg WM, Albers GW, Barnett HJM, et al. Guidelines for the management of transient ischemic attacks: from the ad hoc committee on guidelines for the management of transient ischemic attacks of the Stroke Council of the American Heart Association. *Stroke* 1994;25:1320–1335.

Nadeau SE. Transient ischemic attacks: diagnosis, and medical and surgical management. *J Fam Pract* 1994;38:495–504.

CHAPTER 55

Cerebral Protection

J.C. Wojak

Cerebral protection refers to protecting the brain from the effects of ischemia. This can be accomplished by decreasing metabolic demand or by interfering with the ischemic cascade. Many different approaches to cerebral protection have been investigated in the past; at the present time, interest has focused on hypothermia and barbiturate therapy (which affect metabolic rate) and various pharmacologic agents that interrupt the ischemic cascade (see Chapter 54).

BARBITURATE THERAPY FOR PRE-EMPTIVE CEREBRAL PROTECTION

Mechanism of Action

The neuroprotective effects of barbiturates are complex. They have a direct effect on cellular metabolic rate and oxygen consumption by decreasing synaptic transmission, neurotransmission, and membrane activity.[1, 2] This effect is dose related until the electroencephalogram (EEG) becomes isoelectric; at this point, further increases in dose do not increase cerebral protection. In addition, there is a decrease in overall cerebral blood flow, producing decreases in cerebral blood volume and thus intracranial pressure. This decrease is not uniform; there is relatively more decrease in normal brain, producing a shunting toward the ischemic regions.[3] Barbiturates may also act as free radical scavengers.[4]

Prophylactic Uses

Barbiturates have been shown to have a protective effect when given prophylactically in a number of settings, particularly before planned temporary focal or global ischemia or irradiation.[1, 3, 5, 6] They have been shown to be more effective than any other anesthetic agent in this regard.[5] Clinically, this technique has been used in the setting of carotid endarterectomy,[3, 7] temporary vessel occlusion during aneurysm clipping,[3] temporary vessel occlusion for extracranial–intracranial bypass,[3, 8, 9] and aneurysm clipping under full cardiac arrest.[3] Barbiturate administration is begun before vessel occlusion and continued until circulation is restored. Barbiturate protection has also been used when unforeseen events necessitate vessel occlusion and revascularization intraoperatively (such as tearing of the neck of an aneurysm during surgery).[8] Barbiturates are administered at the time of occlusion of the vessel and continued until bypass is completed.

No study has evaluated the usefulness of barbiturate therapy as an adjunct to temporary vessel occlusion during endovascular procedures. This approach, however, might be considered in the case of a patient whose treatment optimally uses (or requires) temporary vessel occlusion and who marginally passes test occlusion.

Rationale for Therapeutic Use

The role of barbiturate therapy in the setting of acute focal cerebral ischemia has been investigated in animal models.[10, 11] The results are complex. If therapy was begun within 30 minutes of the onset of occlusion, and if revascularization was successful, then barbiturates appeared to offer nearly complete protection. If the onset of therapy was delayed for 2 hours, there was still a beneficial effect, but increased intracranial pressure and neurologic deficits were observed. If therapy was not begun until 4 hours after onset of ischemia, there was a *detrimental* effect, with worsened intracranial pressure elevation and ischemic damage. If circulation was not restored, then the outcome was worse when barbiturate therapy was used, even when it was initiated within 30 minutes. In all cases, therapy was continued for 96 hours, considered beyond the peak of cerebral edema (and intracranial pressure elevation) after acute ischemia (72 hours).

These studies have significant implications regarding the use of barbiturate therapy as an adjunct to fibrinolytic or mechanical revascularization in patients with acute ischemic stroke. If barbiturate therapy can be instituted within 2 hours of the onset of symptoms, its use may lead to decreased edema and intracranial pressure and may extend the time window for revascularization. If attempts at revascularization are unsuccessful, however, then the use of barbiturate therapy actually may worsen the situation. The use of barbiturates therefore requires careful consideration of the situation.

Technical Aspects of Barbiturate Coma

Intraoperative (Prophylactic) Technique

Thiopental generally is used for intraoperative barbiturate therapy because of its rapid central nervous system uptake. Standard general anesthesia technique is used, with direct arterial pressure and end-tidal CO_2 monitoring. Anesthesia is maintained with nitrous oxide, oxygen, and an inhalation agent such as isoflurane. EEG monitoring with compressed spectral analysis is established before administration of barbiturates. At the appropriate time, bolus doses of thiopental are given intravenously (generally 125 to 250 mg) until burst suppression (15 to 30 seconds) is demonstrated on the compressed spectral analysis of the EEG recording.[7] Thiopental is then continued, either by small boluses or by constant infusion at a rate that maintains burst suppression (this may require anywhere from 0.14 mg/kg/min to 0.63 mg/kg/min[9]). Adequate intravascular volume is maintained, and blood pressure is supported with phenylephrine if needed. Isoflurane administration is decreased or stopped during barbiturate administration.

Barbiturate infusion is stopped when circulation is restored (except in patients in whom barbiturate administration was begun in response to the need to clamp a vessel emergently during surgery; if cerebral edema is expected because of a period of ischemia before establishing barbiturate therapy, then maintaining barbiturate coma during the postoperative period [about 96 hours] should be considered). The use of barbiturate therapy generally results in patients being slower to waken after surgery, they may require intubation for up to 1 hour. Brainstem function and withdrawal to noxious stimuli are still present, however, permitting a rudimentary neurologic examination in the immediate postoperative period.

Barbiturate Coma for Control of Cerebral Edema and Intracranial Pressure

When prolonged administration of barbiturates for the management of cerebral edema and intracranial pressure is used, pentobarbital is generally the agent of choice. It is easier to titrate than thiopental and is associated with a more delayed onset of cardiovascular side effects.[1] The initial loading dose is about 10 mg/kg over 30 minutes (adjusted to maintain mean arterial pressure >70 mm Hg), followed by 5 mg/kg/hr for 3 hours. A maintenance dose of about 2.5 mg/kg/hr is then instituted. This is titrated to maintain burst suppression and intracranial pressure control. Volume expansion and pressor support (dopamine infusion) should be used if needed to maintain adequate mean arterial pressure and cerebral perfusion pressure (mean arterial pressure minus intracranial pressure). Any patient maintained in barbiturate coma should have an arterial line and a Swan-Ganz catheter placed to allow accurate assessment of volume status and cardiovascular function. An intracranial pressure monitor should be inserted, and EEG monitoring should be undertaken. The patient's temperature should be maintained at 33° to 39°C. Intake and output should be carefully monitored.

Neurologic assessment of patients in barbiturate coma is limited. Generally, deep tendon reflexes and brainstem functions are suppressed. However, pupils are generally constricted and nonreactive; a dilated pupil may indicate deterioration and herniation.

HYPOTHERMIA

Temperature has a significant effect on cerebral metabolism. Over the clinically relevant range of temperatures, the relation between change in temperature and change in cerebral metabolic rate of O_2 consumption is about 5% per degree Celsius.[12] Thus, even mild hypothermia (core temperature of 34° to 35°C) results in a 10% to 15% reduction in metabolic demand. Likewise, hyperthermia significantly increases metabolic demand.

The cerebroprotective effect of hypothermia has been used in the surgical approach to giant and other difficult aneurysms. In these cases, prolonged temporary occlusion of the parent vessel is required to decompress the aneurysm and provide adequate exposure to the neck, or otherwise the neck would not be accessible. By combining profound hypothermia with circulatory arrest and cardiopulmonary bypass, collapse of the aneurysm can be achieved, allowing adequate surgical exposure. The time constraints imposed by normothermic temporary vessel occlusion are relaxed in this setting. The major drawbacks to this technique are hematoma formation due to intraoperative heparinization, continued oozing of heparinized blood at the operative site during rewarming (until the patient is no longer on bypass and heparin can be reversed), and the standard problems associated with institution and reversal of cardiopulmonary bypass and circulatory arrest (e.g., arrhythmias).[13, 14]

Although hypothermia is not used in the clinical management of cerebral ischemia, there has been much research on this topic. Early reports demonstrated benefits,[15, 16] but others indicated detrimental effects.[17, 18] More recent studies have shown that even very modest lowering of the temperature of the brain (to about 34°C) can provide significant reduction of ischemic injury, even when the temperature is lowered after the insult.[19–22] For instance, if the middle cerebral artery of the rat is occluded for prolonged periods (90 to 120 minutes), the volume of resultant infarct can be reduced by 50% or more by 2° to 3°C reduction of the brain temperature during ischemia. If this temperature is lowered early and long enough, the damage can be reduced by 70% or more.[23–25] Specifically, when the rat brain was cooled down to 33°C, virtually all neuronal necrosis caused by temporary occlusion of the middle cerebral artery was prevented. This level of hypothermia has been used in the treatment of cerebral edema and increased intracranial pressure in head-injured patients and is relatively easy to achieve clinically with cooling blankets supplemented by iced saline gastric lavage if necessary.[26] Ongoing research may suggest a clinical role for mild hypothermia in the treatment of acute stroke.

Alternatively, even very small increases in brain temperature are markedly deleterious, and efforts should certainly be made to keep patients from becoming hyperthermic from any cause. If brain temperature is raised from 37° to 39°C, the pathologic process of ischemic change is accelerated, there is a marked increase in the size of the injury, and there is blood-brain barrier breakdown.[27, 28] Even when hyperthemia occurs more than 24 hours after the original insult, the eventual damage is greatly increased.[29, 30] It has been shown that a modest increase in temperature has effects similar to an increased duration of ischemia.

REFERENCES

1. Shapiro HM. Barbiturates in brain ischaemia. *Br J Anaesth* 1985;57:82–95.
2. Steen PA, Newberg L, Milde JH, Michenfelder JD. Hypothermia and barbiturates: individual and combined effects on canine cerebral oxygen consumption. *Anesthesiology* 1983; 58:527–532.
3. Spetzler RF, Hadley MN. Protection against cerebral ischemia: the role of barbiturates. *Cerebrovasc Brain Metab Rev* 1989;1:212–229.
4. Flamm ES, Demopoulos HB, Seligman MD, Ransohoff J. Possible molecular mechanisms of barbiturate-mediated protection in regional cerebral ischemia. *Acta Neurol Scand* 1977;56(Suppl. 64):152–153.
5. Nehls DG, Todd MM, Spetzler RF, et al. A comparison of the cerebral protective effects of isoflurane and barbiturates during temporary focal ischemia in primates. *Anesthesiology* 1987;66:453–466.
6. Olson JJ, Friedman R, Orr K, et al. Cerebral radioprotection by pentobarbital: dose-response characteristics and association with GABA agonist activity. *J Neurosurg* 1990;72:749–758.
7. Spetzler RF, Martin N, Hadley MN, et al. Microsurgical endarterectomy under barbiturate protection: a prospective study. *J Neurosurg* 1986;65:63–73.
8. Spetzler RF, Selman WR, Roski RA, Bonstelle C. Cerebral revascularization during barbiturate coma in primates and humans. *Surg Neurol* 1982;17:111–115.
9. Wilkinson E, Spetzler RF, Carter LP, Raudzen PA. Intraoperative barbiturate therapy during temporary vessel occlusion in man. In Cerebral Revascularization for Stroke. New York: Theime-Stratton, 1985, pp. 397–402.
10. Selman WR, Spetzler RF, Roessmann UR, et al. Barbiturate-induced coma therapy for focal cerebral ischemia: effect after temporary and permanent MCA occlusion. *J Neurosurg* 1981;55:220–226.
11. Selman WR, Spetzler RF, Roski RA, et al. Barbiturate coma in focal cerebral ischemia: relationship of protection to timing of therapy. *J Neurosurg* 1982;55:685–690.
12. Siesjö BK. Brain Energy Metabolism. New York: Wiley, 1978.
13. Drake CG. Ligature of the vertebral (unilateral or bilateral) or basilar artery in the treatment of large intracranial aneurysms. *J Neurosurg* 1975;43:255–274.
14. Silverberg GD, Reitz BA, Ream AK. Hypothermia and cardiac arrest in the treatment of giant aneurysms of the cerebral circulation and hemangioblastoma of the medulla. *J Neurosurg* 1981;55:337–346.
15. Frost EA. Brain preservation. *Anesth Analg* 1981;60:821–832.
16. Leonov Y, Sterz F, Safar P, et al. Mild cerebral hypothermia during and after cardiac arrest improves neurologic outcome in dogs. *J Cereb Blood Flow Metab* 1990;10:57–70.
17. Steen PA, Milde JH, Michenfelder JD. The detrimental effects of prolonged hypothermia and rewarming in the dog. *Anesthesiology* 1980;52:224–230.
18. Selman WR, Spetzler RF. Therapeutics for focal ischemia. *Neurosurgery* 1980;6:446–452.
19. Weinrauch V, Safar P, Tisherman S, et al. Beneficial effect of mild hypothermia and detrimental effect of deep hypothermia after cardiac arrest in dogs. *Stroke* 1992;23:1454–1462.
20. Sterz F, Safar P, Tisherman S, et al. Mild hypothermic cardiopulmonary resuscitation improves outcome after prolonged cardiac arrest in dogs. *Crit Care Med* 1991;19:379–389.
21. Minamisawa H, Smith ML, Siesjö BK. The effect of mild hyperthermia and hypothermia on brain damage following 5, 10, and 15 minutes of forebrain ischemia. *Ann Neurol* 1990;28:26–33.
22. Minamisawa H, Nordström CH, Smith ML, Siesjö BK. The influence of mild body and brain hypothermia on ischemic brain damage. *J Cereb Blood Flow Metab* 1990;10:365–374.
23. Zhang RL, Chopp M, Chen H, Garcia JH, Zhang ZG. Postischemic (1 hour) hypothermia significantly reduces ischemic cell damage in rats subjected to 2 hours of middle cerebral artery occlusion. *Stroke* 1993;23:1235–1240.
24. Zhang ZG, Chopp M, Chen H. Duration dependent post-ischemia hypothermia alleviates cortical damage after transient middle cerebral artery occlusion in the rat. *J Neurol Sci* 1993;117:240–244.
25. Karibe H, Chen J, Zarow GJ, Graham SH, Weinstein PR. Delayed induction of mild hypothermia to reduce infarct volume after temporary middle cerebral artery occlusion in rats. *J Neurosurg* 1994;80:112–119.
26. Robertson CS, Cormio M. Cerebral metabolic management. *New Horizons* 1995;3:410–422.
27. Dietrich WD, Busto R, Valdes I, Loor Y. Effects of normothermic versus mild hyperthermic forebrain ischemia in rats. *Stroke* 1990;21:1318–1325.
28. Dietrich WD, Halley M, Valdes I, Busto R. Interrelationships between increased vascular permeability and acute neuronal damage following temperature controlled brain ischemia in rats. *Acta Neuropathol* 1991;81:615–625.
29. Baena RC, Busto R, Dietrich WD, et al. Hyperthermia delayed by 24 hours aggravates neuronal damage in rat hippocampus following global ischemia. *Neurology* 1997;48:768–773.
30. Kim Y, Busto R, Dietrich WD, et al. Delayed postischemia hyperthermia in awake rats worsens the histopathologic outcome of transient focal cerebral ischemia. *Stroke* 1996; 27:2274–2281.

Current Directions in Emergency Stroke Therapy

J.J. Connors III / J.C. Wojak

In the interventional neuroradiology field, current efforts have been directed at revascularization of the area of the brain that may be suffering hemodynamically (e.g., blocked by a clot). In addition, other therapeutic agents, such as neuroprotectant drugs, are being evaluated by neurologists and other clinical specialists involved in the care of stroke patients.

Strategies of neuroprotection that appear to have promise include:

- Therapeutic hypothermia
- Antagonism of neutrophil activation or binding
- Free radical antagonism
    Agents affecting nitric oxide
    21-Aminosteroids
    Superoxide dismutase
- Antagonism of excitatory amino acids
    N-methyl-D-aspartate (NMDA) antagonists
    Non-NMDA antagonists
- Calcium channel antagonism
- Sodium channel antagonism of glutamate release
- Immunosuppressive agents
- Adenosine agonists
- Cytokine receptor antagonists

Classes of pharmaceuticals that are currently being investigated for treatment or prevention of ischemic stroke include:

- Thrombolytic agents (urokinase, prourokinase, tissue-type plasminogen activator [t-PA])
- Fibrinogen depleting agents (ancrod)
- Anticoagulants (warfarin, heparinoids)
- Phospholipid precursor (citicoline)
- Antiplatelet agents (aspirin, clopidogrel; in addition, Integrelin and abciximab are currently being considered for investigation)
- Glutamate or channel blockers (remacemide, glycine site antagonists, nimodipine)
- Voltage-gated channel blockers (lubeluzole, riluzole, fosphenytoin)
- Oxygen radical scavengers (tirilazad)
- Neutrophil activation blockers (anti-ICAM-1)
- Glycine site antagonists (ACEA 1021)

Ultimately, the acute management of stroke patients may involve a combination of these modalities. This discussion is based on the fundamental belief that active endovascular intervention is more effective as acute stroke therapy than the currently available intravenous techniques utilizing t-PA or other fibrinolytic agents.

The delivery of emergency services to these patients requires a degree of cooperation, dedication, and sacrifice by emergency room personnel, nurses, neuroscientists, radiology technologists, transportation personnel, computed tomography (CT) technologists, "stat" laboratory personnel, vascular laboratory technologists, and interventional neuroradiologists. This amount of cooperation and speed, however, may render satisfactory care impossible in many locations.

Emergency personnel will have to recognize the clinical situation and be able to coordinate a rapid assessment, "stat" laboratory work, and a CT scan. Simultaneously, an endovascular therapy laboratory will have to spring into action so that by the time the assessment is done, the laboratory is ready.

This discussion attempts to clarify concepts related to emergent revascularization therapy, but with the clear understanding that the knowledge in this field is inadequate at this time. It is emphasized that this procedure carries a significant risk and should be performed by an operator who is specifically familiar with this procedure, its variable nature of presentation, and the risk-benefit patterns.

Fibrinolytic therapy often reveals the proximate cause of the problem to be an underlying stenotic lesion requiring angioplasty as part of the emergency therapy. The separation of these two treatment modalities is artificial, and depending on clinical and pathophysiologic circumstances, either or both therapeutic responses may be necessary.

EARLY RESULTS OF NEUROPROTECTANT AGENT TRIALS

Lubeluzole

An ongoing clinical trial of the neuroprotectant lubeluzole (Prosynap) is now in its phase III portion. A neuroprotectant is any drug that slows the death of a brain cell caused by hypoxemia. In two trials, both of which were placebo-controlled, phase II, single-blind studies of ischemic stroke patients, the safety and efficacy of this drug was evaluated.

Lubeluzole is a benzothiazole intended to offer neuroprotection in the event of an ischemic event. Its activity is based on the inhibition of the glutamate-activated nitric oxide pathway, on inhibition of the release of glutamate, and on subsequent cell membrane–related effects, such as blockage of voltage-operated Na^+ and Ca^+ channels that may regulate excessive ion shifts (thus causing cell damage). This agent is not an NMDA receptor antagonist.

Both of the phase II trials of lubeluzole were aimed at a population of stroke victims reached within 6 hours of the acute onset of a focal neurologic deficit, fulfilling the criteria for enrollment (described later). Different doses were used over varying periods of time, but the eventual result led to the conclusion that the doses were safe and effective in improving the outcome for a stroke victim, if only modestly.

The late phase II trial gave conflicting results but still seemed to indicate at least a possible beneficial response associated with the use of this agent. The eventual analysis of the data yielded enough positive information to proceed with a phase III trial, which is now underway. The inclusion criteria for this trial include the following:

- The *clinical* diagnosis of a cerebral hemispheric stroke (not angiographic, CT, or otherwise)
- A motor deficit of the arm or leg resulting in a score of >2 on the National Institutes of Health Stroke Scale (NIHSS, a detailed assessment of neurologic function).[1] A detailed version of the NIHSS is given in Table 56–1.
- A total NIHSS score of >7
- Institution of therapy within 6 hours or less, after fulfilling all the supplementary criteria

The exclusion criteria are typical: no major previous stroke, no evidence of intracranial hemorrhage as the cause of the symptoms, no conflicting neurologic findings, no concurrent terminal illness, no heart failure or other severe debilitating condition, and no other experimental stroke treatments.

The initial phase III trial results are promising.[2] Patients with mild to moderate stroke severity who received lubeluzole had a 51% lower risk of dying within the first 3 months than did patients receiving placebo; there was no significant reduction in death rate among patients with severe strokes. Lubeluzole administration also resulted in a 22% increased chance of decreased dependency among patients with mild to moderate strokes.

Clomethiazole

A trial of the neuroprotectant clomethiazole is in progress. This agent has been used for many years as an anticonvulsant, sedative, and hypnotic agent. In addition, it has been used to treat the symptoms of alcohol withdrawal. This drug acts at the γ-amino-butyric acid (GABA) receptor both to potentiate the effects of GABA and to regulate ion-channel openings.

In the initial part of the clinical trial, patients were classified according to the type of insult (total or partial anterior circulation, lacunar, or posterior circulation).[3] They were then randomized to receive either a 24-hour infusion of clomethiazole or placebo. Patients were followed for 3 months, and outcome was assessed using grading systems including the Barthel Index (an assessment of the patient's inde-

pendence in performance of activities of daily living).[4] The initial results indicate that among patients in the total anterior circulation group (large vessel occlusion in the anterior circulation), 40.8% of those receiving clomethiazole attained a Barthel Index score of at least 60, whereas only 29.8% of patients receiving placebo attained this score (a 37% relative improvement). This suggests that clomethiazole is of some benefit in patients with large strokes.

Citicoline

Citicoline acts to reduce free fatty acid accumulation during ischemia and stabilizes cell membranes. It also aids in acetylcholine synthesis. This drug recently underwent a phase III dose-escalation, placebo-controlled, double-blind trial to evaluate its effectiveness in the treatment of acute ischemic stroke. A total of 259 patients with ischemic stroke of less than 24 hours' duration were enrolled. The average time to enrollment was 14 hours. Patients were randomized to receive placebo or citicoline 500 mg/day, 1000 mg/day, or 2000 mg/day for 6 weeks; all patients were followed for an additional 6 weeks.

The primary outcome determinant was improvement in Barthel Index score.[4] Of patients receiving citicoline, 500 mg/day, 53% achieved independence at 12 weeks, as did 33% of patients in the placebo group ($P < 0.04$). The groups receiving 500 and 2000 mg/day demonstrated significantly greater improvement in Barthel Index scores overall than did the placebo group ($P < 0.05$). Recovery was also significantly faster in the treatment groups.

When the Mini-Mental Status examination was used to evaluate patients, a significantly higher number of patients in the 500 and 2000 mg/day groups had normal or near-normal scores than in the placebo group ($P < 0.04$). Patients in the 500 mg/day group were more than twice as likely to have normal scores or minimal residual deficit on the NIHSS than those in the placebo group (34% versus 16%; $P < 0.04$). Scores on the Modified Rankin Scale (a measure of the degree of disability) were significantly improved in the 500 mg/day group when compared with the placebo group.[5]

The group receiving 1000 mg/day failed to show statistically significant improvement. One possible explanation is that the patients randomized to this group had a statistically significant higher mean body weight than the other groups, which may have led to significantly lower drug concentrations.

A small subgroup of patients were studied with various imaging techniques. The results imply that citicoline acts to reduce infarct size.

There was no significant difference in mortality between the groups. Among the reported adverse effects, the only statistically significant difference between the groups was an increased incidence of dizziness and falls in the patients receiving citicoline; this did not reach statistical significance in the 500 mg/day group.

The conclusions reached as a result of this trial

T A B L E 5 6 - 1 **Detailed Version of the NIH Stroke Scale**

Administer stroke scale items in the order listed. Record performance in each category after each subscale exam. Do not go back and change scores. Follow directions provided for each exam technique. Scores should reflect what the patient does, not what the clinician thinks the patient can do. The clinician should record answers while administering the exam and work quickly. Except where indicated, the patient should not be coached (i.e., repeated requests to patient to make a special effort).

If any item is left untested, an explanation must be clearly given in the discharge summary. All untested items will be reviewed by the medical monitor and discussed with the examiner.

Instruction	Scale Definition
1a. Level of Consciousness: The investigator must choose a response, even if a full evaluation is prevented by such obstacles as an endotracheal tube, language barrier, orotracheal trauma/bandages. A 3 is scored only if the patient makes no movement (other than reflexive posturing) in response to noxious stimulation.	0 = Alert; keenly responsive. 1 = Not alert, but arousable by minor stimulation to obey, answer, or respond. 2 = Not alert, requires repeated stimulation to attend, or is obtunded and requires strong or painful stimulation to make movements (not stereotyped). 3 = Responds only with reflex motor or autonomic effects, or totally unresponsive, flaccid, areflexic.
1b. LOC Questions: The patient is asked the month and his/her age. The answer must be correct—there is no partial credit for being close. Aphasic and stuporous patients who do not comprehend the questions will score 2. Patients unable to speak because of endotracheal intubation, orotracheal trauma, severe dysarthria from any cause, language barrier or any other problem not secondary to aphasia are given a 1. It is important that only the initial answer be graded and that the examiner not "help" the patient with verbal or non-verbal cues.	0 = Answers both questions correctly. 1 = Answers one question correctly. 2 = Answers neither question correctly.
1c. LOC Commands: The patient is asked to open and close the eyes and then to grip and release the nonparetic hand. Substitute another one-step command if the hands cannot be used. Credit is given if an unequivocal attempt is made but not completed due to weakness. If the patient does not respond to command, the task should be demonstrated to them (pantomime) and the result scored (i.e., follows none, one, or two commands). Patients with trauma, amputation, or other physical impediments should be given suitable one-step commands. Only the first attempt is scored.	0 = Performs both tasks correctly. 1 = Performs one task correctly. 2 = Performs neither task correctly.
2. Best Gaze: Only horizontal eye movements will be tested. Voluntary or reflexive (oculocephalic) eye movements will be scored but caloric testing is not done. If the patient has a conjugate deviation of the eyes that can be overcome by voluntary or reflexive activity, the score will be 1. If a patient has an isolated peripheral nerve paresis (CN III, IV, or VI) score a 1. Gaze is testable in all aphasic patients. Patients with ocular trauma, bandages, preexisting blindness or other disorder of visual acuity or fields should be tested with reflexive movements and a choice made by the investigator. Establishing eye contact and then moving about the patient from side to side will occasionally clarify the presence of a gaze palsy.	0 = Normal 1 = Partial gaze palsy. This score is given when gaze is abnormal in one or both eyes, but where forced deviation or total gaze paresis is not present. 2 = Forced deviation, or total gaze paresis not overcome by the oculocephalic maneuver
3. Visual: Visual fields (upper and lower quadrants) are tested by confrontation, using finger counting or visual threat as appropriate. Patient must be encouraged, but if they look at the side of the moving fingers appropriately, this can be scored as normal. If there is unilateral blindness or enucleation, visual fields in the remaining eye are scored. Score 1 only if a clear-cut asymmetry, including quadrantanopia, is found. If patient is blind from any cause score 3. Double simultaneous stimulation is performed at this point. If there is extinction patient receives a 1 and the results are used to answer question 11.	0 = No visual loss. 1 = Partial hemianopia. 2 = Complete hemianopia. 3 = Bilateral hemianopia (blind including cortical blindness).

Table continued on following page

T A B L E 5 6 - 1   Detailed Version of the NIH Stroke Scale *Continued*

Instruction	Scale Definition
4. Facial Palsy: Ask, or use pantomime to encourage the patient to show teeth or smile and close eyes. Score symmetry of grimace in response to noxious stimuli in the poorly responsive or non-comprehending patient. If facial trauma/bandages, orotracheal tube, tape, or other physical barrier obscures the face, these should be removed to the extent possible.	0 = Normal symmetrical movement. 1 = Minor paralysis (flattened nasolabial fold, asymmetry on smiling). 2 = Partial paralysis (total or near total paralysis of lower face). 3 = Complete paralysis (absence of facial movement in the upper and lower face).

5 & 6. Motor Arm and Leg:
The limb is placed in the appropriate position: extend the arms 90 degrees (if sitting) or 45 degrees (if supine) and the leg 30 degrees (always tested supine). Drift is scored if the arm falls before 10 seconds or the leg before 5 seconds. The aphasic patient is encouraged using urgency in the voice and pantomime but not noxious stimulation. Each limb is tested in turn, beginning with the nonparetic arm. Only in the case of amputation or joint fusion at the shoulder or hip may the score be "9" and the examiner must clearly write the explanation for scoring as a "9."
	0 = No drift, arm holds 90 (or 45) degrees for full 10 seconds.
	1 = Drift, arm holds 90 (45) degrees, but drifts down before full 10 seconds; does not hit bed or other support.
	2 = Some effort against gravity, arm cannot get to or maintain (if cued) 90 (or 45) degrees, drifts down to bed, but has some effort against gravity.
	3 = No effort against gravity, arm falls.
	4 = No movement.
	9 = Amputation, joint fusion.
	   explain:
	   5a = Left Arm
	   5b = Right Arm

	0 = No drift, leg holds 30 degrees position for full 5 seconds.
	1 = Drift, leg falls by the end of the 5 second period but does not hit bed.
	2 = Some effort against gravity, leg falls to bed by 5 seconds, but has some effort against gravity.
	3 = No effort against gravity, leg falls to bed immediately.
	4 = No movement.
	9 = Amputation, joint fusion.
	   explain:
	   6a = Left Leg
	   6b = Right Leg

7. Limb Ataxia:
This item is aimed at finding evidence of a unilateral cerebellar lesion. Tests with eyes open. In case of visual defect, ensure testing is done in intact visual field. The finger-nose-finger and heel-shin tests are performed on both sides, and ataxia is scored only if present out of proportion to weakness. Ataxia is absent in the patient who cannot understand or is hemiplegic. Only in the case of amputation or joint fusion may the item be scored "9," and the examiner must clearly write the explanation for not scoring. In case of blindness, test by touching nose from extended arm position.
	0 = Absent.
	1 = Present in one limb.
	2 = Present in two limbs.
	If present, is ataxia in
	   Right arm 1 = Yes 2 = No
	      9 = amputation or joint fusion.
	      explain:
	   Left arm 1 = Yes 2 = No
	      9 = amputation or joint fusion.
	      explain:
	   Right leg 1 = Yes 2 = No
	      9 = amputation or joint fusion.
	      explain:
	   Left leg 1 = Yes 2 = No
	      9 = amputation or joint fusion.
	      explain:

8. Sensory: Sensation or grimace to pinprick when tested, or withdrawal from noxious stimulus in the obtunded or aphasic patient. Only sensory loss attributed to stroke is scored as abnormal and the examiner should test as many body areas [arms (not hands), legs, trunk, face] as needed to accurately check for hemisensory loss. A score of 2, "severe or total," should only be given when a severe or total loss of sensation can be clearly demonstrated. Stuporous and aphasic patients will therefore probably score 1 or 0. The patient with brainstem stroke who has bilateral loss of sensation is scored 2. If the patient does not respond and is quadriplegic, score 2. Patients in coma (item la = 3) are arbitrarily given a 2 on this item.	0 = Normal; no sensory loss. 1 = Mild to moderate sensory loss; patient feels pinprick is less sharp or is dull on the affected side; or there is a loss of superficial pain with pinprick but patient is aware he/she is being touched. 2 = Severe to total sensory loss; patient is not aware of being touched.

T A B L E 5 6 - 1 **Detailed Version of the NIH Stroke Scale** *Continued*

Instruction	Scale Definition
9. Best Language: A great deal of information about comprehension will be obtained during the preceding sections of the examination. The patient is asked to describe what is happening in the attached picture, to name the items on the attached list of sentences. Comprehension is judged from responses here as well as to all of the commands in the preceding general neurological exam. If visual loss interferes with the tests, ask the patient to identify objects placed in the hand, repeat, and produce speech. The intubated patient should be asked to write. The patient in coma (question 1a = 3) will arbitrarily score 3 on this item. The examiner must choose a score in the patient with stupor or limited cooperation but a score of 3 should be used only if the patient is mute and follows no one-step commands.	0 = No aphasia, normal. 1 = Mild to moderate aphasia; some obvious loss of fluency or facility of comprehension, without significant limitation on ideas expressed or form of expression. Reduction of speech and/or comprehension, however, makes conversation about provided material difficult or impossible. For example, in conversation about provided materials examiner can identify picture or naming card from patient's response. 2 = Severe aphasia; all communication is through fragmentary expression; great need for inference, questioning, and guessing by the listener. Range of information that can be exchanged is limited; listener carries burden of communication. Examiner cannot identify materials provided from patient response. 3 = Mute, global aphasia; no usable speech or auditory comprehension.
10. Dysarthria: If the patient is thought to be normal, an adequate sample of speech must be obtained by asking patient to read or repeat words from the attached list. If the patient has severe aphasia, the clarity of articulation of spontaneous speech can be rated. Only if the patient is intubated or has other physical barrier to producing speech may the item be scored "9," and the examiner must clearly write an explanation for not scoring. Do not tell the patient why he/she is being tested.	0 = Normal. 1 = Mild to moderate; patient slurs at least some words and, at worst, can be understood with some difficulty. 2 = Severe; patient's speech is so slurred as to be unintelligible in the absence of or out of proportion to any dysphasia, or is mute/anarthric. 9 = Intubated or other physical barrier. explain:
11. Extinction and Inattention (formerly Neglect): Sufficient information to identify neglect may be obtained during the prior testing. If the patient has severe visual loss preventing visual double simultaneous stimulation, and the cutaneous stimuli are normal, the score is normal. If the patient has aphasia but does appear to attend to both sides, the score is normal. The presence of visual spatial neglect or anosagnosia may also be taken as evidence of neglect. Since neglect is scored only if present, the item is never untestable.	0 = No abnormality. 1 = Visual, tactile, auditory, spatial, or personal inattention or extinction to bilateral simultaneous stimulation in one of the sensory modalities. 2 = Profound hemi-inattention or hemi-inattention to more than one modality. Does not recognize own hand or orients to only one side of space.
12. Distal Motor Function: The patient's hand is held up at the forearm by the examiner and the patient is asked to extend his/her fingers as much as possible. If the patient can't or doesn't extend the fingers the examiner places the fingers in full extension and observes for any flexion movement for 5 seconds. The patient's first attempts only are scored. Repetition of the instructions, or of the testing, is prohibited.	0 = Normal (no flexion after 5 seconds). 1 = At least some extension after 5 seconds, but not fully extended. Any movement of the fingers that is not to command is not scored. 2 = No voluntary extension after 5 seconds. Movements of the fingers at another time are not scored. a. Left arm. b. Right arm.

were that citicoline produces a statistically significant improvement in recovery of patients from acute ischemic stroke and that the window of treatment is 24 hours. The drug is given orally and is well-tolerated. At a dose of 500 mg/day, it is both safe and probably effective. In addition, there is evidence of a decrease in size of infarct volume in citicoline-treated patients.

An additional trial was then undertaken to assess the efficacy of citicoline, using the 500 mg dose.[6] Patients with acute (24 hours or less) middle cerebral artery strokes and NIHSS scores of 5 or greater were randomized to receive either citicoline or placebo for 6 weeks. There was a significant improvement in full recovery (Barthel Index ≥95) associated with citicoline administration among patients with baseline NIHSS scores of 8 or greater (33%, compared with 21% of patients receiving placebo). There was no significant difference among patients with baseline

NIHSS scores <8. Citicoline, like clomethiazole, may be beneficial in patients with moderate to large strokes.

Other Neuroprotectant Agents in or Nearing Clinical Trials

Several other potentially neuroprotective drugs are either in clinical trial or nearing trial. These agents act at varying levels to halt the ischemic cascade. These include the NMDA receptor ion-channel blocker aptinogel (Cerestat), the NMDA receptor glycine-site blockers ZD9379 and GV150-526A, the sodium-channel blockers fosphenytoin (Cerebyx) and BW619C89, the calcium-channel blocker SNX-111, and the free radical scavenger tirilazad (Freedox).[7] Others include prostaglandins, estrogen, nalmefine, selfotel and several other nitric oxide–supplying compounds, and several other NMDA-receptor antagonists.

These trials appear to indicate at least a possibility of some neuroprotectant effect. This is good for interventional neuroradiology. As those in this field know, the true cure for an occlusive stroke is revascularization, but time to treatment is critical. Any drug that may be able to yield a few more minutes (or hours!) during which definitive endovascular revascularization can be performed safely is welcomed with open arms. It is the general feeling of the interventional neuroradiology community, however, that a neuroprotectant drug alone, without a timely re-establishment of blood flow, will have only limited effect. It is hoped that this belief may be at least partially incorrect.

FIBRINOLYTIC AGENTS

Several different types of fibrinolytic agents are available, with relatively similar properties. These can be divided into those of endogenous origin and those manufactured artificially (or by bacteria or similar means). Agents normally present in the human body include urokinase, tissue plasminogen activator (t-PA), and prourokinase. Exogenous agents include streptokinase, acylated plasminogen streptokinase activator complex (APSAC), and other variants.

All currently available fibrinolytics work by converting plasminogen to plasmin. It would be nice to have bottled plasmin, but it does not store well. Plasmin is the active agent that cleaves fibrin (as well as fibrinogen, and other clotting factors). Too much plasmin can yield a deficiency of these other substances that can result in a systemic anticoagulant effect. There has been much concern and debate concerning the implications of the systemic lytic effect of the various fibrinolytic agents. Nonstatistical analysis, however, appears to indicate that this effect does not predict efficacy or danger of therapy.

Streptokinase

Streptokinase is an exogenous activator of the fibrinolytic system. It is an enzyme produced by *Streptococcus hemolyticus*, which activates plasminogen by complex kinetics. Circulating plasmin, fibrin-associated plasmin, and streptokinase–plasmin complexes are formed, all of which are capable of cleaving fibrin and fibrinogen.[8] Streptokinase is not fibrin specific. This agent was used in several early studies but has largely been replaced by urokinase and newer agents because of multiple problems, including a high rate of hypersensitivity reactions, inactivation of the enzyme by antistreptococcal antibodies, and difficulties with dose-rate adjustments as a result of the complex kinetics.

Urinary-type Plasminogen Activator

At least two physiologic activators of the fibrinolytic system are found in human plasma. One is urinary-type (urokinase and prourokinase) and the second is tissue-type plasminogen activator; the latter is described in a separate section.

Urokinase

Urokinase is a glycoprotein isolated from renal tissue and urine. It converts plasminogen to plasmin by first-order kinetics, and its thrombolytic activity is not fibrin specific.[8] It is available from cell culture and other sources and has been shown to be effective at all forms of thrombolytic therapy. Its half-life is on the order of 9 to 12 minutes, and because it is an endogenous enzyme, it does not yield an immune response.

One million international units of urokinase is equivalent to about 10 mg of t-PA.

Prourokinase

Prourokinase (Prolyse) is a recombinant single-chain form of urokinase. It is converted to urokinase by hydrolysis of a peptide bond (lysine[158]–isoleucine[159]) by plasmin. Prourokinase preferentially activates fibrin-bound plasminogen. The plasmin formed as a result locally activates more prourokinase. This activation cycle is localized primarily to the clot surface. Theoretically, this drug should have less systemic fibrinolytic activity than urokinase or streptokinase.[9] It is currently undergoing clinical evaluation (discussed later).

Tissue-type Plasminogen Activator

Tissue-type plasminogen activator (or t-PA) is an enzyme that converts plasminogen to plasmin. It is found in human plasma but is available in recombinant form (Activase).

The capacity of t-PA to convert plasminogen to plasmin strongly depends on the presence of fibrin; there is about a 100-fold increase in the speed of this conversion if the plasminogen is bound to fibrin as opposed to circulating freely.[10] It is also activated by binding to specific sites on platelet membranes and soluble fibrin-degradation products. As with prourokinase, this should result in limited systemic fibrinolysis. This topic is discussed further, later.

Ancrod

Ancrod is the principal active ingredient of the venom of the Malayan pit viper. It cleaves fibrinogen and results in a circulating ancrod–fibrin product that appears to stimulate the release of t-PA from vessel walls. This would appear to give a generalized fibrinolytic effect, but only rarely does it lead to any bleeding complications.[11, 12] It cannot be given rapidly because of its potential to cause generalized fibrinogen breakdown and so is administered slowly intravenously. A double-blind, placebo-controlled trial in 1990 showed its fibrinolytic ability as well as a positive influence on the outcome of stroke patients, even though it was administered at an unknown time after the ischemic insult and daily thereafter for 6 days. Proof of its fibrinolytic activity was shown by serial hematologic tests. The Scandinavian Stroke Score improvement for severe strokes measured at 90 days was three times greater in the ancrod group than in the placebo group.[13]

Acylated Plasminogen Streptokinase Activator Complex

Acylated plasminogen streptokinase activator complex (APSAC) is an acylated combination of streptokinase and human plasminogen. The acyl group protects the plasminogen until hydrolytic activation in the presence of fibrin. This delay in activity would appear to prolong its activity slightly over that of streptokinase alone. Its lytic effect has been shown to be greater than that of streptokinase as well.[14] APSAC has been shown to be effective in recanalization of coronary arteries in the treatment of acute myocardial infarction.[15]

Because of the presence of streptokinase, the possibility of allergic reaction to APSAC exists, as does the possibility that the drug may not be maximally effective secondary to being bound by antistreptococcal antibodies.

Other Artificial Fibrinolytic Agents

Numerous other combinations of streptokinase, t-PA, prourokinase, antifibrin antibodies, and other related agents are being developed. No large-scale studies have been performed, and there is no indication that any of these agents is better than those available.

RESULTS OF EARLY INTRAVENOUS FIBRINOLYTIC THERAPIES

Numerous trials have been performed over the years attempting to benefit the patient having an acute ischemic infarct. These trials have used fibrinolytics, anticoagulants, volume expanders, and neuroprotectants. Amazingly, urokinase was used intravenously for treatment of acute stroke at least as far back as 1960. Hanaway et al.[16] reported its use in four patients treated between 1972 and 1975 who had acute neurologic deficits; at that time, however, it was not possible to determine accurately whether the insult was hemorrhagic. Additionally, neither the correct dose of urokinase, nor the optimal time frame for treatment, was known.

After the advent of CT, intravenous studies have been carried out using streptokinase, t-PA (most commonly), and urokinase.

Intravenous Tissue-Type Plasminogen Activator

Only one prior study[17] hinted at the possibility of rapid recanalization at any dose range for any fibrinolytic agent administered intravenously (until the National Institute of Neurological Disorders and Stroke [NINDS] trial, discussed later). This study used cerebral blood flow measurements with later confirmation by angiography; there was no direct demonstration of effectiveness. Patients with acute ischemic stroke received 100 mg of t-PA over 1 hour, begun within 78 to 355 minutes after onset of symptoms.[17] Regional cerebral blood flow was measured using ^{99m}Tc-HMPAO single-photon emission computed tomography before and after treatment, with later correlation with angiography. The second scan was performed as late as 24 hours after the insult, thus reducing the validity of a direct relation between t-PA administration and recanalization as well as its speed of action. There was an indication of increased recanalization in the t-PA group in this study.

At least three separate intravenous dose regimens were evaluated by the National Institutes of Health in the Very Early rt-PA Study.[18] Seventy-four patients were treated within 90 minutes of the acute neurologic insult. Increased dosage, up to 87 mg, was not associated with any clinical benefit.

At least three studies using angiography for evaluation of occlusion with administration of t-PA from a peripheral intravenous location have been performed. Mori et al.[19] reported on 31 patients randomly assigned to one of three groups and given placebo, 20 mega-international units (MIU) of t-PA, or 30 MIU of t-PA. Reperfusion appeared to be more common in the t-PA group, but was less than 50%, and the difference was not statistically significant. Three of 12 placebo patients (25%) also had early recanalization, not much different from the t-PA–treated group reported below by von Kummer and Hacke[20] using 100 mg t-PA (34%).

Del Zoppo et al. (the rt-PA/Acute Stroke Study Group)[21] reported on a dose-escalation trial of peripherally administered t-PA. Of 139 patients, 80% had complete occlusion of the primary vessel of concern at a mean of 5.4 hours after the neurologic insult. No relation between dose and recanalization was observed in 93 patients who completed the t-PA infusion. Middle cerebral artery (MCA) branch occlusion was more likely to undergo recanalization than internal carotid artery (ICA) occlusion. Of interest, there appeared to be no relation between recanalization and subsequent hemorrhagic transformation. The study appeared to indicate that site of occlusion, time to treatment, and response to treatment (i.e., recanalization) were the important factors.

Of 93 patients with an angiographically proven occlusion, only 4 had complete recanalization; only 28 patients had any recanalization at all. These are astounding numbers for the only study with direct evidence of vascular occlusion and direct evaluation of the efficacy of intravenous t-PA therapy.

Von Kummer and Hacke[20] reported on the intravenous administration of 100 mg t-PA in 32 patients, with angiographic monitoring of the occlusion. Recanalization was assessed by digital subtraction angiography and transcranial Doppler ultrasound immediately after treatment and again with a third angiogram 12 to 24 hours later. Complete or partial reperfusion was achieved in only 34% of patients at 90 minutes and in 53% within 12 to 24 hours. Good clinical outcome, however, correlated with reperfusion and the presence of good collateral flow. In agreement with other studies, it was possible to achieve reperfusion in distal MCA branches more frequently than in main trunk M1 occlusions. Of eight patients with M1 occlusions and distal ICA occlusions (thus effectively lowering hemispheric perfusion other than through the anterior communicating artery), seven died.

Australian Streptokinase Trial

The Australian Streptokinase Trial was designed to evaluate the safety and efficacy of intravenous streptokinase in the treatment of acute ischemic stroke. Patients who presented within the first 4 hours after the onset of symptom, who had no evidence of bleeding or infarction on CT scan, and who had no contraindications to thrombolysis were randomized to receive placebo or 1.5 million units of intravenous streptokinase over 60 minutes.[22] Patients were assessed using the Modified Canadian Neurological Score (a measurement of neurological function)[23] and the Barthel Index.[4] The study was terminated because of the unacceptably high rate of hemorrhagic transformation and hematoma formation, with a high rate of fatal hematomas.[24, 25]

Multicenter Acute Stroke Trial—Europe (MAST-E)

The MAST-E study was designed to evaluate the efficacy and safety of intravenous streptokinase in the treatment of acute ischemia in the territory of the MCA.[26] Patients were randomly assigned to receive streptokinase (1.5 million units over 1 hour) or placebo. All patients were treated within 6 hours of the onset of symptoms. Outcome was determined by the presence or absence of death or severe disability at 6 months, using the Rankin scale.[5] In the study, 156 patients received streptokinase and 154 received placebo. There was no significant difference in Rankin scale between the treated and untreated groups; however, the mortality rate was higher in the treated group at 10 days and at 6 months, mostly because of hemorrhagic transformation, and the trial was halted.

European Cooperative Acute Stroke Study (ECASS)

This study enrolled 620 patients with acute ischemic stroke who presented within 6 hours of onset of symptoms.[27] All patients had moderate to severe neurologic deficit at presentation. The patients were randomly assigned to two groups; one received placebo, and the other received intravenous t-PA (1.1 mg/kg,

of which 10% was given as a bolus and the rest given over 60 minutes; the maximal dose was 100 mg). No anticoagulant, antiplatelet, cerebroprotective, or volume-expanding agents were administered during the first 24 hours. Outcome was measured at 90 days using the Modified Rankin Scale[5] and the Barthel Index.[4]

Major protocol violations were uncovered involving 17% of patients enrolled, leaving 511 patients who actually met the entry criteria ("target population"). The study data were analyzed with respect to the entire study population as well as the group who satisfied the entry criteria. There was a significant difference in the Modified Rankin Scale scores between the t-PA and placebo groups, but only when the target population alone was evaluated (2 versus 3, $P = 0.035$). Speed of neurologic improvement was greater in the t-PA group when either population was analyzed; this difference was significant up to 7 days in the study population and up to 30 days in the target population. Patients receiving t-PA were hospitalized an average of 17 days, compared with 21 days for the patients who received placebo.

Although the results indicated a potential beneficial effect of t-PA, there was a down side. The 30-day mortality rates were 17.9% in the t-PA group and 12.7% in the placebo group, but this difference was not found to be statistically significant. Although the total incidence of intracranial hemorrhage was the same for the t-PA and placebo groups, the incidence of different types of hemorrhage in each group differed significantly. The incidence of hemorrhagic conversion of infarct was higher in the placebo group (29.9% versus 24.3%, $P < 0.001$ in the target population), whereas frank parenchymal hemorrhage or hematoma occurred more frequently in the patients treated with t-PA (19.4% versus 6.8%, target population).

The investigators came to the conclusion that, although t-PA administration improved some functional measures in properly selected patients, the degree of improvement did not outweigh the risk of increased mortality and parenchymal hemorrhage.

Retrospective evaluation of the results of the ECASS trial revealed that there is a very wide range in the results and risks of fibrinolytic therapy. If a stroke involved more than one third of the MCA territory, the mortality rate for treatment was 24%, compared with a rate of only 4% if the stroke involved less than one third of the MCA territory. If there was CT evidence of edema, the mortality rate associated with therapy was 17%, compared with only 2% if there was no evidence of edema. It should be noted that CT evidence of edema is far more common in patients evaluated more than 3 hours after the acute event than in those studied in less than 3 hours.

NATIONAL INSTITUTE OF NEUROLOGICAL DISORDERS AND STROKE TISSUE-TYPE PLASMINOGEN ACTIVATOR STROKE TRIAL

The NINDS t-PA Stroke Trial was a two-part, randomized, double-blind, placebo-controlled trial evaluating the safety and efficacy of t-PA in the treatment of acute stroke.[28] Criteria for enrollment included clinical evidence of ischemic stroke based on the presence of a measurable deficit on the NIHSS (see Table 56–1),[1] absence of hemorrhage on CT scan, and presentation and treatment within 180 minutes. Exclusion criteria included stroke or head trauma within the previous 3 months, previous intracranial hemorrhage, systolic blood pressure > 185 mm Hg or diastolic blood pressure > 110 mm Hg despite standard therapy, and seizure associated with the onset of symptoms.

Patients who met the criteria and were enrolled received either placebo or 0.9 mg/kg of intravenous t-PA (10% as a bolus and the remainder over 60 minutes, up to a maximum of 90 mg). Patients were further stratified by time to treatment (0 to 90 minutes and 91 to 180 minutes). A total of 624 patients were enrolled. Of these, 291 were in part 1 of the study, and 333 were in part 2. Part 1 was designed to assess the 24-hour results (efficacy); the criteria for favorable outcome were complete resolution of neurologic deficit or improvement of 4 or more points on the NIHSS.

Even though there was *no efficacy demonstrated* in part 1, a retrospective analysis appeared to show some benefit in 3 months. Therefore, part 2 was designed to study the outcome at 3 months rather than any benefit in 24 hours, based on four separate measures. These included the Barthel Index,[4] the Modified Rankin Scale,[5] the NIHSS, and the Glasgow Outcome Scale (a global assessment of function).[29] The scales were arbitrarily stratified to identify patients with favorable outcomes, which included patients with complete independence and minimal or no deficit. In both part 1 and part 2, results were analyzed as a function of time to treatment (0 to 90, 91 to 180, and 0 to 180 minutes). Additionally, factors such as mortality, intracranial bleeding and systemic bleeding were evaluated.

The results of part 2 demonstrated that the t-PA group included significantly more patients with favorable outcomes across all four indices, but only at 3 months (50% versus 38% on the Barthel Index [$P = 0.026$], 39% versus 26% on the Modified Rankin Scale [$P = 0.019$], 44% versus 32% on the Glasgow Outcome Scale [$P = 0.025$], and 31% versus 20% on the NIHSS [$P = 0.033$]). This improvement was constant across age, baseline stroke type, stroke severity, and use of aspirin (this is discussed further below; aspirin and streptokinase have been shown to be a deadly combination). There was no statistically significant difference in mortality rates between the placebo and t-PA groups (21% placebo versus 17% t-PA).

When the patients in parts 1 and 2 were combined, early (presenting within 36 hours) symptomatic intracranial hemorrhage was far more common in the t-PA group (6.4% versus 0.6%, $P < 0.001$), but the incidence still was not overwhelmingly high. After 36 hours, another 1.3% of t-PA and 0.6% of placebo patients developed symptomatic intracranial hemor-

rhage. Patients who developed early symptomatic hemorrhage had a higher mean NIHSS score at presentation (more severe deficit) than those who did not (20 versus 14). These patients also had a higher incidence of cerebral edema on the baseline CT scan (9% versus 4%). This makes intellectual sense; areas with a more severe depth of ischemia would be more prone to hemorrhage.

Asymptomatic intracranial "hemorrhage" (not intraparenchymal hematoma) was noted in 4.5% of t-PA patients and 2.9% of placebo patients. There was no significant difference in the incidence of major systemic bleeding. Minor external bleeding within 10 days of treatment was seen in 23% of t-PA patients and 3% of placebo patients.

The overall results indicate that carefully selected patients who present with signs and symptoms of ischemic stroke of 3 hours' duration or less who receive intravenous t-PA have at least a 30% increased likelihood of favorable outcome in 3 months compared with untreated patients, without increased mortality. This is actually an absolute increase in favorable outcome of about 11% to 14%. Although there is an increase in the incidence of symptomatic intracranial hemorrhage, the mortality or residual deficit in surviving patients was included in the outcome analysis using each of the four indices; the improvements described above are overall figures for each group, including those patients with bleeds. As a result of the findings of this study, t-PA received Food and Drug Administration approval for intravenous administration within 3 hours of the onset of symptoms of an acute stroke. The exclusion criteria for treatment remain unchanged, and the recommended dose is, as given previously, 0.9 mg/kg (10% as a bolus and the remainder over 60 minutes).

The effect of t-PA administration on infarct volume was analyzed separately.[30] The median infarct volume at 3 months after treatment in patients receiving t-PA was 15.5 cm³; the median infarct volume in patients receiving placebo was 25.5 cm³ ($P = .039$).

In separate analysis, patients enrolled in the study were reassessed at 6 months and 1 year, using the Barthel Index, Modified Rankin Scale, and Glasgow Outcome Scale.[31] The patients in the t-PA group demonstrated a sustained benefit and were 30% more likely to have a favorable outcome at 1 year.

Analysis of Results

The results of part 1 indicated a trend toward better outcome at 24 hours in the t-PA group based on the study criteria, although this did not reach statistical significance. In fact, analysis of the actual data indicates that it is *only* the 0- to 90-minute group that actually benefited within 24 hours from the time of onset. The 91- to 180-minute group showed essentially no benefit in 24 hours. These results are summarized in Table 56–2.

Early Improvement Associated With Thrombolytic Therapy

This raises an interesting point. Although the results of the NINDS trial of intravenous t-PA demonstrated

T A B L E 5 6 - 2 **Percentage of Patients with Four-Point Improvement on the National Institutes of Health Stroke Scale in the National Institute of Neurological Disorders and Stroke Tissue Plasminogen Activator Trial***

Trial Part	Time to Treatment From Onset of Symptoms (min)	Percentage With Improvement	
		t-PA Group	*Placebo Group*
Part 1	0–90	51	46
	91–180	42	33
Part 2	0–90	59	39
	91–180	35	40
Combined	0–90	55	42
	91–180	39	37

*Based on 157 patients treated within 90 minutes and 155 patients treated after 91 to 180 minutes.

a statistically significant difference in outcome between the treated and untreated (placebo) groups only at 3 months and beyond, other studies of intra-arterial and intravenous thrombolytic therapy indicated that a significant number of patients improve within 24 hours and that there is a correlation between this early improvement and eventual outcome.

The results of the NINDS trial indicated: "In Part 1, there was no significant difference between the group given t-PA and that given placebo in the percentages of patients with neurological improvement at 24 hours. . . ." In other trials with angiographic evidence of recanalization and evaluation of clinical improvement, however, there is a statistically significant difference between the group with recanalization and that without. If the patient shows clinical improvement at the end point of the trial and has angiographic evidence of recanalization, the improvement is dramatically apparent within the first 24 hours.

Brott et al.,[32] in the pilot study of intravenous t-PA (on which the NINDS trial was based), reported on 74 patients with ischemic strokes treated within 90 minutes of the onset of symptoms. Major neurologic improvement was seen in 22 patients at 2 hours and 34 patients at 24 hours (46%). This constituted most of the 69% of patients with partial or complete recovery at 3 months. In 20 patients treated between 91 and 180 minutes after the onset of symptoms, significant improvement was seen in 3 (15%) at 24 hours; 5 patients had no or mild limitations at 3 months (including 2 of the early improvers, the third was lost to follow-up).[33] These data indicate a poor response to intravenous therapy if given more than 90 minutes after the onset of symptoms.

Mori et al.[34] reported on 22 patients with MCA occlusions treated with intracarotid urokinase. Recanalization was successful in 10 patients; 8 showed improvement in symptoms within the first day, with continued improvement over the next several days, and represented two thirds of the 12 patients with good or excellent long-term outcomes.

In an open trial of intravenous t-PA in acute carotid territory stroke reported by Trouillas et al.,[35] 43 patients were treated within 7 hours of the onset of symptoms. Of these, 20 demonstrated major neuro-

logic improvement at 24 hours (17 at 3 hours). Seventeen of these patients were among the 25 patients with excellent outcomes at 90 days (total or near-total recovery); 2 patients with early improvement subsequently suffered from hemorrhages, and a third experienced reinfarction.

Another study was designed to assess the correlation between early CT findings and outcome after treatment with intravenous t-PA.[36] Ten patients with anterior circulation strokes were treated within 6 hours of onset. Four patients experienced significant improvement within 24 hours (including both patients with demonstrated recanalization on angiography); these four were among the five patients with good or excellent outcome at 1 month.

Overgaard et al.[17] treated 23 patients with anterior circulation ischemic strokes using intravenous t-PA. Angiography obtained in 17 patients at 16 to 24 hours revealed complete recanalization in 12 cases and partial recanalization in 3 cases. There was a strong correlation between recanalization, improved neurologic examination at 24 hours, and improved outcome at 35 days.

The Prolyse for Acute Cerebral Thromboembolism (PROACT) trial has not concluded its investigation, but early anecdotal reports indicate a correlation between recanalization and early positive response.

All these data indicate that if there is recanalization and ultimate improvement, there is high correlation with significant improvement within 24 hours. In the current NINDS trial of intravenous t-PA, this correlation is lacking. Interestingly, there does appear to be improvement in the subgroup of patients treated within the first 90 minutes. This raises the question of exactly what the t-PA is doing. In an independent study by Alexandrov et al.,[37] patients at their institution who were enrolled in the NINDS study underwent single-photon emission computed tomography (SPECT) at the time of treatment and 24 hours after treatment. All patients had perfusion defects on their baseline scans; the defects were comparable in the t-PA and placebo-treated patients, using a standardized grading system. At 24 hours, the patients receiving t-PA had significantly greater reperfusion (although some reperfusion was seen in patients receiving placebo).

What does this imply in terms of the mechanism of action producing the improvement with the use of t-PA, in light of the fact that there was no significant improvement in 24 hours despite evidence suggesting reperfusion? Interestingly, in the part 1 trial, there was a statistically significant difference in the t-PA group versus the placebo group in patients thought to have small vessel as opposed to large vessel embolic disease, with the small vessel group favoring t-PA. This exact statistical difference pattern was duplicated in the part 2 trial. Could this difference account for the slight difference in outcome, including the differences in reperfusion at 24 hours and infarct size at 3 months?

Another fascinating point is that although these data are supposed to be statistically valid, the rate of symptomatic bleed in the control group is at least *one entire order of magnitude* different from almost every other trial evaluating the natural history of stroke (<1%, compared with 6% to 20%). Does this imply that the control group is not statistically accurate? And if the control group is not accurate, is the sample group accurate?

Middle Cerebral Artery Thrombus Treated With Intravenous Tissue-Type Plasminogen Activator

An additional separate post hoc analysis of the data from the NINDS t-PA trial evaluated the presence or absence of the dense MCA sign.[38] On CT scan, if thrombus is present within the MCA, it can make this vessel appear abnormally white (dense). In this separate analysis, the severity of symptoms on the NIHSS was correlated with the presence or absence of this sign as well as the response to therapy.

This analysis indicated that if this sign was positive (i.e., indicative of thrombus within the MCA), the average NIHSS score was significantly higher than if this sign was absent. In addition, almost without exception, *patients in whom this sign was positive were not helped at all by intravenous therapy with t-PA* (only 1 of 18 patients was neurologically normal after 3 months). This is in contrast to the finding that 17 of 37 patients who entered into the study with a negative dense MCA sign were essentially normal.

These data have profound implications. If patients who had clear evidence of MCA thrombus were not being helped, what patients were?

Additional analysis revealed that all patients with dense MCA signs had NIHSS scores over 15, a severe insult. Comparison of all patients with NIHSS scores over 10 with and without dense MCA signs showed that if clot could be seen, intravenous therapy would not help, but if clot could not be seen, there was a chance that intravenous therapy might help. The documented presence of thrombus in the MCA is almost a guarantee that intravenous therapy will not work.

Unfortunately, this sign is insensitive to the presence or absence of MCA thrombus. A subgroup analysis of MCA thrombus in the Emergency Management of Stroke (EMS) trial described later revealed that

immediate follow-up angiography demonstrated thrombotic occlusion in 70% of patients treated with intravenous t-PA but in only 56% of patients who did not receive t-PA.

Trouillas et al.[39] reported on 100 consecutive patients undergoing treatment with intravenous t-PA for carotid territory strokes in a continuation of their study described earlier.[35] Angiography was performed after treatment, and outcome was assessed at 30 days using the Modified Rankin Scale. The proportion of excellent outcomes varied significantly with the location of the occlusion. Smaller vessel occlusions were associated with a high percentage of good outcomes (75.5% in choroidal artery occlusions and 68.8% in MCA branch occlusions), while larger vessel occlusions were associated with fewer excellent outcomes (48% in M1 trunk lesions, 28% in M1 origin lesions, and 10% in internal carotid bifurcation lesions involving both the anterior cerebral artery and the MCA).

These studies have yielded evidence of minimal if any effect on large vessel intracranial thrombo-occlusive disease from therapy with intravenous t-PA.

Patients with MCA thrombus are the specific target of the intra-arterial therapeutic trials and have been shown to benefit from direct local therapy. For this reason, these two modes of therapy (intravenous and local intra-arterial) are not mutually exclusive but will probably be shown to be complementary.

RESULTS OF EARLY INTRACRANIAL LOCAL INTRA-ARTERIAL FIBRINOLYSIS

Early Intra-arterial Prourokinase Trial (PROACT-I)

The first phase of the trial organized by Abbott Laboratories demonstrated the safety of prourokinase infusion in thromboembolic occlusions of the M1 segment of the MCA and successful angiographic recanalization when compared with placebo, but clinical efficacy was not proved (the trend appears to be positive, however).[40] Patients were entered into the double-blind trial only if angiographically demonstrable occlusion could be identified and local intra-arterial therapy could be begun within 6 hours after the acute event.

The results of this trial are encouraging. Placebo (saline) was compared with the active agent (prourokinase) using the identical delivery method (local intracranial infusion), with analysis of not only the radiographic results and complications but also the clinical efficacy. There was also an attempt to analyze the usefulness of adjuvant heparinization (and how much to use). (It is well known in the peripheral interventional radiology community that the use of heparin appears to increase the effectiveness of urokinase exponentially.)

Vascular occlusion was measured by the Thrombolysis in Myocardial Infarction (TIMI) perfusion criteria, ranging from 0 to 3 (0, no perfusion; 3, normal flow). Entry into the study required a TIMI grade of

0 or 1 (no distal opacification). Demographics for the placebo and trial patients were closely matched. The mean NIHSS scores were 17.0 for the prourokinase patients and 16.9 for the placebo patients.

The primary variable measured was recanalization at 120 minutes. In the placebo group, only 14% of patients had any recanalization with the infusion of saline, compared with 58% of patients having either a complete or partial response to the infusion of prourokinase.

Two different heparin doses were used in the study. When high-dose heparin was used, 82% of the prourokinase patients had either partial or complete response, compared with 0% in the placebo group (quite dramatic!). When symptomatic intracranial hemorrhage was analyzed, however, the high-dose heparin patients had a four times higher rate of bleed within 24 hours than the low-dose heparin patients. (This has led the phase II prourokinase study to use a lower dose of heparin than many would prefer.) Later analysis of the data from t-PA trials has not confirmed a higher bleed rate with increasing heparin dose. Therefore, this relation is yet to be proved.

At 90 days after treatment, the NIHSS, Modified Rankin score, and Barthel Index all showed a tendency toward a better outcome with prourokinase. Indeed, 31% of treated patients, compared with only 21% of placebo patients, had a Rankin score of 1 or less at 90 days. This was confirmed when analyzing the data concerning recanalization. *Those who did not recanalize in either group had poorer clinical outcomes.*

The PROACT trial had the best safety record of any of the thrombolytic agents yet reported. This, combined with the positive results, is encouraging for future efforts.

The report of the PROACT trial also provided data regarding the source of the occlusion (one of the few studies to do so). The source of the occlusive thrombus was shown to be cardiac in 54% of patients receiving prourokinase and 64% of placebo-treated patients; angiographic (procedure-related) in 8% and 0% of patients, respectively; carotid artery atherosclerotic in 8% and 7%, respectively; and unknown in 31% and 29%, respectively. Although the patients with unknown sources of occlusion had negative cardiac evaluations, this is the most likely origin.

Intra-arterial Tissue-Type Plasminogen Activator Trials

Most of the trials evaluating the usefulness of t-PA in acute ischemic stroke have focused on intravenous therapy. Zeumer et al.[41] compared the efficacy of local intra-arterial t-PA and urokinase. They found that t-PA, despite being fibrin specific, offered no advantage over urokinase.

In a trial of thrombolytic therapy for basilar artery thrombosis, patients were treated with intra-arterial urokinase, intra-arterial t-PA, or intravenous t-PA. The subgroup of patients treated with intra-arterial

t-PA was too small to draw any valid conclusions about the relative effectiveness of this agent and route of delivery.[42]

EMS Bridging Trial

The EMS trial was a combined intravenous and intra-arterial t-PA trial that used a slightly lower dose of t-PA for the intravenous portion (0.6 mg/kg, as compared with 0.9 mg/kg in the NINDS trial), followed by active aggressive intra-arterial t-PA infusion. Only recently have the results been presented (at the Joint Conference on Stroke and Cerebral Circulation of the American Heart Association, Anaheim, CA, February 1997). The lower dose of t-PA for the intravenous component was administered with the same regimen used for the NINDS trial of 10% bolus followed by infusion. The infusion was given in 30 minutes, however, so that the rate of infusion was actually higher than in the NINDS trial.

The intra-arterial dose was administered by giving 1 mg distal to the clot, 1 mg within the clot, and 9 mg/hr proximal to the clot; the total dose was not to exceed 20 mg. Even so, partial or complete clot dissolution occurred in only 60% to 70% of cases.

At the time the patients underwent angiography (on average about 45 minutes later), there was still thrombus present in 70% of patients treated with intravenous t-PA, compared with only 56% of patients receiving saline. This could be partially explained by the fact that the initial NIHSS scores of the intravenous treatment group were somewhat worse than those of the untreated group. Also seen in this study was a linear rise in the percentage of clots discovered with rising NIHSS scores. The higher the NIHSS score, the higher the chance of having thrombus. This finding has profound implications and is consistent with the results of other studies involving intravenous therapy, as discussed earlier.

Spontaneous recanalization appears to occur in about 14% of cases.[41] With intravenous therapy, there may be true lysis in an additional 0% to 10% of cases. Intra-arterial therapy, with t-PA, urokinase, or prourokinase, may yield recanalization rates up to 70% to 80%. Combined intravenous and intra-arterial therapy may result in *earlier recanalization* in a few patients, but the total recanalization rate is still only about 80%; there appears to be a certain group of patients with thrombus that is resistant to fibrinolysis, at least in the short time allowable for emergency stroke treatment. *Early results of combined intravenous and intra-arterial t-PA appear to indicate that emergency administration of intravenous t-PA does not decrease the detection of thromboembolic occlusion or change the indication for intra-arterial fibrinolytic therapy.*

The only adverse events that occurred in this trial were in the patients treated with intravenous t-PA. There were no adverse bleeding events at all in the intra-arterial arm of the study. The combined therapy group received a fivefold greater total dose than the local intra-arterial therapy group, owing to the large amount given in the intravenous portion, possibly explaining the adverse events. The combined group (patients who received intra-arterial therapy) also demonstrated the best overall response to therapy.

Long-Term Results After Intra-arterial Urokinase

Weschler et al.[43] showed that treatment of acute intracranial thrombo-occlusive disease with intra-arterial urokinase results in sustained benefit. Of 57 patients treated, they were able to follow 49 (mean follow-up 34 months with a range of 1 to 7 years). Nineteen patients died. The 30 survivors were classified according to the Barthel Index and location of occlusion. In agreement with the studies discussed earlier, the percentage of patients with minimal or no disability varied with location: 4 of 5 (80%) patients with MCA branch occlusions, 10 of 19 (53%) with M1 occlusions, 6 of 15 (40%) with ICA or ICA and MCA occlusions, 0 of 2 (0%) with MCA and anterior cerebral artery occlusions, and 1 of 6 (17%) with basilar artery occlusion. Overall, 45% of patients had minimal or no deficit, 8% had moderate deficit, 8% had severe deficit, and 39% died (14 within the first month). These results suggest that a substantial number of patients who survive their acute event experience long-term benefit from this therapy.

ONGOING LOCAL INTRA-ARTERIAL FIBRINOLYSIS TRIALS
PROACT Trial

The largest ongoing protocol for intracranial local intra-arterial infusion of a fibrinolytic agent is the Abbott trial of prourokinase. As discussed previously, this is a recombinant, single-chain form of urokinase that is fibrin specific.

Entry criteria for this protocol are rigorous but generally fall under the standard categories (e.g., time constraints, target constraints, physical constraints). The exclusion list is commensurately long.

This trial has attempted to be specific, with a small therapeutic window, to acquire data of a rational scientific nature. Even though these investigators have received abundant criticism for the decision to use an intracranial placebo infusion (saline) in the first stage of this trial, they are to be commended for achieving the first scientifically rigorous analysis of the natural course and potential treatment of an angiographically proven type of stroke.

The new stage of the trial still requires essentially no manipulation of the occluding embolus. The microcatheter is to be placed just into the clot without disturbing it in any other way (i.e., poking a hole through it to establish some antegrade flow is specifically forbidden). The infusion must be maintained at a given rate for 1 hour (as opposed to the prior 2-hour requirement). This appears to be a major improvement in technique.

After 1 hour, it is possible (with the new protocol) to perform an angiogram to check the results (i.e., see if there is anything left to be treated at all!). If the clot has drifted downstream, it can be chased, as opposed to the prior requirement of continued infusion into an open M1 segment supplying a potentially injured territory (the lenticulostriate arteries).

Termination of the procedure is invariable in most protocols; the PROACT protocol is no exception. After making exquisitely difficult decisions in some cases, this mandate may be a relief. Clinical decisions during a case can be especially difficult, and if a "cookbook" is used for guidance, thinking and worrying are greatly reduced. In one case (see Figs. 59–68 to 59–74), it was difficult to decide just when to stop (see the narrative pertaining to this case).

The PROACT study is designed to be extremely rigorous in the collection and analysis of data. The NIHSS is being used, as well as the Barthel Index, to assess outcome. The early clinical results are encouraging (but nonstatistical at present, and proprietary).

North American Cerebral Local Intra-arterial Fibrinolysis Register

The North American Cerebral Intra-arterial Fibrinolysis Register (NACLIFR), under the direction of Drs. Robert and John Ferguson (Baptist Hospital, Memphis, Tennessee), is a cohort-based registry that was designed to acquire data on treated patients to help guide the planning of future trials as well as modifications in therapeutic technique. It is a phase II study. It was the feeling of the organizers that a phase III trial was not feasible due to the fact that this is a rapidly evolving therapy and that no group of patients large enough to produce statistically significant data was available to guide the design of such a trial.

The NACLIFR is a multicenter registry of patients treated with local intra-arterial urokinase. All patients enrolled have angiographic evidence of intravascular clot and have experienced an acute neurologic event. The main questions are whether restoration of flow correlates with amelioration of symptoms and, therefore, whether this therapy warrants further study in a prospective, randomized trial. Specific points to be addressed include the effectiveness of local intra-arterial therapy in restoring flow, the incidence of improvement of the clinical examination in patients with successful reperfusion, quantification of adverse effects (including iatrogenic vessel injury and hemorrhage), stratification of responses to therapy by time from onset of symptoms to treatment, presence or absence of underlying stenosis, suitability of current techniques, and possible effect on morbidity and mortality in vertebrobasilar occlusion. This study was well conceived and is one of the first attempts to examine this subject in detail and with scientific method.

Inclusion criteria for the registry are ability to obtain informed consent from the patient or family, onset of symptoms within 7 hours of beginning therapy, and angiographic evidence of intravascular clot (vessel cutoff or filling defect) in the target artery (appropriate to symptoms). Exclusion criteria include evidence of hemorrhage on CT scan, fibrinogen level < 80 mg/dl, prothrombin time (PT) > 25 seconds or activated partial thromboplastin time (aPTT) > 55 seconds despite attempts at correction, platelet count < 60,000, active internal bleeding, prior reaction to urokinase, and systolic blood pressure > 200 mm Hg or diastolic blood pressure > 120 mm Hg despite medical therapy.

The parameters to be analyzed include procedural mortality (within 24 hours of therapy), late mortality (1 to 30 days), intraprocedural neurologic changes as determined by clinical testing (within 24 hours, quantified using the NIHSS), late neurologic changes (within 1 to 7 days, also quantified by NIHSS), incidence of hemorrhage on CT (within 7 days, including intracerebral [petechial or hemorrhagic infarct and parenchymal or space-occupying], subarachnoid, subdural, epidural, and intraventricular), incidence of non–central nervous system bleeding, effect of the thrombolytic agent on systemic coagulation (fibrinogen, PT or aPTT, or activated clotting time (ACT), measured serially), change in vessel lumen diameter, presence or absence of residual clot, and procedural non-neurologic morbidity (within 24 hours).

RETROGRADE VENOUS NEUROPERFUSION

Retrograde venous neuroperfusion is a novel technique for maintaining cerebral viability. Superficially, this technique appears to be counterintuitive. The concept is this: both the venous system and the arterial system connect to the capillary tree (by venules and arterioles, respectively). If blood is forced backward (retrograde) in the venous system, it can reach the target location (capillary level, parenchyma) eventually. Therefore, if arterial (oxygenated) blood is pumped in a retrograde direction, it can conceivably maintain tissue viability for a short period of time (and possibly indefinitely).

Exerting this retrograde force is not a simple matter. The best way to accomplish this task is to pulse the arterialized (oxygenated) blood at the same rate as the patient's pulse, but at *diastole rather than systole*. This allows the blood to flow at the time of lowest arterial pressure, not meeting the antegrade arterial pulse pressure head-on. The blood and pulsatile force is supplied by a large catheter system placed through the jugular vein into the sigmoid sinus or transverse sinus regions bilaterally. These catheters have balloons that are nearly occlusive in the sinuses, and they must be large catheters capable of carrying a significant volume of blood. This blood is supplied by a proprietary pump hooked to a large-bore catheter that obtains blood from the femoral artery and then supplies it to the venous catheters. The blood is then forced backward into the brain. Pressure is the regulating and monitoring factor.

The interesting thing about the theory of this generalized "shotgun" perfusion distribution (i.e., forcing blood in a backward manner into the entire hemisphere) is that the parenchyma with the lowest capillary pressure is that with the occluded inflow. The parenchyma receiving its normal blood supply (and arterial pressure) will resist retrograde flow, whereas the parenchyma not receiving its normal supply (i.e., affected by the embolic occlusion) is under low pressure and thus can allow this retrograde flow. This may even dislodge (or loosen) the embolus or allow intrinsic fibrinolysis to proceed at an increased pace.

Early results indicate that if this mechanism is placed rapidly enough, normal electrical activity and neuronal function can return rapidly (in 30 to 60 minutes). Current practice for this technique calls for therapy within 7 hours, but the initial series of patients had a good response even at this late time, in a manner similar to some of the responses to arterial reperfusion even at such a late time. It is far too early to determine if this will have a place in acute stroke intervention, but these early results are encouraging.

HYPERBARIC OXYGEN

Treatment of cerebral ischemia with hyperbaric oxygen is in some ways difficult and in other ways simple. The goal is to increase the PaO_2 in the interstitial tissues that permeate the entire body, thus eventually reaching the ischemic tissue. The therapy involves placing the patient in a pressurized chamber similar to that used for decompressing a deep sea diver with the bends, and pumping in oxygen to a pressure of about 2 to 3 atmospheres. For tissues with borderline metabolic supply, this can yield positive results. It is necessary to have a hyperbaric chamber, however, but these are not as rare as they might seem. Hyperbaric oxygen has been shown to be effective in the treatment of cerebral ischemia in animal models[44]; its clinical use is controversial[45] but early results are promising.[46]

HYPOTHERMIA

The role of hypothermia in cerebral protection is described in Chapter 55. In a pilot clinical study,[47] moderate hypothermia (33°C) was induced and maintained for 48 to 72 hours in 25 patients with severe MCA territory ischemic strokes. Intracranial pressure (ICP) and cerebral perfusion pressure were monitored. Hypothermia was well tolerated, with no severe side effects. It appeared to assist in the control of the elevated ICP produced by severe edema. These are encouraging results, and additional studies are ongoing.

REFERENCES

1. Brott T, Adams HP, Olinger CP, et al. Measurements of acute cerebral infarction: a clinical examination scale. *Stroke* 1989;20:864–870.
2. Hantson L, Wessel T. Therapeutic benefits of lubeluzole in

ischemic stroke. Paper presented at the 23rd International Joint Conference on Stroke and Cerebral Circulation, Orlando, February 1998.

3. Wahlgren NG, for the Clomethiazole Acute Stroke Study Collaborative Group. The Clomethiazole Acute Stroke Study (CLASS). Efficacy results in a subgroup of 545 patients with total anterior circulation syndrome. Paper presented at the 23rd International Joint Conference on Stroke and Cerebral Circulation, Orlando, February 1998.

4. Mahoney FI, Barthel DW. Functional evaluation: the Barthel index. *Maryland State Med J* 1965;14:61–65.

5. Van Swieten JC, Koudsteil PJ, Visser MC, et al. Interobserver agreement for the assessment of handicap in stroke patients. *Stroke* 1987;19:604–607.

6. Clark WM, Williams BJ, Selzer KA, et al., for the Citicoline Study Group. Randomized efficacy trial of citicoline in acute ischemic stroke. Paper presented at the 23rd International Joint Conference on Stroke and Cerebral Circulation, Orlando, February 1998.

7. The RANTTAS Investigators. A randomized trial of tirilazad mesylate in patients with acute stroke (RANTTAS). *Stroke* 1996;27:1453–1458.

8. Pessin MS, Del Zoppo GJ, Estol CJ. Thrombolytic agents in the treatment of stroke. *Clin Neuropharmacol* 1990;13:271–289.

9. Pannell R, Gurewich V. Pro-urokinase: a study of its stability in plasma and of a mechanism for its selective fibrinolytic effect. *Blood* 1986;67:1215–1223.

10. Hoylaerts M, Rijken DC, Linjen HR, Collen D. Kinetics of the activation of plasminogen by human tissue plasminogen activator: role of fibrin. *J Biol Chem* 1982;257:2912–2919.

11. Kim S, Wadhwa N, Kant KS, et al. Fibrinolysis in glomerulonephritis treated with ancrod, renal functional, immunologic, and histopathologic effects. *QJM* 1988;69:875–895.

12. Latallo ZS. Retrospective study on complications and adverse effects of treatment with thrombin-like enzymes. *Thromb Haemost* 1983;50:604–609.

13. Pollak VE, Glas-Greenwalt P, Olinger CP, et al. Ancrod causes rapid thrombolysis in patients with acute stroke. *Am J Med Sci* 1990;299:319–325.

14. Smith RAG, Dupe FJ, English PD, Green J. Acyl-enzymes as thrombolytic agents in a rabbit model of venous thrombosis. *Thromb Haemost* 1982;47:269–274.

15. AIMS Trial Study Group. Long-term effects of intravenous anistreplase in acute myocardial infarction: final report of the AIMS study. *Lancet* 1990;335:427–431.

16. Hanaway J, Torack R, Fletcher AP, Landau WM. Intracranial bleeding associated with urokinase therapy for acute ischemic hemispheric stroke. *Stroke* 1976;7:143–146.

17. Overgaard K, Sperling B, Boysen G, et al. Thrombolytic therapy in acute ischemic stroke: a Danish pilot study. *Stroke* 1993;24:1439–1446.

18. Brott TG, Haley EC, Levy D, et al. Safety and potential efficacy of tissue plasminogen activator (tPA) for stroke [Abstract]. *Stroke* 1990;21:181.

19. Mori E, Yoneda Y, Tabuchi M, et al. Intravenous recombinant tissue plasminogen activator in acute carotid artery territory stroke. *Neurology* 1992;42:976–982.

20. von Kummer R, Hacke W. Safety and efficacy of intravenous tissue plasminogen activator and heparin in acute middle cerebral artery stroke. *Stroke* 1992;23:646–652.

21. del Zoppo GJ, Poeck K, Pessin MS, et al. Recombinant tissue plasminogen activator in acute thrombotic and embolic stroke. *Ann Neurol* 1992;32:78–86.

22. Donnan GA, Davis SM, Chambers BR, et al. Australian Streptokinase Trial (ASK). In del Zoppo GJ, Mori E, Hacke W (eds). Thrombolytic Therapy in Acute Ischemic Stroke II. Berlin: Springer-Verlag, 1993, pp. 80–85.

23. Côté R, Battista RN, Wolfson C, et al. The Canadian Neurological Scale: validation and reliability assessment. *Neurology* 1989;39:638–643.

24. Donnan GA, Davis SM, Chambers BR, et al. Trials of streptokinase in severe acute ischemic stroke [Letter]. *Lancet* 1995;345:579.

25. Donnan GA, Hommel M, Davis SM, for the Steering Committees of the ASK and MAST-E Trials. Streptokinase in acute ischemic stroke [Letter]. *Lancet* 1995;346:56.

26. The Multicenter Acute Stroke Trial-Europe. Thrombolytic therapy with streptokinase in acute ischemic stroke. *N Engl J Med* 1996;335:145–150.

27. Hacke W, Kasto M, Fieschi C, et al. Intravenous thrombolysis with recombinant tissue plasminogen activator for acute hemispheric stroke: the European cooperative acute stroke study (ECASS). *JAMA* 1995;274:1017–1025.

28. The National Institute of Neurological Disorders and Stroke rt-PA Stroke Study Group. Tissue plasminogen activator for acute ischemic stroke. *N Engl J Med* 1995;333:1581–1587.

29. Jennett B, Bond M. Assessment of outcome after severe brain damage: a practical scale. *Lancet* 1975;1:480–484.

30. The NINDS rt-PA Stroke Study Group. Effect of rt-PA on ischemic stroke lesion size by computed tomography: preliminary results from the NINDS rt-PA Stroke Trial. Paper presented at the 23rd International Joint Conference on Stroke and Cerebral Circulation, Orlando, February 1998.

31. Kwiatkowski TG, Libman R, Frankel M, et al., for the NINDS rt-PA Stroke Study Group. The NINDS rt-PA Stroke Study: sustained benefit at one year. Paper presented at the 23rd International Joint Conference on Stroke and Cerebral Circulation, Orlando, February 1998.

32. Brott TG, Haley EC, Levy DE, et al. Urgent therapy for stroke. Part I. Pilot study of tissue plasminogen activator administered within 90 minutes. *Stroke* 1992;23:632–640.

33. Haley EC, Levy DE, Brott TG, et al. Urgent therapy for stroke. Part II. Pilot study of tissue plasminogen activator administered 91–180 minutes from onset. *Stroke* 1992;23:641–645.

34. Mori E, Tabuchi M, Yoshida T, Yamadori A. Intracarotid urokinase with thromboembolic occlusion of the middle cerebral artery. *Stroke* 1988;19:802–812.

35. Trouillas P, Nighoghossian N, Getenet JC, et al. Open trial of intravenous tissue plasminogen activator in acute carotid territory stroke. *Stroke* 1996;27:882–890.

36. Okada Y, Sadoshima S, Nakane H, et al. Early computed tomographic findings for thrombolytic therapy in patients with acute brain embolism. *Stroke* 1992;23:20–23.

37. Alexandrov AV, Bratina P, Grotta JC. T-PA associated reperfusion after acute stroke demonstrated by HMPAO-SPECT. Paper presented at the 23rd International Joint Conference on Stroke and Cerebral Circulation, Orlando, February 1998.

38. Tomsick T, Brott T, Barsan W, et al. Prognostic value of the hyperdense middle cerebral artery sign and stroke scale score before ultraearly thrombolytic therapy. *AJNR Am J Neuroradiol* 1996;17:79–85.

39. Trouillas P, Nighoghossian N, Derex L, et al. rt-PA thrombolysis in acute carotid territory stroke: causative, topographical and radiological correlations in a series of 100 cases. Paper presented at the 23rd International Joint Conference on Stroke and Cerebral Circulation, Orlando, February 1998.

40. del Zoppo GJ, Higashida RT, Furlan AJ, et al. PROACT: a phase II randomized trial of recombinant pro-urokinase by direct arterial delivery in acute middle cerebral artery stroke. *Stroke* 1998;29:4–11.

41. Zeumer H, Freitag H-J, Zanella F, et al. Local intra-arterial fibrinolytic therapy in patients with stroke: urokinase versus recombinant tissue plasminogen activator (r-TPA). *Neuroradiology* 1993;35:159–162.

42. Brandt T, von Kummer R, Müller-Küppers M, Hacke W. Thrombolytic therapy of acute basilar artery occlusion: variables affecting recanalization and outcome. *Stroke* 1996;27:875–881.

43. Weschler LR, Jungreis CA, Massaro LM, et al. Long term followup of patients treated with intraarterial urokinase for acute stroke. Paper presented at the 23rd International Joint Conference on Stroke and Cerebral Circulation, Orlando, February 1998.

44. Konda A, Baba S, Iwaki T, et al. Hyperbaric oxygenation prevents delayed neuronal death following transient ischaemia in the gerbil hippocampus. *Neuropathol Appl Neurobiol* 1996;22:350–360.

45. Nighoghossian N, Trouillas P. Hyperbaric oxygen in the treat-

ment of acute ischemic stroke: an unsettled issue. *J Neurol Sci* 1997;150:27–31.

46. Nighoghossian N, Trouillas P, Adeleine P, Salord F. Hyperbaric oxygen in the treatment of acute ischemic stroke: a double-blind pilot study. *Stroke* 1995;26:1369–1372.
47. Schwab S, Schwarz S, Keller E, et al. Moderate hypothermia in the treatment of patients with severe middle cerebral artery (MCA) territory infarction: a pilot study. Paper presented at the 23rd International Joint Conference on Stroke and Cerebral Circulation, Orlando, February 1998.

ADDITIONAL READING

Bell WR, Royall RM. Heparin-associated thromobocytopenia: a comparison of three heparin preparations. *N Engl J Med* 1980;303:902–907.

Fibbi G, Magnelli L, Pucci M, Del Rosso M. Interaction of uroki-nase A chain with the receptor of human keratinocytes stimulates release of urokinase-like plasminogen activator. *Exp Cell Res* 1990;187:33–38.

Fleury V, Lijnen HR, Anglés-Cano E. Mechanism of the enhanced intrinsic activity of single-chain urokinase-type plasminogen activator during ongoing fibrinolysis. *J Biol Chem* 1993;268:18554–18559.

Peltz SW, Hardt TA, Mangel WF. Positive regulation of activation of plasminogen by urokinase: differences in K_m for (glutamic acid)-plasminogen and lysine-plasminogen and effect of certain α, ω-amino acids. *Biochemistry* 1982;21:2798–2804.

Plow EF, Felez J, Miles LA. Cellular regulation of fibrinolysis. *Thromb Haemost* 1991;66:32–36.

Prentice CRM. Pathogenesis of thrombosis. *Haemostasis* 1990;20:50–59.

Quimet H, Freedman JE, Loscalzo J. Kinetics and mechanism of platelet-surface plasminogen activation by tissue-type plasminogen activator. *Biochemistry* 1994;33:2970–2976.

CHAPTER 57

Radiology of Emergency Stroke Therapy

P. Mohanakrishnan / J.J. Connors III / J.C. Wojak

INITIAL COMPUTED TOMOGRAPHY SCAN

Certain radiographic requirements are necessary before emergency stroke treatment can be instituted, and certain radiographic findings are unique to this pathology and therapy. It is imperative that the initial computed tomography (CT) scan show no evidence of bleeding. Findings consistent with acute infarct involving more than one third of the distribution of the middle cerebral artery (MCA) territory are also a contraindication. A modest amount of loss of definition of the gray matter–white matter interface or effacement of sulcal markings is not a contraindication, and successful fibrinolysis has been performed even in the face of such early signs of edema. The current Prolyse for Acute Cerebral Thromboembolism (PROACT) protocol requires that there be no significant mass effect with midline shift, acute hypodense parenchymal lesion, or effacement of cerebral sulci in more than one third of the affected MCA territory. These requirements appear reasonable. As more experience is gained, the knowledge of what signs to look for improves. Subtle signs of MCA infarction can be determined in most cases within the first 6 hours, and a reasonable estimate of the volume of affected tissue can be made.[1]

FOLLOW-UP COMPUTED TOMOGRAPHY SCAN

A CT scan should be obtained immediately after conclusion of treatment to evaluate for signs of bleeding, infarction, contrast extravasation, or intravascular clot.

Ischemic cortex commonly demonstrates areas of either low density (edema) or high density (extravasated contrast).[2] The increased density in the cortex often is not as striking as in the basal ganglia. The hyperdensity clears rapidly (usually in less than 1 to 2 days) and is thought to represent capillary leakage of contrast material. There is no associated dramatic mass effect with simple capillary leakage, as compared with a true intraparenchymal bleed. An actual bleed can be more inhomogeneous and has a true mass effect (usually impressive). In addition, fluid-fluid levels are frequently apparent in intraparenchymal hematomas, and multiple compartments can be seen. This is an ominous sign, with severe neurologic deterioration or death occurring in more than half of patients suffering from postfibrinolytic hematomas.

We have observed that residual thrombus within a vessel at the conclusion of treatment (usually thrombus within a distal branch that was not pursued) can absorb contrast and can be visible on the postprocedure CT scan. This very high density also demonstrates clearing within 1 to 2 days.

MAGNETIC RESONANCE IMAGING

Early magnetic resonance imaging (MRI) studies indicated that it took about 8 to 12 hours for acute ischemic changes to become apparent, but acute changes (increased signal on T2-weighted images) now can be seen 2 to 6 hours after ischemic insult, particularly in the basal ganglia and internal capsule regions (those supplied by the deep perforators, the lenticulostriates; see Fig. 58-50). It is unclear what this implies, but caution should be taken if the CT is negative and the MRI is positive, particularly if in a deep area supplied by perforators, where it may indicate a greater degree of ischemic damage to a vessel and therefore greater risk. This is not a recommendation for obtaining an MRI in every case, but in some institutions, this has been performed while the vascular laboratory is getting ready and the information gained may prove to be of significance. In the future, an MRI with a magnetic resonance angiogram (MRA) may replace the mandatory CT scan. Early changes in the deep structures of the brain not visible by CT may be revealed by MRI, and MRA may demonstrate that the actual site of occlusion is in an inappropriate location for therapy, thus obviating the need for an angiogram.

Magnetic Resonance Imaging and Spectroscopy of Acute Stroke

Older Methods

Early, correct diagnosis of the nature of the stroke (i.e., hemorrhagic versus ischemic) is the key in making a decision to treat a patient with thrombolytics or nonthrombolytics. Both CT and MRI (especially when gradient echo sequences are used) are highly sensitive to acute parenchymal hemorrhage. MRI is not as sensitive to subarachnoid hemorrhage, thus making CT an integral part of the acute stroke work-up.

Conventional MRI adds increased sensitivity and specificity in the visualization of the ischemic damage, thereby improving the clinical diagnosis and evaluation. Yet, the time course of the pathologic development is such that the normal MRI scans are not helpful in the earliest hours. The region of stroke appears to be normal in the conventional T2-weighted images for the first few hours. Cytotoxic edema, occurring early after an ischemic insult,[3, 4] does not cause sufficient accumulation of water to effect any changes in T1 or T2.[5] At this stage, subtle morphologic changes with sulcal effacement and early mass effect may be seen on T1-weighted spin-echo images.[6]

Vasogenic edema that develops later (typically 4 to 8 hours after infarction) causes a substantial increase in tissue water content.[3, 4, 7] This leads to high signal intensity of the stroke region on T2-weighted spin-echo images. Some patients with significant ischemic symptoms never show detectable changes. On proton-density–weighted spin-echo images, the lesions appear more conspicuous (the infarcts are bright), thus adding more specificity. Subcortical low signal intensity, sometimes seen on proton-density–weighted spin-echo images of patients with acute stroke, may be a consequence of iron accumulation from microscopic hemorrhage.

In acute stroke, paramagnetic contrast agents cause the enhancement of the vessels supplying the infarct region.[7, 8] This effect is dose related and may be seen in the first 24 hours after ictus. In an acute infarct, the cytotoxic edema water molecules can exchange between the free and bound (to cell bodies accumulated) states, permitting the application of magnetization transfer contrast (MTC) imaging. The lower intensity of the background tissue in MTC images allows increased definition of the lesion. A combination of MTC and contrast enhancement may be useful in the earlier detection of acute stroke.[9] In acute stroke, vascular information (e.g., occlusion, stenosis) can be obtained noninvasively using MRA.

Newer Methods

Newer magnetic resonance (MR) techniques, such as diffusion-weighted MRI (DW-MRI), MR perfusion imaging, MR spectroscopy (MRS), and MR spectroscopic imaging (MRSI) have enhanced the ability to understand the pathophysiology of acute stroke and to diagnose the earliest stages.[10] The application of these techniques in the early diagnosis and management of stroke is increasing. It is anticipated that these newer methods will play a significant role in the routine work-up and stroke management schemes, and thus a brief outline of these methodologies is warranted.

Diffusion-Weighted Imaging

The signal intensity in MRI is dependent on both T1 and T2. During the time interval between the application of excitation pulse and the signal detection, the water molecules may undergo coherent motion due to perfusion or blood flow or random motion (or diffusion) in their microenvironments. Such motion can cause a reduction in signal intensities of the images. The molecular diffusion is dependent on the microviscosity of the environment. In neat liquids of low viscosity (like pure water) and gases the diffusion is facile and occurs at random (isotropic). In more viscous liquid samples and in biologic tissues, the diffusion is more restricted and can be direction-oriented (anisotropic).

In DW-MRI protocols, images are obtained in the presence and absence of an extra pair of identical (the diffusion-sensitizing) gradients symmetrically placed around the observation (refocusing) pulse. The use of the extra pair of gradients results in diffusion-weighted images. In such images, the regions where water molecules can diffuse less freely appear brighter. Diffusion is usually expressed in terms of an exponential constant called the *apparent diffusion coefficient* (ADC).

A pixel-by-pixel computation of ADC also can be performed from a set of diffusion-weighted images, recorded at different amplitudes or duration of diffusion-sensitizing gradients. This results in an ADC map (an image). In a typical gray-scale rendition of an ADC map, the regions of hyperintensity correspond to reduced freedom of diffusion. High signal intensity in DW-MRI and MR perfusion imaging (see below) accurately localizes ischemic changes much earlier than does T2-weighted imaging (Fig. 57–1).[11–13] Because diffusion can be anisotropic, it is necessary to obtain the ADC maps along the three principal axes for meaningful characterization of tissue pathology.

In both animal models and human strokes, the general finding is that the apparent diffusion coefficient has an initial rapid decrease. This is believed to be secondary to conversion of relatively freely diffusing extracellular water to more constrained intracellular water (cytotoxic edema).[14a] This occurs within minutes, whereas blood-brain barrier breakdown, which leads to vasogenic edema, takes several hours. This is why DW-MRI demonstrates ischemia sooner than conventional T2-weighted imaging. This initial decrease in ADC is followed by a gradual return to normalcy and a further increase (above the baseline) that is thought to be indicative of tissue necrosis.[11] This means that DW-MRI may be used to differentiate acute stroke from chronic lesions.[12] For example, the mean ADC values for ischemic lesions reported in a recent study[14] were as follows:

$0.41 \pm 0.20 \times 10^{-3}$ mm²/sec   at <8 hr (n = 6)

$0.57 \pm 0.13 \times 10^{-3}$ mm²/sec   at 8 to 24 hr (n = 7)

$0.49 \pm 0.10 \times 10^{-3}$ mm²/sec   at 1 to 4 days (n = 12)

$2.10 \pm 0.29 \times 10^{-3}$ mm²/sec   beyond 11 days (n = 11)

In comparison, the ADC values were $0.88 \pm 0.12 \times 10^{-3}$ mm²/sec and 0.3 to 1.2×10^{-3} mm²/sec, respectively, for normal gray matter and white matter, dependent on orientation within the studied group. The early drop in ADC lasts for about 3 to 4 days. On the basis of this information, one can differentiate old ischemic regions from new stroke.

The combined use of diffusion and T2-weighted imaging has been proposed to be of use in predicting the histopathology of ischemia.[15] According to this scheme, the normal tissue is characterized by normal T2 and ADC values; tissue with normal T2 and low ADC values has a possibility of recovery. Other (high, low, or normal) permutations are indicative of necrosis or transformation to necrosis.

Because of the need to acquire at least two sets of images (with different gradients) in each of the three principal axes in order to produce an accurate ADC map, DW-MRI is time-consuming and subject to patient motion artifact. To compensate for this artifact, single-shot (high-speed) echo planar imaging (EPI) techniques can be employed for diffusion imaging. The use of EPI decreases the scan time but requires extensive modification of the clinical MR hardware (and hence additional costs). Under current conditions, such images may exhibit magnetic susceptibility artifacts. In 1995, there were only 100 clinical MR units with EPI capability, but this number has steadily increased. In addition, manufacturers are providing software for the suppression of image artifacts. These changes are increasing the practicality of using DW-MRI for routine diagnosis of acute stroke.

In conventional clinical scanners, DW-MRI can be carried out with the application of navigator echoes to measure and correct for bulk motion.[16] A double-echo technique is used. The first, fast echo carries

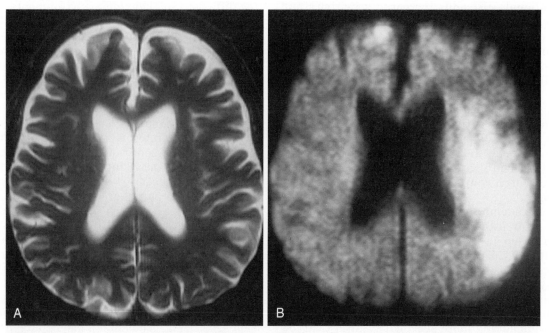

Figure 57-1 The sensitivity of diffusion-weighted magnetic resonance imaging (DW-MRI). These images were obtained 3.5 hours after onset of dense right hemiparesis. *A,* Axial T2-weighted image shows no definite area of signal abnormality. *B,* Axial DW-MRI image obtained at the same time and slice position reveals a large region of abnormally increased signal in the posterior left middle cerebral artery (MCA) distribution. The patient underwent emergency angiography and intra-arterial thrombolysis.

the imaging information and the second spin echo, which has no spatial phase-encoding, is used to correct phase errors in the first echo (any variations in phase of the second echo are due to motion).

Perfusion Imaging

An additional advantage with fast scanners is that one can perform dynamic susceptibility contrast (DSC)-based MR perfusion imaging. After a bolus administration of contrast, images are acquired rapidly (every 10 seconds or less) up to a minute and a half. Thus, one can conduct an entire perfusion study in about 1 to 1.5 minutes. The $T2^*$-shortening effect of the contrast causes transient signal loss in the normal parenchymal tissue around capillary bed and a delayed or attenuated loss of signal in hypoperfused (stroke-affected) regions. The region of stroke appears relatively brighter in DSC-based MR perfusion images (see Fig. 57–2). Intensity measurements can be made in a small region of interest in such images as a function of time after contrast administration, and the data can be fit to an appropriate kinetic equation to obtain quantitative information of blood flow.

Perfusion imaging may also be carried out noninvasively (i.e., without the use of contrast agents) using spin-tagging. In this case, the operator tags (inverts) the magnetization caused by arterial spins. Qualitative cerebral blood flow mapping is then obtained from differences between tagged and untagged images.

Animal studies show that the tissue damage depends on both the degree and duration of the ischemic episode.[17] It thus appears logical that the additional use of a nonhemodynamic marker of cellular status (e.g., DW-MRI) can differentiate between reversible ischemia (the ischemic penumbra) and infarction. It has been hypothesized that DW-MRI changes represent damaged tissue unlikely to recover without intervention and that MR perfusion changes represent the total affected volume.[18] The difference between the two may represent the tissue at risk or ischemic penumbra (Fig. 57–2). From a blood volume map obtained using MR perfusion imaging, regions of hypoperfusion can be identified. Those regions of brains that are hypoperfused below a threshold level are irreversibly damaged, and it has been argued that this threshold may vary among individual patients and within the same patient as a function of time from the onset of stroke.[19] More studies should clarify this.

Practical Implications of Perfusion and Diffusion Imaging

It is rare that a significant abnormality is seen on T2-weighted images 6 hours after the onset of symptoms, but one is always present on DW-MRI. If an abnormality is present on DW-MRI at 6 hours, there is a high probability that a true infarct will appear in this location.

The volume of perfusion abnormality is almost always larger than the volume of diffusion abnormality. Perfusion imaging also shows abnormalities sooner and areas are consistent with the clinical deficits. The final infarct volume is almost always smaller than the area of perfusion abnormality.

Early imaging has been performed using both DW-MRI and MR perfusion images. The perfusion image not only is abnormal sooner but also is more accurate at predicting the ultimate outcome. Additionally, the smaller DW-MRI defect almost invariably grows to reach the larger perfusion defect, unless the area is reperfused in an expeditious fashion.

Spectroscopic Methods

Localized in vivo MRS permits monitoring of the changes in brain chemicals in ischemic regions. Localizing information is obtained from scout images. Until recently, MRS was deemed mostly a research tool. The Food and Drug Administration (FDA) gave permission for routine marketing of the proton MRS packages provided by most manufacturers. In addition, General Electric Medical Systems, Siemens, and Phillips Medical Systems also received FDA approval of their ^{31}P MRS packages for clinical use.

The detection limit of MRS is in the millimolar (mM) range. The proton MRS spectrum of a normal human brain has signals due to N-acetyl moieties (mostly N-acetyl aspartate, or NAA), the methyl group of creatine–phosphocreatine, choline trimethyl-amino groups, methylene and methine hydrogens of aspartate and glutamate–glutamine, ring-attached hydrogens of inositol, the S-methyl group of taurine, and the lactate methyl group, if present.[20] With special techniques, γ-aminobutyric acid (GABA) and glucose also can be monitored, and glutamate and glutamine can be separated. The concentration of NAA in the normal adult brain is about 6 to 8 mM; the concentration in gray matter is about 2 mM higher than that in white matter.[21] NAA is a putative marker of neuronal and axonal loss and dysfunction. Normal adult human brain concentration of glutamate is about 11 to 13 mM, about 11 mM of creatine, 5 to 6 mM of glutamine, about 2 mM of free choline-containing compounds, and 1 to 2 mM of GABA.[23–27]

Two classes of methods are used commonly to obtain volume-localized in vivo spectroscopic information: single-voxel methods and spectroscopic imaging. Single-voxel techniques employ frequency-selective radiofrequency pulses (as in slice selection in MRI) to define a localized volume. In spectroscopic imaging, N phase-encoding gradients are applied during a free precession or the acquisition delay resulting in N simultaneous spatial experiments and consequently N spectra from N voxels. A typical display has the N spectra superimposed over the image so that each spectrum corresponds to the region of its origin. Each method has its own advantages and drawbacks. Finally, an image can be reconstructed based on spatial variation of intensities of each signal. Such a chemical shift image superimposed over a normal image furnishes a pictorial representation of the spatial distribution of each metabolite.

As expected, early proton MRS studies of human

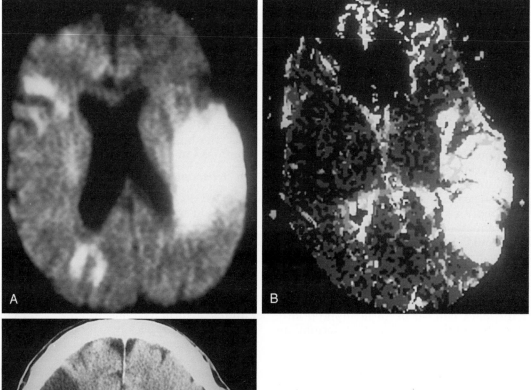

Figure 57-2 The predictive value of magnetic resonance (MR) perfusion imaging in acute stroke. The MR images were obtained 12 hours after onset of dense right hemiparesis. *A*, Axial DW-MRI image shows abnormally increased signal in the left MCA distribution. *B*, Axial time-to-peak-effect map calculated for the same slice position demonstrates abnormal lack of contrast delivery in the same distribution and more posterior tissue compared with the DW-MRI image. Although this suggested additional tissue at risk for infarction, the delayed presentation precluded safe thrombolysis. *C*, Axial noncontrast computed tomographic scan obtained several days later confirmed infarction, including the more posterior tissue.

brains after stroke have shown a decrease in metabolites, especially the NAA and creatine–phosphocreatine levels.[28, 29] Long-term, steady elevation of lactate is observed within or near the infarct region.[28, 30] This may be due to the initial insult, ongoing ischemia, or infiltrating leukocytes. Choline levels may show increases,[31] decreases,[32] or not much change.[30] Choline increases are localized in ischemic white matter, possibly because of the liberation of free choline groups from myelin breakdown.[31] Choline decreases probably reflect a more chronic phase of a cortical or subcortical gray matter stroke.[32] NAA, creatine, and choline levels in contralateral regions are significantly lower than normal.[31]

The Yale group[33] performed a spectroscopic imaging study of the brain of a patient with a 2-week-

old stroke just 1 week before death and correlated the findings with histopathology. The voxels in infarct regions showed a decrease in NAA and elevated (7 to 14 mM) levels of lactate in vivo, whereas postmortem sections showed sheets of foamy macrophages in the infarct.[33] The macrophage cell density at the infarct medial margin was nearly four times that at the surface.

The power of visualizing the physiologic changes in stroke using spectroscopic methods was clearly demonstrated in a study by the Johns Hopkins group.[31] Serial spectroscopic imaging was carried out on a patient 24 hours, 8 days, 22 days, and 5 months after a stroke. The intensity of the NAA and creatine signals progressively decreased, and the lactate signal initially increased in the stroke region (the right basal ganglia, in this case). Relative to the NAA level of the corresponding anatomic region in the contralateral region (defined as 1), the NAA levels in the gray and white matter regions, respectively, were 0.82 and 0.64 at 24 hours after stroke, 0.29 and 0.89 after 8 days, 0.37 and 0.71 after 22 days, and 0.33 and 0.57 after 5 months. The choline levels (relative to contralateral choline) for the same patient were 0.56 and 0.61 after 24 hours, 0.54 and 0.53 after 8 days, 0.71 and 0.60 after 22 days, and 0.75 and 1.0 after 5 months. The choline signal intensity also increased in the adjacent white matter. The corresponding values for lactate were 0.60 and 0.57 after 24 hours, 0.71 and 0.00 after 8 days, and 0.49 and 0.00 after 22 days. The authors also reconstructed the chemical shift images due to NAA, choline, and lactate, and such images give a pictorial representation of the changes. If the affected region has both lactate and significant amounts of NAA, then such a region should have viable neurons. Thus, chemical shift images of lactate and NAA enable the monitoring of the ischemic penumbra.[33]

Having a patient scanned within the early hours (particularly <6 hours) after the onset of symptoms is extremely difficult. This, obviously, is an inherent limitation resulting in a scarcity of data. MRS should be used increasingly in stroke management, and more early data should become available.

The regions that have only neuronal dysfunction and no neuronal loss should revert back to normal on appropriate treatment within the therapeutic window; the recovery should be characterized by metabolite levels returning to near-normal levels. Thus, MRS offers a noninvasive means to monitor the efficacy of therapeutic interventions.

In this account, no attempt has been made to outline the ^{31}P MRS findings. ^{31}P MRS can furnish information on changes in the levels of phosphorylated compounds (such as adenosine triphosphate and phosphocreatine) and the pH. In MR spectroscopy, the sensitivity for ^{31}P is about 6.63 (if the sensitivity for protons is set at 100). Thus, within the operating limits of most clinical scanners, the resolution of small voxels (about 1 ml) is extremely difficult. One solution is to perform studies at higher fields (>2T). Studies at high fields ensure improved resolution and better signal-to-noise ratios, even for proton spectra. Consequently, the number of academic medical centers with 3T and 4T whole-body systems is steadily increasing. Such systems are available for investigational use only, and patient care reimbursements cannot support their routine use and maintenance.

Magnetic resonance imaging has a superior role over other modalities in the early assessment of stroke and may help guide management. Using a single instrument, with the availability of the required packages, the operator can perform almost noninvasively such diverse and necessary examinations as angiography, DW-MRI, MR perfusion imaging, and spectroscopic examinations. With such versatility, MRI is emerging as an integral part of stroke management.

ANGIOGRAPHY

Angiographic Diagnosis of Cerebrovascular Occlusion

Angiographic identification of embolus is not the same in the head as it is in the periphery. If the entire carotid artery is absent or the MCA totally occluded, it may be readily apparent. If occlusion of a major branch of the middle cerebral artery is present, the missing group of distal branches and defect in the capillary blush will usually be obvious. If a proximal M2 branch occlusion is present, however, this may be difficult to identify. The presence of the main MCA (M1) and some branches may distract from the complete absence of another, perhaps vital, branch or division. Occasionally, a stub of a vessel is seen and the actual "clot" is outlined in the artery, but most often, the only evidence of vascular occlusion is slow flow in a vessel, with the remaining vasculature demonstrating normal arteriovenous transit time. Thorough knowledge of intracranial vascular anatomy and normal hemodynamics is therefore necessary for adequate diagnosis and treatment. This is particularly true once therapy has begun; the thrombus may move downstream. The angiogram must be watched for a stagnant vessel or an arterial branch that is still present in the venous phase. This leads the observer to the point of occlusion. The clot may not be where the vessel apparently ends angiographically; this is only where the contrast-filled blood flow exits this vessel into a side branch.

Other signs of acute vascular occlusion include slow antegrade flow in a vessel (as noted previously), collateral or retrograde filling, nonperfused regions (seen best with high-contrast digital subtraction images), and vascular blush consistent with luxury perfusion.

The figures for this chapter were provided by Drs. Robert W. Tarr, Jeffrey L. Sunshine, Jonathan S. Lewin, and C.F. Lanzieri of the neuroradiology section, University Hospitals of Cleveland and Case Western Reserve University, Cleveland, Ohio.

REFERENCES

1. von Kummer R, Holle R, Grzyska U, et al. Interobserver agreement in assessing early CT signs of middle cerebral artery infarction. *AJNR* 1996;17:1743–1748.
2. Komiyama M, Nishijima Y, Nishio A, Khosla VK. Extravasation of contrast medium from the lenticulostriate artery following local intracarotid fibrinolysis. *Surg Neurol* 1993;39:315–319.
3. Schuier F, Hossman K. Experimental brain infarcts in cats. II. Ischemic brain edema. *Stroke* 1980;11:593–601.
4. Gotoh O, Asano T, Koide T, Takakura R. Ischemic brain edema following occlusion of the middle cerebral artery in the rat: the time courses of the brain water, sodium and potassium contents and blood-brain barrier permeability to I-125 albumin. *Stroke* 1985;16:101–109.
5. Yuh W, Crain M. Magnetic resonance imaging of acute cerebral ischemia. In Weingarten K, Zimmerman RD (eds). Neuroimaging Clinics of North America: Stroke. Philadelphia: WB Saunders, 1992.

6. Hossman K, Schuier F. Experimental brain infarcts in cats: pathophysiological observations. *Stroke* 1980;11:593–601.

7. Yuh WTC, Crain MR, Loes DJ, et al. MR imaging of cerebral ischemia: findings in the first 24 hours. *AJNR* 1991;12:621–629.

8. Eisner AD, Moody DM. Early cerebral infarction: gadopentate dimeglumine enhancement. *Neuroradiology* 1990;177:627–632.

9. Mathews VP, King JC, Elster AD, Hamilton CA. Cerebral infarction: effects of dose and magnetization transfer saturation at gadolinium-enhanced MR imaging. *Radiology* 1994;190:547–552.

10. Fisher M, Prichard JW, Warrach S. New magnetic resonance techniques for acute ischemic stroke. *JAMA* 1995;274:908–911.

11. Warrach S, Gaa J, Stewart B, et al. Acute human stroke studied by whole brain echo planar diffusion weighted MRI. *Ann Neurol* 1995;37:231–241.

12. Parks MP, de Crespigny A, Lentz D, et al. Acute and chronic stroke: navigated spin-echo diffusion-weighted MR imaging. *Radiology* 1996;199:403–408.

13. Sorensen AG, Buonanno FS, Gonzales RG, et al. Hyperacute stroke: evaluation with combined multisection diffusion-weighted and hemodynamically weighted echo-planar MR imaging. *Radiology* 1996;199:391–401.

14. Lutsep H, Albers G, de Crespigny A, Moseley M. Diffusion imaging of human stroke. *Proc Int Soc Magn Reson Med 4th Scientific Meeting*, 1996, p. 89.

14a. Spielman DM, Butts K, de Crespigny A, Moseley ME. Diffusion-weighted imaging of acute stroke. *Int J Neuroradiol* 1995;1:44–55.

15. Welch KMA, Nagesh V, D'Olhaberriague L, et al. Diffusion and T2-weighted MRI of human stroke: a model to predict the histopathology of ischemia. *Proc Int Soc Magn Reson Med 3rd Scientific Meeting*, 1995, p. 86.

16. de Crespigny AJ, Parks MP, Enzmann DR, Moseley ME. Navigated diffusion imaging of normal and ischemic human brain. *Magn Reson Med* 1995;33:720–728.

17. Crowell RM, Marcoux FW, DeGirolami U. Variability and reversibility of focal cerebral ischemia in unanesthetized monkeys. *Neurology* 1981;31:1295–1302.

18. Sorensen AG, Koroshetz WJ, Buonanno FS, et al. Diffusion/perfusion mismatch of acute human stroke. *Proc Int Soc Magn Reson Med 4th Scientific Meeting*, 1996, p. 91.

19. Yuh WTC, Maeda M, Wang A-M, et al. Fibrinolytic treatment of acute stroke: are we treating reversible cerebral ischemia? *AJNR* 1995;16:1994–2000.

20. Frahm J, Bruhn H, Gyngell ML, et al. Localized high resolution proton NMR spectroscopy using stimulated echoes: initial applications to human brain *in vivo*. *Magn Reson Med* 1989;9:79–93.

21. Bilken DL, Oldendorff WH. N-acetyl aspartic acid: a literature review of a compound prominent in ¹H-NMR spectroscopic studies of brain. *Neurosci Biobehav Rev* 1989;13:23–31.

22. Rothman DL, Hanstock CC, Petroff OAC, et al. Localized 1H NMR spectra of glutamate in human brain. *Magn Reson Med* 1992;25:94–106.

23. Petroff OAC, Spencer DD, Alger JR, Prichard JW. High-field proton magnetic resonance spectroscopy of human cerebrum obtained during surgery for epilepsy. *Neurology* 1989;39:1197–1202.

24. Michaelis T, Merboldt KD, Bruhn H, et al. Absolute concentrations of metabolites in adult human brain *in vivo*: quantification of localized proton MR spectra. *Radiology* 1993;187:219–227.

25. Hennig H, Pfister H, Ernst T, Ott D. Direct absolute quantification of metabolites in human brain with *in vivo* localized proton spectroscopy. *NMR Biomed* 1992;5:193–199.

26. Christiansen P, Henriksen O, Stubgard M, et al. In vivo quantification of brain metabolites by ¹H-MRS using water as an internal standard. *Magn Reson Imag* 1993;11:107–118.

27. Kreis R, Ernst T, Ross BD. Absolute quantitation of water and metabolites in the human brain II. Metabolite concentrations. *J Magn Reson Ser B* 1993;102:9–19.

28. Graham GD, Blamire AB, Howseman AM, et al. Proton magnetic resonance spectroscopy of cerebral lactate and other metabolites in stroke patients. *Stroke* 1992;23:333–340.

29. Gideon P, Henriksen O, Sperling B, et al. Early time course of N-acetylaspartate, creatine and phosphocreatine, and compounds containing choline in the brain after acute stroke. *Stroke* 1992;23:1566–1572.

30. Mathews VP, Barker PB, Blackband SJ, et al. Cerebral metabolites in patients with acute and subacute strokes: concentrations determined by quantitative proton MR spectroscopy. *AJR* 1995;165:633–638.

31. Barker PB, Gillard JH, van Zijl PCM, et al. Acute stroke: evaluation with serial proton magnetic spectroscopic imaging. *Radiology* 1994;192:723–732.

32. Duijn JH, Matson GB, Maudsley AA, et al. Human brain infarction: proton MR spectroscopy. *Radiology* 1992;183:711–718.

33. Barker PB, Gillard JH, van Zijl PCM, et al. Proton magnetic resonance spectroscopic imaging in acute stroke: identification of the ischemic penumbra. *Proceedings of the Society of Magnetic Resonance 2nd Scientific Meeting*, 1994, p. 186.

CHAPTER 58

Strategic Considerations Concerning Emergency Stroke Treatment

J.J. Connors III / J.C. Wojak

GENERAL CONSIDERATIONS REGARDING FIBRINOLYSIS

The ultimate strategy and specific technique of stroke intervention is yet to be determined. It will most likely be a combination of societal education and medical care delivery. The general populace will have to be trained to recognize the onset of a stroke and the need for emergency evaluation and possible treatment. Effective cytoprotective drugs should allow more time until definitive revascularization therapy is begun. Unfortunately, one recent trial of a neuroprotectant agent has been discontinued because of a lack of efficacy, but others show promise.

Much of what is presented concerning intracranial fibrinolysis has not been proved. There are no large series yielding accurate information about the best fibrinolytic agent, the optimal time window for treatment, the specific technique to be used (intra-arterial or intravenous, much less the specific method of intra-arterial delivery), or even the ideal patient population. In addition, there is no clear understanding of the specific cause (or causes) of the primary severe complication (intraparenchymal hemorrhage or hematoma). For these reasons, this therapy is still evolving. The choices pertaining to technique are made from fundamental experience combined with early results reported by pioneers in the field, and they vary depending on the location of thrombus and the neurologic deficit. The worldwide ongoing trials and registries are giving early indications of usefulness and risks, but it will be years before any hard facts are available concerning optimal therapy. In addition, new cytoprotective and new fibrinolytic agents should render even some of these early conclusions premature or erroneous (see below).[1, 2] Certainly, within a few years, knowledge of this field will be vastly better than it is now.

The available fibrinolytic agents work solely by activating the intrinsic fibrinolytic system of the body, changing plasminogen to plasmin. This fact dictates the delivery technique and subsequent results. If the vessel to be opened is totally occluded and contains a proximal stagnant segment of blood, local infusion simply fills this segment with "water" and fibrinolytic agent. Any activity of the fibrinolytic drug is restricted to only the amount of plasminogen bound in the thrombus. From a practical standpoint, this is probably a small percentage of the plasminogen necessary for effective thrombolysis. If there is no available source of fresh plasminogen (i.e., from free circulating blood), the activity is limited. This has been shown repeatedly in peripheral thrombolysis and by Zeumer et al.[3] in intracranial applications.

Some trials appear to indicate that tissue-type plasminogen activator (t-PA) is more likely to cause remote bleeding than streptokinase or urokinase, agents with supposedly less fibrin specificity than t-PA. A recent study has shown that t-PA is not as fibrin specific as first thought and that reduction in systemic fibrinogenolysis also reduces remote site bleeding.[4] This induction of the systemic plasmin effect is probably part of the local effectiveness of t-PA; that is, plasminogen in the blood also is being activated and greatly aids in effective fibrinolysis. This systemic plasmin formation, however, is the cause of remote site bleeding.

Prourokinase and recombinant t-PA are more specific for activation of plasminogen bound to fibrin. At the clinically administered doses, however, recombinant prourokinase also is less than perfectly clot specific, with subsequent systemic activation of the fibrinolytic mechanism.

This *systemic* activation may, as suggested previously, be part of the effectiveness even of the more fibrin-specific agents. Zeumer et al.[3] compared the effectiveness of urokinase and t-PA. The premise was that a higher dose of a more fibrin-specific activator

might reduce recanalization time. This did not prove to be the case.

These results, combined with repeated observations in the peripheral vasculature that infusion of a thrombolytic agent into a flowing stream of blood appears to produce much more rapid results, suggest that there may be a plasminogen shortage in the clot, due to either aging of the thrombus with loss of plasminogen, some intrinsic chemical change within the fibrin or plasminogen, or the fact that there cannot be enough plasminogen trapped in any thrombus to dissolve the entire mass. Zeumer et al.[3] argued that this may be why t-PA is less effective in treating intracranial thrombus than coronary thrombus: coronary thrombus tends to be "fresh" (formed in situ), whereas anterior circulation intracranial thrombus tends to be "old" (embolic).

These observations support the impression that *fresh blood is needed for rapid effective fibrinolysis,* even with t-PA. This gives a ready supply of fresh plasminogen. It has been shown peripherally that a dead-end tube, such as an occluded graft, can be infused for days with minimal results, but once some antegrade flow is established through the thrombus, the progress of dissolution can be rapid. What is not known specifically, however, is how much systemic plasminogen (i.e., that supplied by fresh blood) is needed for rapid thrombolysis of the intended target thrombus under clinical conditions (i.e., middle cerebral artery [MCA] thrombus).

RATIONALE FOR INTRAVENOUS VERSUS INTRA-ARTERIAL FIBRINOLYTIC THERAPY

In interventional radiology, it is a well-established and universally accepted fact that local intra-arterial, intrathrombus delivery of fibrinolytic agent works immensely better than intravenous delivery. Various techniques have been developed to aid in this process of direct perithrombus or intrathrombus drug delivery, including multifocal infusion, mechanical agitators, pulse-spray delivery, balloons, and brushes. It is obvious that saturation of the microclimate around the clot will increase the absolute level of agent to a tremendous degree relative to infusion from a peripheral location.

Details of previous studies are presented in Chapter 56. Data from multiple intra-arterial and intravenous studies indicate that recanalization and ultimate improvement correlate highly with significant improvement within 24 hours. In the National Institute of Neurological Disorders and Stroke (NINDS) trial of intravenous t-PA,[5] this correlation is lacking, raising the question of what exactly the t-PA is doing. Interestingly, there appeared to be improvement in the subgroup of patients treated within the first 90 minutes. Close analysis of the data from the NINDS study, however, reveals that, in the two groups given t-PA during the 91- to 180-minute time window (from the first and second parts of the study), there was no significant difference in the number of patients with improvement at 24 hours. Indeed, in the second part of the trial, *a higher percentage in the placebo group improved at 24 hours than in the t-PA group!*

This contradiction, combined with the more than 50% difference in small vessel occlusive disease in *both parts of the trial* (33 patients in the two t-PA groups versus 20 patients in the two placebo groups) and corresponding reversed difference in the large vessel occlusive subgroups, brings into question a statement released by the Special Writing Group of the Stroke Council of the American Heart Association in its guidelines[6] that there was a "significant increase in improvement at twenty four hours. . . ." Although there was numeric improvement in the mean National Institutes of Health Stroke Scale (NIHSS) score in the 91- to 180-minute statistics (8 versus 13), the percentages of patients with actual improvement were only 39% and 37%, respectively. This implies large improvements in relatively few patients and again points out the potentially misleading nature of post hoc analysis.

Although the mechanism of action is unclear, intravenous t-PA does appear to be of some benefit in the subgroup of patients with small vessel disease. Further refinement in patient selection may increase the percentage of patients with improvement.

The Target Population of Middle Cerebral Artery Thrombi

How were the patients with large vessel occlusive disease and small vessel occlusive disease distributed in the subcategory of patients with improvement in the 91- to 180-minute group in the NINDS trial? An analysis of the data from this trial has yielded some interesting results.[7] Evaluation of the initial computed tomography (CT) scans of these patients for the presence or absence of the hyperdense MCA sign revealed that 18 of 55 patients were positive for this sign, with a median baseline NIHSS score of 19.5. This was compared with patients who were negative for this sign, who had a median score of 10. After acute intravenous t-PA therapy, at the end of 3 months, only 1 of 18 patients with the hyperdense MCA sign (6%) was completely neurologically normal, compared with 47% of the patients without the hyperdense MCA sign.

The results of the Emergency Management of Stroke (EMS) bridging trial (presented at the 22nd International Joint Conference on Stroke and Cerebral Circulation, Anaheim, CA, February 1997, by the EMS Investigators) are equally disturbing. Patients in this trial were randomized within 3 hours to receive either 0.6 mg of t-PA over 30 minutes or a placebo (saline). Immediate cerebral angiography was then performed. If clot was found, patients from both groups received up to 20 mg of t-PA over 120 minutes. Of 35 patients randomized, clot was found in 19 of 23 with an NIHSS score greater than or equal to 10. Of patients treated with intravenous t-PA, 70% had thrombus found at the clinically appropriate site *after t-PA infusion* (angiography was performed an average of 45 minutes after institution

of therapy). Of those patients receiving saline, thrombus was demonstrated by angiography in only 56% of cases. This is a clear indication of the lack of efficacy of peripheral (intravenous) t-PA in this trial.

These two studies have profound implications!

If patients with MCA thrombus are not helped with intravenous t-PA, the procedure of direct attack of the clot by intra-arterial means must be employed. These patients with thrombus in the MCA are the same patients that make up the target population for treatment by intra-arterial means, with preliminary outstanding results.

Post hoc analyses may give some interesting results, but some unanswered questions may remain concerning the intravenous method of treatment for stroke. Although administration of t-PA in the first 2 hours after stroke is desirable, actually trying to identify the offending lesion and trying to dissolve an appropriate thrombus by direct superselective intra-arterial means also are important.

Direct superselective local infusion works better *intracranially* than peripheral infusion for clot dissolution.[8] If the neuroscience community loses sight of the fact that direct intra-arterial thrombolysis has been proved to work far better than intravenous thrombolysis in numerous studies concerning thrombolysis in general, they, as medical professionals, may be neglecting the most beneficial form of therapy available for intracranial large vessel occlusive disease. The real question then becomes whether the ability to administer a dose of a thrombolytic agent peripherally at an earlier time is sufficient to make this a completely adequate therapy. The answer appears to be "no." The ultimate role of intravenous t-PA may be as an initial therapy. Emergency angiography would then be performed; patients with demonstrable thrombus would then undergo local intra-arterial thrombolysis.

TIMING OF THERAPY

In animal models, early thrombolytic therapy increases the degree of reperfusion and reduces cerebral infarction and related edema, clinical deficits, and mortality.

Early clinical data suggest that when total occlusion of the M1 segment (i.e., including the lenticulostriate arteries) extends beyond 3 hours, the chance of significant recovery diminishes sharply,[9] but striking recovery in other occlusions lasting longer has been observed (see the detailed strategic case analysis, below). Some additional early data indicate that when there is total occlusion of the M1 segment of the MCA and thus the lenticulostriate arteries after 6 to 9 hours, the risk of devastating postfibrinolytic intracerebral hemorrhage may increase. Theron et al.[10, 11] have reported that occlusion of the lenticulostriate arteries for longer than 4 to 5 hours causes an increased incidence of hemorrhage. More peripheral (M2) branch cortical occlusions eventually may be shown to be treatable long past this time period because of the presence of pial collaterals and the lack of critical deep distribution originating from these vessels (e.g., internal capsule, see Fig. 59–75). In the report by Theron et al.,[11] if the lenticulostriate arteries are occluded, the time period for rescue is grossly shorter (6 hours) than if only cortical vessels are occluded (12 hours). This is a tremendous difference but makes sense when the concept of pial collaterals is added to the equation.

Additional modalities may be shown to prolong the window for safe and effective thrombolysis. As discussed previously, infarct-limiting effects have been demonstrated for certain neuroprotectant agents as well as for hypothermia, when employed in a timely fashion.[12] Hypothermia decreases the speed of thrombolysis. Even with this handicap, the eventual result of treatment with hypothermia is better than without hypothermia.[12]

Patient variability is a major confounding factor. Some patients have been treated as long as 2 to 3 days after ictus with no untoward events (and perhaps with no benefit either, but see the exception to this in the case presented below), whereas others have been treated within the specified time frames for the studies with resultant devastating intracranial hemorrhage. Suffice it to say that treatment of acute anterior circulation stroke (typical MCA occlusion) should begin as early as possible, hopefully within about 3 to 5 hours from the acute event, and should terminate by about 6 to 8 hours after ictus. These numbers are not cast in stone and can certainly vary from patient to patient, but it should be emphasized once again; speed is absolutely of the essence. It would be ideal if the procedure could end by 5 hours after onset of symptoms, or even before. Collateral supply via pial vessels is tremendously variable from patient to patient and can be evaluated by a skilled practitioner with good digital subtraction angiographic equipment fairly accurately. This variability renders therapy unsuitable for a cookbook approach; good judgment should be exercised.

Territorial, Hemispheric, and Systemic Hypoperfusion

There is a vast difference between the effect of cardiac-induced vascular stasis and that of a small occlusive thrombus impacted, for instance, at the MCA bifurcation. Evidence has shown repeatedly that hypoxemia from generalized vascular stasis results in neuronal death in as few as 10 minutes. Additionally, in cases of generalized hemispheric vasospasm, the lack of collateral supply can render apparently adequate supply to the MCA territory inadequate.

The limited time window for treatment of cases of vascular stasis is not the same as that for certain embolic and thrombotic occlusions that involve only one vascular territory. This is because of the presence of pial-to-pial collaterals and at least some blood flow in surrounding tissues yielding a minimal amount of perfusion and diffusion. These combined factors can keep astounding amounts of cerebral tissue alive for

considerable periods of time (but perhaps without electrical or functional activity).

The magnitude of superficial cortical collateral (pial) supply from one territory to another can have a powerful influence on the brain's ability to withstand proximal occlusions of large intracranial vessels and is extremely variable among patients. This can affect not only the time available for therapy but also the margin of safety and results of therapy. For example, the case presented later in this chapter describes a patient with a hemiparesis for longer than 48 hours, which was associated with total mutism for more than 12 hours. The patient was returned to complete neurologic normalcy by reperfusion. Although this may be an extreme example of the ischemic continuum, commonly encountered clinical cases can have nearly the same wide range of severity and outcomes.

Even when total occlusion of the main trunk of the MCA has occurred and there is no good collateral supply from the superficial cortical branches of the anterior or posterior cerebral arteries to the occluded branches of the MCA, these occluded cortical vessels still do not tend to hemorrhage or to cause a devastating intraparenchymal hematoma as often as do the lenticulostriate arteries. This may be due to at least a trickle of perfusion reaching these cortical vessels, whereas the lenticulostriate arteries get absolutely none. In addition, although the cortex may have a relatively high metabolic rate, the deep white matter beneath this has a much lower rate. Therefore, the need for high perfusion of the cortex is not as great as that for the area supplying the basal ganglia (the lenticulostriate arteries). Further results on this topic will come out of the ongoing trials. It will be years or even decades, however, before definitive proof of cause and effect related to these bleeds is determined.

Watershed Zones

The location of occlusion can affect the watershed area, that is, the area of greatest ischemic depth (Cases 1 and 2, Figs. 58–1 to 58–5). These watershed zones can influence the outcome of a stroke significantly. (e.g., involvement of Wernicke's area).

Excellent collateral supply from the posterior cerebral circulation can supply the posterior parietal lobe, sensory cortex, and Wernicke's area well. Total occlusion of the distal internal carotid artery therefore can yield an area of maximal ischemia in the anterior lateral region surrounding the insula, such as Broca's region. Alternatively, for the same occlusion, if the anterior communicating artery is good and there is poor supply to the posterior fossa and posterior cerebral artery territory, the area of maximal ischemia may well be the same posterior parietal and Wernicke's area, not the peri-insular region. The same insult therefore can have dramatically different implications.

Lenticulostriate Arteries

The lateral lenticulostriate arteries are among the small perforating vessels that arise directly from cir-

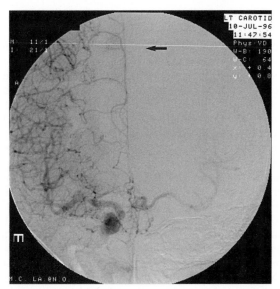

Figure 58-1 Case 1. Shifting watershed zones. Anteroposterior (AP) right carotid injection in a patient with total occlusion of the internal carotid artery on the left. Note the small right A1 segment of the anterior cerebral artery in this later arterial phase image, which illustrates limited cross-filling to the opposite hemisphere, with poor perfusion of the anterior cerebral territory indicated by the small amount of contrast in the left pericallosal artery *(arrow)*.

Implications of this appearance are (1) very poor (or no) inflow from the left internal carotid artery; (2) hypoplastic left pericallosal artery (unlikely), good inflow from the posterior supply to the pericallosal artery relative to the demand from the middle cerebral artery (MCA) territory on the left, or a combination of both; (3) probably a small amount of supply from either the posterior communicating artery or the internal carotid artery; and (4) the territory of the left anterior cerebral artery is more in jeopardy than that of the MCA.

Case 1 continues

cle of Willis vessels at the base of the brain. These are true end arteries that have minimal or no intrinsic collateral connections to other vessels and are thus subject to intense immediate ischemia when directly occluded. Other groups of perforating vessels arise from the basilar artery (pontine perforators), posterior communicating arteries (thalamoperforating arteries), and anterior cerebral arteries (recurrent artery of Heubner, medial lenticulostriate arteries). The critical location of the origin of the lateral lenticulostriate arteries along the M1 and M2 segment of the MCA renders these vessels crucial in planning treatment of anterior circulation ischemia.

Not only are these vessels vulnerable because of vascular anatomy; they also supply small but critical territories (specifically the basal ganglia and internal capsule). These structures contain fibers carrying motor and sensory signals between the cortex and the spinal cord, and even a small infarct in their territory can result in major disability (e.g., hemiplegia). Acute awareness of the status of these vessels is warranted for both these reasons.

In agreement with Theron et al.,[11] we believe that the degree and duration of ischemia of the lateral lenticulostriate arteries and their territory are key to both the success and the safety of treatment in many cases. Direct occlusion of the origin of these

vessels probably results in infarction of the supplied territory in as few as 2 to 4 hours; attempted rescue after this time is therefore probably ineffectual and possibly dangerous. Accurate analysis of the status of the lenticulostriate arteries at the initiation of therapy yields important strategic and prognostic information

Even when the lenticulostriate arteries are not visualized because of a proximal M1 segment occlusion, the distal M1 segment may still be receiving a trickle of blood, either through the apparent occlusion (radiographically invisible) or retrograde through collateral pathways (see Fig. 59–75). Alternatively, even when they are supposedly seen, there could be an unsuspected distal lenticulostriate branch that remains occluded, causing a small (perhaps clinically inconsequential) infarct in a lateral territory that could result in a devastating bleed secondary to therapy.

A major confounding factor in the management of occlusion of the MCA therefore is the variable anatomy of these lenticulostriate arteries (Fig. 58–6). At least a few branches of the lenticulostriate arterial system arise at the bifurcation of the MCA or beyond in about 40% of the population. These can be occluded easily by a typical embolus at the MCA bifurcation and thus can be unseen and probably unsuspected. Even under normal circumstances and with good angiographic equipment, some of these branches are nearly invisible. In Theron's study,[11] one of the significant bleeds was caused by delayed treatment in a patient not thought to have occluded lenticulostriate vessels; an erroneous conclusion.

This variability in the origin of the lenticulostriates, along with subsequent occlusion, may be the root cause of at least some of the "idiosyncratic" complications seen to date (e.g., posttherapy hemorrhages and hematomas). It will take years, if not decades, to prove or disprove this hypothesis, but this is a problem, and when possible, the operation should *actively* try to avoid infusing a possibly damaged lenticulostriate artery.

This also makes it imperative to clear the M1 segment of the MCA, as well as the first few millimeters of the M2 segments, as rapidly as possible. Once this is done, there may be more time for therapy.

TIME VERSUS DIAGNOSTIC INFORMATION

Time is brain.

A choice has to be made between speed and knowledge. The current Prolyse for Acute Cerebral Thromboembolism (PROACT) trial (of treatment of main trunk MCA occlusions) requires initial evaluation to be of the suspected occluded vessel only, with immediate access to the affected vessel and rapid positioning of the microcatheter into the thrombus to begin institution of fibrinolysis at that time. For a recipe-type method of therapy, this is good. For an interventionist with a biplane digital subtraction angiography suite, ignoring the rest of the intracranial vasculature may not be ideal. For the investment of

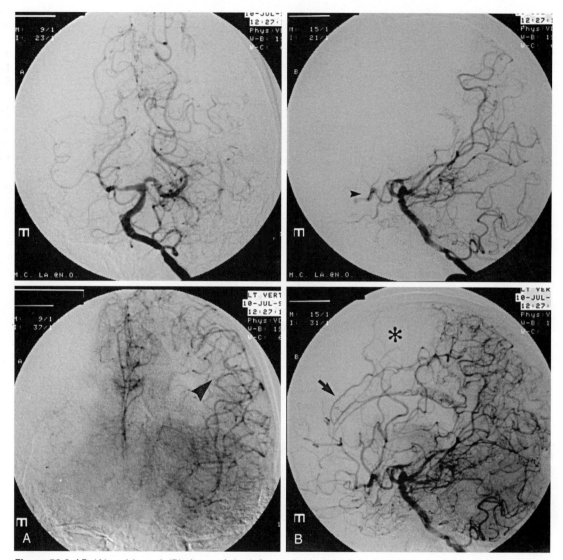

Figure 58-2 AP *(A)* and lateral *(B)* views of the left vertebral artery injection. Note the extensive filling of the territory of the middle cerebral and anterior cerebral arteries. This is accomplished by three different routes: (1) through the posterior communicating artery into the internal carotid artery, and thence into the MCA distribution *(small arrowhead);* (2) through the splenial branches of the posterior cerebral artery into the posterior portion of the pericallosal artery and thence into the posterior portion of the anterior cerebral artery *(arrow);* and (3) through typical superficial pial collaterals from the posterior cerebral branches to the MCA branches *(large arrowhead).*

Note the relative dearth of vascularity in the anterosuperior frontal lobe region *(asterisk).* In this hemodynamic situation, this is the terminal vascular watershed zone, farthest from the supply from the anterior and posterior communicating arteries and the pial collaterals. Typically, the terminal watershed would be slightly more lateral in the peri-insular region of the MCA with an M1 occlusion, which is not the case here.

Case 1 continues

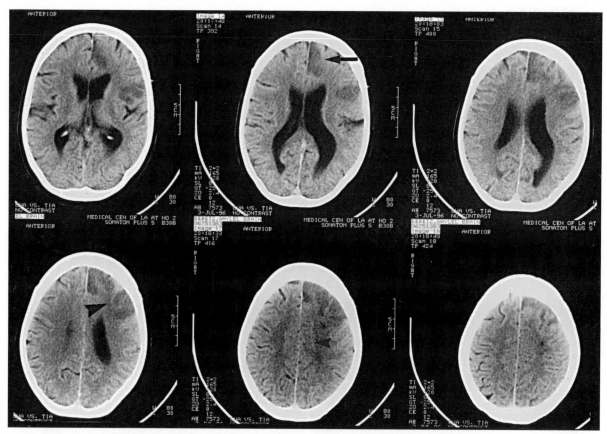

Figure 58-3 CT scan demonstrating the result of the hemodynamic situation. Note that the deep pericallosal territory is spared *(small arrowhead on fifth image)* but that the anterior callosomarginal region *(small arrow)* and anterior watershed zone *(large arrowhead)* are not. This pattern of infarct illustrates the shift in overall watershed zones from the more typical posterior region associated with *hypoperfusion* secondary to typical internal carotid artery stenosis or occlusion.

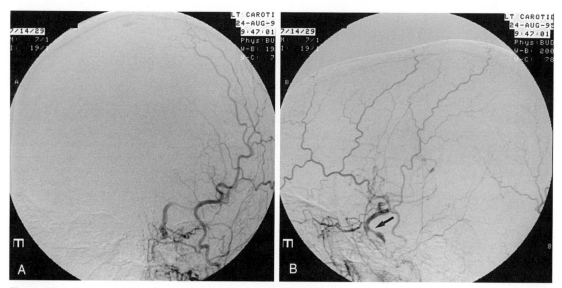

Figure 58-4 Case 2. Shifting watershed zones. Posteroanterior (PA) *(A)* and lateral *(B)* left common carotid angiogram reveals minimal flow in the internal carotid artery, with the predominant supply coming from retrograde flow in the ophthalmic artery. This vessel can supply only the proximal MCA territory, however, and even this supply is poor, as evidenced by the fact that the rate of flow in the external carotid artery branches is significantly faster than the intracranial flow rate. The residual segment of cavernous internal carotid artery *(arrow)* may be filling from petrous branches.

Case 2 continues

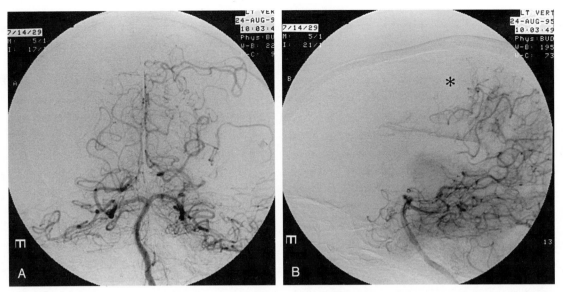

Figure 58-5 PA *(A)* and lateral *(B)* left vertebral artery injection. Note the shift in the watershed zone from a posterior location (Wernicke's area) to a more anterior location, the midparietal lobe region *(asterisk)*, but *not* the MCA trifurcation region. This is as opposed to an MCA *occlusion,* in which the watershed (or most ischemic) zone *is* shifted to the lenticulostriate–insular trifurcation region of the MCA, the farthest from any collateral supply. Also note on the lateral view that the posterior circulation is supplying a portion of the pericallosal territory, confirming the lack of flow from the internal carotid artery and implying that the supply from the opposite anterior cerebral artery is not as robust as would be desirable. This could be because the available perfusion from the anterior communicating artery is being requisitioned by the sump of the MCA territory, leaving a minimal amount for the anterior cerebral artery.

3 or 4 minutes, there is the potential of obtaining valuable, if not vital, information. It already has been shown that patients with good collaterals to the affected territory have better outcomes than those without. When the procedure is not standardized, this knowledge can be important. This was specifically the situation in the case discussed later. Knowing when to chase an embolus or persist in fibrinolysis may be learned by observation of intracranial hemodynamics. The discovery of additional thrombus elsewhere or of an unruptured aneurysm can complicate possible intervention.

In agreement with Higashida et al.,[13] we perform a complete cerebral angiogram, starting with the nontarget vessels and ending with the vessel in question. The posterior cerebral artery collateral supply has been as important as the anterior cerebral artery in many cases because of the importance of Wernicke's area, the posterior watershed zone, and the collaterals between the posterior cerebral artery and the MCA branches (see the case analysis below and Figs. 59–49 to 59–62).

HEART VERSUS BRAIN (RATIONALE FOR DIFFERENT THERAPIES FOR CORONARY AND CEREBRAL VASCULAR OCCLUSIONS)

The brain is not similar to the heart. It has been shown that reperfusion therapy in the heart is beneficial even when performed *at least* up to 12 hours after symptom onset.[14] In patients with ongoing chest pain, benefits from thrombolytic therapy can occur even up to 24 hours. If a thrombotic occlusion is

cleared in the coronary circulation within 30 minutes, generally there is no tissue loss and there is 100% salvage.[15] These results differentiate these two end organs (heart and brain).

Superficially, it would appear that an occlusive lesion in a major coronary vessel would be similar to that in a cerebral vessel, on a 1 to 10 scale for degree of seriousness concerning life and the quality of life. Additionally, *superficially* it would appear that the specific therapy, necessity for rapidity of rescue, and strategy of rescue would be similar. Both of the above conclusions, however, are incorrect.

A key differentiating factor between the heart and the brain is that the heart is essentially a bulk operating unit. As long as some significant portion of the heart can function, its overall task can be completed, albeit perhaps neither as efficiently nor as strongly. This is patently not the case with the brain; for example, elimination of a small but crucial portion of cerebral tissue may result in the entire right side of the body not working *at all.* The *exact* site of vascular occlusion has far more profound implications in the brain than in the coronary vessels. In general, in the coronary vessels, the more proximal the occlusion, the worse the situation; the more distal the occlusion, the less is the total volume of territory threatened.

In the cardiovascular field, it has been shown that reestablishing most of the flow to an occluded area (e.g., opening the main trunk of the left anterior descending coronary artery) by angioplasty of thrombus results in overall benefit. Downstream embolic events are less consequential, and small infarcts ad-

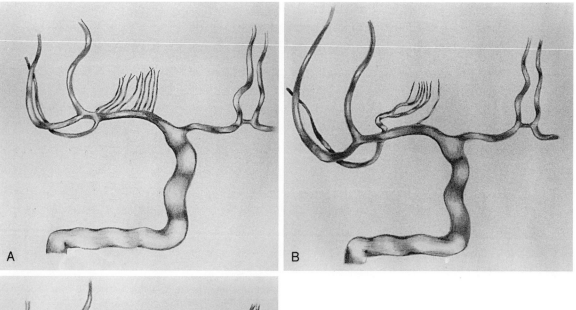

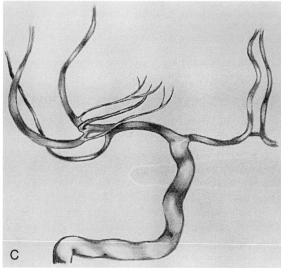

Figure 58-6 Drawings demonstrating the possible variations in the origins of the right lateral lenticulostriate arteries. In *A*, they arise as multiple small, individual vessels. In *B*, the proximal lenticulostriate arteries arise individually; the origin of the distal group is a common trunk. In *C*, potential sites of origin of lateral lenticulostriate arteries from points *distal* to the M1 segment of the MCA are shown.

jacent to the angioplastied thrombus are less consequential. Small distal infarcts may occur, but most of the cardiac tissue is rescued (Figs. 58–7 and 58–8).

The implications for occlusive lesions in the coronary circulation are nearly completely dependent on *the total volume of cardiac tissue damaged,* irrespective of the exact location of the insult. Even when conduction defects result, these almost always can be treated. Certain areas of the heart yield slightly different symptoms; the patient's exercise tolerance is affected more or less, and there are implications concerning ankle swelling and other clinical features. The heart, however, can continue to perform its primary function even if weakened overall. Indeed, after a myocardial infarct, most patients have few if any symptoms on a day-to-day basis and can resume a normal existence.

This is not the case with the brain. An infarct in the frontal lobe may be practically asymptomatic, whereas a small infarct in the motor strip can have major implications. A small infarct in the internal capsule (supplied by a lenticulostriate artery) can be devastating. Parenchymal lesions as small as a pea

can produce permanent hemiplegia, or even death, depending on the location of the infarct. For this reason, errant sacrifice of some eloquent territory is unacceptable in the cerebral circulation.

Collateral perfusion through cerebral pial collaterals can keep some tissue alive long enough for the proximal thrombus to be dissolved slowly (Figs. 58–9 and 58–10 and the case analysis below). The key is whether the end arteries are occluded. Specifically, the most vulnerable and eloquent territory for an anterior circulation ischemic insult is that supplied by the most medial of the lateral lenticulostriate vessels, arising from the proximal portion of the MCA. There are no vessels comparable to these in the coronary circulation. Mashing thrombus downstream in the brain can potentially block collateral perfusion pathways and shorten the period of time that is available for rescue, which has been shown to be detrimental[12] (see Fig. 58–10).

In the coronary vasculature, the exact site of vascular occlusion has fewer implications concerning the blockage of collateral circulation. Most collateral circulation to other coronary territories arises from the

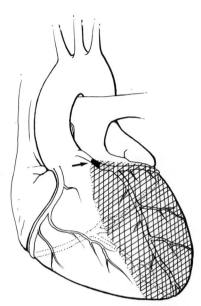

Figure 58-7 Distribution of coronary ischemia. If an occlusion blocks the left anterior descending (LAD) artery at its origin *(arrow)*, a huge area of heart is ischemic. The primary collateral supply to this area is through terminal collateral vessels. If these are not robust, the entire territory of the LAD artery is in jeopardy.

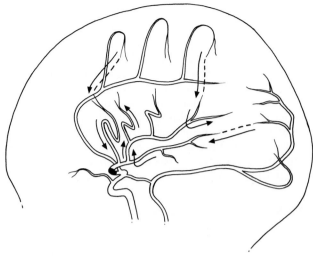

Figure 58-9 Potential collateral supply to cerebral structures. Occlusion of the MCA trunk *(black band)* allows retrograde flow in scattered branches of the MCA *(arrows),* supplied by pial collaterals from the anterior cerebral artery. Note the ability of blood to flow retrograde down to a branch point and then antegrade out into other branches that have no pial collaterals.

distal terminal anastomoses of each primary coronary artery with the other (see Figs. 58–7 and 58–8). In the cerebral circulation, the potential collateral pathways are multiple and are extremely varied. In addition, in the brain, some of these collateral pathways involve proximal main branches that can resup-

ply other branches of the same primary trunk. If these branch points in the cerebral circulation are occluded, the alternate pathways for collateral supply are blocked, with resultant profound implications concerning the depth and breadth of the cerebral ischemia. It is imperative to keep these proximal branch points open while the occluding thrombus is being dissolved.

For these reasons, the approaches to reperfusion in the heart and brain are different. For the heart, reperfusing the greatest total volume of territory,

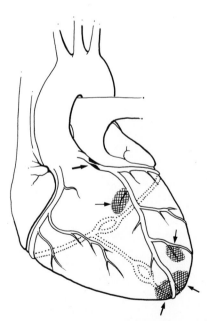

Figure 58-8 Coronary ischemia (continued). If the LAD artery is forcefully opened, the chunks of thrombus may dislodge and embolize, causing scattered infarcts, but the overall picture is improved. These scattered infarcts in the heart are apparently of less consequence than scattered infarcts in the brain. The bulk function of the heart is preserved even with these insults, whereas in the brain, these scattered insults would result in disseminated symptoms.

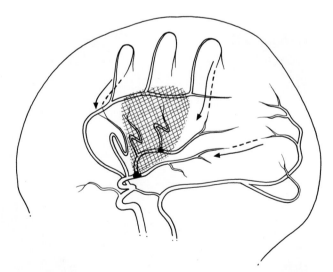

Figure 58-10 Potential collateral supply to cerebral structures (continued). If occlusion is more distal in the MCA *at the branch points,* flow cannot travel retrograde down a distal branch and then back out into other branches. This also results in the absence of a pressure gradient so that flow will not even come back to the branch point at all, the distal column of blood being a stagnant tube. This produces an even greater area of stagnation owing to absence of even retrograde flow.

opening flow in the largest vessel and the bulk of its distribution, and letting this large flow go where it may makes sense. Salvage of the greatest amount of tissue possible is of primary concern; various modest distal infarcts in the heart all have nearly the same implications. When dealing with the intracranial circulation, however, attention must be paid to the specific location of the occlusion; this can alter the therapeutic approach. Reperfusing the bulk of the MCA territory while flow is blocked to the specific vessels supplying the motor cortex or Wernicke's area would appear to be grossly counterproductive.

The No-Reflow Phenomenon

The strategy of reperfusion is influenced directly by two factors: (1) the pattern and extent of potential collateral circulation, and (2) the implications of emboli to the distal capillary beds.

In the interventional cardiology field, there is a phenomenon called *no-reflow*. No-reflow originally was observed in experimental models of myocardial infarction as a failure of restoration of normal perfusion despite removal of a proximal bulk-obstructing lesion.[16, 17] Since that time, no-reflow has been associated with thrombolytic therapy and mechanical revascularization techniques.[18, 19] Angiographically, it is characterized by the lack of antegrade flow despite the absence of proximal dissection, stenosis, thrombus, or spasm. In other words, the main vessel is open, but there is no runoff.

No-reflow is associated primarily with atherectomy devices, percutaneous transluminal coronary angioplasty, and transluminal extraction catheter atherectomy (TEC).[20, 21] Although its cause is not clear, it is thought to occur secondary to blockage of the microvasculature by debris, arising either from the proximal lesion (e.g., thrombus, plaque) or locally from sloughed epithelium in the capillaries. Spasm may play a role because symptoms can be relieved somewhat by vasodilators.[22]

No-reflow is more common after manipulation of thrombus-containing lesions, but a myocardial infarction is not necessary for this to occur. No-reflow most commonly is observed after the use of Rotablator atherectomy devices,[23] but is worst after the use of TEC, in which case the effect may be irreversible.[19]

Therapy is aimed at clearing the distal capillary bed by forceful injection of saline, fibrinolytics, vasodilators, or calcium channel blockers; the last appear to have the best success rate.[19] In one study, no-reflow was associated with a 10-fold increase in death, indicative of the serious nature of this pathology.[19]

In the heart, this is a major problem, but in the brain, it would be an absolute disaster. As stated previously, a shower of downstream emboli may be tolerated in the heart, with eventual return to an asymptomatic status if the patient survives, but it would not be tolerated in the brain. The strategy of primary angioplasty of thrombi or emboli therefore may be a poor choice for cerebral vessels.

In the brain, the mass of thrombus should not be greatly disturbed and certainly should not be intentionally smashed downstream. It should be either *dissolved* as quickly as possible in the optimal, most expeditious fashion or removed (e.g., with a clot retriever; see "Clot Retrieval" below and Chapter 60.)

THE NEED TO REESTABLISH FLOW: MECHANICAL VERSUS FIBRINOLYTIC MEANS

Although it appears in direct contradistinction to the previous discussion, establishing at least some

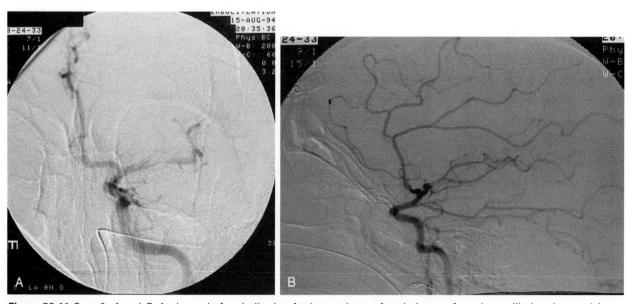

Figure 58-11 Case 3. *A* and *B,* At the end of embolization for hemorrhage after drainage of a submandibular abscess (shown in Fig. 15–1), a routine control evaluation of the intracranial distribution of the left common carotid artery reveals a nearly occlusive thrombus in the MCA (M1) trunk. The superior division of the MCA is absent. The patient exhibited right hemiparesis (arm greater than leg).

Case 3 continues

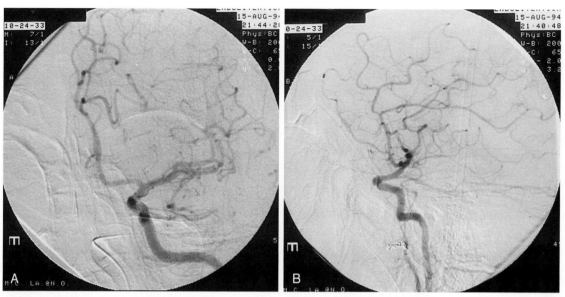

Figure 58-12 *A* and *B,* It was not possible to obtain consent from the attending service for the use of urokinase to treat the thrombus. In the belief that the lenticulostriate arteries are of overwhelming importance, it was thought that trying to displace the clot downstream past the M1 segment would be beneficial. This was done with a microwire. The patient's neurologic status improved on the table. Note the truncated inferior division of the MCA.

degree of antegrade flow may be of benefit for two reasons: (1) the action of fibrinolysis is accelerated tremendously in a flowing vessel because of delivery of fresh plasminogen, and (2) distal ischemic structures can get some relief with the reestablishment of even a trickle of flow through the occlusion (see "General Considerations Regarding Fibrinolysis" above). Manipulation of the thrombus too aggressively, however, can break it up into fragments that can occlude multiple vessels—a worse situation than a simple, large, proximal occlusion. This is particularly true if there is a large bulk of thrombus, a situation that may not be apparent.

Contradictory anecdotal reports have been made. Displacement of clot in the M1 segment by an 0.014″ guidewire with subsequent clearing of the M1 segment (Case 11, Figs. 58–11 to 58–14) has been performed, resulting in almost instant (if partial) clinical improvement (obviously a desperate maneuver; simple fibrinolytic infusion was not possible in this particular clinical circumstance). Alternatively, a forceful injection through a 5.5-Fr. diagnostic catheter with its tip in the distal internal carotid artery has shoved an M1 segment thrombus downstream into an M2 branch, again with almost immediate clinical improvement (see Figs. 59–63 to 59–67). It is not known whether this ultimately complicates thrombolysis by "packing" the clot or producing multiple branch occlusions. Alternatively, an anecdotal report has been made of fragmentation of a large proximal occlusion, with resultant inability to clear all the branch occlusions, and with a devastating outcome.

From a strategic standpoint, it is the belief of many interventional neuroradiologists that clearing of the segment occluding the lenticulostriate arteries as quickly as possible is imperative. Fibrinolytic infu-

sion can then be performed downstream in a cortical branch rather than in the main trunk of the MCA.

Clot Retrieval

There are four techniques for mechanically reestablishing flow, the first of which, probing, is our pre-

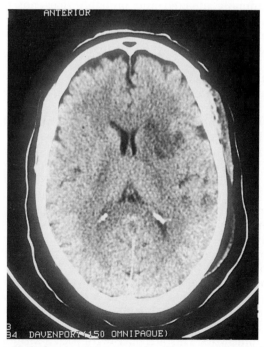

Figure 58-13 Computed tomographic (CT) scan obtained 4 days later reveals an infarct in the far lateral lenticulostriate territory sparing the majority of the internal capsule and cortex. No cortical infarct is seen.

Case 3 continues

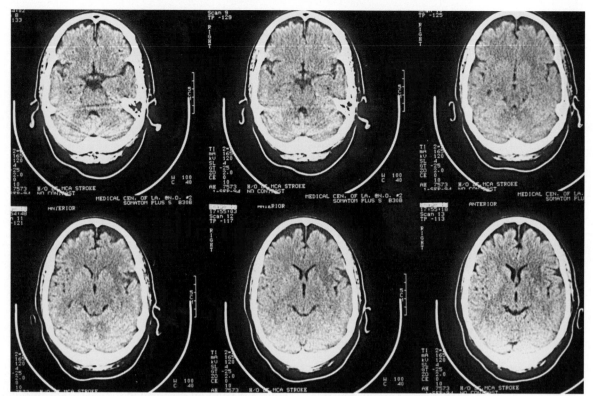

Figure 58-14 CT scan obtained 2 weeks later reveals maturation of the small infarct (essentially asymptomatic at that time). There is no cortical ischemic component.

ferred method. Probing can establish antegrade flow, allowing more effective thrombolysis while allowing more time for the rescue because some nutrients are making their way to the ischemic area. The thrombus is minimally affected and probably does not move much in this instance. This is usually successful. Sometimes, however, this maneuver is unsuccessful, and other means may be required to achieve this goal, particularly for an embolus that is old and resistant to thrombolysis.

The second technique, angioplasty of the thrombus, is inelegant and unpredictable. As stated previously, it is not known where the thrombus will be smashed (i.e., into lenticulostriate vessels, the superior branch of the MCA, or fragmented into several vital vessels). The mass could be compacted and even more resistant to thrombolysis, or it could be smashed into a side branch of limited usefulness. It has not been clearly proved that angioplasty is uniformly counterproductive; in some cases, it may be beneficial.

The third method involves actually removing the embolic mass by means of a snare (described in Chapters 3 and 60). This can remove a firm embolic mass and has been shown to be a useful maneuver.

The fourth method also mechanically removes the clot. This entails the use of a clot removal device from Medtronic/MIS. This is a microwire with a nitinol coil at its distal end in the shape of a spiral with a radius of about 4 mm, tapering to 2 mm at the distal end, similar to the Tornado fibered embolic coils from Cook, Inc. The clot removal device is deployed from a microcatheter placed *distal* to the embolic mass.

The wire is slowly extruded from the end of the catheter (as the catheter is being slowly withdrawn) and allowed to form into a basket in a conical shape that cups the embolus and pulls it out when the entire unit is withdrawn. Although we have not used this device, it appears to have promise.

Detailed Strategic Case Analysis of Acute Mechanical Revascularization Alone

Several cases presented in this chapter are examples of the potential validity of the hypothesis concerning the need for a mechanical means to aid revascularization, including the following case (Case 4, Figs. 58–15 to 58–54).

Day 1

A 29-year-old man had undergone resection of a left frontal lobe microglioma followed by radiation therapy 10 years earlier. He now presented with the acute onset of right arm motor dysfunction (4/5 strength) combined with worsening dysarthria. A CT scan showed no acute change but did reveal the expected postoperative change in the patient's left frontal lobe.

Day 2

The patient's speech and motor deficits (arm) worsened the next day. In addition, he began to suffer

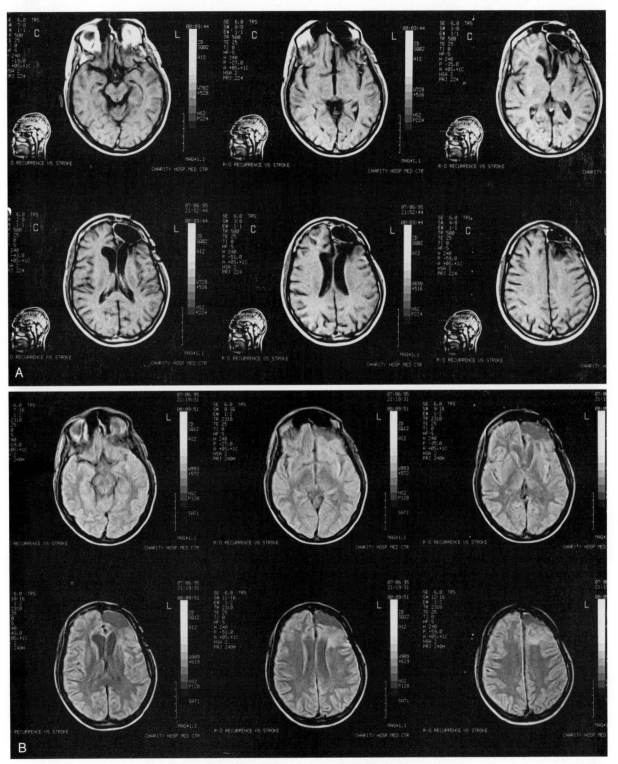

Figure 58-15 *See legend on following page*

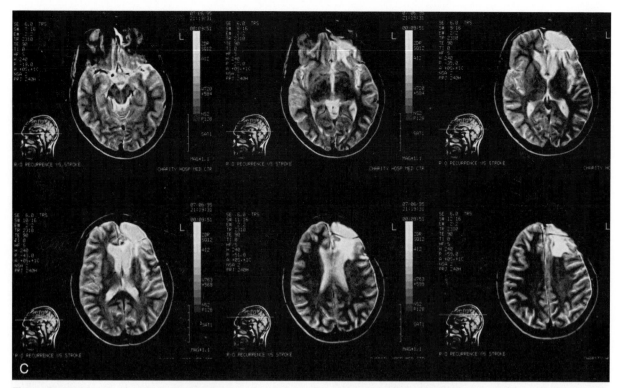

Figure 58-15 Case 4. *A* to *C*, A 29-year-old man who presented to the emergency room with acute right-sided weakness (4/5 arm strength) and increasing dysarthria. Magnetic resonance imaging (MRI) was performed more than 36 hours after onset of symptoms. Note the remarkable lack of pathologic change in any territory that could explain the clinical status (the postoperative, postradiation changes are very apparent). Note also the abnormal appearance of the M1 segment of the MCA on the left, of questionable but unknown significance. The insular cortex is slightly abnormal compared with the opposite side.

Specifically, note the lack of any signal change in the normal distribution of the lateral lenticulostriate arteries. This is of *paramount* importance, offering the hope that a revascularization effort could have a reasonable chance of success without an unreasonable risk of devastating hemorrhage. If the lenticular nucleus or internal capsule had looked similar to the insular cortex, the modest confidence felt in the prospects of successful therapy would have vanished completely.

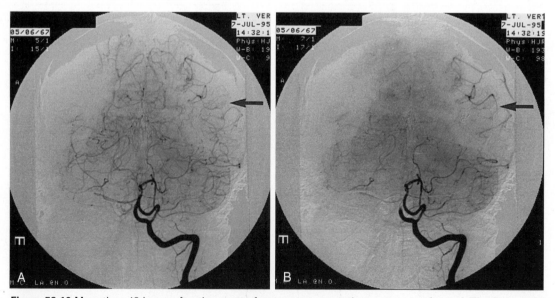

Figure 58-16 More than 48 hours after the onset of symptoms, an angiogram was performed. The first vessel selected by the routine cerebral angiography team was the left vertebral artery. The early phase *(A)* reveals extensive supply to an unusual area for the posterior cerebral artery to supply (the far lateral area on the left—in the usual distribution of the left MCA), while an early parenchymal blush is noted in the standard posterior cerebral artery territory. The peripheral branches on the left *(arrow)* are slightly late to fill and have no parenchymal blush. *B,* The later image demonstrates a normal capillary blush in the cerebellum and posterior cerebral artery territories, but continued slow filling of MCA branches *(arrow)*. Note the unfortunate stasis in the left vertebral artery, probably due to spasm at the catheter tip.

Case 4 continues

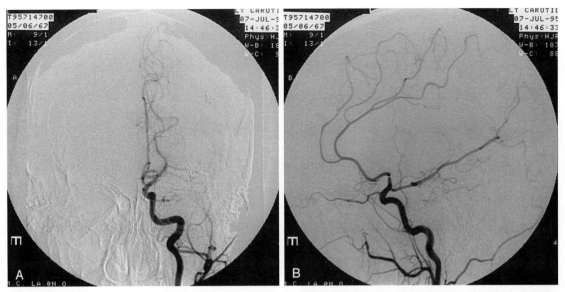

Figure 58-17 *A* and *B,* PA and lateral views of the left common carotid injection reveals absence of the left MCA. Note the prominent filling of the posterior cerebral artery, apparently to supplement the supply to the entire hemisphere, and possibly related to hemodynamic deficiency of the left vertebral artery (spasm?).

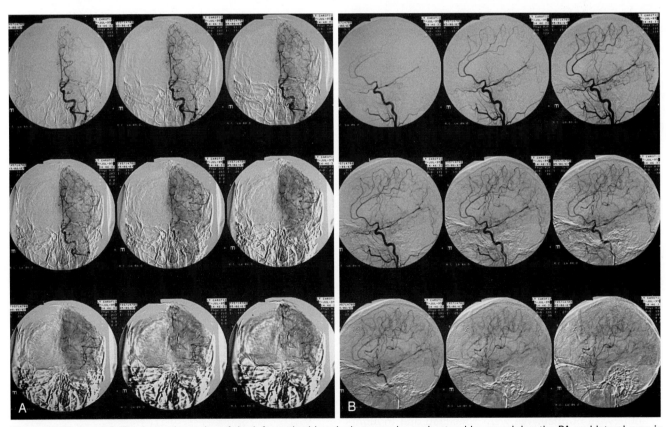

Figure 58-18 *A* and *B,* The hemodynamics of the left cerebral hemisphere can be understood by examining the PA and lateral runs in their entirety. Although motion artifact obscures the subtle detail, it is readily apparent that there is an incredible amount of slow flow into the entire left MCA distribution. On the lateral view, note the slow percolation of blood into even the most proximal portion of the MCA trunk.

Analysis of these images allowed these conclusions. First, there is at least some supply not only to the distal MCA territory, but also to the proximal MCA territory. Second, the retrograde flow to this proximal point can be caused only by hemodynamic demand; i.e., the capillary bed in this proximal location must still be actively drawing blood back to this point, and thus presumably at least a portion is still viable. Third, any antegrade flow from the MCA trunk must be nonexistent (in all likelihood) or minimal, or else there would not be any impetus for the blood to flow in a retrograde fashion all the way back to the bifurcation of the M1 segment of the MCA *(small arrow* in the last image in *B).*

Case 4 continues

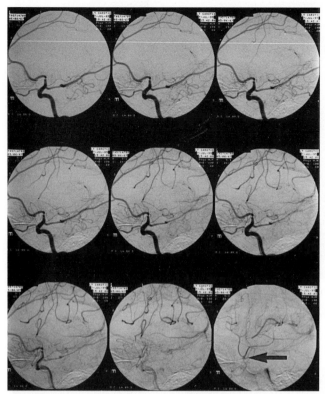

Figure 58-19 A repeat angiogram with magnification of the left common carotid artery clearly demonstrates the extensive but very slow retrograde filling of the main cortical branches of the MCA. Note the eventual opacification of the actual bifurcation of the MCA *(arrow)*.

leg weakness. Carotid Doppler examination was unrevealing, and an MRI scan was performed that evening (more than 36 hours after the onset of these symptoms). This was surprisingly unremarkable (other than what was thought to represent changes consistent with prior partial frontal lobectomy and radiation). *No MRI findings were seen that explained the patient's current clinical condition.*

Day 3

The patient awoke totally mute. His right arm was now 2/5 to 3/5 strength and his leg 4/5 strength. A cerebral angiogram was performed that afternoon, nearly 16 hours after the MRI and more than 48 hours after the onset of symptoms. The patient had now been mute for 8 hours. This study demonstrated total occlusion of the left MCA (intracranial vascularity was otherwise normal). We were consulted and thought that good pial collateral supply from the anterior and posterior cerebral arteries with a considerable amount of extremely slow retrograde filling of distal MCA branches was present.

More important, there appeared to be a striking lack of damage to the area of the lenticulostriate vessels on the MRI scan, implying that at least *some blood flow had to be reaching these vessels.* This raised a question about the actual status of the entire M1 segment of the MCA, which appeared to be totally

occluded. The "normal" MRI scan in this region and the "total" occlusion of the MCA appeared to be mutually exclusive. Perhaps just the origin of the MCA was occluded, with some remaining, invisible perfusion of the lenticulostriate arteries.

After further careful analysis, it was thought that some filling of the main trunk of the MCA could be seen on the lateral view (owing to the concentration of the contrast achieved when looking down the barrel of the vessel), even though it was never visible on the various posteroanterior projections obtained. (The imaging equipment used was a state-of-the-art, 1024 × 1024 matrix, high-resolution Siemens Neurostar.) This filling could have been from retrograde branch flow (M2, but doubtful) or from some invisible flow through the apparent occlusion.

The decision was made to present the information to the family and to obtain the necessary informed consent to proceed with a rescue attempt. If some patency of the M1 segment of the MCA artery was present, the lenticulostriate territory was viable, and the MRI findings were still valid, there was the potential for rescue of the entire hemisphere, even though there had been a motor deficit for more than 48 hours and the dysarthria had progressed to complete mutism (now present for over 8 hours). The strategy (and anxieties) at this point concerned the *current* intracranial status, as opposed to the status shown on the MRI scan that was now more than 16 hours old. We hoped that most of the lenticulostriates (and their territory) were still viable; if even a few were not, their rupture could devastate all the surrounding rescuable tissue, if not kill the patient.

Reestablishment of antegrade flow by mechanical means (a guidewire followed by a microcatheter) was

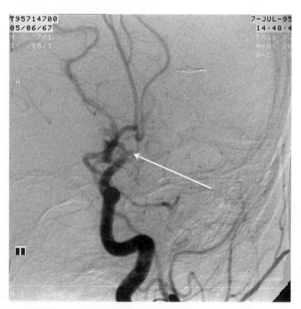

Figure 58-20 A slightly oblique magnification PA view demonstrates the truncation (occlusion) of the left MCA approximately 1 mm from its origin *(arrow)*. The posterior communicating artery and posterior cerebral artery overlie the anterior cerebral artery in this projection.

Case 4 continues

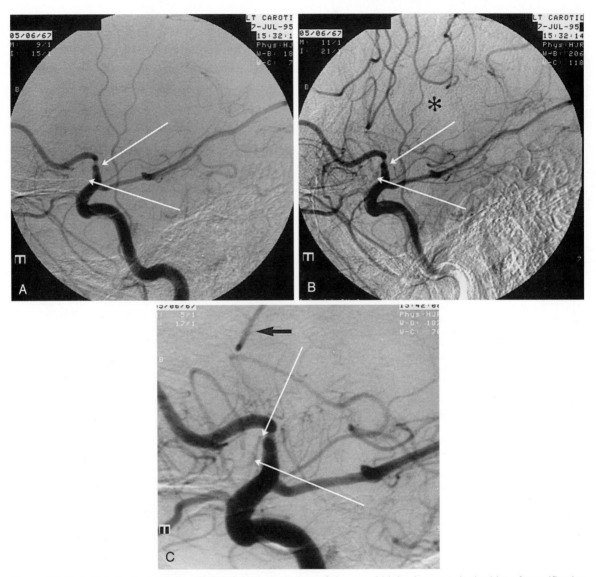

Figure 58-21 *A,* Extremely careful analysis of the lateral view of the carotid injection reveals the hint of opacification of an unknown structure. The top arrow shows the stub of the MCA. The lower arrow is apparently aimed at nothing, but late in the run there is the appearance of some vague density *(B).* This vague density appears even after the MCA branches have filled in a retrograde fashion down to the sylvian fissure level *(asterisk).* The vague shadow is the same appearance that the cavernous sinus might make, but is too high (cephalad) for this structure, it was believed to represent the main trunk of the MCA.

Confirmation could not be obtained on multiple PA views and injections, however. This was thought to be due to the fact that the density was much more visible when looking "down the trunk" of the M1 segment of the MCA rather than from the side (i.e., from the front—PA).

The extreme magnification in *C* reveals the vague shadow somewhat more clearly. The upper white arrow points to the origin of the MCA; the lower arrow points to the vague opacification of the (supposed) trunk of the vessel. Note the very late appearance of the posterior frontal branch of the MCA at the top of the picture *(black arrow).*

Case 4 continues

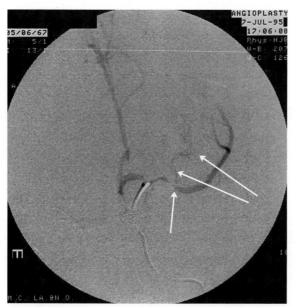

Figure 58-22 The use of urokinase in this situation was considered too risky, there being a fixed neurologic deficit more than 24 hours old. It was also thought that there was probably only a short segment occlusion and that "poking" a catheter through this hole might be possible.

This was done by advancing the microcatheter while being led by a very tight P curve on a Seeker Standard guidewire (Target Therapeutics) (a P curve is an overdone J). The P curve collapsed at the occlusion, but this blunt curve rendered forceful advancement of the catheter possible. This was advanced through the occlusion.

Once downstream a few centimeters, the wire was *very slowly* withdrawn, the hub of the catheter being filled with saline the entire time. This was to prevent inadvertent admission of air into a closed system (if the catheter was in an occluded or clotted vessel). After it was very slowly rinsed, the catheter was infused with contrast while being slowly withdrawn.

The image demonstrates the appearance of the MCA after the catheter had been withdrawn into the region of the bifurcation of the internal carotid artery. Note the very narrow M1 segment of the MCA, but more important, note the abrupt widening of the main trunk of the MCA *(inferior arrow)* just proximal to the origin of at least a few incredibly important lenticulostriate arteries *(superior arrows)*. These could have been kept alive by the pitiful amount of blood flow demonstrated on the previous angiograms (their origin appears to be within a segment of "normal" vessel).

Note also the near-normal appearance of the distal MCA branches.

considered reasonable if for no other reason than to determine the hardness and distance of the occlusion; angioplasty might then be performed if a lesion was found. Fibrinolysis, although feasible, was considered an unknown risk at this late time and therefore contraindicated under the circumstances.

It was possible to advance a guidewire, followed by a microcatheter, past the occlusion, but with significant difficulty. Instead of advancing the guidewire with a typical angled curve on its tip, a tight P curve was used. This is considered far safer for blind probing and tends to follow the true lumen. Once the catheter had been advanced through this stenosis, extremely careful injection through the catheter revealed that the distal branches of the MCA were normal in appearance. A tight stenosis underlying the

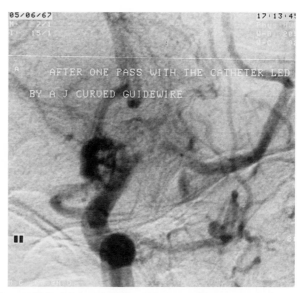

Figure 58-23 After one pass with the catheter, this was the appearance of the proximal trunk of the MCA; barely visible but patent.

occlusion in the proximal M1 segment was encountered. This was dilated with a 2 mm × 10 mm Fas-STEALTH microangioplasty catheter, again advanced through the stenosis with great difficulty.

Although the initial postangioplasty result was far less than ideal, fibrinolytic agents were not used because of the duration of the occlusion and the unknown status of the downstream microvasculature. Infusion of papaverine resulted in improvement in the appearance, indicating that at least part of the residual narrowing and irregularity was due to spasm.

Text continued on page 681

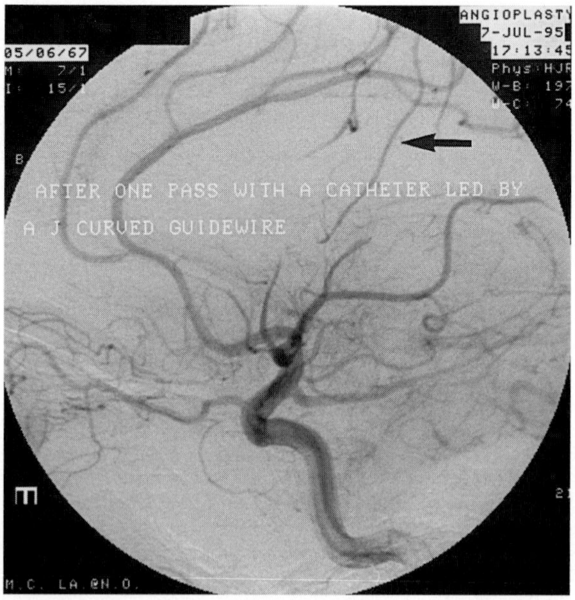

Figure 58-24 The lateral view of a subsequent injection reveals some minimal branch filling of the MCA, but far slower than the normal anterior distribution, and retrograde filling of MCA branches is still present *(arrow)*.

Case 4 continues

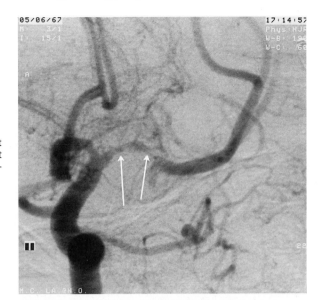

Figure 58-25 Because of the fear of using urokinase, the best attempt at establishing antegrade flow had to be mechanical. The arrows point at the lumen after the catheter had been passed again. Note the irregular lumen and extremely small size.

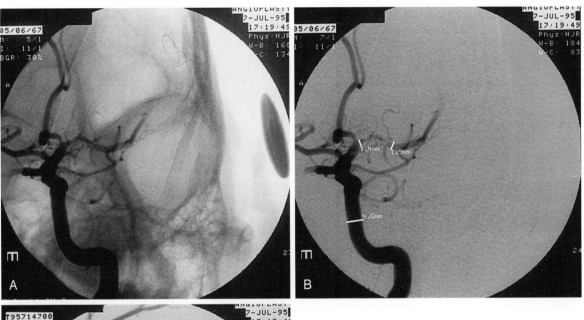

Figure 58-26 In anticipation of the possibility of angioplasty, specific vessel measurement was performed by placing a quarter on the side of the head and performing another injection. This revealed the apparent size of the MCA to be less than 2 mm. Note in *C* that the coin overlies the area of interest, thus indicating that on the orthogonal view, the PA projection (*A* and *B*), the "object-screen" distance would be the same for the coin and lesion (*A* and *B* are the same; one is subtracted and the other is not).

Case 4 continues

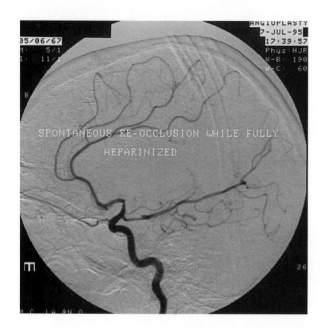

Figure 58-27 In view of continuing worry about the use of urokinase under these circumstances, it was thought that a period of watchful waiting was indicated; antegrade flow had been established by the passage of the catheter, and that might be all that was necessary. Even while the patient was fully heparinized, the vessel reoccluded.

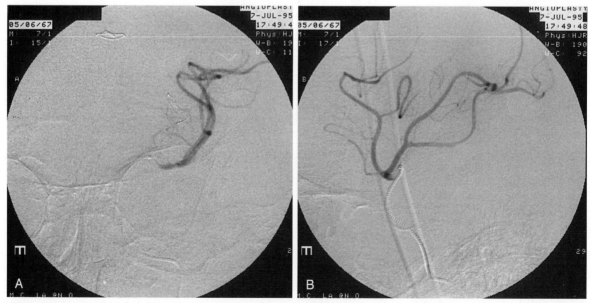

Figure 58-28 *A* and *B,* The catheter was readvanced through the lesion (with a tightly curled P guidewire leading the way). Again, injection revealed good flow into the MCA branch vessels.

Case 4 continues

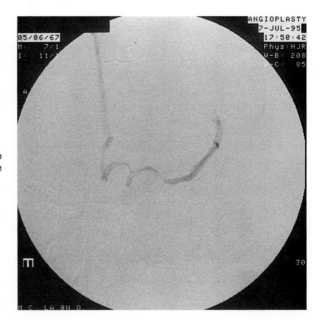

Figure 58-29 The catheter was again withdrawn and the follow-up injection revealed continuing stenosis in the M1 segment, but the vessel looked a little better (maybe?).

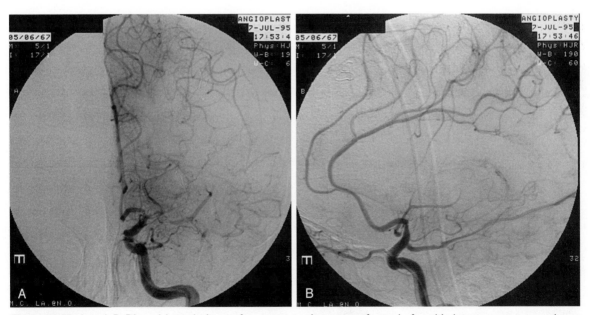

Figure 58-30 *A* and *B,* PA and lateral views of a repeat angiogram performed after this latest passage reveal very slow flow through the "lumen" of the MCA trunk. Note on the PA view that there is extensive filling of the anterior cerebral branches with minimal filling through the stenotic segment. On the lateral view, the MCA again appears almost occluded.

Case 4 continues

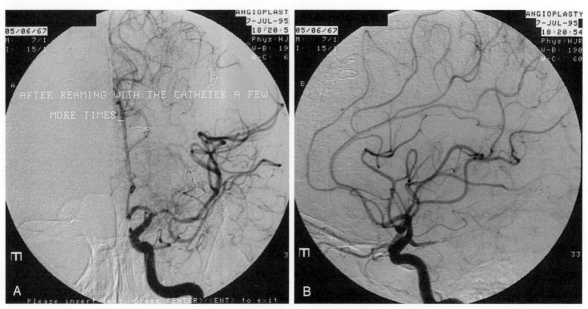

Figure 58-31 *A* and *B,* Still fearful of using any fibrinolytic agent, we performed more vigorous mechanical disruption ("reaming" is how it is described on the angiographic film). This resulted in far better antegrade flow. Note that the MCA branches are not only filling almost as quickly as the anterior cerebral branches, but are at least as dense, if not more so (on both PA and lateral views). Could this be ischemic steal?

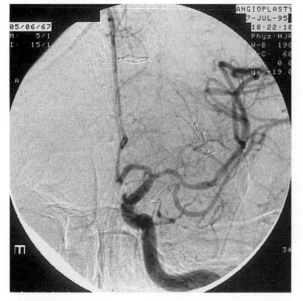

Figure 58-32 Further watchful waiting was undertaken. Everything looked good for the first 2 minutes.

Case 4 continues

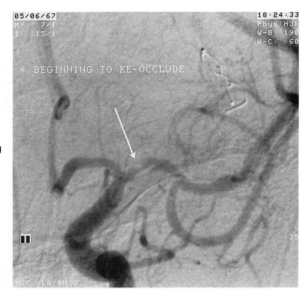

Figure 58-33 Two minutes later the vessel appears to be narrowing *(arrow)*.

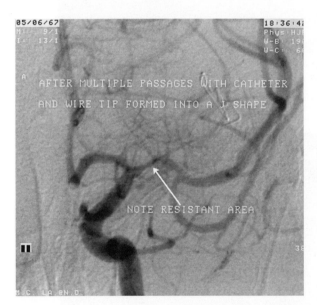

Figure 58-34 Multiple passes with the microcatheter have now convinced us of the vessel's natural tendency to reocclude. Note the apparently resistant region of the vessel *(arrow)*.

Figure 58-35 Angioplasty was considered necessary to keep this vessel open. However, the pathologic status of the vessel was not known (it was believed that previous radiation was the cause of the apparent focal pathology). Was it "tissue paper" (secondary to radiation), or scarred? Again, the options were put to the family and the decision to proceed was made.

Our decision was to use the smallest angioplasty balloon available, for two reasons: (1) the native vessel appeared to be small, although this might be artifactual; and (2) it was felt that, initially, any permanent significant increase in lumen size would be beneficial, and the last thing anyone wanted was an intimal dissection. The smallest intracranial angioplasty catheter available was the 2-mm STEALTH (Target Therapeutics). This was advanced through the internal carotid artery with the occluding valve wire leading the way. This impacted at the stenosis.

When this catheter and wire met the stenosis, it was apparent that any additional force only buckled the catheter. Remembering work in the periphery, it was decided that inflation where the balloon lay would possibly begin the dilation process at the proximal portion of the stenosis.

Case 4 continues

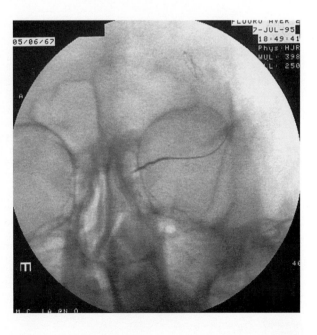

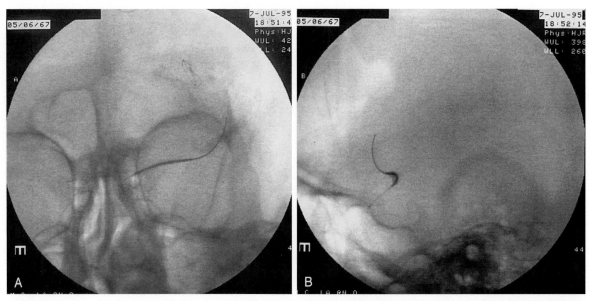

Figure 58-36 *A* and *B,* Once the balloon had been inflated once, it was possible to advance the STEALTH through the stenosis and place it in the position shown, and inflate it as shown best on the lateral view *(B)*.

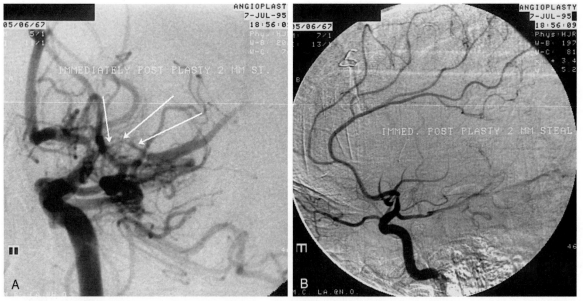

Figure 58-37 *A* and *B,* The angioplasty was performed and a follow-up angiogram was done with the catheter in place. The typical poor results were thought to be due to the STEALTH still being in place. Inevitably, the results of the angioplasty were unobservable and underappreciated. For this reason, the STEALTH was removed and a follow-up angiogram obtained, revealing almost total occlusion of the entire angioplastied segment (arrows in *A*). Very poor flow is seen in the MCA and its branches.

At this point in this type of procedure, urokinase would normally be infused. Owing to the clinical circumstances, however, this was again considered inadvisable.

Faced with this situation, the only active interventional therapeutic option available appeared to be infusion of a vasodilator, as recrossing an angioplastied vessel is considered very risky. Papaverine was the drug that came to mind, but nitroglycerin could possibly have given a more powerful and immediate response.

Case 4 continues

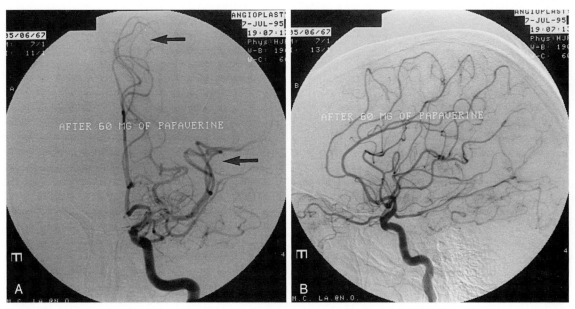

Figure 58-38 *A* and *B,* After 60 mg papaverine had been infused in the internal carotid artery just proximal to the bifurcation, PA and lateral views of a repeat angiogram reveal significantly increased flow in the branches of the MCA previously occluded; however, this flow is still somewhat slower than in the anterior cerebral artery *(arrows).*

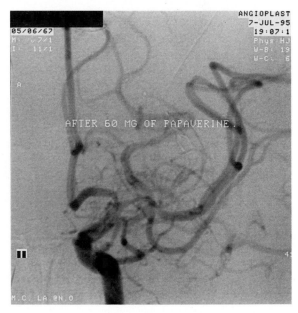

Figure 58-39 High-resolution magnification of the angioplastied area after administration of 60 mg papaverine reveals some improvement in the appearance of the angioplastied vessel, but it is still suboptimal.

Case 4 continues

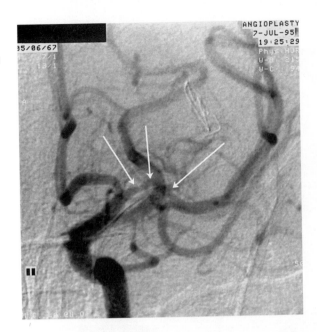

Figure 58-40 Another 60 mg papaverine has been infused over 30 minutes and a repeat angiogram performed. High-magnification, high-resolution imaging is employed and demonstrates the angioplastied segment to be widely patent (although less than the natural lumen of the vessel). This lumen (judged to be approximately 1 mm, *arrows*) is thought to be adequate under the current clinical circumstances.

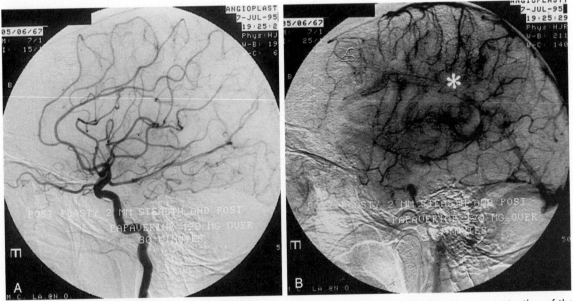

Figure 58-41 *A* and *B,* The lateral view (displayed in the capillary phase with intentional contrast accentuation of the computer window width and level in order to accentuate any region of hypervascularity) can be used to evaluate any abnormal capillary blush ("perfusion") secondary to infarct. It has been observed that any area that does not blush at all (with the extreme window settings used in this image) is usually dead tissue with no requirement for perfusion. Conversely, any capillary blush that is more than usual is probably due to reactive hyperperfusion of a previously ischemic region, which is potentially salvageable. Note that there is some evidence of hypervascularity in the midparietal region in the capillary phase *(asterisk),* but nothing extreme. This is far better than no capillary blush in this region, which could be indicative of regional neuronal/vascular/endothelial anoxia (no demand for perfusion) and probable regional cell death.

Case 4 continues

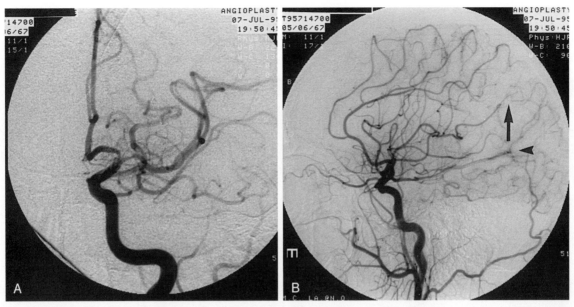

Figure 58-42 *A* and *B,* After a delay of 25 minutes of watchful waiting, a repeat angiogram reveals a widely patent MCA with good flow to the distal distribution of its territory. Note that the speed of flow and density of the MCA branches compared with the anterior cerebral artery branches is now about the same. In particular, the vessels in the typically most severely affected watershed zone (the terminal branches of the angular branch of the middle MCA *[arrow]*) are no slower than the posterior cerebral branches in the same region *(arrowhead)*. This implies that the capillary bed of the two areas may be similar; that is, normal.

At this time, while still on the angiogram table, the patient's arm strength was gradually increasing, but he was still mute.

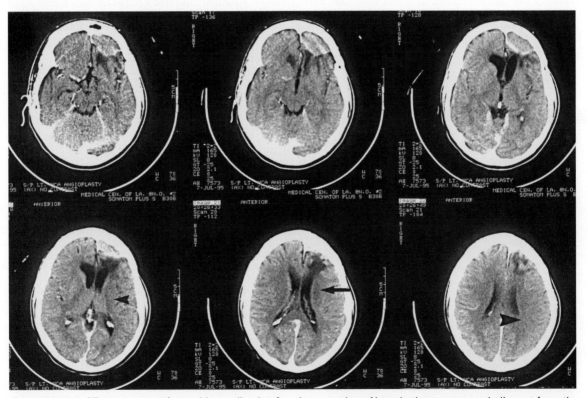

Figure 58-43 A CT scan was performed immediately after the procedure. Note the large porencephalic cyst from the previous tumor resection and surrounding blush (probably postoperative glial scar). Also note the lack of any blush in the distribution of the MCA. This may be important; to our minds the lack of blush, much less the lack of hemorrhage, in the lenticulostriates is the most reassuring aspect of the study. There is some very vague low density in the corona radiata *(arrow)* and loss of definition of the lenticular nucleus on the slice just below this *(small arrowhead)*. In addition, there is loss of the gray-white interface on the topmost slice in the posterior parietal lobe compared with the opposite side *(large arrowhead)*.

Case 4 continues

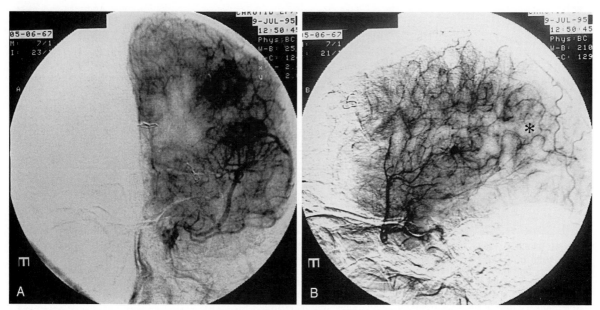

Figure 58-44 *A* and *B*. In view the nature of the procedure and the patient's current status, it was decided to leave him on anticoagulation (heparin); therefore, the sheath could not be withdrawn immediately. If a hyperdense area (leakage of contrast) had been seen on postprocedure CT, the heparin would have been immediately stopped. Two days later, a follow-up angiogram confirms what had been seen before. The PA view demonstrates a hypervascular reaction in the midparietal lobe. The lateral view is not nearly so dramatic but still shows a hypervascular reaction in the midportion of the MCA distribution. Note the patchy blush in the very peripheral territory of the angular branch of the MCA *(asterisk);* is this a region of poor capillary or neuronal viability?

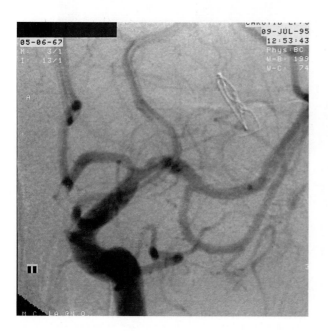

Figure 58-45 Final close-up view of the region of angioplasty. Even though the result looks acceptable, the residual lumen is still less than 1 mm. Is this large enough? What is the natural history of these lesions? It is not known what the actual course would be in every case, but early work at the University of Pittsburgh indicates that critical intracranial stenoses have a high rate of occlusion within 1 to 2 years. It is our feeling that any lesion less than 1 mm should be seriously considered for angioplasty.

The plan was to switch the anticoagulation to warfarin (Coumadin), follow this man every 3 months for at least 1 year, and then decide whether to lengthen the interval.

Case 4 continues

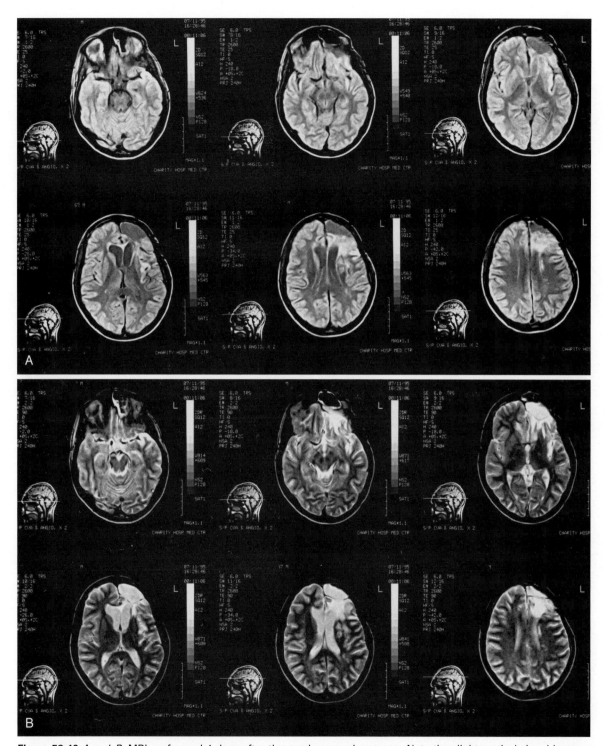

Figure 58-46 *A* and *B,* MRI performed 4 days after the cerebrovascular rescue. Note the slight cortical signal increase in the insula, as well as a patchy increased signal in the corona radiata. There is also the suggestion of some increased signal in the deep white matter in the posterior watershed region. The patient's clinical condition was nearly back to baseline at this point. It had taken more than 2 days for the dysarthria to mostly clear, and an additional 2 days for the residual motor deficit to clear. He was now neurologically intact.

Case 4 continues

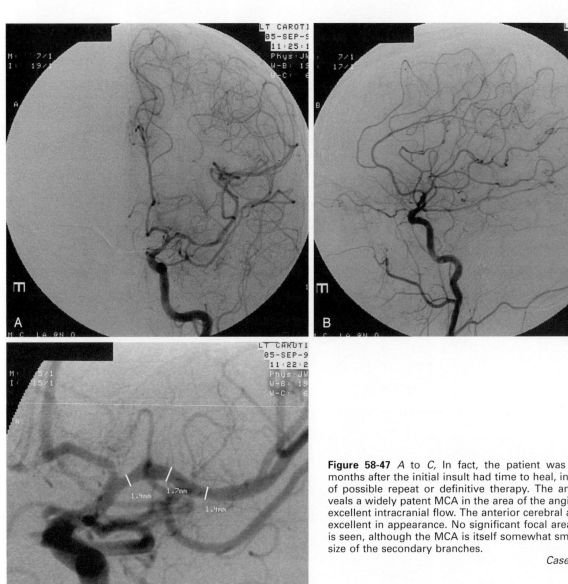

Figure 58-47 *A* to *C,* In fact, the patient was restudied 2 months after the initial insult had time to heal, in anticipation of possible repeat or definitive therapy. The angiogram reveals a widely patent MCA in the area of the angioplasty with excellent intracranial flow. The anterior cerebral artery is also excellent in appearance. No significant focal area of stenosis is seen, although the MCA is itself somewhat small. Note the size of the secondary branches.

Case 4 continues

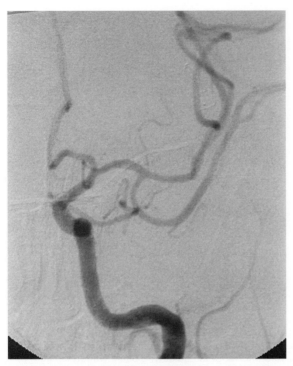

Figure 58-48 Nine-month follow-up angiogram. The patient was doing well and was asymptomatic. He had now been off warfarin for 4 months because the appearance of the MCA had been good on the previous follow-up study and it was felt that anticoagulation was no longer necessary. The lumen of the M1 segment looks excellent, similar to its appearance on every study since the procedure the summer before.

The next day, the patient could speak, but with significant word-finding problems, dysarthria, and complete inability to express certain things. His motor skills were improved but still diminished. Over the next 2 to 4 days, he regained all of his lost functions. His speech was completely normal. His strength was 5/5 throughout. Although he claimed to be completely neurologically normal, there was some subtle loss of fine motor skill and quickness of the hand. The delayed MRI scan revealed some deep lateral lenticulostriate territory damage (see Fig. 58–46), but this apparently affected only a minimal volume of radiating fibers.

Lessons of the Case

This case represents by far the longest duration, fixed neurologic deficit that has been reversed. This example epitomizes the range of potential underlying pathologies and the possible therapeutic results achievable by endovascular techniques. If the decision had been made to use fibrinolytics alone from the start, the patient may have done well. The fact that an area of true cell death in a deep perforator (lenticulostriate) distribution was later demonstrated, however, suggests that there also may have been the possibility of inducing a true intraparenchymal hemorrhage, which, even if arising from a small area, could have caused massive cerebral destruction or even death.

Conversely, the use of a fibrinolytic may have *prevented* this small area of infarct from occurring by cleaning the vessel lumen more thoroughly!

The cause of this patient's underlying stenosis was thought to be a focal area of radiation-induced vasculitis secondary to the previous radiation treatment of the glioma. The pathophysiologic result was fibrosis in this short segment. Due to the desire to achieve the goal of the therapy (rescue of the vascular distribution of this vessel), we did not attempt a complete and thorough treatment (i.e., dilation to a normal MCA size); our hands had been tied by the clinical circumstances. In other words, any time an intracranial angioplasty is performed, the use of a fibrinolytic agent may become necessary, but this was not possible in this case. Because of the small caliber of the new channel, it was deemed appropriate and necessary to keep the patient on anticoagulant therapy, wait for the parenchyma to recover from the insult, and restudy the patient later with the thought of performing definitive therapy at that time.

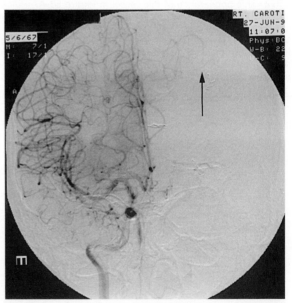

Figure 58-49 The patient returned only 6 weeks later with a transient ischemic attack (TIA) that, although only 5 minutes in duration, was enough to get his attention (he immediately went into the house and took two warfarins and an aspirin). The symptoms were weakness in the right hand only and a facial palsy. There was a questionable difficulty with speech. In our experience, in addition to speech difficulties, focal weakness of the hand has been a recurrent symptom associated with focal M1 stenoses.

The initial portion of any nonemergent but potentially interventional examination should be to evaluate the vessels *not in question*. Once the vessel of interest has been selected, there is a tendency to stop at this location and not go to the others. Injection of the opposite (right) carotid artery affords a good view of the exact distribution of the anterior cerebral artery on the affected side, the left. This reveals a worrisome shift of the watershed zone on the left from the anterior cerebral artery to the MCA *(arrow)*. The watershed zone appears to now be somewhat more lateral than usual, indicative of probable poor inflow from the MCA on the left.

Case 4 continues

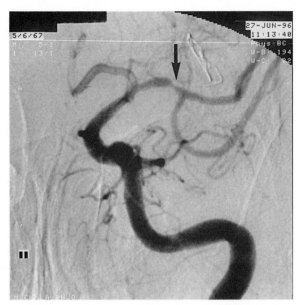

Figure 58-50 Now that the catheter is on the side of interest (the left), it is seen that there is a narrowing in the distal M1 segment *(arrow)* not seen on the previous angiogram just 6 weeks earlier. Is this truly significant? The shift in the watershed zone, combined with the recent event, and the change from the previous angiographic appearance of the vessel in Figure 58–47 indicates that it is! (The patient now admitted to beginning smoking again within the previous 2 weeks.)

What does this narrowing represent? He had been in the hospital on heparin for the 3 days before the study (we had been out of town); it was therefore considered that this did not represent a minute amount of thrombus, but a true stenosis.

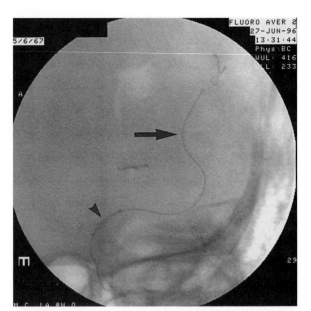

Figure 58-52 After the distal lesion had been angioplastied, the guidewire was advanced up the distal MCA branch *(arrow)* and the angioplasty catheter withdrawn to the internal carotid artery bifurcation region *(arrowhead)*. This maneuver was performed to avoid the risk of the guidewire being withdrawn back through the previously angioplastied site. One would not want to risk recrossing this location if the wire accidentally migrated too proximally, a maneuver that has been associated with enlarging a small intimal flap into a large one with resultant occlusion of the vessel.

A repeat angioplasty was performed at the proximal M1 segment because this region also looked somewhat narrow on the initial image.

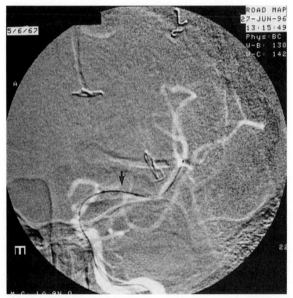

Figure 58-51 An angioplasty was performed without difficulty, utilizing a Stratus angioplasty balloon (Medtronic/MIS) and an Envoy guide catheter (Cordis Corp.). Roadmapping was used for accurate placement of the balloon across the lesion. Note the guidewire/occlusion wire in the superior division of the MCA. A 2 × 10 mm balloon was used. The stenosis is just proximal to the inferior branch and seen as an area of absence of white contrast *(arrow)*.

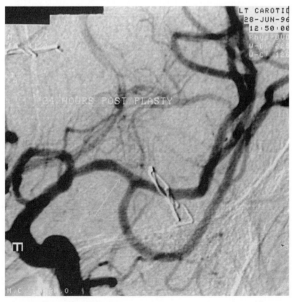

Figure 58-53 The angioplasty site was repeatedly watched for the next hour with the patient on the table and anticoagulated. After it is seen that there is no aggressive thrombus formation, the procedure can be terminated, but the patient still remains anticoagulated and the sheath is left in the patient's leg.

Case 4 continues

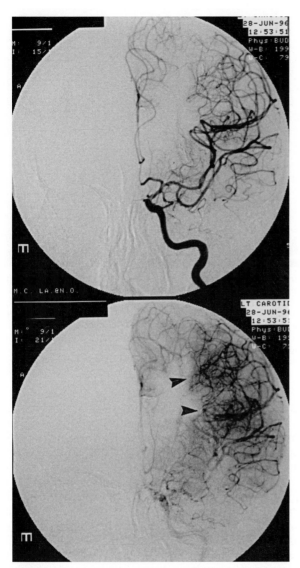

Figure 58-54 A global hemodynamic view demonstrates an intense reactive hyperemia in the main territory of the MCA, the result of the increased flow to this previously ischemic area *(arrowheads)*. The patient was again asymptomatic and again swore he will never smoke another cigarette. A follow-up angiogram performed 24 hours later demonstrated an excellent remodeling result.

Follow-Up

After 2 months, the patient returned for repeat angiography with possible angioplasty. The angiogram (see Fig. 58–47) revealed an amazing recovery of the vessel. The patient was taken off anticoagulants after 5 months. Follow-up angiography 6, 9, and 12 months after his acute event revealed a stable appearance.

Surprisingly, however, the patient returned 6 weeks after his 9-month follow-up after suffering a transient ischemic attack (TIA) in the left MCA distribution (temporary arm weakness associated with dysarthria). Angiography at that time revealed a small but tight area of recurrent stenosis that was not present on the most recent angiogram, even on close review. When questioned carefully, the patient admitted to resuming smoking 2 weeks before this admission. The patient underwent an uneventful repeat MCA angioplasty and was again neurologically intact. Close angiographic follow-up will be maintained for a period of time, with continued follow-up for the patient's entire life.

FACTORS AFFECTING SUCCESS OF FIBRINOLYTIC THERAPY FOR ACUTE STROKE

Aspirin Inhibits Fibrinolysis

Studies indicate that aspirin inhibits the effectiveness of t-PA and probably urokinase as well. One trial demonstrated that, at physiologic doses, and measured by two different techniques, fibrinolysis is inhibited significantly by aspirin.[24] These findings have been at least partially confirmed by others.[25, 26]

Specifically, when aspirin was administered at the dose of 20 mg/kg 18 hours before insult, the pretreatment antagonized the rate and extent of t-PA–induced clot lysis by up to 70%. The positive point of this study was that it also showed that this suppression effect could be reduced or reversed by administration of the prostacyclin analog iloprost (10 mg/kg/hr) directly into the cerebral circulation. This may imply that the aspirin effect is due to the result of a loss of endothelial prostacyclin production.

This is a most disturbing finding and brings into question the results of several other trials. Specifically, in the Multicenter Acute Stroke Trial as well as others, aspirin was part of the therapy. In addition, a large percentage of the population is either on a chronic aspirin regimen or had a recent dose before the time of therapy. This may have distorted the results of many trials.

Data presented by Bednar et al. at the Joint Section on Cerebrovascular Surgery of the AANS and CNS (22nd International Joint Conference on Stroke and Cerebral Circulation, Anaheim, CA, February 1997) confirm the antagonistic effect of aspirin on t-PA thrombolysis and indicate that nitroprusside (1 mg/kg/hr given intravenously), nitroglycerin (10 µg/kg/min given intravenously), or L-arginine appeared to reverse these effects. These are all sources of nitric oxide. The simple vasodilatory effect of nitroglycerin, for instance, was not the cause of this response (a control using another vasolidator that is not a nitric oxide source confirmed this); however, the hypotensive effects of intravenous nitroglycerin could be detrimental to the outcome of an ischemic stroke. The full implications of these facts and possible alterations in treatment required in response have not been worked out, but the implications are that the effects of t-PA would be seriously compromised by the concomitant administration (or recent ingestion) of aspirin.

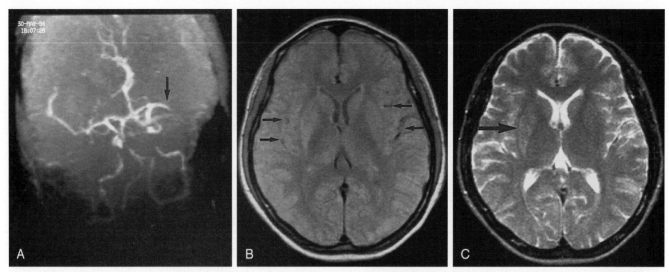

Figure 58-55 Case 5. *A to C,* A 44-year-old woman experienced abrupt onset of left-sided weakness and speech impairment during an aerobics class. Her history was significant for mitral stenosis secondary to rheumatic fever. She presented to an outlying hospital, where CT, MRI, and magnetic resonance angiography (MRA) were performed before involvement of interventional neuroradiology. The T2-weighted image *(C)* reveals subtle increased signal intensity in the right basal ganglia *(arrow),* with implications unknown at that time. Note the isointense signal in the right MCA branches (rather than flow voids), particularly on the balanced image *(small arrows, B).* The MRA (three-dimensional time-of-flight) reveals occlusion of the right MCA at the level of the distal M1 segment *(small arrow, A).* This study was obtained approximately 3 hours after the onset of symptoms.

Case 5 continues

Ultrasound Speeds Fibrinolysis

Ultrasound may accelerate thrombolysis by accelerating the distribution of thrombolytic agents deep inside the clot by a phenomenon known as an acoustic stream. In an experiment performed by Akiyama et al. (Jikei University, Tokyo, Japan: presented at the Neurosonology meeting, August 1997, Winston-Salem, NC), the combination of low-frequency, low-intensity transcranial ultrasound and urokinase was twice as effective at clot dissolution as the drug alone, requiring only 4 hours to dissolve a clot, whereas urokinase alone took 8 hours. This already was shown with high-frequency and high-intensity ultrasound in prior studies. The more recent work was applied to intravascular thrombus without active pharmacologic fibrinolysis; if active fibrinolysis was ongoing, the rate of dissolution could conceivably be rapid. Further research should reveal whether this technique should be applied to standard intravenous t-PA therapy or combined with intra-arterial therapy. Superficially, it would appear that supplying transcranial ultrasound would have no detrimental effects and might render appreciable aid.

FACTORS ASSOCIATED WITH INTRAPARENCHYMAL HEMATOMA AND POOR OUTCOME

Intraparenchymal hematoma is the primary significant complication of local intracranial fibrinolysis (Cases 5 and 6, Figs. 58–55 to 58–67). If there were no major life-threatening bleeds after therapy, there would be less hesitancy concerning emergency therapy.

In intravenous trials of t-PA for myocardial infarction, there is an incidence of 1% to 3% of sponta-

neous intracranial hemorrhage secondary to therapy.[27] This pervading rate is troublesome and confounds accurate analysis of procedures. There may be an underlying 1% to 3% of stroke patients who would bleed no matter what was done, or when.

Although the rate of symptomatic bleeds in the NINDS trial was 6%, the rate varied greatly in other trials. This was probably because the other trials used different fibrinolytic agents (e.g., streptokinase), dosages, and time to treatment. The rates of intraparenchymal hematoma formation were 20% for the European Cooperative Acute Stroke Study (ECASS), 18% for the Multicenter Acute Stroke Trial–Europe, and 13% for the Australian Streptokinase Trial. All these trials were terminated early because of these results.

Although no firm data exist to support the following hypothesis, we believe that the primary risk of local intracranial fibrinolytic therapy is related to the condition of the lenticulostriate arteries and their territory (as mentioned previously). These are true end arteries that have poor collateral supply and thus are subject to severe injury from an ischemic insult. Although bleeds can and do arise from cortical branches, they are not as common or severe as deep hemorrhages. Superficial oozing is a relatively common occurrence (hemorrhagic conversion). It has been shown repeatedly that, after a stroke, up to 20% to 43% of patients suffer "hemorrhagic transformation."[28–30]

The rationale for therapy for acute stroke consists of the belief that reestablishment of antegrade flow can rescue redeemable tissue. If the act of revascularization alone was the cause of these devastating intraparenchymal bleeds, then even a magical cure for the thrombotic occlusion would be *contraindi-*

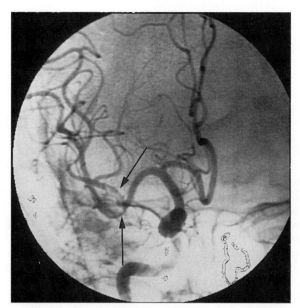

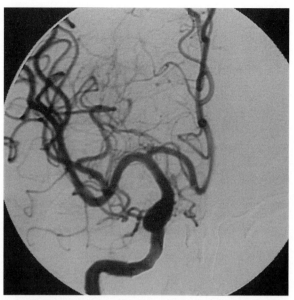

Figure 58-56 Owing to the initial location of the patient at an outlying hospital, angiography was not performed until approximately 6 hours after the acute event. The initial angiogram confirmed total occlusion of the MCA in the middle to distal portion of M1 consistent with the MRA, and failed to demonstrate the distal group of lateral lenticulostriate vessels. A bolus of 5000 units of heparin was administered and a microcatheter was advanced into the clot. After 30 minutes of infusion of urokinase at 6000 U/min, the main trunk of the MCA (M1) was completely clear, but residual clot *(arrows)* was seen in both MCA (M2) branches.

Figure 58-58 The infusion was continued through the microcatheter at the bifurcation of the MCA until its main (M2) branches were clear. The final image reveals these vessels to be free of thrombus. The total infusion time was approximately 110 minutes (with completion of therapy by about 8.5 hours after the insult). The total amount of urokinase infused was 730,000 units. Heparin had been continued at 1000 U/hr.

cated. It is therefore not the re-establishment of perfusion that is the primary problem, but rather the infusion of a fibrinolytic agent for a prolonged period into a damaged and vulnerable territory, the timing

of this maneuver, and the subsequent reperfusion. Additional complicating maneuvers can coexist, such as the infusion of large amounts of hypertonic contrast into the same damaged territory. Reestablishment of perfusion to injured capillaries during a critical time window probably is the most dangerous factor, that is, *after a certain period of time and before a satisfactory interval.*

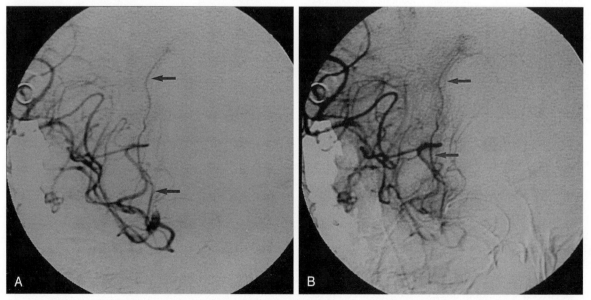

Figure 58-57 *A* and *B,* After repositioning the microcatheter, contrast injection revealed a large ascending lateral lenticulostriate artery *(arrows),* which was not visible on the prethrombolysis injection and poorly visible on the previous injection through the guide catheter after initial thrombolysis (Fig. 58–56). This striate artery arose from the actual bifurcation, not from the M1 segment. Note the reactive hyperemic anteriovenous shunting with a parenchymal blush around this vessel; again, this is of uncertain significance.

Case 5 continues

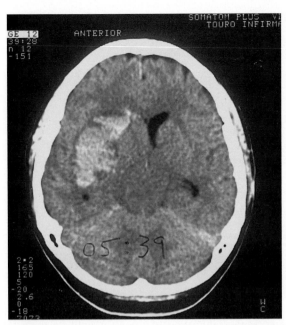

Figure 58-59 At the termination of the procedure, while the patient was still on the table, her neurologic status was significantly improved. Her motor strength was 3/5 in the upper extremity and 3/5 to 4/5 in the lower extremity. Her speech was slow but clear and the facial palsy had almost completely resolved. The attending neurosurgeon desired that she be transferred to the intensive care unit (ICU) and maintained on intravenous heparin with the goal of maintaining the activated partial thromboplastin time at 1.5 times normal. (At that time, the association between high heparin doses and later intraparenchymal bleeds was not known.)

Approximately 5 hours after treatment, the patient experienced a sudden, dramatic neurologic deterioration. An emergency CT scan revealed a 3 × 5 cm basal ganglia hemorrhage (lateral to the internal capsule and putamen) in the territory of the large hyperemic lateral lenticulostriate artery revealed on the microcatheter injection described above. The patient remained comatose, with enlargement of the intraparenchymal hemorrhage, and died 7 days later.

It is believed that it was the previously identified vessel that hemorrhaged, probably because of its distal location in the M1 segment of the MCA and the resultant duration and depth of ischemia sustained.

Data indicate that post-treatment systemic hypertension is correlated with subsequent parenchymal hematoma and therefore that active blood pressure management is indicated. Although no definite upper limits of pressure are known, some data indicate that elevated pulse pressure or simply elevated diastolic pressure (100 mm Hg) may be a critical factor.[9] According to Brott (verbal communication), for patients treated with intravenous t-PA, intravenous labetalol should be used to treat systemic pressures above 185/110. Treatment of hypertension is indicated only for patients treated with fibrinolytic therapy. Blood pressure elevation should not be actively managed in patients not treated with fibrinolytic agents.

Early predictors of subsequent bleeding are difficult to come by; early focal hypodensity or mass effect appears to be a predictor of subsequent hemorrhagic transformation, but does not differentiate oozing from hematoma.[30] This is not really useful information, however, because simple oozing is not clinically significant. In one series, 43% of patients had "hemorrhagic" transformation, and 11% of these cases were hematomas (4.6% overall). An analysis of the NINDS trial indicated that these early CT changes yield an odds ratio of 7.8 for a subsequent symptomatic intracranial bleed. An additional factor associated with an increased incidence of intracerebral hemorrhage was an NIHSS score greater than 20, which resulted in an 11-fold increase in the rate of bleed. Interestingly, a history of tobacco use was associated with a lower incidence of symptomatic bleed.

The dose of t-PA appears to affect this outcome. It must again be remembered that no absolute value is available; although some trials have administered more than 1.0 mg/kg of t-PA (e.g., 1.1 mg/kg with an upper limit of 100 mg in the ECASS trial), the most recent t-PA trial (NINDS) reduced this to 0.9 mg/kg. In a previous study,[9] 4 of 22 patients (18%) had intraparenchymal hematomas at this dose level and above, whereas below this dose level, only 1 in 72 had an intraparenchymal hematoma. The symptomatic hematomas occurred early (usually about 1 hour after treatment). Interestingly, the bleeds were not in the acutely infarcted area in a significant percentage of cases, but rather were widely distributed, similar to the incidental bleeds associated with t-PA use in acute myocardial infarctions. This may have implications concerning the presence of prior silent infarcts rather than the acute infarct in progress. It

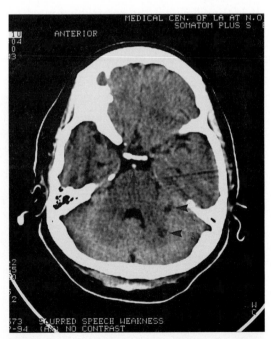

Figure 58-60 Case 6. This 56-year-old woman came to the emergency room with increasing weakness; while there, she had a respiratory arrest. A CT scan demonstrates hyperdensity of the basilar artery *(arrow)* and at least two lacunar infarcts in the left cerebellar hemisphere *(arrowheads)*. These findings, suggestive of basilar artery thrombosis, were not appreciated by the emergency personnel and the patient was admitted to the Neurosurgical ICU for observation and evaluation.

Case 6 continues

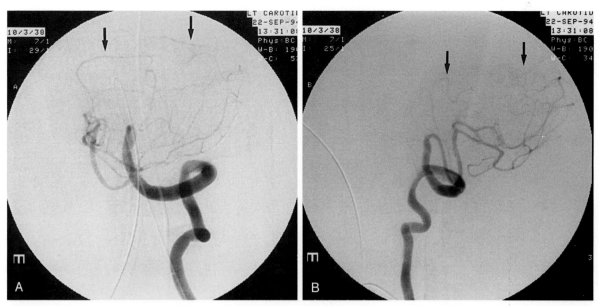

Figure 58-61 *A* and *B,* After the neuroradiologist correctly interpreted the CT scan the next morning (about 12 hours later), there was unfortunately an additional long delay before the attending neurologist could be contacted, thus postponing the emergency angiogram. The patient, who had demonstrated 2/5 quadriparesis with response to verbal stimuli that morning, had deteriorated to a comatose state with only minimal response to pain by the time the angiogram was performed. The left vertebral injection reveals total occlusion at the level of the posterior inferior cerebellar artery. The remainder of the four-vessel cerebral angiogram confirmed total occlusion of the basilar artery with very poor supply to the posterior fossa from any collateral supply. Note the attempts of the posterior inferior cerebellar artery to fill the superior cerebellar artery territory *(arrows).*

also should be a signal to obtain a thorough history of any recent TIAs before the stroke in question is to be treated; these prior TIAs actually may be a small infarct waiting to bleed.

Vascular reperfusion did not appear to be associated with an increase in the number of bleeds.[9] Once

again, if this were the case, even a magical removal of thrombus would be contraindicated.

There appears to be a lack of data supporting a risk of bleeding associated with hypofibrinogenemia. Support for the argument against increased risk comes from the lack of an increased incidence of

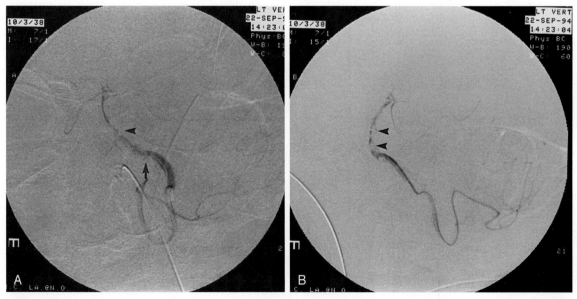

Figure 58-62 *A* and *B,* In the realization that the patient's chance of survival was essentially zero with the current status, recanalization by fibrinolytic therapy was requested, even though this still offered only a slim chance for survival. After institution of intra-arterial urokinase infusion, early clearing reveals abundant thrombus in the distal vertebral artery *(arrow)* and basilar artery *(arrowheads).* Note the minimal filling of the anterior inferior cerebellar artery. Urokinase infusion was continued.

Case 6 continues

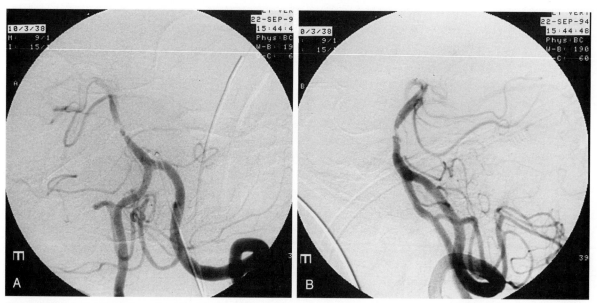

Figure 58-63 *A* and *B,* After completion of infusion, a severe stenosis in the midbasilar artery was identified. Even though the patient was fully heparinized, watchful waiting revealed reocclusion of the basilar artery *within minutes.* The severity of the underlying stenosis is underscored by the fact that most of the injected contrast refluxed down the opposite vertebral artery rather than flowing in a normal antegrade fashion through the basilar artery. Fibrinolysis was again able to clear the vessel, but angioplasty now became mandatory.

bleeds in the prior trial of ancrod versus placebo.[31-34] The primary mode of action of ancrod is fibrinogen depletion, and there was no evidence of increased incidence of bleeding associated with its use.

Data are conflicting, however, concerning the association between heparin use and subsequent bleeding. This was reported in the Gruppo Italiano per lo studio della sopravivenza nell'Infarto Miocardio (GISSI-2), Third International Study of Infarct Survival International Study Group, and intracranial urokinase administration trials for the treatment of stroke.[35-37] In these last studies, there was a significant increase in the incidence of intraparenchymal hematoma in the high-dose heparin group.

Data released from the NINDS and ECASS trials appear to indicate that heparin use does *not* increase the incidence of symptomatic bleed, but the ECASS data were based on a large percentage of patients receiving subtherapeutic doses of heparin (56%). Therefore, these data should not be taken as proof of safety.

The association of heparin with hematoma is un-

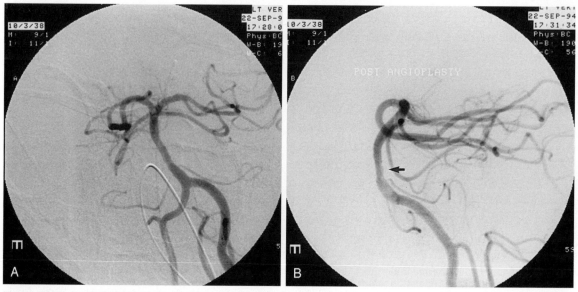

Figure 58-64 *A* and *B,* Angiogram obtained immediately after angioplasty. A near-pristine appearance of the basilar artery is now seen, typical of our very slow inflation technique of angioplasty (see text). Note a small intimal irregularity on the posterior wall *(arrow).*

Case 6 continues

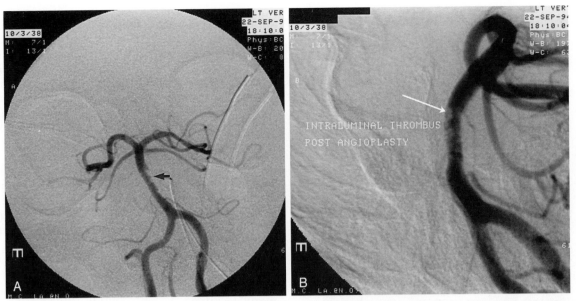

Figure 58-65 *A* and *B,* A period of 39 minutes later, thrombus is seen to be forming on the wall at the angioplasty site *(arrows).* This should not be confused with intimal dissection, and reangioplasty should be avoided. This was seen to progress, and repeat urokinase infusion was performed, although with great trepidation. We were not yet using abciximab at the time of this case. Although we do not routinely use this drug when performing angioplasty as part of acute stroke therapy, in the situation of recurrent thrombus formation and a dire outcome if patency is not maintained, its use should be considered.

fortunate because heparin is synergistic with urokinase for clot dissolution. For this reason, a happy medium for heparin use had to be reached for the recent PROACT trial (April 1996). Some heparin had to be used, but not too much. It is for this reason that the prescribed dose is 2000 units as an initial bolus followed by 500 U/hr for 4 hours only (the intra-arterial infusion of prourokinase has a 2-hour maximum duration). This amount of heparin may be adequate to ensure effectiveness of the infusion

without increasing the incidence of intraparenchymal hematoma (as confirmed in the previous trial).

We use a bolus of 5000 units of heparin followed by infusion of 1000 U/hr intravenously *during the fibrinolysis procedure only.* The heparin is terminated when the fibrinolysis procedure is stopped. This regimen is used to achieve adequate heparinization during active fibrinolysis, but not too high a level after the procedure (see Chapter 60).

In summary, it appears that patients with the

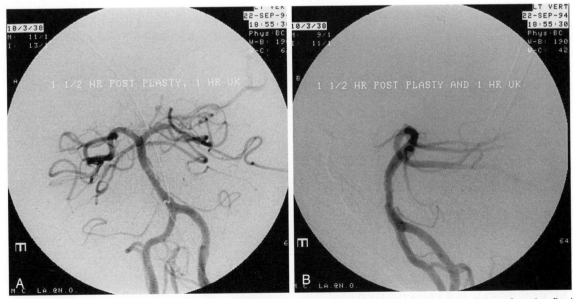

Figure 58-66 *A* and *B,* Final angiographic appearance (1½ hours after angioplasty and 1 hour after the final urokinase infusion). Watchful waiting confirms that the thrombotic cascade has ceased and the luminal appearance has stabilized. Unfortunately, the status of the pontine perforators is questionable at best.

Case 6 continues

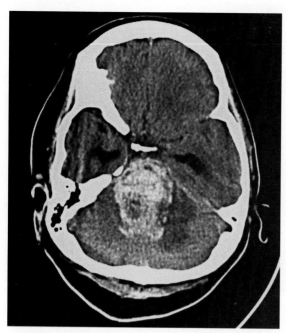

Figure 58-67 Follow-up CT scan reveals multiple intraparenchymal hematomas. Obviously the delay in treatment had been too great. The patient's status rapidly deteriorated and she died several hours later. This procedure currently has only a 50% rescue rate, but progress is being made regarding patient selection (see text).

largest (worst) strokes and vessels that are not reopened expeditiously are the most likely to develop a devastating intraparenchymal hematoma.

OTHER PREDICTORS OF POOR OUTCOME

Several factors that may worsen the neurologic deficit (and outcome) associated with acute cerebral ischemia are discussed in Chapter 54. Additional factors of a functional vascular nature influence the rapidity and depth of ischemia and the response to emergency revascularization efforts. These include the initial location of the occlusion and the presence or absence of functional collateral supply, mostly pial collaterals. These can be seen on the initial angiograms if searched for carefully.

This collateral supply can be identified indirectly by comparing perfusion-weighted MRI scans with diffusion-weighted MRI scans. The dichotomy in the size of the lesions using these two techniques is an indirect indicator of the depth of ischemia. These techniques are not available in many locations, particularly on an emergency basis.

Additionally, if the MCA appears dense on CT, there is little chance of a good response to intravenous therapy (only 1 of 18 patients with this sign was normal after 3 months in the NINDS trial). This situation was described in more detail under "Rationale for Intravenous Versus Intra-Arterial Fibrinolytic Therapy" above.

OPTIMAL EMERGENCY STROKE THERAPY

In accordance with the reasons presented in the previous discussions, we believe that the best available therapy for acute stroke is a combination of ultraearly intravenous therapy and direct local intracranial revascularization. As the results of trials evaluating various neuroprotectant agents become available, use of such agents may be incorporated. Even with the recent Food and Drug Administration approval of intravenous t-PA for stroke therapy, we believe that this therapy has only limited application in and minimal benefit to a small subset of patients. Although the ideal fibrinolytic agent may not be known, it is clear that local intracranial infusion of any fibrinolytic agent works far better than systemic application for an occluded vessel of any significant size. This is supported by the findings presented in "Rationale for Intravenous Versus Intra-Arterial Fibrinolytic Therapy" above.

The treatment of stroke eventually will involve a "multipronged" attack, similar to how aggressive myocardial infarction therapy is handled now in many locations. It will include intervention by the general community, emergency medical technicians, emergency room personnel, CT technologists (possibly, later, MRI technologists), laboratory personnel, neurologists, radiologists, and angiography personnel. The steps involved in this emergency therapy probably will include the following:

1. Undertake clinical screen for acute stroke; confirm positive screen and onset in less than about 5 hours. Administer oxygen by mask (4 L/min.)
2. Activate an in-hospital stroke team.
3. Transport patient to hospital; administer safe and effective cytoprotective agents during transit.
4. Obtain preliminary laboratory work, electrocardiogram, and other tests as indicated.
5. Obtain CT scan for exclusion purposes (or ultrafast MRI and magnetic resonance angiography). CT angiography eventually will be routinely available.
6. Confirm no rapid improvement in symptoms, satisfy inclusion and exclusion criteria, confirm postictus time.
7. If time is still less than 3 hours after ictus, administer intravenous t-PA or other proven fibrinolytic agent.
8. Perform immediate angiogram. If postictus time is still less than about 6 hours, and an appropriate target is found, perform superselective thrombolysis. (An angiogram can be done safely, using adequate technique and a micropuncture set, even when the patient is receiving heparin or has received t-PA.)

REFERENCES

1. Maruki Y, Koehler RC, Kirsch JR, et al. Effect of the 21-aminosteroid tirilazad on cerebral pH and somatosensory evoked potentials after incomplete ischemia. *Stroke* 1993;24:724–730.
2. Leach MJ, Swan JH, Eisenthal D, et al. BW619C89, a glutamate release inhibitor, protects against focal cerebral ischemic damage. *Stroke* 1993;24:1063–1067.

3. Zeumer H, Freitag H-J, Zanella F, et al. Local intra-arterial fibrinolytic therapy in patients with stroke: urokinase versus recombinant tissue plasminogen activator (r-TPA). *Neuroradiology* 1993;35:159–162.

4. Weitz JI. Limited fibrin specificity of tissue type plasminogen activator and its potential link to bleeding. *J Vasc Interv Radiol* 1995;6:19S–23S.

5. The National Institute of Neurological Disorders and Stroke rt-PA Stroke Study Group. Tissue plasminogen activator for acute ischemic stroke. *N Engl J Med* 1995;333:1581–1587.

6. Adams HP Jr., Brott TG, Furlan AJ, et al. Guidelines for thrombolytic therapy for acute stroke: a supplement to the guidelines for the management of patients with acute ischemic stroke. A statement for healthcare professionals from a special writing group of the Stroke Council, American Heart Association. *Stroke* 1996;27:1711–1718.

7. Tomsick T, Brott T, Barsan W, et al. Prognostic value of the hyperdense middle cerebral artery sign and stroke scale score before ultraearly thrombolytic therapy. *AJNR* 1996;17:79–85.

8. Sasaki O, Takeuchi S, Koike T, et al. Fibrinolytic therapy for acute embolic stroke: intravenous, intracarotid, and intra-arterial local approaches. *Neurosurgery* 1995;36:246–253.

9. Levy DE, Brott TG, Haley C Jr, et al. Factors related to intracranial hematoma formation in patients receiving tissue-type plasminogen activator for acute stroke. *Stroke* 1994;25:291–297.

10. Theron J, Courtheoux P, Casasco A, et al. Local intraarterial fibrinolysis in the carotid territory. *AJNR* 1989;10:753–765.

11. Theron J, Coskun O, Huet H, et al. Local intraarterial thrombolysis in the carotid territory. *Intervent Neuroradiol* 1996;2:111–126.

12. Overgaard K. Thrombolytic therapy in experimental embolic stroke. *Cerebrovasc Brain Metab Rev* 1994;6:257–286.

13. Higashida RT, Halbach VV, Barnwell SL, et al. Thrombolytic therapy in acute stroke. *J Endovasc Surg* 1994;1:4–15.

14. LATE Study Group. Late assessment of thrombolytic efficacy (LATE) study with alteplase 6–24 hours after onset of acute myocardial infarction. *Lancet* 1993;342:759–766.

15. Fibrinolytic Therapy Trialists' (FTT) Collaborative Group. Indications for fibrinolytic therapy in suspected acute myocardial infarction: collaborative overview of early mortality and major morbidity results from all randomized trials of more than 1000 patients. *Lancet* 1994;343:311–322.

16. Kloner RA, Ganote CE, Jennings RB. The "no-reflow" phenomenon after temporary coronary occlusion in the dog. *J Clin Invest* 1974;54:1496–1508.

17. Kloner RA. No-reflow revisited. *J Am Coll Cardiol* 1989;14:1814–1815.

18. Piana RN, Paik GY, Moscucci M, et al. Incidence and treatment of no-reflow after percutaneous coronary intervention. *Circulation* 1994;89:2514–2518.

19. Abbo KM, Dooris M, Glazier S, et al. No-reflow after percutaneous coronary intervention: clinical and angiographic characteristics, treatment and outcome. *Am J Cardiol* 1995;75:778–782.

20. Kitazume H, Iwama T, Kubo H, et al. No-reflow phenomenon during percutaneous transluminal coronary angioplasty. *Am Heart J* 1988;116:211–215.

21. Ellis SG, Popma JJ, Buchbinder M, et al. Relation of clinical presentation, stenosis morphology, and operator technique to the procedural results of rotational atherectomy and rotational atherectomy-facilitated angioplasty. *Circulation* 1994;89:882–892.

22. Pomerantz RM, Kuntz RE, Diver DJ, et al. Intracoronary verapamil for the treatment of distal microvascular spasm following PTCA. *Cathet Cardiovasc Diagn* 1991;24:283–288.

23. Warth DC, Leon MB, O'Neill W, et al. Rotational atherectomy multicenter registry: acute results, complications and 6-month angiographic follow-up in 709 patients. *J Am Coll Cardiol* 1994;24:641–648.

24. Thomas GR, Thibodeaux H, Errett CJ, et al. Intravenous aspirin causes a paradoxical attenuation of cerebrovascular thrombolysis. *Stroke* 1995;26:1039–1046.

25. Overgaard K, Sereghy T, Pederson H, Boysen G. Dose response of t-PA and its combination with aspirin in a rat embolic stroke model. *Neuroreport* 1992;3:925–928.

26. Clark WM, Madden KP, Lyden PD, Zivin JA. Cerebral hemorrhagic risk of aspirin or heparin therapy with thrombolytic treatment in rabbits. *Stroke* 1991;22:872–876.

27. Stone GW, Grines CL, Browne KF, et al. Comparison of in-hospital outcome in men versus women treated by either thrombolytic therapy or primary coronary angioplasty for acute myocardial infarction. *Am J Cardiol* 1995;75:987–992.

28. Okada Y, Yamaguchi T, Minematsu K, et al. Hemorrhagic transformation in cerebral embolism. *Stroke* 1989;20:598–603.

29. Ott BR, Zamani A, Kleefield J, Funkenstein HH. The clinical spectrum of hemorrhagic infarction. *Stroke* 1986;17:630–637.

30. Toni D, Fiorelli M, Bastianello S, et al. Hemorrhagic transformation of brain infarct: predictability in the first 5 hours from stroke onset and influence on clinical outcome. *Neurology* 1996;46:341–345.

31. Duke RJ. IV heparin for prevention of stroke progression in acute partial stable stroke. *Ann Intern Med* 1986;105:825–828.

32. Kim S, Wadhwa N, Kant KS, et al. Fibrinolysis in glomerulonephritis treated with ancrod, renal functional, immunologic, and histopathologic effects. *Q J Med* 1988;69:875–895.

33. Latallo ZS. Retrospective study on complications and adverse effects of treatment with thrombin-like enzymes. *Thromb Haemost* 1983;50:604–609.

34. Pollak VE, Glas-Greenwalt P, Olinger CP, et al. Ancrod causes rapid thrombolysis in patients with acute stroke. *Am J Med Sci* 1990;299:319–325.

35. Gruppo Italiano per lo studio della sopravvivenza nell'Infarto Miocardio. GISSI-2: a factorial randomized trial of alteplase versus streptokinase and heparin versus no heparin among 12,490 patients with acute myocardial infarction. *Lancet* 1990;336:65–71.

36. Third International Study of Infarct Survival, Collaborative Group. ISIS-3: a randomized comparison of streptokinase vs. tissue plasminogen activator vs. anistreplase and of aspirin plus heparin vs. aspirin alone among 41,299 cases of suspected myocardial infarction. *Lancet* 1992;339:753–770.

37. The International Study Group. In-hospital mortality and clinical course of 20,891 patients with suspected acute myocardial infarction randomized between alteplase and streptokinase with or without heparin. *Lancet* 1990;336:71–75.

ADDITIONAL REFERENCES

Bruetman ME, Fields WS, Crawford ES, DeBakey ME. Cerebral hemorrhage in carotid artery surgery. *Arch Neurol* 1963;9:458–467.

Hornig, C, Dorendorf W, Agnoli A. Hemorrhagic cerebral infarction; a prospective study. *Stroke* 1986;17:179–185.

Kim JS, Lee JH, Lee MC. Small primary intracerebral hemorrhage: clinical presentation of 28 cases. *Stroke* 1994;25:1500–1506.

Molinari GF. Lobar hemorrhages: Where do they come from? How do they get there? *Stroke* 1993;24:523–526.

Wijdicks EFM, Jack CR. Intracerebral hemorrhage after fibrinolytic therapy for acute myocardial infarction. *Stroke* 1993;24:554–557.

CHAPTER 59

Specific Stroke Situations, Territories, and Guidelines for Therapy

J.J. Connors III / J.C. Wojak

VERTEBROBASILAR STROKE

Mechanism of Insult

As noted in Chapter 53, posterior circulation vascular occlusion is more commonly due to *intrinsic* thrombus formation and subsequent vascular occlusion (associated with an underlying lesion) than to migratory embolus. The cases illustrated in Figures

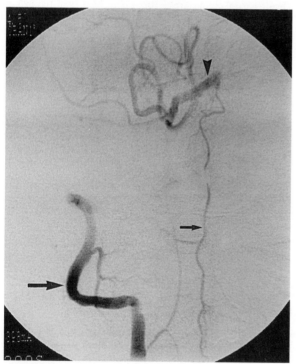

Figure 59-1 Case 1. This 67-year-old man presented with sudden onset of somnolence and generalized weakness. He survived in a somnolent and/or poorly arousable state for 1 week. The left vertebral artery ended in the posterior inferior cerebellar artery (PICA). This right vertebral artery injection reveals a large vessel *(large arrow)* with slow flow. This is obviously not a chronic condition. Retrograde flow in the anterior spinal artery *(small arrow)* leads up to the distal right vertebral artery *(arrowhead)*, which then supplies the right PICA. The implications of this are as follows: (1) there is absolutely no supply from the proximal vertebral artery to the distal intracranial vertebral artery, (2) the density in the distal vertebral artery indicates that there is absolutely no supply from the opposite (left) vertebral artery (no wash-in of unopacified blood), and (3) the fact that the anterior spinal artery is supplying as much flow as it is to the vertebrobasilar junction implies that basilar artery supply is extremely tenuous.

Case 1 continues

59–1 to 59–41 (Cases 1 and 2) are examples of in situ thrombus formation. Embolic occlusions of the vertebrobasilar system do occur, however, as shown in Figures 59–42 to 59–48 (Cases 3 and 4). As noted in the discussion of "Vertebral Artery Origin Stenosis" in Chapter 47, the vertebral artery *origin* can serve as a source of emboli in the presence of stenosis in this location. Vertebral origin stenoses, however, more typically are symptomatic on the basis of hemodynamic insufficiency than because of emboli. (The embolic consequences of this pathology, however, are extreme). The case presented in Figures 59–45 to 59–48 is an example of this.

Clinical Manifestations: General

In general, most posterior fossa hypoperfusion problems occur in patients with an isolated posterior fossa. The exceptions are associated with emboli to the posterior inferior cerebellar artery (PICA), the basilar tip, and the posterior cerebral arteries. From a diagnostic standpoint, however, prediction of hemodynamic insufficiency often is not possible from simple angiographic observation; some patients appear to have adequate supply but improve with an increase in perfusion. As opposed to carotid ischemic disease, nausea and vomiting are early indicators of posterior fossa ischemia; indeed, these symptoms are practically pathognomonic.

A significant portion of the time (more frequently than in anterior circulation events), *posterior fossa strokes have a gradual onset,* manifested by increasing weakness (commonly asymmetric quadriparesis), dizziness, and nausea, followed by somnolence and coma. Dysarthria is an underappreciated part of the presentation. Ataxia, cranial nerve palsy, and respiratory distress are variable. Visual disturbances are more typical of embolic phenomena or *severe* vascular compromise of the vertebrobasilar system.

An eventual midbasilar occlusion can result in a "locked-in" syndrome, with total-body paralysis but a normal level of consciousness. These symptoms may progress over a period of minutes to days with occasional hints (transient ischemic attacks, or TIAs) for several hours or days in advance.

Basilar tip occlusions produce well-described syndromes, rarely found without a decrease in level of consciousness. Visual hallucinations or disturbances, ocular movement disorders or skewed gaze, and somnolence typically are present. Occlusion of one or both posterior cerebral arteries may occur subse-

Text continued on page 706

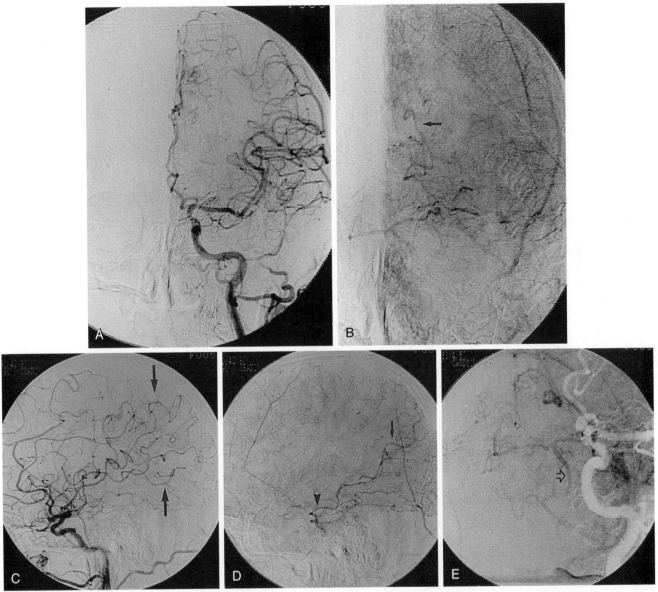

Figure 59-2 *A* to *E,* Posteroanterior (PA) and lateral views of the left common carotid injection with delayed imaging reveal a remarkable finding. Very late pial collateral supply from the posterior branches of the middle cerebral artery (MCA) (including the angular branch *[large arrows* in *C]*) to the posterior cerebral artery *(small arrows* in *B* and *D)* flows retrograde back down this vessel *(arrowhead* in *D).* Very late images reveal the basilar artery filling in a slow retrograde fashion all the way down to the region of the vertebrobasilar junction (the reason this patient is alive) *(open arrow* in *E).* This has powerful implications. The basilar artery is not full of clot; thus, reestablishing supply to this vessel may rescue the situation. Magnetic resonance imaging (MRI) confirmed no true infarct in the pons. The fact that the basilar artery was not directly affected has implications concerning rescue, in that angioplasty of the basilar artery for acute occlusion has a significantly higher complication rate than angioplasty of the intracranial vertebral artery.

Case 1 continues

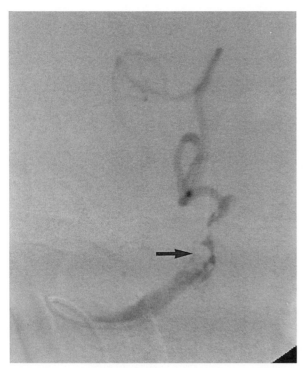

Figure 59-3 A microcatheter was placed into the distal right vertebral artery. Infusion of urokinase was performed at the rate of 250,000 U/hr, slower than usual for intracranial fibrinolysis. There was thought to be no immediate urgency since the patient had survived for more than 1 week. Saturation of the cerebral parenchyma was considered more dangerous than a modest delay in fibrinolysis. After infusion of 250,000 units of urokinase in 2 hours, the vessel had this appearance. Slight antegrade flow has been established by poking a hole with the guidewire and catheter. Residual thrombus is seen *(arrow)*.

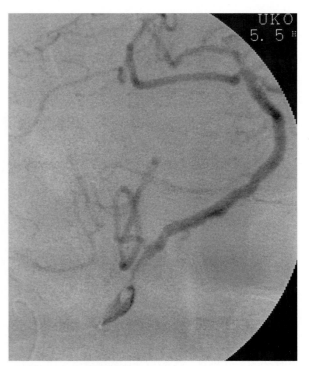

Figure 59-5 Final appearance after 5 hours of urokinase infusion. The mass in the center of the lumen remains.

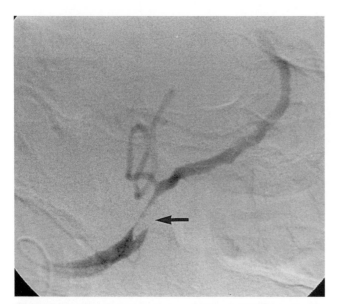

Figure 59-4 After infusion of an additional 250,000 units, the vessel has cleared further and antegrade flow is now better. The filling defect *(arrow)* remained stable in appearance for the next hour with continued infusion, and it was determined that this did not represent thrombus, but actually an island of plaque attached to the rear wall.

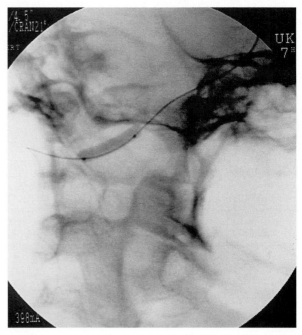

Figure 59-6 A 3.5-mm Stratus balloon (Medtronic/MIS) is in place across the stenosis.

Case 1 continues

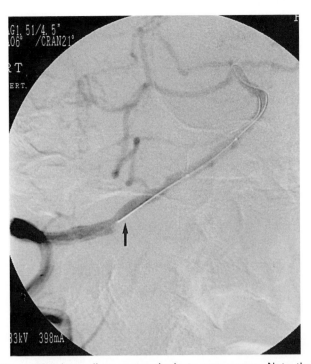

Figure 59-7 Immediate postangioplasty appearance. Note that the mass of plaque has been pressed against the wall *(arrow)*. Also note that the distal balloon occlusion guidewire (Quicksilver, Medtronic/MIS) has formed a safe "buckle" loop downstream. Antegrade flow is excellent. The patient became more alert on the table at this point.

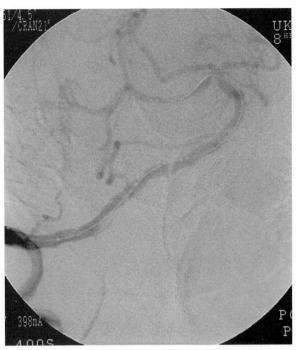

Figure 59-9 Repeat angioplasty was performed, yielding this appearance. The vessel slowly began to close again.

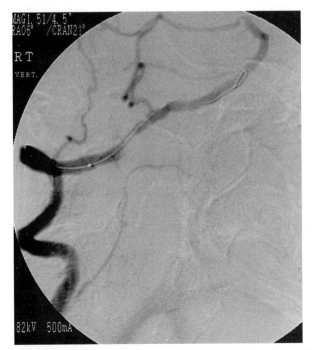

Figure 59-8 Fifteen minutes later, the vessel began to close. The patient had received a bolus of 10,000 units of heparin followed by 1000 U/hr as well as the standard abciximab (ReoPro) infusion (see Chapter 4). The appearance of the closing vessel was more consistent with rebound plaque than with fresh thrombus.

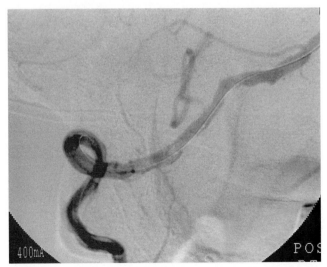

Figure 59-10 Repeat angioplasty yielded this result. Antegrade flow is again excellent. This process was repeated five times.

Case 1 continues

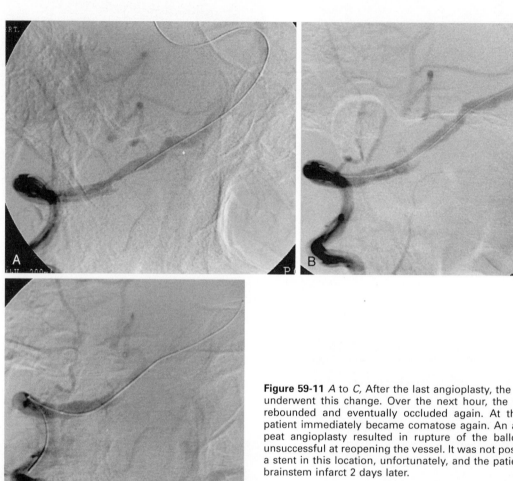

Figure 59-11 *A* to *C,* After the last angioplasty, the vessel slowly underwent this change. Over the next hour, the vessel slowly rebounded and eventually occluded again. At this point, the patient immediately became comatose again. An attempt at repeat angioplasty resulted in rupture of the balloon and was unsuccessful at reopening the vessel. It was not possible to place a stent in this location, unfortunately, and the patient suffered a brainstem infarct 2 days later.

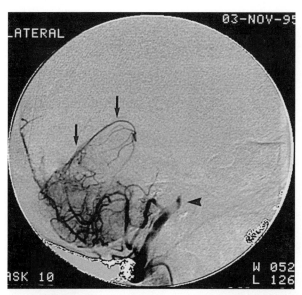

Figure 59-12 Case 2. A 49-year-old man presented with gradual onset of weakness, somnolence, and double vision. The initial computed tomographic (CT) examination was unremarkable. Angiography revealed a totally occluded left vertebral artery. The right vertebral artery supplied only the right PICA *(arrowhead)*. Note the retrograde supply to the superior cerebellar artery via PICA–superior cerebellar artery collaterals *(arrows)*. Anterior circulation (carotid) injection revealed very late and slow trickling perfusion of the basilar artery via a small posterior communicating artery.

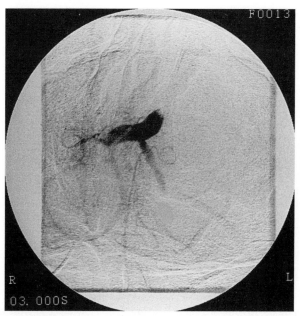

Figure 59-14 After 2 hours of thrombolysis, there was minimal change; perhaps 1 mm has been gained, but certainly nothing significant. At this rate, there would be no hope at all. It was decided to attempt to find the lumen by probing with a guidewire.

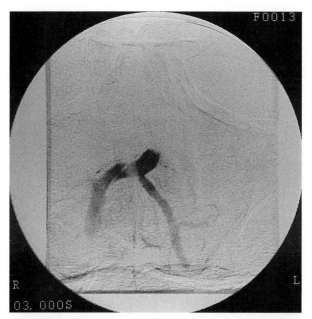

Figure 59-13 Endovascular intervention was requested. Owing to the clinical situation and the knowledge that the mental status of patients can fluctuate during these procedures, general anesthesia was undertaken for this procedure. It is most distressing and inconvenient if an emergency intubation has to be performed while delicate intracranial manipulations are being undertaken.

Initial microcatheter injection demonstrates the problem for the first time: an abrupt occlusion in the proximal basilar artery. Fibrinolysis was begun at the rate of 250,000 U/hr of urokinase, along with a bolus of 5000 units of heparin followed by a 1000 U/hr drip.

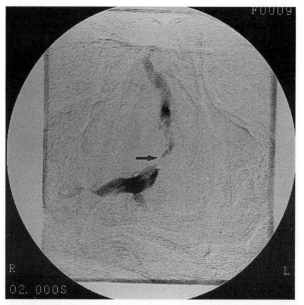

Figure 59-15 After gentle probing with a guidewire, no lumen could be found. More forceful probing with a guidewire was then done to no avail (all guidewires kept curling back on themselves or buckling). Substituting a gold-tipped Glidewire (Medi-Tech, Inc.) did not help, although this wire is usually capable of penetrating anything! A guidewire was then advanced to the end of the catheter and the two together were very forcefully advanced while probing. Suddenly the catheter shot forward 3 or 4 cm (just what was wanted, but frightening!). A very slow injection after withdrawal of the catheter revealed a nearly invisible stenotic lumen *(arrow)* with a trail of contrast flowing more distally, and the suggestion of intraluminal thrombus. Fibrinolysis was resumed.

Case 2 continues

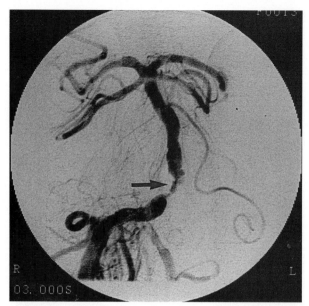

Figure 59-16 After 1½ hours and approximately 300,000 units of urokinase, a repeat angiogram reveals a widely patent distal vessel with good intracranial flow. The stenotic segment is very irregular in appearance and still very tight *(arrow)*. A full intracranial image was then attempted to evaluate the posterior cerebral vessels (see Fig. 59-17).

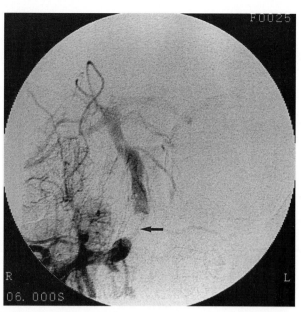

Figure 59-18 After the urokinase was restarted (the microcatheter was still in place), this is the appearance. Obviously, the lumen will not stay open on its own, and an angioplasty was planned. Note that the distal end of the stenosis is now nearly full of thrombus and only a thread is left *(arrow)*.

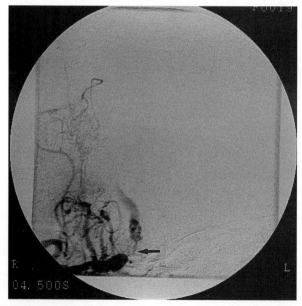

Figure 59-17 Three minutes later, this is the appearance of the basilar artery. The flow is now nearly stagnant and the stenotic segment *(arrow)* nearly occluded. Three minutes, fully heparinized!

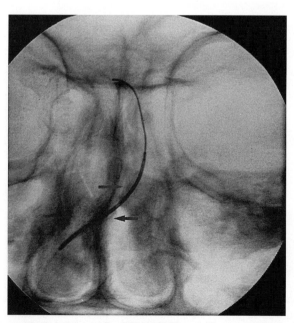

Figure 59-19 A 2.5-mm FasSTEALTH (Target Therapeutics) angioplasty catheter is now in place and slowly being inflated *(arrows)*. The goal is to obtain an adequate lumen capable of supplying the necessary cerebral structures and remaining open without risking a devastating intimal dissection. For this reason, we tend to undersize balloons in this location (the vessel measured slightly more than 4 mm). A good 2-mm vessel should supply plenty of flow, if it stays open. The patient remained fully heparinized.

Case 2 continues

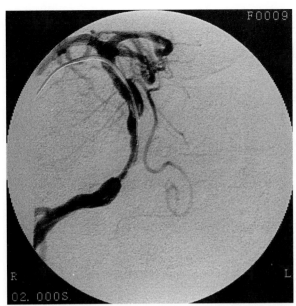

Figure 59-20 Postangioplasty result, with the balloon still in the vessel. To get the balloon out of the angioplastied site and maintain a wire across the lesion, it is necessary to advance the entire unit forward. This is because if the occlusion wire used with the STEALTH is loaded in the routine fashion, the bead on the end of the wire prevents the wire from being advanced out the end of the balloon catheter; thus, the balloon cannot be pulled back. (It is possible to place another wire through the STEALTH while it is still across the lesion, but this is time consuming in a vessel that may be occluded with the balloon.)

The injection reveals a modest lumen with excellent downstream flow, but surely less than 2.5 mm! There is no evidence of gross dissection necessitating reinflation. The shaft of the catheter probably covers some of the angioplastied lumen, and it will improve in appearance after the catheter is removed.

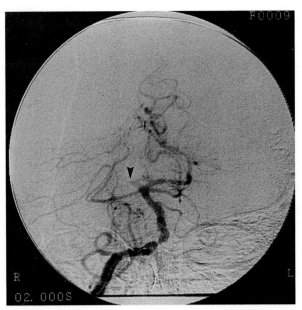

Figure 59-22 One hour later the vessel is again patent, but the flow is poor and there is no right posterior cerebral artery *(arrowhead)*. While this could simply reflect hemodynamics (the vessel being predominantly supplied by the posterior communicating artery, which is known to be open), embolic occlusion has to be considered in this situation. What does one do? The urokinase infusion was continued, with a plan for repeat angioplasty of the lesion with a larger balloon to try to increase flow through the vessel and prevent rethrombosis.

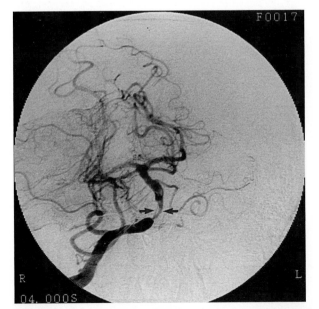

Figure 59-21 A full intracranial image was obtained to assess the downstream structures and hemodynamics. It appears that the right side of the cerebellum is well perfused, but the left less so (no PICA filling). Both posterior cerebral arteries are filling, with no gross filling defects. The stenotic segment is not looking as good as it did a few minutes earlier. The "2.5-mm" lumen is beginning to look very small *(arrows)*. A few minutes later, it reoccluded. Another bolus of 3000 units of heparin was given and the hourly dose was increased to 1500 units.

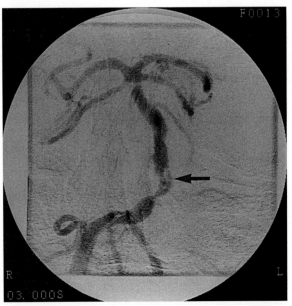

Figure 59-23 Fifteen minutes later, before the second angioplasty, a repeat angiogram demonstrates the suboptimal result of the first angioplasty with evidence of new thrombus *(arrow)*.

Case 2 continues

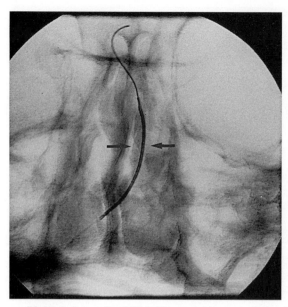

Figure 59-24 A 3-mm FasSTEALTH angioplasty catheter (the largest in the hospital) is in place across the lesion, with what looks like adequate width *(arrows)*.

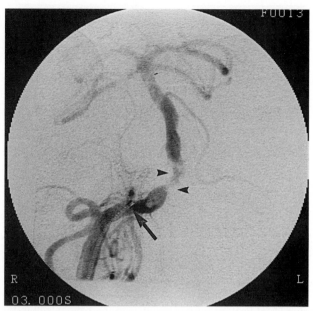

Figure 59-26 For all intracranial angioplasties (and many others), we always wait to see what happens, keeping the patient on the angiography table and obtaining delayed images. As explained in Chapter 48, there is a malignant platelet cascade that usually peaks fairly rapidly (within the first 10 to 30 minutes). This reaction will not even be seen if it is not watched for, and is the reason that many angioplasties seem to fail in the recovery room. This is the appearance of this lesion *32 minutes later.* The patient had remained fully heparinized. Platelet cascade is the problem *(arrowheads* on fresh thrombus). Note the microcatheter, which has been repositioned *(arrow);* we planned to restart urokinase.

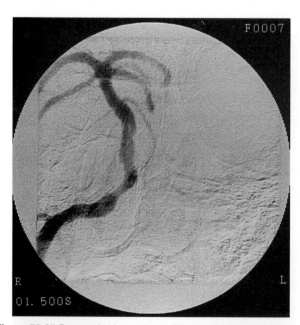

Figure 59-25 Postangioplasty result. The basilar artery looks gorgeous and the stenotic segment finally looks big enough. Note the rapidity of flow out into the major distal vessels, before any right PICA branches are even filling. The patient remains fully heparinized.

Is this the end of the procedure? No!

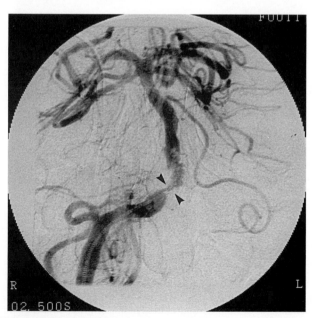

Figure 59-27 This image was obtained 1 hour and 12 minutes later. What is going on? There is minimal improvement; the vessel is still open, but there is still a large amount of thrombus *(arrowheads).* This would be a good time for abciximab (see Chapter 4), but unfortunately it was not available at the time. The stenosis even looks worse. This procedure has now lasted 8 hours. More urokinase and more heparin are needed.

Case 2 continues

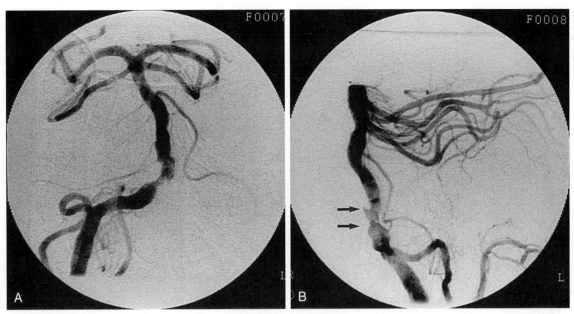

Figure 59-28 *A* and *B,* After 30 minutes the urokinase was stopped and another 30-minute wait was undertaken. These are the PA and lateral views obtained after the wait. The vessel is still patent and essentially clean, but on the lateral view the angioplasty site looks very irregular *(arrows);* luckily, this was a very localized process and did not extend further. We were very hesitant to angioplasty this lesion again; simply attempting to advance a guidewire past the flap seen on the lateral view would be dangerous. It appeared that the site would stay open on its own (as indicated by the fact that it had done so now for 30 minutes). The decision was made to terminate the procedure and take the patient for a CT evaluation for a bleed.

The patient did not wake up on the angiography table and was transported to the CT unit comatose. The patient's family was ready for the worst, but after the CT, which was unremarkable, he started to move. By the third postprocedure day, he was nearly recovered, but there were some visual deficits, later shown to be due to small bilateral occipital infarcts. He was placed on warfarin (Coumadin) and was ambulatory when he left the hospital 1 week later.

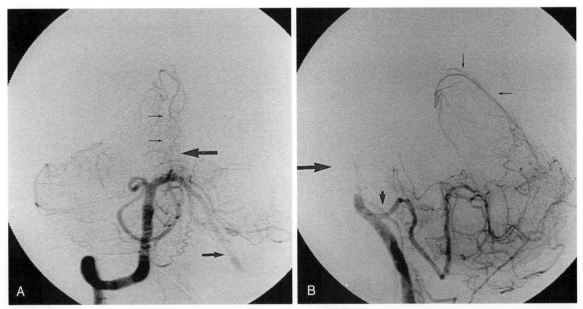

Figure 59-29 *A* and *B,* The patient was scheduled to return to the hospital 3 months later for a follow-up evaluation of the stenosis. After he stopped the Coumadin, his insurance company refused to cover his admission to the hospital. Within the week, he became weak again, could not get out of bed, cried episodically (pseudobulbar palsy), and could not talk clearly. He was urgently admitted to the hospital after communication with his insurance company. After the angiogram was finally approved, this was the appearance. Note the reflux down the opposite vertebral artery *(small arrows),* the absent basilar artery *(large arrows),* and the retrograde flow in the distribution of the superior cerebellar artery from peripheral PICA branches *(thin arrows).*

Case 2 continues

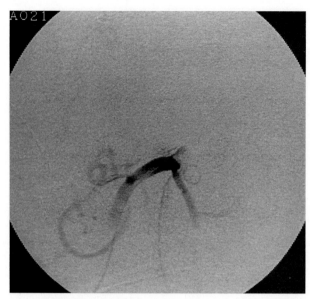

Figure 59-30 Initial appearance of the distal vertebral artery during a microcatheter injection. The proximal basilar artery looks even worse now than it did previously. It is amazing that the patient is still alive. A bolus of 5000 units of heparin was administered intravenously, and urokinase infusion started through the microcatheter.

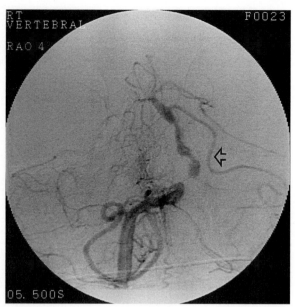

Figure 59-32 Forty-five minutes later (2¼ hours after the start of the urokinase infusion), there is some improvement, but minimal. What is happening to any perforators arising from the basilar artery? How about the anterior inferior cerebellar artery *(open arrow)*? What has been supplying this vessel? PICA? Superior cerebellar artery? Where *are* the superior cerebellar arteries? Presumably, they were receiving some supply from the PICA (at least the right one was, as seen on the initial injection [Fig. 59–29]). The basilar tip is seen to receive some blood from the anterior circulation, as it had before the original proximal basilar occlusion, and is keeping some of the superior cerebellar territory viable. The basilar thrombus, seen on the initial portion of the study (Fig. 59–30), did not totally fill the basilar artery and presumably spared the basilar tip.

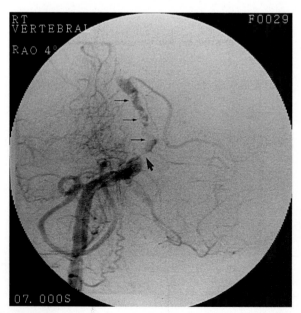

Figure 59-31 After 1½ hours of urokinase infusion at 250,000 U/hr, the vessel now looks like this. There is a trickle of antegrade flow through the hairlike lumen *(small arrow),* but an abundant amount of thrombus is seen in the basilar artery *(thin arrows).*

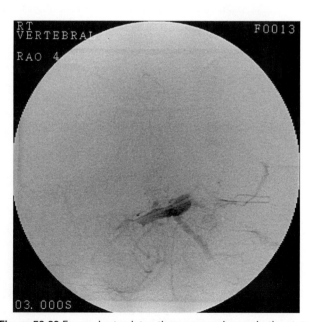

Figure 59-33 Four minutes later, there was a change in the status of the patient and a repeat angiogram reveals reocclusion of the basilar artery. Again, the patient was fully anticoagulated and urokinase was still being infused. At this hospital, administration of ReoPro, which was undergoing clinical trials for use during cardiovascular therapies, was not allowed.

Case 2 continues

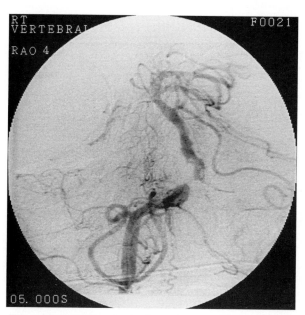

Figure 59-34 Thirty minutes later the vessel has reopened.

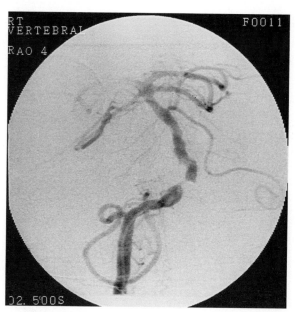

Figure 59-36 This image was obtained 2 minutes later! Apparently there had been a small plug in the hairlike stenosis, which was now gone. Distal perfusion is still poor.

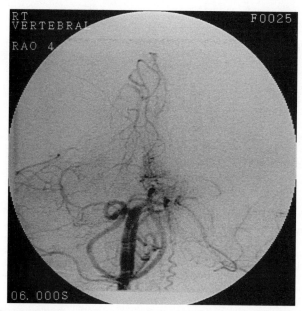

Figure 59-35 Ten minutes later, it looked like this. Another bolus of heparin was given.

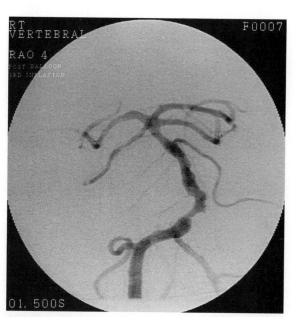

Figure 59-37 A 3-mm FasSTEALTH angioplasty balloon was used, resulting in this appearance. Still not good, and not acceptable this time.

Case 2 continues

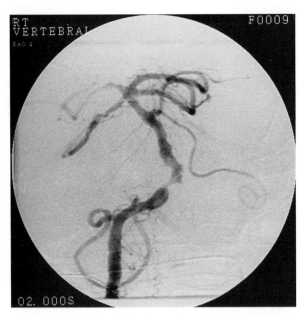

Figure 59-38 Indeed, 16 minutes later, it looked like this.

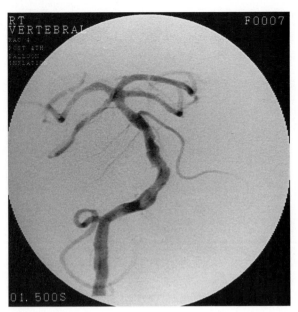

Figure 59-40 Final postangioplasty result. The vessel looks excellent, but time will tell.

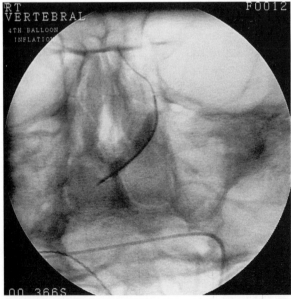

Figure 59-39 A 4-mm FasSTEALTH angioplasty balloon is now in place (inflated gradually to 8 atmospheres). Again, this looks as if it will yield a huge lumen size!

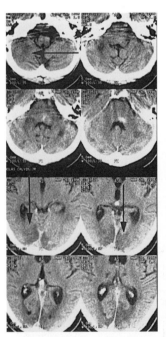
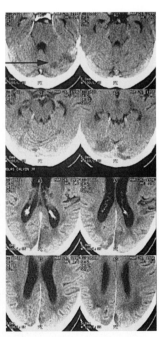

Figure 59-41 A postprocedure CT scan was obtained. Most of the hypodense changes are old *(arrows),* but the posterior pontine hyperdensity is new. This is contrast, which cleared. The left occipital lobe ischemic change is new and is presumably secondary to the abundant thrombus in the basilar artery, which embolized to the posterior cerebral arteries.

What did we learn? Use more heparin. Try ReoPro. Have an adequate supply of balloons in stock. Coumadin should be continued until the patient is in the hospital!

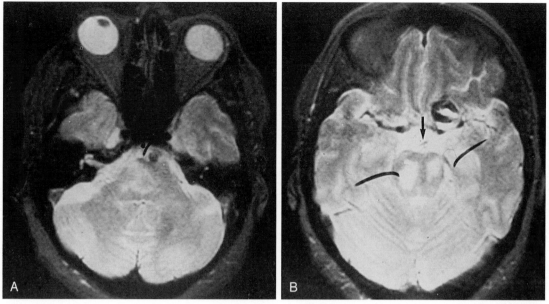

Figure 59-42 Case 3. *A* and *B,* A 43-year-old woman presented to the emergency room (ER) with slight generalized weakness. Four days later she was quadriplegic, able to move only her eyes, and wide awake. An early MRI scan reveals high signal in the pons and medulla *(large marks on images).* Note the absence of flow void in the basilar artery *(arrow).* The attending neurologist had read a German paper on intracranial fibrinolysis and, in view of the patient's condition, this was requested (this was in 1988).

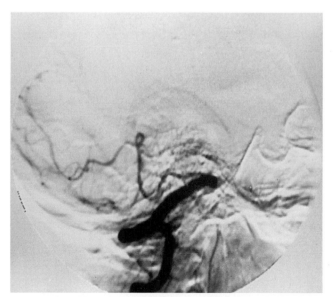

Figure 59-43 The initial angiogram revealed an isolated posterior fossa with a totally occluded basilar artery. Owing to the unavailability of microcatheters capable of intracranial work (no TRACKER-type catheters were then available), a cardiology microcatheter not capable of reaching the basilar artery was used. There was no experience with this procedure, and thus a grossly inadequate dose of urokinase was given (120,000 units over 2 hours) and was not continued as long as we would now.

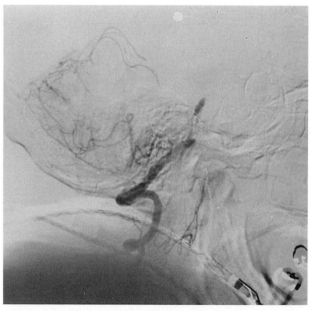

Figure 59-44 After the slow infusion, this angiogram was obtained and the procedure was stopped. Note the antegrade flow in the basilar artery to the distal tip. The patient was continued on heparin, and over the next week improved to the point that she left the hospital using a walker. She gradually returned to normal. At that time, it was believed that she had suffered an embolus secondary to a hypercoagulable state, and that reestablishing any flow at all had allowed her to recanalize the basilar artery. Now, we would consider the possibility of an underlying basilar artery stenosis. The areas of pathology seen on MRI were apparently reversible areas of edema.

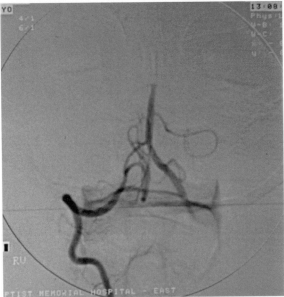

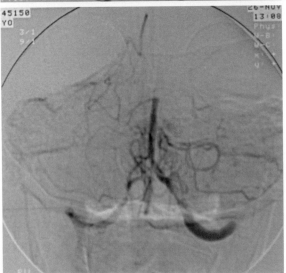

Figure 59-45 Case 4. This young woman presented to the ER with sudden onset of blindness. An emergency angiogram reveals a small distal right vertebral artery with complete basilar occlusion at the tip. The posterior cerebral arteries do not fill from the basilar artery at all, and the left superior cerebellar artery is also gone. Note the large distal left vertebral artery, with evidence of poor antegrade flow (because of the retrograde flow in the left vertebral artery to this degree).

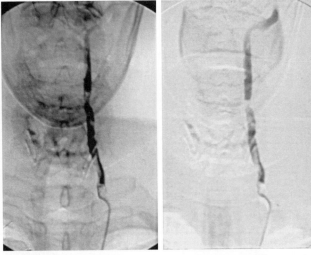

Figure 59-46 Catheterization of the left vertebral artery reveals a thrombus-filled vessel, the obvious origin of the emboli to the posterior cerebral arteries.

pain and temperature sense, ipsilateral Horner's syndrome, hoarseness, and usually some degree of ataxia, nausea, vomiting, nystagmus, dysphagia, diminished taste, and ipsilateral facial sensory disturbance.

Occlusion of both vertebral arteries yields basilar occlusion. Often, one vertebral artery is chronically occluded; the second vertebral artery occlusion is the precipitating event (see Figs. 59–1 to 59–11). Alternatively, the basilar artery can have a severely stenotic segment that progresses to occlusion; this classically occurs at the junction of the proximal and middle thirds, but recent data indicate a more uniform distribution.

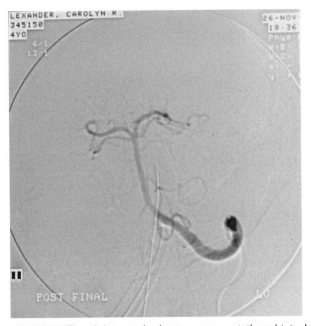

Figure 59-47 The right vertebral artery was not thought to be large enough to catheterize, and therefore the left vertebral artery was cleared of thrombus with urokinase, along with the posterior cerebral arteries. The postinfusion angiogram reveals good flow into these vessels.

quently, depending on the status of the posterior communicating arteries. This yields a homonymous hemianopia of the contralateral field. Again, dysarthria is an underappreciated symptom.

The ascending reticular-activating system usually is supplied by the thalamoperforators, arising from the P1 segments of the posterior cerebral arteries. Coma, in general, can be caused by either lack of perfusion to this system or total bilateral anterior circulation ischemia (rare). Reestablishment of perfusion to one P1 segment after the basilar artery is cleared usually is enough to awaken the patient.

Distal vertebral artery occlusion with occlusion of the PICA results in the lateral medullary (Wallenberg's) syndrome, which includes loss of contralateral

Case 4 continues

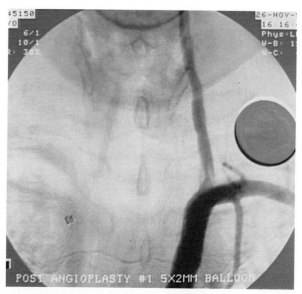

Figure 59-48 The cause of the thrombus was a tight stenosis at the origin of the left vertebral artery. This stenosis was not clinically evident because enough flow was supplied by the opposite vertebral artery to prevent posterior circulation hemodynamic insufficiency. However, it did not prevent sludging of flow in the left vertebral artery, with subsequent embolization. This was corrected with an angioplasty at this site. Note the classic intimal tear in this early example of angioplasty.

Specific Infarct Locations and Their Presentation

Brainstem Infarcts

Brainstem infarcts were poorly understood in the past because of lack of specific imaging capability. Magnetic resonance imaging (MRI) has changed this. Dysarthria, vertigo, and transient or persistent gait disturbance can implicate the pons as a site of infarction.[1] Pontine infarction may herald with crescendo TIAs, similar to impending internal capsular infarcts, and is associated with tonic limb spasms or pure hemiparesis in 4% to 28% of cases.[1, 2]

Cerebellar Infarcts

The mechanism of infarction in posterior fossa stroke and the degree of aggressiveness pertaining to therapy are determinants of the prognosis. Cerebellar infarction, although it represents only about 5% of all strokes, has several causes and not a terribly grim prognosis. The mechanism of infarction is predominantly large vessel occlusion; this is the vertebral artery in half of cases, the intrinsic cerebellar arteries in about one fifth of cases, and the basilar artery in about one fourth of cases.[3] Cardiogenic emboli account for about 25% of these insults, and local atherothrombotic occlusion (vertebral and basilar artery origin) accounts for a large portion of cerebellar infarcts.[4]

Superior cerebellar artery infarcts are mostly due to cardiogenic embolic events, whereas PICA infarcts are due to cardiogenic emboli and local atherothrombotic disease equally.[5] Anterior inferior cerebellar artery (AICA) infarcts ordinarily are due to local atheromatous occlusion; patients commonly have hypertension or diabetes.[3, 5]

Young patients with posterior fossa infarcts often have vasculitis or vertebral artery dissection at or above the level of C2. Other intrinsic vascular pathology may be present as well (e.g., fibromuscular dysplasia or vertebral insufficiency). As stated previously, cardiogenic causes should be sought.

Posterior Cerebral Artery Infarcts

Visual symptoms are the classic manifestation of occipital lobe infarct secondary to posterior cerebral artery occlusion. Hemianopia is the predominant finding, but partial field defects can be present. Strokes producing amnesia can be caused by occlusion of the posterior cerebral artery with involvement of the posterior medial temporal lobe (the amygdala and hippocampus). Interestingly, a syndrome almost indistinguishable from a middle cerebral artery (MCA) stroke can be caused by a posterior cerebral artery stroke.[6] Symptoms include hemiplegia, hemisensory loss, aphasia, hemianopia, and eye and head deviation. This is due to the involvement of the temporal and occipital lobes, the pyramidal tracts, and medial lemniscus and thalamus.

Thalamic Infarcts

The findings in patients with thalamic infarcts are variable, depending on the specific nuclei involved. Hemisensory disturbance, weakness, movement disorders, pain and temperature sensation loss, proprioception loss, aphasia, visual gaze disturbances, and visual field defects may occur. The common causes are intrinsic small vessel disease, intrinsic large vessel atheromatous lesions that primarily occlude the small thalamic perforators, and emboli. Thromboembolic insult may cause thalamic infarct secondary to occlusion of the top of the basilar artery.

Prognosis of Posterior Circulation Infarcts

The prognoses for these pathologies are diverse. The extent and mechanism of occlusion appears to be the primary predictive factor, with the presence or absence of subsequent reperfusion determining the outcome. If there is only a small embolus to any limited *intracerebellar* territory, the prognosis is fairly good. In one study of intracerebellar infarcts,[7] as many as 40% of patients had minimal or no disability at the time of discharge. In this same study, however, nearly 20% died soon after the insult. Isolated cerebellar infarcts had the best prognosis, with only a 3% death rate, whereas brainstem infarction yielded a 19% death rate. In brainstem infarcts, disturbances of hearing may herald a poor prognosis, with incipient locked-in syndrome.[8]

Occlusion of the main trunk of the basilar artery or of both vertebral arteries carries a much different prognosis. Acute occlusion of the basilar artery carries a nearly certain death sentence unless the vessel can be reopened. In the largest series reported to date,[9] only 3 of 22 patients who received conventional anticoagulant therapy survived, all with a moderate clinical deficit. Of those receiving aggressive fibrinolytic therapy, if no recanalization was achieved, all died (24 of 24). If recanalization was obtained, 14 of 19 patients survived, but only 10 had a favorable outcome.

A retrospective analysis of a consecutive series of 51 patients treated with intra-arterial urokinase or tissue-type plasminogen activator (t-PA) for basilar artery occlusion further defines this grim situation.[10] Sites of occlusion were the caudal (23 of 51), middle (18 of 51) and distal (10 of 51) segments of the basilar artery. The mechanism of occlusion was thought to be embolic in most (35 of 51) patients and intrinsic local thrombosis in the remainder (16 of 51). This large number of emboli is surprising in a site "known" for local thrombosis.

Interestingly, collateral circulation appeared to be good in 32 of the 51 patients, but this did not prevent poor outcomes in most patients. Recanalization was achieved in 26 of the 51 patients, but 12 of these 26 still died (46%). If recanalization was not achieved, 23 of 25 died (92%). This left 14 survivors in the group that was successfully recanalized and only 2 survivors in the group in whom recanalization failed. Of these 2 survivors without recanalization, the best outcome was moderate disability, with a Modified Rankin Scale score of 3. The only other survivor of the 25 patients who had no recanalization was severely disabled.

In a recent series,[11] the development of the need for intubation was a fatal prognostic sign, but this was without aggressive revascularization efforts. In a series reported by Cross et al. (Interventional Neuroradiology meeting, Val d'Isère, France, 1997), there was an overall survival rate (with aggressive intracranial therapy) of only 35% in patients with basilar artery occlusion. Distal basilar artery occlusions resulted in a 71% survival rate, whereas proximal occlusions allowed only a 15% survival rate. Of the survivors of distal basilar artery occlusion, however, only 27% had a good outcome. Factors that did not predict outcome were age, delay of therapy, and computed tomography (CT) scan appearance. Delay in instituting therapy, however, is difficult to measure in many patients with this disease because of the slow or stuttering progression and resultant slow presentation and work-up.

Kellogg, Nesbit, Kuenther, et al. (American Society of Therapeutic and Interventional Neuroradiology/World Federation of Therapeutic and Interventional Neuroradiology Scientific Conference, New York, September 1997) reported that even delayed treatment of basilar artery thrombosis can produce a good outcome. Urokinase therapy was started a mean of 12 hours after onset of symptoms in 12 patients with a mean age of 57 years and mean baseline National Institutes of Health Stroke Scale (NIHSS) score of 30 (range, 7 to 40) and infused over 1 to 2 hours (average dose 500,000 U). The three patients in whom vessel recanalization could not be achieved

died within 48 hours. Of the nine patients in whom recanalization was achieved, two died and the other seven had moderate to good outcomes. The resultant mean NIHSS of these survivors was 4.5 (range, 0 to 10) at 1 month.

In the analysis by Brandt et al.,[10] recanalization of an occluded basilar artery was achieved in only 26 of 51 patients and was associated with an embolic occlusion to a significant degree. The mortality rates were 46% in the recanalization group and 92% in the nonrecanalization group.

There is a reciprocal relationship between the AICA and PICA regarding supply to the brainstem. As long as one is open, there is usually enough flow to supply this structure, but if both are eliminated, there is a high likelihood of ischemia of the brainstem. The posterior portions of the PICA collateralize with the superior cerebellar artery around the periphery of the cerebellar hemisphere. This helps to supply the distal basilar artery past an occlusion but usually does not help the midbrain and pons.

In the basilar artery, a proximal location for occlusion is far worse than distal occlusion. This is possibly due to multiple factors:

1. The main trunk of the basilar artery is still perfused if the occlusion is distal.
2. The PICA and AICA can supply practically the entire cerebellum and brainstem if the occlusion is distal.
3. A distal occlusion is more likely due to an embolus, implying a potential lack of intrinsic vascular disease in the vertebrobasilar arterial system. (This factor has direct implications pertaining to therapy as well. Occlusions secondary to underlying plaque in the basilar artery are resistant to reperfusion with fibrinolytics, and angioplasty in this diseased artery is difficult and fraught with risks. Pontine perforators also may be involved in the vasculopathy, with resultant borderline perfusion of the brainstem and pons.)

Factors Affecting Recanalization and Outcome

Analysis of the factors relating to recanalization and clinical outcome in the series of patients reported by Hacke et al.[9] indicates that some factors help predict clinical outcome but not the success of recanalization. Specifically, the presence of good collateral supply correlated with a good outcome but did not correlate with increased likelihood of recanalization. This seems reasonable.

Recanalization was more successful with embolic occlusions than with local atherothrombotic occlusions. This is consistent with our small number of cases (see Figs. 59–1 to 59–48). Atherothrombotic occlusions do not appear to contain much material that dissolves (i.e., thrombus). There is progressive formation of atheroma to the point at which only a pinpoint-sized hole remains, which then occludes. In these cases, the vessel must be opened forcefully and dilated in association with fibrinolysis (as suggested by Brückman et al.[12] and by our own experience; see Figs. 59–1 to 59–41).

Opening the basilar occlusion may be extremely difficult, necessitating a forceful puncture of the occlusion in the basilar artery with the combined microcatheter and microwire after direct urokinase infusion yields no response. Also, just as with vascular occlusions in the periphery, angioplasty of a previously occluded vessel has a poorer result than angioplasty of a still-patent stenosis, even if tight. In the periphery, this commonly requires the use of a stent for a successful result (not currently available for intracranial vessels).

The length of the occluded segment of the basilar artery is an independent predictor of outcome, presumably because there is a greater chance of pontine perforators surviving if the amount of basilar artery that is occluded is minimal. As opposed to MCA occlusion, the downstream structures (occipital lobe, distal pons, basilar apex) are not necessarily in immediate jeopardy because of potential collateral supply from the posterior communicating arteries, pial collaterals from the MCA to the PCA, and flow around the occlusion from the PICA to the superior cerebellar artery by cerebellar pial collaterals. The status of the posterior communicating arteries and other collaterals impacts greatly on the eventual clinical outcome; the presence of these arteries is an asset that the anterior circulation (MCA) does not have.

Inclusion Criteria for Intracranial Fibrinolytic Therapy of Posterior Circulation Stroke

Inclusion criteria for fibrinolytic therapy of posterior circulation stroke include stroke in progress with increasing or incomplete deficit or both. Deep coma for more than 6 hours has a poor prognosis but does not necessarily exclude a patient from treatment. Angiographic evidence of basilar artery occlusion (or bilateral vertebral artery occlusion) with symptoms of basilar insufficiency is a requirement for therapy.

Exclusion Criteria for Intracranial Fibrinolytic Therapy of Posterior Circulation Stroke

There is no absolute time limit for intracranial fibrinolytic therapy because of the variable speed of progression of posterior circulation stroke and the almost uniformly grave prognosis. We have treated a patient 4 days after initial presentation and another after 2 days. The patient with the 4-day history (who was quadriparetic at the time of therapy) had an excellent outcome with minimal permanent deficit, whereas the patient with the 2-day history had a fatal brainstem hemorrhage.

Evidence on CT scan of hemorrhage or infarct is a contraindication to this therapy, as it is for all intracranial thrombolysis. It may be difficult, however, to differentiate edema from infarct in the poste-

rior fossa after the slow progression has had time to render signal changes on MRI.

Any setting in which systemic anticoagulation or fibrinolysis is contraindicated is a relative cause for exclusion; this includes uncorrectable clotting abnormality, recent intracranial surgery, uncontrollable hypertension, and active gastrointestinal or other internal bleeding. History of sensitivity to urokinase (or whichever agent is being used) is also a contraindication to use of that agent, but another agent may be used.

Guidelines for Treatment

The choice of technique and method of infusion of thrombolytic agents are discussed in Chapters 58 and 60. The following is a discussion of the application of these techniques to specific lesions.

Basilar Artery Occlusion

Rationale for Therapy

The overall prognosis for patients with basilar artery occlusion appears to be grim. The data presented above reveal the extremely high mortality rate and poor neurologic outcome associated with this disease. It appears that recanalization is nearly mandatory for survival of basilar occlusion. For a patient presenting with a clinical picture and radiographic findings suggestive of acute basilar occlusion, emergency angiography is mandatory. If occlusion is found, the best hope is local intra-arterial fibrinolysis. If incomplete occlusion with antegrade flow is present, watchful waiting with systemic anticoagulation (heparinization) may be in order, with a rescue planned if the clinical picture deteriorates.

Because of the almost invariably poor prognosis described above (death or locked-in syndrome), the decision to treat a basilar artery thrombus is made relatively easily by the clinician. In addition, the delayed completion of full occlusion can result in a minimal actual preexisting infarct, potentially providing a greater window of opportunity for therapy. This is important because the slow presentation may delay aggressive diagnostic evaluation or therapy while it delays completion of the infarct. A preexisting infarct seen on CT, however, indicates the increased likelihood of a devastating bleed occurring after fibrinolytic therapy.

Diagnostic Evaluation

Accurate evaluation requires a true four-vessel angiogram to assess the intracranial hemodynamics and area of ongoing vascular insult and its most likely origin, possible consequences, complications of therapy, and most appropriate therapeutic target.

The angiogram typically reveals a vertebral artery ending in a large (or healthy) PICA. Both vertebral arteries may or may not be present. The posterior fossa usually is essentially isolated, with minimal supply from the posterior communicating arteries. On digital subtraction angiography, minimal retrograde slow trickle may be observed down the occluded basilar artery. Other lesions that may alter or complicate therapy may be identified. It may be necessary, for example, to perform angioplasty of a vertebral origin stenosis before dissolution of a basilar tip embolus.

Occasionally, evaluation of the status of the posterior communicating arteries shows that the basilar artery occlusion is compensated nearly or completely by collateral flow; this may alter therapy. A well-collateralized occlusion can be watched, depending on the clinical circumstances. If well compensated by anterior circulation collateral supply, these patients may maintain an essentially asymptomatic existence. Because the presence of symptoms generally is what led the patient to seek treatment, however, the prognosis may be guarded at best.

Alternatively, an embolus to the top of the basilar artery may be present. This yields a completely different radiographic picture and requires a different approach to therapy. The embolus can be from a proximal vertebral artery stenosis with subsequent thrombus formation or can be cardiogenic in origin.

Fibrinolytic Therapy Procedure

The underlying pathology usually is a focal stenosis at the junction of the proximal and middle thirds of the basilar artery that has progressed to occlusion. This can lead to thrombus formation in the proximal stagnant section, in the segment of basilar artery distal to the occlusion or both. It may not be until fibrinolysis is complete that the reason for the basilar artery occlusion is found.

Midbasilar stenosis is a difficult and dangerous entity to treat, more so than an embolus to the top of the basilar artery. All thrombus that has accumulated around a stenosis should be removed as best as possible by fibrinolysis. The infusion should follow the guidelines outlined in Chapter 60. Some of the underlying thrombus may have formed well before the final insult and may be relatively resistant to thrombolysis or may simply be hard plaque. First, the proximal lumen should be cleaned up; that is, any thrombus is present should be dissolved. Establishment of antegrade flow by poking a hole in the occluded segment may or may not be readily accomplished but speeds thrombolysis. Any thrombus distal to the occlusion should be dissolved as best as possible because of risk of downstream propulsion once antegrade flow is reestablished.

If the causative lesion was not identifiable before fibrinolysis, it may become evident after therapy and be revealed as a stenotic plaque. Identification of an underlying plaque does not necessarily imply that it must be treated, at least not at that particular time. Intracranial angioplasty can be a dangerous procedure (particularly of the midbasilar artery) and can add one more risk to an already dangerous situation. It may be possible to maintain the patient on anticoagulants, remove any causes of hypercoagulability (e.g., smoking), and thus preclude any further trouble from the site in question. It may be possible to maintain heparinization and anticoagulation for a few weeks to allow parenchymal healing before further intervention is performed. This can be tested by observing the site for a prolonged period with the patient on the angiography table.

After the thrombus has been dissolved and the area cleaned up, however, thrombosis can recur, even while the patient is heparinized in the angiography suite. The basilar artery under these circumstances appears to be extremely thrombogenic. As discussed in Chapter 48, the addition of abciximab may aid in deterring rethrombosis and reocclusion, but even this may not be enough. Reinstitution of fibrinolytic therapy can again open the vessel, but treatment of the underlying lesion (angioplasty) is now mandatory.

Angioplasty of the midbasilar artery is dangerous. Although the postangioplasty radiographic appearance may be acceptable (or even spectacular), any intimal damage in the basilar artery can result in the occlusion or sloughing of vital direct perforators originating from the basilar artery, with dire results. These perforators generally supply small areas of major consequence. In the case of a previously occluded basilar artery, the results of emergency basilar artery angioplasty are unpredictable. Even if the angioplasty does not disrupt any perforators, there are usually some at the basilar apex, and these may have been ischemic for a prolonged period. Luckily, the midbasilar artery often is a bare segment, with a leash of perforators originating from a more distal position and coursing inferiorly to supply the pons.

If angioplasty has to be performed, it is important remember that stretching is better than tearing and that "good enough" is better than great. It eventually will be proved that gentle minimal improvement is good enough when basilar artery angioplasty is necessary. A thread of residual lumen in a 3-mm vessel that is increased to 1.5 mm is sufficient to supply the downstream territory. If this can be achieved without a significant intimal disruption, it is a major success.

Bilateral Vertebral Artery Occlusion

Strategy for Therapy

As stated previously, one vertebral artery generally has been occluded for some time either at the vertebrobasilar junction or at the site of entrance of the vertebral artery into the dura. The other vertebral artery then undergoes occlusion at the mirror image site, precipitating the clinical event that brings the patient to treatment. Some flow either is trickling past the obstruction or, more likely, circumventing the obstruction by collateral circulation through the PICA-to-superior cerebellar artery collaterals.

Some flow may be reaching the posterior fossa through the posterior communicating arteries, or even retrograde through the anterior spinal artery. In one case (see Figs. 59–1 to 59–11), perfusion was observed through pial collaterals from the MCA to the posterior cerebral artery, then retrograde back down P1 to the basilar artery, and then retrograde down the basilar artery. In general, if the posterior communicating arteries are large (i.e., if the posterior fossa is not isolated), a symptomatic event may not occur; however, this is unpredictable.

Depending on when the initial event occurred, the speed of progression, and the presence or absence of a completed infarct, the initial therapy may be aggressive heparinization in an effort to stabilize the situation or allow the intrinsic fibrinolytic system to reopen the stenosis or occlusion. This may work to some degree (see Figs. 48–39 to 48–48). Reopening one vertebral artery, combined with continued anticoagulation, may be enough to maintain the status quo.

If a tenuous hemodynamic situation has been maintained, and there is no true basilar artery thrombus, minimal infarct may be present. If this is the case, a slow infusion of fibrinolytic agent can be performed to clean thoroughly the vessel to be opened while avoiding establishment of a systemic fibrinolytic state (thereby decreasing the risk of perfusing remote ischemic tissue with the fibrinolytic agent).

Fibrinolytic Therapy Procedure

Because of the possible slow-motion nature of the event, a frantic, aggressive fibrinolysis maneuver may not be necessary. Particularly with posterior fossa occlusions, there may still be some perfusion present; that is, the incident is related to progressive stenosis with some perfusion provided by the collateral vessels described previously. The degree of ischemia may be sufficient to cause electrical dysfunction without the presence of a completed infarct. A lower-dose and slower infusion of fibrinolytic agent, followed by angioplasty, may suffice.

To avoid infusion of damaged cerebellar tissue with excessive amounts of fibrinolytic agent, initial establishment of antegrade flow is beneficial. This allows downstream flow of the drug *through the occlusive thrombus* rather than through collateral pathways, such as the PICA-to-superior cerebellar artery.

There may not be a large volume of thrombus to dissolve in this particular pathologic situation. The primary task may be to perform angioplasty of the critically stenotic distal segment of the vertebral artery. Because the underlying pathology in this condition is progression of the stenosis of the second vertebral artery either to occlusion or near occlusion, in combination with an isolated posterior fossa, the treatment may be angioplasty alone, and going directly to this form of therapy may be the correct maneuver. This depends completely on the degree of secondary thrombosis. This topic is covered more fully in Chapter 48.

ANTERIOR CIRCULATION STROKE
Clinical Manifestations

In contrast to the variable and often gradual onset of posterior fossa stroke, the presentation of anterior circulation stroke usually is far more dramatic (Cases 5 to 7, Figs. 59–49 to 59–74). As described later in "Strategic Hemodynamic Considerations for Specific Anterior Circulation Occlusions," the severity of symptoms usually depends on the amount of thrombus and the territory affected. Some TIAs are thought to represent small occlusions of branches of

Text continued on page 719

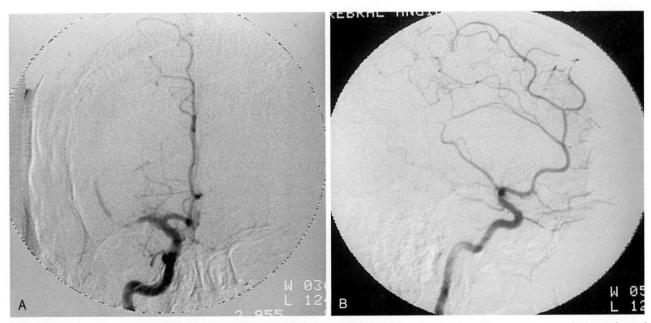

Figure 59-49 Case 5. *A* and *B,* PA and lateral right internal carotid angiograms performed in a 34-year-old man who experienced sudden onset of hemiparesis while eating lunch. The initial CT scan was totally unremarkable. The angiograms reveal almost total occlusion of the right MCA in the mid-M1 segment. The inferior division is seen to fill slightly on the lateral view. Note the absence of perfusion of a large portion of the hemisphere; almost all visualized vasculature is the anterior cerebral artery and its branches.

Case 5 continues

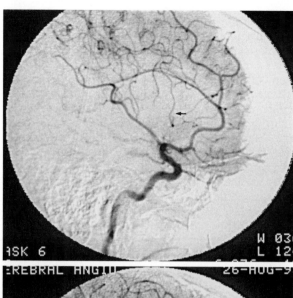

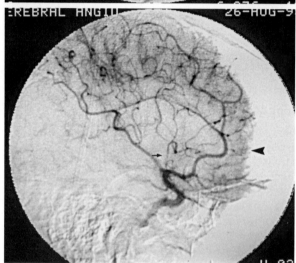

Figure 59-50 Later filming reveals a slow trickle of perfusion toward the MCA bifurcation *(arrows),* a good sign. The MCA territory is still in its arterial phase while the anterior cerebral artery territory is in the capillary phase *(arrowhead).*

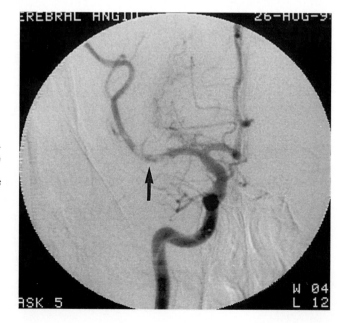

Figure 59-51 After poking through the thrombus with the guide-wire and catheter, a repeat angiogram reveals some flow past the occlusion *(arrow).*

Case 5 continues

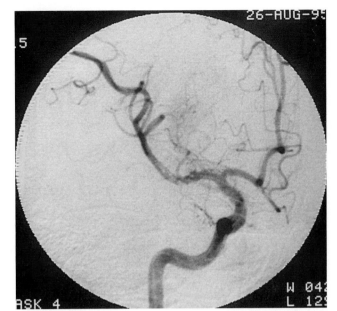

Figure 59-52 After infusion of urokinase at the rate of 500,000 U/hr for 20 minutes, a repeat angiogram reveals increased flow in the MCA.

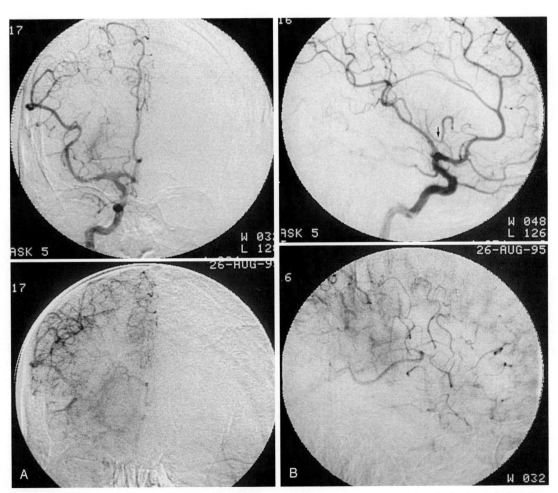

Figure 59-53 *A* and *B,* Further urokinase infusion produced some improvement in hemispheric perfusion, best seen on the lateral view. Note that the flow is predominantly in the inferior division, however *(arrow).* The patient could now barely move his arm.

Case 5 continues

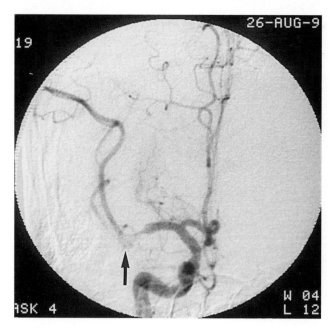

Figure 59-54 Several minutes later, the patient became plegic again and the repeat angiogram revealed worsening of the occlusion. Note the unusual appearance of the MCA at its trifurcation *(arrow)*. Poor antegrade flow is now present.

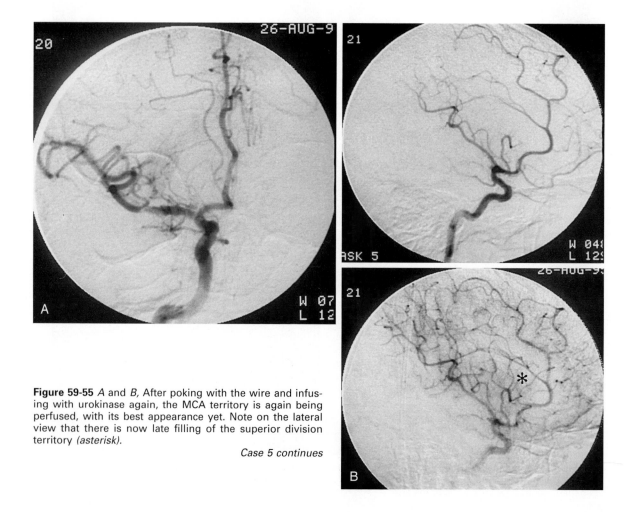

Figure 59-55 *A* and *B*, After poking with the wire and infusing with urokinase again, the MCA territory is again being perfused, with its best appearance yet. Note on the lateral view that there is now late filling of the superior division territory *(asterisk)*.

Case 5 continues

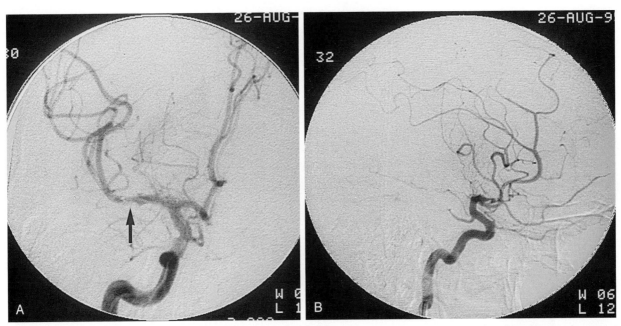

Figure 59-56 *A* and *B,* After infusion at the rate of about 8000 U/min (500,000 U/hr) for another 20 minutes, the repeat angiogram again reveals occlusion of MCA branches, but now there is predominant filling of the superior division with no perfusion of the inferior division. Infusion was continued. Note the unusual appearance of the inferior portion of the M1 segment *(arrow).*

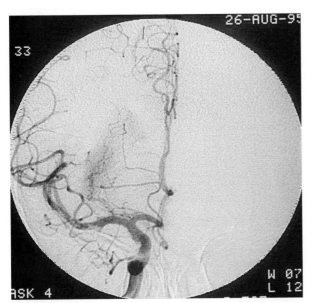

Figure 59-57 Twenty minutes later, the repeat angiogram reveals improved flow in two large MCA branches. The inferior portion of M1 really looks strange and suggests the (occluded) origin of another branch, the anterior temporal branch.

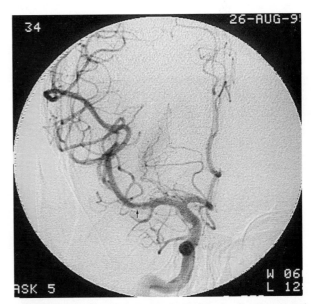

Figure 59-58 Further poking with the guidewire finally opened a small entry to this branch (never before seen). The infusion had now been maintained over a period of 2 hours. Additional infusion was now performed for another 15 minutes in an attempt to clear the distal main trunk of the MCA. Note the residual thrombus within the anterior temporal branch *(arrow).*

Case 5 continues

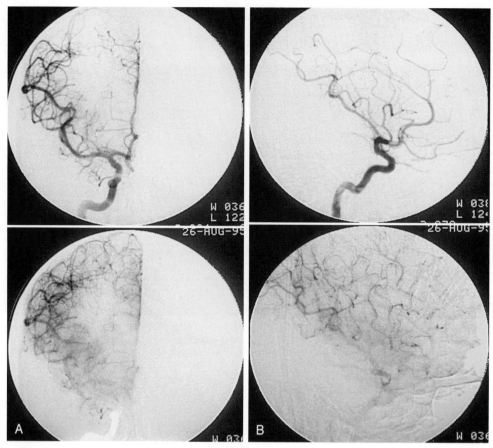

Figure 59-59 *A* and *B,* Final PA and lateral arteriograms. There is good perfusion of the bulk of the MCA distribution. The temporal lobe region is poorly perfused. Note the now *slightly* patent anterior temporal artery. The infusion was thought to be reaching a point of maximal benefit-risk ratio at this time, the interval from insult now almost 8 hours.

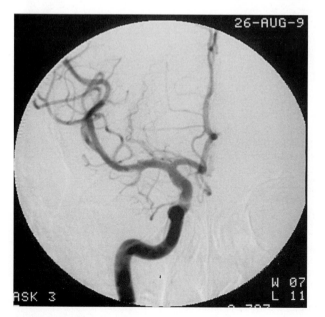

Figure 59-60 Final appearance of the previously occluded MCA. There is still some minimal thrombus in the main trunk as well as nearly complete occlusion of the anterior temporal branch.

Case 5 continues

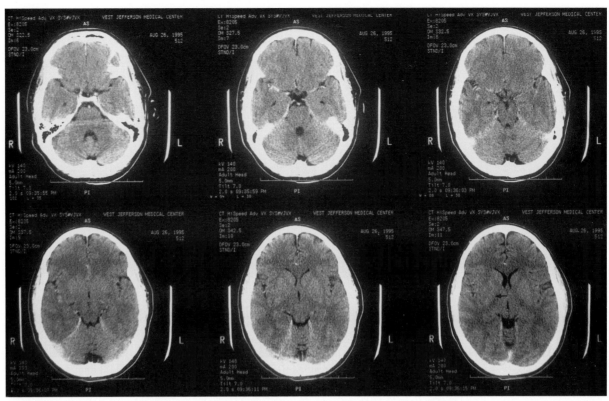

Figure 59-61 Postinfusion CT scan reveals some hyperdensity in the region of the occluded main temporal branch as well as a subtle change in the posterior portion of the putamen *(arrow)*.

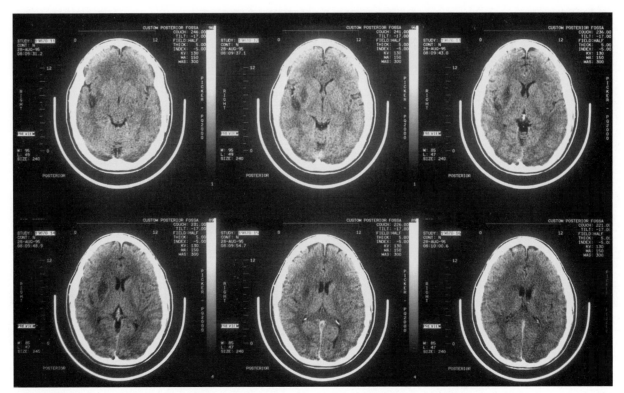

Figure 59-62 Two days later, the putamen displays edematous changes and the perisylvian area displays an infarct. The patient was completely intact neurologically.

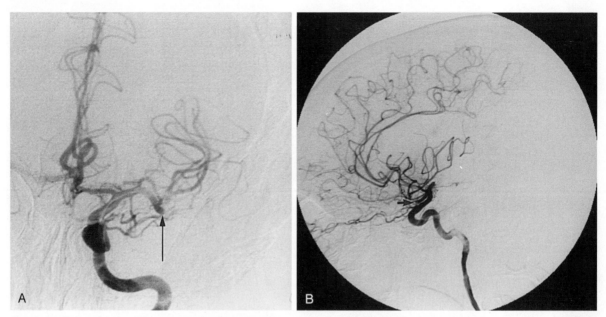

Figure 59-63 Case 6. *A* and *B,* A 54-year-old man with a history of atrial fibrillation presented to the ER after acute onset of right hemiparesis and aphasia. The ER physician obtained a CT scan and called the attending cardiologist. We were then contacted. Initial injection of the left internal carotid artery during an emergency angiogram reveals abrupt occlusion of the upper division of the MCA (although it initially courses downward) *(short arrow).* Note the truncated appearance on the magnified PA view *(long arrow).* On the lateral view, there is absence of filling of parietal branches, whereas the anterior cerebral artery branches and the inferior division (temporal lobe branches) of the MCA are well filled.

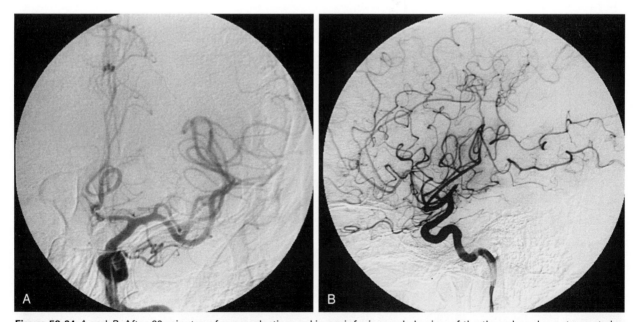

Figure 59-64 *A* and *B,* After 60 minutes of superselective urokinase infusion and chasing of the thrombus downstream twice, the proximal trunk of the upper division is now clear. Residual occlusion is present in a more distal branch. The patient had begun to try to talk, although with meaningless noises. His arm and leg strength had improved. It was now approximately 7 hours from the onset of symptoms.

Case 6 continues

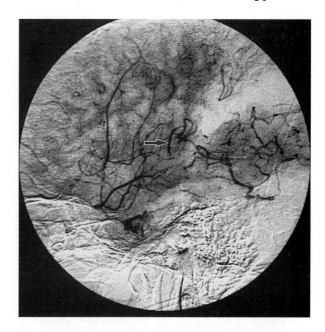

Figure 59-65 Final lateral left internal carotid angiogram reveals good parenchymal blush in most of the parietal and temporal lobes, but a distinct wedge of unperfused tissue in the posterior parieto-occipital region (Wernicke's area). The thrombus was very resistant to mechanical (wire poking) and chemical (urokinase) disruption, and this area unfortunately did not perfuse from any other source.

Note the slow flow in the angular artery *(arrow)* proximal to the occlusion. The other distinct vessels seen in the parietal lobe in this capillary phase are veins.

the MCA (which can clear rapidly) rather than M1 trunk occlusions.

Occlusion of the proximal main (M1) trunk of the MCA produces severe cerebral ischemia and results in contralateral hemiplegia and hemianesthesia, stupor, and deviation of head and eyes to the affected side. If the insult is to the dominant hemisphere, global aphasia results; hemineglect results if the nondominant side is affected. MCA trunk occlusion results in an immediate (1-month) mortality rate that approaches 30% and in severe long-term disability in 40% to 65% of the survivors.[13]

If the main trunk of the MCA is spared and the insult is to the superior-division M2 branch, the sensorimotor deficit is denser in the arm and face, with some possible sparing of the leg. The initial global aphasia may become primarily expressive at a later time. The long-term prognosis is much more favorable for branch occlusions of the MCA than for main trunk occlusions.

When the angular branch of the MCA is affected (the usual supply to the posterior parietal lobe), Wernicke's aphasia can be seen if the insult is in the dominant hemisphere (see Figs. 59–63 to 59–67). If the nondominant side is involved, contralateral neglect is present. Wernicke's aphasia is devastating, and it can be argued that hemiparesis with preservation of communication skills is better than normal motor function with loss of a significant degree of comprehension and speech. Unfortunately, these two functions are usually lost together, but if the supply to Wernicke's area originates from the inferior division of the MCA or posterior circulation, these functions can be affected separately.

Inclusion Criteria for Intracranial Fibrinolytic Therapy of Anterior Circulation Stroke

Inclusion criteria were discussed previously with regard to ongoing trials. In general, they include the presence of angiographically demonstrable occlusion

of the distal internal carotid artery (ICA) or MCA and the onset of a severe, clinically appropriate neurologic event. This neurologic event usually includes one or more of the following: hemiplegia, visual deficit, aphasia or dysphasia, and neglect. The onset should be within a period allowing completion of therapy by 6 to 9 hours after the event. (Theron et al.[14] believe that up to 12 hours may be permissible for branch occlusion of the MCA; this may be reasonable, as discussed under "Timing of Therapy" in Chapter 58.)

These criteria are further outlined in Tables 59–1 and 59–2.

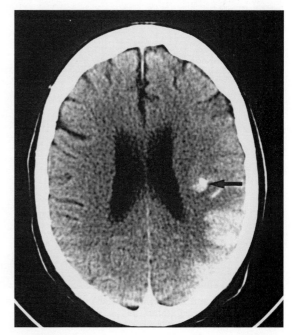

Figure 59-66 Immediate postprocedure CT scan reveals typical "extravasation" of contrast from distal ischemic territory (see text) as well as the actual nidus of the residual embolus *(arrow)*. This distal territory evolved a true infarct.

Case 6 continues

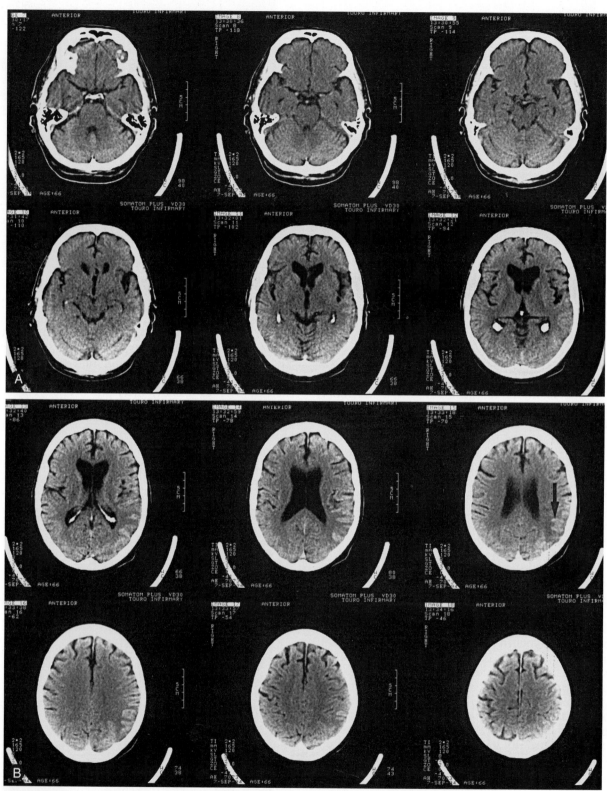

Figure 59-67 *A* and *B,* Follow-up CT scan 2 weeks later reveals minimal ischemic change in the left posterior parietal region *(arrow)*. However, as stated, this is in Wernicke's area. The patient retired after this event and is very functional from a motor standpoint (he still plays golf), but his functionality from a communicative standpoint is greatly affected.

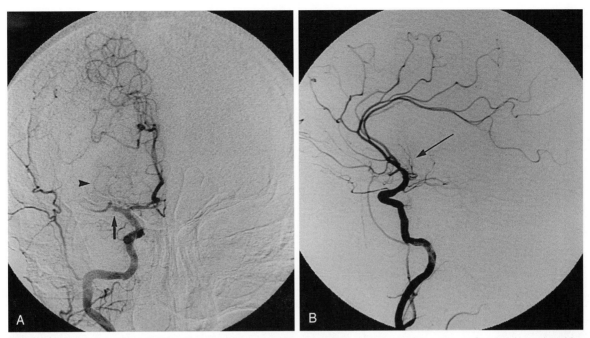

Figure 59-68 Case 7. *A* and *B,* This 58-year-old woman, status post coronary artery bypass graft, experienced sudden onset of left hemiplegia, dysarthria, and hemineglect (see Chapter 6). The PA and lateral right carotid angiograms demonstrate total absence of the MCA *(short arrow)*, but with some filling of lenticulostriate vessels *(arrowhead)*, along with blush in the region of the basal ganglia and internal capsule. This renders this occlusion a type M1-B (MCA occlusion, without lenticulostriate occlusion, with the embolus near or at the MCA bifurcation). Note the posterior communicating artery, the anterior choroidal artery, and the leash of lenticulostriate vessels *(long arrow)* on the lateral view.

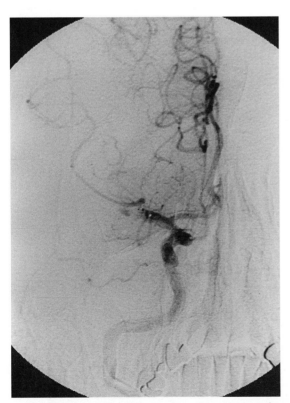

Figure 59-69 Magnification view with a microcatheter now in place. The clot is outlined by contrast, with some penetration through the embolus into two branches due to passage of the microwire.

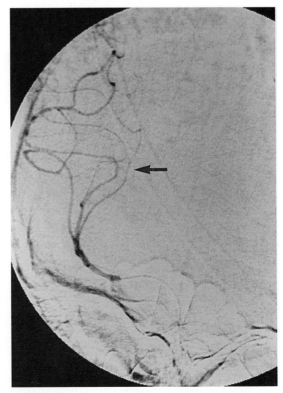

Figure 59-70 The microcatheter has now been advanced through the embolus into a main MCA branch, apparently a superior division branch. Careful injection of contrast reveals a clear downstream distribution *(arrow).*

Case 7 continues

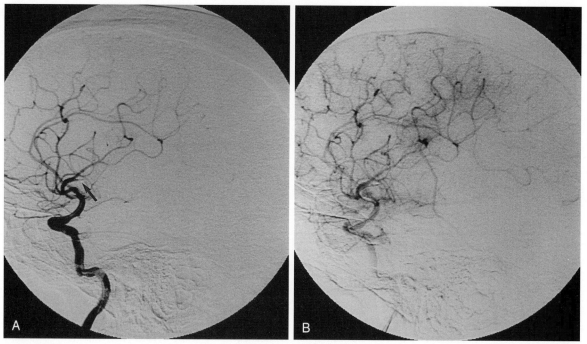

Figure 59-71 *A* and *B,* The microcatheter was withdrawn into the main trunk of the MCA and urokinase was infused for 45 minutes. These are early and late images from a lateral view after the urokinase infusion. Note the excellent flow into the anterior half of the superior division of the MCA (supplying primarily the posterior frontal lobe). The microcatheter has been advanced into an occluded stub of a major branch headed posteriorly *(arrow).* This branch will probably supply a large portion of the motor strip as well as Wernicke's area.

The fact that the main trunk of the MCA is now clear, and the lenticulostriate arteries were mostly if not totally clear to begin with, slightly decreases the intense urge to finish the procedure. An increased margin of safety now exists. The newly opened branch leading to the posterior frontal and parietal lobes displays some hyperemic blush typical for a previously occluded vessel that has been reopened.

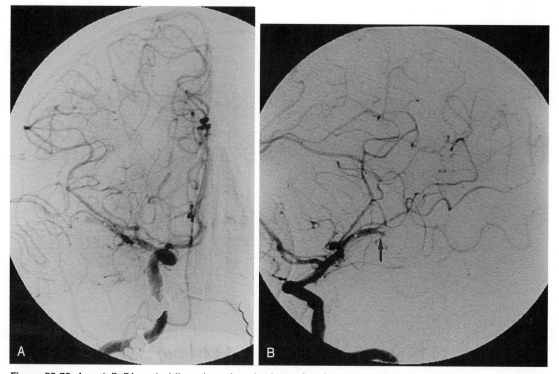

Figure 59-72 *A* and *B,* PA and oblique lateral projections after further infusion of urokinase into this branch vessel stub. It has opened to some degree, with some supply now going to an additional branch, but a new stub is now seen *(arrow),* probably representing the angular branch to Wernicke's area.

Case 7 continues

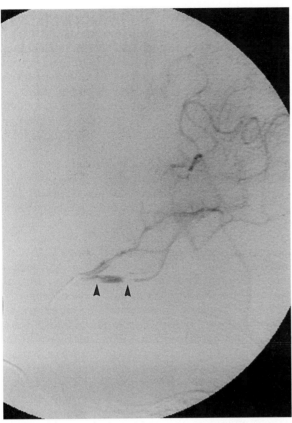

Figure 59-73 Magnification view of contrast injection through the microcatheter in the region of the tertiary branch occlusions. Note the thrombus within the lower of the two branches *(arrowheads)*. The upper branch does not look pristine, either. Continued infusion was maintained in this peripheral location.

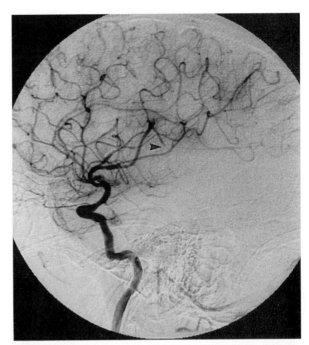

Figure 59-74 Final lateral view after 3 hours of infusion (7½ hours after the original insult). Most supply to the MCA territory is now intact. Note the residual stub of a distal branch still occluded *(arrowhead)*. This could not be dissolved even with prolonged superselective infusion, indicative of a mature embolus. Most of the hemisphere is now perfused adequately. The procedure was terminated because of increasing concern over the length of the procedure and the amount of urokinase infused.

Exclusion Criteria for Intracranial Fibrinolytic Therapy of Anterior Circulation Stroke

The exclusion criteria also were discussed in association with various trials. In general, they include CT scan evidence of hemorrhage or infarct, sensitivity to the thrombolytic agent, recent surgery (especially intracranial), uncontrollable hypertension, and uncorrectable clotting abnormalities. These criteria are further outlined in Tables 59–3 and 59–4.

Strategic Guidelines for Treatment

This topic is covered to some extent in Chapters 58 and 60. Accurate angiographic evaluation should start with evaluation of the normal side. Time constraints, clinical condition, and vascular anatomy may make this impractical. The Prolyse for Acute Cerebral Thromboembolism (PROACT) protocol requires angiography of the pathologic side only, with prompt superselection and infusion.

Evaluation of the normal side (opposite carotid artery) and vertebral arteries first allows some degree of understanding of collateral supply to the affected side. Theron et al.[14] emphasize the concept of a global

---

T A B L E   5 9 - 1   Inclusion Criteria for Emergency Direct Intracranial or Fibrinolytic Infusion for Stroke Treatment

---

Clinical

1. The signal stroke must be acute and the most recent significant, acute worsening of serial neurologic events, or related to a diagnostic radiographic procedure but not an interventional procedure
2. Clinical signs consistent with the diagnosis of ischemic stroke, including impairment of motor function, language, cognition, vision, and gaze or neglect
3. Onset of new neurologic signs of a stroke within 6 hours of the time to initiation of treatment
4. No prior neurologic event that would obscure the interpretation of the signal neurologic deficits
5. Minimal score of 4 on the NIHSS, except for isolated aphasia or isolated hemianopia

Cerebral CT Scan

1. Normal study or early findings that do not meet CT scan exclusion criteria

---

T A B L E   5 9 - 2   Inclusion Criteria for Intravenous Tissue-Type Plasminogen Activator Treatment of Acute Ischemic Stroke

---

1. Focal neurologic deficit, including aphasia (expressive, receptive, or global), ataxia, cranial nerve palsies, diplopia, dysarthria, hemianopia, hemiparesis, loss of sensation, quadriparesis, visual field disturbances
2. Presentation within 3 hours of onset of symptoms

T A B L E 5 9 - 3 Exclusion Criteria for Emergency Direct Intracranial Fibrinolytic Infusion for Stroke Treatment

Clinical

1. Coma
2. Neurologic signs that are rapidly improving by the time of randomization
3. Major stroke symptoms (>30 on the NIHSS)
4. History of stroke within the previous 6 weeks
5. Seizure at the onset of stroke
6. Clinical presentation suggestive of subarachnoid hemorrhage, even if the initial CT scan is normal
7. Previous known intracranial hemorrhage or subarachnoid hemorrhage at any time
8. Known neoplasm or intracranial arteriovenous malformation or aneurysm with any evidence of associated hemorrhage
9. Presumed pericarditis related to recent acute myocardial infarction
10. Suspected lacunar stroke
11. Recent (within 30 days) surgery, biopsy of a parenchymal organ, or lumbar puncture
12. Recent (within 30 days) trauma, with internal injuries or ulcerative wounds
13. Recent (within 90 days) head trauma
14. Known active inflammatory bowel disease, ulcerative colitis, or diverticular disease
15. Any active or recent (within 30 days) hemorrhage
16. Known hereditary or acquired hemorrhagic diathesis (e.g., activated partial thromboplastin time or prothrombin time greater than normal; unsupported coagulation factor deficiency)
17. Baseline laboratory values that reveal platelets <100,000/µl, hematocrit, or packed cell volume <25 volume %, or international normalized ratio >1.7
18. Pregnancy, lactation, or parturition within the previous 30 days
19. Known serious sensitivity to contrast agents
20. Any condition in which angiography is contraindicated
21. Presumed septic embolus
22. Uncontrollable hypertension; hypertension is defined as systolic blood pressure >180 mm Hg or diastolic blood pressure ≥100 mm Hg

Cerebral CT Scan

1. Early CT scan changes
    High-density lesion consistent with hemorrhage of any degree
    Evidence of significant mass effect with midline shift due to a large infarct
    Acute hypodense parenchymal lesion or effacement of cerebral sulci in more than one third of the MCA territory
2. Other CT scan findings:
    Evidence of an intracranial tumor (except small coincidental meningioma)
    Subarachnoid hemorrhage

parenchymal phase obtained by digital subtraction imaging of the brain with an arch aortogram to demonstrate the current ischemic situation; this is a quick method of obtaining valuable information.

Demonstration of a clinically appropriate vascular occlusion is then necessary before institution of therapy. The details of infusion are covered in Chapter 60.

Clearing of the M1 segment of the MCA as quickly as possible is the initial goal of treatment. This is done to clear rapidly any obstruction to the lenticulostriate vessels. Initial establishment of antegrade

flow by puncture of the thrombus with the microcatheter can aid in this goal. Angioplasty of the M1 segment thrombus may just pack clot into the tiny orifices of the lenticulostriate arteries, potentially rendering reperfusion of these vessels impossible. Further discussion of the rationale for therapy of this situation is presented in Chapter 58, specifically concerning the rationale for clearing the origins of the lenticulostriate arteries as rapidly as possible.

Once clearing of the main trunk of the MCA is achieved, the clot should be followed wherever it goes as long as time and dose permit. The question of what should be done in each circumstance is yet to be answered, and it will probably be years before specific strategies are known for every situation.

The variability in the preexisting vascular anatomy and the possible subsequent damage to the lenticulostriate territory, combined with the unknown intrinsic collateral perfusion elsewhere, results in a degree of uncertainty that may never be resolved fully (see "Strategic Hemodynamic Considerations for Specific Anterior Circulation Occlusions," below). It is for this reason that advancing the microcatheter past the M1 segment of the MCA (and the lenticulostriate arteries) as soon as possible is considered desirable.

Once the embolus has moved downstream, it is more difficult to visualize and to follow with the catheter. The clot is radiolucent; the farther it migrates, the more normal vessels are seen on each injection, which can confuse the evaluation. (We have observed thrombus that apparently soaked up con-

T A B L E 5 9 - 4 Exclusion Criteria for Intravenous Tissue-Type Plasminogen Activator Treatment of Acute Ischemic Stroke

Absolute

1. Evidence of intracranial hemorrhage on pretreatment CT
2. Suspicion of subarachnoid hemorrhage
3. Recent intracranial surgery or serious head trauma or recent previous stroke
4. History of intracranial hemorrhage
5. Uncontrolled hypertension at time of treatment (e.g., >185 mm Hg systolic or >110 mm Hg diastolic)
6. Seizure at the onset of stroke
7. Active internal bleeding
8. Intracranial neoplasm, arteriovenous malformation, or aneurysm
9. Known bleeding diathesis, including but not limited to:
    Current use of oral anticoagulants (e.g., warfarin sodium) with prothrombin time >15 seconds
    Administration of heparin within 48 hours preceding the onset of stroke and an elevated activated partial thromboplastin time at presentation
    Platelet count <100,000/mm³

Relative

1. Patients with severe neurologic deficit (e.g., NIHSS >22) at presentation; there is an increased risk of intracranial hemorrhage in these patients
2. Patients with major early infarct signs on a CT scan (e.g., substantial edema, mass effect, or midline shift)

trast and was dense on the postprocedure CT scan, but later returned to radiolucency within 24 hours.)

The ability to chase the clot extremely distally is limited. The catheter should not be placed in a stagnant branch vessel for a prolonged period without adequate heparinization. Checking its position and results more often, and perhaps moving it, should be performed.

There comes a point when further pursuit and heroic efforts become counterproductive. Total infusion dose, elapsed time from the ischemic event, and the patient's clinical status dictate when to stop (see Figs. 59–68 to 59–74). Infusion in an occluded M1 segment should not be done past 7 to 9 hours at the *maximum* (and preferably not after 5 to 6 hours), but peripheral cortical branches probably have a much greater window of opportunity. Each clinical circumstance is different. The PROACT trial does not directly address these situations, whereas the North American Cerebral Local Intra-Arterial Fibrinolysis Register allows adaptation according to circumstances and is recording the results for current and later analysis. In a distal small branch, the dose of urokinase necessary for effective action is smaller and can be decreased from the dose used in more proximal locations. This also decreases the systemic activity and thus increases safety.

For a particular case, the interventional neuroradiologist should let his or her conscience be the guide. Remember the statement often repeated throughout this book, however; this is not the time to learn intracranial catheter use, superselection technique, nor cerebral hemodynamics.

Strategic Hemodynamic Considerations for Specific Anterior Circulation Occlusions

Intrinsic vascular design, combined with luck regarding where the clot goes, determines to a tremendous degree the ultimate outcome of an embolic event as well as the result of emergency treatment. The initial angiogram can in large measure give an idea of the chance of success and of the length of time available for therapy. Some ischemic insults may demand therapy within minutes (not possible), whereas others may allow many hours, if not days, for a rescue (see the case presented in Chapter 58 [Figs. 58–15 to 58–54]).

Pioneers in the emergency intra-arterial treatment of stroke have supplied an approach to the analysis of the severity of insult produced by acute cerebrovascular events.[15–18] Their conclusions and our own have implied that the status of the deep perforators (primarily the lateral lenticulostriate arteries) has tremendous implications concerning prognosis, time for rescue, and safety of therapy. Zeumer et al.[15] have classified various types of insult by location as types I, II, III, IV, and M type. This method of analysis is rational and is one of the first truly intellectual considerations of this subject. Theron et al.[17] have used a classification system stratified by worsening prognosis, from group 1 to group 3, with various

subgroups. Theron's recent work is fundamentally based on the concept that it is the status of the lenticulostriate arteries that determines the outcome and the length of time for rescue.[14]

We agree with this fundamental concept and prefer to think of cerebrovascular insults based on where the occlusion is located, progressing from proximal to distal locations, with specific consideration given to any threatened deep perforators. The analysis then incorporates the status of adequate superficial pial collaterals and the connections in the circle of Willis.

Most of this information is apparent on analysis of the diagnostic angiogram; the site of occlusion is revealed, and with high-quality modern digital subtraction angiographic equipment, an accurate estimate of the quality of pial collaterals can be made if evaluation of the correct angiographic injections is made. There always will be a degree of uncertainty relative to the origin of unseen lenticulostriate vessels, however (see Fig. 58–6). These potential sites of occlusion are presented below along with a method of reasoning for evaluation of the depth of ischemia, the prognostic implications concerning neurologic outcome, and the time available for therapy (Table 59–5 and Fig. 59–75).

Location of Occlusion

As stated previously, it is the status of the deep perforators that will ultimately affect the length of time available before therapy will no longer be effective and at which point therapy may become dangerous. Thus, simple progression from proximal to distal (concerning where the occlusion is located) does not necessarily correlate directly to the severity of the insult. In addition, the status of the pial collaterals in each instance of occlusion determines to a significant degree whether the outcome of rescue will be positive, not to mention less dangerous.

Type ICA-O (ICA-Origin)

The ICA is occluded at the level of its origin from the common carotid artery. The posterior and anterior communicating arteries can be open, as is the anterior choroidal artery. The carotid bifurcation is open. **Implications.** The most typical, but worst, presentation of occlusion of the cervical ICA is caused by an embolus to the intracranial circulation from the stagnant ICA. If this occurs, the symptoms are typical for the particular occlusion, as described later. The most important thing to realize is that the cervical ICA can contain a large volume of thrombus and that the more thrombus enters the intracranial circulation, the more difficult it is to reestablish enough flow to prevent a large infarct. The real problem is *not* the occlusion of the cervical ICA or the thrombus that remains in this vessel, but the intracranial embolus. It is crucial that no additional thrombus be displaced intracranially.

If there is no embolus to the intracranial circulation, then more than in any other occlusion, the status of the circle of Willis determines the clinical situation. These patients present secondary to borderline

T A B L E   5 9 - 5   Strategic Hemodynamic Considerations for Treatment of Specific Anterior Circulation Location Occlusions

Type of Occlusion	Angiographic Appearance	Time for Rescue	Functionally Most Critically Threatened Area	Most Critical Portion of Occlusion to Clear	Risk of Fibrinolytic Hemorrhage	Prognosis (almost always dependent on the pial collaterals)
ICA-O ("origin"; ophthalmic and anterior and posterior communicators may be open)	Entire ICA is occluded at the common bifurcation; retrograde flow in the ophthalmic keeps the distal ICA open; collateral supply to the anterior circulation may be present through communicators	Possibly prolonged; perhaps no need to treat at all; depends on symptoms	Watershed area usually is Wernicke's area, sensory and motor cortex	Point of ICA occlusion (could be ICA origin or siphon), but bulk of thrombus may be prohibitive (see discussion)	Low to moderate; no deep perforators are occluded; but clot can be displaced downstream into cerebral arteries (see discussion)	Good, depending on etiology of occlusion, any ongoing emboli, and status of circle of Willis
ICA-B ("bifurcation")	ICA is open to supraclinoid segment, usually supplies the ophthalmic artery	Limited	Internal capsule, putamen	ICA bifurcation and M1 (see discussion)	Moderate to high; ? volume of thrombus; ? ischemia of lenticulostriates	Usually poor, possibly too much thrombus; totally dependent on volume of pial collateral supply, which may be seen on diagnostic angiogram
M1-O ("origin")	Flow is rapid through the ICA into the anterior cerebral	Minimal to moderate	Internal capsule, putamen	M1 trunk; may mechanically re-establish flow to M1 to give time for rescue (poke a hole in the clot)	Questionable; may be low depending on state of pial collaterals	May be revealed on diagnostic angiogram; totally dependent on status of lenticulostriates and amount of retrograde pial collateral supply to M1
M1-T ("trunk")	Angiographically indistinguishable from M1 origin	Very short	Internal capsule, putamen	M1 trunk; origin of lenticulostriate arteries; may mechanically re-establish flow to M1 to give time for rescue (poke a hole)	High; perhaps the worst case for fibrinolysis due to almost assured lenticulostriate death	Poor; limited time to re-establish perfusion to lenticulostriate arteries
M1-B ("bifurcation")	Lenticulostriate arteries are seen to fill from the ICA and M1 trunk	Long; potentially up to 12 hours	Motor and sensory cortex	Upper division of MCA	Low	Fair to good; may be revealed on diagnostic angiogram; totally dependent on amount of retrograde pial collateral supply to MCA branches
M2	M1 fills as well as the M1 bifurcation region	Long; potentially up to 12 hours	Territory of occlusion	Thrombus	Low	Good

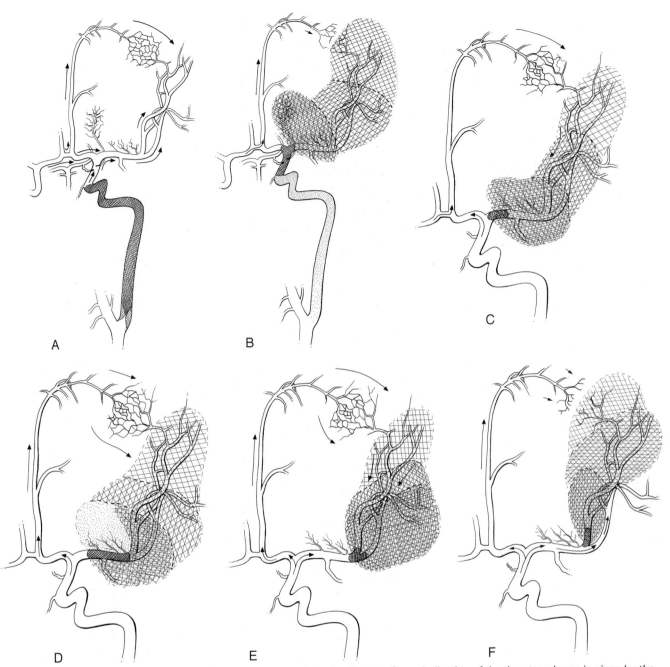

Figure 59-75 Locations of anterior circulation occlusions and their significance. Some indication of the threatened area is given by the shading—the darker the shading, the more threatened is the area. The degree of threat is almost always determined by the extent of the pial cortical collateral vessels, represented by the small anastomotic channels between the MCA branches and the anterior cerebral artery branches. Arrows indicate the path of collateral supply. See the detailed discussion in the text for additional information.

A, Type ICA-O (origin) occlusion. Note the absence of any shading indicating threatened areas. This is potentially a totally asymptomatic situation, compensated by the anterior and posterior communicating arteries.

B, Type ICA-B (bifurcation). In the illustrated example, nearly the entire MCA territory is immediately in jeopardy. This is one of the more dangerous and difficult therapeutic situations. Even with very good pial collaterals, the sheer volume of ischemic tissue is so great that rescue has to be so fast it may be impossible.

C, Type M1-0 (origin). The lenticulostriate arteries are the most threatened area, possibly irredeemably so. In the illustrated case, however, the fact that these vessels are not directly occluded makes a huge difference.

D, Type M1-T (trunk). Note the stippling over the lenticulostriate arteries. These vessels are basically forfeit, with severe clinical implications.

E, Type M1-B (bifurcation). The pial collaterals in this situation can potentially support the ischemic territory in jeopardy more readily than in most other situations. The anterior and posterior cerebral arteries, as well as the lenticulostriate arteries, are supplied normally.

F, Type M2; the best situation to have. These patients may be able to survive the insult long enough for intrinsic fibrinolysis to recanalize the occluded vessel, and these same patients are likely to be those who suffer severe transient ischemic attacks (TIAs) but eventually recover without therapy.

hemodynamics, with either recurrent or crescendo TIAs or a chronic neurologic deficit (with or without a true infarct at the time of presentation). Alternatively, they may present incidentally (asymptomatically) with adequate collateral supply to the occluded hemisphere. If the occlusion is well compensated by the posterior communicating artery or the anterior communicating artery, it may be completely silent, and no therapy is necessary.

The mechanism of occlusion usually is progression of stenosis at the common carotid bifurcation. The external carotid artery also may display evidence of atherosclerotic disease. Alternatively, the stenosis could be at the siphon of the ICA, with retrograde thrombosis back to the bifurcation of the common carotid artery at the origin of the ICA. The appearance of the ICA at its origin suggests the cause but is not definitive.

The posterior communicating artery and the anterior communicating artery are both high-flow, low-resistance vessels. Either or both can supply the MCA territory alone. In this type of occlusion, the path for supply from the anterior communicating artery to the MCA territory is directly antegrade through the main trunk of M1, unlike in the case of occlusion of M1, whereby the supply from the anterior communicating artery has to traverse the pial collaterals from the anterior cerebral branches to the MCA branches.

The manner of presentation suggests the degree of emergency, threatened areas, and time for therapy. If the patient presents with symptoms referable to hemodynamic factors (e.g., state of hydration, orthostasis), the time for therapy may be prolonged. True occlusion of deep perforators may not be present; indeed, no real infarct even will be forthcoming if the blood pressure is kept up.

Therapeutic Choices. If there is no intracranial embolus, therapy for a carotid occlusion usually is not necessary. If therapy is necessary, the time for rescue can be prolonged. The deep perforators (lateral lenticulostriate arteries) are not immediately threatened; *it is the distal watershed areas of the MCA territory that are threatened* (e.g., Wernicke's area, motor and sensory strip), owing to lack of pressure head.

If emergency rescue is necessary, however, this usually implies inadequate hemodynamic reserve, and a large area of cerebral tissue can be threatened. Also, the symptoms may be secondary to emboli to the MCA from the carotid artery stump. This has very different implications.

The bulk of thrombus in the ICA can be prohibitive. Mechanical thrombectomy maneuvers may aid in this task but are difficult to control.

This is often the situation seen when the carotid bulb finally occludes as a result of atheromatous process. There may be some question about occlusion of the ICA on carotid Doppler. An angiogram can be performed to evaluate for a "string sign." If a string sign is present, surgical endarterectomy should be performed.

If the occlusion is distal (the siphon), slow fibrinolysis can be performed with relative impunity until the distal lesion is opened. (If a *proximal* stenosis is opened too rapidly, however, a large mass of thrombus can be displaced downstream into the MCA trunk, with disastrous consequences.) Once the carotid lumen is clear, angioplasty of the distal stenosis can be performed.

If the stenosis is at the bifurcation of the common carotid artery (the origin of the ICA) and there is thrombus downstream, the acute symptoms may be due to an embolus to the MCA territory. The thrombus in the ICA greatly impairs an effective approach to the intracranial thrombus. There is no good way to get there; trying to advance a standard catheter through the ICA thrombus invites disaster (more thrombus can embolize). It may be possible (and necessary) to advance a microcatheter through the thrombus in the cervical ICA to treat the intracranial thrombus, effectively ignoring the ICA thrombus.

If time is not critical, patient clearing of the ICA followed by an angioplasty can be totally curative. Placement of a flow control guide catheter (e.g., the Zeppelin) in the common carotid artery during therapy to prevent sudden migration of the entire mass downstream into the MCA may be helpful. After all, the ICA has been occluded all this time.

If the occlusion is at the level of the siphon, the stenosis protects the intracranial vasculature from emboli. The main trunk of the ICA can be cleared and the siphon then dilated.

Type ICA-B (ICA-Bifurcation)

The ICA-B class represents occlusion (generally embolic) of the distal ICA at its bifurcation into the anterior and middle cerebral arteries, with or without occlusion of the anterior choroidal artery or posterior communicating artery. This has been referred to by other authors as the "T" lesion because of its shape (extending from the ICA into the MCA and anterior cerebral artery).

Implications. Even without the involvement of the anterior choroidal artery, this is a severe problem. This type of occlusion has been shown to be one of the worst, if not *the* worst, in previous studies.[19] There is severe hemispheric ischemia with resultant severe and massive cerebral edema after reperfusion.

If the thrombus is at the ICA bifurcation alone and not filling the main trunk of the MCA (M1), then the lenticulostriate arteries are not directly occluded and therefore not *immediately* threatened (but only if there is excellent retrograde perfusion of the MCA territory).

With a true ICA bifurcation thrombus or embolus, the occlusion of the ICA supply to the *anterior cerebral artery* has major implications concerning the ischemic insult involving the MCA territory. The anterior cerebral artery is the primary source of collateral circulation to the MCA territory through the pial collaterals (along with the posterior cerebral artery). Occlusion of the normal supply to the anterior cerebral artery therefore decreases the pressure head to this vessel, and thus to the pial collaterals *and the entire anterior* (supratentorial) *circulation*. The ipsilateral anterior cerebral artery territory can be supplied by the anterior communicating artery, however. As opposed to proximal occlusion of the ICA, there is now no good direct path to supply any of the MCA territory (through either the posterior or anterior communicating arteries).

In particular, with ICA bifurcation occlusion, the lateral lenticulostriate arteries (arising from the nonoccluded M1 trunk) are at the farthest extent of any collateral circulation to the ischemic territory. Wernicke's area and the motor and sensory cortex are no longer the watershed zones. Indeed, even though their normal supply is gone, their territory is the *closest to receiving any auxiliary collateral supply* (through the pial collaterals from the posterior and anterior cerebral arteries).

For this reason, how good the pial collaterals are between the anterior and middle cerebral arteries is critical in this setting. Rarely is there enough of a pressure head (or flow) through the anterior communicating artery to perfuse the entire territory of the anterior cerebral artery *and* the MCA. Even if there is, there rarely is enough to supply the bulk of the MCA territory cortex and the lenticulostriate arteries arising from the main trunk of the MCA. (This has been observed, however, in a case presented previously, which was recanalized with direct angioplasty of the MCA. It was not an embolic occlusion, however. See Figs. 58–15 to 58–54.)

Typically, with robust pial collaterals, the watershed zone shifts down slightly to a more lateral and inferior position in the parietal lobe, but the lenticulostriate arteries probably are still lost (they are the farthest from any supply), with resulting drastic consequences. The rescue of these lenticulostriate vessels therefore is of primary importance.

In addition, the bulk of the MCA territory probably eventually is still lost, even with an excellent anterior communicating artery, and there is always the possibility with this insult that the anterior choroidal artery also is occluded (the embolic mass may have covered its origin). Reestablishment of antegrade flow in the MCA must occur rapidly if it is to be of any benefit.

The posterior cerebral artery can supply a significant amount of flow to the posterior portion of the MCA territory through pial collaterals similar to those from the anterior cerebral artery. Even though the ipsilateral anterior cerebral artery is supplied only by the anterior communicating artery, the posterior cerebral artery has its normal supply from the vertebral arteries and therefore its normal pressure head. This has direct implication for a major important cerebrovascular zone—Wernicke's area. Wernicke's area is in the watershed between the MCA and the posterior cerebral artery and also is at the most posterior extent of the upper or lower division of the MCA, depending on where the angular branch of the MCA originates and how dominant it is. (This posterior distal territory commonly is a victim of embolic branch occlusion.) If the posterior cerebral artery can supply this posterior MCA territory, some major disability is spared. Sparing of this territory may or may not make much of a difference, however, if the rest of the hemisphere is infarcted, including the radiating fibers through the internal capsule.

It is unusual, however, for the posterior cerebral artery to be able to supply the motor and sensory areas of the MCA. The direct collateral communication between the posterior cerebral territory and Wernicke's area is not present between the more anterior branches of the MCA (motor strip) and the posterior cerebral artery. For the posterior cerebral artery to be able to supply this territory, flow has to enter the posterior angular branch of the MCA, travel retrograde back to the region of the MCA bifurcation or trifurcation, and then travel antegrade to the motor and sensory territories. This is difficult.

Supply can, however, traverse the anastomotic branch from the splenial branch to the posterior portion of the pericallosal artery, thus aiding in rescue of the caudal portion of the anterior cerebral artery territory.

Occlusion at the ICA bifurcation therefore results in therapeutic and prognostic implications that are extremely poor. It is not possible to know the exact volume of thrombus present, but that volume may be too large for effective therapy. Clot may extend all the way down M1 into the branches of M2. Even if only a slight amount of thrombus is present in M1, it can occlude the valuable, most medial set of lateral lenticulostriate arteries, which supply an extremely vital part of the internal capsule.

This type of occlusion, although successfully treated in the past in a few patients, more often than not has yielded a poor outcome after therapy, can result in a deep bleed from the lenticulostriate territory or cerebral edema from reperfusion, and should be approached with great trepidation.

Therapeutic Considerations. If a small amount of clot is impacted at the ICA bifurcation, it may be possible to dislodge this mechanically to the MCA bifurcation and thus reperfuse the anterior cerebral artery and lenticulostriate artery territories immediately. Alternatively, a microcatheter with side holes can be placed past the occlusion, flushed, infused, and allowed to carry a small trickle of blood past the occlusion by acting as a stenting catheter. This can allow a slight reprieve while therapy is aimed at the primary problem. Speed is of the essence to save the lenticulostriate arteries.

If a large bulk of thrombus is present, dissolution may take longer than is practical under the circumstances of having both the anterior and middle cerebral arteries occluded, with resultant deep ischemia. Aggressive mechanical actions may be indicated in this case, including thrombectomy. This is discussed in Chapter 58, and the snares and clot retrieval device are described in Chapter 1.

Type M1-O (M1-Origin)

In type M1-O, thrombus occludes the orifice of the MCA but spares the origin of the anterior cerebral artery. In this particular instance, the lenticulostriate arteries are *not* occluded. The cause can be stenosis secondary to atherosclerotic (or other) occlusive disease of the M1 origin, or the occlusion may be embolic in origin.

Implications. It may be practically impossible to differentiate this type of occlusion from the next type—that of total thrombotic filling of the MCA trunk. Careful analysis of the angiogram or CT may provide useful information (see Figs. 58–15 to 58–54). The best information may be obtained by trying carefully to traverse the occlusion with a guidewire and catheter and slowly injecting contrast as the catheter is withdrawn. If thrombus extends all the way out into branches, then the lenticulostriates have had a most severe insult and may be unrescuable, depending on the time frame. If the M1 trunk (and thus the lenticulostriate arteries) is open, the occlusion is this in type, and there may be more time for rescue.

The prognosis depends completely on the condition of the pial collaterals between the anterior and posterior cerebral arteries and the MCA. With only the origin of the MCA occluded, both the posterior and anterior cerebral arteries can work together to supply the MCA territory. All major sources of intracranial vascular supply (the vertebral and carotid arteries) are still present, even if the route is changed (i.e., the anterior cerebral artery has its normal pressure head from the ICA, and the posterior circulation is supplied normally). It is conceivable for these pial collaterals to supply the entire MCA territory for a time (see Figs. 58–15 to 58–54).

The most endangered vessels (and their territories) are the lateral lenticulostriate arteries, especially the most medial of these (which are perhaps the most important of this group because they supply the internal capsule, corona radiata, putamen, and a variable portion of the globus pallidus). These lenticulostriate arteries are now at the extreme limit of the vascular distribution of the hemisphere and do not usually survive for long. The small amount of circulation that M1 receives, however, may allow these lenticulostriate arteries to survive for a longer period than if they were directly occluded by thrombus.

As noted previously, we have performed a rescue on a patient with a complete occlusion of the MCA origin for over 48 hours, who recovered completely. This was entirely due to the fact that his pial collaterals were excellent, and the diagnostic procedures were analyzed carefully enough to indicate the possibility of this rescue.

If the pial collaterals are poor, the prognosis is considerably worsened. If excellent flow is present, the consequences of this scenario may be minimal. *If collaterals are absent, the outcome will be the same as if the entire MCA trunk (M1) was filled with thrombus (i.e., the typical total MCA infarct with profound neurologic deficit).*

Type M1-T (M1-Trunk)

Thrombus commonly occludes the entire M1 segment of the MCA and most of the lenticulostriate arteries.

A variable number (or all) of the lenticulostriate arteries may be occluded, with variable results. Typically, an embolus impacts at the bifurcation of the MCA and occludes the two main divisions, some or all lenticulostriate vessels, and a temporal or frontal branch.

Implications. There are essentially two different aspects of this implication to analyze: *time* until cerebral tissue death (and thus the window for rescue) and *danger* of fibrinolysis. Any direct occlusion of lenticulostriate vessels has two direct consequences. First, the time allowed for rescue is shortened tremendously. No adequate tests have been done, but we believe that direct complete occlusion of these deep perforators will result in irreparable harm in a short period of time (15 minutes to 4 hours at the two extremes; more likely 30 minutes to 3 hours). This is not long enough to provide a real chance of direct rescue.

The magnitude of pial collaterals has essentially no effect on directly occluded lenticulostriate arteries; therefore, the clock is ticking from the moment of the original insult, and rescue of this territory is ineffective after a relatively brief time.

The risk of hemorrhage from reperfusion of the lenticulostriates is another matter, however. It may be futile to reopen these vessels after a certain period of time, but still not too dangerous until an additional period of time has passed. This information is not known, but Theron[14] believes that about 6 hours is the magic time beyond which this danger increases, in basic agreement with the ongoing trials in the United States. We believe that differentiation of cases based on occlusion of the lenticulostriates (or lack thereof), as Theron does, is correct. The rounded-off number of 8 hours for completion of therapy is just that—an estimated number for all circumstances—and occasionally invites disaster.

In Theron's recent article,[14] the time limit for therapy for occlusion that affected these vessels either directly or indirectly was 6 hours. No accurate analysis was made, however, about the exact location of occlusion and degree of potential ischemia. Even in those patients in whom fibrinolysis was performed before 6 hours, there was no clear indication of what percentage actually recovered from the ischemic insult to the lenticulostriate territory.

Several of the classes of occlusion discussed previously involved the lenticulostriate arteries indirectly and thus also should have as rapid a rescue as possible. This scenario (M1 trunk occlusion), however, is the most critical, has the highest risk, and allows the shortest time for therapy.

The amount of thrombus in this instance is not known, just as in type M1-O; it could be more than is feasible to attempt to clear. The status of the pial collaterals is not nearly as important as in other situations, in which the lenticulostriate arteries are preserved. If the lenticulostriate arteries are eliminated totally, the functional neurologic effect is similar to a global MCA infarct. Whether the pial collaterals are good or bad may make little difference.

If only the distal, most lateral, branch of the lateral lenticulostriate arteries is occluded, it may be only the extreme capsule that is lost, with resultant minimal symptoms if rescue is successful. The hemisphere may be salvageable, depending on the pial collaterals. Therefore, active intervention is indicated. The danger of active fibrinolysis remains unchanged, however, independent of the neurologic importance of these particular vessels. They can still hemorrhage later.

Type M1-B (M1-Bifurcation)

In type M1-B, there is occlusion of the MCA at its bifurcation. No lenticulostriate arteries are occluded (unless the last branch or two arise from a proximal M2 branch; see Fig. 58–6). This situation is one of the more common types of embolic occlusion, and can be one of the more gratifying to treat.

Implications. If one were going to have an embolic occlusion with a rescue, this is what one would want. The lenticulostriate arteries are being fed directly by their normal source (the ICA and M1). Although the distal MCA branches may be occluded, this is not the entire hemisphere. The most threatened area is the proximal M2 area, the insular region (Broca's region). The typical distal watershed areas are now the closest of any of the MCA territory to any collateral supply (the pial vessels of the anterior and posterior cerebral arteries).

Again, if the pial collaterals are nonexistent, the territory of the particular MCA branches does not last long (perhaps 2 hours or so). If the pial collaterals are good, however, the amount of tissue they have to supply is as minimal as possible. Each pial collateral only has to supply a small area of the MCA territory; they do not have to supply any of the lenticulostriate arteries, only the MCA branch territory. It may be possible for this area to survive for a considerable period even with poor direct perfusion.

Therefore, in a type M1-B occlusion, the condition of the pial collaterals is of primary concern. If they are good, it is possible that the entire hemisphere is viable and rescuable for a prolonged period, perhaps many hours. The worst that can happen during therapy is that the thrombus breaks up, migrates distally, or does not dissolve at all. If there is no progress made on dissolution, there could be an MCA infarct, but this is the probable outcome without therapy, and less than a total M1 occlusion infarct.

Whether or not there is any return of function after this prolonged period of occlusion depends entirely on the status of the preexisting pial collaterals, but at least the danger is lessened. We agree with Theron[14] that rescue in this territory can be performed safely up to 12 hours after occlusion (but perhaps not effectively).

Type M2

In type M2, occlusion of an MCA branch is present, and no deep perforators are occluded.
Implications. The difference between this and type

M1-B is minimal. There is no involvement of the lenticulostriate arteries, and the prognosis depends entirely on the state of the pial collaterals, the extent of vascular deficiency, and which specific territory is involved. Although the various sites of occlusion (which branch) may be distinct in their functional implications, the hemodynamic implications are similar.

The difference between this type of occlusion and that of the entire bifurcation of the MCA is in quantity, not quality. In other words, the other pial collaterals may have an easier time supplying just one branch occlusion that has a smaller total territory to perfuse. The collaterals and adjacent branches may be able to help each other to supply the absent vessel's territory.

As stated previously in the discussion of type M1-B occlusion, we agree with Theron[14] in that rescue in this territory can be performed safely up to 12 hours after occlusion.

DURAL SINUS THROMBOSIS

Clinical Manifestations

The clinical presentation of intracranial venous thrombosis may be either sudden or insidious. Most patients present with headaches of variable severity or of a crescendo nature. Nausea and vomiting or a change in mental status may be present, along with papilledema. Focal deficits are less common but, when present, are more ominous. Not infrequently, the initial presentation is as described above, but by the time the radiographic work-up is truly underway, the symptoms may be focal, representing a developing venous infarct (Figs. 59–76 to 59–93).

A confounding point is that meningitis is a common cause of sinus thrombosis and can have its own set of nonspecific signs and symptoms. Other common causes are dehydration, pregnancy, meningioma, any hypercoagulable cause, and birth control pills.

Diagnosis

Early intracranial venous thrombosis may be difficult or impossible to detect on standard CT examination. The pathology may be present only in cortical veins, which are poorly appreciated (if at all) on routine CT scan. As the disease progresses, the sinuses may become abnormal in appearance before the brain parenchyma does. A thrombosed sinus may appear as a high-density spot or line on a noncontrast CT scan (see Fig. 59–76); after contrast administration, the clot within the sinus may appear as a low-density center outlined by contrast. This yields the so-called delta sign in the thrombosed superior sagittal sinus. With further progression of venous hypertension and focal backpressure, a noncontrast CT scan may show a poorly marginated peripheral area of low attenuation in the parenchyma. This vasogenic edema tends to spread along the white matter tracts, giving an irregular pattern not generally

Text continued on page 737

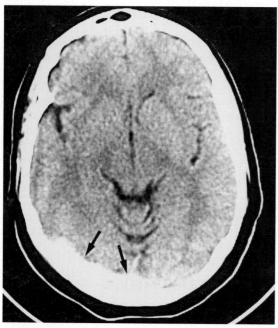

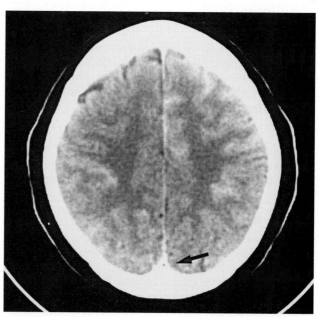

Figure 59-76 Case 8. This patient presented to the ER with increasing headache and vague sensorimotor changes. CT demonstrates a hyperdense right transverse sinus and superior sagittal sinus *(arrows).*

Figure 59-77 Later the same day, she developed increasing arm weakness. A repeat CT scan demonstrates a bilateral high-density gyral pattern, probably representing subarachnoid oozing. Hyperdensity of the superior sagittal sinus is again seen *(arrow)*; the windowing setting makes this particular image difficult to read—the sinus looks like bone.

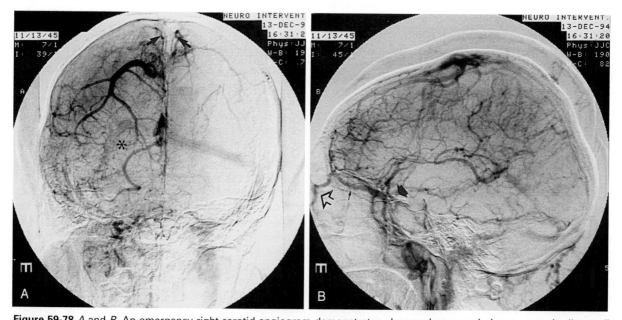

Figure 59-78 *A* and *B,* An emergency right carotid angiogram demonstrates abnormal venous drainage; note the "empty" superior sagittal sinus *(arrows, PA view)*, absent right transversesinus *(asterisk)*, and increased drainage through the cavernous sinus *(fat arrow, lateral view)* and the superior ophthalmic vein (seen best on the lateral view) *(small arrow)*, and then out through the facial vein *(open arrow)*. Note the prominence of the deep medullary perforating veins.

Case 8 continues

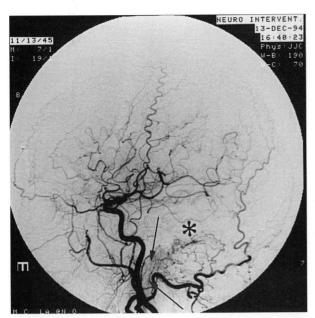

Figure 59-79 Very interesting "whole head" lateral view right carotid angiogram (obtained at the same time as the images in Fig. 59–78). Superficially this is unremarkable, but note the abnormal vascular supply to the region of the right transverse and sigmoid sinuses *(asterisk)*, as well as the slight blush of the jugular vein *(arrows)*. This probably represents a dural arteriovenous fistula in evolution. Whether this evolves into a true fistulous state may depend on the rapidity of clearance of the involved sinus. Note also that the external carotid branches are filling more rapidly than the intracranial vessels.

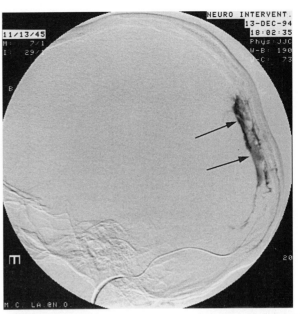

Figure 59-81 Lateral angiogram through the microcatheter with its tip in the posterior portion of the superior sagittal sinus (after reaming with the buckled wire and catheter). Note the large amount of residual thrombus *(arrows)*.

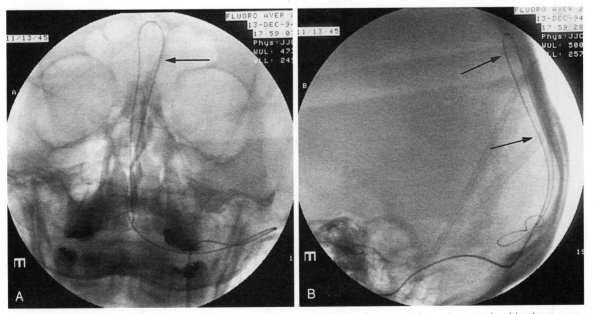

Figure 59-80 *A* and *B,* PA and lateral unsubtracted views demonstrating the use of the catheter and guidewire to try to break up and move the indwelling thrombus. The catheter-guidewire combination had been buckled into the superior sagittal sinus *(arrows)*.

Case 8 continues

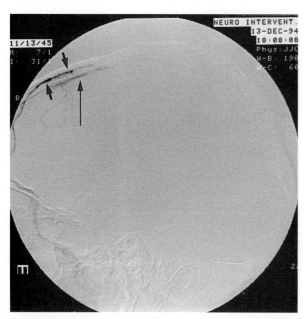

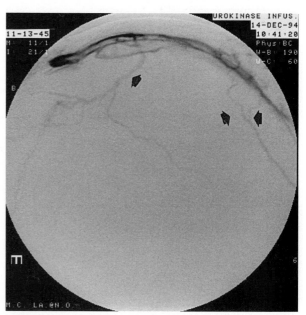

Figure 59-82 Injection through the microcatheter with its tip *(long arrow)* in a far distal (anterior) position in the superior sagittal sinus. Note the transosseous venous flow (small "hairs" between intracranial and extracranial veins), with venous drainage almost exclusively extracranial from this location *(short arrows)*.

Figure 59-84 Direct injection through the microcatheter reveals antegrade flow down the superior sagittal sinus, but owing to potential major inflow from unopacified cortical veins, this is difficult to interpret. The angiogram appears to show considerable restriction of the lumen as well as an abnormal drainage pattern (small veins) *(arrows)*. Compare this with the previous arterial injection (Fig. 59–83).

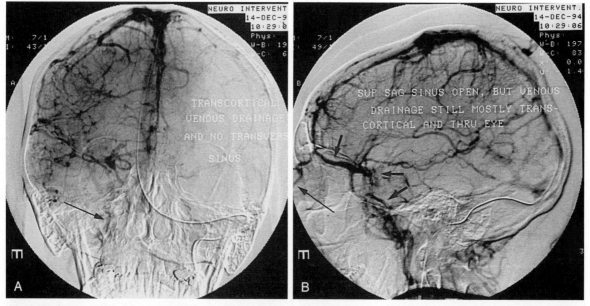

Figure 59-83 *A* and *B,* After overnight infusion with the microcatheter in the superior sagittal sinus, there is some normal venous drainage through this sinus (opacification of the previously "empty" sinus), but the intracranial hemodynamics are still abnormal. Note the prominence of the deep medullary veins as well as the predominant anterior drainage pattern *(short arrows, lateral view)* through the cavernous sinus, inferior petrosal sinus, superior ophthalmic vein, and facial vein *(long arrows)*. The superior sagittal sinus is not acting as if it is open. The right transverse sinus is still not seen.

Case 8 continues

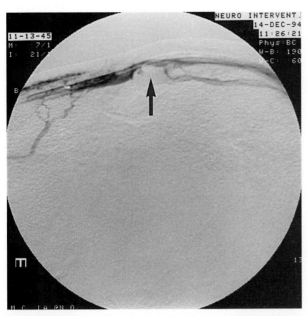

Figure 59-85 A magnified view of injection through the microcatheter with its tip in a more distal (anterior) location in the superior sagittal sinus appears to show significant flow restriction *(arrow)* in the sinus as well as major transosseous drainage (small "hairs" leading to extracranial veins; not a normal finding).

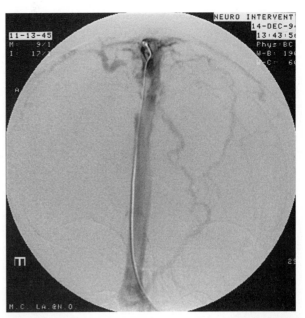

Figure 59-87 A 4-mm STEALTH balloon angioplasty catheter (the largest available) has been placed over a guidewire into the superior sagittal sinus and the entire sinus "reamed" a few times. The post-"reaming" venogram shows much improved flow in the superior sagittal sinus.

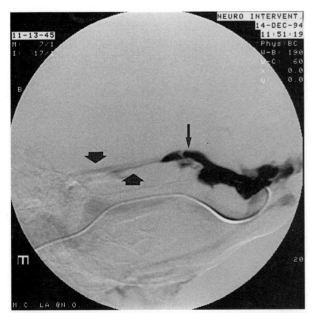

Figure 59-86 Evaluation of the right transverse sinus via a left sigmoid and transverse sinus approach, with the tip of the catheter in the right transverse sinus *(thin narrow)*, reveals additional abundant thrombus with essentially no antegrade flow *(fat arrows)*. It was determined that more aggressive mechanical thrombodisruption was indicated. This maneuver is necessary because the hemodynamics render infusion of urokinase difficult in such a broad area of clot, and the flow is directing the urokinase away from the area to be treated (right transverse and sigmoid sinuses).

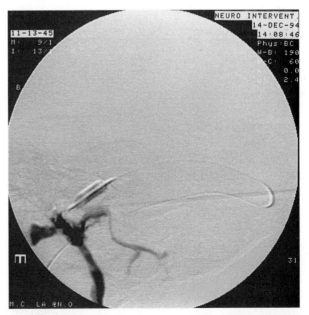

Figure 59-88 The STEALTH angioplasty balloon is in the anterior transverse or sigmoid sinus. Note that the injection through the STEALTH catheter inflates the balloon as it flows out of this mono-lumen catheter. Note also the lack of filling of a normal jugular bulb-sigmoid sinus confluens.

Case 8 continues

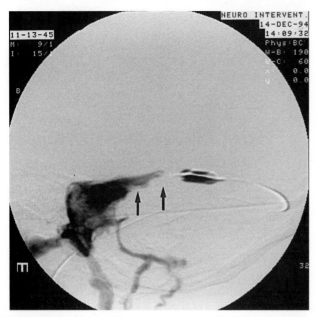

Figure 59-89 After partial clearing of the confluens by maceration with the balloon and wire, there is better antegrade flow, but the transverse sinus is still largely occluded by residual thrombus *(arrows)*. Again note the balloon inflated by the injection (to the right of the arrows).

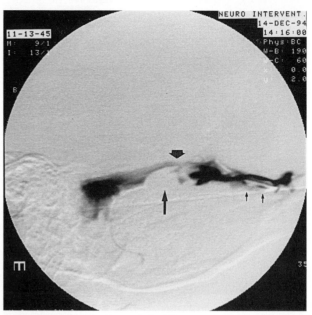

Figure 59-91 After further withdrawal of the catheter, the ability of the soft elastic thrombus to rebound is seen *(thin arrow)*. Note the worse than previously seen compromise of the residual lumen *(fat arrow)* and the well-demonstrated lump of thrombus. There is probably more thrombus coating the wall of the posterior transverse sinus *(small arrows)*.

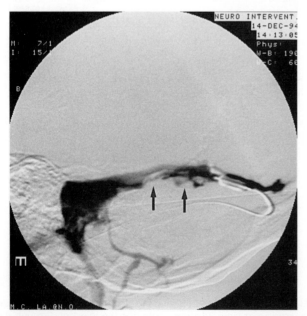

Figure 59-90 Further maceration clears more of the midtransverse sinus, but huge lumps of thrombus remain *(arrows)*. Note that most of the flow is now physiologic.

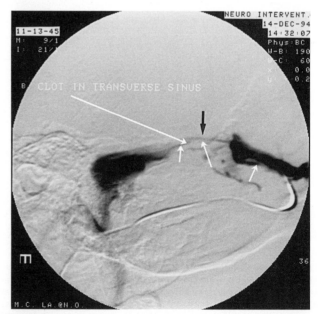

Figure 59-92 Fifteen minutes later, the residual lumen is even smaller. Note the true lumen of the transverse sinus with clot laying on the inferior wall *(white arrows* and *black arrow)*.

Case 8 continues

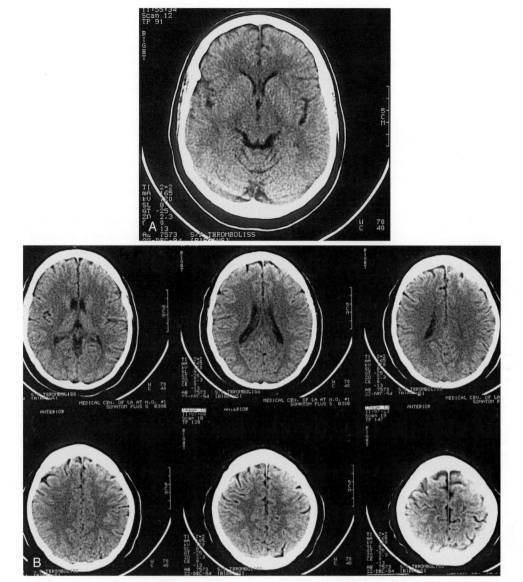

Figure 59-93 *A* and *B,* The catheter was left in the transverse sinus for overnight infusion. However, the patient developed bleeding at the puncture site, resulting in a large retroperitoneal hematoma. The infusion was therefore stopped and the catheter withdrawn. A follow-up CT scan obtained 1 week later was normal.

matching an arterial vascular distribution. Mass effect may be present.

Early hemorrhage is more common with venous infarcts than with arterial infarcts but is more of a "superficial ooze" variety in this setting and not as dangerous. This may correlate with focal clinical symptomatology. *It is often distinctive in that the hemorrhage, like the edema described previously, may not follow a clear arterial distribution* (see Fig. 59–77).

To compound the diagnostic problem, angiography can be slightly confusing. Some cortical veins may be present, but some may be absent. Because of their normally variable anatomy, it may not be readily apparent that some veins are missing; this is nonspecific in any event. There may be flow toward the

crown of the head, but if high-dose contrast and perfect centering are used, it can be seen on the posteroanterior view that the superior sagittal sinus is not truly filling; the dura is hypervascular, but there is an empty center where the opacified superior sagittal sinus should be (see Fig. 59–78).

Absence of one transverse sinus commonly is seen; but again, asymmetry is a normal variant. In addition, a transverse sinus normally can fill preferentially from one side or the other, or preferentially from the anterior circulation or the posterior circulation.

More important for diagnosis of this pathology is evaluation and recognition of the intracranial hemodynamics. If a true acute vein or sinus thrombosis is present, there is an overall unusual drainage pattern. The cavernous sinus and inferior petrosal sinus may be carrying more venous drainage than usual, and the superior ophthalmic vein may be recruited to help drain the intracranial structures (see Fig. 59–78). In addition, there often is more use of the paravertebral plexus than typically seen (to get around an occluded sigmoid sinus). On review of real-time digital subtraction images, the arteriovenous transit time is longer than usual if there is a significant back-up, such as that caused by thrombosis of the superior sagittal sinus. The visualized cortical veins also may appear denser than usual because the patent veins are carrying more blood, albeit to a point without an exit.

Strategy of Treatment

For many years, the only treatment for dural sinus thrombosis has been hydration and heparinization. Even heparinization can be tricky in the setting of an already oozing infarct. The increasing use of fibrinolytics, however, has opened the door for more aggressive therapy.

Treatment of intracranial venous thrombosis is similar to that of venous thrombosis in the calf. There is no practical way to get the fibrinolytic agent to the many small veins that need it.

There are basically two pathways to attack the problem: from the arterial side and from the venous side. The venous approach appears more reasonable because that is where the clot is, but only the large veins (i.e., the sinuses) can be accessed easily. Clearing these may not help the still occluded cortical veins, which are the actual site of blocked drainage from the brain. These blocked cortical veins usually are not seen on the angiogram because they are occluded (although slight filling may be seen, or the clot may be outlined by contrast).

For this reason, arguments have been presented to infuse the arterial side in the hope of bathing the venous drainage with the fibrinolytic agent. This technique, however would appear to invite a bleed because the arterial and capillary systems are already under increased pressure and there already may be evidence of oozing (although on the venous side). In addition, it is known by those who have performed calf vein thrombolysis by infusing the arterial side that the fibrinolytic agent tends to drain out the path of least resistance, that is, where there is no clot obstructing normal arteriovenous flow. For these two reasons, current active interventional strategy is aimed primarily at the venous side, although there is a movement underway to attack both sides simultaneously.

The volume of thrombus usually is far greater with intracranial venous thrombosis than with arterial thrombosis. In addition, the direction of flow is a handicap to treatment. The intracranial veins also are technically more difficult to work in, because of their size, variability, pattern of branching, and the possible presence of webs or synechiae.

Typically, a symptomatic dural sinus occlusion involves either a large segment of one transverse sinus or both a transverse sinus and the superior sagittal sinus. If a transverse sinus is occluded, the occlusion typically extends down to the next large venous inflow channel, at which point flow is re-established; this inflow usually is from occipital, petrosal, clival, paravertebral, or other veins. If the inflow from the vein of Labbé also is occluded by the indwelling thrombus, this may be of dire consequence.

Attempts to cannulate the occluded sigmoid or transverse sinus in a retrograde manner are difficult because of the unknown exact anatomy, preexisting tortuosity of the sigmoid sinus, and presence of the occluding thrombus. Any probing of the blind pouch should be done with either a J-tip hydrophilic guidewire (such as the new Connors J wire, Cook, Inc.) or a microguidewire with a large curve, *not an angle-tip hydrophilic guidewire*. This latter guidewire perforates or dissects the vessel too easily, although the dural sinuses are tough. It often is necessary to access the occluded sinus from the opposite internal jugular vein–sigmoid sinus–transverse sinus approach.

Need for Mechanical Disruption

Once in place, initial mechanical disruption of any kind probably helps because of the large volume of clot and its critical location. It has been shown with endovascular dialysis graft rescue that the amount of thrombus (3 to 5 ml at most) displaced to the lung in fragments is tolerated in the setting of ongoing fibrinolytic therapy. Specifically, this small amount of clot is less acutely life-threatening in the pulmonary circulation than in the brain. A larger volume can be dangerous, however, and in the presence of compensated high-output cardiac failure or preexisting pulmonary hypertension, any amount of thrombus could be deadly.

Maceration of the clot can be performed by repeatedly probing with the guidewire, passing a loop snare, or placing a balloon distally and pulling it back. The loop snare is the easiest method but is not nearly as effective as a balloon catheter. This balloon can be either an Endeavor (Target Therapeutics), requiring a guide catheter of some sort, which is difficult if not impossible in some cases; STEALTH (Target Therapeutics); Solstice (Medtronic/MIS); Stratus (Medtronic/MIS); or Grapevine (Medtronic/MIS). The STEALTH, Solstice, Stratus, and Grapevine can be advanced over a leading guidewire and thus usually can be placed where needed. The STEALTH and Stratus are stiff balloons and limited to 4-mm maximal diameter. In the dural sinuses, a 6- to 8-mm balloon would be ideal, preferably latex or silicone (the Solstice is silicone, but is only 3.5 mm when inflated).

Perhaps the best technique to place a 9-Fr. Brite-Tip guide catheter (Cordis Corp.) or Lumax Neuroguide (Cook, Inc.) into the jugular vein in question (using the technique described in "How to Introduce a Guide Catheter" in Chapter 3), and then to place a small (0.042″ lumen, 5.4-Fr.) Zeppelin (Medtronic/MIS) in the internal jugular vein and *through this* to select the superior sagittal sinus, opposite transverse sinus, ipsilateral sigmoid sinus, or other sinus with a microguidewire followed by a microcatheter. Once the microcatheter is in place, a Platinum Plus (Medi-Tech, Inc.) wire can be placed, allowing advancement of the Zeppelin to its intended distal location. This may be difficult because of the stiffness of the Zeppelin (this problem is being addressed by Medtronic/MIS); the sigmoid sinus is tortuous and resistant to passage of the catheter. At this point, the soft silicone balloon can be inflated (up to about 10 mm) and withdrawn (while inflated), thus removing a significant portion of the thrombus.

Fibrinolytic Infusion

After as much mechanical removal of thrombus as feasible has been performed, fibrinolytic infusion can be performed. A potential reason for all thrombus not being removed by the balloon withdrawal maneuver or some difficulty being encountered in the treatment is the possible presence of an underlying venous stenosis, typically in the sigmoid sinus.

If the attack is undertaken on the venous side, the most ideal point of infusion of the fibrinolytic agent must be determined. During the entire process of fibrinolytic infusion, repeated evaluation of hemodynamics must be made to see where the drug actually flows. This determines where the tip of the catheter should be placed. A position as far distal as possible (e.g., in the superior sagittal sinus) would appear to be the correct location for infusion; however, a very slow injection during a prolonged digital subtraction angiogram may reveal that the flow from this point is all transcranial (through the skull) or toward the anterior sagittal sinus, cavernous sinus, and ophthalmic vein, and not actually back through the thrombus. (A blast of contrast will *not* show where the fibrinolytic agent will actually go during the extremely slow infusion; it will go everywhere.) Moving the catheter tip repeatedly may be required to chase the dissolving thrombus or allow perfusion of the area of thrombus causing the most problems.

If a multisidehole catheter, such as a Softstream (Target Therapeutics), is used, then a pulse spray technique should be used, which is more effective under these circumstances (i.e., a large volume of thrombus in a large diameter vessel).

If the superior sagittal sinus is involved, this should be the area attacked first. Clearing of this may have a more global and important result than clearing an occluded transverse sinus first, unless both transverse sinuses are occluded. If the superior sagittal sinus can be opened, it can then drain by way of the already open transverse sinus, thus relieving pressure on both hemispheres. The residual occluded transverse sinus can be attacked later. Also, infusion into this sinus allows the agent to flow back along the clot for a greater distance.

Preparation and infusion of the fibrinolytic agent is discussed in Chapter 60. Because of the volume of thrombus, the infusion may be long. During any long fibrinolytic procedure, all standard monitoring and supportive measures should be undertaken.

The rate of infusion is not determined. Because of the desire to keep systemic fibrinolysis to a minimum, a low-dose infusion is recommended (60,000 to 120,000 U/hr). This can be achieved by mixing 1,000,000 units in 500 ml of normal saline and infusing at a rate of about 30 to 60 ml/hr. If combined infusion in both the arterial and venous sides is planned, the dose should be half in each side.

As stated previously, the large volume of thrombus, combined with the inefficient delivery technique, renders this a long procedure. Reported times for recanalization are 3 to 10 days, with an average of about 100 hours. Maceration and displacement of as much clot as possible at the beginning of this procedure by mechanical means greatly speeds the process.

Heparinization

The issue of the use of heparin during treatment of a dural sinus thrombosis has not been resolved. Heparinization is usually the treatment of choice, however, even without active fibrinolytic therapy. In addition, fibrinolysis without heparin repeatedly has been shown to be a losing battle; thrombus stimulates more thrombus. Even in the typical situation of dural sinus thrombosis with superficial oozing of blood associated with venous infarction, heparinization is recommended for the entire duration of the procedure (the activated partial thromboplastin time should be kept at 1.5 to 2 times control).

Procedural Evaluation

Because accurate evaluation is best performed from the arterial side, it will be necessary to maintain both arterial and venous catheters. An injection on the venous side may reveal an apparent filling defect that in fact may be the wash-in from a high-flow, unopacified (and unobstructed) venous structure. Therefore, follow-up evaluation of the efficacy of the procedure is best performed by arterial injections with careful attention to arteriovenous hemodynamics.

Evaluation of efficacy of treatment and working from the venous side are the limitations of this procedure. Attempting to recanalize a draining network in a retrograde fashion is strategically unsuitable because of flow dynamics. Trying to find the individual occluded cortical veins to work on is technically difficult, if not impossible, because of the size of the vessels and the inherent difficulty of trying to catheterize a vessel that may not be visible and that is filled with thrombus. In addition, the angle of entry for these veins into the sagittal or transverse sinus commonly is not ideal for catheterization (i.e., a very acute angle).

Computed tomography scans can be of value for following the progress of the disease, particularly if there has been a neurologic change. The greatest fear associated with a procedure such as this is that of an intracranial bleed.

Now for the good news. Often, because of the ongoing systemic heparinization and effects of the fibrinolytic agent, at least some of these cortical veins become fully patent on their own, or at least better than they were (if the interventionalist is lucky).

If the situation does not improve, and the patient still has symptoms, there are three choices: (1) continue on systemic heparin and hope for the best, (2) attempt to find the occluded cortical veins and work on them individually, or (3) infuse the fibrinolytic agent from the arterial side as well as the venous side. The correct strategy for treatment of these occluded cortical veins is not known, but we believe that given the opportunity (i.e., patent major sinuses, some systemic fibrinolytic activity, adequate hydration, and systemic heparinization), these cortical veins probably will reopen. Simultaneous local intra-arterial fibrinolytic infusion may increase the likelihood of complete recanalization. Once the main sinus is open, simply continuing heparinization is the best choice.

Underlying Venous Stenosis

Occasionally, an underlying cause can be found for the original condition, such as a stenosis at some point in the intracranial venous drainage system (the dural sinuses). This stenosis has already revealed itself to be capable of creating a major problem (the thrombus); however, direct treatment at this time may be unnecessary. Long-term anticoagulation may suffice, as might removal of the cause of the hypercoagulable state (if present). Any possible predisposing factor should be treated (e.g., dehydration, polycythemia). If treatment of an underlying stenosis is necessary, angioplasty of the sinus should be possible, with the recognition that any minimal improvement should be adequate for a time.

Veins notoriously are thrombogenic when dilated; therefore, caution and delicacy should be used if intervention is contemplated, and the angioplasty site should be observed for 30 to 60 minutes, until the site stabilizes. If an angioplasty is performed, a dural sinus is a truly high-flow location, unlike most other typical peripheral veins, which have slow flow and a propensity to thrombose. These sinuses can be extremely tough and can behave in a manner similar to a stricture at the venous anastomosis of a dialysis graft; that is, they can require considerable pressure to achieve any dilation.

Open surgical correction of a stenotic area in a sinus (a patch graft) also is possible and has been performed successfully. Implantation of a stent also has been performed, but the long-term results of a stent implanted in this location are not known.

When to Stop Treatment of Dural Sinus Thrombosis

Knowing when to stop is difficult with any acute stroke therapy, but this is particularly true when the procedure is intrinsically long and evaluation of the results difficult.

The best way to examine results is by injecting contrast in the artery and observing the anatomy of the venous drainage and the hemodynamics of the situation. In this way, speed of flow can be compared not only between each hemisphere but also within each hemisphere. Abnormal patterns of drainage can be observed (see Case 8, Figs. 59–76 to 59–93).

Intrasinus pressure also can be measured. A pressure of less than 17 mm Hg is compatible with no further parenchymal injury or clinically significant symptoms.[20]

TREATMENT OF A STROKE DURING OR SUBSEQUENT TO AN ANGIOGRAPHIC PROCEDURE

A stroke that occurs during or after angiography usually is caused by thrombus, probably from the catheter or catheterized vessel; intracerebral hemorrhage also may be the cause if a major branch occlusion is not seen. The possibility of a seizure also should be considered. Immediate anticoagulation and aggressive fibrinolysis may appear to be the obvious treatment, but this depends on the clinical circumstances (Case 9, Figs. 59–94 to 59–98). Was the patient on the table for evaluation of a recent aneurysmal bleed? Was the study being performed for evaluation of recent TIAs? If so, there could be a recent silent infarct that would *contraindicate fibrinolysis* and lead to a massive problem (intraparenchymal bleed) if fibrinolysis were undertaken.

The possibility of a recent silent infarct cannot be ignored! If the procedure was done for TIA evaluation, an immediate CT scan should be performed and closely scrutinized (unless done before the procedure). In other words, move the patient off the angiography table and get a CT! The information gained makes the short delay worthwhile.

If the procedure was unrelated to TIA evaluation or an aneurysm hunt, the immediate worries may be lessened. Immediate steps for therapy can then be instituted.

General Goals for Therapy of a Stroke on the Table

1. Physical and neurologic evaluation
2. Acquisition of appropriate auxiliary medical aid (e.g., anesthesiology, internal medicine, neurology, neurosurgery, attending physicians)
3. Oxygenation of cerebral tissue
4. Cerebral perfusion
   a. Direct (open a vessel)
   b. Indirect (increase systemic blood pressure)
5. Neuroprotection (see "Neuroprotectant Agents" in Chapter 54). This may include steroids at the very least. See specific recommendations below.

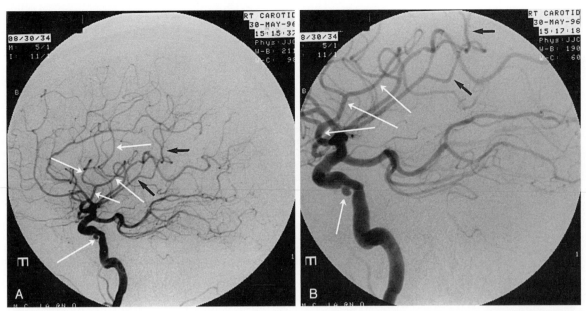

Figure 59-94 Case 9. *A* and *B,* This 61-year-old woman presented with repeated TIAs and diffuse atherosclerotic disease. The initial right common carotid injection, lateral view, reveals an unremarkable intracranial distribution other than the huge ulcerated plaque in the cavernous portion of the internal carotid artery *(lowest white arrow).* Note the MCA vessels *(white arrows* and *black arrows).* During attempted catheterization of the left common carotid artery, these will become occluded.

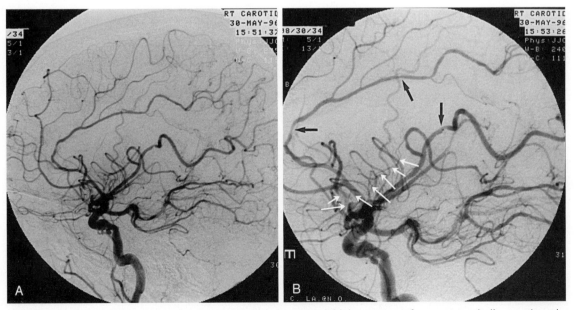

Figure 59-95 *A* and *B,* The patient became agitated (a common initial symptom of an acute embolic event), and a repeat angiogram demonstrates occlusion of the upper division of the MCA *(white arrows).* Note also that the branch indicated by black arrows in Figure 59–94 is not seen. Extensive intracranial atherosclerotic disease is identified in other locations *(black arrows).* We were consulted, heparin was immediately administered, and a microcatheter was placed into this upper division.

Treatment at this time is not as straightforward as would be presumed. The immediate nature of the institution of therapy gives an increased degree of safety if there has not been a recent significant ischemic event. This is crucial. Even though a patient may be neurologically intact, the history of TIAs raises the possibility that there may have been a silent infarct in the danger period (within the last 4 to 6 weeks). If this is the case, there is the possibility that intracranial fibrinolysis could cause a major intraparenchymal bleed. A preprocedure CT scan is not always obtained, but had been in this patient and was negative.

Case 9 continues

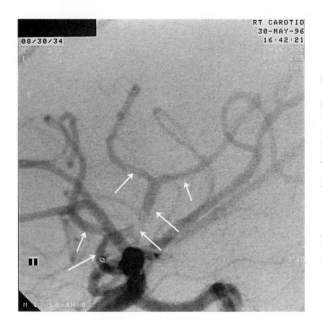

Figure 59-96 A superselective infusion of urokinase was begun and a heparin drip was continued at the rate of 1000 U/hr. This is high from the standpoint of the Abbott Prolyse for Acute Cerebral Thromboembolism (PROACT) trial, but that trial assumes a possible delay of several hours, allowing the damage to the brain to "ripen." Additionally, bleeds almost always occur a matter of hours after the urokinase infusion has been stopped (typically, after about 8 hours). For this reason, it is believed that for a truly acute occlusion, standard anticoagulation during urokinase infusion can be given up to about 5 hours after the event. At that time, the dose is cut to 500 U/hr and ceased at 8 hours after the event (2 hours before the allowed maximum for the PROACT trial).

After 45 minutes of infusion at the rate of 500,000 U/hr (about 8000U/min), this angiogram was performed by injecting through the guide catheter. Note the microcatheter tip (just below the *lowest arrow*). The injection reveals partial clearing of the branches of the occluded vessel; note the retained thrombus in the recanalized vessel *(arrows)*.

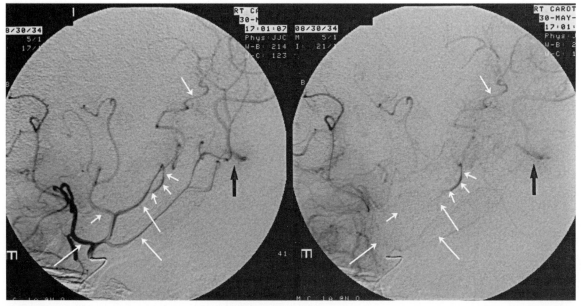

Figure 59-97 After 1 hour of infusion, the superselective injection reveals normal patency of the M2 branches (a laminar flow defect is seen but no thrombus), but there is a delay in one of the distal (M3–M4) branches of the posterior division *(small white arrows)*. This usually indicates an occlusion even if the stub or intraluminal thrombus is not seen. A separate distal offshoot of this same branch is patent *(uppermost large white arrow)*. In addition, there appears to be a delay in a far posterior branch (postcentral) with an intense blush at its end *(black arrows)*. Infusion was continued. Time from occlusion is now about 1½ hours.

Case 9 continues

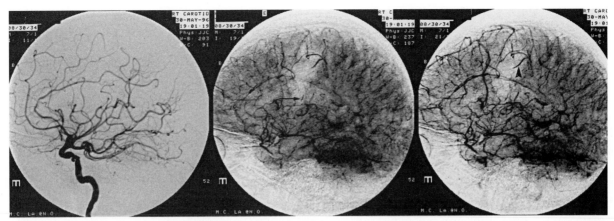

Figure 59-98 After 2½ hours, the catheter was advanced to the clot itself (which felt very hard and had not changed in appearance since Fig. 59–97) and the infusion was continued. After 3½ hours, a repeat angiogram was performed. There is no change in the apparent point of occlusion *(arrow)*. Note that with the artificially enhanced capillary blush, areas of hypoperfusion can be easily identified. There is now slow retrograde flow from a distal branch back into the hypovascular area *(arrowhead)*. By this time in the procedure the patient was asymptomatic, but there was no way to predict whether this area would go on to clear or become a small infarct. The procedure was terminated at this point. There were no clinical sequelae to this event.

6. Auxiliary systemic support and monitoring (e.g., heart, lungs)
7. Consideration of barbiturate coma (see "Barbiturate Therapy for Pre-emptive Cerebral Protection" in Chapter 55).
8. Evaluation of etiology (specifically, rule out bleed)
9. Consideration of definitive therapy
   a. Intravenous t-PA
   b. Heparin
   c. Local intra-arterial urokinase
   d. Angioplasty
   e. Craniotomy, intracranial pressure monitoring

These maneuvers can be performed at the appropriate time, depending on the circumstance.

Specific Guidelines for Treatment of a Stroke on the Table

Phase I

1. Perform neurologic examination; localize the insult. Make sure the insult is consistent with the vessel suspected as the cause. Talk to the patient; this not only yields a quick evaluation of speech and comprehension but also reassures the patient.
2. Check vital signs, electrocardiogram, and pulse oximetry.
3. Administer supplemental oxygen by facemask at 5 to 12 L/min.
4. Increase systemic pressure by running intravenous fluids "wide open"; consider the substitution of plasmanate or other volume expanders after a central venous line is placed. Pressor support should also be considered. The goal is a systolic pressure in the range of 160 to 180 mm Hg.

5. Call a code, or at least alert anesthesiology, the attending clinical service, other auxiliary medical personnel, and possibly neurosurgery.

Phase II

6. *Don't panic.* There should be adequate time to eradicate any thrombus that formed during the procedure. Indeed, this material commonly dissolves on its own if the inciting material is removed. As stated elsewhere in this text, intact endothelium is a hostile environment to thrombus.
7. Establish auxiliary medical supportive measures and monitoring, including electrocardiogram, blood pressure, central venous line, and arterial line.
8. Perform repeat angiogram to evaluate for definitive cause. The inciting cause most likely is a catheter-related thrombus or embolus.
9. If there is thrombus or embolism and anticoagulation is not contraindicated, administer a bolus of 10,000 units of heparin, followed by 1000 U/hr. (After 4 hours, this will be an effective level of only 1000 to 1500 units but will saturate the stagnant intracranial blood more effectively initially than a more modest dose).
10. Administer dexamethasone, 24 mg by intravenous bolus.
11. Administer nimodipine, 60 mg given orally (consider other neuroprotectant agents as they become available).
12. If there is an identifiable and accessible thrombus, the heparin bolus should be followed by direct local infusion of urokinase to eradicate the thrombus (see Chapter 60). If the lesion is a dislodged plaque and proves to be resistant to fibrinolysis, angioplasty may be necessary. If the blockage is caused by coil or balloon

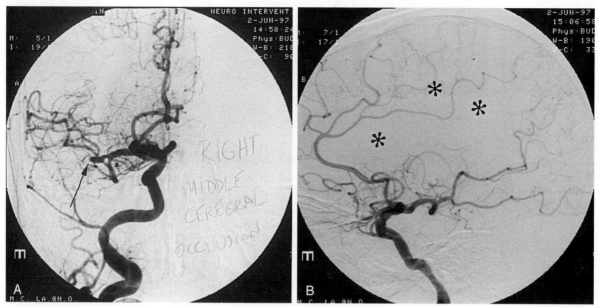

Figure 59-99 Case 10. PA *(A)* and lateral *(B)* right common carotid artery injection reveals an MCA bifurcation occlusion *(arrow)*. The vascular territory was supplied mostly by pial collaterals from the anterior and posterior cerebral arteries, but there was significant neurologic deficit (4/5 strength of both the arm [proximal muscle group] and leg). The patient's grip was excellent. Note the huge perfusion deficit in the territory of the MCA *(asterisks)*.

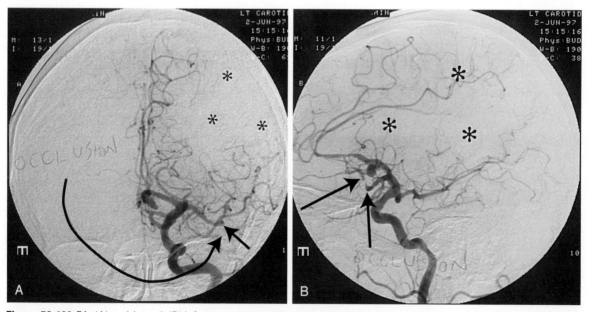

Figure 59-100 PA *(A)* and lateral *(B)* left common carotid artery injection reveals a mirror-image occlusion of the left MCA bifurcation *(arrows, A)* along with an aneurysm at the anterior communicating artery. A single residual frontal branch remains, also with a severe stenosis *(arrows, B)* on the lateral view. The patient had a recent reversible ischemic neurologic deficit with nearly total recovery but still with repeated episodes of aphasia, usually in the morning and never lasting longer than 2 hours. Again note the large perfusion deficit *(asterisks)*. Note the stenosis of the pericallosal artery. This vessel supplies most of the anterior circulation on this side.

Case 10 continues

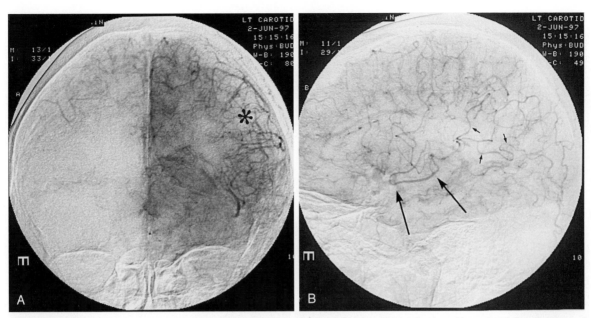

Figure 59-101 PA (*A*) and lateral (*B*) delayed images of a left common carotid injection. Note the delayed filling of most of the MCA territory through pial collaterals in a fashion similar to that on the contralateral side (*asterisk* on PA view). The flow extends retrograde all the way down the angular branch (*short arrows*) to the MCA bifurcation (*long arrows*) and then turns to head back up to the region of the central sulcus (but not yet completely opacified on this image). It is amazing that there had not been a major infarct yet, but it is unknown how long it will be before one occurs.

Case 10 continues

malposition, retrieval (endovascular or surgical) should be considered.

Phase III

13. Consider barbiturate coma. This must be performed quickly if it is to have any use (see the discussion in "Barbiturate Therapy for Preemptive Cerebral Protection" in Chapter 55).

Sudden Ischemic Neurologic Deficit on the Table Without Major Branch Occlusion

If during an angiogram or interventional procedure, there is a sudden focal change in the neurologic status of the patient without an intracranial bleed and *without a major vascular occlusion,* an accurate determination of the cause of this change is required before any rescue can be performed. A sudden neurologic change is not likely to be secondary to metabolic cause and is almost certainly secondary to vascular obstruction or a seizure. Although differentiating a seizure from a sudden vascular deficit should be straightforward, in certain rare circumstances, this may be difficult (e.g., an akinetic seizure may be inapparent, leaving a residual focal motor deficit [Todd's paralysis]). Headache (stroke) or a brief episode of unconsciousness (seizure) may help differentiate the two in this instance.

Numerous ischemic strokes have been caused by microemboli. When bleed and major vessel occlusion have been excluded and the patient has a significant deficit, the possibility of a small, strategic lacunar deficit should be considered. Although no controlled trials have been performed for this maneuver, a small embolus could be amenable to fibrinolysis even if administered in a regional infusion (e.g., in the ICA rather than directly in the MCA). Indeed, we believe that a large percentage of patients who responded to the National Institute of Nervous Disorders and Stroke t-PA trial were patients with microemboli. Therefore, if a true ischemic catastrophe has occurred and a large branch occlusion is not seen, *regional* low-dose fibrinolytic infusion in addition to heparinization should be considered.

Case Studies

The examples of "strokes on the table" presented in Figures 59–99 to 59–112 (Cases 10 and 11), here yield additional insight into the reasoning for therapy and the exact steps taken.

We gratefully acknowledge the aid given by Dr. Charles Kerber with "Specific Guidelines for Treatment of a Stroke on the Table."

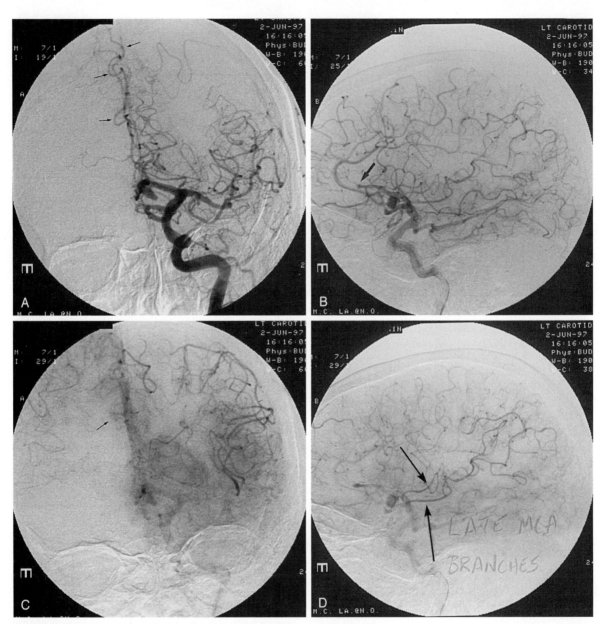

Figure 59-102 Early and late PA (*A* and *C*) and lateral (*B* and *D*) views after an exchange for a guide catheter had been made to treat the aneurysm with Guglielmi detachable coils. The patient became mute at this time, with paresis of the right arm and leg. The angiogram superficially appears unremarkable, but the anterior cerebral artery seen on the lateral view is actually the right anterior cerebral artery (*arrows* on PA views). Note the stub of the occluded pericallosal branch of the left anterior cerebral artery (*arrow* on early lateral view, *C*). Note also that the previously identified MCA branch is still present, filling from the same pial collaterals from the posterior cerebral artery as it had previously (*arrows* on late lateral view, *D*).

Note also, however, the large area of poor capillary blush (*C*). This is the area at most immediate risk, but essentially the entire motor and sensory strips of both the middle and anterior cerebral distributions are threatened by this single occlusion.

Heparin was given immediately. While an infusion of urokinase was being prepared for superselective administration using a pump, a slow infusion of 250,000 units of urokinase was administered through the guide catheter. This urokinase will bathe all that it touches and flow retrograde to areas that may have received embolic material.

Case 10 continues

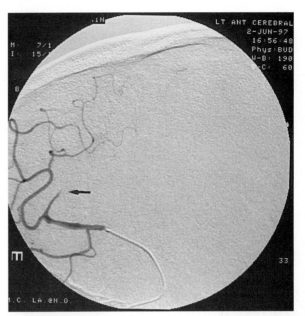

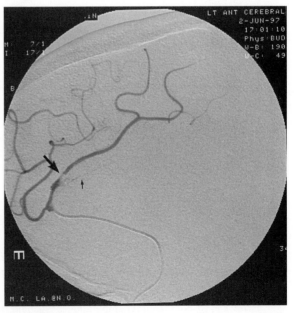

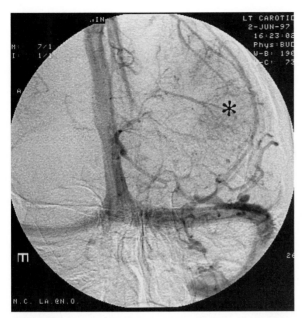

Figure 59-103 Very delayed PA image of the left common carotid artery injection after 5000 units of heparin had been administered. Note the blush in the MCA territory (*asterisk*), an indication that this territory may survive for some period.

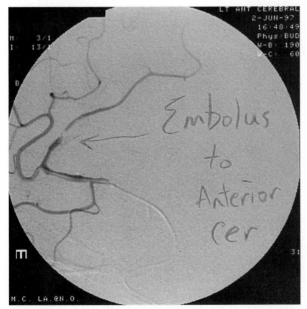

Figure 59-104 Superselective catheterization of the involved vessel (the left anterior cerebral artery) has been performed. Injection reveals that the embolus totally occludes the pericallosal artery, but flow is making it past this point into a callosomarginal branch. Infusion of urokinase had been ongoing for several minutes at a rate of 500,000 U/hr, certainly adequate for a vessel this small and for a bulk of thrombus so small.

Figure 59-105 Follow-up image 8 minutes after Figure 59–104 reveals a common situation: the embolus has shifted and now is occluding the entire artery (*arrow*). The urokinase infusion is continued, but a guidewire is used to poke a hole through the occlusion to reestablish antegrade flow.

Figure 59-106 Five minutes later, flow is again brisk in the callosomarginal artery (*large arrow*), but the pericallosal artery, the primary supply to vital anastomoses with the MCA territory, is still occluded (*small arrow*).

Case 10 continues

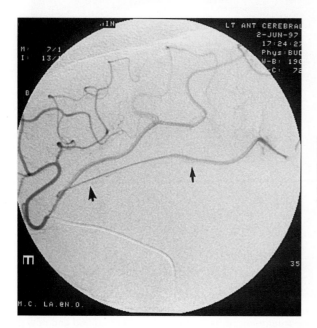

Figure 59-107 After more poking with a guidewire, 25 minutes later there is flow in the pericallosal artery *(arrows)*. This is not only good for the territory in question but also buys some time for further rescue. Downstream, there is still probably some residual debris to clean up; therefore, the infusion is continued. Some branches probably still contain thrombus.

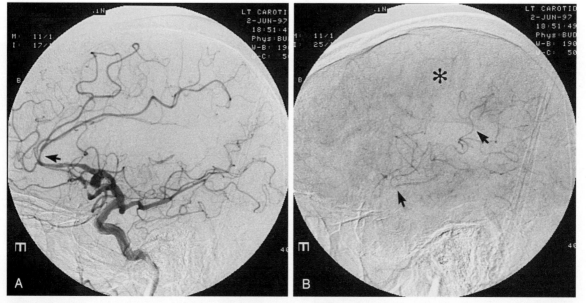

Figure 59-108 Early *(A)* and late *(B)* lateral views of the final injection after infusion had been maintained for about 2½ hours. The angiogram is back to baseline (note the stenosis again seen in the pericallosal artery, *arrow in A*). On the delayed lateral view, the same retrograde angular branch is seen filling from the posterior cerebral collaterals *(arrows in B)*, but the motor strip region is blushing *(asterisk)*. The patient could now speak normally and could move his hand with 3/5 strength, but his leg and proximal arm were still plegic. Because of the reasonably rapid rescue, the lack of involvement of the lenticulostriate vessels, and the reestablishment of normal flow, it appeared that the patient would regain all function. This did occur but took 2 weeks.

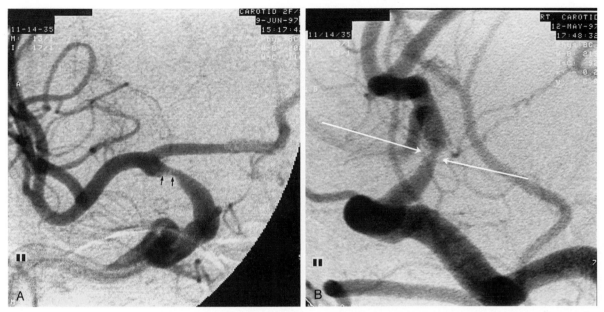

Figure 59-109 Case 11. PA *(A)* and lateral *(B)* views of a tight stenosis of the right internal carotid artery in a patient with a previous transient episode of left-hand weakness associated with speech difficulty. Note should be made of the irregular appearance of the stenosis (just at the *arrows* in *A*); this should have been a warning of the potential for embolus from this lesion (not to mention the history!).

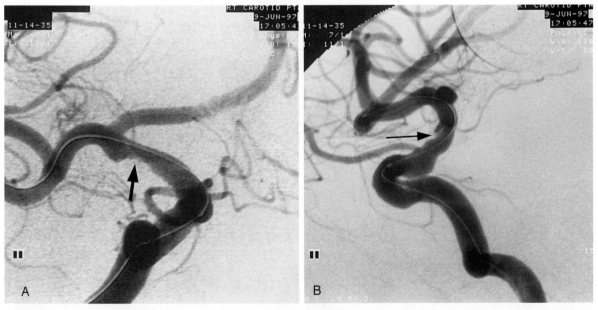

Figure 59-110 *A* and *B*. After careful measurement (with an external quarter, as described in Chapter 3), the vessel was determined to be between 2.9 and 3.7 mm in diameter. The decision was made to use a 2.5-mm angioplasty balloon to deliberately undersize the balloon. The PA *(A)* and lateral *(B)* views show the appearance of the vessel after angioplasty: excellent flow with good morphologic appearance. Note, however, the appearance of the vessel on the lateral view (intimal tear, *arrow* in *B*).

Case 11 continues

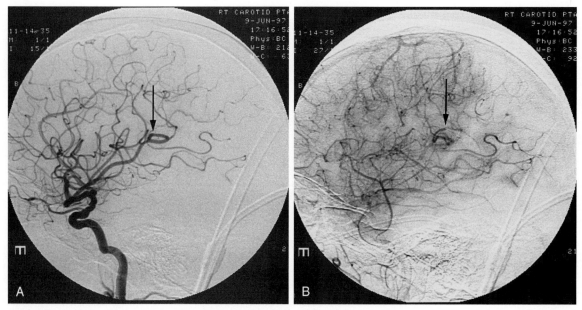

Figure 59-111 Early *(A)* and late *(B)* views of the postangioplasty carotid injection. Note the stagnant artery *(arrows)* and the absent capillary blush in the peripheral distribution of this vessel. An embolus has traveled to the distal angular branch, with resultant branch occlusion. This is an example of failure of simple anticoagulation to clean a lesion and of the need to evaluate the preangioplasty appearance carefully. It was decided that flow to the occlusion site was reasonable and that the occlusion was in a branch that could withstand a period of ischemia. Rather than try to pass a catheter past the angioplasty site (and potentially create a dissection or make a small one worse), it was determined that infusion of urokinase in the internal carotid artery in all likelihood would be successful.

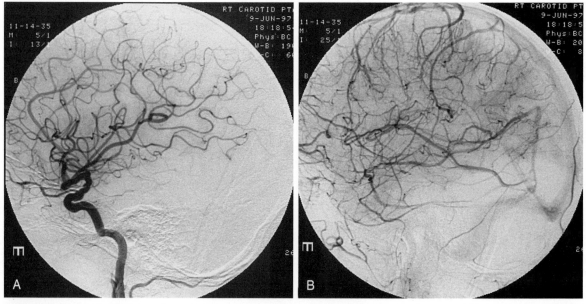

Figure 59-112 *A* and *B,* One hour later, the angiogram reveals that the vasculature is now normal (note the homogeneous capillary phase). The patient was totally neurologically intact and remained so.

REFERENCES

1. Nighogassian N, Ryvlin P, Trouillas P, et al. Pontine versus capsular pure motor hemiparesis. *Neurology* 1993;43:2197–2201.
2. Melo TP, Bogousslavsky J, Van Melle G, Regli F. Pure motor stroke: a reappraisal. *Neurology* 1992;42:789–798.
3. Barth A, Bogousslavsky J, Regli F. The clinical and topographic spectrum of cerebellar infarcts: a clinical-magnetic imaging correlation study. *Ann Neurol* 1993;33:451–456.
4. Toghi H, Takahashi S, Chiba K, Hirata Y, for the Tohuku Cerebellar Infarction Study Group. Cerebellar infarction: clinical and neuroimaging analysis in 293 patients. *Stroke* 1993;24:1697–1701.
5. Kase CS, Norrving B, Levine SR, et al. Cerebellar infarction: clinical and anatomic observations in 66 cases. *Stroke* 1993;24:76–83.
6. North K, Kan A, De Silva M, Ouvrier R. Hemiplegia due to posterior cerebral artery occlusion. *Stroke* 1993;24:1757–1760.
7. Hornig CR, Buttner T, Hoffman O, Dorndoff W. Short-term prognosis of vertebrobasilar ischemic stroke. *Cardiovasc Dis* 1992;2:273–281.
8. Huang MH, Huang CC, Ryu SJ, Chu NS. Sudden bilateral hearing impairment in vertebrobasilar occlusive disease. *Stroke* 1993;24:132–137.
9. Hacke W, Zeumer H, Ferbert A, et al. Intra-arterial thrombolytic therapy improves outcome in patients with acute vertebrobasilar occlusive disease. *Stroke* 1988;19:1216–1222.
10. Brandt T, von Kummer R, Müller-Küppers M, Hacke W. Thrombolytic therapy of acute basilar artery occlusion: variables affecting recanalization and outcome. *Stroke* 1996;27:875–881.
11. Wijdicks EF, Scott JP. Outcome in patients with acute basilar artery occlusion requiring mechanical ventilation. *Stroke* 1996;27:1301–1303.
12. Brückmann HJ, Ringelstein EB, Buchner H, Zeumer H. Vascular recanalizing techniques in the hind brain circulation. *Neurosurg Rev* 1987;10:197–199.
13. Furlan AJ. Natural history of atherothrombotic occlusion of cerebral arteries: carotid versus vertebrobasilar territories. In: Hacke W (ed). Thrombolytic Therapy in Acute Ischemic Stroke. Heidelberg: Springer-Verlag, 1991.
14. Theron J, Coskun O, Huet H, et al. Local intraarterial thrombolysis in the carotid territory. *Interven Neuroradiol* 1996;2:111–126.
15. Zeumer H, Freitag H-J, Zanella F, et al. Local intra-arterial fibrinolytic therapy in patients with stroke: urokinase versus recombinant tissue plasminogen activator (r-TPA). *Neuroradiology* 1993;35:159–162.
16. Mori E, Yoneda Y, Tabuchi M, et al. Intravenous recombinant tissue plasminogen activator in acute carotid artery territory stroke. *Neurology* 1992;42:976–982.
17. Theron J, Courtheoux P, Casasco A, et al. Local intraarterial fibrinolysis in the carotid territory. *AJNR* 1989;10:753–765.
18. Overgaard K, Sereghy T, Pederson H, Boysen G. Dose response to t-PA and its combination with aspirin in a rat embolic stroke model. *Neuroreport* 1992;3:925–928.
19. Toni D, Fiorelli M, Gentile M, et al. Progressing neurological deficit secondary to acute ischemic stroke: a study on predictability, pathogenesis, and prognosis. *Arch Neurol* 1995;52:670–675.
20. Tsai FY, Wang A, Matovich VB, et al. MR staging of acute dural sinus thrombosis: correlation with venous pressure measurements and implications for treatment and prognosis. *AJNR* 1995;16:1021–1029.

ADDITIONAL REFERENCES

Scott JA, Pascuzzi RM, Hall PV, Becker GJ. Treatment of dural sinus thrombosis with local urokinase infusion. *J Neurosurg* 1988;68:284–287.
Vogl TJ, Bergman C, Villringer A, et al. Dural sinus thrombosis: value of venous MR angiography for diagnosis and follow-up. *AJR* 1994;162:1191–1198.
Yuh WTC, Simonson TM, Wang A-M, et al. Venous sinus occlusive disease: MR findings. *AJNR* 1994;15:309–316.

CHAPTER 60

Specific Technical Procedure of Emergency Intracranial Fibrinolysis

J.J. Connors III / J.C. Wojak

Available data concerning specific details of therapy in this field are inadequate. Therefore, many of the specific procedural techniques presented here are based on accumulated knowledge combined with what has been learned in trials of acute stroke therapy by any means, specifically local intracranial fibrinolysis.

GETTING STARTED

No glucose-containing fluids are ever administered during any part of treatment of an ischemic stroke.

Oxygen is continuously administered by facemask (2 to 4 L/min) A hyperbaric oxygen chamber would be ideal but an interventional neuroradiology suite so equipped currently is impractical.

All inclusion and exclusion criteria are confirmed (see Tables 59–1 and 59–3). Blood work is performed, including complete blood count, blood urea nitrogen, creatinine, chemistries, glucose, electrolytes, platelets, activated partial thromboplastin time (aPTT), and prothrombin time or international normalized ratio.

A micropuncture set (see Chapter 1) is used to gain access. This simplifies entry and prevents errant punctures of an artery from being a problem later during fibrinolysis (i.e., bleeding or hematoma). Immediately, a 6-Fr. neuro sheath (see Chapter 1) is placed. All diagnostic and interventional work is then done through this access.

The initial angiogram should be performed with the goal of discovering the hemodynamics of cerebral perfusion and the exact location of occlusion as quickly as possible. In cases of anterior circulation stroke, we quickly perform a vertebral artery angiogram, followed by a contralateral common carotid injection. The target vessel is *catheterized last;* this is to ensure gaining crucial information about the collateral supply to the region in question.

Alternatively, a pigtail catheter can be placed within the aortic arch, and a large volume can be injected while performing digital subtraction imaging over the head. Theron advocates this procedure for global perfusion evaluation (see Chapter 45), and we think is reasonable.

If technical difficulty limits access to any of the brachiocephalic vessels, only a regional injection is performed (i.e., proximal common carotid or arch aortogram.) This is a good reason to have started off with a neuro sheath (i.e., it makes switching catheters quick and easy). An ideal injection is not necessary. Using a state-of-the-art biplane digital subtraction system, simply placing the tip of the catheter in the origin of any of these vessels and hand injecting a bolus of 10 to 20 ml of contrast is adequate for visualizing the main branches of the intracranial vasculature. Actually advancing the catheter up the vessel is not absolutely necessary. This is particularly true when using the new diagnostic catheters from Cook, Inc., which are large-lumen, nontapering selective 6-Fr. catheters with a 4.8-Fr. lumen and four sideholes at the distal end, allowing a huge bolus injection in the origin of these vessels from the aorta. This catheter is introduced percutaneously over the matching dilator, which is then removed.

These injections provide valuable information concerning the state of the collateral circulation in the affected hemisphere. This information is useful in planning the strategy of rescue, knowing how much time is available, and determining the risk of the procedure.

DOSE OF HEPARIN

Most interventional radiologists use heparin during the active phase of any fibrinolysis. Fresh thrombus stimulates more thrombus, and it is counterproductive to have to dissolve continually forming thrombus. Early results from the trial of intracranial pro-urokinase therapy for stroke intervention have confirmed that at least some heparin is beneficial for adequate thrombolysis. Conflicting early anecdotal evidence, however, suggests that even though heparin is useful during the procedure, postprocedure heparinization may be associated with an increased incidence of hemorrhage and hematoma formation. Other data appear to refute this conclusion, however.

A bolus of 5000 units of heparin given after vascular access when an occlusion is detected, followed by infusion of 1000 U/hr, is typical of the amount used for a long-term fibrinolysis case in the peripheral vasculature. The goal of this heparinization during fibrinolysis is to maintain the aPTT at about 1.5 to 3 times normal (50 to 90 seconds) while a catheter is sitting in a stagnant vessel or in clot. Checking these results and maintaining an accurate level during an emergency intracranial fibrinolysis case is difficult in most settings (if not impossible); therefore, the rough guidelines for heparin administration (adjusted according to laboratory evaluations) used in the periphery are not ideal for this clinical situation.

In the Prolyse for Acute Cerebral Thromboembolism (PROACT) trial, a bolus of 2000 units is given, followed by an infusion of 500 U/hr for 4 hours. We consider this regimen to be suboptimal.

We prefer a bolus of 5000 units followed by 1000 U/hr for 2 hours or until the end of the procedure. This provides an effective heparin level of less than 1000 units by the 3-hour mark and less than 500 units by the 4-hour point, while providing a therapeutic dose during the active phase of thrombolysis when the catheter is in a vessel with stagnant flow. The heparin level can thus be tapered rapidly once acute fibrinolysis is stopped.

A microcatheter sitting for prolonged periods of time in a vessel with slow flow (or no flow) can cause a thrombus to develop. In no other type of intracranial work does a catheter sit for prolonged periods in a small vessel without being manipulated. It is an unfortunate combination of circumstances to have prescribed suboptimal heparinization along with static placement of a catheter, as in the PROACT trial. We recommend that during emergency intracranial fibrinolysis, either adequate heparinization is maintained as we suggest (5000 unit bolus followed by 1000 U/hr until the thrombolytic infusion is stopped) or the ongoing therapeutic situation is checked more frequently than once per hour and the catheter tip is slightly moved. This is particularly important if the clot is chased downstream into a secondary or tertiary branch past the high flow of the middle cerebral artery (MCA) main trunk. The catheter tip should not sit for a prolonged period in a stagnant vessel.

CHOICE OF MICROCATHETER

A standard end-hole microcatheter is the catheter of choice for these procedures; we choose any of the current third-generation variety with some wall braiding to prevent kinking. The Intime catheter by Boston Scientific is an interesting design (it has a built-in microwire), but the inability to aspirate or inject contrast is a disadvantage. Placing a standard microcatheter and microwire and removing the wire to institute therapy is not significantly time-consuming.

Multisidehole infusion microcatheters are available, such as the Softstream (Target Therapeutics); Cordis Corp. and Medtronic/MIS are developing others. In the periphery, these may require pulsed delivery rather than infusion by a pump. In certain circumstances, these multisidehole catheters can aid in the fibrinolytic procedure, particularly if there is a large volume of thrombus in the internal carotid artery (ICA). In general, however, intracranial thrombi are small (less than 1 cm long) and more selectively infused with a simple end-hole catheter.

This multisidehole infusion catheter, however, also can act as a stenting catheter. Theoretically, it can be placed *through* the thrombus, with its tip in the unoccluded MCA, and flow can be maintained past the thrombus in the ICA. Alternatively, fresh arterial blood can be injected past the occlusion while an infusion is maintained in a more proximal location. This is heroic endovascular gymnastics.

MICROCATHETER TIP AND GUIDE CATHETER LOCALIZATION

After determining the location of occlusion, the diagnostic catheter is exchanged for an adequate guide catheter. This guide catheter should be one with a soft tip capable of sitting in the vessel for a prolonged period and supplying adequate support for deployment of a microcatheter (FasGUIDE, Target Therapeutics, is our choice). The guide catheter does not have to be as stiff as an ideal interventional guide catheter; the microcatheter only has to be capable of advancing to a relatively proximal location for infusion without any other form of aggressive intervention (e.g., angioplasty). The guide catheter is advanced into an appropriate location in the ICA and taped to the skin and sheath. Final diagnostic images with magnification are obtained.

The microcatheter of choice (e.g., Jetstream, Medtronic/MIS; Transit, Cordis Corp.; Turbo TRACKER, Target Therapeutics) is then advanced to the thrombus.

ESTABLISHING ANTEGRADE FLOW

Establishment of antegrade flow is extremely helpful for two reasons: (1) it supplies blood to downstream ischemic structures, and (2) it speeds the process of fibrinolysis substantially. This is discussed further in Chapter 58. A hole is poked through the thrombus with the microwire and then followed by the catheter, if this can be done easily. Distal infusion of 125,000 units of urokinase in 10 ml of heparinized saline is then performed as the microcatheter is withdrawn to the proximal thrombus interface. (The remainder of the vial of 250,000 units is saved for possible use later.)

In the Abbott trial of prourokinase (PROACT), the microcatheter is advanced only into the proximal third of the thrombus, but a hole is not poked through the occlusion, and no antegrade flow is actively established. No mechanical manipulation of thrombus is permitted. As opposed to the exacting procedure specified in the PROACT trial, more variation in technique is permitted in the North American Cerebral Local Intra-Arterial Fibrinolysis Register.

Mechanical disruption of clot is permitted to establish antegrade flow.

A final microcatheter placement angiogram is performed by very slow injection of contrast and injection through the side port of the Y-adapter on the guide catheter.

We prefer to check the results every 15 to 30 minutes, readjusting the catheter position if necessary.

DOSE OF FIBRINOLYTIC AGENT

Once the microcatheter is in place, the urokinase (or fibrinolytic agent of choice) is infused. Infusion of the fibrinolytic agent in a concentrated form prevents washing out all blood products by a large volume of fluid (water). The fibrinolytic solution should be mixed to deliver the intended amount of agent in 30 to 50 ml of fluid per hour. There formerly was no "magical" amount of drug to use, but recent work has narrowed down the appropriate amount. The exact amount of tissue-type plasminogen activator (t-PA) nearly has been worked out, but only for intravenous administration begun in the first 3 hours.

Direct local intracranial infusion of a fibrinolytic agent requires *far less agent* than does systemic infusion. This may partially explain why the incidence of intracranial bleeding appears to be less with intra-arterial therapy than with intravenous therapy.

For intra-arterial urokinase, the dose should be about 250,000 to 750,000 U/hr, or 4000 to 12,000 U/min. For prourokinase, this dose would be 4.5 mg/hr (the current PROACT trial uses 9 mg in 2 hours). The approximate equivalent dose of t-PA would be 5 mg/hr. Zeumer et al.[1] infuse up to 750,000 units of urokinase or 20 mg of t-PA in 2 hours, mixed in 50 ml of normal saline.

If too high an infusion *volume* is administered into an occluded main trunk of the MCA, it refluxes out into the anterior cerebral artery. This fibrinolytic water also prevents any fresh blood, and therefore new plasminogen, from reaching the proximal thrombus.

We use 1,000,000 units of urokinase in 100 ml of normal saline infused over 2 hours; in other words, 50 ml/hr containing 500,000 units of urokinase, in addition to the initial 125,000 units administered by hand. This mixture can be infused using a standard intravenous-type pump or a Harvard-type syringe pump.

In recent years, the trend has been to increase the rate of administration of urokinase; problems related to therapy have appeared to be more closely associated with *duration* of infusion and *lateness* of infusion rather than with total dose or rate of infusion. This is not true with peripherally (intravenously) administered t-PA, however, of which an exponentially higher dose is used and for which an upper limit appears to be established (see "Results of Early Intracranial Local Intra-Arterial Fibrinolysis" in Chapter 56).

Increasing the amount of urokinase above the amounts previously described does not appear to increase local fibrinolytic efficiency but can produce more systemic effects and affect the fibrinogen level adversely.

CHOICE OF CONTRAST MATERIAL

During the procedure, it is vital to cause no further damage to the vascular endothelium or brain parenchyma; therefore, iso-osmolar nonionic contrast is recommended for the repeated brachiocephalic and intracranial injections during the case (see Chapter 1). A normal, nonionic contrast material that has been diluted with sterile water (*not* saline) can be used. Alternatively, the newer isotonic nonionic contrast material Visipaque (Nycomed) can be used. Even when this contrast is used, an intense stain of the basal ganglia on CT is common immediately after the procedure, without mass effect. This is indicative not of bleeding but of extravasation of contrast in the area of endothelial damage.

Contrast diluted with saline yields a hypertonic, hyperosmolar solution. The viscosity may be lower, but who cares? Plain sterile water should be used to dilute regular contrast to yield a nearly isotonic nonionic agent (but it will be less dense on angiography).

Leakage of contrast from vessels into the brain parenchyma after local intra-arterial thrombolytic therapy has been described (see Chapter 57). This is thought to be due to a combination of factors, including ischemia, endothelial damage, direct toxic effect of hypertonic contrast material on the already damaged vessel, and overpressurization of perforating arteries.[2] The smaller the volume of hypertonic extravascular material deposited, the better. Extravascular hypertonic material can suck water out into the interstitium, increasing the forces causing edema. Repeated contrast injections are required during fibrinolysis procedures; therefore, use of an iso-osmolar nonionic contrast material is recommended. For example, 4 ml of iso-osmolar nonionic contrast material can be injected through the guide catheter every 15 minutes for a total of only 32 ml, spread over the entire 2-hour period. This limited amount of isotonic iso-osmolar material is preferable to continued prolonged infusion of a fibrinolytic agent into a damaged vessel (which can occur if the intracranial hemodynamic situation is not checked). Therefore, we prefer to check results and move the catheter downstream when possible.

DEALING WITH RESISTANT THROMBUS

Some embolic material may be resistant to thrombolysis. This makes sense considering that these emboli can originate from cardiac sources and can be very old. Usually, however, at least some portion of the thrombus dissolves, and the mass shrinks.

If the embolus does not respond to simple fibrinolysis, it may be possible to remove this material by mechanical means. As stated in Chapter 58, there are four methods for establishing antegrade flow mechanically and removing embolic material: poking a hole, using a snare, performing angioplasty, and using a loop basket (a new device from Medtronic/MIS). The typical means to achieve this is with a microsnare (see Chapter 1). This can grab the hard mass and pull it from the intracranial location.

A recent development is the coil embolus grabber from Medtronic/MIS (the Gobin device, also described in Chapter 1). This is a nitinol wire with a small, spiral-shaped, tapering coil at the end that can be deployed into the thrombus and then withdrawn while the coil holds the thrombus. It is not yet commercially available but appears promising.

Grabbing a resistant thrombus and removing it can yield a dramatic correction of the hemodynamic occlusion, but, this task may be difficult. An additional means of removing the occlusive mass is by angioplasty of this obstruction. This is not nearly as elegant a solution as removal by snare. The mass is displaced into an unpredictable branch, which may worsen the problem. In addition, some of this mass may be smashed into a small lenticulostriate artery, with devastating consequences. See the detailed discussion of the rationale for therapeutic techniques in Chapter 58.

An alternative method for dealing with resistant thrombus is not to deal with it, to circumvent it. It is possible to advance a multisidehole catheter past the occlusion and allow this to carry some blood past the clot, as well as to infuse some blood through it. The multisidehole Softstream catheter can be used for this purpose.

CHASING THE CLOT

Avoiding Infusion of Vulnerable Vasculature

As the clot dissolves, it either shrinks in place or migrates distally. After clot migration, continued infusion in the same proximal location can be ineffective because of the fibrinolytic agent now exiting the first available side branch (this principle is well demonstrated in the periphery). Additionally, continued proximal infusion can be dangerous because of infusion of injured perforators (lenticulostriate arteries). Therefore, it is desirable to reposition the microcatheter, that is, to chase the thrombus and get the microcatheter tip past any injured lenticulostriate arteries, as soon as possible.

Zeumer et al.[1] check their results every 30 minutes, a reasonable frequency.

The Danger of Pericatheter Thrombus Formation

One danger inherent in pursuing clot fragments into distal arterial branches is that as the branches become smaller, blood flow around the catheter becomes slower (or even stagnant if there are no patent side branches distally). There is a significant risk of pericatheter thrombus formation if the microcatheter is left in place in these small vessels for prolonged periods during infusion of thrombolytic agent. This is a good argument for the use of adequate intraprocedural heparin. This also is a strong argument for frequent monitoring and repositioning of the catheter. The microcatheter must not be placed too far downstream in a stagnant vessel, nor allowed to sit there for a prolonged period. For this reason, there has to be a practical limit to how far distally the catheter should be advanced to pursue thrombus. Also, if chasing the thrombus into a distal branch becomes necessary, exchanging the catheter for a smaller catheter is probably wise (such as the Prowler from Cordis Corp.).

If all other branches are clear, infusion into a single tertiary branch should be done with caution, and infusion into the main division of the MCA supplying this branch probably is adequate. This means placing the catheter tip into the superior division of the MCA, for example, no farther than 2 to 4 cm past its origin. This strategy of proximal infusion assumes that at least a slight amount of flow reaches the embolus. Then, it does not take much urokinase to dissolve a small clot, and any clot this small is obstructing flow to only a small territory, with the ischemic area receiving some collateral flow from the nearby vascular territory.

It is reasonable, however, to try to establish antegrade flow in this occluded vessel while infusing from a more proximal location. This can be done with the guidewire (carefully) or with both the guidewire and microcatheter before pulling the microcatheter back to a more proximal location for the infusion.

WHEN TO STOP

This is a good question. In the various trials, the stopping point is well defined (i.e., 8 hours after the acute ischemic event in the current PROACT trial). In reality, and for optimal therapy, a well-defined stopping point is not spelled out; good clinical judgment is better than a "recipe." The duration of infusion and persistence of fibrinolytic therapy are totally dependent on the time of presentation (how long the ischemia has persisted), the location of the occlusion, and the depth of ischemia.

This is why the original diagnostic approach described previously included injection of the vertebral artery and the opposite carotid artery: these injections allow analysis of the total vascular supply to the brain and provide information concerning collateral pial supply to the ischemic area. This, combined with the vital information concerning the lenticulostriate arteries, allows judgment concerning how much time is available for therapy and when the anxiety level associated with duration of therapy will rise to an intolerable degree. After performing this procedure a number of times, the interventionist will be able to appreciate this worry.

Remember, if the lenticulostriate arteries have been occluded, the possibility of a posttherapeutic bleed is increased. If therapy is aimed simply at a cortical vessel, the time for rescue is more prolonged, and the danger is decreased (see Chapter 58). For directly occluded lenticulostriate arteries, the time for rescue is about 3 hours, whereas for indirectly occluded lenticulostriate arteries (e.g., M1 origin occlusion without occlusion of the lenticulostriate arteries), there may be up to 6 to 8 hours. For cortical vessels, the time for rescue can be 8 to 12 hours or even longer. The key question, however, is: Were the lenticulostriate arteries occluded before the procedure began, or were there some lenticulostriate branches occluded that were unseen?

Another key to deciding when to stop is how vital the vessels are that are still occluded; is a temporal branch of the MCA (e.g., inferior division) occluded, or is the main angular branch to Wernicke's area occluded? This decision is based on knowledge of neurovascular anatomy.

POSTPROCEDURE MANAGEMENT

At the termination of the procedure, the arterial sheath is left in place; the heparin is not reversed. It is, however, terminated, as stated previously, and allowed to wear off. Some neurologists prefer to continue heparin.

The patient's blood pressure is monitored actively and kept below 160 to 180/100 mm Hg. A labetalol drip can be started or continued if necessary (see Chapters 4 and 7). Aggressive "normalization" of blood pressure is not undertaken. The body is attempting to perfuse ischemic regions of the brain by elevating the pressure. No aspirin or nonsteroidal anti-inflammatory agents are administered. No volume expanders are permitted. The patient is then transferred to the computed tomography scanner, and a follow-up scan is obtained.

ASPIRIN AND ACUTE STROKE THERAPY

The role of aspirin is another unknown variable, but as stated previously (see "Aspirin Inhibits Fibrinolysis" in Chapter 58), aspirin should *not* be administered during fibrinolysis or is administered only after it has been *proved* beneficial. The current evidence suggesting significant hindrance of fibrinolysis has to be countered before aspirin can be associated with a procedure.

REOPRO (ABCIXIMAB) AND ACUTE STROKE THERAPY

The question of the use of abciximab (ReoPro) has not been answered; we are sure that it will be investigated at some point.

REFERENCES

1. Zeumer H, Freitag H-J, Zanella F, et al. Local intra-arterial fibrinolytic therapy in patients with stroke: urokinase versus recombinant tissue plasminogen activator (r-TPA). *Neuroradiology* 1993;35:159–162.
2. Komiyama M, Nishijima Y, Nishio A, Khosla VK. Extravasation of contrast medium from the lenticulostriate artery following local intracarotid fibrinolysis. *Surg Neurol* 1993;39:315–319.

Technique of Superselective Intraophthalmic Artery Fibrinolytic Therapy Using Urokinase for Central Retinal Vein Occlusion

J.N. Vallee / H.S. Jhaveri / M. Tovi / P.Y. Santiago / P. Paques / A. Gaudric / J.-J. Merland

Central retinal vein occlusion (CRVO) is a vascular retinal problem caused by significant reduction in venous flow, which leads to progressive loss of visual acuity (sometimes rapid and significant), with reduction in light perception. CRVO often is seen in patients with atherosclerosis, an associated risk factor. The presence of thrombosis as the cause of CRVO, although controversial, has been well documented by anatomic and pathologic examination.[1] The spontaneous evolution of this condition usually is prolonged, typically 6 to 12 months, with recovery of visual acuity (>5/10) in only 15% of cases.[2]

We have infused urokinase intra-arterially in the ophthalmic artery with the object of treating recent and severe cases of CRVO. This therapy immediately improved visual acuity as well as arteriovenous retinal circulatory time, and no other effective therapy is available.

INCLUSION CRITERIA

Inclusion criteria for intra-arterial therapy include recent and edematous occlusion of the central retinal vein with (1) fundoscopic examination showing dilation and tortuosity of all the retinal veins, superficial retinal hemorrhage of "dots" or "dashes" appearance, diffuse retinal and papillary edema, and rare or absent nodular cotton-wool avascular zones; (2) reduction in visual acuity; and (3) fluorescein angiography revealing slow venous flow (as judged by arteriovenous transit time) and absence of diffuse retinal ischemia (absent or rare zones of nonperfusion).

EXCLUSION CRITERIA

Exclusion criteria for intra-arterial therapy include ischemic CRVO, with fundoscopic examination showing deep, flame-shaped hemorrhages and several nodular, cotton-wool avascular zones, or fluorescein angiography showing diffuse capillary nonperfusion.

TECHNIQUE
Setting

This therapy requires collaboration between the interventional neuroradiologist, ophthalmologist, and anesthesiologist. An angiography room, with digital angiography equipment if possible, is required. Patients are premedicated; if neuroleptic anesthesia is necessary, the anesthesiologist should be present. The entire procedure is performed under sterile conditions.

Materials Used

For this procedure, we use a 5-Fr. introducer (Terumo, Japan), 5-Fr. vertebral curve catheter (Terumo, Japan), 0.035″ hydrophilic-coated guidewire (Terumo, Japan), 1.8-Fr. or 1.5-Fr. Magic microcatheter (Balt Extrusion), nonionic contrast media (Omnipaque 300, Nycomed), and 300,000 units of urokinase (Hoeschst, France).

Procedural Technique

The steps of the procedure are as follows:

1. The femoral artery is punctured under local anesthesia using Seldinger's technique, and the 5-Fr. Terumo introducer is placed. The introducer is connected to a continuous flush of normal saline.
2. The internal carotid artery is catheterized using the 5-Fr. Terumo vertebral curve catheter and 0.035″ Terumo guidewire (Fig. 61–1).
3. Selective internal carotid angiography is performed in the lateral projection, with centering for intracranial vessels, using Omnipaque. This provides a pretherapeutic reference. We evaluate the geometry of the carotid siphon as well as the caliber of the ophthalmic artery.
4. Heparin (2000 units) is injected as an intravenous bolus just before the microcatheter is introduced into the system to avoid thrombus formation related to the catheter.
5. Using the 1.8-Fr. or 1.5-Fr. Magic microcatheter, the ophthalmic artery is superselectively catheterized (Fig. 61–2). The tip of the Magic microcatheter is given an S-shaped curve using steam before superselective intra-arterial navigation is undertaken.
6. During the entire procedure, normal saline is

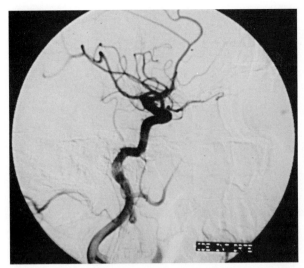

Figure 61-1 Selective right internal carotid angiogram using the 5-Fr. Terumo vertebral curve catheter.

infused constantly through the guide catheter through a Y hemostatic valve to prevent thrombus formation in the system and to avoid intra-arterial air embolism. This also greatly facilitates gentle manipulation of the microcatheter in the guide catheter.

7. Superselective ophthalmic angiography is performed to verify the stability of the microcatheter at the origin of the ophthalmic artery and to assess the different branches of the ophthalmic artery and the choroidal blush (see Fig. 61–2).
8. The microcatheter is flushed with normal saline before use of urokinase to avoid contact of urokinase with contrast media, which may cause precipitation.
9. Urokinase (300,000 units prediluted in 60 ml of normal saline) is infused at a constant slow rate over 40 minutes using an electric syringe.
10. At the end of the intra-arterial urokinase infusion, superselective ophthalmic angiography and selective ipsilateral internal carotid angi-

ography are performed to verify choroidal blush and the status of the ophthalmic artery, and various intracranial branches of the internal carotid artery.

Postprocedure Management

The patient is observed in the recovery room for 3 to 4 hours. The 5-Fr. introducer is removed after the coagulation profile is assessed and hemostasis of the femoral arterial puncture is obtained. Intravenous heparin is continued for 48 hours to maintain the activated partial thromboplastin time at two times control.

The patient is transferred from the recovery room to the ophthalmology service for 2 to 3 days. Visual acuity testing, fundoscopic examination, and fluorescein angiography to measure arteriovenous transit time are performed 24 hours after therapy. Arteriovenous transit time normally is less than 2 seconds. This is judged by the difference in time (in seconds) between the appearance of color in the retinal artery and the appearance of laminar flow in the retinal vein of the papilla.

Continuing Management

Subcutaneous low-molecular-weight heparin (5000 U/day) is continued for 4 weeks. One tablet of aspirin is given daily for 3 months. Long-term follow-up includes fundoscopic examination, visual acuity, and fluorescein angiography at 7, 15, 30, 90, and 180 days and at 1 year.

RESULTS

During the past 3½ years, we have treated 13 patients (11 were men and 2 women) in the interventional neuroradiology department at Hôpital Lariboisière (Paris). The average age was 58 years (range, 35 to 75 years). The average delay in starting therapy was 10 days (range, 12 hours to 30 days).

Among these 13 patients, 5 patients showed sig-

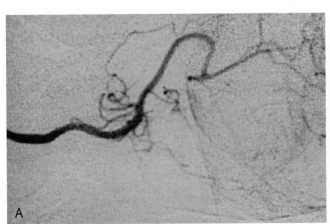
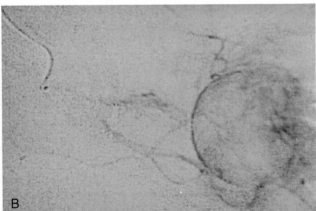

Figure 61-2 Superselective right ophthalmic angiogram through the 1.8-Fr. Magic microcatheter. The ophthalmic artery *(A)* and choroidal blush *(B)* are shown.

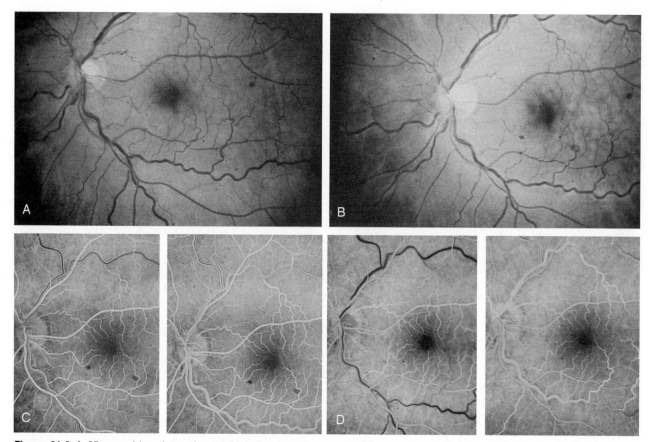

Figure 61-3 A 35-year-old patient whose initial visual acuity was <1/50 seen 24 hr after the onset of visual disturbance. *A,* Fundoscopic retinal photograph obtained during the initial evaluation shows moderate dilation of the vascular network and occasional hemorrhages. The gray appearance of the posterior pole *(right)* is due to secondary slowing down of the arterial flow. *B,* Fundoscopic evaluation 24 hr after fibrinolytic therapy. The caliber of the veins did not change, and the retinal hemorrhages increased. *C,* Fluorescein angiography of the fundus of the eye obtained during the initial evaluation revealed that the arteriovenous transit time is significantly prolonged (55.9 sec). The image on the left is an early image and that on the right is later. Note that the fluorescein has not entered the veins at all in the left image. The venous network did not completely fill until after 85 sec. *D,* Fluorescein angiography of the fundus of the eye, 24 hr after in situ fibrinolytic therapy. Again, the left image is an early image and the right image was obtained a few seconds later. This reveals significant improvement in arteriovenous transit time (35.5 sec). The venous network is almost completely filled by 43 sec (left image). At this time, the patient's visual acuity had improved significantly to 20/20.

nificant improvement in visual acuity within 24 hours after the fibrinolytic therapy, with 2 patients returning to completely normal vision (Fig. 61–3). Four of these 5 patients showed significant improvement in arteriovenous circulatory time in the first 24 hours after the fibrinolytic therapy, with 1 patient having a completely normal arteriovenous transit time. These 5 patients showed significant improvement in their fundoscopic examination in 2 to 4 weeks, with completely normal fundoscopic examinations in 4 patients. No complication due to fibrinolytic therapy was observed in this series.

CONCLUSION

These preliminary results have shown that it is possible to rapidly and spectacularly improve visual acuity and arteriovenous circulatory transit time in certain cases of recent and severe CRVO by this minimally invasive therapy, with long-lasting results. These results are better if patients are treated as soon as possible. We propose this as an emergency treatment. No alternative therapy for this condition is available.

Editor's note: There have been institutions that treat CRVO with intravenous tissue plasminogen activator, with mixed but poor results. Obviously, direct infusion of the retinal or ophthalmic artery would yield a much higher local dose. In addition, many chronic (old) occlusions of the lower extremity have been treated with prolonged low-dose urokinase infusion, with eventual success. Perhaps a slightly longer infusion may be warranted in these cases, in which the occlusion may be more mature than would be wished and in which the failure of therapy can be so devastating.

REFERENCES

1. Green WR, Chan CC, Hutchins GM, Terry JM. Central retinal vein occlusion: a prospective histopathologic study of 29 eyes in 28 cases. *Retina* 1981;1:27–55.
2. Quinlan PM, Elman MJ, Bhatt KA, et al. The natural course of central retinal vein occlusion. *Am J Ophthalmol* 1990;110:118–123.

ADDITIONAL READINGS

Annonier P, Sahel J, Wenger JJ, et al. Traitement fibrinolytique local dans les occlusions de l'artère centrale de la rétine. *J Fr Ophthalmol* 1984;7:711–716.

Brown G, Duker J, Lehman R, Eagle R. Combined central retinal artery and central vein obstruction. *Intern Ophthalmol* 1993;17:9–17.

Cohen D, Gaudric A. Occlusions veineuses rétiniennes. *Sang Thrombose Vaisseaux* 1992;4:105–112.

Elman MJ, Bhatt AK, Quinlan PM, Enger C. The risk for systemic vascular diseases and mortality in patients with central retinal vein occlusion. *Ophthalmology* 1990;97:1543–1548.

Fong A, Schatz H. Central retinal vein occlusion in young adults. *Surv Ophthalmol* 1993;37:393–417.

Glacet-Bernard A, Chabanel A, Coscas G, et al. Elévation de l'agrégation érythrocytaire au cours des occlusions veineuses rétiniennes. *J Fr Ophthalmol* 1990;13:500–505.

Glacet-Bernard A, Coscas G. Actualités sur les occlusions veineuses rétiniennes. *J Fr Ophthalmol* 1993;16:685–695.

Gutman FA. Evaluation of a patient with central retinal vein occlusion. *Ophthalmology* 1983;90:481–483.

Iijima H, Tsumura T. Combined occlusion of the central retinal artery and vein. *Jpn J Ophthalmol* 1994;38:202–207.

Jorizzo PA, Klein ML, Shults WT, Linn ML. Visual recovery in combined central artery and central retinal vein occlusion. *Am J Ophthalmol* 1987;104:358–363.

Keyser BJ, Duker JS, Brown GC, et al. Combined central retinal vein occlusion and cilioretinal artery occlusion associated with prolonged retinal arterial filling. *Am J Ophthalmol* 1994; 117:308–313.

Kohner EM, Cappin JM. Do medical conditions have an influence on central retinal vein occlusion? *Proc R Soc Med* 1974;67:1052–1058.

Laatikainen L. Management of retinal vein occlusion. *Curr Opin Ophthalmol* 1992;3:372–378.

Levinger S, Zauberman H, Eldor A. Prevention of clot formation in cat retinal vein by systemic and subconjunctival urokinase. *Arch Ophthalmol* 1987;105:554–558.

Rath EZ, Frank RN, Shin DH, Kim C. Risk factors for retinal vein occlusions. *Ophthalmology* 1992;99:509–514.

Schmidt D, Schumacher M, Wakhloo AK. Microcatheter urokinase infusion in central retinal artery occlusion. *Am J Ophthalmol* 1992;113:429–434.

Vine AK, Samama MM. The role of abnormalities in the anticoagulant and fibrinolytic systems in retinal vascular occlusions. *Surv Ophthalmol* 1993;37:283–292.

CHAPTER 62

Management of Intracranial Hemorrhage During Thrombolysis

J.C. Wojak

Intracranial hemorrhage is the most serious complication of thrombolytic therapy for stroke. Indeed, it is considered to be the most dreaded complication of *any* form of thrombolytic therapy, and many of the exclusion criteria for thrombolytic therapy of acute myocardial infarction are meant to lessen the risk of this particular complication.

Intracranial hemorrhage usually occurs during or shortly after therapy (hours to days). If hemorrhage is suspected on clinical grounds (e.g., deterioration in neurologic status, severe headache, nausea and vomiting, acute elevation of systemic blood pressure), then the following steps should be taken:

1. Stop infusion of:
   - Thrombolytic agent.
   - Anticoagulant (heparin).
   - Abciximab (ReoPro), if being administered.
2. Draw blood.
   - Send for prothrombin time (PT), activated partial thromboplastin time (aPTT), platelet count, and fibrinogen level.
   - Type and cross-match for 6 to 8 units of platelets and cryoprecipitate (containing fibrinogen and clotting factors).
3. Obtain computed tomography scan.
   - If hemorrhage is present, then continue with the following steps (4 to 9).

- If hemorrhage is not present, then reassess the patient and continue management as indicated.
4. Consult neurosurgery and hematology:
   - To assist in patient management.
   - If immediate surgical intervention is indicated, the following steps can be carried out while the patient is being prepared for surgery and during surgery.
5. Evaluate hematologic results.
   - Evaluate PT and aPTT, platelet count, and fibrinogen level when available.
   - If not immediately available, begin administration of cryoprecipitate while awaiting results.
   - If fibrinogen level is >100 mg/dl, stop cryoprecipitate administration.
6. Consider platelet replacement.
   - If the platelet count is <100,000 or platelet dysfunction is suspected, administer 6 to 8 units of platelets.
7. Draw additional blood samples.
   - Repeat fibrinogen level and PT and aPTT after infusing cryoprecipitate (if initial level <100 mg/dl).
   - If fibrinogen level remains <100 mg/dl, administration of fresh frozen plasma (2 units) should be considered.

- If the aPTT remains elevated once the fibrinogen level is >100 mg/dl, protamine sulfate (1 mg for every 100 units of heparin administered over the previous 4 hours) may be given by slow intravenous infusion.
8. Transfer patient to the intensive care unit for observation:

- If immediate surgery is not indicated.
9. Repeat the computed tomography scan:
  - Within 4 hours to evaluate for expansion of the hematoma.
  - Sooner if further deterioration in the patient's clinical status occurs.

CHAPTER 63

Treatment and Prevention of Acute Ischemic Stroke by Endovascular Techniques:
A Network-Based Community Model

B.L. Berger / A.S. Callahan III

BACKGROUND

Previous chapters have developed the scientific rationale for endovascular treatment of acute ischemic stroke and included scientific studies of safety and efficacy. Recent publications have put surgical treatment of atherostenosis at the carotid bifurcation on a scientific basis.[1, 2] Despite these advances, stroke remains a formidable clinical opponent and a major public health issue. More than 550,000 strokes occur annually, and about 85% of these are ischemic. Stroke is the leading cause of adult disability and the third leading cause of death. Estimates of the annual cost of stroke approach $30 billion, but such a number does not indicate the impact that having a stroke has on the patient and the family. No other illness creates such dread and fear in everyone.

In 1994, we decided to develop an approach to stroke prevention and treatment at the community level; this included efforts in screening, acute treatment, and aftercare. From the onset, this approach was marked by cooperation between patient care (neurology) and intervention (neuroradiology).

SCREENING

Exit surveys indicated that the illness most feared by inpatients was stroke. When free community screenings were held, large turnouts overwhelmed the volunteer staff. Yet the yield from the screenings was extremely low; fewer than 3% of screened patients had either carotid bruits or atrial fibrillation. Although those who attended the screenings were a captive audience and were fascinated with new treatments, it seemed that this was not an effective

means for stroke prevention. At best, such initial screenings were an educational forum and a time to showcase new efforts.

More effective programs of screening would include a wider search for the two areas where there is proof of efficacy of treatment: carotid atherostenosis and atrial fibrillation. New areas of potential effective treatment, such as plaque stabilization by pharmaceutical means, require the incorporation of serologic studies into any screening program. Because of the potential for dropout after screening, it appears reasonable to include as much imaging assessment as possible at the time of screening. This serves to focus the patient's attention on the problem, especially if the patient is given a photographic reminder of plaque.

A step that occurs before screening and that is implicit in any discussion of screening is the education of the public. This is an enormous issue that requires vast exertions to get those who should be screened to come in. Patients do not understand these issues and often resort to denial when warning symptoms of threatened stroke (transient ischemic attacks, or TIAs) occur. Although denial may be an important defense mechanism and not modifiable, the pessimism concerning stroke can be changed. We have worked to educate patients and physicians so that stroke is not seen as an inevitable part of aging and that once it occurs there is nothing to do. It is for this reason that our outreach programs have used our younger patients to send the message subliminally that stroke can occur at any age. Older patients are included in such programs so that age does not become an exclusion criterion or pejorative.

Although national efforts can be led by organized

bodies, such as the American Heart Association and the National Stroke Association, eventually the response has to trickle down to a community level. Everyone must be educated if any headway with prevention is to be made. Regardless of how advanced the science of treatment becomes, prevention always will be stronger medicine than treatment.

ACUTE TREATMENT

Patient Evaluation

With the publication of the National Institute of Neurological Disorders and Stroke (NINDS) recombinant tissue-type plasminogen activator trial in December 1995,[3] further emphasis was added to the two essential components of stroke treatment: time and team. In his editorial,[4] del Zoppo stated the following:

> For patients with acute myocardial infarction, the length of time before the initiation of thrombolytic therapy has an important bearing on clinical outcome. This is probably also true for stroke. The ability to perform a neurologic evaluation and computed tomography (CT), obtain informed consent, and carry out randomization in a period as short as three to six hours underscores the unusual efficiency of patient care in these clinical trials. It is unlikely that this level of efficiency could be easily duplicated in routine clinical practice. The NINDS results indicate that if any recovery is to be expected, very early intervention is necessary.

Our presentations from 1994 on emphasized that early intervention was the only intervention. After the appearance of the NINDS article, there followed letters to the editor in May 1996. In his reply, Marler added further emphasis[5]:

> This trial provides a basis for developing an acute care response to stroke. Further research may lower risks and increase benefits. In the meantime, we urge the development of the teams needed to treat stroke as the true emergency that it is.

These papers verified that there was something to do, that it should be done early, and that there needed to be an acute response team. For our study, the initial step in care was the patient or family recognizing that there was a problem. That recognition has to be coupled with a call to an emergency service (911) rather than to a physician's office. Once the patient was transported to a peripheral center, a checklist of inclusion and exclusion criteria had to be worked through (Table 63–1). Assuming that the inclusion criteria were met, the patient was transported to us *without any imaging study*. Obtaining imaging at a peripheral facility would take time, and scanners at those facilities did not provide the needed data to establish whether treatment could be considered. Once the patient was at our facility, we worked through our own list of inclusion and exclusion criteria (Table 63–2). Having established the concept of a therapeutic or treatment window, we asked that all our referring facilities not lose time while the window was open. The availability of air transport by helicopter did not provide any quicker yield of patients,

although when an outlying area's only ambulance was away on another call, air transport was used. Generally, we could get patients within 100 miles to our hospital quicker by ground transport than air.

The basis for an intervention-based program such as this was to move the patient as quickly as possible through the diagnostic arteriogram. Only after the angiographic data were available was it possible to begin to consider the type of endovascular treatment that would be presented to the patient and family for consideration. With continued fine tuning, we were able to reduce the elapsed time from the emergency room door to completion of diagnostic angiography to 45 minutes. This time included obtaining a noncontrast CT and neurologic examination.

Choice of Treatment

For patients screened angiographically, there were several clinical paths, including immediate revascularization or thrombolysis, arterial reconstruction (surgical or endovascular, without or with endovascular prosthesis [i.e., a stent]), a combination of revascularization and reconstruction, or conservative care. This algorithm is depicted in Table 63–3.

T A B L E 6 3 - 1   Peripheral Center for Criteria for Acute Ischemic Stroke

1. Stroke with submaximal deficit.
2. Known time of onset. If the patient awakens with deficit, duration of deficit is time from going to sleep.
3. Blood sugar greater than 50 mg/dl; can be performed with fingerstick method.

If these three criteria are met and the patient is receptive to treatment, then the patient is transported emergently and without obtaining imaging data.

T A B L E 6 3 - 2   Stroke Center Criteria for Acute Ischemic Stroke

Inclusion Criteria

1. Stroke with submaximal deficit
2. Known time of onset
3. Lack of contraindication

Contraindication/Exclusion

1. Coma
2. Maximal deficit (hemiplegia, sensory loss, field loss, and gaze paralysis)
3. Hypoglycemia (serum glucose <50)
4. Treatment unable to begin within time window
5. Bleeding disorder: hematologic, peptic ulcer disease, coagulopathy (prolonged prothrombin and activated partial thromboplastin times)
6. Recent transmural myocardial infarction (within 2 weeks)
7. Recent surgical procedures (including laparoscopic, within 2 weeks)
8. Trauma or puncture in a noncompressible site
9. Sensitivity to anticoagulants or thrombolytic agents
10. Uncontrolled hypertension (systolic >185 mm Hg)
11. Seizure at onset of stroke
12. Recent major stroke without satisfactory recovery

T A B L E 6 3 - 3	**Treatment Algorithm for Acute Ischemic Stroke Defined by Vascular Territory**

Revascularization by local thrombolysis
  Anterior circulation: 6-hour window
  Posterior circulation: longer window
Arterial reconstruction
  Carotid territory
    Bifurcation
      1. Small stroke—early reconstruction: CEA or PTA with stent
      2. Large stroke—delayed reconstruction: CEA or PTA with stent
    Surgically inaccessible
      1. Small stroke—early reconstruction: PTA
      2. Large stroke—delayed reconstruction: PTA
  Vertebrobasilar territory
    1. Vertebral origin: end-to-side reconstruction, PTA
    2. Distal vertebral, vertebrobasilar junction, basilar: PTA

CEA, carotid endarterectomy; PTA, percutaneous transluminal angioplasty.

Management of Transient Ischemic Attacks

Another large volume of patients seen through outpatient or emergency referral were those with TIAs. Although occasional patients underwent solely noninvasive investigation, angiographic delineation of the vascular anatomy usually permitted selection of treatment. This approach is outlined in Table 63–4.

RESULTS

Thrombolysis

We have used our algorithm in the treatment of 61 patients with stroke from thrombus or embolus in all

T A B L E 6 3 - 4	**Treatment Algorithm for Transient Ischemic Attack**

Carotid Territory

Bifurcation: CEA and PTA with endovascular prosthesis
Surgically inaccessible: PTA

Vertebrobasilar Territory

Vertebral origin: end-to-side reconstruction, PTA
Distal vertebral, vertebrobasilar junction, basilar: PTA

CEA, carotid endarterectomy; PTA, percutaneous transluminal angioplasty.

territories and vessels, primarily by intra-arterial thrombolysis with angioplasty (11 patients) or without angioplasty (50 patients). An example of our technique is shown in Figures 63–1 to 63–3. The method used for local thrombolysis in acute ischemic stroke is reviewed in Table 63–5.

In this population, we saw clinical improvement to a National Institutes of Health Stroke Scale (NIHSS) score of 0 to 1 in 70% of treated patients, without complicating hemorrhage.[6] These results exceed those reported with peripheral thrombolysis. An initial NIHSS score of more than 20 was associated with poor outcome. Immediate postprocedure CT was performed to ensure that there was no hemorrhage. This generally showed the treated area to be heavily stained with angiographic contrast. When staining was absent, this suggested a lack of reestablishment of flow. Separating contrast staining from reperfusion hemorrhage was challenging early in our series. Delayed magnetic resonance imaging (MRI) (at 72 to 96 hours) confirmed that there had been no reperfusion hemorrhage and showed that petechial

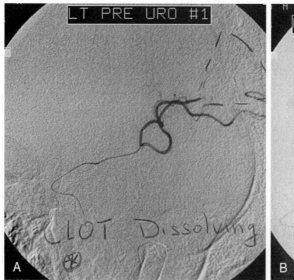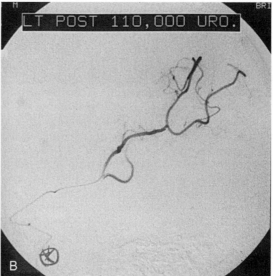

Figure 63-1 Case 1. Thrombolysis of occluded distal branch of the left middle cerebral artery (MCA). *A,* Lateral view obtained at the beginning of thrombolysis during injection through the microcatheter reveals abrupt cutoff of a branch. The parenchyma supplied by this branch *(dashed lines)* is not being perfused, and there is reflux of contrast into an adjacent branch. *B,* After thrombolysis, a repeat injection through the microcatheter reveals filling of the vessel and its distal branches, with minimal reflux into the adjacent branch.

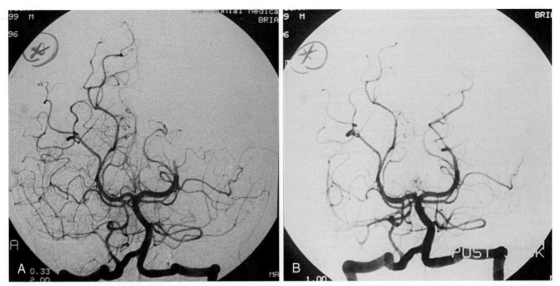

Figure 63-2 Case 2. Patient with left posterior cerebral artery occlusion treated with thrombolysis. *A,* Posteroanterior (PA) view (vertebral artery injection) before thrombolysis reveals abrupt cutoff of the posterior cerebral artery. *B,* After thrombolysis, there is restoration of flow in the artery and its branches distally.

change at the cortical periphery of ischemic change was lacking.

During the past 3 years, we have found that the dose of thrombolytic (urokinase) administered has declined steadily. There was more than a log drop from the often 2 million units to 250,000 units. This decrease was due to further refinement of catheter placement.

Of the 61 patients treated acutely, 14 had large-vessel (internal carotid artery, vertebral artery, basilar artery) occlusion. These cases were more challenging because clot volumes typically were large. Often, early arterial reconstruction by balloon angioplasty permitted reduction in thrombolytic dose; however, complicating hemorrhage occurred in 6% to

8% of the cases. Good outcomes were achieved in only two patients. Three patients died, and three patients' conditions worsened. Refinement of selection criteria is critical in these cases, especially with early access to the patient. This is an area in which new technologies in endovascular technique should presage clinical progress.

Angioplasty

A subset of patients with acute ischemic stroke or TIAs consisted of patients who had known symptomatic vascular stenosis but in whom treatment with sodium warfarin (Coumadin) failed. This cohort provided a basis for the balloon angioplasty series. The

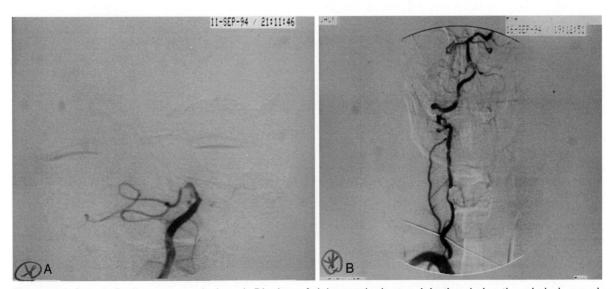

Figure 63-3 Case 3. Basilar artery occlusion. *A,* PA view of right vertebral artery injection during thrombolysis reveals occlusion of the basilar artery distal to the anterior inferior cerebellar artery. *B,* A right vertebral injection obtained during follow-up angiography 5 days later reveals the basilar artery and its distal branches to be patent. Note the dissection in the vessel proximally, the probable embolic source.

T A B L E   6 3 - 5   Method for Local Thrombolysis

1. The infusion catheter is placed firmly against the proximal clot face, and a hand infusion of thrombolytic agent (urokinase) is begun.
2. Systemic anticoagulation with intravenous heparin is begun before the use of thrombolytics. The heparin is given as a 5000-unit bolus and an infusion at 1000 U/hr.
3. Urokinase is mixed as 250,000 units in 50 ml of normal saline, providing a concentration of 5000 U/ml. A 50,000-unit bolus injection is made through the microcatheter, and a hand infusion of 5000 U/min is begun.
4. A digital angiogram run is made every 125,000 units to confirm catheter placement into the proximal thrombus and to verify the progress of thrombolysis.
5. Clot is lysed proximally to distally, and all angiographically identified clot is "chased." When the catheter cannot be advanced suitably, then a final infusion is made from the most distal accessible site. Generally, 250,000 units have been a total dose tolerated without hemorrhage. A ceiling of 2 million units is never exceeded.
6. After the procedure, the sheath is left in the groin, and systemic anticoagulation with heparin is continued until the sheath can be removed. A noncontrast head CT is obtained, and blood is sent immediately for platelet count, fibrinogen level, fibrin split products, and prothrombin and activated partial thromboplastin times.

CT, computed tomography.

general angioplasty procedure is given in Table 63–6.[7]

A total of 79 patients underwent angioplasty. Of these, 11 were performed acutely in combination with thrombolysis, as noted previously. As the series has grown, we have had the opportunity to treat patients in all vascular territories (see Table 63–7). Illustrative cases are shown in Figures 63–4 through 63–8.

AFTERCARE

Once endovascular treatment was complete, inpatient stays were limited. With effective re-establishment of flow, patients often improved to the point at which inpatient rehabilitation stays were brief or limited. The clinical pathway was modified to omit floor care for some cases of acute ischemic stroke, permitting patients to go from the intensive care unit to rehabilitation or home.

Because many patients came from many miles away, an effective program was necessary to include the referring physicians in the treatment and information exchange. As patients returned to their own communities for continued care, this program involved outpatient therapies and services, serologic monitoring of anticoagulation, and continued surveillance of identified atherostenotic lesions.

Programs for plaque stabilization using pharmacologic and adjunctive therapies have become increasingly important. The ability to provide information to patients about lifestyle issues and dietary change became a means of empowering them to participate in their care. Further scientific study of the efficacy of 3-hydroxy-3-methylglutaryl-coenzyme A (HMG-CoA) reductase inhibitors in normolipemic patients with

T A B L E   6 3 - 6   Method for Balloon Angioplasty

1. Pretreatment with aspirin, 325 mg, for 48 to 72 hours before the procedure.
2. Arteries are measured using a guidewire marked in millimeters (Medi-Tech Magic Torque calibrated hydrophilic guidewire). Once positioned, Philips digital measuring software is used, and the result is rounded down to the nearest 0.5 mm.
3. During the procedure, patients are given sublingual nifedipine and a 5000-unit bolus of heparin followed by a continuous infusion of 1000 U/hr.
4. Through a 6-Fr. Medi-Tech Pinnacle sheath, a 6-Fr. Cordis guide catheter is advanced to the C2 to C3 level.
5. A 0.016″ hydrophilic-coated microwire is used to cross the stenotic segment using digital roadmapping. A Stealth balloon angioplasty microcatheter (Target Therapeutics) is advanced to midstenosis. The 0.016″ microguidewire is then exchanged for a 0.0 cm valve wire, and the balloon is inflated to 8 atmospheres for 10 seconds. Alternatively, a 0.5- or 1-cm length Stratus (Medtronic/MIS) balloon angioplasty catheter can be used with a properly sized microwire.
6. After balloon deflation, angiography is performed through the guide catheter. If significant stenosis remains and there is no evidence of dissection or extravasation, one or two serial reinflations are performed using the same procedure. Generally, the angioplasty site is not recrossed with larger-sized balloons at the same sitting.
7. After the procedure, patients are admitted to the intensive care unit and maintained on heparin for 24 hours. Generally, patients are discharged on sodium warfarin (Coumadin) with or without antiplatelet agents.
8. For patients at high risk for hyperacute occlusion, abciximab (ReoPro) is administered intravenously at the conclusion of the diagnostic angiogram, before angioplasty.

atherostenosis may permit biochemical modification of existing plaque.

TECHNICAL PROBLEMS, COMPLICATIONS, AND SOLUTIONS

The overall complication rate has been low. There were three deaths out of 79 angioplasties (two due to arterial rupture) and a single complicating stroke. The low complication rate is due to several factors. First, it is not necessary to reconstruct the artery perfectly. Often, flow can be improved by mild

T A B L E   6 3 - 7   Distribution of Lesions in Patients Undergoing Angioplasty

Location	No. of Cases
Intracranial	41
Vertebral artery	7
Basilar artery	6
Petrous internal carotid artery	3
Cavernous internal carotid artery	10
Middle cerebral artery	15
Extracranial	38
Carotid artery bifurcation	28
Distal cervical internal carotid artery	1
Vertebral artery origin	2
Other miscellaneous locations	7

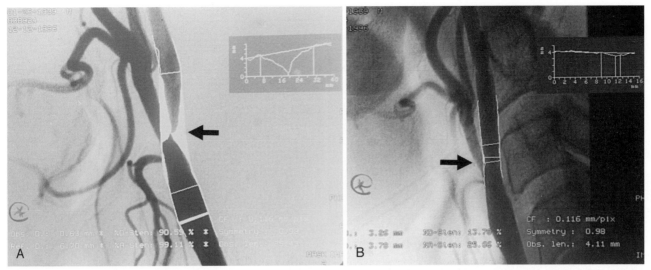

Figure 63-4 Case 4. Stenosis of the internal carotid artery (ICA) at the bifurcation. *A,* Injection of the common carotid artery demonstrates a high-grade stenosis *(arrow).* The measurements reveal 91% reduction in diameter and 99% reduction in area. *B,* A repeat view obtained after angioplasty and stent placement demonstrates the stent crossing the bifurcation. There is 14% residual reduction in diameter and 25% residual reduction in area at the level of the arrow.

changes in cross-sectional diameter. The average postprocedure stenosis in this series was about 30%. Oversizing the balloon can prove disastrous, whereas undersizing the balloon can be efficacious. Often, further remodeling occurs after completion of angioplasty, and this may be amenable to pharmaceutical manipulation.

Second, hyperacute thrombosis can be treated by

local thrombolysis and may be preventable with the use of abciximab (ReoPro). We used this agent when treating an isolated circulation, that is, one for which we did not have identifiable angiographic collateral.

Third, once a lesion was angioplastied, we tried to not recross the treated segment for additional treatment with a larger-sized balloon.

Fourth, generally we avoided using balloons of 3

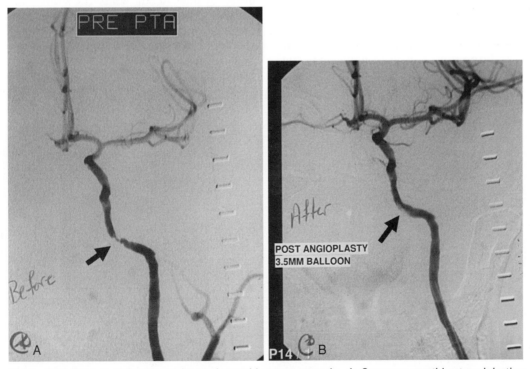

Figure 63-5 Case 5. Left petrous internal carotid artery stenosis. *A,* Common carotid artery injection reveals an irregular, high-grade stenosis *(arrow).* *B,* After angioplasty, there is still mild residual stenosis *(arrow),* but there is markedly improved distal runoff (note the improved filling of MCA branches and visualization of the ophthalmic artery and opposite MCA). This patient had a contralateral ICA occlusion.

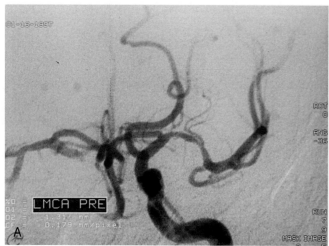 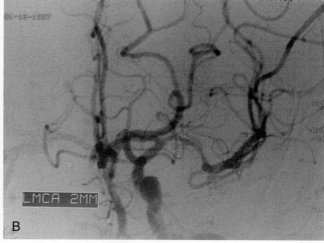

Figure 63-6 Case 6. Left MCA stenosis. *A,* PA view during left carotid artery injection reveals stenosis of the mid M1 segment just proximal to the origin of a group of lenticulostriate arteries. Note the filling of the basilar artery and the opposite anterior and middle cerebral arteries and distal internal carotid artery. This patient obviously has severe disease in multiple vessels! *B,* After angioplasty, the stenotic segment has a near-normal diameter. The lenticulostriate arteries continue to fill (an important observation).

mm or larger in the intercranial circulation to ensure undersizing. The two ruptures in this series occurred with a 3-mm balloon.

BENEFITS OF A DEDICATED ENDOVASCULAR SERVICE

Another collateral benefit from the endovascular service was the ability to identify patients with peripheral vascular disease, some of whom became candidates for peripheral angioplasty. Some patients were wrongly referred and were rerouted to other types of care, including treatment of subdural hematoma, brain tumor, central nervous system infection, or cardiac disease. The penumbra effect of the endovascular service was large and embraced additional specialty care, including neurosurgery, cardiology, general surgery, and vascular surgery.

REFERRALS

Successfully treated patients become ambassadors for further referrals. Additionally, they may become active in educational efforts in their own communities. We have had patients who have met with hospital officials to emphasize the time window for referral. Others started their own educational efforts, including one who started his own Web site for stroke.

We traveled frequently to speak to physicians or other groups about what they were doing in their centers. This permitted building a 14-hospital network of potential referrers. As other hospitals in their communities saw what we were doing, they began their own centers and hired interventional specialists. The development of many centers should prove to be a rising tide that will lift all the boats.

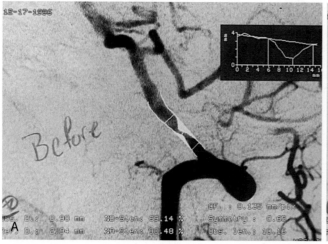 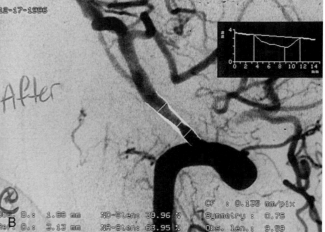

Figure 63-7 Case 7. Distal vertebral artery stenosis. *A,* Lateral view obtained during initial injection of the vertebral artery reveals a severe stenosis near the craniocervical junction. Measurement of the lesion reveals 69% reduction in diameter and 90% reduction in area. *B,* After angioplasty, there is 40% residual reduction in diameter and 64% residual reduction in area. These are not perfect results, but adequate flow has been restored (this is the goal, not a pretty postprocedure picture).

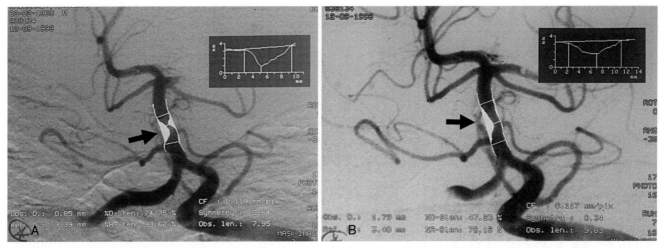

Figure 63-8 Case 8. Midbasilar artery stenosis. *A,* PA view during initial left vertebral artery injection reveals severe stenosis *(arrow),* resulting in 75% reduction in diameter and 93% reduction in area. These numbers do not truly represent the critical nature of this lesion—the residual diameter is at most 1 mm, and in situ thrombosis with occlusion is certainly a possibility. The appearance of the left posterior cerebral artery is due to inflow of unopacified blood from the posterior communicating artery rather than an occlusion. *B,* After angioplasty, there is still a moderate stenosis *(arrow)* with 47% reduction in diameter and 72% reduction in area, but there is significantly improved distal perfusion (note that the left posterior cerebral artery is now visualized—there is enough contrast-containing blood mixing with the unopacified blood to allow the vessel to be seen). The risk of thrombosis at the site of stenosis is greatly reduced, and there has been no potentially disastrous dissection of the vessel.

FUTURE TRENDS

Three years into our experience, we have seen dramatic growth in our clinical services. The angiographic volume that used to be performed in a month is now seen in a week. Imaging demand has resulted in acquisition of another high-field MRI scanner. Neurosonology volumes have increased by 250%. More than 130 patients have been treated with endovascular techniques. About half of patients screened go on to intervention, two thirds of which is surgical endarterectomy.

Reimbursement for new techniques restrains acute intervention in many centers. The low reimbursement for stroke makes acute intervention costly until reimbursement is changed to reflect today's treatment possibilities. The better outcomes occasioned by treatment reduce the subsequent expenses of caring for the patient with a completed stroke. Returning a patient to functional status permits that patient to contribute to society rather than becoming its ward. The lack of reimbursement for angioplasty above the aortic arch has prevented its wider use. With clinical proof of efficacy in stroke prevention, economic restraint will not prove successful or cost-effective. Patients demand better and expect better.

With the advent of better biochemical therapies for plaque stabilization, the medical profession is poised at the threshold of a revolution in cerebrovascular disease care. With an aging population, such a revolution will be essential in keeping health care in the United States the standard for the world.

REFERENCES

1. North American Symptomatic Carotid Endarterectomy Trial Collaborators. Beneficial effect of carotid endarterectomy in symptomatic patients with high-grade stenosis. *N Engl J Med* 1991;325:445–453.
2. Executive Committee for the Asymptomatic Carotid Atherosclerosis Study. Endarterectomy for asymptomatic carotid artery stenosis. *JAMA* 1995;18:1421–1428.
3. The National Institute of Neurological Disorders and Stroke rt-PA Stroke Study Group. Tissue plasminogen activator for acute ischemic stroke. *N Engl J Med* 1995;333:1581–1587.
4. del Zoppo GJ. Acute stroke-on the threshold of therapy? *N Engl J Med* 1995;333:1632–1633.
5. Marler JR. Authors reply. *N Engl J Med* 1996;334:1406.
6. Berger BL, Callahan AS, Weindling SM. Treatment of acute ischemic stroke from embolism [Abstract]. Proceedings of the 34th Annual Meeting, American Society of Neuroradiology, New York, 1992, p 115.
7. Callahan AS, Berger BL. Intracranial balloon angioplasty for stroke prevention. *J Neuroimag* 1997;7:232–235.

PART VII

COMPLICATIONS OF INTERVENTIONAL NEURORADIOLOGIC PROCEDURES AND THEIR TREATMENT

CHAPTER 64

Problems, Complications, and Solutions in Embolization

J.J. Connors III / J.C. Wojak

Perhaps the most important assets of a responsible and successful interventional neuroradiologist are knowledge of and respect for the myriad possible technical difficulties, procedural complications, and adverse reactions that may be encountered in any of these procedures. In addition, a thorough knowledge of the immediate maneuvers that may be necessary if difficulty arises during a case is an absolute necessity. In this way, it is hoped that the old ABCs of complications will not have to be relived (**a**ccuse, **b**lame, and **c**riticize).

Having all the necessary materials on hand before the case begins should be the rule. There may not be time to find items such as a temporary stenting catheter, urokinase, vasodilators, thrombin-coated fibered coils, or a snare when urgently needed during a case.

There are certain intrinsic risks involved with interventional neuroradiological procedures that are poorly defined or quantified at this time. For the novice practitioner or clinician, the most easily understood risks are those related to embolization, most particularly when using "glue" (cyanoacrylates). This has been performed for a number of years, and the general medical community has had at least some exposure to this procedure and its risks. Perhaps more difficult to quantitate (and perhaps underappreciated, as well) is the risk associated with working inside intrinsically diseased vessels.

The original work performed in interventional neuroradiology was not aimed specifically at degenerative vascular disease or sick vessels per se but rather at tumors or vascular anomalies (e.g., arteriovenous malformations [AVMs], arteriovenous fistulae). These vessels not only were relatively young (in their owners) but sometimes were even tougher than normal vessels because of their workload. These vessels could be manipulated in a manner that, in retrospect, appears amazingly aggressive. Recent endeavors in the field of interventional neuroradiology have intruded into "repair work" rather than "demolition." Demolition work is far simpler than repair work, and the early lessons learned by pioneers in the field concerning catheterization and manipulation of diseased vessels need to be taken to heart. Simply advancing a guidewire in a diseased vessel can have unforeseen consequences, and angioplasty has become one of the more dangerous procedures performed.

Note should be made that there are far more complications than can be mentioned here; indeed, many other complications have been mentioned in the text during the discussion of various pathologies. Those discussed in this chapter are some of the major and more common ones that potentially are treatable rather than simply lamentable.

As opposed to other fields of interventional radiology, the complications of interventional neuroradiology procedures usually are not directly treatable. Knowledge of these therefore is necessary from the standpoint of prevention rather than treatment. Luckily, however, some complications can be addressed.

Most complications related to embolotherapy are related to inadequate knowledge rather than to accidents or poor technique. Accidental reflux of material can and does occur, as do other mishaps, but it is the incorrect choice of embolic material, the incorrect use of such, the incorrect choice of embolic location, poor fluoroscopic visualization, or other strategic errors that are the primary causes of significant complications. Once again, simply being capable of performing a procedure should not constitute certification of competence to perform that procedure.

In general, particulate emboli are less dangerous than liquids, but flow dynamics and location can alter danger parameters considerably. In addition, there probably exists a certain degree of good and bad luck concerning some poor outcomes when embolizing certain vessels; sometimes, a complication occurs even when everything is done according to plan (i.e., a cranial nerve deficit can result from the use of routine embolic particles in 1 patient but not in 20 others). Intimate knowledge of vascular territories, dangerous collaterals, particular dangerous vessels (see Chapter 5), and hemodynamics is absolutely necessary. The following is an overview of the more common complications of neurointerventional embolotherapy.

MICROPARTICULATE PULMONARY EMBOLISM

It is almost axiomatic that in any microparticulate embolization procedure there is at least some embolization to the lungs. This is of concern to the interventional neuroradiologist because not many other endovascular embolizations (i.e., peripheral) are performed, and when they are, they commonly involve use of coils. Almost exclusively, it is interventional neuroradiologic cases that require extensive use of microparticles. Care has to be taken to prevent an inadvertent amount of pulmonary embolization.

When this occurs, it is due to lack of appreciation of the hemodynamics of the embolization procedure and the possible need for adaptation (i.e., use a larger size particle, proximal flow control, or another technique).

When extensive pulmonary embolization has occurred, it may be difficult to detect by standard laboratory means, even if significantly symptomatic. In particular, standard ventilation–perfusion radionuclide scans are either nondiagnostic, nonspecific, or normal. Pulmonary angiography is unremarkable other than potentially revealing increased pulmonary artery pressure. Usually, no focal defects are seen. The clinical findings are more suggestive of chronic (or acute) pulmonary hypertension than acute embolus, except for the acute onset of symptoms.

Increased pulmonary artery pressure can affect cardiac function to a varying degree. The degree of pulmonary hypertension that develops is dependent on the degree of loss of cross-sectional area of the pulmonary vascular bed. In addition, prolonged increased flow through the remaining channels may incite secondary hypertensive changes in these vessels, further increasing vascular resistance and contributing to increased right ventricular workload.

The hallmark of this process is dyspnea. This may be exertional or at rest, depending on the severity of the capillary occlusion and hypertension. Other symptoms include fatigue and occasionally acute pleuritic chest pain. In the extreme case, there is a progressive increase in hypertension, and cor pulmonale can develop. The chest radiography and electrocardiography (ECG) findings are nonspecific and reflect the degree of pulmonary hypertension and resultant right ventricular and atrial enlargement,[1] but these findings may not be present because of the acuteness of the situation.

The treatment of pulmonary hypertension secondary to embolization of the vascular bed is supportive. If the patient is hypoxic, oxygen is administered. As previously noted, anticoagulation is indicated to prevent propagation of capillary plugs and further vascular occlusion. Digoxin combined with low salt intake and possibly a loop diuretic may be helpful.

In the long term, the lungs can compensate to some degree, but a certain amount of loss of pulmonary vascular bed probably is permanent. It appears that this symptomatology requires a massive amount of microparticulate embolization. Current techniques combined with the trained interventional neuroradiologist's knowledge of correct technique appear to have decreased the incidence of inadvertent symptomatic pulmonary embolization.

When a fulminant situation is present, the use of intrapulmonary artery nitroglycerin may decrease vascular resistance for a short time, allowing for acute adaptation. This is an unproved but possibly useful maneuver. The nitroglycerin can be titrated to the point of inducing systemic hypotension. Another agent that can be used in this setting is prostacyclin (Flolan). This drug is approved for the treatment of acute and chronic pulmonary hypertension and is administered through a central venous catheter or through a Swan-Ganz catheter. It acts as a pulmonary and systemic arterial vasodilator and inhibits platelet aggregation (an ideal combination in this setting). It can be administered for a longer time than nitroglycerin, allowing the patient's system more time to adapt.

If a patient has preexisting high-output cardiac failure that has been physiologically compensated, even a small amount of polyvinyl alcohol (PVA) particles may cause an acute decompensation; therefore, care should be maintained during embolization in a patient of this type.

CRANIAL NERVE DAMAGE

Any procedure involving the skull base, cavernous sinus, or vessels of the neck can cause a cranial nerve palsy. This usually is temporary, unless a toxic liquid agent has been used (e.g., alcohol or glue). In the cavernous sinus, mass effect or increased venous pressure can cause cranial nerve palsies that improve slowly, particularly if the underlying insult has been corrected.

Rarely does particulate arterial embolization result in cranial nerve palsy, but it has occurred. It can be due to mass effect rather than to the direct effect of the embolization (devascularization with subsequent nerve death). Mass effect or hypoperfusion usually results in temporary deficits. Although no therapy has been proved successful, treatment with steroids is indicated.

When embolizing with particulate matter in the region of the skull base, even presumably "safe" vessels can cause problems (see Chapter 5). In general, particles greater than 150 to 250 microns in diameter usually do not cause serious or permanent problems related to cranial nerve palsy or tissue necrosis, although such problems have been reported. Note should be made that agents such as Avitene or Gelfoam powder can contain particles smaller than 50 microns in diameter and thus can penetrate to a distal location and cause true cell death.

Liquid embolic agents are far more dangerous than particulate agents. The exception to this may be Ethibloc, a more viscous substance not capable of the rapid distal micropenetration of ethanol and cyanoacrylates (see Chapter 1). These agents should be used with extreme caution in the vicinity of the skull base and cavernous sinus.

CARDIOPULMONARY COLLAPSE AFTER ETHANOL EMBOLIZATION

Reports have been made of an unusual syndrome related to ethanol use. For unknown reasons, after even minor amounts of ethanol have been used, some patients have been noted to become bradycardic and appear to suffer an acute pulmonary hypertensive event. Some practitioners have begun to place a Swan-Ganz catheter in the main pulmonary artery to monitor central pulmonary artery pressure during an ethanol embolization case, with the goal of ceasing embolization if a rise in pulmonary artery pressure is seen. Depending on the patient's preexisting cardiopulmonary status, a rapid though minimal rise may be significant.

Treatment

If a transient significant increase in pulmonary artery pressure is noted, instillation of nitroglycerin directly through the Swan-Ganz catheter and into the main pulmonary artery may help to lower the pulmonary artery hypertension. No controlled trials have been performed, but some practitioners familiar with this potential disaster routinely use 200 µg/ml of nitroglycerin infused at a "wide-open" rate. The goal of this therapy is to relieve what is believed to be spasm of the precapillary arterioles in the pulmonary

tree, and this can be of overriding importance. The massive amounts of nitroglycerin can cause systemic effects and drop the systemic blood pressure, at which point the infusion has to be slowed. Conversely, when the pulmonary hypertension begins to respond to the infusion of nitroglycerin, the infusion can be slowed. This is a balancing act that requires trained anesthesiologic skills.

Another agent that can be used in this setting is prostacyclin. This produces direct vasodilation of the pulmonary and systemic arterial beds and inhibits platelet aggregation. The agent is infused through a central venous catheter or through the Swan-Ganz catheter, beginning at a rate of 2 ng/kg/min. The dose can be increased in 2 ng/kg/min increments; doses above 8 ng/kg/min generally produce dose-limiting side effects, such as bradycardia and hypotension. Again, the use of this agent is best left in the hands of the anesthesiologist.

TISSUE NECROSIS

The term *tissue necrosis* generally applies to death of tissue that is not of vital importance (e.g., skin); otherwise, another term for this complication would be used (e.g., *stroke*). Usually, tissue necrosis involves damage to scalp, face, or neck structures or causes impaired postoperative healing. It can be caused by ischemic insult or direct toxic effect.

Generally, tissue necrosis is not a significant problem unless territories of known vascular overlap are all embolized with material capable of penetrating to the anastomotic arteriole level, thus precluding collateral recruitment. Certain areas are more vulnerable than others, with more or less significant consequences. Territories that are at the extreme limits of distribution of only two vessels are more vulnerable than those that may be reached by several vessels. The tip of the nose is an example of a region that may be supplied by up to six or eight different vessels, whereas the occipital scalp may have a surprisingly limited collateral supply in some people.

In general, it is possible to embolize both sides of overlapping territories if very small particles (150 to 250 microns) are used on only one side and medium to large particles (350 to 750 microns) are used on the other. If small particulate embolization is used in a patient with intrinsically deficient collaterals or capillaries, however, necrosis or (more commonly) hair loss or poor healing can result.

Treatment

By the time this complication manifests, treatment usually is late and ineffective. Therapy is aimed at creating conditions that increase local perfusion. This can include local warmth, with or without anticoagulation, or the use of a peripheral vasodilator. Depending on location, surgical repair may be possible with a flap. Secondary infection is a potential threat that is difficult to treat in a devascularized area; this problem is rare.

COIL MALPOSITION

Deposit of a coil in an incorrect location can occur; more commonly, a portion of coil may protrude into a vital parent vessel. Although this can have disastrous consequences depending on coil location, this is not necessarily the case. Although this frequently is an unforeseeable technical problem, as more cases are performed by the practitioner, more experience is gained and fewer problems occur.

Malposition of a coil can be due to poor coil choice, poor catheter position, or poor technique. For instance, as a coil is deposited, it may be necessary to advance the catheter slightly to hold the tip in position (i.e., place some downstream force on the tip of the catheter to help prevent reflux of the tip of the catheter during forceful coil extrusion). The skills necessary to perform microcoil embolization are beyond the scope of this discussion and require not only training but also practice.

A straight coil should never be placed just within the orifice of the feeder from the normal branch. There is nothing to hold it in position, and any change in pulse or gravity, or even a cough, can jar the coil loose and eject it back into the flowing vessel. Any coil placed just within the orifice should have an intrinsic curl and should be self-retaining (e.g., a small BOD coil [Target Therapeutics]).

Treatment

If a small microcoil embolizes to a normal distal cortical branch, immediate anticoagulation is required. If the coil truly "blew" downstream, it must have been very small and therefore should not cause a major vessel occlusion. Typically, a cortical branch can tolerate a small peripheral occlusion; in this case, distal reconstitution or collateral supply occurs. In fact, a small coil displaced by a cough has been seen to enter a middle cerebral cortical branch with no sequelae whatsoever. Heparinization allows time for hemodynamic adaptation and prevents formation or propagation of thrombus.

Thrombosis can occur despite heparinization, but this can be readily treated by fibrinolysis. Once cleared, it remains clear with heparin administration and potentieally without. Once a surface layer of platelets has adhered to the coil surface, no further stimulation to thrombotic cascade is present, and the situation should stabilize. Therefore, a period of watchful waiting after an inadvertent coil embolization should be maintained; 1 hour is probably enough.

If a microcoil has embolized to the lung, no specific treatment is necessary. Typically, the pulmonary artery branch involved is small, and the insult is asymptomatic. Attempt at retrieval is difficult, should be unnecessary, and adds risk. The branch may not even become permanently occluded. The coil can become endothelialized, and a lumen can persist past it.

If the tail of a coil is protruding into the lumen of an intracranial parent vessel, immediate heparinization is indicated. In addition, aspirin therapy should be instituted (its antiplatelet effect can begin to work in a matter of hours, if not minutes). Abciximab (ReoPro) is an intravenously administered drug with strong and immediate platelet aggregation inhibitory effects and would probably be of more immediate use in this situation than aspirin (see Chapter 4).

Most commonly, if the tail of the coil is in a high-flow vessel and occludes only a small portion of the lumen, complete occlusion of the vessel does not occur. Thrombi can form and embolize distally, however. If thrombus does begin to form around the coil in a vital vessel, fibrinolysis can dissolve this, usually without difficulty. As stated previously, once the initial thrombus has been lysed, the platelet coat can stabilize, and clot tends not to reform. Abciximab would appear to be the ideal agent for use in this situation as well as aspirin. Aspirin or ticlopidine should be instituted for 3 months.

Commercially available microsnares are available from Target Therapeutics and Microvena (see "How to Use a Snare" in Chapter 3), but their use is difficult and can make a bad situation worse. They can, however, succeed in retrieving a coil if truly necessary. In addition, the patient can be referred to a clinician experienced in microcoil retrieval and the use of microsnares.

BALLOONS

Premature Detachment

Balloons can have dramatic results when used for occlusion, but they are difficult and dangerous to use. Untoward detachment can result in migration to a hazardous location. It cannot be emphasized enough how much help a flow control guide catheter can be when using detachable balloons (see "Flow Control Catheters" in Chapter 1).

If accidental detachment occurs when treating a large arteriovenous fistula, the inflated balloon can embolize to the lungs. This typically occurs when the balloon has been detached in essentially the correct location, but owing to pulse pressure or lack of adequate friction between the wall and the vessel, the balloon migrates. For this reason, it is wise to have a long Chiba-type needle available to puncture the balloon emergently. A punctured or deflated balloon in the lung is of minimal consequence, whereas an occluded main or lobar pulmonary artery may be life-threatening.

Secondary effects of balloon occlusion of large arteriovenous fistulae are discussed in Chapter 15. Suffice it to say that total cessation of flow through a large fistula leaving a huge residual venous pouch can be the source of a large pulmonary embolus.

Accidental detachment and migration of a balloon to an intracranial location should be addressed by immediate anticoagulation and induction of arterial hypertension. Premature detachment should not be a problem if a flow control guide catheter is used, but postdetachment migration can occur secondary to the force of a fistula. An open embolectomy can be performed by a neurosurgeon. If this is not possible, anticoagulation and hypertension can allow whatever physiologic hemodynamic adaptation is possible to occur. Retrieval of a balloon by a snare may be feasible but technically difficult if not impossible in the small vessels in the brain. Once again, use of a flow control guide catheter during initial placement of the balloon is helpful. The detached balloon remains in place until another balloon (or coils) can be placed to hold it.

Nondeflating Balloon

If the balloon does not deflate while in an intracranial position, it should not be moved. Initially, a guidewire should be placed through the catheter into the balloon. This tends to stent the catheter and balloon neck open, so that aspiration can be performed. (The guidewire has to be placed through a Y-connector, so that aspiration can be performed around the wire.) The wire should be uncoated and have a coil at the end, not a monofilament; the uncoated coil does not seal as tightly as a monofilament.

If this maneuver does not work, the balloon should be overinflated and ruptured where it sits. This is safer than trying to remove it if there is any question about it binding or becoming dislodged.

A ruptured but nondetached balloon is not a significant problem so long as the balloon was prepared properly (i.e., there was no air bubble in it) and there is no attempt to withdraw the balloon and delivery catheter back into the guide catheter. The entire unit should be withdrawn into the descending aorta before further manipulation is attempted. An attempt at withdrawal of the delivery catheter and balloon remnant into the guide catheter can be made carefully (see Chapter 3).

Invisible Balloon

If a balloon cannot be seen with injection of contrast, it is either detached, deflated (popped), or filled with saline instead of contrast. The operator should aspirate slightly and constantly on the syringe for a minute. If blood returns, it is either popped or detached, and the catheter can be withdrawn safely as described previously.

If blood does not return on aspiration, the balloon probably is still attached, whether inflated or not. In the rare circumstance, it could be inflated and not deflating even with aspiration (i.e., the balloon could be occluding the tip of the catheter); therefore, it is necessary to determine if the balloon is still there.

If there is some concern that the balloon is still on the catheter (but not deflating), but it is still invisible, there are two options. First, an attempt should be made to *advance* the catheter slightly (do not try to withdraw it, even slightly); this should indicate if the balloon is inflated. If the catheter doesn't advance correctly, the balloon is possibly inflated. Alterna-

tively, contrast can be injected through the guide catheter and observation made for a filling defect at the end of the catheter.

If the balloon is inflated and there is trouble with deflation, this may be helped by advancing a guidewire to the tip of the catheter and out the end slightly (through a rotating hemostatic valve on the hub of the microcatheter). Care should be taken because advancing this wire too far can dislodge the balloon. This maneuver can help to "stent open" the catheter tip, allowing deflation of the balloon by having contrast come back around the wire.

Conversely, it is also possible to burst the balloon intentionally by overinflating it. This allows safer withdrawal of the catheter. *A balloon that possibly is even slightly inflated should never be withdrawn.*

POSTEMBOLIC SYNDROME

A constellation of signs and symptoms, including local pain, elevation of peripheral leukocyte count, and fever has been described by interventional radiologists after embolization of tumors (such as renal cell carcinomas, giant cell tumors, and aneurysmal bone cysts) and solid parenchymal organs (such as the spleen).[2–5] These findings have been noted to vary somewhat depending on the type of embolization performed. When particulates are used, pain typically begins 30 to 60 minutes after embolization; symptoms may last 24 to 72 hours. When absolute ethanol is used, pain is immediate, and the full-fledged postembolic syndrome may not develop.

The same signs and symptoms can be seen after embolization of tumors such as meningiomas, paragangliomas, and juvenile nasopharyngeal angiofibromas. Ketorolac tromethamine (Toradol), a potent, injectable nonsteroidal anti-inflammatory drug, controls the pain and fever well. It is important to administer a loading dose immediately on onset of symptoms (60 mg intramuscularly for a typical adult patient) and continue with 30 mg every 6 hours (*not* prn) to maintain an adequate serum level and symptomatic relief. This is generally continued for 48 hours.

HYPERTENSIVE CRISIS

Hypertensive crisis usually is precipitated (in interventional neuroradiology) by the manipulation or embolization of paragangliomas (glomus tumors). They can be vasoactive in up to 5% of cases. Patients typically have symptoms related to catecholamine or serotonin release, producing episodic palpitations, sweating, flushing, or headaches.

Studies have shown that the risk of embolization producing a hypertensive crisis is small.[6] When it happens, however, it gets the interventionist's attention.

Premedication with an α-adrenergic blocker is useful; phentolamine or phenoxybenzamine typically is used. If a reaction occurs during the procedure, 5-mg intravenous boluses of phentolamine mesylate are given, up to 20 mg in an adult male. If needed, labetalol can be given concurrently; 10 mg/min can be given, up to a total of 300 mg.

If tachycardia is also present, a β-adrenergic blocker usually effectively addresses this, such as propranolol, 2 to 10 mg given intravenously over a 10-minute period.

If the hypertensive crisis is unresponsive to the above measures, an anesthesiologist should be contacted to manage a nitroprusside drip (anywhere up to 600 to 800 μg/min). The latter can deal effectively with the most severe reaction, but if the reaction has gone this far, an entire team of physicians usually is necessary to manage the patient.

NORMAL PERFUSION PRESSURE BREAKTHROUGH

Areas of chronically decreased perfusion pressure may be present in patients with occlusive atherosclerotic disease or with large, high-flow AVMs, which steal from the surrounding brain. When normal pressure is restored to these regions, there may be edema or frank hemorrhage. This has been termed *normal perfusion pressure breakthrough*.[7] In regions with chronic hypoperfusion, there is little or no cerebrovascular reserve. The arterioles in these regions lose their normal pressure sensitivity. When normal pressure is restored suddenly, there is vascular disruption, leakage of blood products, edema, or hemorrhage. The changes are similar to hypertensive encephalopathy but occur at normal pressure.

This phenomenon has been recognized as a possible complication of carotid endarterectomy for many years.[8] In patients undergoing endarterectomy who are suspected on the basis of clinical or angiographic findings to be at risk, the acetazolamide challenge test (as described in Chapter 3) may be helpful in identifying areas of impaired vasoreactivity. It also has been described in patients undergoing treatment for high-flow arteriovenous fistulae (carotid and vertebral) with chronic ischemia distal to the fistula secondary to steal.[9]

Normal perfusion pressure breakthrough also is suspected to occur in the region surrounding high-flow AVMs. Early evidence, however, indicates that *hyperreactivity* of the surrounding vessels in response to acetazolamide challenge is associated with poor outcome; the implications of this are not clear.[10]

Once normal perfusion pressure breakthrough occurs, there is little that can be done to treat it, except for vigorous antihypertensive therapy (systemic hypertension only worsens the situation; there is already too much flow). In the case of large AVMs, staged embolization (allowing for a more gradual shift in hemodynamics) may be helpful, but this is not always feasible.

Steroid use would appear to be of use, if for no other reason than membrane stabilization, but this is unproved.

FAILURE OF RESIDUAL TRUNK PATENCY: RETROGRADE THROMBOSIS

Occlusion of the distal portion of a large vascular pedicle to a high-flow AVM that leaves the large trunk patent to supply some small residual side branches may not be successful. The high flow going to the AVM is what kept the large trunk open. If most of the flow is stopped, the trunk may thrombose back to the first large side branch, thus occluding any small side branches that were meticulously spared. This can be a significant problem for both a surgeon and an endovascular therapist, either of whom would occlude the large feeder in the same location. Staging the embolization may help to circumvent this problem by allowing the large pedicle to shrink to a size appropriate to the demand of the remaining side branches.

CATHETER OCCLUSION

During an embolization procedure with a microcatheter, it is not unusual for the microcatheter to become clogged, either by particulate agents or by coils. The best way to deal with this problem is to prevent it from happening.

If the catheter is clogged by particulate agents, the problem could occur at any point along the length of the catheter. Most commonly, however, the problem is at the hub. The large lumen of the syringe funnels down to the small lumen of the catheter, and at that point, the particles can become jammed. This can be prevented by judicious flushing of the funnel of the hub with saline between syringes of embolic agents. Frequent shaking of the particle-containing syringe (and therefore continual mixing of the particles) during injection also should be employed. Be sure to choose a brand of PVA that mixes well with water (hydrates) and stays suspended well. In addition, careful attention to this funneling region of the hub should be maintained while embolizing to watch for particle clumping.

The original mixture of embolic material also can be made more dilute, thus causing less crowding in the funneling region of the hub. This is particularly true for the larger particles. The larger the embolic particles, the more dilute the particles need to be. Practice makes perfect. Also, certain embolic materials tend to clump more readily than others. This clumping may be an advantage for the intravascular result of embolization but a liability for the actual delivery process.

If jamming has occurred in the hub, clearing can be obtained with a small-gauge intravenous catheter or needle attached to a syringe, which is slowly inserted while vigorously flushing through it. A small guidewire (0.009″) may be used (butt end) to try to poke a hole in the jam and help loosen the particles. If the jam actually is down in the hub or distal in the catheter, pressure from a 1-cc syringe can clear the clog, at the risk of catheter rupture. The risk is dependent on the specific make of catheter.

If the problem is at the hub and simple clearing is not successful, replacement of the catheter is the correct choice.

If particles are clogged near the distal end of the catheter, clearance with a guidewire smaller than the lumen may work (e.g., 0.009″). If there are abrupt curves in the catheter near its end (due to tortuous vascular anatomy), there may be a change from a round lumen to an oval one, as frequently occurs. If this is the case, ramming with a guidewire may invite perforation of the catheter just proximal to or at the kink. In addition, any clogged particles can become even more completely packed by this maneuver. Slow infusion with a 1-cc syringe is the best bet, recognizing that a forceful injection may rupture the catheter. A 1-cc syringe can develop tremendous force in these microcatheters. Slight withdrawal may change the location of the oval lumen, freeing the clog. Again, replacement of the catheter probably is the correct decision.

If the catheter is clogged by a coil, an attempt can be made to flush the coil with a 1-cc syringe filled with saline. This can dislodge the jammed coil or flush any red blood cells away from the coil, thus freeing it. This also can rupture the catheter proximal to the jam point. Caution is indicated. If the coil cannot be freed easily and is completely within the catheter, withdrawal of the entire unit is the correct option. Again, the coil usually is jammed at a point of constriction of the catheter lumen because of ovaling. Withdrawal as a unit usually can be done without difficulty.

If a portion of coil is protruding from the end of the catheter, the situation is more complex, but slow withdrawal usually is successful. The protruding coil is soft and tends not to grab the vessel as much as would be thought. A note of caution is in order, however. The reason the coil became jammed usually is that the catheter had a tight curve at some point and the lumen became oval, thus decreasing its luminal diameter. When the catheter is withdrawn, this decreased lumen returns to normal, which can free the coil. Constant aspiration during the slow withdrawal is recommended.

Retrieval of a coil that becomes dislodged is covered under "Coil Malposition" and "How to Use a Snare" in Chapter 3.

During any embolization procedure, frequent flushing between embolization syringes or coils is needed. This is to prevent any thrombus from forming in the catheter, to keep it filled with only saline, and to appreciate the intracatheter flow dynamics. It is possible to "feel" when there is an early problem developing—the force needed to flush the catheter changes subtly.

Frequent evaluation of the embolization results with repeat contrast injections also is needed. This requires only 1 to 2 ml of contrast per test. After a contrast injection, clearance with saline is necessary before repeat embolization is performed with either particles or coils. This is to maintain low viscosity in the catheter and to allow visualization of when the embolic particles start to exit the catheter during the injection. If the catheter is full of contrast, it is not possible to see when the particles start to exit the catheter because plain contrast is followed by the contrast and particle suspension.

PROBLEMS ASSOCIATED WITH FLOW-DIRECTED CATHETERS

The 1.5-Fr. Magic (Balt Extrusion) catheters tend to ball up and migrate distally when broken off but 1.8-Fr. Magic catheters do not. When a catheter is broken off, thrombus tends to form at its *end*, not along the sides; fibrin is seen along the sides. Thrombus/fibrin will tend to form a tail.

During withdrawal of the microcatheter, pulling the *guide catheter* simultaneously with the microcatheter tends to not let the microcatheter stretch as much. The pulling force may be transferred to the end of the guide catheter more effectively than by just pulling the microcatheter; it applies tension more distally on the microcatheter, as if the microcatheter were being pulled at the point where it exits the guide catheter. It will be more likely to break distally or come out.

Stuck Flow-Directed Catheters

It is rare for an over-the-wire microcatheter to become stuck in a distal intracranial vessel; this almost always occurs with flow-directed microcatheters without hydrophilic coating. In this rare circumstance, several maneuvers can be performed. There are three common causes of inability to remove a microcatheter: (1) vasospasm actively holding the catheter, (2) simple friction, or (3) gluing of the catheter into the vessel. If the catheter is stuck and it is anticipated that it will remain within the vessel for a prolonged time, the patient should be anticoagulated to prevent thrombus from forming.

Flow-directed catheters can become stuck before glue is injected because of vasospasm around the distal portion. Once the microcatheter is in position, backing it out slightly and allowing it to readvance on its own before rinsing it and injecting glue will confirm the absence of spasm and the free nature of its distal position. If the catheter is stuck because of vasospasm, nitroglycerin or papaverine can be infused through the guide catheter. Alternatively, a very slow gradual traction can be placed on the catheter and patiently held for a few minutes. This may allow the catheter to gradually withdraw.

Slow, gentle traction may also free a catheter that is stuck because of simple friction between the catheter and the vessel walls if the vessel is tortuous. If traction does not free the catheter, a more aggressive maneuver can be attempted. Slight kinks are placed at 5- to 10-mm intervals along the distal portion of a hydrophilic-coated microwire (e.g., the 0.010″ Quicksilver-10 [Medtronic/MIS]). The wire is advanced through the catheter until it is about 1 cm from the tip of the catheter. The wire is then rotated while the catheter is slowly withdrawn. This rotating, contorted wire tends to pull the catheter off the wall of the vessel and tends to release any points of friction. This system of removal works very well for any situation other than true spasm clamped tightly on one spot of the catheter.

A final, last-ditch effort to free the stuck catheter may be undertaken by anticoagulating the patient fully, probably utilizing antiplatelet agents as well, and placing a fixed traction force on the catheter overnight. The catheter may be freed when the patient is re-examined the next day.

If the catheter is actually glued in place with cyanoacrylates, the only way to release this is to break the catheter or the glue. The management of broken catheters is discussed in Chapter 66.

REFERENCES

1. Viner SM, Bagg BR, Auger WR, Ford GT. The management of pulmonary hypertension secondary to chronic thromboembolic disease. *Prog Cardiovasc Dis* 1994;37:79–92.
2. McLean GK, Meranze SG. Embolization techniques in the urinary tract. *Radiol Clin* 1986;24:671.
3. Chuang V, Wallace S, Swanson D, et al. Arterial occlusion in the management of pain from metastatic renal carcinoma. *Radiology* 1979;133:611–614.
4. Chuang V, Soo C-S, Wallace S, Benjamin R. Arterial occlusion: management of giant cell tumor and aneurysmal bone cyst. *AJR* 1981;136:1127–1130.
5. Keller FS, Rösch J, Bird CB. Percutaneous embolization of bony pelvic neoplasms with tissue adhesive. *Radiology* 1983;147:21–27.
6. Kretzschmar K, Milewski C, Dienes HP. The risk of endocrine activation in interventional procedures on paraganglioma of the head and neck. *Radiologe* 1988;28:497–502.
7. Spetzler RF, Wilson CB, Weinstein P, et al. Normal perfusion

pressure breakthrough theory. *Clin Neurosurg* 1978;25:651–672.
8. Sundt TM Jr. The ischemic tolerance of neural tissue and the need for monitoring and selective shunting during carotid endarterectomy. *Stroke* 1983;14:93–98.
9. Halbach VV, Higashida RT, Hieshima GB, Norman D. Normal perfusion pressure breakthrough occurring during treatment of carotid and vertebral fistulas. *AJNR* 1987;8:751–756.
10. Batjer HH, Devous MD. The use of acetazolamide-enhanced regional cerebral blood flow measurement to predict risk for arteriovenous malformation patients. *Neurosurgery* 1992;31:213–217.

ADDITIONAL REFERENCES

Coils

Chuang V, Wallace S, Gianturco C, Soo C-S. Complications of coil embolization: prevention and management. *AJR* 1981;137:809–813.

Embolization

Eskridge JM, Harris AB, Finch L, Alotis MA. Carotid sinus syndrome and embolization procedures. *AJNR* 1993;14:818–820.
Martins IP, Baeta E, Paiva T, et al. Headaches during intracranial endovascular procedures: a possible model of vascular headache. *Headache* 1993;33:227–233.
Partington CR, Graves VB, Rufenacht DA, et al. Biocompatibility of 1-French, polyethylene catheters used in interventional neuroradiology procedures: a study with rats and dogs. *AJNR* 1990;11:881–885.

Normal Perfusion Pressure Breakthrough

Powers AD, Smith RR. Hyperperfusion syndrome after carotid endarterectomy: a transcranial Doppler evaluation. *Neurosurgery* 1990;26:56–60.
Wilson CB, Hieshima G. Occlusive hyperemia: a new way to think about an old problem. *J Neurosurg* 1993;78:165–166.

CHAPTER 65

Rupture of a Vessel, Aneurysm, or Arteriovenous Malformation

J.J. Connors III / J.C. Wojak

First and foremost, when any intracranial hemorrhage occurs, anticoagulation must be reversed immediately.

INTRACRANIAL VASCULAR PERFORATION

Perforation of a vessel is a rare occurrence during intracranial work and usually is related to microguidewire manipulation. This infrequently requires treatment, but the decision to treat should be rapid.[1] A microwire makes a 29- to 30-gauge hole; this

should be self-sealing if in a nondiseased vessel, particularly if it is a puncture rather than a tear. High-flow intracranial hemorrhage can last for only a matter of minutes; the exact duration depends on the rate and location of bleeding (e.g., subarachnoid, intraparenchymal), among other factors. Flow eventually stops, either because of a platelet plug or because the intracranial pressure equilibrates with the mean arterial pressure. This effectively stops *all* intracranial blood flow and results in brain death.

Most perforations from guidewires are extremely small and almost uniformly self-seal quickly. If the patient is anticoagulated at the time, this equation is changed.

As noted previously, a hole produced by a guidewire is tiny (about 0.014″, or 0.09 mm^2; about 29 to 30 gauge), and the leak is slow. Plugging the hole with a small coil has been advocated, but we think this is not indicated. To get a coil through the hole, it is important to realize that the guidewire is extravascular and not to withdraw it. The catheter must then be advanced forcefully over the guidewire and through the hole, thus making the hole tremendously larger (increasing the cross-sectional area to about 0.45 mm^2). The difficult task of placing a coil half in and half out is then necessary. This coil is only about 0.014″ (i.e., about 0.09 mm^2), which now is smaller than the hole; this would leave four fifths of the hole still open (about 0.35 mm^2, more area than the original hole!). In addition, a good portion of the coil would remain intravascular, possibly occluding the vessel. Far simpler and more effective would be to occlude the vessel over the hole or just proximal to it with a small coil.

The rate of bleeding from a micropuncture can be extremely slow; the bleeding can start and stop and last for hours. If there is any indication of recurrent bleeding, a neurosurgeon should be contacted and consideration given to performing an open craniotomy to stop the bleeding with a small amount of Gelfoam, with a microstitch, or by other means.

RUPTURED ARTERIOVENOUS MALFORMATION

A ruptured arteriovenous malformation (AVM) represents a worse situation. Rupture of an AVM during a case usually is due to overinjection before occlusion or before significant reduction of flow is obtained, thus causing intralesional rupture (possibly because the tip of the catheter is wedged), or to overinjection of the feeder after partial or complete embolization, causing rupture of the feeder. The latter is the better situation.

If the extravasation is due to vessel rupture, the hole is a linear tear rather than a round puncture and is larger than a guidewire hole. In addition, the probable abnormal vascular wall most likely does not have a good muscular component capable of contracting and thus decreasing or terminating the flow.

Immediate occlusion of the vessel by means of a coil therefore is necessary. If cyanoacrylate is available, this can be used. If no collateral supply is present, the leak is terminated. If the AVM has been occluded and it is the feeder that is leaking, this approach usually works well. If the hemorrhage is intralesional, simple occlusion of the feeder that the catheter is in may not stop the hemorrhage, but at least the pressure will be decreased. Continued supply may be present, allowing the bleed to continue.

Depending on the clinical circumstances, after the hemorrhage has ceased, it may be necessary to raise the systemic pressure until the intracranial pressure can be lowered; this is a risky maneuver. Systemic arterial pressure can be raised pharmacologically or by means of rapid intravenous volume expansion. In addition, decrease of intracranial pressure can be achieved by evacuation or drainage of the hematoma (if intraparenchymal), by simply draining the subarachnoid fluid and blood, or by placing a ventriculostomy. Other methods of lowering intracranial pressure, such as hyperventilation, may be employed as well. This is a neurosurgical decision based on the patient's clinical status and intracranial hemodynamics and another reason for close cooperation between the interventional neuroradiologist and neurosurgeon.

ANEURYSM RUPTURE

Rupture of an aneurysm during a case is a situation similar to rupture of an AVM. There is no normal vascular wall, and the tear commonly is large. If occlusion of the hole is not achieved, the situation can be terminal.

If Guglielmi detachable coils (GDCs) are used, continued rapid placement of additional coils may suffice. These coils, however, are less thrombogenic than standard coils and thus may not occlude flow in time. In addition, it may be possible to place only one additional GDC before intracranial pressure has equilibrated with systemic pressure, thus ending normal intracranial perfusion. For this reason, a small standard fibered coil would be our first choice to achieve as rapid cessation of flow as possible.

Early experimental work has been done to evaluate the use of small amounts of hydrogel to plug a hole. This material forms a mass rapidly (immediately) that is too large to go through a hole and could terminate any extravasation. In addition, dipping a fibered coil in thrombin to promote rapid clot formation has been employed.[2] As can be surmised, however, there are no controlled trials evaluating the best means to deal with the potential disaster of a ruptured aneurysm.

Coil occlusion of the parent vessel may be the easiest practical solution, but depending on aneurysm location, this usually is not a viable option. More appropriate would be to have in place a guide catheter capable of temporary occlusion (see "Flow Control Catheters" in Chapter 1). Indeed, for coil occlusion of aneurysms, the use of a guide catheter capable of temporary occlusion probably would be routine if one were available with the correct characteristics. Temporary occlusion not only can facilitate additional coil placement but also permits thrombus formation and may be all that is necessary to achieve a satisfactory result without the risk of additional forceful coil placement. Even without a rupture of the aneurysm, temporary occlusion or reduction of flow in the parent vessel may aid performance of the procedure.

REFERENCES

1. Halbach VV, Higashida RT, Dowd CF, et al. Management of vascular perforations that occur during neurointerventional procedures. *AJNR* 1991;12:319–327.
2. McLean GK, Stein EJ, Burke DR, Meranze SG. Steel occlusion coils: pretreatment with thrombin. *Radiology* 1986;158:549–550.

CHAPTER 66

Other Problems, Complications, and Solutions

J.J. Connors III / J.C. Wojak

UROKINASE CHILLS

In the early years of urokinase use, it was unusual to see a patient develop any untoward effects from the use of urokinase. After the passage of time, some scattered reports of chills (rigors) were received by Abbott Laboratories. No cause-and-effect relationship has been established, and there is no link to a particular batch of the drug. Usually, the patient who experiences this symptom has received a bolus dose.

Urokinase is still the fibrinolytic agent of choice for most interventional radiologists and interventional neuroradiologists. In a small percentage of patients, an uncontrollable shaking chill (sometimes severe) develops that is not amenable to simple tranquilization. These chills usually appear within 5 to 10 minutes of urokinase administration and subside within 20 to 30 minutes, either after temporary cessation of therapy or with continued therapy.

When faced with this reaction, the anesthesiologist or attending interventionist tends to overmedicate the patient with α-adrenergic blockers, neuroleptics, or paralytics, unaware that this reaction is not uncommon and responds well to narcotics, specifically 25 to 50 mg of meperidine. Prophylaxis has been attempted with acetaminophen, diphenhydramine, and hydrocortisone, but the efficacy of these treatments has not been shown by a controlled clinical trial. Alternatively, an H_2-receptor blocker has been tried. We have had good success with meperidine.

BROKEN CATHETER

Catheter breakage usually is caused by the use of too much force, either when pushing a coil or when injecting fluid, and typically does not result in complete detachment of the piece of catheter. The fracture usually is at a junction point between segments of catheter of different composition or is a longitudinal tear at the point of maximal force. If the catheter fragment is not totally separated, slow withdrawal of everything (e.g., guide catheter, microcatheter, and microguidewire) as a unit usually moves the broken catheter into the aorta. If there is simply a hole in the side of the microcatheter, the microcatheter can be withdrawn into the guide catheter.

If the microcatheter is truly fractured (i.e., angled), it is not possible to withdraw it into the guide catheter in use. Again, withdrawal of everything as a unit is necessary, certainly down into the descending aorta. Retrieval can then be performed using a much larger sheath (see "Preparing a Large Lumen Intravascular Withdrawal System for a Foreign Body" in Chapter 3).

INTRAPROCEDURAL VASOSPASM

Prophylaxis can be obtained to some degree using a strip of nitroglycerin paste on the chest. A length of 1″ to 5″ may be used (5″ almost guaranteeing a headache for the patient).

When working in extracranial vessels, vasospasm can greatly hinder evaluation or embolization. The best way to deal with vasospasm is to avoid inducing it; this is accomplished by careful catheter and guidewire manipulation. The most common cause of vasospasm in an extracranial location is stimulation by the guide catheter or guidewire (Fig. 66–1). It is far better to have vasospasm than an intimal dissection, however. The simplest method of dealing with this problem is to withdraw the offending item and wait. The spasm eventually will resolve.

Treatment of extracranial vasospasm is possible by

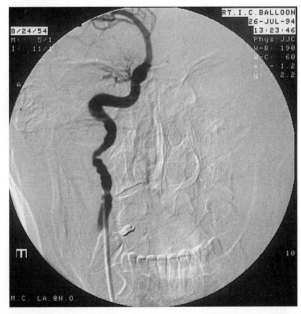

Figure 66-1 Case 1. An example of the difficulty in placing a temporary occlusion balloon (as well as a diagnostic catheter) into a tortuous and sensitive internal carotid artery. The tip of the temporary occlusion balloon appears to be in adequate position, but spasm is present. This was caused by the *exchange* wire. As stated in the text, a good, safe, benign exchange wire is essential, but does not currently exist.

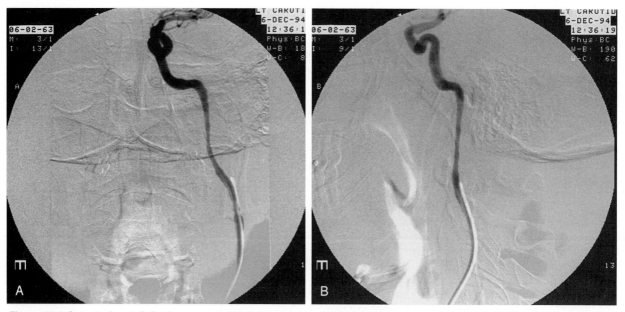

Figure 66-2 Case 2. *A* and *B,* During an embolization procedure for a glomus tumor, severe spasm was inadvertently caused in the internal carotid artery (ICA). This angiogram reveals poor flow in the cervical ICA with no filling of the anterior cerebral artery.

Case 2 continues

injecting nitroglycerin (50 μg is usually sufficient)[1] or papaverine (30 to 60 mg *over 3 to 15 minutes*),[2] or more simply, by having the patient inhale several breaths of amyl nitrite (Figs. 66–2 and 66–3). When injecting a vasodilator through the working catheter, giving short, rapid bursts ensures adequate mixing of the drug in the blood, rather than simply infusing the agent, with the possible result of streaming of the material without adequate vessel wall contact. A large bolus injection of papaverine is painful and runs the risk of precipitating when it exits the catheter. Bolus papaverine injections also have been asso-

ciated with transient intracranial pressure increases and brainstem dysfunction.

Amyl nitrite comes in small, breakable vials (15 or 30 ml) for nasal inhalation for the treatment of angina. It has immediate and profound coronary and peripheral vasodilatory effects. These are short-lived but generally sufficient to relieve the vasospasm in the area of work. (Inhaled amyl nitrite also can be used to induce a hyperemic response in the nose for evaluation of nosebleed or to allow embolic particles to flow more distally.) It is administered by breaking the vial and having the patient take deep breaths

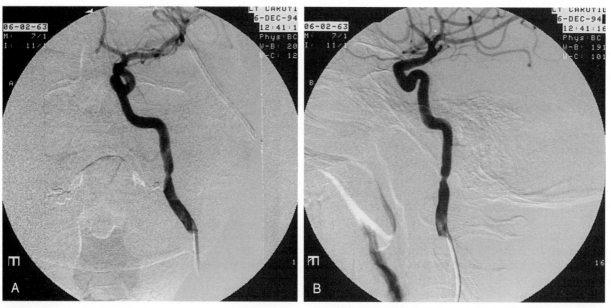

Figure 66-3 *A* and *B,* After several breaths of amyl nitrite from an ampule, there is prompt response of the ICA with only minimal focal stenosis and with greatly increased flow to the intracranial distribution (note the anterior cerebral and middle cerebral artery distribution).

while the broken vial is held under the nose. This method is easy to use and works well, but the patient may become restless because of the profound physical effects (i.e., the subsequent "rush" that is experienced with any nitrate). Amyl nitrite also induces a generalized systemic reaction rather than a focal one.

DISSECTION

Dissections are prone to occur at the vertebral artery origin, but owing to the relative frequency of catheterization, they are probably more common in diseased carotid arteries. A truly benign guide catheter and guidewire are absolutely needed, as well as extreme care during placement (see "Safe Catheterization of Difficult and Tortuous Vessels" in Chapter 3).

Any guide catheter with a tip stiff enough to maintain a shape (suitable for selecting vessels) is too stiff to be placed in a vulnerable location for an extended period of time. Movement of the guide catheter tip during the procedure secondary to heartbeat, respiration, or manipulation of the microcatheter *always occurs* and has been known to cause delayed dissections, occlusions, and death. For this reason, truly distal placement of the guide catheter is discouraged for any guide catheter stiff enough to have a curve or for any guide catheter without a truly blunt and benign tip.

Intimal flaps can be no problem or a major problem. In either case, immediate heparinization is indicated to keep any subintimal blood from clotting. Depending on location, there is probably no further therapy indicated; intimal dissections usually are self-limited and self-healing. Spiral dissections with almost total occlusion have been seen to heal in a matter of minutes, but others have progressed to occlusion in a matter of minutes.

Depending on location, it may be possible to "tack" the intima back down. This maneuver is dangerous, however, particularly if there is a need to recross the original area of injury. If tacking down is considered necessary, a soft balloon (i.e., silicone) is preferable to a hard angioplasty balloon, but some practitioners would debate this. The angioplasty balloon should not be oversized. Balloon dilation suffices to flatten the intima without damaging the underlying muscularis or causing more intimal damage. New balloon choices are becoming available for this purpose (such as the Solstice and Grapevine microangioplasty catheters made by Medtronic/MIS; see Chapter 1).

In almost all situations, however, any attempt at manipulation can worsen the situation, and anticoagulation combined with hopeful restraint is probably the best tactic.

If the dissection is heading toward the skull base and appears to be progressive, total occlusion of the vessel can stop this progression. Collateral intracranial supply can be tested before occlusion with a temporary occlusion balloon, but usually loss of one major brachiocephalic vessel is well tolerated. Once a propagating dissection reaches the intracranial subarachnoid level, vital side branches can be torn or occluded, with devastating results. In addition, a subarachnoid bleed can occur.

CLOT

Thrombus is perhaps the most insidious problem in interventional neuroradiology procedures. In various situations, it can have a different origin and potential solution. When thrombus formation can be reasonably expected because of the nature of the procedure, intraprocedural heparinization should be considered.[3] Many skilled interventional neuroradiologists almost never use heparin during cases, whereas others use heparin in almost all cases. The early fears of vascular perforation due to the extreme forces exerted on the microcatheters and microwires has eased to some degree in recent years because of better catheter technology, allowing more finesse. It was this fear of bleed that discouraged the use of heparin during a case. The fear of thrombus is now more worrisome than that of vascular perforation; therefore, there may be a trend toward more use of heparin. Additionally, the instigating pathology is now related more frequently to clot and vascular disease than it was in the past, and more patients with an underlying hypercoagulable state are being treated than in the past, hence, the more frequent need for heparin.

The classic case of thrombus forming around a diagnostic catheter does not appear to be a significant problem if proper technique is used, if the extracranial vessel is not traumatized, and if the patient is not abnormally hypercoagulable. Instead, the most common pericatheter thrombus problem appears to be related to the newer, large-lumen guide catheters; thrombus can form around the microcatheter *inside* the guide catheter. Compared with the previous use of 0.042″ catheters to deliver the microcatheter, there is such a large volume of dead space around the microcatheter in the large-bore guide catheters that the flush solution has to be turned up to a much higher flow rate than previously used to prevent a column of stagnant blood from developing inside the lumen of the guide catheter. Meticulous attention to flush rate through the guide catheter, therefore, has to be maintained throughout the case.

If thrombus does occur, it can manifest in several ways. If exterior to the guide catheter, it may be noted that the runoff from the injections through the microcatheter is slower than would be expected (the excellent filling of the vascular tree when injecting the microcatheter could be attributed simply to the force of the injection; it is important to observe the runoff *after* the injection). This implies poor inflow, and suspicion should be raised concerning either spasm or clot formation around the guide catheter; either possibility decreases vascular inflow. If thrombus forms around the microcatheter distal to the guide catheter, the hemodynamics may be the same: slow runoff after an injection through the microcatheter. Thrombus within the guide catheter may manifest as an inability to aspirate through the catheter before contrast injection.

After a diligent attempt at therapy of an intracranial lesion, it is most discouraging to discover that thrombus has formed around the shaft of the microcatheter, which is revealed when the microcatheter is withdrawn, leaving a beautiful silhouette of its former location. Fresh thrombus such as this is easily addressed by infusion of thrombolytics (specifically, urokinase) but is probably not what was originally intended. Amazingly, the few times this has been personally observed, there was no tendency for the mass to migrate, and fibrinolysis simply dissolved the material in place.

A thrombus that has formed around the guide catheter is a different situation. Frequently, it is not until the end of the case that this situation is discovered (unless a change in runoff of contrast is noted, as described previously). In addition, the mass of thrombus may be much larger and is in a location inviting movement (i.e., a large vessel, usually with good flow and large caliber, and usually in the neck—a flexible object). This situation can be most disturbing. In our experience, this occurs more frequently in the vertebral artery than in the internal carotid artery, probably because the vertebral artery is closer in size to the guide catheter, producing slower flow of blood around the catheter.

If suspicion is raised concerning the presence of thrombus because of the flow rate, extremely careful injection after slight withdrawal of the guide catheter should be performed; caution is used to avoid propelling potential thrombus downstream. If it is determined that there is a mass of thrombus, a choice of action must be made. The decision tree is different, depending on whether the thrombus is in the vertebral artery or in the internal carotid artery.

Vertebral Artery Thrombus

There are no large controlled trials comparing outcome of adaptive maneuvers for vertebral artery thrombus. The best choice must be made under the circumstances. If there is a long intravascular "noodle" of thrombus in the vertebral artery that is worrisome, the consideration of purposeful total proximal occlusion of the vertebral artery should be made (as opposed to thrombolysis). Total proximal occlusion ensures that the mass does not embolize downstream. This choice cannot be made if the opposite vertebral artery has not been previously evaluated and determined to be adequate to supply the intracranial structures as well as the posterior inferior cerebellar artery on the affected side.

An alternative approach is to occlude the subclavian artery with a flow control guide catheter (reversing the flow in the vertebral artery) while infusing a fibrinolytic from a distal location. Careful initial placement of the microcatheter is made so as not to displace any thrombus, but if flow reversal has already been established, the danger of this is lessened considerably. This permits gradual dissolution of thrombus in the vertebral artery without the risk of downstream embolization to the basilar artery or its branches.

Many practitioners would simply place the patient on oral anticoagulants without interventional treatment. We believe that this can be risky. Any movement (e.g., cough) can dislodge a portion of this thrombus, with devastating results. We have seen this policy of "benign neglect" result in posterior inferior cerebellar artery infarcts (and worse).

Internal Carotid Artery Thrombus

The equation is considerably different if the "long noodle" is in the internal carotid artery. Purposeful occlusion of this vessel is not generally performed, and a temporary test occlusion could make the situation worse (i.e., the new thrombus can grow even if the patient is fully anticoagulated). Generally, pericatheter thrombus is not occlusive, allowing time for deliberation and therapy. As a large thrombus dissolves or just sits in the vessel, however, any number of portions could break off and travel downstream, becoming occlusive in any branch they lodge in. This is a significant therapeutic challenge.

A thrombus that is inside the guide catheter surrounding the microcatheter may only be discovered on withdrawal of the microcatheter, followed by vigorous aspiration of the guide catheter before any fluid (saline or contrast) is instilled into this guide catheter. During certain cases, it is a common practice to inject contrast around the microcatheter that is still within the guide catheter, using a three-way stopcock on the side of the rotating hemostatic valve. This maneuver does not convey to the operator an adequate feel for the intraguide catheter hemodynamics, and it may be possible to aspirate some blood through the side port of the rotating hemostatic valve (unless the thrombus truly is occlusive) and then propel any clot out of this catheter with the subsequent forceful injection. This situation has been reported to have occurred.

The optimal therapy is to place a flow control guide catheter in the common carotid artery (not the internal carotid artery). This allows retrograde flow in the internal carotid artery rather than stagnation. Once this is done, fibrinolysis can be performed without the risk of material breaking up and embolizing to an intracranial location.

STROKE ON THE TABLE

When a patient suffers a sudden change in neurologic status during a procedure, there are several steps to be taken. First, *the nature of the insult must be determined.* Is this an ischemic event (e.g., thrombus or embolism, errant vessel occlusion by a coil or balloon) or a hemorrhagic event (e.g., rupture of a vessel, arteriovenous malformation, aneurysm, or hypertensive bleed)? Was it a seizure? The management of hemorrhagic events is described in Chapter 65.

Acute Intraprocedural Ischemic Events

If there is any question about the nature of the insult, the patient must be moved to the computed tomography scanner for evaluation. Additional questions that should be answered are: Why was the patient on the table to begin with? For evaluation of transient ischemic attacks? Could there be a recent silent infarct (thus precluding the use of fibrinolytic agents)? Was this an aneurysm hunt? Once it has been determined that the change in the patient's neurologic status is not due to vascular rupture and hemorrhage, certain steps should be followed. Although some obvious causes of blockage may be identified (e.g., balloon or coil malposition), medical therapeutic measures should be instituted before any attempt at specific therapy.

The steps we take are presented under "Stroke During or Subsequent to an Angiographic Procedure" in Chapter 59. The reader is referred to this section for a complete discussion.

CERVICAL RADICULOPATHY AND PERIPHERAL NEUROPATHY

Cervical radiculopathy (and occasionally myelopathy) is a known complication of surgical procedures performed under general anesthesia in patients with underlying cervical spondylosis or cervical disc disease. Careful questioning of the patient before the procedure often yields this information. In patients with known or suspected disease, care should be taken during induction and intubation not to hyperextend the patient's neck. The patient's head also should be placed in as neutral a position as possible; the imaging apparatus should be maneuvered rather than the patient's head. If necessary, a soft cervical collar may be placed on the patient. In any patient with preexisting cervical radiculopathy or myelopathy, the physical examination and any available computed tomography and magnetic resonance imaging findings should be documented in the chart as a baseline before the procedure.

The most common peripheral neuropathies associated with prolonged procedures are ulnar (due to pressure on the ulnar nerve at the elbow) and peroneal (due to pressure at the head of the fibula). Careful positioning of the patient, padding of the angiography table, and padding of any potential pressure sites (especially elbows and heels) should be routine. Heel and elbow protectors are readily available in most hospitals; they should be ordered, and the patient should arrive at the angiography suite with them. Alternatively, foam padding can be used not only to pad the table but also to pad heels and elbows (and any other potential pressure sites).

Generally, these palsies are self-limited and respond to time. A short course of corticosteroids may help hasten recovery.

REFERENCES

1. Halbach VV, Hieshima GB, Higashida RT, David CF. Endovascular therapy of head and neck tumors. In: Vinuela F, Halbach VV, Dion JE (eds). Interventional Neuroradiology: Endovascular Therapy of the Central Nervous System New York: Raven Press, 1992, pp. 17–28.
2. Isomura T, Hisatomi K, Hirano A, et al. Use of the right gastroepiploic artery as a pedicled arterial graft for coronary revascularization. *Eur J Cardiothorac Surg* 1993;7:38–41.
3. Fujii Y, Takeuchi S, Koike T, et al. Heparin administration and monitoring for neuroangiography. *AJNR* 1994;15:51–54.

ADDITIONAL REFERENCES

Arteriography

Davies KN, Humphrey PR. Complications of cerebral angiography in patients with symptomatic carotid territory ischaemia screened by carotid ultrasound. *J Neurol Neurosurg Psychiatry* 1993;56:967–972.

Dion JE, Gates PC, Fox AJ, et al. Clinical events following neuroangiography: a prospective study. *Stroke* 1987;18:997–1004.

Mani RL, Eisenberg RL. Complications of catheter cerebral arteriography: analysis of 5,000 procedures. II. Relation of complication rates to clinical and arteriographic diagnosis. *AJR* 1978;131:867–869.

Mani RL, Eisenberg RL. Complications of catheter cerebral arteriography: analysis of 5,000 procedures. III. Assessment of arteries injected, contrast medium used, duration of procedure, and age of patient. *Am J Roentgenol* 1987;131:871–874.

Mani RL, Eisenberg RL, Pollock JA, Mani JR. Complications of catheter cerebral arteriography: analysis of 5,000 procedures. I. Criteria and incidence. *Am J Roentgenol* 1978;131:861–865.

McIvor J, Rhymer JC. 245 transaxillary arteriograms in arteriopathic patients: success rate and complications. *Clin Radiol* 1992;45:390–394.

Shunaib A, Hachinski VC. Migraine and the risk from angiography. *Arch Neurol* 1988;45:911–912.

Contrast

Baxter A. Management of adverse reactions to iodinated contrast media. *Appl Radiol* 1993;(suppl):9–16.

Cohan RH, Dunnick NR, Bashore TM. Treatment of reactions to radiographic contrast material. *AJR* 1988;151:263–270.

Parfrey PS, Griffiths SM, Barrett BJ, et al. Contrast material-induced renal failure in patients with diabetes mellitus, renal insufficiency, or both. *N Engl J Med* 1989;320:143–149.

Index

Note: Page numbers in *italics* refer to illustrations; page numbers followed by t refer to tables.

ISBN 0-7216-7147-0

90038